Get the MOST from this book!

Watch the DVD!

Companion DVD

Will Chapleau, EMT-P, RN, TNS; and Peter T. Pons, MD, FACEP

Containing 44 skill demonstrations, this unique DVD brings a new dimension to learning. Demonstrations in real time give you unlimited exposure to seeing the skills performed the right way by real practitioners. Plus, you'll also **discover medical animations** that clearly demonstrate core functions in anatomy and physiology!

Go online. Get more! *evolve*

Evolve

With this free Internet resource site, you'll have access to hundreds of additional learning opportunities, including: anatomy challenges, body spectrum, a talking glossary, lung sounds, links to the National Registry Skills Sheets, and more! Simply go to **http://evolve.elsevier.com** to get started today.

Apply what you're learning!

Virtual Patient Encounters

ISBN: 0-323-04923-0 • ISBN-13: 978-0-323-04923-8

This study guide and CD-ROM package provides realistic, challenging simulations that you may never otherwise encounter in your education. These unique cases will take you from the classroom to the field by allowing you the opportunity to make crucial clinical decisions in the prehospital setting as you progress through this textbook. Be sure to ask your instructor about **Virtual Patient Encounters** — it's the ultimate interactive learning experience in critical thinking!

Reinforce key concepts!

Workbook

Will Chapleau, EMT-P, RN, TNS; and Peter T. Pons, MD, FACEP
2007 • 375 pp.
ISBN: 0-323-04008-X • ISBN-13: 978-0-323-04008-2

Featuring approximately 1,500 questions in a variety of formats, this workbook is your source for complete comprehension of the material covered in the text. You'll be able to check your answers quickly and easily with the answers in the back of the book, as well as build upon the knowledge gained from EMS experts.

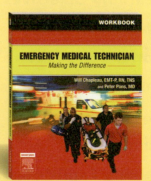

Get your copy today! Call toll-free 1-800-545-2522,
order online at www.mosbyjems.com or visit your local bookstore.

ELSEVIER

evolve

- To access your Student Resources, visit:

http://evolve.elsevier.com/Chapleau/EMT

Evolve® Student Resources for *Chapleau and Pons: Emergency Medical Technician: Making the Difference* offer the following features:

Instructor Resources

- **Chapter Pre-test**
- **Lecture Outline**
- **Classroom Activities**
- **Power Point Presentation**
- **ExamView Test Bank**

Student Resources

- **Learning Objectives**
- **Chapter Summary**
- **Power Point Lecture Notes**
- **Anatomy Challenges**
- **Body Spectrum**
- **Lung Sounds**
- **Talking English/Spanish Glossary**
- **Link to the National Registry Skill Sheets**
- **Weblinks**

EMERGENCY MEDICAL TECHNICIAN

Making the Difference

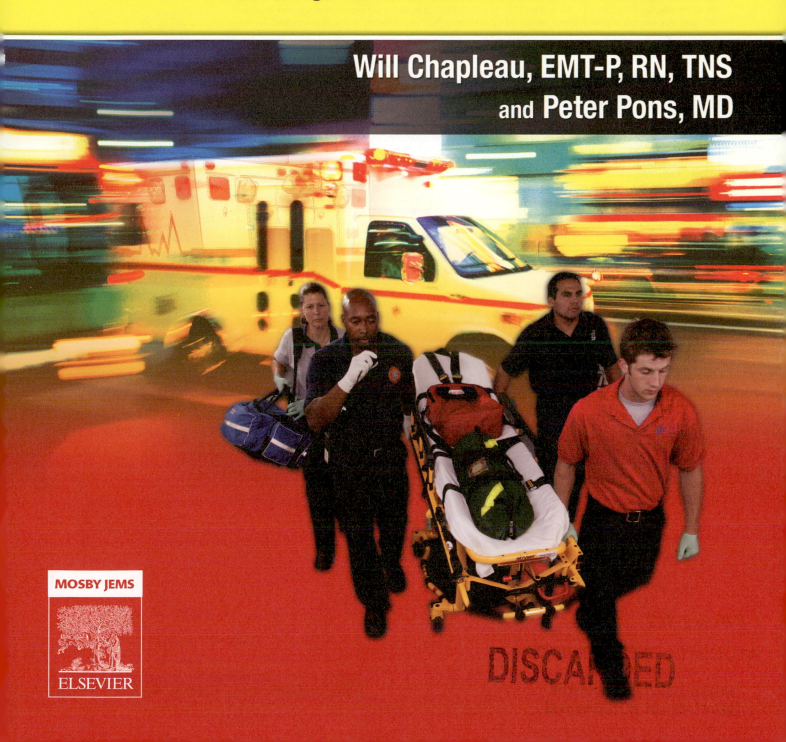

EMERGENCY MEDICAL TECHNICIAN
Making the Difference

Will Chapleau, EMT-P, RN, TNS
and Peter Pons, MD

MOSBY JEMS

ELSEVIER

MOSBY JEMS
ELSEVIER

11830 Westline Industrial Drive
St. Louis, Missouri 63146

EMERGENCY MEDICAL TECHNICIAN: MAKING THE DIFFERENCE   ISBN-13: 978-0-323-03272-8
ISBN-10: 0-323-03272-9

Notice

Knowledge and best practice in this field are constantly changing. As new research and experience broaden our knowledge, changes in practice, treatment and drug therapy may become necessary or appropriate. Readers are advised to check the most current information provided (i) on procedures featured or (ii) by the manufacturer of each product to be administered, to verify the recommended dose or formula, the method and duration of administration, and contraindications. It is the responsibility of the practitioner, relying on their own experience and knowledge of the patient, to make diagnoses, to determine dosages and the best treatment for each individual patient, and to take all appropriate safety precautions. To the fullest extent of the law, neither the Publisher nor the [Editors/Authors] [delete as appropriate] assumes any liability for any injury and/or damage to persons or property arising out or related to any use of the material contained in this book.

ISBN-13: 978-0-323-03272-8
ISBN-10: 0-323-03272-9

Acquisitions Editor: Linda Honeycutt
Developmental Editor: Laura Bayless
Publishing Services Manager: Julie Eddy
Project Manager: Rich Barber
Designer: Julia Dummitt

Printed in China

Last digit is the print number: 9 8 7 6 5 4 3 2 1

About the Authors

Chief Will Chapleau has 32 years of emergency care experience including 30 as a paramedic. He has 17 years of experience as a Trauma Nurse Specialist and 15 years in Fire Service.

For more than 22 years, students have had the benefit of Chief Chapleau's educational expertise in a variety of settings. As an international faculty member for Prehospital Trauma Life Support (PHTLS) since 1984 and as a board member of the National Association of EMS Educators, and National Association of EMTs, Chief Chapleau is well respected by students and peers worldwide.

Chief Chapleau has contributed to numerous textbooks and journal articles over the course of his career. He serves on the editorial board for EMS Magazine.

As the Fire Chief of a busy department and the Chairperson for the Prehospital Trauma Life Support (PHTLS) program since 1996, Board of Directors of the Society of Trauma Nurses, Chief Chapleau's experiences lend a perspective and credibility second to none.

Peter T. Pons, MD is a senior physician in the emergency department, Denver Health Medical Center (Denver General Hospital). Dr. Pons also serves as professor of emergency medicine in the Department of Surgery, University of Colorado Health Sciences Center in Denver Colorado. He completed his M.D. at New Jersey Medical School, Internship at Martland Hospital in Newark, New Jersey and Residency at Denver General/St. Anthony/St. Joseph Hospitals in Denver. Dr. Pons also contributes as an associate medical director for PHTLS.

Dr. Pons is certified by the American Board of Emergency Medicine and has been the recipient of several awards for teaching, clinical excellence, and leadership. He has contributed to over 100 books, chapters, journal articles, editorials and abstracts, holds several editorial and consulting positions and has lectured extensively nationally and internationally.

He served on the board of directors and as senior examiner for the American Board of Emergency Medicine, the advisory council on First Aid and Safety for the American Red Cross, ABEM representative for the American College of Emergency Physicians, task force on Weapons of Mass Effect, chair of the Disaster Committee, Denver Health Medical Center, and board of directors for the Colorado Trauma Institute.

Dedication and Author Acknowledgements

This book is dedicated to all EMS providers, educators and medical directors. We have made a career of working in EMS and it is a rewarding and fulfilling endeavor. In dedicating this book to all of you, we would like to thank all of the providers we have worked with and the students who have sat in our classrooms or read something we have written. We would like to thank the educators we have worked beside in designing curricula and educational materials. We are grateful for the things we have learned from educators all over the world so far in our careers and look forward to more rewarding exchanges. We look forward to continued input from the students and educators using this book and support materials. We are also thankful to the visionary medical directors that have helped EMS grow and the gifted next generation that will lead us into the future of EMS.

As you have seen, we've been at this for a while. It would be impossible for us to keep up with the demands of our careers and the work of getting this book and its ancillaries done without the support of our wives, Kathryn and Kathryn (yes, they have the same name). Not only have they tolerated the bizarre hours our jobs call for, the travel to teach and work on the future of EMS, but they have also tolerated our temper when we worked to meet deadlines writing and reviewing manuscripts. They have endured much and we are indebted.

The people we work with at the Hospital and Fire Department have been great supporters of this project as well. Many of our co-workers have contributed chapters and/or participated in photo shoots, videos or reviews. Their participation was crucial to the work and their enthusiasm to support us in this project was humbling. It has been a pleasure to work for administrators and city officials who have supported and shown enthusiasm for our work.

Lastly, I would like to thank our editor Laura Bayless for her patience in working with us and for Linda Honeycutt who signed us to the project and believed in our concept.

And finally thank you, the readers of this text. May it be of good use to you as you begin your career in EMS.

How to Use This Book

Lesson Goals and *Objectives* have been provided to help students in identifying key content. Throughout the chapters, *Ask Yourself, Special Considerations, and Special Populations* boxes will help EMTs become familiar with the variety of situations they may encounter in the field. These boxes should be used to generate discussion with classmates and the instructor.

Each chapter ends with a review in *Nuts and Bolts*. This section includes critical points, a learning check-list, key terms, and objectives. Special skills, such as pediatric CPR and spinal immobilization, are explained in detail for review in the *Step-by-Step Skills* pages. *DVD icons* 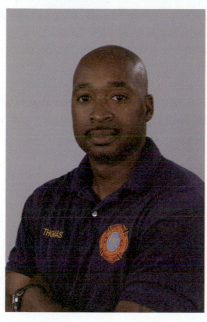 appear throughout the text, whenever a skill is available on video for review. The DVD of skills is available at the back of this book.

Detailed, three-part *Case Scenarios* follow four EMTs throughout the book:

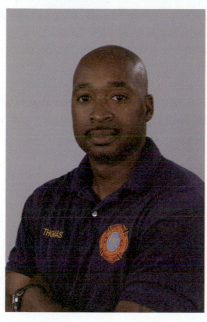

Jack Thomas
Jack is near the end of his EMT training. Growing up in a Baltimore neighborhood, Jack received CPR and basic first aid training during a health education class in high school. The information seemed so interesting that he signed up for an EMT class during his first semester at the local community college.

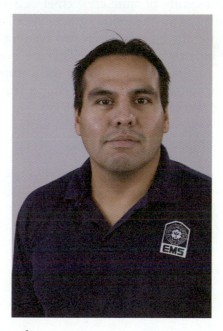

Rafael Gonzales
Rafael is a 35-year-old firefighter working in Los Angeles County Fire Department. On the job for just over a year, Rafael is halfway through his probation period as an EMT-firefighter on Engine 32. He feels fortunate that he is working with a friendly crew, especially his officer, Captain José Alvarez. A former paramedic, the Captain takes special care to ensure that Rafael provides medical assistance with care and compassion.

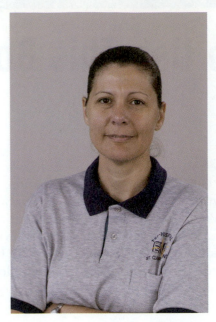

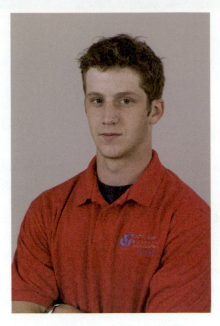

Elizabeth Stafford
Elizabeth recently became crew chief at a volunteer rescue squad. A mother of two grade-school children, she leads her three-person crew two evenings a week, and responds via pager as a backup crew every other weekend. An EMT for many years, she is respected by her fellow squad members as being a very experienced and resourceful care provider.

Ray Barnes
Ray has been working at the County hospital ambulance service for nearly 3 years, in a mostly rural service area. Calls are few but are often serious. Between calls, Ray and his partner work inside the emergency department with the hospital staff, assisting the nurses and physicians with the care of ambulatory patients. A gregarious young man, Ray is able to establish trust quickly with his patients and is considered to be a compassionate care provider.

Publisher Acknowledgements

Contributors

Katherine Bakes, MD
Denver Health Medical Center
Denver, Colorado

Augie Bamonti, EMT-P, FF
EMS Training Officer
Chicago Heights Fire Department
Chicago Heights, Illinois

Ann Bellows, EdD, NREMT-P
Training Specialist
New Mexico State University
Las Cruces, New Mexico

Cheryl Blazek, EMT-P
EMS Training Program Coordinator
Southwestern Community College
Creston, Iowa

Stephen Cantrill, MD
Denver Health Medical Center
Denver, CO

Will Chapleau, EMT-P, RN, TNS
Fire Chief
Chicago Heights Fire Department
Chicago Heights, Illinois

Clark Christenson, Paramedic
Logistics Officer/DMAT Coordinator
Iowa Department of Public Health
Des Moines, Iowa

Chris Colwell, MD
Denver Health Medical Center
Denver, Colorado

Peter Connick, EMT-P, EMT-I/C
Captain/Adjunct Faculty
Chatham Fire-Rescue/Cape Cod Community College
Chatham, MA/West Barnstable, Massachusetts

John Elder, CCEMT-P, EMT-P
Director of Education
Careflite
Fort Worth, Texas

Jeffrey S. Guy, EMT-P, FACS, MD
Director, Regional Burn Center/Associate Professor
of Surgery
School of Medicine
Vanderbilt University
Nashville, Tennessee

Kennon Heard, MD
University of Colorado Health Sciences Center
Denver, Colorado

Art Hsieh, MA, NREMT-P
San Francisco Paramedic Association
Hospital Consortium Education Network
Piedmont, California

Andrew Knaut, MD
Porter Adventist Hospital
Denver, Colorado

Jon Krohmer, FACEP, MD
Kent County EMS
EMS Physician Certification Ad Hoc Committee
Grand Rapids, Michigan

Bob Loftus, EMT
Doctors Hospital
Springfield, Illinois

Tom Martello
Captain
Chicago Heights Fire Department
Chicago Heights, Illinois

Dean Martin, AS, Paramedic
Division Chief
Columbia Fire Department
Columbia, Missouri

Michelle McLean, MD
Medical Doctor, Emergency
Covenant Hospital
Saginaw, Michigan

Valerie J. Phillips, FACEP, MD
Medical Director Emergency Services and Emergency
Medical Services
Advocate Good Samaritan Hospital
Downers Grove, Illinois

David Stilley, BCEM, CMPE, FAAFP, MD
Medical Director, Emergency Department
Mercy Medical Center
Des Moines, Iowa

David M. Tauber, NREMT-P, CCEMT-P, I/C
Paramedic
Advanced Life Support Institute
Conway, New Hampshire

Jamie Temple, BS, REMT-P
Quality/Education Manager
Medic EMS
Davenport, Iowa

Robert Vroman, BS, NREMT-P
Paramedic
HealthONE EMS
Lakewood, Colorado

Steve Wirth, Esq.
Attorney
Page, Wolfberg & Wirth, LLC
Mechanicsburg, Pennsylvania

Lynn Yancey, MD
University of Colorado Health Sciences Center
Denver, Colorado

Reviewers

David K. Anderson, BS, EMT-P
Director, Paramedic Education Program
Northwest Regional Training Center
Vancouver, Washington

Jeffrey K. Benes, BS, NREMT-P
jeff benes company
Antioch, Illinois

Chip Boehm, RN, EMT-P/FF
EMS Educator
Portland Fire Department
Falmouth, ME

Kristen D. Borchelt, NREMT-P
Cincinnati Children's Hospital
Cincinnati, Ohio

Lisa Kaye Cannada, MD
Parkland Hospital
University of Texas-Southwestern
Dallas, Texas

Robert Joseph Carter, NREMT-P
Law Enforcement Instructor/Paramedic
Emergency Services Section
U.S. Secret Service
Washington, DC

Peter Connick, REMTP, EMT I/C
Adjunct Faculty
Cape Cod Community College
West Barnstable, Massachusetts
Captain, Chatham Fire Rescue
Chatham, Massachusetts

Jon S. Cooper, NREMT-P
EMS Training Division
Baltimore City Fire Academy
Baltimore, Maryland

Ken Davis, NREMT-P, CCEMT-P, FP-C
Eastern New Mexico University
Roswell, New Mexico

Douglas Alan deBest, AS, BS, MPA, EMT
Firefighter/EMT
University of Notre Dame Fire Department
Notre Dame, Indiana
Adjunct Professor
EMT and EMS Instructor Coordinator
Kalamazoo Valley Community College
Kalamazoo, Michigan

Steven Donald Dralle, BA, LP, EMSC
Director of Clinical and Education Services
American Medical Response-Texas/Oklahoma
Division
San Antonio, Texas

Ann Maureen Dunphy, BS, EMT-I, Wilderness EMT-I
Instructor
Eagle River Memorial Hospital
Eagle River, Wisconsin
Nicolet Area Technical College
Rhinelander, Wisconsin
Wilderness Medicine Associates
Portland, Maine

Dennis Edgerly, EMT-P
Program Coordinator
HealthONE EMS
Englewood, Colorado

Keith Ervin, NREMT-P, CCEMT-P
Eastern New Mexico University
Roswell, New Mexico

Jacqueline Evans, NREMT-P
Southwest Ambulance, Pima Operations
Tucson, Arizona

Thomas E. Ezell III, NREMT-P, CCEMT-P, EMT-T
Center for Emergency Health Services
James City County Fire Department
Williamsburg, Virginia

Gregory T. Friese, MS, NREMT-P, WEMT
President, Emergency Preparedness Systems, LLC
Plover, Wisconsin

Fidel O. Garcia, EMT-P
St. Mary's Hospital
Grand Junction, Colorado

Rudy Garrett, AS, NREMT-P, CCEMT-P
Training Coordinator
Somerset Fire/EMS
Somerset, Kentucky

Gerry Goodale, EMT-I
Barrick Underground ET
American MedFLight
Elko County Ambulance
Elko, Nevada

John Gosford, AS, EMT-P
State EMS Training Coordinator
Florida Department of Health
Tallahassee, Florida

Thomas James Gottschalk, NREMT-P, I/C, CCEMT-P
Platinum Educational Group, LLC
Jenison, Michigan

Seth Collings Hawkins, MD
Mountain Emergency Physicians
EMS Coordinator and Disaster Management Chair
Blue Ridge HealthCare
Morganton, NC

Chad S. Kim, BA, NREMT-P, I/C
University of New Mexico EMSA?
Eastern New Mexico University
Roswell, New Mexico
Albuquerque Fire Department
Albuquerque, New Mexico

Shannon Lizer, DNSc, APN, CNP
University of Illinois–Chicago
School of Nursing
Chicago, Illinois

Dean Martin, AAS, EMT-P
Division Chief
Columbia Fire Department
Columbia, Missouri

Reylon Ann Meeks, RN, BSN, MS, MSN, EMT
Blank Children's Hospital
Des Moines, Iowa

Mark Milliron, MS, MPA, EMT
EMS Instructor
Pennsylvania State University
University Park, Pennsylvania

Laraine Yakowich Moody, RN, MSN, CPNP
Children's Hospital of Michigan
Detroit, Michigan

Greg Mullen, BS, MS, NREMT-P
National EMS Academy
Lafayette, Louisiana

Dennis Nothnagel, NREMT-P
Medical Training Incorporated
Coon Rapids, Minnesota

Roy Ramos, NREMT-P
Heart EMTS
Pueblo, Colorado

William E. Rich, AAS, EMT, EMT-P, CEM
Emergency Medical Educator
Orise Fellow
Centers for Disease Control and Prevention
Atlanta, Georgia

Larry Richmond, AS, NREMT-P, CCEMT-P
EMS Education Manager
Mountain Plains Health Consortium
Ft. Meade, South Dakota

Janet L. Schulte, AS, BS, NR-CCEMTP
Director of Continuing Education
IHM Health Studies Center
St. Louis, Missouri

Maureen Shanahan, RN, BSN, MN
Health Care Technology Department
City College of San Francisco
San Francisco, CA

Douglas R. Smith, MAT, EMT-P, I/C
Platinum Educational Group, LLC
Jenison, Michigan

Gilbert N. Taylor, NREMPT-P, I/C
Director, Institute for Emergency Medical Education
Bourne, Massachusetts

Robert Vroman, BS, NREMT-P
Paramedic
HealthONE EMS
Lakewood, CO

Justin W. Witt, JD, NREMT-P
EMT Instructor
Center for Emergency Health Services
Williamsburg, Virginia

The publishers and authors also wish to thank the following for their active participation in the photographs for this book:

Demonstrations and Patients
Carolyle Borner
Tracy Borner
Alex Chapleau
Cameron Chapleau
Joe Chapleau
Kyle Chapleau
Matt Chapleau
Ryan DeBergh
Frank Enright
Doug Fisher
Juan Garcia
Nathan Garcia
Phil Giannattassio
Alan Graber
Job Gunn
George Hartman
Cody Hogeveen
Kyle Hogeveen
John Hogeveen
Page Hogeveen
Ethan Jones
Brian Kowalski
Ron Lucarini
Kalvin Lueder
Angie Pacetti
Mark Perez
Wendell Thomas
Dave Troiani

Special Thanks
Chicago Heights Fire Department
Ingalls Memorial Hospital
Mama Mary's Restaurant
Minto Research and Development, Inc.
Prarie State College
Ridgeview Towing
St. James Hospital

Moulage make-up provided by Graftobian Make-Up Company, makers of the EMS Makeup/Severe Trauma Kit. For more information, please visit www.graftobian.com.

Contents

■ **DIVISION FOUR MEDICAL AND BEHAVIORAL EMERGENCIES**

16 Pharmacology, 314

17 Respiratory Emergencies, 324

18 Cardiovascular Emergencies, 346

■ DIVISION SIX
SPECIAL POPULATIONS

CHAPTER

1

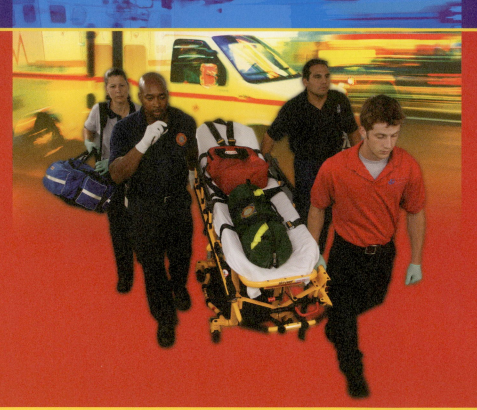

LESSON GOAL

This chapter provides a brief introduction to the EMS system. You will learn about the administrative elements of an EMS system and how EMS systems are composed of individuals and institutions that combine various skills and resources to form an effective team with a single purpose—to provide the best medical care for the emergency patient. As an **emergency medical technician (EMT),** you have a major role in this system. ■

Introduction to Emergency Medical Services (EMS) Systems

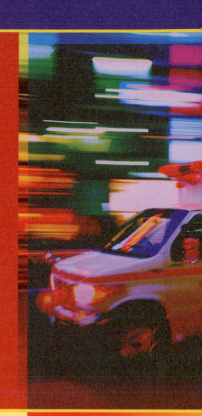

CHAPTER OBJECTIVES

After completing this chapter, the EMT student will be able to do the following:

1 Define the EMS system.

2 Differentiate the roles and responsibilities of the EMT from those of other prehospital care providers.

3 Describe the EMT's roles and responsibilities with regard to personal safety.

4 Discuss the EMT's roles and responsibilities with regard to the safety of the crew, the patient, and bystanders.

5 Define quality improvement and discuss the EMT's role in this process.

6 Discuss medical direction and the EMT's role in this process.

7 Identify how a patient's race, gender, age, and socioeconomic status can affect an EMT's judgment.

8 Discuss the rationale for maintaining a professional appearance when on duty and when responding to calls.

9 Identify a resource for statutes and regulations pertinent to EMS systems in your state.

OBJECTIVES

CASE SCENARIO

Jack is excited as he gets out of his car. He is in front of the Community Rescue Squad, a two story brick building with graceful columns framing the main entrance. Through the three bay doors, he can see that two of the bays house white and orange ambulances. The third bay is empty, the electrical charging cord and exhaust ejector tubing dangling from the ceiling. "Must be out on a medical event," he thinks to himself as he joins a growing group of fellow students gathering in front of the main doors. His EMT instructor is already there, talking to the group.

"Please be respectful of the ambulance crews and other folks working right now," the instructor reminds the students. "This is essentially their second home, and we are invited guests." With that a woman in a squad uniform opens the main door and steps out into the warm light of the setting sun. "Hello, everyone, my name is Elizabeth Stafford, and I am one of the crew chiefs on duty today. Chief McFadden asked me to take you on a tour of the facility, and I am more than happy to do so. Does everyone have an identification badge on? Good. Come with me and let's take a look at the EMS system."

Question: What are some of the components of an EMS system? What roles does an EMT play in the EMS system?

Few things are more exciting or rewarding than answering a call for help. As an EMT in the **emergency medical services (EMS) system,** you will be a professional trained to render basic life support at the scene of an emergency and during transport to the hospital. Your skills will also enable you to assist your neighbors, coworkers, friends, and others when they need help the most. By serving your community, you will become a public asset. Strangers will look to you for help in their darkest hours, and years later you may find out how you touched their lives. The lessons you learn while providing prehospital care can also benefit you for the rest of *your* life. You will learn to be organized in the midst of chaos, to communicate effectively, to lead others, and to meet challenges. These personal assets are valuable not only at the scene of an emergency, but also in most professions and careers. EMS providers hold a respected and privileged position in our society.

The EMS system consists of a sophisticated team of emergency care providers. An EMT is a prehospital professional trained to render basic life support at the scene and during transport to medical facilities. The EMS system is part of the continuum of care that encompasses the prehospital environment to the hospital environment. Moreover, each team member fulfills a unique role. Often emergency interventions are needed within the first minutes of an emergency. The care given in those few minutes can be vital to the patient's survival and outcome. The overall goal of EMT training is to produce an emergency medical provider skilled at securing the airway, breathing, and circulation; controlling bleeding, and immobilizing fractures.

EMERGENCIES

When an **emergency** occurs, the first step involves someone recognizing that an emergency has occurred and activating the EMS system. Bystanders at the scene of an emergency may call 911, for example, or a person may call 911 to seek aid for a family member in the home. As an EMT, you may happen upon the scene first and may be the one who calls for additional help, or you may be the first medical responder who is dispatched to a scene. Making sure that the scene is safe before you enter is important. You must also look after the safety of your partner, the patient, and any bystanders.

When you arrive at the scene, inform the patient that you are a trained EMS provider. In addition, ask the patient or bystanders what happened. You may be surrounded by well-meaning but untrained bystanders. Sometimes you may need to enlist their help. Give your instructions respectfully and clearly and then ask the person assisting you to repeat them to make sure he or she understands.

Bystanders often assist EMS providers by calling for additional emergency care personnel if the EMS system has not yet been contacted when you arrive at the scene. The most important information the emergency operator needs is your location. Therefore, ask someone who can give detailed, accurate location information to make the call. If the emergency has occurred in a remote or industrial setting or anywhere that cannot easily be seen from the street, ask someone to meet the ambulance at the main road and direct the crew to the scene.

You may have responded to a scene where trained first responders, the first level of prehospital care, are delivering care as they wait for your arrival. They should be prepared to give you a report on what they found and what has happened. They also should be prepared to assist you. You may find yourself assigned not to an ambulance, but to a police, fire, or industrial nontransport team that interacts with other EMTs or paramedics (the role of paramedics is described in greater detail later in the chapter). These teams provide additional emergency medical care at the scene and transport the patient to a receiving facility by ground or air ambulance. The patient then is transferred to the in-hospital care system (Figure 1-1).

■ COMPONENTS OF AN EMS SYSTEM

A person in the community who needs emergency assistance often expects immediate, state of the art care. This level of service is the ideal. However, considerable organization, planning, and support are required for a community to provide emergency medical services. As a member of the EMS system, you need to understand its fundamental components (Figure 1-2). EMS systems consist of 10 basic organizational elements:

- Regulations, policies, and protocols
- Resource management
- Human resources and training
- Transportation
- Medical facilities
- Communications
- Public information and education
- Medical oversight
- Trauma systems
- Evaluation

Regulations, Policies, and Protocols

EMS regulations and policies are developed on the national, state, and local levels for many emergency treatment issues. Guidelines vary in different areas for training requirements, equipment standards, and treatment regimens. As an EMT, you need to know your state and local EMS regulations and policies. This information generally is available from the state EMS office.

Medical protocols govern the level and type of care administered by trained EMS providers. Protocols outline the standard operational procedures (SOP) for EMS providers based on community standards of care specific to the authority with jurisdiction over the area.

Resource Management

Delivery of state of the art prehospital care requires training programs, specialized instructors, equipment, vehicles, communication networks, and buildings to house these resources. The system of cost assessment, acquisition, maintenance, and replacement of these resources is known as *resource management*. Resource management involves determining the equipment requirements of the local EMS system in light of the needs of the particular service and community.

Human Resources and Training

As with any organization, the greatest asset of the EMS system is its people. A large number of EMS providers are volunteers. The work of EMTs can be physically and emotionally challenging, yet it is also rewarding. The human resources and training element of an EMS system ensures recruitment, training, and retention of talented individuals.

Transportation

Transportation is the process of moving the patient from the emergency scene to an appropriate medical facility. Either a ground or an air ambulance may be used. The priority is to transport the patient quickly while ensuring the safety of the patient, the driver or pilot, the EMS personnel, the public, and the vehicle or aircraft.

Medical Facilities

Most patients are transported to the emergency department of a local general hospital. Some patients may require treatment in specialized medical centers, such as burn units or pediatric hospitals (these specialized centers are described later in the chapter).

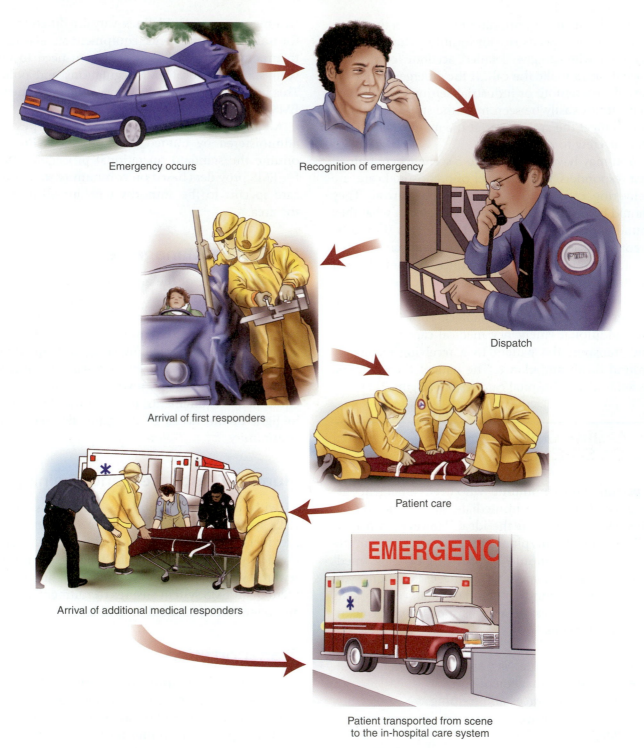

Emergency occurs

Recognition of emergency

Dispatch

Arrival of first responders

Patient care

Arrival of additional medical responders

Patient transported from scene
to the in-hospital care system

Figure 1-1. Continuity of care in an EMS system.

EMS personnel must be knowledgeable about the capabilities and locations of different facilities. This helps ensure the best and most complete patient care.

Communications

The communications element of the EMS system includes public access to emergency care and communication between EMS providers and hospitals. It also includes interagency communication.

Effective crisis management requires the coordination of several groups of people. EMS, police, and fire personnel usually are present at the scene to help with this coordination. To control the scene and provide the best medical care to patients, various agencies must be able to communicate with each other.

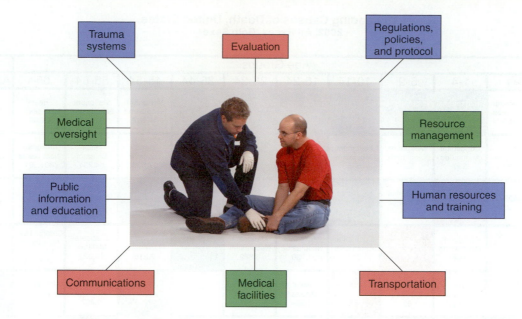

Figure 1-2. Ten organizational elements of an EMS system.

Communication problems could result in duplication of efforts or lack of needed resources. They may even result in additional injury to patients or rescue personnel. Sophisticated communications networks have been established to coordinate the activities and movements of large groups of rescuers and equipment.

Typically, a unified command system is used to coordinate the efforts of many assisting agencies in crisis situations. This type of system, called an incident command management system, is discussed further in Chapter 35.

Public Information and Education

One of the most important components of the EMS system is public information and education. As an EMT, you can best ensure proper use of EMS resources by helping to educate the community you serve about emergency medical services and how to access them.

Education should include providing information about preventing injury. Trauma is a leading cause of death in people between the ages of 1 and 44 years (Figure 1-3), but in many cases death caused by traumatic injury can be prevented. EMTs can save lives by participating in and leading injury prevention programs. As an EMT, you should talk to groups about seat belts, bicycle safety, fire prevention, and smoke detectors (Figure 1-4). Many injury prevention programs have been organized by EMS systems.

Cardiopulmonary resuscitation (CPR), first aid, and other training programs can also help prepare the community to recognize and respond appropriately to emergencies. Public information and community education efforts are rewarding because even small efforts can have a big impact.

Medical Oversight

Medical oversight is the process by which a physician directs and monitors the medical care provided by an EMS system. This is discussed in greater detail later in the chapter.

Trauma Systems

Care for a patient with multiple injuries often requires a variety of health care specialists. Immediate access to surgical care may also be needed. Trauma systems have been developed because few general hospitals can provide these resources. A **trauma system** ensures that patients with life-threatening injuries are transported quickly to the most appropriate hospital or specialized center for lifesaving interventions and surgical care.

Evaluation

Evaluation is important for the continuing success of any EMS system. It helps to identify both the elements of a service's care that excel and those that

15 Leading Causes of Death, United States
2002, All Races, Both Sexes

Rank	<1	1-4	5-9	10-14	15-24	25-34	35-44	45-54	55-64	65+	All Ages
						Age Groups					
1	Congenital Anomalies 5,623	Unintentional Injury 1,641	Unintentional Injury 1,176	Unintentional Injury 1,542	Unintentional Injury 15,412	Unintentional Injury 12,569	Unintentional Injury 16,710	Malignant Neoplasms 49,637	Malignant Neoplasms 93,391	Heart Disease 576,301	Heart Disease 696,947
2	Short Gestation 4,637	Congenital Anomalies 530	Malignant Neoplasms 537	Malignant Neoplasms 535	Homicide 5,219	Suicide 5,046	Malignant Neoplasms 16,085	Heart Disease 37,570	Heart Disease 64,234	Malignant Neoplasms 391,001	Malignant Neoplasms 557,271
3	SIDS 2,295	Homicide 423	Congenital Anomalies 199	Suicide 260	Suicide 4,010	Homicide 4,489	Heart Disease 13,688	Unintentional Injury 14,675	Chronic Low. Respiratory Disease 11,280	Cerebro-vascular 143,293	Cerebro-vascular 162,672
4	Maternal Pregnancy Comp. 1,708	Malignant Neoplasms 402	Homicide 140	Congenital Anomalies 218	Malignant Neoplasms 1,730	Malignant Neoplasms 3,872	Suicide 6,851	Liver Disease 7,216	Diabetes Mellitus 10,022	Chronic Low. Respiratory Disease 108,313	Chronic Low. Respiratory Disease 124,816
5	Placenta Cord Membranes 1,028	Heart Disease 165	Heart Disease 92	Homicide 216	Heart Disease 1,022	Heart Disease 3,165	HIV 5,707	Suicide 6,308	Cerebro-vascular 9,897	Influenza & Pneumonia 58,826	Unintentional Injury 106,742
6	Unintentional Injury 946	Influenza & Pneumonia 110	Benign Neoplasms 44	Heart Disease 163	Congenital Anomalies 492	HIV 1,839	Homicide 3,239	Cerebro-vascular 6,055	Unintentional Injury 8,345	Alzheimer's Disease 58,289	Diabetes Mellitus 73,249
7	Respiratory Distress 943	Septicemia 79	Septicemia 42	Chronic Low. Respiratory Disease 95	Chronic Low. Respiratory Disease 192	Diabetes Mellitus 642	Liver Disease 3,154	Diabetes Mellitus 5,496	Liver Disease 6,097	Diabetes Mellitus 54,715	Influenza & Pneumonia 65,681
8	Bacterial Sepsis 749	Chronic Low. Respiratory Disease 65	Chronic Low. Respiratory Disease 41	Cerebro-vascular 58	HIV 178	Cerebro-vascular 567	Cerebro-vascular 2,425	HIV 4,474	Suicide 3,618	Nephritis 34,316	Alzheimer's Disease 58,866
9	Circulatory System Disease 667	Perinatal Period 65	Influenza & Pneumonia 38	Influenza & Pneumonia 53	Cerebro-vascular 171	Congenital Anomalies 475	Diabetes Mellitus 2,164	Chronic Low. Respiratory Disease 3,475	Nephritis 3,455	Unintentional Injury 33,641	Nephritis 40,974
10	Intrauterine Hypoxia 583	Benign Neoplasms 60	Cerebro-vascular 33	Septicemia 53	Diabetes Mellitus 171	Liver Disease 374	Chronic Low. Respiratory Disease 1,008	Viral Hepatitis 2,331	Septicemia 3,360	Septicemia 26,670	Septicemia 33,865
11	Atelectasis 400	Cerebro-vascular 53	Anemias 29	Benign Neoplasms 45	Influenza & Pneumonia 167	Influenza & Pneumonia 345	Influenza & Pneumonia 971	Septicemia 2,074	Influenza & Pneumonia 2,987	Hypertension 17,345	Suicide 31,655
12	Neonatal Hemorrhage 387	Acute Bronchitis 23	Perinatal Period 15	Diabetes Mellitus 29	Septicemia 118	Septicemia 314	Septicemia 856	Influenza & Pneumonia 1,918	Hypertension 1,526	Parkinson's Disease 16,577	Liver Disease 27,257
13	Necrotizing Enterocolitis 352	Anemias 21	Meningitis 10	Anemias 24	Anemias 111	Chronic Low. Respiratory Disease 301	Nephritis 749	Homicide 1,915	Aortic Aneurysm 1,460	Pneumonitis 16,236	Hypertension 20,261
14	Birth Trauma 345	Meningitis 19	Nephritis 9	HIV 21	Complicated Pregnancy 89	Nephritis 269	Viral Hepatitis 740	Nephritis 1,893	HIV 1,347	Athero-sclerosis 13,085	Homicide 17,638
15	Chronic Respiratory Disease 314	Nephritis 14	Two Tied 7	Meningitis 21	Benign Neoplasms 87	Anemias 180	Congenital Anomalies 572	Hypertension 923	Benign Neoplasms 1,193	Aortic Aneurysm 12,187	Pneumonitis 17,593

Produced By: Office of Statistics and Programming, National Center for Injury Prevention and Control, CDC

Data Source: National Center for Health Statistics (NCHS) Vital Statistics System.

Figure 1-3. Fifteen leading causes of death in males and females.

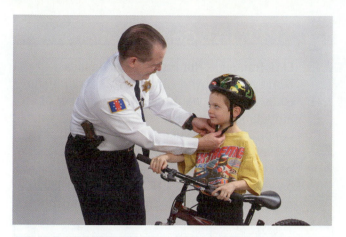

Figure 1-4. Injury prevention programs are important and can have a positive effect on the community.

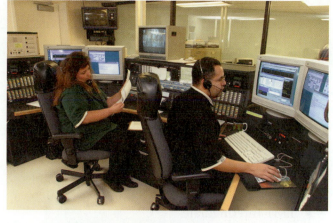

Figure 1-5. 911 Dispatch center.

need improvement. This assessment is often called *quality assurance* or *quality improvement.*

■ ACCESS TO THE EMS SYSTEM

As an EMT, you may be sent to a scene involving an injured or ill patient, or you may be at the scene and providing patient care before the EMS system is activated. In the latter situation, you or someone else will need to call for additional medical help. The 911 system and the popularity of cell phones have greatly simplified calling for help. Before the 911 emergency system was developed, each community had separate phone numbers for police, fire, and ambulance services. Many communities now have access to either basic or enhanced 911 systems.

In the basic 911 system, calls to the emergency number are routed to a central **dispatch center** (Figure 1-5). To dispatch help, the operator must learn the exact location of the emergency from the caller. In the enhanced 911 system, the caller's location is immediately displayed on the dispatcher's computer monitor. Thus the caller doesn't need to know or provide that information. Much of the country is now moving toward phase II cellular capability. As a result, the caller's location can be pinpointed to within a few feet. However, some systems still have drawbacks. A glaring problem (at the time this text was published) is the Internet-based phone. The caller's ability to contact 911 is intermittent at best with these phones. Other problems also have been documented; for example, some callers get either a delayed response or no response at all. Of course, the enhanced system can display only the location of the

ASK YOURSELF

As you embark on your new career, you must be wondering, "When do we learn about trauma and medical emergencies?" Before you begin, you should ask yourself several questions. For example, have you thought about your role in the EMS system and about the responsibilities you will face? How will you provide the best possible care for your patients? Why is the uniform an important part of your equipment?

telephone, not the location of the emergency. Always give the location of the emergency when calling for emergency assistance. A caller using a cell phone should also give the dispatcher the details of the emergency location.

In some emergency situations, a victim who calls 911 might not be able to talk to the dispatcher. The person's injury may affect the ability to speak, or the person may feel threatened by a possible attacker at the scene. In such cases, when the enhanced 911 system provides the dispatcher with the location, police may be dispatched first to determine the nature of the emergency. The investigating police officer may then request additional medical help.

Not all areas have 911 dispatch centers, and some may still have different phone numbers for police, fire, and EMS. A nonunified system may cause communication and dispatch delays and ultimately may delay patient care. As an EMT, it is important that you understand the dispatch system used for all emergency response agencies in your area.

LEVELS OF TRAINING FOR PREHOSPITAL CARE PROVIDERS

Training for prehospital care providers in the United States currently has four nationally recognized levels. At each subsequent level, additional training is required and the prehospital care provider gains additional skills. The four levels of training are

- First responder
- EMT
- EMT-Intermediate
- Paramedic

First Responder

The **first responder** usually is defined as the first person arriving at the scene who has emergency medical training. A first responder may be a firefighter, a police officer, a neighbor, a schoolteacher, or an industrial first aid worker. First responder also is the first designated level of professional emergency medical care, as outlined by the National EMS Scope of Practice skills taught to a first responder include the following:

- Assessment for life-threatening conditions in both medical and trauma patients
- Provision of initial airway care
- Assistance with breathing
- Provision of CPR
- Use of automatic external defibrillators (AEDs)
- Control of bleeding
- Stabilization of spinal and extremity injuries

First responders also are taught other skills and the use of a limited amount of equipment as determined by local and state regulations. They are expected to control a scene initially and to activate the EMS system. In addition, first responders are trained to assist other prehospital care providers.

Emergency Medical Technician (EMT)

The EMT provides many of the same skills as the first responder, but also offers additional skills for managing medical and trauma emergencies. EMTs are trained in more advanced airway skills, the use of pneumatic antishock garments (PASGs), spinal immobilization, the management of fractures, the administration of some medications, and the transport

---

SPECIAL Considerations

EMT Training – Not just for ambulances
Not everyone who starts EMT training finishes the class wanting to be a member of an ambulance crew. However, numerous other opportunities to use your EMT skills are available. For example, in many large companies EMTs work in the health office or as on-site responders. EMTs' skills and knowledge are also in demand at 911 call centers, hospitals, prisons, and lifeguard agencies.

---

of patients. In most jurisdictions EMT is the minimum training level required to work on an ambulance. EMT knowledge and skills are the foundation for the more advanced EMS provider levels.

EMT-Intermediate

In addition to the skills of an EMT, the EMT-Intermediate (EMT-I) has the skills to establish intravenous (IV) lines and administer IV fluids and certain drugs. The EMT-I also may be taught more advanced airway management techniques. Currently, the EMT-I level is one of the most variable in the EMS training program. Different jurisdictions have different training and skill expectations.

Paramedic

In the United States, a **paramedic** provides the highest level of prehospital care. In addition to having the skills of the three preceding levels, paramedics are trained in advanced airway procedures (e.g., endotracheal intubation), administration of medications, and management of cardiac emergencies.

IN-HOSPITAL CARE SYSTEMS

As mentioned previously, most patients who receive EMS care are transported to the emergency department of a local community hospital. Emergency department staff members handle a wide spectrum of emergencies and medical conditions with little or no advance notice. They may treat a bleeding nose one minute and then manage a major trauma or medical emergency the next (Figure 1-6).

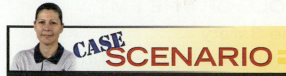

Elizabeth takes the students though the station, pointing out various areas and equipment the ambulance service uses during the course of the shift. Rounding a corner, they meet a gentleman who is talking to other members of Elizabeth's crew. "Excuse me," Elizabeth says, "Dr. Jameson, I'd like to introduce you to some local EMT students, who are touring the station." Turning to the group, Elizabeth explains, "Dr. Jameson is our service's medical director."

Dr. Jameson shakes hands with several of the students. "I'm glad you came by to visit. This service depends on the community college to provide well-trained and enthusiastic EMTs to staff the units. I hope you will consider spending some time with us. Right now, I am reviewing a call Elizabeth and her crew had a week ago. It was a great learning experience, and I wanted to provide some follow-up information about how well she and her team did, based on the care provided by the ambulance crew."

Question: The reason for Dr. Jameson's visit to the station is an example of which critical concept in EMS? As an EMT, what other steps can you take to further improve the quality of your care for patients?

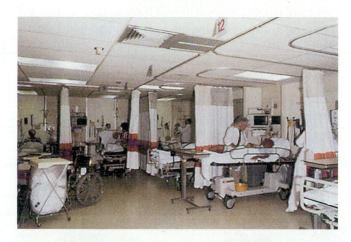

Figure 1-6. Most patients receiving EMS care are transported to the emergency department of a local community hospital.

Some types of emergencies require more resources than are available in the local emergency department and hospital. For this reason, specialized emergency centers have been established around the country. In some cases, a patient first may be transported to the local emergency department, where staff members begin treatment and stabilize the person's condition; the patient then may be transported to a specialized center. In other cases, the patient may be transported directly to the specialized center.

A **trauma center** is a specialized hospital committed to maintaining a state of readiness to care for patients with serious multiple injuries (Figure 1-7). This

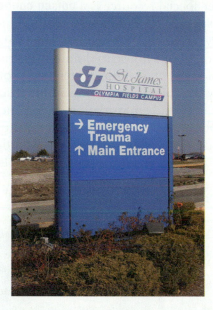

Figure 1-7. Trauma centers are specialized hospitals that are ready to care for patients with serious multiple injuries.

type of care is demanding for the hospital staff and requires special resources. Specialized surgeons and nurses must be prepared 24 hours a day to perform complex surgery at very short notice. These centers have dedicated intensive care units, computed tomography (CT) scanners, blood banks, specialty physicians, and support staff.

Burn centers provide specialized care for victims of thermal, chemical, electrical, and radiation burns. Staff members at these centers also have special expertise for treating smoke inhalation injuries. Because there is only one burn center for every six trauma centers in the United States, a patient may first be transported to a trauma center and later transferred to a specialized burn center.

A child with a severe injury or sudden illness also presents unique challenges. It often is said that children are not just small adults, and this is true in important ways. The medical emergencies of children are rarely similar to those seen in adults. Even with the same kind of trauma, the injuries in a child are different from those in an adult. Specialized pediatric emergency centers and hospitals have been established to meet the special needs of children.

Complications of childbirth also require specialized care. For example, a woman in preterm labor may be transported from a community hospital to a center specializing in perinatal care (a center that can care for both the mother and the baby).

Another special resource is a **poison control center,** which responds to individuals with a poisoning emergency. These centers maintain large databases of information about household and industrial toxins. The people who staff these centers are proficient in toxicology. Poison control centers play a supportive role and can provide information on a particular poisonous substance. The nationwide phone number for Poison Control is 800-222-1212. In addition, each state may have its own poison control center phone number.

■ ROLE OF THE EMT
Scene Safety

EMTs save lives because they are well-trained professionals who may get to the patient first. A child who chokes on a peanut or an elderly man in cardiac arrest has only a few minutes to live unless someone intervenes. A teenager with a head injury from a vehicle collision may suffer irreversible brain damage very quickly unless someone opens the airway. The lifesaving skills that you as an EMT will use with these patients are often simple and do not require specialized equipment.

Personal safety must always be a primary responsibility. As an EMT, you should never jeopardize your own safety for that of a patient. This principle at first may seem selfish or even cowardly. Keep in mind, however, that your objective is to help the patient, and the most immediate threat to the patient is the loss of your care if you are injured at the scene. If you are injured while rushing to a patient in an unsafe situation, your partner or other EMS personnel then will have two patients and will have to divide their efforts and resources between you and the first patient (Figure 1-8).

You should also be mindful of bystanders and make sure that they are safe. Having to care for an injured bystander complicates an already difficult task. Bystanders who try to assist you may actually block your access to the patient or may cause confusion at the scene with emotional outbursts. Relatives of patients are understandably anxious and emotional. However, when their presence promotes chaos or dis-

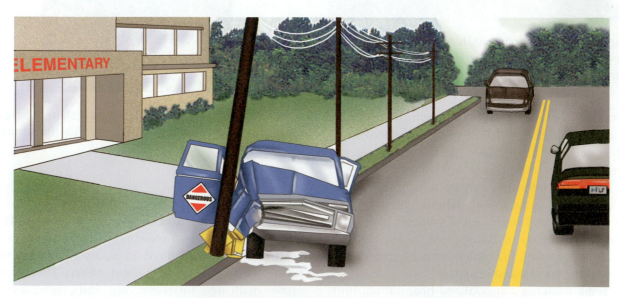

Figure 1-8. An EMT must be aware of potential hazards at a scene.

rupts care, the situation quickly can become dangerous and patient care can become ineffective. If the presence of family members becomes a problem, you should ask another bystander to help move them out of the immediate area. EMTs should always maintain control of the scene until a more advanced health care provider or an incident command officer relieves them.

Patient Care

In some situations the patient may not be readily accessible. As a general rule, if the scene is unsafe, wait until it is made safe for you to enter. Even if the scene is safe, the patient may need to be moved before patient assessment can begin.

Once at the patient's side, you perform a systematic evaluation for any life-threatening conditions. This is the initial part of patient assessment. In emergency care, patient assessments should always be performed in the same organized manner, as you will learn in the following chapters. No matter how chaotic a situation might become, you can always use the techniques you will learn and practice in this course (Figure 1-9).

After the assessment, the patient is treated, or managed, based on your assessment findings. Once you have begun treatment, periodically reevaluate the patient to determine whether the person's condition is improving or worsening.

If you are not part of the transport team, when the ambulance or more advanced medical care arrives on the scene, identify yourself as a trained EMT and re-

SPECIAL Considerations

Patient Advocacy
Patient advocacy is a critical part of patient care. Not all patients who call 911 require the services of an emergency department, particularly patients in end-stage terminal illness. EMTs may provide the best care for patients and their families by helping the family contact hospice care, home health care agencies, and community resources (e.g., agencies for the elderly).

port the details of the emergency, your physical assessment, and the treatment you have given. Document this information in the prehospital care record according to your local or state requirements for documentation. Details about the first few minutes after the occurrence of an emergency can be very helpful to physicians in the diagnosis and treatment of the patient's condition. When emergency personnel with more advanced training arrive, they become responsible for the care of the patient. However, even then a first responder remains a valuable team member and can still render assistance.

Personal Traits

As an EMT your responsibilities involve more than just your actions at the scene of an emergency.

Personal Health and Well-Being
Emergency care can be physically, emotionally, and psychologically draining. To deal with these stresses, you should strive to maintain your own health. Regular exercise helps prevent personal injury. Moreover, it has proved to be an effective tool for preventing the adverse effects of emotional stress. As a prehospital care provider, you can have a positive impact on the lives of people in your community, but only if you stay fit and prevent injury to yourself. Chapter 2 more fully addresses ways to maintain your health and well-being.

Personal Behavior
Your personal behavior is also important. Consider for a moment the role you play as a prehospital care provider. People in crisis allow you, a stranger, to care for their sick or dying loved ones. Few other

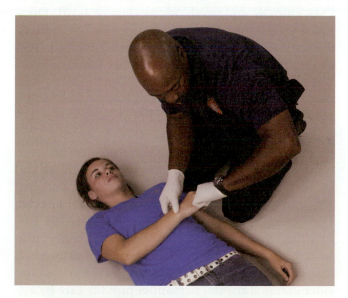

Figure 1-9. Patient assessment.

individuals in society share this privilege. You should never betray the public's trust by making rude, crass, or insensitive remarks. Remember that what might be a routine situation for you may be a frightening and foreign one to a patient. Every patient deserves your empathy and compassion; sometimes the most important service you can perform is just to hold the patient's hand and provide emotional support.

Changing your care based on a patient's race, religion, gender, age, or socioeconomic status is inappropriate. All patients have the right to the best care you can provide.

Self-Composure

Self-composure is essential whenever you are dealing with an emergency. The patient, family members, and bystanders expect you, the EMT, to be in control of the situation. How you react to the emergency affects how they react. If you panic, bystanders also may panic, and the scene may become chaotic. This is a dangerous situation in which either the patient or you (or both) may be hurt. Feeling some anxiety when you face a life-threatening situation is normal, but you must contain this anxiety and project calm confidence. A technique for accomplishing this is to remember to Stop, Think, and Act. Stop for a brief moment to think about what you are doing and what you have been trained to do, and then perform your duties.

Professional Appearance

A professional appearance contributes to your credibility. People formulate their initial impressions based on your appearance. When you respond to an emergency as part of an EMS agency, you essentially represent that entire service. If your appearance is unprofessional, people may falsely assume that your assessment and care will be below par. Your clothes or uniform should be clean and neat and fit well. Your shoes should be comfortable yet professional and should have good traction for wet surfaces. Remember that you will be kneeling, squatting, and lifting when you wear these clothes, so make sure they are not too tight or constrictive. Health care workers usually refrain from wearing fragrances, which sometimes can aggravate a patient's nausea or allergies. Remember that you are most effective as an EMT when you have total control of the scene. An EMT is a very visible individual; you should take advantage of this visibility by making the best possible impression with your behavior and appearance.

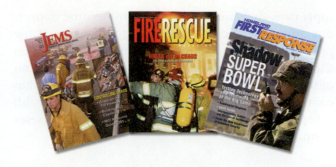

Figure 1-10. EMTs can keep up-to-date on national issues by subscribing to EMS journals.

Maintenance of Knowledge and Skills

As an EMS professional, you are responsible for the welfare of your patients. People expect that when they call for help, they will receive state-of-the-art emergency care. Therefore all prehospital care providers are responsible for maintaining their knowledge and skills by attending continuing education programs and practicing their skills. Continuing education courses generally are offered at hospitals, fire departments, community colleges, and conferences. Your local EMS system is only as good as its members, so get involved and take an active role in your continued training. Participation in EMT refresher courses also helps you maintain your skills.

Current Knowledge of Local and National Issues

As an EMT, make an effort to be aware of issues affecting your community. You can maintain your knowledge of national issues by staying involved in national or state organizations and subscribing to EMS journals and publications (Figure 1-10). Organizations in which you can become involved include the National Association of Emergency Medical Technicians (NAEMT) and your state EMS association.

■ MEDICAL OVERSIGHT

Every EMS system has some form of medical oversight. Usually a physician develops guidelines and protocols for the emergency treatment of patients. This physician is referred to as the **medical director.** The exact responsibilities of medical directors vary in different areas, but the medical director ultimately is responsible for the prehospital medical care delivered by that EMS service. Many states consider that prehospital personnel provide care by acting as an agent for the medical director. Because, as a prehospital care provider, you are a surrogate for the physician, both you and the medical director may be held responsible in the event of a problematic outcome.

The two common types of medical oversight are direct medical control and indirect medical control. With **direct medical control** (also called *online* or *immediate control*), the prehospital team communicates with the physician before providing a specific treatment. This communication usually occurs by radio or telephone (Figure 1-11).

Indirect medical control (also called *offline* or *prospective control*) involves clear protocols, or standing orders, for the treatment of various emergencies. The medical director develops these protocols and ensures that prehospital care providers are well trained in them. This allows prehospital care personnel to provide care in some emergency situations by following the protocols, without first having to communicate directly with the medical director. A continuous quality improvement (CQI) program is needed to evaluate how well the protocols are being carried out. If problems are found, the protocols might need revision or additional training might be required.

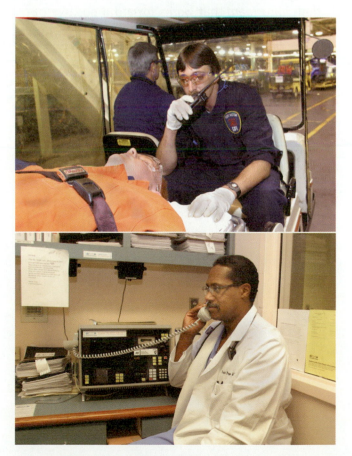

Figure 1-11. Direct medical control.

Many EMS systems use a combination of these two types of medical control. For example, written protocols may be in place for many emergencies, but the physician's orders may be required for administration of a particular medication.

As an EMT, you are considered an agent of the physician who is the medical director. Frequent and open communication between you and the medical director is in everyone's best interest.

■ SPECIFIC STATUTES AND REGULATIONS

Every state has its own laws regarding how prehospital care is provided, but the important issues generally are the same from state to state. Legal issues affecting EMS include Good Samaritan laws, consent for treatment, consent for refusal of treatment, abandonment, and confidentiality.

Good Samaritan laws cover the liability of an individual who volunteers assistance in an emergency. These laws protect licensed health care providers who give emergency assistance in good faith, as long as they do not commit negligent, willful, or wanton acts of misconduct or omission, or charge for their services. In general, this means that if you volunteer your assistance and act in accordance with your training, you cannot be held liable. If you attempt a technique you are not trained to perform or if you intentionally harm a patient, you may be held liable for any resulting injuries. Once you begin emergency treatment, you are obligated to continue to give care until you have transferred that care to someone of equal or higher training. Failure to continue treatment until you are appropriately relieved is called *abandonment.*

Before giving treatment, you need consent from the patient. With a minor, consent comes from the child's parent or guardian. Consent need not be written; verbal consent is acceptable. In life-threatening emergencies or situations in which the patient is unconscious or otherwise unable to give consent, the consent is said to be implied. Competent patients, however, are allowed to refuse help. If a patient refuses help, you may disagree with that decision but must respect the patient's legal rights. In such a case, you must first ensure that the patient understands the risks of refusing care and explain to the patient what might happen without timely medical attention. You should also inform patients that if they change their mind or their condition worsens, they should call EMS or go to a local emergency department. Chapter 3 covers these and other legal topics in more detail.

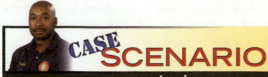

CASE SCENARIO
conclusion

Jack was fascinated by what he saw and heard during the tour. It was so much more than just the ambulance with its flashing lights and loud siren! Elizabeth was very knowledgeable, friendly, and patient as Jack asked his questions about EMS. At the end of the tour, she pulled Jack aside. "You seem very interested in the profession, Jack. When you have the time, come on down during our duty shifts and ride along. You'll get to see a lot of what you learn in action!"■

References

NHTSA Documents
– National Scope of Practice
EMS Agenda for the Future
EMS Education Agenda for the Future

TEAMWORK

As we saw in this chapter, EMTs work in a variety of settings. You may be on a team at an industrial site or school, or you may be part of a sophisticated rescue team. Wherever you are employed, you will be working with police officers, firefighters, rescue teams with specialized training in medical and nonmedical areas, and others. As an EMT you must familiarize yourself with agencies likely to respond in your service area and plan ways of working with them. You need to work closely with police and fire personnel to ensure scene safety for yourself and your patient. Rescue and EMS personnel depend on you for the initial history of the patient's emergency. It is important to work within the limits of your certification or licensure and to assist other health care providers when called upon to do so. Your patients certainly benefit from your ability to give an accurate account of their medical history, the results of your examination, and any treatment you may have provided. EMTs should always remember that they are part of the patient care *team* that works toward a positive patient outcome.

NUTS AND BOLTS

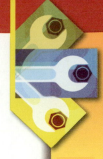

Critical Points

The EMT student must be able to describe an EMS system and explain the role an EMT plays in that system. EMTs require both adequate training to fulfill their roles and a knowledge of how to interact with other members of the health care team.

Learning Checklist

Having completed this chapter, the EMT student should now be able to:

❏ List the steps involved in an emergency: initial recognition of the emergency, activation of the EMS system, arrival of the EMT, patient care, arrival of additional responders, transport of the patient, and transfer of the patient to the in-hospital care system.

❏ Name the 10 components of an EMS system: (1) regulations, policies, and protocols; (2) resource management; (3) human resources and training; (4) transportation; (5) medical facilities; (6) communications; (7) public information and education; (8) medical oversight; (9) trauma systems; and (10) evaluation.

❏ Explain how access to the EMS system usually is achieved through the basic or enhanced 911 system. In both systems, calls are routed to a central 911 dispatch center. In the basic system, the caller must identify the location to which help should be sent. In the enhanced system, ideally the caller's location is immediately displayed on the dispatcher's computer monitor.

❏ Give the four levels of training for prehospital care: (1) first responder, (2) EMT, (3) EMT-I, and (4) paramedic.

❏ Discuss the skills needed by an EMT who is first on the scene of an emergency and who provides medical attention to the patient. Necessary skills include immediate assessment and management of life-threatening conditions, control of a scene, activation of the EMS system, and assistance to other prehospital care providers.

❏ Discuss the skills utilized for managing an airway and shock management. Necessary skills for managing an airway would include the use of oral and nasal airways, bag-mask device, and mouth-to-mask ventilation. Shock management skills include conserving body heat, controlling hemorrhage, use of supplemental oxygen, and application of anti-shock garments.

❏ Describe the skills of an EMT-I. The EMT-I has the skills of an EMT and also can establish IV lines and more advanced airways and can administer some medications.

❏ Explain the role of paramedics. Paramedics are the highest level of prehospital care. For example, they are trained in endotracheal intubation and other advanced airway techniques and in the administration of medications.

❏ Explain the course of action when a patient is transferred to the in-hospital system. The patient may go to a local general hospital or to a specialized center. Specialized centers include trauma centers, burn centers, pediatric emergency centers and hospitals, and perinatal centers.

❏ Describe the responsibilities of an EMT. These include personal safety, patient care, personal health and well-being, professional and courteous personal behavior, self-composure in an emergency, a professional appearance, current knowledge and practice of skills, and awareness of local and national issues.

❏ Describe the role of the medical director. The medical director is the physician who maintains medical oversight over an EMS system.

❏ Define direct medical control. With direct medical control, the prehospital team communicates directly with the physician before giving treatment to a patient. This communication usually occurs over the radio or the telephone.

❏ Define indirect medical control. With indirect medical control, protocols, or standing orders, outline the care to be provided in a given situation.

❏ Explain the importance of keeping up-to-date on legal issues involving prehospital

15

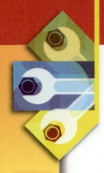

care. Every state has its own laws regulating prehospital care. It is important for a first responder to know the local laws.

Key Terms

Direct medical control: Real-time communication between prehospital care personnel and medical control. This can take place in person, on the phone, or over the radio; also called *online medical control.*

Dispatch center: A central location where personnel obtain information about an incident and assign resources and EMS workers to manage it.

Emergency: An unexpected, life-threatening situation.

Emergency medical services (EMS) system: The network of services that handles prehospital medical and trauma emergencies. EMS systems can be organized at the local, regional, state, or national level.

Emergency medical technician (EMT): A medical provider who performs prehospital care; the term typically refers to the EMT level of qualification but may be used to denote any level of prehospital care. EMTs are part of the organized EMS system.

First responder: The first person at the scene of a medical or trauma emergency who is trained in medical care. First responders are part of the organized EMS system.

Indirect medical control: The use of standing orders, or written protocols, to provide care. This type of medical control does not involve actual communication with a medical director at the time of the incident; also called *offline medical control.*

Medical director: A physician who develops guidelines and protocols for prehospital treatment of patients. The medical director is responsible for the prehospital medical care delivered by EMS providers.

Paramedic: The most advanced level of prehospital emergency medical care. Paramedics are part of the organized EMS system.

Poison control center: A service that provides data on all aspects of poisonings, keeps records of poisonings, and refers patients to treatment centers.

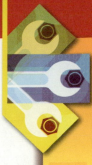

Trauma center: A specialized hospital equipped with the personnel and resources to provide immediate advanced level care for a critically injured trauma patient.

Trauma system: A system that helps identify the appropriate hospital or specialized center to which a trauma patient should be transported.

National Standard Curriculum Objectives

Cognitive Objectives
After completing this lesson, the EMT student will be able to:

- Define the EMS system.
- Differentiate the roles and responsibilities of the EMT from those of other prehospital care providers.
- Describe the EMT's roles and responsibilities with regard to personal safety.
- Discuss the roles and responsibilities of the EMT with regard to the safety of the crew, the patient and bystanders.
- Define quality improvement and discuss the EMT's role in the process.
- Define medical direction and discuss the EMT's role in the process.
- State the specific statutes and regulations governing the EMS system in his or her state.

Affective Objectives
After completing this lesson, the EMT student will be able to:

- Assess areas of personal attitude and conduct of the EMT.
- Characterize the various methods used to access the EMS system in the community.

Psychomotor Objectives
No objectives identified.

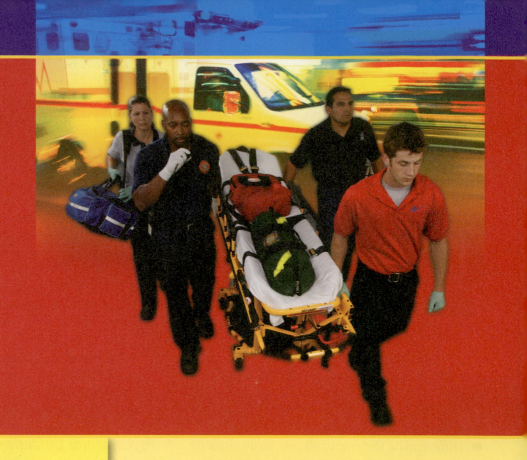

CHAPTER

2

OUTLINE

GOAL

LESSON GOAL

As an emergency medical technician (EMT), you will find yourself in many stressful situations involving physical and emotional hazards. EMTs must be prepared to protect themselves from the potentially harmful physical and psychologic effects of such situations. Many of the risks of the job involve hazards at the scene. These hazards require the EMT to take measures to make the scene safe for operations. Therefore EMTs must have the assessment skills to determine whether they can enter a scene safely. Furthermore, patients often have diseases that can be transmitted to the EMT providing care. To reduce this risk, EMTs must be protected by vaccines and personal protective equipment.

This chapter addresses the orientation to prehospital care required by EMTs so that they are physically and mentally prepared for the job. The very nature of this work compels individuals to rush in when others are rushing out. Consequently, the work holds certain risks. However, these risks can be minimized to promote a safe, healthy career in prehospital care. ■

Well-Being of the Emergency Medical Technician (EMT)

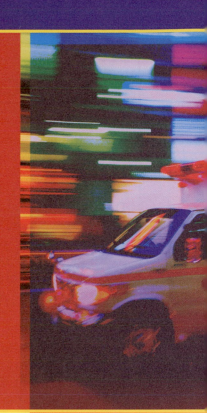

2

CHAPTER OBJECTIVES

After completing this chapter, the EMT student will be able to do the following:

1 Discuss the emotional reactions the EMT may experience when faced with trauma, illness, death, and dying.

2 Discuss the reactions a family member may show when confronted with death and dying.

3 Describe the steps in the EMT approach to a family confronted with death and dying.

4 Describe the reactions the EMT's family may experience as a result of their outside involvement in emergency medical services (EMS).

5 Describe the signs and symptoms of critical incident stress.

6 Describe the steps an EMT may take to minimize or alleviate stress.

7 Explain the need to determine scene safety.

8 Discuss the importance of body substance isolation.

9 Describe the steps EMTs should take to protect themselves from airborne and blood-borne pathogens.

10 List the personal protective equipment necessary for each of the following situations:

- Hazardous materials
- Rescue operation
- Violent crime
- Crime scene
- Exposure to blood-borne pathogens
- Exposure to airborne pathogens

Thick, angry smoke is pouring out of the upper floors of the six unit apartment building as Engine 32 pulls up. Captain Alvarez and his crew had already seen the glow of the fire from several blocks away, as they came in on the second assignment. The first-in companies had already reported that "numerous injuries" had occurred and that rescues were taking place. Over the noise of the diesel motor, Captain Alvarez yells to his crew to hook up to the hydrant down the street and begin to set up another attack line on the house. He spots the rescue crews carrying out limp bodies and laying them on the driveway in front of the building. He taps Rafael Gonzales on the back and directs him to head to the scene with the medical bag and airway kit. Rafael hesitates briefly, his attention drawn to the fire, but then rushes to follow the captain's order.

Other EMS crews are also heading over to the growing scene. Some are using scissors to cut open nightgowns and pajamas. Rafael joins an EMT who is working on a young girl about 5 or 6 years old. Rafael can feel his heart pounding as he begins his own assessment. The child does not appear to be breathing, and she has no pulse. While the other EMT ventilates her with a bag-valve-mask, Rafael begins performing chest compressions. The child seems so small beneath his hands. Sweat gathers on Rafael's forehead as he pumps the little girl's chest methodically and quickly. Looking up briefly, he sees other firefighters performing cardiopulmonary resuscitation (CPR) on other children nearby.

Question: An EMT may become involved in situations that cause undue stress. Can you give some other examples? If you were friends with Rafael, what are some things you might do if you learned about this event?

I n deciding to become an EMT, you have made a decision to help others at the potential risk of danger or injury to yourself. This is a commendable decision, but it is also a serious commitment. You must become skilled at coping with the emotional and physical stress of the job. Also, you must learn to understand and assist others as they endure the stress of an emergency situation. When you arrive at the scene of an emergency, you will assess risks, prepare yourself, and intervene to help victims of injury and illness. You will be able to perform procedures that can save a patient's life. Therefore, even in the midst of chaotic situations, you must remember your training. However, your first priority must always be to protect your own safety and well-being. You can be the best help to others when you are safe, healthy, and emotionally strong.

The work of an EMT is rewarding, but it is not easy. Sometimes the scene is dangerous, and the EMT encounters a variety of hazards. You must prepare yourself to minimize the risks. This chapter explores ways to help you maintain your well-being on the job.

■ STRESSFUL SITUATIONS

The horrible things that happen to people can be difficult to witness and to live with (Box 2-1). For instance, mass casualty incidents (MCIs), which may involve many people, can be confusing. The cumulative impact of dealing with all the casualties and pain can be overwhelming. Working with pediatric patients also can be particularly difficult, partly because children are expected to be bright and playful, not sick or seriously hurt. Moreover, violent situations make little sense, whether the perpetrator is a stranger or a family member. Abuse of children, spouses, or the elderly can evoke anger or sadness in the EMT. Amputations of limbs can be challenging to witness and difficult to deal with emotionally. The death of a patient can be a jolting experience. When you work hard to keep a patient alive, it may be difficult not to take it as a personal failure if the patient dies. If a coworker or another public safety officer is injured or killed, you may feel the fear or loss more keenly. These are just a few examples of the stressful

BOX 2-1

Examples of Stressful Situations

- Mass casualty incident (MCI)
- Pediatric patient
- Death
- Amputation
- Violence
- Abuse
- Death or injury of a coworker or other public safety worker

situations an EMT may face. However, everyone has different triggers and thresholds for stress. The trigger that causes stress for you may not be the same for another person.

As an EMT, you must be aware of, understand, and plan to manage stress. Stress can come from your patients or from other aspects of your life. The hours and environments of your work can induce stress. Furthermore, you will experience not only your own stress but also the stress of patients, families, and bystanders. You must find ways to cope with these stresses, or they will have a detrimental effect on your personal and professional life. The recognition of stress and the use of coping mechanisms are addressed in greater detail later in the chapter.

■ EMOTIONAL ASPECTS OF EMERGENCY CARE

Death and Dying

Death affects EMTs, other health care team members, the families and friends of patients, and bystanders. The way people respond to death is highly individual, shaped by their culture and experience. You may see responses that vary from a family quietly crying, to a room full of inconsolable people wailing and throwing themselves on the floor, to a mob yelling angrily at you. A large part of how individuals respond to death is learned from their parents and family members or others involved in their upbringing. What you are or are not exposed to as you grow up greatly affects your ability or inability to handle the stress of death and dying. Yet no matter what your life experiences may be, as an EMT you must be able to respond professionally

and compassionately to dying patients and those affected by death. Some adults may not have experienced the death of someone close to them. Without past experiences from which they have recovered, their sense of loss can be overwhelming. As an EMT, you will probably encounter scenes involving death, you will treat dying patients, and you will provide support to the families and friends of those who have died. You must try to understand the concerns of the dying patient, communicate empathetically with family members after the death of a loved one, and manage your own feelings about death and loss.

Signs of Death

Only a physician can determine the cause of death. However, there are universally accepted signs that can indicate death. In many situations, death is defined as the absence of circulatory and respiratory function. Many states have adopted *brain death* provisions. These provisions define death as irreversible cessation of all functions of the brain and brainstem. As an EMT, you may need to determine whether a patient is dead or requires emergency medical care. By most current standards, EMTs must resuscitate all patients unless they are obviously dead or a *do not resuscitate (DNR)* order is presented. Terminally ill patients may not want to be resuscitated. (The EMT's rights and responsibilities with regard to resuscitation and DNR orders are discussed in Chapter 3.) If a DNR order is unclear or does not seem authentic or if some other question exists, you should provide emergency medical care in the absence of definitive signs of death. You should provide this care until the DNR order is clarified or you transfer care to another health care provider.

As a general rule, you should begin emergency medical care if the body is warm and intact. In cases of cold temperature emergencies in which the patient may have hypothermia, you should always begin emergency medical care.

Presumptive signs of death are indications of death that, in combination, are accepted by most medical and legal authorities. These presumptive signs carry even more weight after severe trauma or in the end stages of a long-term illness, such as cancer. These signs *are not considered adequate* in cases of extremely cold body temperature (hypothermia), poisonings, or heart attack (cardiac arrest). Box 2-2 presents some of the presumptive signs of death.

BOX 2-2
Presumptive Signs of Death

- Lack of response to painful stimuli
- Absence of breathing
- Absence of a pulse or heartbeat
- Absence of deep tendon or corneal reflexes
- Absence of eye movement
- Absence of blood pressure
- Dependent lividity (blood settling to the lowest point of the body, causing discoloration of the skin)
- Profound cyanosis (bluish coloration)
- Lowered body temperature

The definitive, or conclusive, signs of death include the following:

- *Clear mortal damage.* This includes such conditions as separation of the body into parts (as with decapitation).
- *Rigor mortis.* This is the stiffening of body muscles caused by chemical changes in muscle tissue. It develops first in the face and jaw and gradually extends downward until the body is in full rigor. The rate of stiffening is affected by the rate at which the body loses heat to the environment. A thin body loses heat faster than one with more body fat. A body on a tile floor loses heat faster than a body wrapped in a blanket in a bed. Rigor mortis can begin 2 to 12 hours after death.
- *Putrefaction.* This refers to the decomposition of body tissues. Depending on temperature conditions, putrefaction begins 40 to 96 hours after death.

Emotions of Critically Ill and Injured Patients

Individuals who are dying as a result of trauma, an acute medical emergency, or a terminal disease may experience a wide spectrum of emotions. They may feel threatened, frightened, hopeless, helpless, peaceful, or resigned. Their emotions also may change rapidly. Common emotional states of injured, critically ill, and dying patients include the following:

- Anxiety
- Pain and anger
- Depression
- Dependency
- Guilt

Often these emotions are related to the normal stages of grieving. (These stages are discussed later in the chapter.) When patients display emotions related to their critical condition, you should communicate honestly and empathetically as you acknowledge their feelings. Stay calm, and comfort and reassure the patient while you wait for additional resources. A familiarity with the common emotional responses of critically ill or injured patients can help you to provide effective care.

Anxiety

Anxiety is a response to the anticipation of danger. Ill and injured patients often are anxious about what will happen to them—whether they will die or become disabled—and about the care you provide. Patients who are anxious may be described as follows:

- Upset
- Sweating and cool (diaphoretic)
- Breathing fast (hyperventilating)
- Tachycardic (a fast pulse)
- Restless
- Tense
- Fearful
- Shaky (tremulous)

Panic is a severe anxiety reaction. It can endanger both patients and EMTs. Your calm and confident care can reduce patients' anxiety and help them maintain their self-control.

Pain and Anger

Pain often occurs with illness or trauma. Patients also may fear anticipated pain and potential injury. You should encourage patients to express their pains and fears. This may help them adjust to the pain and accept your emergency medical care.

In addition, patients may complain, express anger, and be demanding. You should understand that this anger may be a display of their fear or anxiety about emergency medical care. Patients who feel anger toward you or other health care providers may express it physically. If a patient or family member gets so emotionally upset that you feel threatened or are physically assaulted, you should remove yourself from the scene and call for law enforcement. Remember, if you cannot make the scene safe, do not enter it. Furthermore, if it becomes unsafe, leave. Your safety must be your first priority.

Depression

Most dying patients experience some degree of depression. Some individuals have many dissatisfac-

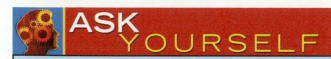

tions and regrets about their lives, whereas others may be concerned about financial, legal, social, or family problems. You should encourage patients to express their feelings and concerns. Support patients and their families in resolving unsettled matters. This helps to ease the patient's feelings of depression.

Dependency

When you provide emergency medical care to patients, they may develop a sense of dependency on you. This occurs because patients often feel that they are no longer in control of their future and their life. They are putting their well-being in the hands of strangers and are depending on the skills and expertise of the many health care providers. As a result, they may become resentful or may feel helpless, ashamed, weak, or inferior.

Guilt

Many dying patients and their family members feel guilty about what has happened or about what they may or may not have done. Often they cannot explain their feelings. Patients or family members who delayed requesting emergency medical care may also feel guilty.

Behavioral Problems

Disorientation, confusion, or delusions may develop in a dying patient. The patient may behave in ways that do not reflect normal patterns of thinking, feeling, or acting. Common characteristics of such behavior include the following:

- Loss of contact with reality
- Distorted perception
- Regressive behavior and attitudes
- Diminished control of basic impulses and desires

- Abnormal mental processes, including delusions and hallucinations
- Generalized personality deterioration

Providing Care for Critically Ill and Injured Patients

As an EMT, you should introduce yourself to all patients and let them know your level of training and your motivation—you are there to help. Moreover, you should let patients know that you are attending to their immediate needs, which are your primary concern. Also, make sure that you continually explain what is happening. This will alleviate the patient's confusion, anxiety, and feelings of helplessness. You, other medical providers, and family and friends should not make any grim comments about a patient's condition. Such remarks may depress the patient, diminish hope, and possibly compromise recovery.

Lights, sirens, smells, and unknown personnel can confuse a patient. You should understand this and help the patient stay oriented to the situation. You can give explanations such as, "Mr. Smith, you are hurt. The police are here, and I'm now treating your arm. My name is John, and I am an EMT trained in emergency medical care. I'm here to help you." You should use your judgment in being honest with patients without unnecessarily shocking or confusing them. If a patient refuses emergency medical care or asks that you leave him or her alone, you should explain the seriousness of his or her condition and your ability to help. You should not express undue alarm to try to persuade the patient. You also should not say, "Everything will be okay," when that is obviously not the case. If a patient refuses emergency care, document this refusal in your report and, if possible, have the patient sign a refusal of care form.

Patients may ask if they are going to die. You may feel at a loss for words if you know that the prognosis is poor. Remember that it is not your responsibility to tell a patient that death is imminent. Instead, make honest but helpful statements, such as, "I know this is scary, but let's fight this together," or "I'm not going to give up on you, so don't give up on yourself." It is appropriate for an EMT to offer hope and to show conviction about doing everything possible to save a patient's life.

Often patients will ask you to contact a family member or someone else. A patient may or may not be able to assist with phone numbers or other information. In these situations, assure the patient that you or someone else will attempt to locate the person.

With critically ill or injured children, calm, comfort, and reassure the patient while waiting for additional responders. You can and should enlist the help of a family member, friend, or accompanying adult to relieve a child's anxiety and assist with care as appropriate.

Grieving helps individuals move through the stages of dealing with death and dying. People progress through these stages to move on with their lives. By becoming familiar with the grieving process, you will be more competent at understanding and helping the people you encounter in each of the stages (Fig. 2-1).

Stages of Grief

Denial
The first stage of the grieving process is denial. People try to tell themselves, "This is not happening to me." This is a self-defense mechanism to create a buffer against the shock of death or illness. You may frequently encounter families in the denial stage. Therefore your understanding of this defense mechanism may help you to deal with this difficult situation. This stage is often characterized by disbelief at the situation or a "not me" response.

Anger
The next stage of grief often is anger. The patient or family may ask you, "Out of all the people in the world, why me/us?" Patients or families also may make you the target of their disbelief and anger. It is important that you do not take this personally or get defensive. Instead, try to be tolerant and listen empathetically, even if you do not fully understand how the patient feels. Attentive listening and genuine communication are deeply appreciated by people in distress.

Bargaining
In the next stage of the grieving process, people bargain. For example, the son of a critically ill mother might reason, "Let her live, and I'll quit smoking," in an attempt to delay death or hold out the chance for a deal to be struck. Again, you can help by listening to the patient and communicating clearly and with empathy. You must be sensitive to the patient and, at the same time, show strength by conveying the reality of the situation to all involved.

Depression
In the next stage, people may begin to express sadness and despair. Crying followed by silent withdrawal is common. Staying involved with desperately sad individuals is difficult, but an EMT must cope with the sorrow and maintain communication with the patient.

Acceptance
In the last stage, a person eventually may accept approaching death even while remaining sad or angry. The friends or family usually require more support during this stage than the patient. Acceptance may or may not be reached during the grieving process. It is important to understand that moving through each of these stages can take time.

Dealing With the Dying Patient and Family Members
Not only the dying patient, but also the family and friends go through some or all of the stages of grief. As an EMT, you, too, may go through a grieving period. It is important to note that different people may be at different stages of their grief at the same time. For example, the patient may have had time to accept death, but the family may be in denial during your entire experience with them. Another family may have reached acceptance while the patient still struggles with denial. Understanding the process of grief can help you to treat those dealing with death appropriately. Ultimately, you need to express compassion and understanding to the patient and family.

You must respect a dying patient's emotions. The patient deserves dignity during this ultimate test. You should try to protect the dying patient's privacy and allow the person any possible control over the care you provide. The patient will want you to listen em-

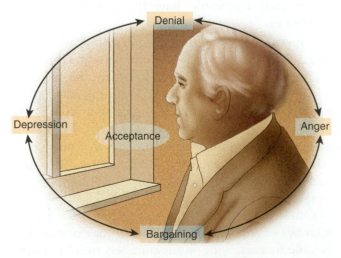

Fig. 2-1. The stages of grief.

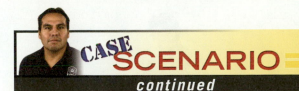

CASE SCENARIO *continued*

Back at the station, Rafael showers and changes his uniform. It smells of smoke from the fire and of vomit from the child they had worked so hard to save. Sadly, the child never regained a pulse and was pronounced dead shortly after arriving at the trauma center. Quietly Rafael goes about the duties of cooking a late dinner for the crew, who also seem to be reflecting on the event.

In his office, Captain Alvarez calls the officers of the other fire crews and finds that several other department members also seem to be stressed. He discusses this situation with the officers, formulating several options that could help these rescuers cope with the stress.

Question: *If you were the captain, what are some tactics you could use to help Rafael and his coworkers deal with this event?*

pathetically and will need you to communicate reassuringly. Avoid distorting the reality of the situation or making false reassurances. In a gentle tone, simply let the patient know that you and others will do everything you can to help. When appropriate, your reassuring touch can be very powerful.

The patient's family and friends may also need to express emotions ranging from rage to despair. In this situation, also listen empathetically and respond in a gentle tone. Express your concern for the patient and the family and be honest about the patient's condition. You must be emotionally available to offer comfort to the family.

■ POST-TRAUMATIC STRESS DISORDER

Post-traumatic stress disorder (PTSD) is a serious condition. It can involve illness, personality changes, and self-destructive behavior. It also can cause disruptive changes in the EMT's life. Review of the cases of some suicide victims has pointed to PTSD. Professional help is needed to treat PTSD effectively. EMTs should be familiar with the warning signs of the disorder so

that they can recognize it and make sure it is treated early. These warning signs include the following:

- Exposure to a critical incident
- Avoiding thinking of, talking about, or being reminded of an incident
- Reliving the incident in thoughts and dreams, possibly even seeing correlations in daily life
- Showing emotional, behavioral, mental, and/or physical changes after the incident
- Dramatic changes that persist for longer than a month

■ BURNOUT

The term *burnout* refers to a situation in which people lose interest in their work. At the very least, people who suffer from burnout become ineffective. At the worst, they leave their profession. Burnout can arise from a number of causes. In all cases, however, it comes from a sense of helplessness and of an inability to change unacceptable situations. EMTs who find themselves confronted with senseless violence every day may "burn out" from this exposure to endless, mindless destruction. Burnout also can arise from poor working conditions with lack of administrative support or lack of a professional work environment. In any event, unacceptable situations without hope of change can cause burnout.

■ STRESS MANAGEMENT

You may have many sources of stress in your life. Relationships, jobs, and certain financial situations all can cause stress. Working as an EMT will add more stress to your life. The various situations you will be called upon to deal with can profoundly affect your life. Consequently, you must identify the root causes of your stress to manage the resulting feelings effectively. Moreover, you should recognize that avoiding stress is not a solution.

Recognizing Warning Signs

To manage the stress in your professional and personal life, you must be able to detect the warning signs of stress:

- Irritability with coworkers, family, and friends
- Inability to concentrate

- Difficulty sleeping and/or nightmares
- Anxiety
- Indecisiveness
- Guilt
- Loss of appetite
- Loss of interest in sexual activities
- Isolation
- Loss of interest in work

The sooner stress and its effects are recognized, the simpler it is to implement techniques that reduce the impact of stress.

Lifestyle Changes

Once you have recognized the sources of stress in your life, you can make changes in your lifestyle to help you recover from its effects. Job burnout is common among EMTs. If you are unable to find healthy ways of dealing with the natural stress of responding to emergencies, you probably will want to stop experiencing emergency situations. You may need to change your diet to help manage stress. Reducing your consumption of caffeine, sugar, and alcohol and balancing your diet will increase your energy level and allow you to think more clearly. Avoiding fatty foods and maintaining an adequate protein intake also will increase your energy stores.

Exercise is important for increasing stamina and energy. You should stay physically active in sports or other recreational pursuits. In addition, you can learn and practice relaxation techniques, such as meditation or visual imagery.

These are only a few methods of handling stress. You must find appropriate ways of distancing yourself from stress to recharge your emotional batteries.

Balance

An EMT's well-being depends on maintaining a balance of work, family, friends, fitness, and recreation (Fig. 2-2). People who undergo heavy stress often lose this balance, which is so important to their physical and emotional well-being. If necessary, you must force yourself to make adequate time to balance the elements essential to your well-being. For example, you can make a schedule and stick to it to ensure time for certain key activities. After engaging in these activities, you will be more relaxed and will think more clearly.

Family and Friends

A common concern of EMTs is that their friends and families do not understand the nature of their work. Such feelings may cause you to withdraw from your

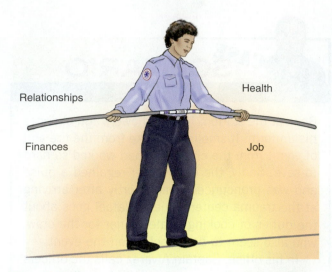

Fig. 2-2. Keeping a balance in your life is an important part of maintaining your well-being.

family and friends and delve even deeper into work. Moreover, the need for EMTs to be on call can add more stress to family relationships. As a result, you may find that coworkers may better understand and share your feelings about the challenging work. However, your family may feel ignored and fear separation. You may be frustrated by your family's apparent lack of understanding, whereas your distance may discourage them. You must work to prevent this cycle from starting or getting out of control. In addition, you should keep the lines of communication open, share things that are important to you, and take the time to listen to the needs of your family and friends.

Work Environment Changes

Any work environment produces stresses that are independent of those expected with EMS work. For instance, your coworkers and supervisors and the way you interact with them can produce work-related stress. For your well-being, it is important that you recognize this. Once recognized, improved communication and/or counseling may help alleviate or otherwise address this type of stress. Shift work is a well-documented cause of stress. Changing shifts and working during hours when the body is used to sleeping disrupts rest, nutrition, and recreation cycles. It can affect your emotional and physical health. You may need to make compromises to balance your work and your family better. For example, you can request a shift that allows you time to relax with family and friends. If you experience warning signs of excessive stress from your work and your personal life, you might request a temporary rotation to a less stressful assignment.

Professional Help

At some point you or a coworker may feel unable to balance the stress of your personal and professional life alone. Mental health professionals, including physicians and social workers, are trained to help you deal with stress and return balance to your life. Clergy may also be helpful. If you had a medical emergency, you would not hesitate to call your EMS system. Likewise, if you have an emotional problem, call on a mental health professional early to prevent serious disruption of your life. Many employees have access to the confidential services of an Employee Assistance Program (EAP) or a Member Assistance Program (MAP). You should take advantage of the many resources available to help you maintain balance in your life.

Critical Incident Stress Management

An overload of stress can come from a single critical event, an accumulation of incidents, or an MCI. Whatever the source, this overload can be overwhelming and damaging to your emotional health. **Critical incident stress** is a normal response to abnormal circumstances. The **critical incident stress management (CISM)** system is a comprehensive program designed to help people deal with work-related stress. The system operates on the premise that you will stay healthier or recover faster if you can discuss your fears, feelings, and reactions arising from critical incidents and feel support from coworkers and professionals. Specially trained teams of peer counselors and mental health workers can provide many essential services, including the following:

- Preincident stress education
- On-scene peer support
- One-on-one support
- Disaster support services
- Follow-up services
- Family and spouse support
- Community outreach programs
- Wellness programs

Critical incident stress debriefing (CISD) is a function of the CISM system. This debriefing uses specific techniques to help people express their feelings and recover more quickly from a stressful incident. Techniques used by the CISD team include **defusing** and **debriefing** (Box 2-3). CISM leaders and mental health personnel listen to individuals, evaluate the information, and offer support and suggestions to reduce stress. Proponents of CISM

BOX 2-3
Defusing and Debriefing

Characteristics of Defusing
- Shorter, less formal, and less structured version of a critical incident stress debriefing (CISD)
- Takes place a few hours after the event
- Lasts 30 to 40 minutes
- Allows initial ventilation
- May eliminate the need for a formal debriefing
- May enhance the formal debriefing

Characteristics of Debriefing
- Takes place 24 to 72 hours after the event
- Includes open discussion of feelings and fears
- Not an investigation or interrogation
- All information kept confidential

SPECIAL Considerations

Family Support for EMS Providers
Critical incident stress debriefing (CISD) often involves training family members of an EMS provider to help in the intervention. Family members are urged to
- Listen carefully
- Spend time with the traumatized person
- Offer assistance with daily tasks
- Reassure the person that he or she is safe
- Give the person some private time
- Avoid taking the individual's anger personally
- Tell the traumatized person that they are sorry the event occurred and they want to help

---

believe that it can be helpful when any of the following occur:

- Line-of-duty death or serious injury
- MCI
- Suicide of a coworker
- Serious injury to or death of children
- Events with excessive media interest
- Events involving victims known to you
- Any event that has an unusual impact on personnel
- Any disaster

Important Points

In recent years critical incident stress management (CISM) has become a controversial concept. Some studies have determined that CISM may not be helpful and in some cases may even be harmful. Studies continue to evaluate CISM and other methods of dealing with critical incident stress. Managers and medical directors should gather as much information on these topics as possible to help determine the best practice, given the information currently available. EMTs should discuss the policies and procedures regarding these events and responses within their agencies and EMS systems.

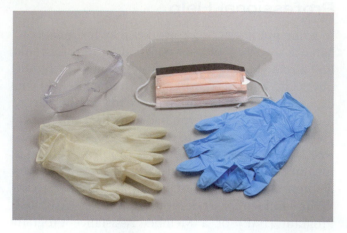

Fig. 2-3. Personal protective equipment (PPE).

Learn how to gain access to your local critical incident stress response team. This team should be within easy reach for the times you or a coworker could benefit from their expertise,.

■ PERSONAL PRECAUTIONS

Risks Facing EMTs

Some of the most serious hazards you will face as an EMT are invisible. You must be constantly aware of the risks associated with your job, including exposure to body substances such as a patient's blood. The **Occupational Safety and Health Administration (OSHA),** an agency of the U.S. government, has developed guidelines to protect health care workers. Protocols for protection against infection from body substances are established by another federal agency, the **Centers for Disease Control and Prevention (CDC).** These guidelines and protocols are referred to as **body substance isolation (BSI)** or as *standard* or *universal precautions.* You must follow the appropriate guidelines to ensure your personal safety.

You can protect yourself from all body substances by using appropriate **personal protective equipment (PPE).** Gloves and eye protection should always be worn; however, PPE may also include a mask and a gown (Fig. 2-3) or other specialty equipment, depending on the event. You should always use a pocket-mask with a one-way valve or other barrier device when ventilating or breathing for a patient. This helps prevent your exposure to any diseases the patient may carry. Always assess the potential risk and be vigilant about taking appropriate precautions. You should be familiar with and use PPE as required by your local system.

In addition, review government regulations with regard to BSI, including OSHA and state regulations. These should be available through your state EMS office.

Infection Control

Many infections and diseases are transmitted by airborne and blood-borne **pathogens,** which are organisms that cause infection. Patients may carry minor viruses, such as those that cause colds or flu, or dangerous ones, such as the human immunodeficiency virus (HIV) or the viruses that cause hepatitis. Blood-borne pathogens can cause a number of serious viral diseases. You may also be exposed to bacteria. Tuberculosis (TB), for example, is transmitted by airborne bacteria. Another airborne pathogen multiplies on food and, when eaten, causes food poisoning. You can limit your risk of exposure by using PPE and sound infection control practices. Good personal hygiene and frequent hand washing, before and after all patient contact, are simple and effective techniques for preventing the transmission of disease (Fig. 2-4). *Hand washing is the most important method of stopping the spread of infection* (Box 2-4). Equipment should be properly discarded, cleaned, or disinfected after each use. A commercially prepared solution can be used for this purpose, or you can make a common cleaning solution by mixing bleach and water (generally 1 part bleach to 10 parts water).

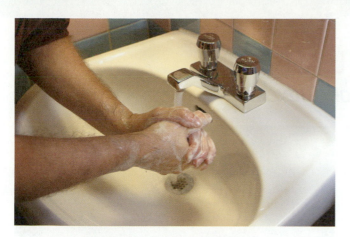

Fig. 2-4. Frequent hand washing is the most important technique you can use to prevent infection.

BOX 2-4
Hand Washing
As an EMT, you should wash your hands before and after every patient contact. To do this properly, remove any jewelry and then lather all surfaces of the hands, fingers, and lower arms. Ten to 15 seconds of vigorous scrubbing with soap removes most contaminants. Rinse thoroughly with water and then dry off, if possible with a disposable towel.

Personal Protective Equipment

Eye Protection

Protective eyewear prevents body substances from reaching the mucous membranes of your eyes. If you wear prescription glasses, goggles may not be required in some cases if removable side shields are used. However, goggles should be worn over prescription glasses in situations such as a motor vehicle crash or when exposure to body fluids is highly likely (e.g., childbirth).

Gloves

EMTs should put on vinyl, plastic, or another type of synthetic gloves before having any physical contact with a sick or injured person. If you are working in an environment in which the gloves are likely to be ripped or punctured, you should wear two layers of gloves and/or wear them inside work gloves. These gloves should be properly discarded after any use. Wearing gloves does not replace washing your hands. Remember to wash your hands before and after every patient treatment. Also remember that both patients

SPECIAL Populations

Immunocompromised Patients

Infection control isn't just about protecting yourself from your patient; sometimes it's about protecting the patient from you. Young children, elderly patients, some patients undergoing chemotherapy, organ transplant recipients, malnourished patients, chronically ill patients, and patients infected with the human immunodeficiency virus (HIV) are likely to be immunocompromised. Immunocompromised patients cannot fight off infection. If you are sick or have a respiratory infection or the flu, you should not be involved in direct patient care. If you think you may be developing a respiratory infection or the flu, use respiratory precautions, such as a face mask, to protect your patient from your illness.

CAUTION!

Many items of personal protective equipment (PPE) are made of latex. A number of health care workers and providers have had serious allergic reactions to latex. If you have a latex allergy, it is important that you identify products containing latex to which you may be exposed and replace them with nonlatex material.

and health care workers may be allergic to the materials in gloves. Skill 2-1 shows the correct way to put on gloves, and Skill 2-2 shows the proper technique for removing soiled gloves.

Gowns

You should wear a gown if you anticipate the possibility of large splashes of body fluids, such as with childbirth, coughing, spitting, vomiting, or massive bleeding. If a gown is unavailable, you should change your clothes after contact with the patient.

Masks

Several types of masks are available. A surgical-type mask protects your mouth and airway against possible blood splatter. A special **high-efficiency particulate air (HEPA)** mask should be worn if a patient is suspected of having TB. HEPA masks are used particularly in enclosed areas (Fig. 2-5). If you believe a pa-

SKILL 2-1
Putting on Gloves

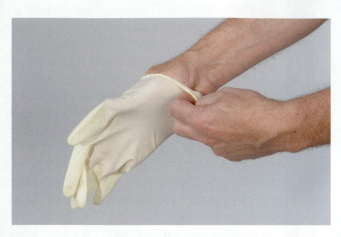

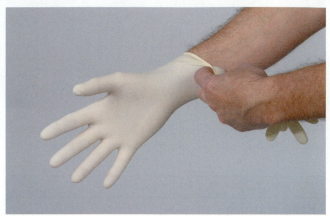

1. Pull glove onto one hand using the fingers of your other hand at the lower cuff area.

2. Pull glove tight without touching your ungloved hand to the fingers or hand area of the gloved hand.

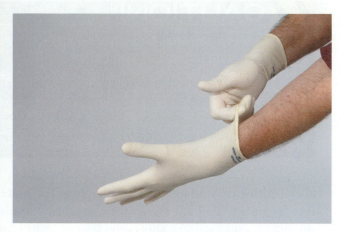

3. Put on the other glove using the fingers of the gloved hand.

SKILLS

SKILL 2-2
Removing Soiled Gloves

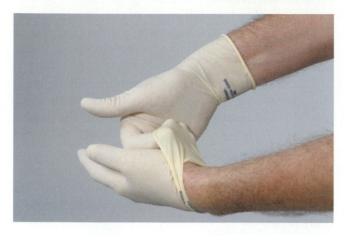

1. Insert a finger from one hand into the glove on the other hand.

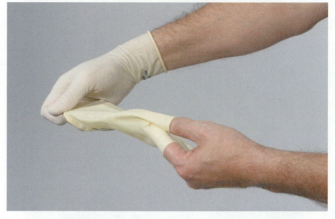

2. Pull the glove off by turning it inside out.

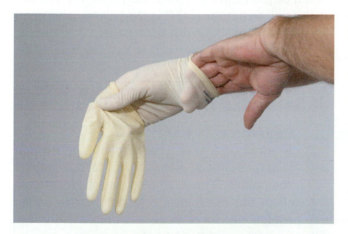

3. Insert your fingers into the other glove.

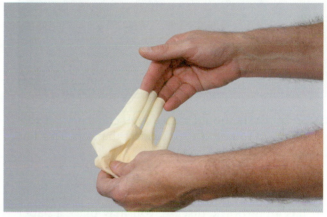

4. Pull the second glove off by turning it inside out.

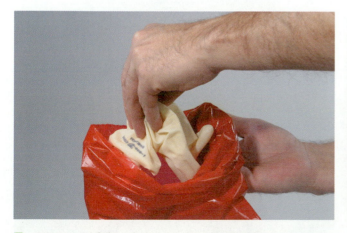

5. Dispose of the gloves in an appropriate container.

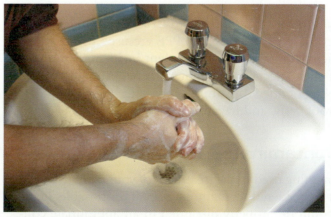

6. Wash your hands.

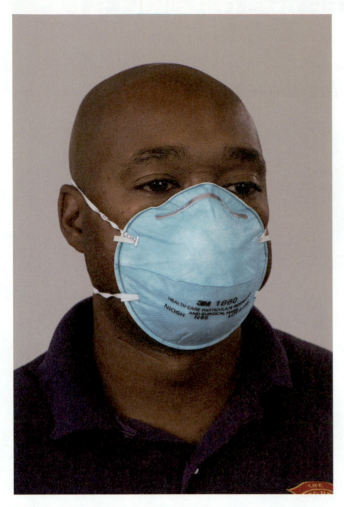

Fig. 2-5. EMTs should wear a high-efficiency particulate air (HEPA) mask if they suspect that a patient has tuberculosis (TB).

tient has an airborne disease, you may place a paper surgical mask on the individual as long as it does not adversely affect the patient's breathing.

Specialty Personal Protective Equipment

Several types of specialty PPE are used in situations such as fires, rescues, or violent incidents. Examples of such specialty equipment include turnout gear, a self-contained breathing apparatus (SCBA), bullet-proof vests, and hazardous materials suits.

Contaminated Equipment

Anything used in the treatment of your patient should be considered contaminated. All disposable items should be properly discarded in an appropriate container. This might include turning over any disposable items to the transport crew or special disposal at your workplace. Your employers or the system in which

you work should have policies in place to guide you in the proper procedures for discarding patient-related disposable equipment.

Cleaning a piece of equipment means washing it with soap and water. **Disinfecting** a piece of equipment means cleaning it and using a substance such as alcohol or bleach to kill many of the contaminants. **Sterilizing** a piece of equipment involves the use of chemicals and aids such as superheated steam to kill *all* contaminants.

Usually your equipment will require only cleaning and disinfecting if it comes into contact with a patient's skin or body fluids (including items the patient may have breathed on directly). You should be sure to wear heavy-duty utility gloves when cleaning and disinfecting equipment. Depending on the manufacturer's recommendations, some equipment requires sterilization if it comes into contact with a patient's body fluids.

Disposable equipment should be used when possible. After use, contaminated disposable equipment should be placed in an appropriate plastic bag (usually labeled as infectious waste) (Fig. 2-6). Disposable items should be double-bagged if your patient is known to have an infectious disease, such as HIV infection.

SPECIAL Considerations

Manufacturer Knows Best
To avoid problems, always follow the manufacturer's recommendations for cleaning equipment. For example, using bleach to clean the clear plastic faceplates on some equipment can damage and permanently fog the surface of the faceplate.

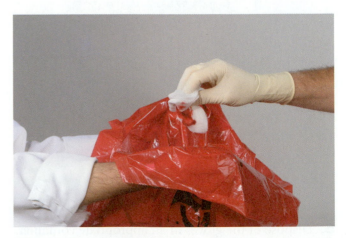

Fig. 2-6. Contaminated equipment should be discarded in appropriate containers.

Both your equipment and your vehicle should be thoroughly cleaned and disinfected after each patient contact.

Specialized Training

You may be called to work in situations that involve a variety of hazards. It is important to learn all that you can about the materials in the community and the environments in which you work. If you work in an area that has specific hazards, such as chemical, electrical, radioactive, biologic, poisonous, or explosive materials, special training in additional necessary precautions should be available to you. Take advantage of specialty training to increase your knowledge and reduce your risk. In addition, special PPE may be required in these situations (Fig. 2-7).

Immunizations

Immunizations can protect you from many serious or fatal diseases that your patients may carry. The following immunizations are recommended for all health care providers:

- Tetanus
- Hepatitis B
- Measles, mumps, and flu (you may have had these when you were a child, but some need to be reassessed)
- Others, as recommended locally or currently

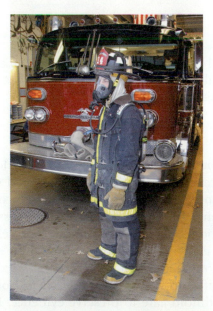

Fig. 2-7. Turnout gear and a self-contained breathing apparatus (SCBA) are examples of specialized protective equipment.

Obtain your immunization history and compare it with your department recommendations. Your EMS system can help you gain access to immunizations in your community. In addition, annual skin testing is recommended to evaluate for TB exposure.

Exposure Notification and Testing

Any possible exposure to a patient's body fluids should be reported to other members of your team and to the receiving hospital. The hospital will include the possible exposure in its record and follow up with your agency if necessary. The report should include the date and time you were exposed, the type and amount of body fluid to which you were exposed, and the source. You should also know your local and state laws concerning reporting requirements and the transfer of patient information. This information usually can be found through your state EMS office.

■ SCENE SAFETY

Whenever an EMT approaches an emergency scene, the first priority is to assess the safety of the scene. If the scene is unsafe and poses a threat to the responder, it should be made safe before the EMT enters. Some hazards that might make a scene unsafe include motor vehicle crashes or rescues, hazardous materials, and violence.

Motor Vehicle Crashes or Rescues

The EMT must determine whether the scene poses a danger of fire, explosion, or collapse, or whether a hazardous material may be present. Motor vehicle crashes present many challenges. The traffic that continues to pass around the crash is a hazard. This traffic must be controlled before rescue can be attempted. Scene safety depends first on controlling the traffic around the scene. The vehicle also may present hazards. Certainly a damaged vehicle with broken glass and jagged metal edges is a hazard to both the patient and the EMT. EMTs on the scene of motor vehicle crashes should wear clothing that protects them from injury from these sharp objects. Other professional rescuers with specialized training may need to secure the scene before the EMT can approach the patient. The EMT must understand how to get special rescue teams and equipment to the scene if needed (Fig. 2-8).

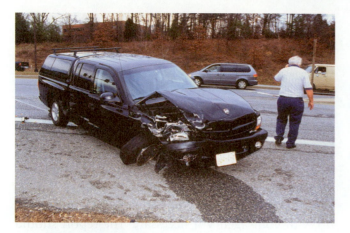

Fig. 2-8. Motor vehicle crashes can present a variety of hazards. Always make sure the scene is safe.

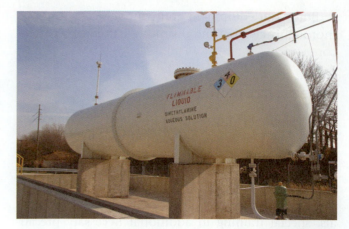

Fig. 2-9. Hazardous materials should be identified with placards.

Hazardous Materials

Toxic substances or hazardous atmospheres might include dangerous liquid, solid, or gaseous chemicals that prevent you from entering the scene. Hazardous materials should be identified with placards that specify the type of hazard (Fig. 2-9). These placards are numbered in order to guide you to a reference in the *Emergency Response Guidebook*, which is published by the U.S. Department of Transportation (Fig. 2-10). Binoculars may be your most important piece of equipment in identifying hazards. They allow you to evaluate the placard or situation at a distance before you risk exposing yourself to unseen hazards. Once identified, hazardous materials incidents are handled by the Office of Hazardous Materials Safety (HAZMAT) teams. These teams consist of rescuers specially trained in identifying and securing hazardous situations and in decontaminating people exposed to these materials. They may have to decontaminate your patient before they can release the person to you for treatment. Fire or other hazardous situations may create toxic gases or severely deplete the amount of oxygen in the air. This is another situation in which rescuers with training specific to these hazards must make the scene safe for the responder to enter. If the scene cannot be made safe, the patient may need to be taken to the EMT by the specially trained rescuers. It is important that you familiarize yourself with these specialty teams in your area. Learn how to contact them and how you might work with them. They probably provide awareness training that will enable you to work with them more closely and prevent you from becoming part of the emergency.

Violence

Crime scenes or violent scenes present another possible hazardous situation and special concerns that

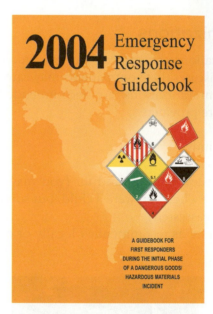

Fig. 2-10. The U.S. Department of Transportation puts out the *Emergency Response Guidebook*, a reference for hazardous materials.

EMTs should address. First, the EMT should not enter the scene until the police have secured the scene for safe entry. Second, if a crime has been committed at the scene, the EMT should avoid unnecessarily disturbing possible evidence. Although preserving the chain of evidence is important, it is even more important to remember that the patient's needs are the priority after the safety of the rescuers. You should never withhold care to preserve evidence. However, you should avoid destroying evidence during the course of care. For example, you can cut around suspected bullet or knife holes when removing clothing from a patient at a crime scene or violent scene.

Physically Unstable Scenes

EMTs may also be called to assist at an emergency scene that is physically unstable. If a patient is found in a ditch, on a slope or if water or ice presents an unstable surface, the EMT should make sure the scene is stable enough to remove the patient without endangering the rescue team. If this is beyond the EMTs' ability, they must wait for specially trained rescuers to stabilize the site.

Patient Protection

Patient protection is your priority. Keep in mind that the environment may pose a threat to your patient. Shield the patient from extremes of temperature and other environmental factors. Also, keep the patient dry and help the person maintain body heat.

Bystander Protection

The protection of bystanders is also a priority. Make sure that the cause of your patient's difficulties does not potentially affect others. Also make sure that your activities in working to help your patient do not harm others who may be crowding around out of curiosity or in an attempt to help.

The rule is clear and important: Scene safety must be determined before you enter. If the scene is unsafe, make it safe. If you cannot make it safe, do not enter.

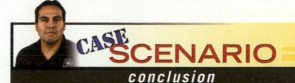

CASE SCENARIO
conclusion

The defusing session goes well. The department chaplain, who is trained in critical stress management, leads the fire crews through a safe process in which members can voice their frustration and anger over their perceived helplessness. The process does not take long, and afterward a couple of crew members thank Captain Alvarez privately for setting up the session. Rafael is relieved to realize that he wasn't alone in his feelings. ■

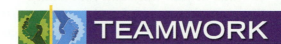

TEAMWORK

An EMT is an important part of the health care team. As a team member, you must learn to recognize the signs of imbalance in physical and emotional well-being, not only in yourself but also in your coworkers, family, and friends. A healthy team requires that its members watch out for one another. An EMT who does not understand the importance of being safe, healthy, and emotionally balanced is the weak link in the chain of prehospital care.

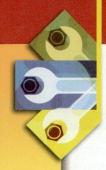

Critical Points

- EMTs must understand the likely reactions to death and dying. You should recognize the stages of the grieving process and be able to listen empathetically and communicate honestly with patients and their friends and family.

- As an EMT, you will experience unusual stress. Find healthy ways to manage that stress and balance your personal and professional needs. Use the resources provided by your EMS system and your local mental health professionals. Your emotional well-being is essential to your work and your family.

- You must be aware of and protect yourself from the risks associated with emergency medical care. Use the established protocols for protective equipment and practices to reduce your risks. Gloves, mask, gown, and eye protection should be worn to isolate body substances.

- The EMT must assess the scene and surroundings of a medical emergency to ensure the safety of all involved. Use your training to protect yourself in scenes involving hazardous materials, motor vehicle crashes, and violence. Remember, if the scene is unsafe, make it safe. Otherwise, do not enter.

Learning Checklist

- ❑ An EMT will face many stressful situations. These may involve MCIs, pediatric patients, violent situations, abuse, amputations, death, and injury or death of a coworker.

- ❑ As an EMT, you will encounter scenes involving death, you will treat dying patients, and you will provide support to the families and friends of those who have died. You must try to understand the concerns of the dying patient, communicate empathetically with family members after the death of a loved one, and manage your own feelings about death and loss.

- ❑ Definitive signs of death include clear mortal damage, rigor mortis, and putrefaction.

- ❑ Common emotional states of dying, critically ill, and injured patients include anxiety, pain and anger, hostility, depression, and guilt.

- ❑ To help alleviate anxiety and confusion in patients, always introduce yourself, let them know you are there to help them, and continually explain what is happening around them.

- ❑ Be honest with patients without unnecessarily shocking or confusing them.

- ❑ The stages of grief are denial, anger, bargaining, depression, and acceptance.

- ❑ Different family members, friends, and patients go through the different stages of grief at different times. As an EMT, you should recognize this fact and also that you, too, may go through stages of grieving.

- ❑ The warning signs of stress may include irritability, inability to concentrate, difficulty sleeping and/or nightmares, anxiety, indecisiveness, guilt, loss of appetite, loss of interest in sex, isolation, and loss of interest in work.

- ❑ To help manage stress, reduce your consumption of caffeine, sugar, and alcohol and balance your diet. In addition, avoid fatty foods and maintain an adequate intake of protein.

- ❑ Stay physically active in sports or other recreational pursuits to stay healthy and help alleviate stress.

- ❑ Family members and friends may not understand the nature of an EMT's work. They may feel ignored or fear separation, and you may unwittingly separate yourself from them.

- ❑ You should recognize the warning signs of stress and make the appropriate changes in your lifestyle or work environment to alleviate the stress as much as possible. This may include seeking professional help from a mental health worker or a member of the clergy.

- ❑ CISM is a comprehensive system designed to help individuals deal with work-related stress. The services offered include preincident stress education, on-scene peer support, one-on-one support, disaster support services, follow-up services, family and spouse support, community outreach programs, and wellness programs.

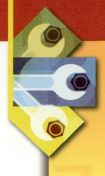

- CISD is a function of CISM. The debriefing involves specific techniques to help individuals express their feelings and recover more quickly from a stressful incident.
- CISM should be used when any of the following occur: line-of-duty death or serious injury, MCI, coworker suicide, serious injury or death of children, events with excessive media interest, events with victims you know, any disaster, and any event that has an unusual impact on personnel.
- BSI (also referred to as *standard* or *universal precautions*) incorporates the protocols set by the CDC for protection against infection from body substances.
- Good personal hygiene and hand washing before and after each patient contact are simple but effective techniques for preventing disease transmission.
- PPE includes gloves, eye protection, gowns, masks, and specialty pieces, such as turnout gear.
- Anything used in treating a patient should be considered contaminated and discarded appropriately.
- All health care providers should be immunized against tetanus, hepatitis B, measles, mumps, and flu. Annual skin testing for TB is also recommended.
- EMTs should report any possible exposure to a patient's body fluids to the EMS transport team.
- Some hazards an EMT may face include motor vehicle crashes or rescues, hazardous materials, violence, and a physically unstable scene. At any scene, your safety, the safety of your patient, and the safety of bystanders are of utmost importance.

Key Terms

Body substance isolation (BSI) Protective equipment worn to prevent exposure to bloodborne pathogens or body fluids.

Centers for Disease Control and Prevention (CDC) An agency of the U.S. government that provides resources and equipment for the investigation, identification, prevention, and control of infectious disease.

Cleaning Washing thoroughly with soap and water.

Critical incident stress A stress reaction that normally occurs after a person has experienced a particularly difficult situation.

Critical incident stress debriefing (CISD) A function of the critical incident stress management system. The debriefing uses specific techniques to help individuals express their feelings and recover more quickly from a stressful incident.

Critical incident stress management (CISM) A comprehensive system devised to help professionals recover from critical incidents.

Debriefing A review of a stressful event that allows discussion among the people involved. It usually is held 24 to 72 hours after the event.

Defusing Another form of review of stressful events that allows discussion among the people involved, but shorter and less formal than a debriefing. It usually is held within a few hours of the event.

Disinfecting In addition to cleaning, using alcohol or bleach to kill contaminants.

High-efficiency particulate air (HEPA) mask A special mask designed to reduce the spread of infectious airborne diseases, such as TB.

Occupational Health and Safety Administration (OSHA) A federal agency that has developed guidelines to protect health care workers.

Pathogens Microorganisms capable of causing disease.

Personal protective equipment (PPE) Equipment used to isolate a health care worker from a patient's body substances. Also refers to specialty equipment used by emergency providers during the course of a rescue or fire.

Post-traumatic Stress Disorder (PTSD) An anxiety disorder caused by exposure to an extremely traumatic event. Affected individuals may relive the event in nightmares or flashbacks. Symptoms may include avoidance of stimuli associated with the trauma, hyperalertness, and difficulty sleeping, remembering, or concentrating.

Sterilizing Using chemicals and superheated steam to kill all microorganisms.

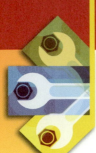

NUTS AND BOLTS

National Standard Curriculum Objectives

Cognitive Objectives

After completing this lesson, the EMT student will be able to do the following:

- List possible emotional reactions that the EMT may experience when faced with trauma, illness, death, and dying.
- Discuss the possible reactions of a family member when confronted with death and dying.
- State the steps of the EMT's approach to a family confronted with death and dying.
- State the possible reactions of the EMT's family prompted by their outside involvement in EMS.
- Recognize the signs and symptoms of critical incident stress.
- State possible steps the EMT may take to help alleviate stress.
- Explain the need to determine scene safety.
- Discuss the importance of BSI.
- Describe the steps the EMT should take to ensure personal protection from airborne and blood-borne pathogens.

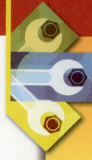
- List the PPE necessary for each of the following:
  Hazardous materials
  Rescue operations
  Violent scenes
  Crime scenes
  Exposure to blood-borne pathogens
  Exposure to airborne pathogens

Affective Objectives

After completing this lesson, the EMT student will be able to do the following:

- Explain the rationale for serving as an advocate for the use of appropriate protective equipment.

Psychomotor Objectives

After completing this lesson, the EMT student will be able to do the following:

- Given a scenario with potential infectious exposure, use appropriate PPE and then properly remove and discard the protective garments.
- Given the above scenario, complete disinfection and cleaning and all reporting documentation.

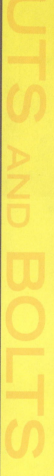

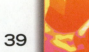

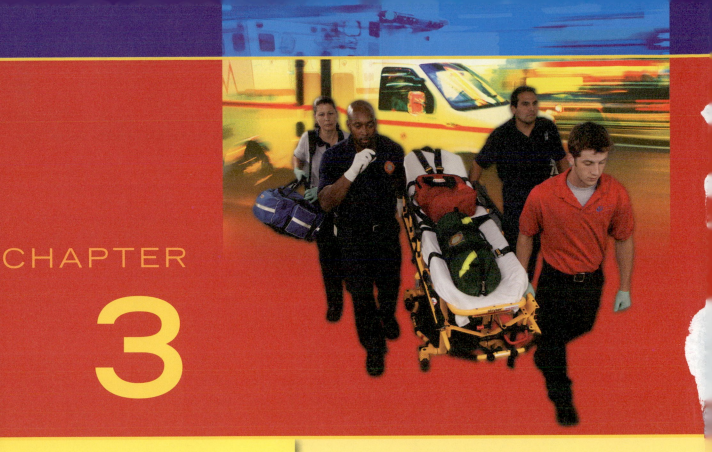

CHAPTER

3

CHAPTER OUTLINE

LESSON GOAL

As an emergency medical technician (EMT), you will be confronted with many ethical dilemmas in your practice. In addition, you will come to appreciate the legal implications and issues involved in your work. Some of the ethical dilemmas will be rather simple and straightforward, whereas others will have no specific solution and will deeply challenge your emotions. How do you resolve these situations while doing what is right for the patient, what is comfortable for you, and what is legal? This chapter outlines ethical dilemmas you may face and attempts to provide a simple approach to resolving them—hopefully, leaving you feeling better about yourself and your career. The legal implications of your work are also identified and defined. The guidance provided by this information will enable you to face the ethical and legal issues that arise in your work with more knowledge, understanding, and confidence. ■

Legal and Ethical Aspects of Emergency Medical Services (EMS)

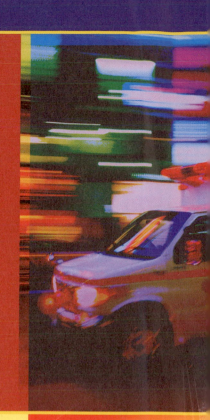

CHAPTER OBJECTIVES

3

After completing this chapter, the EMT student will be able to do the following:

1 Define the EMT standard of care.

2 Discuss the importance of do not resuscitate (DNR) orders and advance directives as they apply to emergency medical services.

3 Define consent and discuss the ways EMS providers receive consent from their patients.

4 List the circumstances that must be in place to establish a duty to act.

5 Explain the difference between competence and decision-making capacity.

6 Discuss the factors the EMT must think about when a patient refuses transport.

7 Explain why it is important to maintain patient confidentiality.

8 Discuss the importance of proper documentation.

9 Discuss the factors the EMT should consider when dealing with a potential organ donor.

10 Define the term *quality of life.*

11 Talk about how the EMT should act when faced with an unethical situation.

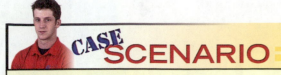

CASE SCENARIO

"Now you can see what I've been going through all day!" exclaims Madeline Walsh, her hands nervously twisting the dishcloth she is holding.

"It's okay, Mrs. Walsh," Ray reassures the anxious woman. "Give me a few more minutes to try to convince your husband that he really needs to go to the emergency department."

Turning back to the kitchen table, Ray looks at the heavyset, white-haired man sitting in front of his now cold lunch. John Walsh is a respected member of the farming community. He often works with the local bankers and farm equipment dealers to help some of his struggling fellow farmers stay afloat financially.

Typically a stoic, no-nonsense individual, John began experiencing chest tightness and indigestion while eating lunch with Madeline. Although that was not unusual, the intensity and duration of the episode made John a bit nervous. Madeline became frightened when John turned very pale and broke out in a cold sweat. At first John refused to let her call the doctor or 911, telling her that the discomfort would go away on its own. However, when the squeezing sensation in his chest had not let up after 10 minutes, he relented and had Madeline call the hospital. After asking a few questions, the emergency department nurse told Mrs. Walsh to hang up and call 911.

On arrival, Ray and his partner quickly assessed Mr. Walsh and placed him on oxygen. Soon he felt much better. The sensation in his chest subsided, and he felt he could breathe normally again. He tells Ray that he feels better and that he doesn't want to go to the emergency department. "It's so expensive," says Mr. Walsh. "Besides, I can see my primary physician, probably tomorrow."

Question: *Should Ray allow Mr. Walsh to stay home and wait to see his doctor? What are the ethical and legal issues involved in Ray's decision?*

As health professionals, EMTs must always conduct themselves in full compliance with the law and the standards of the profession. In addition, they face the challenge of confronting and dealing effectively with ethical dilemmas. Medical care has significant consequences, and as an EMT, you have the highest responsibility imaginable—a life entrusted to your hands. This chapter describes the legal and ethical contexts of providing prehospital care, the legal basis for a negligence lawsuit, and issues related to patient rights, such as protecting patient information and dealing with consent and refusal of care. The top liability areas associated with prehospital care are discussed, along with strategies for minimizing the two key risks: harm to the patient and the likelihood of a lawsuit.

Avoiding liability often comes down to the basics: skill, knowledge, good judgment, and adherence to protocols and procedures. These factors can help reduce the chance of a bad patient outcome or a lawsuit. Your job is to minimize the chance of such a result whenever possible. You can best do that by better understanding the risks and by following all procedures designed as safeguards to help you avoid them.

In addition to liability, you must consider the ethical issues you will face on the job. What exactly is an ethical dilemma? All EMTs have experienced them, but they may not have fully understood their consequences. For example, if a 90-year-old nursing home patient with advanced cancer and dementia is a full code status and has a cardiac arrest, would you be uncomfortable with the possibility that you may break her ribs performing cardiopulmonary resuscitation (CPR)? Should you let an obnoxious intoxicated patient sign a refusal of transport? What should you do when a police officer won't let you evaluate a patient with carbon monoxide poisoning because a crime scene is involved (Box 3-1), even though you think resuscitation may be indicated?

These situations are not uncommon. How do repeated episodes such as these affect you as a professional and as a person? By addressing ethical dilemmas in advance, you may be able to make your life easier, prevent burnout, and provide better care for your patients.

SCOPE OF POTENTIAL LEGAL LIABILITY

On a national scale, errors in patient care are a very serious problem, even in the more controlled environment of a hospital. Statistics from the Institute of Medicine[1] (IOM), a subdivision of the National Academy of Sciences, show that

- Approximately 50,000 to 100,000 Americans die each year as a result of general medical errors.
- Medical errors are the eighth leading cause of death, ranking higher than breast cancer and human immunodeficiency virus (HIV) infection.

EMS systems are not immune to this problem. In fact, in many EMS cases the problem can be even worse because of environmental conditions or other situational factors that are not present in a hospital.

Ironically, most lawsuits against EMS agencies do not deal directly with alleged negligence in patient care. Rather, they are the result of the most common area of EMS liability—vehicle accidents. Estimates indicate that nearly 90% of all litigation against an EMS agency has to do with injuries sustained when an ambulance is involved in a motor vehicle accident. This underscores the importance of good driving habits, strict adherence to motor vehicle laws, and use of common sense when operating an ambulance.

The root cause of an EMS lawsuit often is related to the behavior and attitude of the EMT in dealing with the patient, family members, or bystanders. Failure to communicate effectively and to reassure the patient in an empathetic way often is the foundation of a lawsuit against an EMS agency. Studies have shown that most lawsuits in personal injury cases are the result of poor communication with the patient.

OVERVIEW OF THE LEGAL SYSTEM

The legal system is the formal manner of resolving disputes in our society. Unfortunately, it is an expensive way of seeking redress of the harm that may be caused by others. The legal system is composed of both federal and state court systems. The federal courts are reserved primarily for violations of federal statutes and for issues involving a possible violation of the Constitution by government agencies. Each state has its own court system, where claims are brought under state law. Most negligence claims are brought in state court, which is the most likely place for any lawsuit involving an EMS agency.

There are two basic types of law. Laws that are "on the books" and authored by legislators are called *statutes*. You can look up a statute and, in most cases, understand what it takes to violate the law. Each state has hundreds of statutes on the books. Also, new laws are added every day, and old laws are constantly amended. A statute begins as a *bill* in the state legislature. After the bill is passed by the elected representatives, the governor signs it into law. The statute is enacted into the laws governing society. A state EMS Act and the law outlining the requirements for certification and recertification as an EMT are examples of statutes.

The other type of law is *common law.* Common law is not written as a statute. Instead, it is legal theory based on years of court decisions in which specific rights have evolved, but no clear statute exists. An example of common law would be a claim for *loss of consortium* (the loss of companionship of the opposite sex) that could be tied to a negligence lawsuit or lawsuit for violating a specific statute.

The two types of court action are civil lawsuits and criminal prosecution. *Civil lawsuits* deal with violation of civil laws that are on the books as statutes or are embodied in the common law. These cases involve claims for money or other damages and do not involve punishment in the form of a prison sentence. Civil lawsuits are typically between private parties, as when one person sues another person or an organization for negligence.

Criminal actions are claims brought by the state to protect society in general. These are cases in which

SPECIAL Considerations

EMTs frequently transport patients who have been restrained by and are in the custody of the police. Police officers often restrain violent individuals by securing their arms behind their back and placing them in a face-down position. Several patients have died from positional asphyxia while transported in this position. In these cases the exertion of the struggle is believed to have tired the individual and depleted the oxygen level. Also, the face-down position placed additional weight on the chest and stomach; this impaired the mechanical respiratory process of inhaling and exhaling, leading to the patient's death. Several court cases have held the EMS providers responsible for the patient's death under these circumstances.

government prosecutors, such as the district attorney, bring an action on behalf of the state (the people) against a person suspected of committing a crime. Jury trials are common in both civil and criminal actions. In fact, the Constitution guarantees a trial by a "jury of one's peers" in any criminal prosecution that is carried to trial.

Administrative actions are a third type of legal action. Every state has an EMS Act that outlines the basic requirements for training of EMS personnel, certification, licensure, and proper conduct. A state agency typically enforces the EMS Act in each state, and the agency usually has the power to grant or deny certification or to pursue an administrative action against an EMT who violates the law. For example, if an EMT is arrested for driving while under the influence of alcohol, in most states this leads to suspension of EMT certification. The EMS regulatory agency in your state may have the authority to suspend or revoke an EMT certification, because that "right" is a function of state law. However, to suspend or revoke a certification or license, the agency must follow certain administrative procedures to ensure that the action is warranted and fair. This means that the state can initiate an adverse action against an EMT or ambulance service only if the person involved has received *due process*. Due process provides basic rights in the law in all cases in which the government tries to discipline or take away something a citizen has earned under the law, such as EMT certification. This essentially means that the action can

be taken only if you are made aware of the charges or accusations against you, have the opportunity to confront your accuser, and have an opportunity to be heard and tell your side of the story. Typically appeal rights also exist. These provide an added safeguard: the option of challenging the administrative decision in court.

■ ANATOMY OF AN EMS LAWSUIT

Litigation can take months or even years before a judge or jury hears the case. Most states have a *statute of limitations* for most legal actions that can be brought against you. This means that the plaintiff must file the lawsuit within a certain period of time after the injury or harm or else the right to file one will be lost. In most states the statute of limitations for a negligence action is 2 years. However, some exceptions may extend this period; for example, if the harm or injury were not discovered until some time after the incident that caused the harm. In such situations the limitations period for filing a lawsuit may be considered to run 2 years from the date the injury was discovered. The following are the basic steps of a lawsuit.

- **The incident.** This is the event that triggers the patient's potential rights and ability to seek recovery. Typically it is the accident or medical call that caused the patient to activate EMS in the first place.
- **The complaint and the answer.** The *complaint* is the formal document filed in court that starts the lawsuit. The complaint includes the parties named, an outline of the "facts" that describe the incident and how the patient was harmed, a list of violations of the law or specific claims against the defendant or defendants, and a request for recovery (e.g., monetary damages). The *answer* is the formal response of the defendant to the complaint. It is typically a short admission or denial of each of the specific allegations in the complaint.
- **Discovery.** After the complaint has been filed but before the trial, the parties involved in the lawsuit exchange large amounts of information. The goal is to get to the real facts of the case and to determine the validity of much of the complaint. Discovery includes deposition testimony by witnesses, answers to written questions (these questions are called *interrogatories*), requests for one party to admit or deny specific questions or allegations in writing, and case evaluation and reports from experts hired by each party.

- **Pretrial motions.** In most lawsuits, motions will be submitted to dismiss the entire case or parts of it based on the information obtained during discovery. Motions to limit certain testimony or to limit the introduction of certain evidence in the case also may be filed. The judge assigned to oversee the case and to preside over it at trial usually rules on the pretrial motions.

- **The trial.** This is the orderly presentation of the evidence of the case and arguments by both sides as to why their side should prevail. The "fact finder" in a trial may be a judge or a jury. Most laws grant the plaintiff the right to a jury trial, but it usually must be requested when the complaint is filed in court. Most negligence cases are tried before a jury, because juries tend to be more sympathetic and more likely to side with the plaintiff.

- **The role of experts.** Experts are important to every negligence trial. They help determine the *standard of care* the jury will use in determining whether the EMS personnel followed the proper procedures. Experts also provide an opinion as to what caused the harm to the patient. Both the plaintiff and the defendant typically hire experts to provide testimony on the standard of care that should apply and on how that standard was met in the case at hand. Sources for determining that standard come from a wide range of material. They may include textbooks such as this one; the United States Department of Transportation national standard curriculum for the EMT-Basic; state, regional, and local treatment protocols; orders from the local physician medical director; and the experts' own experience in dealing with patient care in the EMS setting.

  Example: Waylon Yelp is an EMT for ABC Ambulance, which is being sued for negligence. The plaintiff was the passenger in a car that was struck from the rear. She complained of neck pain at the scene, but EMT Yelp decided not to use a short backboard or Kendrick Extrication Device (KED) when extricating the patient. After movement on the long spine board, the patient experienced a sharp pain in the back of her neck and began to have a tingling sensation in her arms. She suffered a fracture of the cervical spine at the C6 and C7 level. She has partial paralysis of her arms, and she alleges that EMT Yelp caused the paralysis because he failed to immobilize her cervical spine properly prior to extrication.

  Dr. Jones is a paid expert for the plaintiff. He is a medical director for a neighboring EMS regional council and was involved in developing the state's

Basic Life Support (BLS) Protocols. He testifies that the proper procedure according to the protocol for management of possible spinal injuries is that patients in the seated position be immobilized with a short backboard or KED. He also testifies that, in his experience as an emergency department physician, patients in situations similar to that experienced by the plaintiff should be immobilized before they are moved from the vehicle onto a long board. He also describes elements of the EMT training program, for which he is an instructor in his home area, and describes how spinal immobilization procedures are taught in accordance with the BLS protocols and the national standard curriculum. The sources for his expert testimony to establish the standard of care in this case include the national curriculum, the curriculum for the EMT training program, the state BLS protocols for spinal immobilization, and his own experience as a physician familiar with EMS.

- **Post-trial motions.** After the trial is over and the jury has spoken, there may be motions in court to disregard the jury's verdict if it is contrary to the law. For example, this may occur in a case in which evidence indicates improper conduct on the part of the jury in reaching its decision. There may be motions to limit or reduce the amount of the jury award or to address the payment of attorneys' fees.

- **Appeals.** In most cases the losing party has the right to appeal the case to an appeals court. An appeals court is usually a panel of judges who review the case to make sure it was decided in accordance with the law. Winning an appeal of a jury verdict is difficult in most cases, because the legal system is based on letting the jury decide the case. However, if the judge made an error in allowing testimony to be heard or evidence to be presented that should not have been presented or if legal counsel made serious errors, the case may be overturned on appeal. The case then usually goes back to the trial court to be retried.

ASK YOURSELF

Think about your last job for a moment: did you ever make a mistake? Did you follow the procedures established by your employer? Did your actions ever have any legal ramifications, whether criminal or civil? How do you protect yourself from becoming a defendant in a legal case?

Key Laws Governing EMS

The fundamental law that governs EMS personnel is the EMS Act for the state in which the EMT is certified. Every state has an EMS Act, which provides the framework within which an individual is permitted to function as an EMT. These laws cover such key areas as the following:

- The levels of EMS certification (e.g., first responder, EMT, EMT-Intermediate [EMT-I], paramedic)
- The training requirements to obtain each level of certification
- The *scope of practice*, or list of specific skills and procedures the EMS professional is legally permitted to perform based on the level of certification
- The procedures for certification, such as prerequisites for becoming certified (most states specify a minimum age and no significant history of convictions for serious crimes)
- Steps for maintaining certification (e.g., continuing education requirements) and procedures for recertification
- Procedures the state will follow to investigate complaints involving the conduct of the EMT or the care rendered
- Procedures for taking disciplinary action against the EMT, such as written reprimand, suspension, or revocation of certification

Many EMS laws also have immunity provisions that provide statutory protection to EMTs in the event

SPECIAL Populations

Mandatory Reporters

In many states, EMS providers, police officers, and firefighters are *mandated reporters* of certain crimes that may have been committed against their patients. Mandated reporting requirements typically extend to children and elderly individuals who have been or may have been neglected or abused. However, in some states the requirements are much broader and include many other crimes (see Box 3-2). A significant fine or other punishment may be imposed for failure to file a mandated report. As EMS providers, you should know what is required of you, both for your protection and that of your patient.

a civil lawsuit is filed against them for performing their duties as EMTs (Box 3-2). In most cases these immunity provisions make it more difficult for a patient to prevail in a lawsuit against the EMT.

Many other laws also affect the role of the EMT. For example, privacy laws protect the confidentiality of patient information (covered later in the chapter), some laws regulate safety in the workplace, and others deal with the operation of emergency vehicles.

■ MAINTAINING CERTIFICATION: A PERSONAL RESPONSIBILITY

The hallmark of a medical professional is personal responsibility in maintaining all necessary certification requirements. Most states have minimum continuing education requirements that must be met during the period of EMS certification. If you have not met these requirements by the end of the certification period, your certification will lapse or you may be required to retake the practical and written examinations.

Many states provide a system for monitoring continuing education status via a web site. Moreover, many states are moving toward a system of online certification courses. These courses make it much easier to fulfill the continuing education requirements. Pennsylvania, for example, uses a system of online continuing education courses to make the programs much more accessible to everyone.

BOX 3-2

Special Reporting Situations

State and local laws may require EMTs to report incidents involving the following circumstances:
- Child abuse or neglect
- Elder abuse or neglect
- Spousal abuse or neglect
- Sexual assault
- Injuries caused by violent crime
- Exposure to certain infectious diseases
- Animal bites
- Patient restraint by forcing the patient to be transported against the person's will
- Transporting a patient considered mentally incompetent (e.g., an intoxicated person with injuries)

Some states require retesting as part of the recertification process. This helps verify that the individual has maintained the skills and knowledge necessary to fulfill the responsibilities of an EMT.

Regardless of the way your state handles the recertification process, it is your professional responsibility to keep apprised of the current process in your state and to plan ahead so that you can achieve recertification as smoothly as possible.

The following steps can help make sure your recertification goes smoothly.

1. Establish a personal file of all your EMS certifications, including letters advising you of completion of the course, the certificates, and records of all continuing education seminars or courses you have taken during the certification period.
2. Make copies of these records and keep them in a separate location just in case you lose the originals or they are inadvertently destroyed.
3. Provide copies of all certification records to your EMS organization's training officer or person assigned to maintain up-to-date records of all EMS personnel for your agency.
4. Don't rely on others, including the state EMS office or your EMS agency, to keep you informed of the status of your recertification. It is up to you to keep close track of this information to avoid the risk of your certification lapsing.
5. Keep up to date with your local EMS regional council or planning agency regarding any changes in the EMS laws or certification requirements for your state.

THE ROLE OF PHYSICIANS AND OTHER MEDICAL PROFESSIONALS

Physicians provide essential oversight of EMS systems. Most states have a statewide physician medical director who is responsible for developing protocols, reviewing training programs, and performing other important advisory functions for the state agency that regulates EMS. Regional medical directors may perform a similar function.

Some states require ambulance services, even those that operate only at the basic life support level, to have a physician medical director to oversee the medical care provided in the field by EMS personnel of the service. The physician may be involved in qual-

ity assurance activities to make sure that patient care is provided according to all standards and protocols and to provide initial and remedial training of EMS personnel when needed.

As part of the total health care team, EMTs also come in contact with a wide range of health professionals. Registered nurses and licensed practical nurses staff the emergency department and other floors of a hospital. When EMTs arrive at the hospital with a patient, it is critically important that they make sure the transfer of the patient to hospital staff goes smoothly. This means that an EMT must stay with the patient until a report can be given to the physician or nurse responsible for the person. A concise, accurate summary of the patient's condition and of the care you have provided assists the hospital staff greatly in those first few minutes after you arrive.

STANDARD OF CARE AND ETHICAL RESPONSIBILITY

The primary ethical responsibility of the EMT is to provide appropriate medical care to a patient for whom the EMT is responsible. This requires timely intervention, in a caring manner, to the level of the EMT's training. This responsibility may be fulfilled while the EMT is on call as a provider or when the EMT acts as a **good Samaritan** in an unexpected situation.

As you have learned, federal guidelines, state laws, and local EMS protocols and **standing orders** provide the framework for the EMT's level of training and scope of practice.

Consider the following: would or should you

- Stop to assist victims at a car crash?
- Help an apparently intoxicated individual staggering on the side of the road on a heavily traveled street?
- Perform CPR on a patient known to be HIV positive?

Would your decision be influenced by whether you are on duty, on call, or just stopping to help while off duty?

The standards are specifically written in formal documents. What you do reflects your personal morality. What would you expect of another EMT if you or your loved one were the victim or patient? The term *standard of care* really implies the prescribed clinical and technical standards you are trained to perform. The standard of "care" defines you as a compassionate human being who has the greater ability to help others.

Ethical decision making can be intimidating and often causes individuals to "shoot from the hip." Although this type of response is common, it can be treacherous. "Because I said so" often does not work. Moreover, legal pronouncements are not always fully understanding of a specific patient's needs. Society expects you to act honorably and morally. Yet, where do you really learn right from wrong?

Therefore, how can you approach this process so that you do the right thing as often as possible? The following principles can serve as a guide.

- *Respect the patient's* **autonomy**. Patients have rights, and even if those rights conflict with your ideas or opinions, they should be honored within obvious societal norms and constraints.
- *Consider the patient's best interest.* This may conflict with autonomy, but you should respect the patient's rights.
- *"First, do no harm."* Don't make the situation worse.
- *Practice fairness in your approach to patient care.* It is not your place to **ration** care based on your own social beliefs.

If conflict between any of these concepts creates an ethical dilemma, you can approach the situation with understanding and shape a reasonable response. Think of situations you have encountered and what created the ethical dilemma. Now, consider what could have been done to lessen the conflict and help resolve the problem, keeping in mind the rights of the patient and that person's needs. Each time you do this, you will make the next dilemma more understandable and less frustrating for all involved.

Quality of Life

What is a good **quality of life?** Who determines it? Most EMTs have witnessed events they consider horrible and frightening. Third-degree burns and spinal cord injuries are among the most upsetting. Advanced cancer and debilitating illnesses also are devastating. You may think, "Don't ever let me be like that," and from your perspective of life, these conditions may be unacceptable. However, you can learn from these patients that there is much more to experience in life than you customarily consider. What you may regard as a poor or worthless quality of life, a patient may still consider a life worth living. Simi-

larly, patients whose lifestyle or socioeconomic condition may be deplorable to your standards may still find value in their existence. Consequently, you must be very careful when you assume an individual's quality of life is poor or nonexistent. If you value all human beings as having purpose, your approach to patient care will be less burdensome for you and more helpful to patients, and your ethics will not be in question.

Organ Donation

With the scarcity of available organs for donation, it is important for you to be aware of this need. All patients should be treated equally. However, what may appear to be an entirely futile situation for a patient (e.g., a gunshot wound to the head) may result in the resuscitation or survival of many other patients (e.g., heart, lungs, liver, kidneys, intestines, and corneas).

Unethical Situations

What should an EMT do if confronted with an unethical situation, whether facing the EMT personally or involving someone else?

You should never be forced to do something you believe is unethical (political and religious beliefs should be clarified well in advance; patient care is not the arena for debate or action). An example of this situation would be an order from a supervisor *not* to document a medication error ("no harm, no foul"). A mechanism must be in place for you to report such an occurrence, such as to your EMS coordinator or chief. If this is not possible, your EMS medical director should be available to discuss this situation in a confidential manner.

If you observe an unethical act on the part of a colleague, you have an obligation to report it. Regardless of who the offender is, if you allow this situation to go unnoticed, you are no different from your colleague. Again, the means of reporting this occurrence should be clear and confidential.

Work with your colleagues, administrators, and medical director to encourage an environment of honesty, integrity, and open communication. This is your ethical responsibility, and you and your patients deserve this type of understanding.

Principles of Negligence

Negligence is the legal claim in this society to seek redress from others who have caused you harm. *Ordinary negligence* (as basic negligence is called) is de-

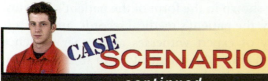

CASE SCENARIO
continued

Mr. Walsh is insistent. "Really, Ray, I think that I will be fine. I hardly feel anything at this point." Ray persists. "Mr. Walsh, I hear what you're saying. I'm glad you're feeling better. I just can't tell you that things are, in fact, better. Just because you're not having any pain doesn't mean that whatever was causing the problem in the first place went away. However, if you really don't want to go to the hospital with us, I need to tell you a few things so that you can make a fully informed decision."

Question: *What should Ray tell Mr. Walsh about this situation? What other actions should Ray take at this point?*

fined in most texts as the failure to exercise the degree of care that another reasonable person in a similar position would exercise in the same or a similar situation, resulting in harm to another person. That is the standard to which the average person or professional normally is held to in a negligence lawsuit.

Applying this concept to medical care, including EMS, courts have stated that actions that would be considered ordinary negligence are acts that caused harm to the patient *and* "deviated from good and acceptable medical standards."[2]

All of the following four elements of negligence must be proved in court for the plaintiff to prevail.

- **Duty to act.** This is generally an easy element for the plaintiff to prove. It is fairly simple: did you have a duty to provide care to the patient? Because your ambulance service or EMS agency promotes itself to the public as responding to emergency ambulance requests, your agency has a "duty" to respond to the patient and provide the care that a reasonable EMT would be expected to provide. However, the duty to act must be a "legal duty." In other words, you must have a legal obligation to respond and treat and transport the patient before you can breach the duty to act. In most cases, this is a given fact.

  Example: Paramedic Waylon Yelp is on his way to start the night shift at ABC Ambulance and Res-

cue. He hears on his scanner that a serious motor vehicle crash (MVC) has occurred just a few blocks away from his location. Waylon chooses not to respond to that call in his private vehicle. He has no duty to act, because he is not legally obligated to respond. However, if Waylon had been at the station and on duty and had failed to respond, he would have violated the duty to act.

- **Breach of the duty to act.** If you fail in any way to provide the care that your agency requires or local protocols require, you may have breached your duty to act. At this point the standard of care comes into play. The issue will be this: If you failed to act, was the failure to act inconsistent with local protocol or other direction to provide care? Expert witnesses are used to testify to the standard of care for EMS personnel in the community you serve. The question will be: *What would a reasonably prudent EMT do when confronted with the same or a similar situation?*

  Example: Waylon is at the end of his shift and is very tired. He is so tired that all he cares about is going home. Right before his shift ends, a call comes in for a possible heart attack. The BLS treatment protocols for the EMT agency require that oxygen be administered in this situation. Waylon simply does not want to turn on the oxygen, because it means he may have to replace the cylinder when the call is over. So he decides not to administer oxygen, even though it is part of the standard treatment protocol for a heart attack patient. Waylon has breached his duty to act by not administering oxygen in this situation.

- **Causation.** The plaintiff has to prove that your conduct was a substantial factor in bringing about the harm to the patient. This is difficult to prove in most EMS cases, because the wheels of harm to the patient have already been set in motion before EMS is even activated. In other words, you are responding to a patient who has already suffered harm. You are merely trying to intervene to lessen the impact of that harm. The question the jury will have to answer is: *Was your conduct the legal cause of the harm to the patient?* That is called *proximate cause.* If the harm the patient suffered can be shown to have come from other sources, and not you, this element of proof would not be met.

  Example: A patient suffering a heart attack calls 911. First responders arrive and find an unconscious patient in cardiac arrest; they begin CPR. The basic life support ambulance arrives quickly. The EMTs apply the automatic external defibrillator (AED), but it does not work because the battery is dead. CPR is continued until the paramedic unit arrives 15 minutes later. The paramedics attach a cardiac monitor and defibrillate the patient. The patient does not respond to several defibrillation attempts. The patient is transported and pronounced dead at the hospital emergency department.

If it can be shown that the 15-minute delay in delivering a shock to the patient (because the AED battery was dead) could have meant the difference between life and death, then proximate causation may be shown. However, as may be apparent from this example, in defending the EMT or EMS agency, the defense attorney would argue that the patient was in an irreversible condition and could not have been saved even if the EMTs were able to deliver a shock with the AED. The attorney would argue that the proximate cause of the patient's death was the heart attack that caused the cardiac arrest and not the 15-minute delay in defibrillation.

In some cases, errors in the field and their effect on the patient can be "isolated out" rather easily from the initial insult to the patient. For example, take the situation of an alcoholic patient who falls asleep on top of a cement wall and subsequently falls about 10 feet to the base of the wall. The patient is seen moving his arms and legs before the ambulance arrives. The EMTs on the ambulance crew treat the patient poorly (recognizing him as a "regular" patient they had seen before) and conduct no patient assessment. They lift the patient to a seated position without spinal immobilization, allowing his head and neck to jerk back. The patient suddenly goes limp. He later describes his arms and legs as "going numb" as soon as the EMTs lifted him to a seated position. He now is a quadriplegic.

In this example, it may be relatively easy for the plaintiff to prove that the action (or inaction) of the EMTs was a substantial factor and the proximate cause of the patient's harm. The question is: *Would the patient have been a quadriplegic* but for *the conduct of the EMTs?* In this situation, the answer clearly is no, because the patient was able to move his arms and legs before the EMTs arrived. Consequently, this element of negligence likely can be shown.

- **Harm to the patient.** A successful lawsuit based on negligence requires that there first must be some harm to the patient. This is usually seen as some sort of physical or emotional injury that has caused some "damage" to the patient. Damage

can be shown in the form of the patient's own testimony, the patient's medical records, and the testimony of expert witnesses and other evidence that can show the extent of harm to the patient. The cost of this harm can be translated into medical costs for treatment, recovery, and rehabilitation and for "pain and suffering," as well as other compensatory damages. To prove negligence, the plaintiff typically must show that the harm was the type that could have been caused by the EMS provider.

Example: ABC Ambulance responds to a motor vehicle accident. Upon arrival, EMS personnel find the driver of the vehicle walking around with no apparent injuries. The vehicle suffered minor damage when it struck a parked car. Waylon approaches the patient, who refuses treatment and says he is fine. Waylon attempts to convince the patient to go to the hospital and explains the risks of refusing treatment and transport. Despite Waylon's efforts, the patient refuses care. Waylon reluctantly asks the patient to sign a refusal of care form, and the patient signs it. The patient goes home and goes to sleep. The next day he wakes up with a throbbing headache and goes to the emergency department. He is admitted with a cerebral aneurysm that requires surgery, and he also has suffered some permanent paralysis as well. He sues the ambulance service because he thinks he should have been transported. He alleges that they were negligent because they did not automatically transport him. In this case, it is likely that no harm to the patient has resulted from the acts or omissions of the EMS personnel, as long as the refusal was informed and the EMTs followed proper procedure in obtaining it.

The Immunity Defense

Many states provide certain "immunities" under the law that make it more difficult for a plaintiff to prove negligence against an EMS provider. These immunities are based on the age-old *good Samaritan* principle. This principle basically is designed to encourage others to assist an ill or injured person to the best of their ability without fear of a lawsuit for mistakes they may make.

Virtually every state has some form of good Samaritan law. Many of these laws merely protect the bystander or person without medical training from being sued for providing assistance in an emergency. Some of these laws protect physicians and nurses outside their work environment if they provide care at the scene of an emergency. These laws are designed to encourage off-duty health professionals to help out in an emergency without the fear of liability that could cloud their judgment.

Other state laws extend the immunity to EMS personnel and other responders. For example, Pennsylvania's immunity statute for EMS personnel states: "*No* first responder, emergency medical technician or EMT-paramedic, or health professional who in good faith attempts to render or facilitate emergency medical care authorized by this act *shall be liable* for any civil damages as a result of any acts or omissions, *unless guilty of gross or willful negligence.*"[3]

If these laws apply to you, does it mean you are completely immune from a negligence lawsuit? Not necessarily. The type of immunity that these laws embody is not a full immunity but rather a *qualified* immunity. The immunity has a restriction; you may not act in a reckless, wanton manner in total disregard of the patient, because acting in this manner would be considered gross negligence. Most immunity statutes provide that you are immune from a negligence lawsuit unless your actions could be shown to constitute gross negligence.

Gross negligence is difficult to prove in many cases. Actions or lack of action must be more than a mere mistake (i.e., more serious than ordinary negligence) to be considered grossly negligent acts. As the Pennsylvania Supreme Court described it, gross negligence is *substantially more* than "ordinary carelessness, inadvertence, laxity or indifference." It is behavior that is *"flagrant, grossly deviating from the ordinary standard of care."*[4] Volunteer EMS personnel often enjoy legal protection for their conduct that may be stronger than the immunity protections for career or paid EMS personnel. The concept is that, if you volunteer to save someone's life or to assist the person in a medical crisis, you should not have to worry about being sued. Otherwise, few "good Samaritans" would be willing to help in an emergency. In many cases these state laws require that you at least have some level of training, such as CPR or first aid training, and that you render assistance only within the level of that certification or training.

These immunity protections often apply to all EMS personnel, but some states have limited this protection to volunteer personnel and do not apply it to paid EMS personnel. Why? Because the lawmakers in some states believe that you owe a higher duty to the people you are obligated to serve as part of your profession. This makes some sense, because responding to an emergency is part of your job, and you should be better prepared for these situations than

the volunteer good Samaritan. You should check your state laws carefully to determine whether the immunity statutes apply to paid or career EMS personnel. If the state does not have an immunity statute, the standard for evaluating your conduct likely will be based on ordinary negligence, which is easier to prove than gross negligence.

How do you avoid committing gross negligence? First and foremost, function within your certification level. Don't perform skills or administer medications that are out of your scope of practice, which is the extent to which you can treat the patient as defined in state law. For example, if you are not authorized under state law and by your medical director to administer paralytic agents to a difficult patient who needs to be intubated, you should not use that medication even if it is available to you or is included in your drug box.

Second, always act in good faith. The best way to do this is always to treat patients as if they were your own close relatives. Function in a reasonable and prudent manner with the interest of the patient in your heart and mind. Common sense often helps you in this area. Ask yourself, "Is this the right thing to do in this situation?" If the answer is no, you should reevaluate your plan of action. For example, failure to provide spinal immobilization for an accident victim with neck and back pain clearly is not the right thing to do and is so blatantly wrong that most jurors would find that failure to be outside the bounds of what a reasonable EMT would be expected to do. This failure likely would be seen as an example of not acting in good faith.

Third, don't do things or fail to do things that could be construed as grossly negligent. Function within your scope of practice and do what the public would expect you to do. Don't commit or omit an action that you are under a recognized duty to another to do or not do, knowing or having reason to know that the act or omission could create a substantial risk of harm to the patient. Remember the first rule of medical care: do no harm. If it is likely your actions could harm the patient, you should not initiate them.

Risk Management: A Personal Responsibility

Mistakes occur every day in the field. It's a tough work environment, and you need to be on top of your game at all times. Even the smallest mistake can lead to serious harm to the patient. However, mistakes do not necessarily mean that you were negligent under the law. The successful plaintiff must prove by a *preponderance of the evidence* that you breached your duty to the patient.

The best way to describe preponderance of the evidence is to look at two equal scales. If you put all the evidence in favor of the plaintiff on one scale and all the evidence in favor of the defendant on the other scale, the direction in which the scale tips (more evidence on one side) points to the *preponderance* (most of the evidence) in favor of that side. Breach of duty usually is demonstrated by showing that you deviated from the standard of care expected of the typical EMT in your area.

Even if the plaintiff can show that you breached your duty to the patient, the most difficult element to prove is that your conduct was a substantial factor in causing the harm to the patient. This element is tough to prove because in the typical EMS response, the patient already is suffering from some sort of immediate harm, such as a heart attack or internal bleeding from trauma. The plaintiff must show that your actions or lack of action harmed the patient beyond the harm that the person already received. It is very difficult to separate these two types of harm; that is, the initial harm from the insult that caused the EMS response and the harm that may have occurred after that event and because of your intervention or failure to intervene.

Proving negligence is difficult, but in many cases juries are going to be sympathetic to the plaintiff or the surviving family members. Many jurors view EMTs as professionals who are no different from nurses or other health professionals in a hospital. In addition, even though proving negligence is difficult, jurors do not always decide cases based on the law. No one knows except the jurors themselves what discussions lead to their decision. Unfortunately, in this society the manner in which a jury decides a negligence case is not subject to review on appeal unless clear errors exist in trial procedures. Examples of clear errors include admission of evidence that the judge should have disallowed and jury instructions that do not reflect the current state of the law. A clear basis for appeal would be tampering with the jury or juror misconduct. However, an appeal rarely is won on these issues.

The point is, a jury that can be influenced by many factors will judge you. Moreover, the jury will make its decision based on many sources of information. Elements that contribute to the decision on liability include the jury's assessment of witness credibility, their like or dislike of the plaintiff or defense counsel, and each juror's life experiences. Other, more tangible factors include the extent of harm to the patient, the life

expectancy of the patient, the impact of the harm on daily living, and other emotional issues that are part of the case. Juries are expected to follow the law and the jury instructions read to them by the judge. However, in this system of justice, the biases, prejudices, and persuasiveness of the attorneys have a lot to do with the final decision. That decision typically cannot be challenged on appeal unless an error in courtroom procedure occurs, as described previously.

In all aspects of your role as a professional EMT, you must take care to avoid conducting yourself in a manner that could be construed as negligent. How is this best accomplished? You can take a number of steps to minimize the risk of a mistake that could harm the patient and result in a lawsuit.

- **Be well educated.** Keep up to date with current trends in EMS treatment and periodically review key areas of the training program materials you received. EMS is developing at an increasingly rapid pace, and the treatment modalities for particular medical situations are constantly changing. Periodic skill practice sessions can help keep your skills sharp, especially with techniques that you don't use very often. For example, errors commonly occur in the management of pediatric patients, particularly airway management. EMTs don't use the smaller pediatric equipment very often. In addition, the procedures for treating small children may be very different from the techniques for treating the same condition in adults.
- **Be well rested.** You are more apt to make a mistake when you are tired and stressed out. In emergency services, failure to be in the best possible physical condition can lead to serious errors. Medication administration is one of the skills that require you to be sharp and at your best more than other skills do. Many aspects of medication administration require an intact thought process and mental skill. Studies have shown that failure to be well rested can lead to mistakes in patient care, and medication errors are more likely to occur when you are tired and unable to think clearly.

In one study involving nurses, researchers at the University of Pennsylvania found that medical mistakes increased threefold after nurses worked shifts stretching beyond $12\frac{1}{2}$ hours. In this study, most of the errors attributed to the long shifts were medication errors, such as administering the wrong medication, giving the wrong dose, or giving the medication beyond scheduled dose times. Working longer than the regularly scheduled shift increased the likelihood that at least one error would be made.[5]

- **Know your protocols and follow them.** The standard of care is examined in negligence cases. The standard of care in a lawsuit is determined by your scope of practice (the legally approved skills you may perform and the medications you are authorized to administer) as described by state law. Other, supplemental sources also establish scope of practice, such as training program curricula, textbooks, the reports of medial experts, and expert testimony. In addition, the standard of care very often is defined by your local medical protocols, which can become direct evidence not only of your legally authorized scope of practice, but also of the standard of medical care for your community. Deviating from these protocols can be seen as deviating from the standard of care.

- **Maintain your knowledge and skills.** You have a professional obligation as an EMT to maintain your knowledge and skills. This means keeping up with recent developments in the field, periodically reviewing your EMT training materials, practicing skills you don't often use, and regularly attending continuing education programs. Regular practice and review can keep you from getting rusty, which can lead to a greater likelihood of making mistakes.

■ BAD ATTITUDES AND POOR COMMUNICATION: THE LIABILITY OF APATHY

Many EMS personnel are surprised to learn that most lawsuits are not directly related to patient care skills. The suits initiated in most cases involve a patient or family members who are unhappy with the manner in which a situation was handled. Bad attitudes and poor communication are the true culprits in the triggering of a lawsuit. The basic point is that patients generally do not sue you if they like you!

Research studies support the proposition that most lawsuits related to patient care are about dissatisfaction with the behavior of the caregivers toward the patient rather than technical errors.

Being well rested, working at the top of your game, and having a positive attitude at all times are the keys to making a positive impression on patients and family members. Some common steps can help you improve communication with patients and family members.

- *Be well rested.* Make sure you get enough sleep and that you are alert and ready to go. If you work more than one EMS job, it is important to remember that you owe a high duty to every patient with whom you come into contact, including those you see at the end of the day.

- *Present a professional appearance.* If you approach the patient looking sloppy and unprofessional, the patient and family will start to question your competence. A professional appearance makes a good first impression. If you are a volunteer responding to calls from a variety of locations, keeping a clean jumpsuit close at hand is a good way of ensuring a professional appearance, even when you are not dressed to respond.

- *Project confidence in your initial approach to the patient.* Most people decide whether or not they like someone in the first few seconds of interaction. Like it or not, the patient's first impression is often the one the person uses to evaluate your competence. It is critically important to be positive and to convey a sense of calm professionalism when you approach the patient. This helps put the person at ease and gets your relationship off on the right foot.

- *Convey your sincere concern and empathy.* Putting yourself in the patient's shoes helps you become a more compassionate and effective care provider.

- *Use verbal and nonverbal techniques to enhance communication.* Use body language, eye contact, and other physical cues that let the patient know you are interested in what the person has to say.

- *Work at the patient's level, both physically and verbally.* This is true of adults and pediatric patients. Make sure you are not towering over the patient, regardless of the person's age (Fig. 3-1).

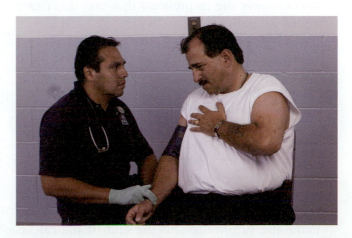

Fig. 3-1 Address patients at eye level.

- *Introduce yourself in a warm, friendly manner.* The first 30 seconds with the patient usually provide a lasting impression. You need to make the first impression a good one to instill confidence in the patient. Look the patient in the eye and speak clearly and in a friendly tone when you introduce yourself.

- *Explain what you are doing and why.* Patients want to know what is going on when you are assessing them and providing treatment. Giving them this information makes them feel more in control and better about what you are doing for them.

- *Reassure but do not make any guarantees.* Be sensitive and careful not to promise specific results. Let the patient know you are doing everything you can and that the individual is in good hands.

- *Follow the basic steps of physical comfort (e.g., provide a blanket and pillow).* Patients often complain about the basics. Put yourself in the patient's shoes; keep alert for times a patient may be uncomfortable and address those issues promptly.

- *Communicate with the family.* The family may be watching with a lot of anxiety. Keep them as involved as you can by letting them know what you are doing for their loved one. This also helps you to get important information you may need from them about the patient.

- *Smile.* Smiling appropriately helps calm the situation and conveys a message that you care about the patient and you like caring for the person. It also helps allay anxiety.

- *Speak in a comforting tone and volume.* Speak in an appropriate tone and volume that the patient can hear and understand, so that the person does not get worked up or upset further.

- *Avoid unnecessary chatter with coworkers.* Pay attention to the patient and the family. Extraneous chatter with others not only is unprofessional, it also conveys the impression that you don't care about the patient.

- *If something doesn't work, don't make it obvious!* Sometimes things break or go wrong. Don't try to hide the problem, but don't make it the focus of the situation, thereby increasing the patient's anxiety.

- *Be time efficient.* Work efficiently at the scene and move with a purpose. Don't run; however, people expect that in an emergency situation, you will at least act as if it's an emergency.

- *Say goodbye.* As they say, first impressions and last impressions are what people remember. They will forget a lot of the bad stuff in the middle if you make the beginning and the end of the call as positive an experience as it can possibly be. In ad-

dition, this is good customer relations and can minimize any bad feelings the patient or family members may have had toward you.

When apathy creeps into your conduct as an EMT, you become a liability. The uncaring attitudes that go with apathy can cause you to become a liability to the patient, your service, other organizations, your coworkers, and yourself! Treat every call as if it were your first call. That way, you can be sure you are providing the best possible care for the patient, and the risk of a lawsuit will be greatly reduced.

Ethical and Legal Consent Issues and Refusal of Care

A highly intoxicated woman involved in a motor vehicle crash refuses medical treatment. Is this person capable of making this decision? You determine that she is not. What are the grounds for your position? The answer is you believe the patient lacks **decision-making capacity.** This is a clinical judgment founded on the patient's ability to make a coherent decision. Now let's say this same individual is involved in a motor vehicle crash but is not intoxicated and is fully lucid. She refuses treatment. This patient is said to have decision-making capacity. Again, this is a medical determination.

Where does **competency** come into play? All people are assumed to be competent. If for some reason a judge declares an individual incompetent, a guardian is appointed to act on the person's behalf. *Competency,* therefore, is a judicial determination, not a medical decision. Examples of such a determination would apply to severely demented patients or individuals who can no longer safely care for themselves.

When one describes a patient's ability to accept or refuse treatment, one is referring to the patient's decision-making capacity, not the individual's competency (unless the person has been judicially declared incompetent).

Ethical Aspects of Refusal of Care

Certain parameters should be met for a patient to refuse medical treatment. Essentially, what goes into decision-making capacity and the ability to decline care? The answer is **informed refusal.**

When the EMT obtains informed refusal from a patient, special care must be exercised to avoid future problems. This may be time consuming and bothersome, but in the long run, it is proper patient care and potentially the best prevention against future litigation.

Informed refusal requires that the patient understand the following:

- What you propose to do and why
- The risks involved
- The alternative treatment possibilities with their potential risks
- The consequences of not being treated and the risks (the worst possible outcomes should be mentioned and documented)

Two additional elements are necessary for informed refusal:

- The patient must comprehend this discussion and demonstrate full understanding.
- The patient's response must be free of **coercion.**

This process should be well documented and appropriately signed as your local protocol dictates.

Of course, you should make all reasonable attempts to convince a patient with decision-making capacity to accept your treatment. The EMT's personal convenience should not be a factor in encouraging a sign-off.

Another consideration is who can sign a refusal of care. A patient with decision-making capacity can; a durable power of attorney for health care can; and a legal guardian can. However, a spouse who is none of these cannot. When the patient lacks decision-making capacity and no legal **surrogate** exists, you (with the help of medical control if needed) must be an advocate for the patient. A family member should not be permitted to refuse care for a patient.

When it comes to consent issues and refusal of care, a safe philosophy is to err on the side of life. Defending why you cared is always easier than trying to justify why you didn't do something for the patient.

Legal Aspects of Refusal of Care

Patient refusal of care is an area that can be fraught with legal liability for ambulance service providers. In fact, it is one of the most significant areas of liability, because leaving a patient can give rise to a claim of abandonment. Often the damages for an abandonment claim can be staggering, particularly if the patient is young and dies after you leave the scene.

Just think; a refusal case that evolves into litigation can leave you and your service in the unenviable position of having to defend yourselves for doing nothing on the patient's behalf. Defending yourself from making a mistake in providing patient care is one thing; it is entirely another to have to defend yourself

in a case in which the patient received no care, potentially because of your failure to determine whether the person was indeed competent to refuse care.

The law recognizes generally that, subject to certain interests of society, a *competent* individual has a right to refuse any and all medical care, even if that care would save the person's life. This is embodied in the common law notion of patient self-determination. However, this concept has evolved from a common law notion into a statutory one. More than a decade ago, Congress enacted the Patient Self-Determination Act.[6] Among other things, this law requires most health care facilities in the United States to inform patients upon admission of their right to execute a living will.

The law takes the concept of self-determination by competent patients very seriously. Therefore a critical element of any refusal situation is an assessment by the EMS providers as to whether their patient is competent. If they determine that the patient is competent, EMS providers should be especially careful to explain fully the specific risks that may result from the patient's refusal and should make sure the patient is informed of alternatives in the event the person persists in refusing care.

The U.S. Supreme Court has upheld the right of every competent patient to self-determination when it comes to medical care and the application of lifesaving or life-sustaining measures.[7] Put simply, each person has the right to determine whether to accept or reject any type of medical care or treatment (including any form of "laying on of hands" by health care providers) as long as the person is capable of making that decision as a competent adult. Although the fact that a patient can refuse care may be difficult to accept, an EMT can be charged with **battery** for touching a person without permission or with **assault** for creating the fear of injury.

This principle of self-determination applies just as clearly in the prehospital environment as it does within the four walls of the hospital. However, in the prehospital setting the patient is less likely to be competent to make that determination because of a variety of factors, such as shock, alcohol use, and decreased level of consciousness. EMS providers must make sure the patient consents to the assessment and treatment that is to be provided. All competent adults have the right to consent to or refuse care and treatment, even in emergency situations. This includes the right to refuse not just the entire care and treatment package, but also portions of it.

Can a patient consent to some treatment and then refuse to consent to certain types of specific treatment? Absolutely. For example, a patient may specifically refuse to consent to the administration of oxygen. What should you do in such cases? First you must make sure the patient understands the importance of the oxygen. A convincing approach usually changes the patient's mind. If not, make sure the patient is competent to make that refusal. All refusals of care must be carefully documented, or you run the risk of a claim of abandonment or negligence. Failure to assess properly the patient's ability to give consent and improper documentation of a refusal of care are crucial areas of liability risk.

A refusal of care can be a complete or a partial refusal. Complete refusals are situations in which the patient refuses all aspects of treatment. This is probably the most common type of refusal. A partial refusal occurs when the patient agrees to some but not all of the treatment you wish to provide. If a patient refuses a portion of treatment, such as the administration of a specific medication, you can still provide other treatment that the patient agrees to allow. In these situations, you should obtain written documentation of the refusal, even if it is just a partial refusal. Documentation of refusals of care is not limited just to complete refusals.

Consent and the refusal of a patient to provide consent must be handled properly to minimize the potential liability that can arise. The attorneys at Page, Wolfberg & Wirth, LLC, a national law firm that counsels and represents private and public EMS agencies, have developed and modified a set of refusal guidelines called *A three, E three, P three* ($A^3E^3P^3$).[8] These guidelines are intended to help EMS providers remember the important things to consider in dealing with refusal situations.

1. **Assess** the patient's legal and mental capacity to refuse care. Is the patient 18 years of age, or does the patient meet your state's exceptions for emancipated minors? The patient must be a legally recognized adult (over the age of 18) or deemed by law to be treated as an adult (as in the emancipated minor and other special circumstances). Only adults can consent to care or refuse it. Most state laws permit minors to consent to treatment, but they usually are not considered legally competent to refuse treatment. Is the patient suffering from any mental condition that might prevent the person from making an informed decision? Examples would include permanent conditions, such as a brain disease (e.g., Alzheimer's disease), or situational conditions, such as shock, alcohol or drug intoxication, or decreased level of consciousness caused by a head injury or other trauma.

2. **Advise** the patient of his or her medical condition and your proposed treatment. Even though you don't diagnose in EMS, you should tell a patient what's going on with his or her condition and how you propose to treat it so that the person's refusal decision is *informed!* Don't be afraid to tell patients what could be happening to them.

   The patient's decision to refuse care should be a conscious one made with all the information a reasonable person would find important to the decision-making process. You should also inform the patient of the potential consequences of refusal, including, if appropriate, the possibility of death or long-term disability. Your handling of a refusal case is much more defensible if you can demonstrate (through effective documentation, of course) that you fully informed your patient of the possible medical implications of the person's decision.

3. **Avoid** the use of confusing terminology when talking to your patient. Make sure you use terms the person can understand! A decision to release a refusal patient is most defensible when the patient made the decision from a position of complete and informed decision making. Your purpose in fully advising the patient of his or her condition is not to impress the person with your grasp of medical terminology but to make sure that the individual's decision on whether to refuse or consent to medical care is an informed one. Therefore terms such as "subdural hematoma," "compound tib/fib fracture," and "anaphylaxis" should have no place in the patient refusal interview. Instead, use terms such as "head injury," "broken leg," or "serious allergic reaction."

4. **Ensure** that the patient's decision to refuse care is the product of the person's own informed decision making and not the result of improper influence or coercion by others. Make sure the patient is not merely parroting what a family member is telling him or her to say. A refusal cannot be the result of incomplete or erroneous information. It should not be the result of undue pressure from a friend or family member, but rather should come from an informed *patient*.

5. **Explain** the alternatives to your patient if the person refuses your care and transport. Some refusal situations that otherwise would be defensible may lead to liability if the providers fail to inform the patient of possible courses of action that can be followed in light of the patient's refusal of care. EMTs must be sure to advise their patients that patients can call 911 again if symptoms persist or

worsen, that they can follow up with their doctor, and/or that care is available 24 hours a day from an emergency department.

6. **Exploit** uncertainty! If you ask the patient for permission to examine her and she appears hesitant, this should be seen as an invitation to engage the patient in additional conversation and be persuasive about recommending further care when necessary. If you ask a patient if it's okay to examine her and her first reaction is, "Gee, I don't know," a prudent EMS provider will say something like, "Well, we're already here; it's no bother. But if you're unsure, why don't we take a look and see what's going on?" Many patients simply are unsure about whether they should really go to the hospital, and that uncertainty should be used to your advantage in advising the patient to obtain the care the person needs.

7. **Persist** in trying to persuade your patient to obtain the care the person needs. Don't accept the first "no" for an answer. Stick around long enough to make it clear to your patient that the person is not being a bother. You may have to make several attempts to convince a patient that he or she needs to consent to EMS treatment and transport to the hospital. In the event you are sued, a well-documented refusal helps demonstrate this persistence.

8. **Protocols**—follow them! If your service or your EMS system has protocols in place regarding patient refusals, be sure to adhere to them. Be sure to follow any applicable policies or protocols your EMS agency may have in place. For example, some systems require advanced life support (ALS) providers to contact medical command before releasing care to a BLS crew. Failure to follow protocols not only can lead to greater civil liability, it also can expose the provider to discipline or a formal action by certification or licensing authorities.

9. **Protect** yourself with adequate documentation of the refusal. Write a thorough narrative explaining all the steps in the process. Whenever possible, obtain the patient's signature to verify the person's understanding of his or her decision. Try to get the names and addresses of witnesses who observed the refusal process. Describe the specifics of any partial refusal of care. The trip sheet on a refusal should say more than "patient refused." At minimum it should have the following:

- A history of the incident
- A description of the patient as you encountered the person
- A description of the scene, witnesses, or others present
- Vital signs and other physical observations
- Specific words used by the patient to indicate understanding and to refuse care or transportation
- A patient signature
- Specific potential consequences of which you informed your patient
- Instructions given to the patient in the event of persistent or worsening symptoms

Every refusal situation should be treated with individualized attention. The actions of the ambulance service provider might be viewed under a microscope several years down the road by a judge or jury. Above all, don't be tempted to blow off a call that at the time seems like "just another patient refusal." This is the complacency that breeds liability.

Thorough and accurate documentation of all aspects of the refusal of care must be included as part of the patient care report. Without it, you could be stuck defending actions without the contemporaneous documentation. This documentation adds the credibility you may need to overcome the critical eye of the fact finder in the courtroom.

Living Wills and Advance Directives Limiting Treatment

Ethical Issues with Advance Directives

An **advance directive** is a document that allows a person to state autonomously his or her desires for what should or should not be done in the event the person cannot speak for himself or herself. This usually relates to concerns over aggressive treatments or end-of-life issues. Advance directives can prove very helpful in the most stressful of situations for families and medical personnel.

The two main types of advance directives are the living will and the durable power of attorney for health care. A **living will** is restrictive, may not address all issues of withholding or withdrawal of treatment, and generally is not relevant in the prehospital emergency setting because, in most cases, the patient has to be incapacitated for a specified period of time before the living will becomes active. A **durable power of attorney for health care** is the person (agent) appointed by the patient to make all medical decisions on the person's behalf if he or she cannot. This document may also contain certain guidelines for the agent. This form of advance directive allows for more latitude on the part of the agent, who is considered to be speaking as the patient. It is important to remember that a family member is not automatically a legal guardian or an agent. These are appointed by a judge or by the patient, respectively.

What happens if a patient does not have a written advance directive? Most states have a health care surrogate law. This law specifically determines the appropriate person or people empowered to make medical decisions for the patient who lacks that ability. The following is an example of this order of surrogacy:

- Court-appointed guardian
- Spouse
- Adult children (may require majority rule)
- Parent
- Adult siblings
- Adult grandchildren
- Close friend

EMTs should become knowledgeable about the laws of their states as they apply to advance directives.

Do Not Resuscitate (DNR) Orders

The issue of **do not resuscitate (DNR)** orders can be a difficult issue and a major frustration for EMTs. Often EMTs are called upon to attempt resuscitation on a patient who appears to have no logical chance for meaningful survival. Yet, on the other hand, a young patient who appears to have a reasonable chance for a successful resuscitation will have a DNR order. This is very difficult for the emergency medical services community.

From an ethical perspective, remember that CPR is presumed for any individual unless specifically declined (DNR). This means that a DNR patient, or the person's appropriate surrogate, has thought out the risks versus benefits of resuscitation and has elected, autonomously or by surrogate appointment, not to be resuscitated. This is the patient's right. A patient may still desire aggressive treatment up until the time of cardiopulmonary arrest.

The area of most concern with a DNR status is comfort care. DNR status does not preclude aggressive treatment for other clinical conditions (e.g., infection, transfusion). Also, a DNR patient should never feel that "do not resuscitate" equals "do not care." You must always strive to alleviate your patient's suffering. A DNR patient who is short of breath can still be given oxygen to keep the person comfortable.

Legal Issues

All states have living will statutes that allow a person to predesignate the level of medical intervention the

person would like to have in the event of a terminal illness. These legal documents provide advance directives, more commonly described as specific orders to the caregiver, as to what level of treatment the patient would like to have in the event of a particular medical situation.

Many advance directives provide limitations on treatment in the event of a cardiac arrest or if the patient lapses into a coma. Typically these directives allow the care provider to treat the patient with palliative or comfort measures and restrict the use of resuscitative measures, such as CPR, endotracheal intubation, or administration of medications.

Most state laws have strict verification requirements to make sure the directive being followed is proper. Some states rely on identification tags that the patient must wear, whereas others require a document signed by the patient's attending physician. Some states require that online medical control be consulted before an advance directive can be recognized. It is important to remember that even if the patient has an advance directive in place, it can be overruled at any time by the patient. A competent patient has the right to void the directive or change his or her mind during the course of treatment.

Scope of Practice Issues

Many ALS systems have worked hard to encourage BLS personnel to participate in the ALS care of the patient through paramedic assist courses and other programs. The EMT-I or paramedic should proceed very cautiously when involving BLS personnel in ALS procedures. Even if you don't have enough hands to do everything at once, it is very risky to assign to basic level personnel any procedures that legally can be performed only by an advanced level caregiver. At all times, BLS and ALS personnel must function within the limitations of their respective scopes of practice, which are defined by the state EMS Act.

The procedure for starting an intravenous (IV) line offers a good example of how scope of practice dilemmas can become a problem. Should a paramedic allow the EMT to set up the IV bag and tubing, including flushing the line of any air? This level of assistance should not be allowed, unless, of course, the basic level personnel are permitted to establish IV lines under state law. Unless the EMS provider is certified to provide that level of care, it would be improper to allow basic level personnel to perform any part of the procedure that would involve advanced training. For example, properly identifying the IV solution, maintaining a sterile field when removing protective covers and hooking up the IV tubing, and flushing the line may seem like simple tasks; however, they usually involve some level of advanced training that only the EMT-I or paramedic may receive. A paramedic who permits a basic level EMS provider who is not certified to perform a skill could be seen as negligent in improperly delegating the skill. The basic level EMS provider may be in violation of the state's EMS Act by performing a skill outside the scope of practice for the provider's level of certification.

What could the basic level provider do in this situation? In a nutshell, everything short of performing a skill that could be seen as restricted to a more advanced care provider. Using the example of starting an IV line, this could include pulling out the solutions and IV start supplies and removing them from their packages (but not exposing sterile surfaces), tearing tape, or preparing other material to be used to secure the IV site and tubing.

■ COMPLETING ACCURATE AND LEGAL PATIENT CARE DOCUMENTATION

The ethical issues involving documentation are rather straightforward:

- Document honestly and in an unbiased manner.
- *If you didn't write it, you didn't do it!*

The patient care report (commonly called the *PCR*) is the foundation of all that you do in the field. It is the official record of the care you provided. The PCR has significant patient care, billing, and liability ramifications. The basic purpose of the PCR is to provide the reader with a "picture" of the continuum of care provided to the patient, from the arrival of first responders to the transfer of care to hospital staff.

In a lawsuit the PCR becomes your substitute memory, because most liability lawsuits end up in trial years after the harm occurred. Most people have trouble remembering what they did on a particular call a year ago, let alone several years ago. Therefore you need a complete and "visual" record of what you found and what you did if you expect to come across as a knowledgeable and credible witness before a jury. Sloppy, incomplete, and poorly constructed patient documentation reflects poorly on the individual EMT or paramedic and on the ambulance service itself. Poor documentation may also be used against you in a lawsuit or federal investigation.

Now more than ever, ambulance services must be vigilant in their documentation efforts. The law of negligence comes into play when a patient sues your service for the care that was provided. The recent focus on the antifraud and abuse laws makes documentation a concern outside of the traditional patient care areas. More than ever, Medicare carriers and the government are closely scrutinizing patient care documentation for false statements, inconsistent information, and other inaccuracies that could lead to a federal false claims act action or other criminal prosecution or civil sanctions.

Clear, accurate documentation is not only required for good patient care, it also is a necessity in this ever-litigious society. Your PCR will be center stage in a malpractice or negligence trial. Therefore make sure your documentation helps you in your defense rather than hurts you. If you are called to the witness stand, you absolutely will be cross-examined by the plaintiff's counsel about the quality of your documentation. Sloppy, incomplete documentation of the patient care you provide reflects on your credibility as a competent caregiver, even if your documentation has no gross errors.

Bruce, Sones, and Peck[9] point out some very important dos and don'ts to consider when documenting patient care.

Do

- Make sure the documentation is an accurate reflection of your prehospital capabilities and your scope of practice.
- Write legibly and in complete sentences, using proper abbreviations so that all personnel can read your report.
- Accurately document the times treatment was provided and give a clear description of that treatment.
- Document any refusal of care by the patient, including instances when a patient refuses only a portion of the treatment you are attempting to provide (e.g., patient refuses oxygen). State why the patient refused the treatment and the steps you took to make this refusal one in which the patient was informed of all the risks of refusing the treatment.
- Document vital signs before and after key treatment and when the patient is moved.
- Document any changes in vital signs, especially if the patient's condition worsens.
- Create a "picture" of the patient's condition so that when others read the PCR, they can actually visualize the patient.

Don't

- Scribble or write illegibly.
- Misspell words or medication names.
- Forget to check the patient's response to any treatments.
- Make up abbreviations or use inappropriate acronyms in your documentation. Use only approved abbreviations.
- Assume that others will take care of your documentation. If you provided the treatment, it is your responsibility to document it.
- Prepare your report late if you can avoid it. Chart any late entries or errors in charting if changes or entries are made after the original report is completed and turned in. And always prepare your documentation as if it will be revealed in a court of law.

Documenting Care Provided to the Patient by Others

A question that often arises is whether an EMT or first responder should document on the BLS patient care report the interventions or assessments performed by the paramedic. This might be an issue in areas where EMS is provided in tiered systems. In other words, it might be an issue in areas where BLS and ALS are provided by separate organizations. In such systems, BLS providers respond in a transporting ambulance and ALS providers respond in a nontransporting paramedic intercept or "fly car" unit.

In some systems the practice may be to document that the ALS provider applied a cardiac monitor and to record the electrocardiographic (ECG) rhythm displayed on the monitor. Some EMTs also document that the paramedic started an IV line, the number of attempts needed to establish the line, the medications and solutions administered through the IV line, and other such information about the ALS care. As a general rule, EMS providers should document according to their scope of practice and should *not* attempt to document skills beyond those for which they are trained and are certified to perform themselves. The risk of inconsistent and inaccurate records is too great when providers document beyond their scope of practice. In addition, such "beyond the scope" documentation may impair the credibility of an EMS provider who ends up on a witness stand defending a lawsuit. For example, EMTs who document a particular cardiac rhythm are left wide open to a stinging and damaging cross-examination about their training and qualifications, or lack thereof, to make such determinations and why they would doc-

ument care beyond their scope of practice. Not being able to answer questions in a deposition or on the witness stand about all the documentation, including the EMT-documented ALS care, could call into question the EMT's quality of BLS treatment by undermining the credibility of the witness.

This is not to suggest that EMTs cannot document anything that happens in regard to ALS. The EMT should certainly document the fact that the paramedic provided patient care and should certainly document the EMT's role in the care. For example, if the paramedic intubates the patient and the EMT handles the bag-valve-mask ventilation, the BLS patient care report certainly should reflect that. Other general observations on a BLS patient care report, such as, "Paramedic performed a patient assessment," "Paramedic intubated the patient," "Paramedic applied a cardiac monitor," and "IV medications administered by the paramedic," likewise wouldn't create any problems, as long as the EMT refrains from describing details, such as the intubation technique or tube size used, the particular cardiac rhythm displayed on the monitor, or the names and dosages of specific medications administered by ALS providers.

The bottom line is this: In many areas, the provision of emergency medical services is a team effort involving BLS and ALS providers, with each group performing specific responsibilities in patient care. Just as EMS providers must render all patient care within their respective scopes of practice, their documentation shouldn't exceed their scopes of practice.

Changing the Patient Care Report

A common misperception seems to prevail among some EMS professionals; that is, once a PCR is completed, it cannot, under any circumstances, be changed, altered, appended, or amended. As a general rule, this is untrue. Unless your specific state law prohibits it (and we are not aware of any that do), PCRs can be amended to correct erroneous information (e.g., name, address, and insurance information).

You can also add to a PCR after it is completed, using an *addendum* or second sheet, in the event you later recall important information that was omitted when you completed the initial record. Of course, changing a PCR is improper and illegal if it is done to falsify or misrepresent information for any reason, particularly for billing or reimbursement purposes. Your EMS agency, in conjunction with their legal counsel, should develop a policy regarding the completion and modification of PCRs.

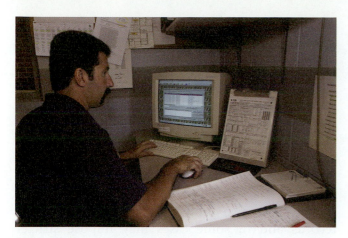

Fig. 3-2 Carefully follow procedure when changing or adding to a patient care report.

This policy should reaffirm the agency's commitment to honesty, accuracy, and ethics in documentation and should include other specific directions for field personnel. For example, the policy should address issues such as the following: (1) only the original author of the PCR should make modifications; (2) all entries made after the PCR is initially completed should be signed and dated; and (3) errors on written PCRs should be corrected by striking out the original information, writing the word "error," and entering the correct information. These same principles apply if you complete the PCR electronically (Fig. 3-2). Most electronic PCR completion software has built-in protections to prevent the original record from being changed without a proper notation. Some programs default to an addendum screen whenever an entry is added after the initial PCR has been completed.

Five Simple Ways to Improve Your Documentation Skills

Good documentation is important to you and your ambulance service for many reasons. Effective documentation can facilitate quality patient care, help protect you from liability, and favorably affect your EMS agency's reimbursement for the services you provide. Here are five quick and easy steps for improving your documentation skills.

1. **Paint a picture.** Think of your documentation as painting a picture of the incident. Instead of using a paintbrush or a camera, you are using words. Set the scene. For instance, at an accident scene: where are the cars? Are there broken glass and tire marks? Is there significant damage to the vehicles and was the passenger compartment compromised? What sights, sounds, and smells are registering on your senses? Documenting these elements can help the reader visualize a patient consistent with the patient about whom you are writing.

2. **Use chronologic narratives.** Avoid the tendency to jump around as things enter your mind. Stay focused; write your narrative so that it flows in chronologic order. Make sure that the steps of your dispatch, assessment, treatment, and transport are documented in a logical fashion. This can be especially problematic when too much time passes between the call and the time the documentation is done. Document when the call is as fresh in your mind as possible.

3. **Stick to the facts.** A well-written PCR is objective rather than subjective. This means that your charts should stick to the facts and should leave out personal interpretations and "spin." For instance, don't simply say that your patient was "intoxicated." Instead, document the facts that led you to that conclusion, such as "Patient's speech was slurred," "Odor of alcohol on patient's breath," "Patient admitted drinking eight beers in the past hour," and other such objective facts.

4. **Do not use "homegrown" abbreviations.** Many EMS providers love to use homegrown abbreviations. Reading their charts is like grading a test—and they're the only ones who have the answer key! Abbreviations are fine, but stick to ones that are common and accepted in the health care professions. Your service can even consider adopting a standard table of abbreviations to be used in your company's PCRs.

5. **Spelling counts.** This can be a tough one. Not everyone has top-notch spelling skills, but proper spelling and good grammar are important. Remember that a jury looks at the PCR you completed, and if it is full of errors, it may lead the jurors to conclude that you are as sloppy at patient care as you are at documentation. That affects your credibility as an EMS professional and could affect the jury's ultimate decision. Nobody's perfect in this department, and medical terms can be especially tricky to spell properly. So, pick up an EMT textbook or get a medical dictionary at the station and commit to learning a new word or two on each shift. This will boost your vocabulary, both in EMS and in life, and also improve your trip sheets.

■ CONFIDENTIALITY AND PRIVACY RIGHTS OF THE PATIENT: A NEW WAVE OF PROTECTION

Patient confidentiality in emergency medical services is important; however, it is violated frequently. Virtually everything a patient shares is confidential. However, consider the many ways this information is inadvertently released. An EMT may discuss an EMS run with colleagues. The colleagues can identify the patient from the address of the call. When the EMT arrives at the emergency department with a patient, invariably a nurse or physician asks across the room, "What do you have?" The EMT may then state the chief complaint back to the nurse or physician. Other patients and families often overhear this statement. Do these bystanders need to know that the patient has chest pain or a urethral discharge? What if a bystander knows the patient or the patient's employer? In these examples, medical information has been given away without patient consent.

The legal requirements for maintaining confidentiality are extensive, and the EMT should be familiar with them. Patients trust EMTs with their inner-most feelings and secrets. Beside the legal requirements, you have a solemn ethical obligation to maintain the integrity of your patients' information.

The federal privacy regulations mandated by the Health Insurance Portability and Accountability Act of 1996 (known as *HIPAA*) went into effect on April 14, 2003.[10] HIPAA is the first comprehensive federal law to protect the privacy of patient information. Its regulations are commonly called the Privacy Rule. These regulations require most health care providers, including ambulance services, to put into place safeguards to protect the use, distribution, and storage of the confidential health information of patients, commonly called *protected health information* (PHI).

The regulations have some cumbersome aspects. For example, organizations covered by the regulations must appoint a privacy officer, have privacy policies in place, develop a Notice of Privacy Practices to give to patients outlining their rights, obtain acknowledgement that patients received this notice, and train all members of their workforce in the organization's privacy practices. Compliance with HIPAA takes time and effort and requires ongoing work (e.g., training required by the Occupational Safety and Health Administration [OSHA] and fulfillment of other legal requirements).

HIPAA places greater restrictions on the release of health information. PHI is defined as any individually identifiable information about a patient's past, present, or future health care or payment for health care. Under the privacy regulations, EMS personnel are permitted to disclose as much information as necessary and to share that information with other health care providers involved in the patient's care without the patient's specific authorization. Other uses and disclosures of a patient's PHI without an authorization are permitted for billing and for certain quality assurance and health care operations purposes.

State laws also protect the privacy of medical records and in some cases may impose stricter rules than the federal regulations. PCRs must be kept strictly confidential. Every ambulance service must protect them to the fullest extent possible. Maintaining patient privacy is an essential legal obligation of the EMT. You should take all reasonable steps to safeguard patient information and to protect it from improper or inadvertent use or disclosure.

The Patient Care Report: A Legally Protected Medical Record

The PCR is considered a medical record, and as such the EMS agency that creates it is the owner of the record. As the owner, your service has a duty to safeguard the documents and protect their confidentiality. This means that you may not release the PCR or its contents without the written consent of the patient, a proper subpoena, or a court order. You also should not discuss the contents of the PCR or anything about the patients you treat and transport with individuals outside your organization. Detailed internal discussions about the specific patients you treat should be kept at a professional level, respecting the patient's dignity. Only those with a "need to know" in your organization should be given details about the patient care you provided in a particular case.

The following are the most common examples in which the PCR may be released to others:

- Insurers and third-party payors, for reimbursement purposes, when the patient has given permission to release the information
- Legally authorized research
- Litigation in which the document has been obtained through proper legal process, as during the discovery phase of a lawsuit
- Law enforcement and other investigative agencies pursuant to a subpoena

Whenever your service receives a request for a PCR or any other documents, you should follow these steps:

1. *Verify the request.* Make sure the request is coming from a legitimate source, such as the patient, or from the patient's official representative or attorney with the patient's approval. You should also verify the identity of the person making the request to ensure that this individual is who he says he is. Some private investigators have been known to misrepresent themselves just to get a copy of a PCR.
2. *Consult with counsel.* Before releasing any records, consult with the agency's legal counsel to make sure that proper procedures are in place for the various types of requests for documents.
3. *Get a written release.* Never release a PCR or any other document without a signed authorization from the patient unless it is pursuant to a court order. Also, make sure the individual signs a receipt acknowledging that she received what you provided to her, should there ever be any question as to whether you released the documents in a timely manner. The receipt also documents exactly what you gave the person, because it may appear as evidence at a trial down the road, and remembering exactly what was provided could prove difficult if you are relying simply on memory.

"Superprotection" for Specific Patient Situations

The importance of confidentiality and of protecting the integrity of a medical record, such as a PCR, cannot be overemphasized. Crews must be trained in the importance of not showing or releasing PCRs and other documentation to others. Legal claims for invasion of privacy frequently can arise when a health care organization does not treat medical records and reports with the highest degree of respect. The state and federal governments recently have increased the legal protection and privacy of medical information, and the ambulance industry is not exempt from many of these new requirements.

Some aspects of an individual's medical history have superprotection under the law. For example, a patient infected with the human immunodeficiency virus (HIV) or who has acquired immunodeficiency syndrome (AIDS) is protected from the release of information about the person's medical status in most states. These laws, often referred to as *Confidentiality of HIV/AIDS Information*, limit the extent to which

health care providers may share information with others about a patient's HIV status. These laws vary from state to state, to an extent. However, most states have adequate safeguards to ensure that ambulance service personnel are adequately informed in case they should come in contact with a patient with HIV or AIDS and exposure to the disease is likely. Beyond that, sharing with others the HIV or AIDS status of a patient you treat or transport generally is improper and may well be illegal.

Does this affect how you document when a person has HIV or AIDS? Absolutely not. The key is to document your observations in an objective way without drawing conclusions. Don't document on the PCR that you "think" the person has AIDS or HIV. However, document it if the patient tells you that he or she has the disease. For example, you can write, "Patient stated, 'I have HIV,' when asked about his past medical history."

As with HIV and AIDS, many states have laws that protect the release of information about an individual's mental health information or past record of drug or alcohol treatment. Many states' laws governing mental health procedures dictate how health care providers may treat this information. In fact, many laws exist to protect individuals from discriminatory treatment based on their particular medical status, such as a history of mental illness or drug or alcohol treatment. In many cases these laws do not specifically include ambulance personnel; however, the general rules of confidentiality should still apply, to minimize your risk of a lawsuit and the inappropriate handling of very sensitive information.

Incident Reporting

Your agency should have a policy on "unusual occurrence reporting." This policy should define what occurrences should be reported and the procedures for reporting them. Once the incident report is completed, it should be submitted to your immediate supervisor. In many cases it is unwise to attach the incident report to the PCR, because anything attached to that document may become part of the medical record and more easily discovered in litigation. Of course, your PCR should clearly indicate any known errors that occurred in patient care and the steps taken to remedy the errors. However, the details of how the errors occurred are best left for the separate incident report.

Appropriate management personnel and the system medical director should promptly investigate the incident. Depending on the situation, appropriate corrective action should be taken when a medication error has been made. Corrective action may include additional continuing education for the individual, as well as disciplinary action in some cases. Many state EMS laws also require that certain medication errors be reported to the EMS office, and a standard incident report format may be in place.

In many cases of medical errors, problems in the system may have contributed to the occurrence of the error. Every medication error should be reviewed from the quality assurance and risk management perspectives. This helps to ensure that system problems are identified and corrected. Otherwise, the risk of a future error may not be reduced, as another care provider in the system may be just as likely to make the same mistake. System-wide education may be required after the error has been closely reviewed. Obviously medication and other treatment errors are not a good thing to have happen because of the potential for harm to the patient and the risk of a lawsuit. When they do occur, these errors provide an opportunity to review the system critically and to make changes for the betterment of overall prehospital patient care.

■ TESTIFYING IN COURT

The moment you've dreaded your entire EMS career has arrived: you are being called as a witness in a lawsuit (Fig. 3-3). In most cases you will be called to testify in a case that does not directly involve the ambulance service. It likely will be a lawsuit between the patient (now also a plaintiff) and a defendant who caused harm to the patient, such as the person who drove recklessly and struck the patient's car. You often will be asked to describe the patient's condition when you found the person, the treatment you provided, and the patient's level of pain or distress.

In rare cases you will be a named defendant in a lawsuit alleging that you were negligent in providing patient care, or you will be a witness in a lawsuit against your EMS agency.

In both situations, preparation is the key to providing effective, professional testimony. In many cases your appearance, your demeanor, and the manner in which you answer questions will be the deciding factors when a juror makes a determination as to your credibility. Here are a few basic do's and don'ts to remember when testifying in court. These pointers also hold true for giving a deposition, an out-of-court discovery tool taken under oath.

- *Tell the truth!* The foundation of this legal system is that once you are placed under oath, you are

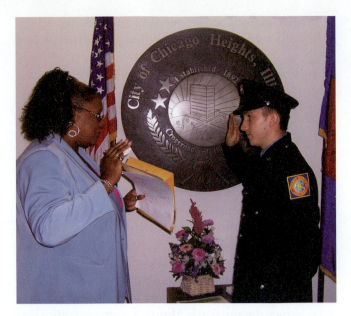

Fig. 3-3 An EMT may be called upon to testify in court.

obligated to tell the truth. Failure to do so could result in the criminal penalty of perjury.

- *Be yourself and use plain language.* Don't try to impress the jury by acting like someone you're not, and don't use medical terminology if you can avoid it.

- *Avoid EMS jargon or slang.* EMS providers use a lot of "terms of art" that have unique meaning to the work. For example, "responding Code 3" or responding to a "Delta call" probably are completely foreign phrases to a jury.

- *Remember to testify, and don't try to persuade the jury.* Your role as a witness is to respond to the questions you are asked and to help get the facts out in the open. You should never appear to be advocating a particular view when you testify.

- *Speak clearly and with proper volume.* Use good diction, and don't mumble. Don't cover your mouth or rest your chin on your hand while you are speaking. Don't talk too fast. The court reporter and the jury need to hear every word.

- *Think before you answer.* Make sure you hear and understand the question. Ask that it be repeated if you don't. Think about your answer before you start to respond to the question. It's all right to say, "I do not know," or "I do not remember," if necessary. Do not hesitate to ask for clarification if you are uncertain about a question.

- *Avoid appearing arrogant or like a "know it all."* Juries are quick to pick up on arrogance and other signs that may indicate you did not really care about the patient as a human being.

- *Don't start to answer a question until the attorney has finished asking it.* This is to ensure that you have the complete question and that you have a chance to think about the answer. Questions in court are usually well thought out, and it is critical that the question be answered as accurately and fully as possible.

- *If your testimony is interrupted for any reason, stop talking.* Often there will be objections to the type or form of the question being asked. As soon as you hear an objection, stop answering and wait for an order from the judge to continue.
- *Don't read from the PCR unless you are specifically asked to do so.* Reading a report makes it seem as if you don't have a good grasp of the facts of the situation. However, at times you may be asked to read a portion of the report so that the jury can hear exactly what was written. Make sure to read it slowly and clearly.
- *Do not be intimidated by the attorneys.* They are simply representing their clients and at times may try to rattle you on the witness stand. This sometimes helps ensure that witnesses give truthful answers.
- *Be objective.* Testify only to what you saw, heard, smelled, tasted, or felt unless you are an expert witness qualified by the court to give your opinion.

■ THE ROLE OF INSURANCE IN EMS

Your EMS agency must have several types of insurance in order to operate. Vehicle insurance provides coverage for damage and injury from a motor vehicle accident. General liability provides coverage for most other potential lawsuits, including whenever the agency is sued because of the acts of its EMS personnel. Directors' and officers' insurance provides protection for the decisions made by key individuals in charge of overseeing the organization.

Anytime a potential claim arises that is likely to end up in litigation, the EMS agency is obliged to report the incident to the insurance company. Most policies require prompt notification whenever a formal complaint is filed against the agency, as well as in cases in which one is likely to be filed. The classic example is dropping a patient. A litter drop case will very likely end up in litigation. Therefore it would be best to report this to the insurance company as soon as possible, before a formal complaint is filed in court.

Insurance companies also have a duty to defend the EMS agency if a claim is made under the policy. The insurance company typically assigns a claims agent to review the case and to make a determination as to coverage. Often an insurance company settles a case for a much lower amount than might be awarded in a trial to avoid the expense of a trial and the potentially high jury award. Settlement agreements usually end up with a "no admission" of liability by the ambulance service.

Do individual EMTs get sued very often? EMTs usually are named in a lawsuit as an agent of the EMS agency. The liability of the organization may flow through the actions of the field provider. This is called *vicarious liability*, which means that the EMS agency can be liable if the patient can show that the EMT was negligent. If no negligence is proved against the EMT, the organization cannot be liable.

On the other hand, more EMS agencies are being sued under what is called the *corporate negligence theory*. According to this theory, the organization itself can be liable for not having the proper personnel, equipment, and policies and procedures in place to provide EMS effectively. Liability of the agency can be proved if the harm to the patient can be attributed to inadequate personnel, equipment, and policies and procedures. Finding affordable insurance is becoming increasingly difficult for EMS agencies. This is why implementation of a risk management program is so important. EMS agencies that minimize the risk of a lawsuit are agencies that insurance companies are most likely to want as a policyholder. Insurance companies look at factors such as the claims history, amount of awards paid out, and other issues in determining whether they will provide coverage for the agency and at what cost.

Some EMTs opt to carry personal liability insurance. This type of insurance provides protection if the EMT is sued individually. However, EMTs are not considered the "deep pockets," therefore there are very few court cases in which an individual EMT has had to pay out any monetary awards as a result of a lawsuit. Personal liability insurance is relatively inexpensive, and some choose to have it for this reason. However, some experts believe it is unwise to carry this insurance, because the fact that you have the coverage may be a factor in naming you in a suit.

■ THE FUTURE OF EMS LAW AND LITIGATION

Increasingly, the public considers EMS a medical profession and compares EMTs to other health professionals. The concept of EMS continues to evolve in the public's eye. The notion that an ambulance service is simply transportation is rapidly being replaced by the concept of EMS as sophisticated health care that is part of a total health care system. As EMS evolves, no doubt regulatory requirements (new laws) will increase to control it, and more lawsuits will be filed against EMS agencies.

Your best bet to avoid litigation as much as possible is to adopt a professional approach in all aspects of your work as an EMT. Two key elements in a successful strategy of risk management are a commitment to preventing mistakes and positive changes to reduce the potential for litigation.

Risk reduction is the key to avoiding liability in all aspects of prehospital care. The two primary goals always should be to eliminate or reduce the risk of harm to the patient and to eliminate or reduce the risk of a successful lawsuit against your EMS organization. Improving overall patient safety generally is the best way to reduce errors.

In 2001 the EMS Division of the National Highway Traffic Safety Administration (NHTSA) sponsored a roundtable discussion of EMS patient safety and error reduction strategies. The participants discussed the types of error reduction activities occurring in other sectors of medicine. They also considered how errors can be reduced and what patient safety activities should be pursued. The participants recognized that EMS providers need greater insight into the human factors that affect patient safety and a better system for reporting errors.[11] Accepting personal responsibility for recognizing the human factors that may affect your own ability to function error free is the key to a professional approach to avoiding mistakes, reducing the risk of harm to your patients, and minimizing the risk of liability for your EMS agency.

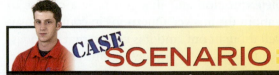

CASE SCENARIO

conclusion

Ray pats Mr. Walsh's hand as they ride to the hospital. "I'm glad you spoke with your private doctor, John. Sounds like he was really concerned." Mr. Walsh replies, "Yeah, he said he couldn't be sure if it was something related to my heart and that he would be more comfortable if I got seen sooner than later." Ray nods. "It's the right thing to do." ■

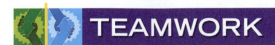

TEAMWORK

As discussed in this chapter, EMTs must understand their responsibilities, both legal and ethical, as they apply to the patient. As members of the health care community working side by side with firefighters, police officers, nurses, and physicians, you are on the front lines, representing your agency. Your actions or lack thereof will affect the entire system, your patient, and you!

References

1. Kohn LT, Corrigan JM, Donaldson MS, editors: *To err is human: building a safer health system.* A report of the Committee on Quality of Health Care in America, National Academy of Sciences, Institute of Medicine, Washington, DC, 2000, National Academy Press.
2. *Hoffman v Brandywine Hospital,* 661 A 2d 397 (Pa Super), 1995.
3. 35 Pa Stat § 6931(j).
4. *Albright v Abington Memorial Hospital,* 696 A 2d 1159 (Pa), 1997.
5. EMS House of DeFrance. Medical mistakes increase threefold after 12-hour days. Available at: www.defrance.org/artman/publish/article_932.shtml.
6. US Congress: Patient Self-Determination Act. Omnibus Budget Reconciliation Act (OBRA), Public Law 101-508, 1990.
7. *Cruzan v Director, Missouri Dept of Health,* 497 US 261, 1990.
8. Page J, Wolfberg D, Wirth S: A³E³P³, Page, Wolfberg & Wirth, LLC. Mechanicsburg, PA. www.pwwemslaw.com/ACTIVE/Tips/TipsArchives/03.16.03.htm
9. Bruce M, Sones S, Peck P: Medication safety: implications for EMS, *EMS Magazine,* 97-106, 2003.
10. Health Insurance Portability and Accountability Act of 1996. Public Law 104-191. Available at: www.access.gpo.gov/nara/cfr/index.html.
11. National Highway Traffic Safety Administration: *Patient safety in emergency medical services: roundtable report and recommendations,* Washington, DC, 2002, NHTSA.

Resources

Chapleau W: *Emergency first responder: making the difference,* St Louis, 2004, Mosby.
Heilicser BH: Ethics. In Zimmermann PG: *Nursing management secrets,* Philadelphia, 2002, Hanley & Belfus.
Iserson KV, Sanders AB, Mathieu D: *Ethics in emergency medicine,* ed 2, Tucson, 1995, Galen Press.

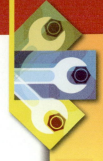

Critical Points

- EMTs must understand the difference between scope of practice and standard of care and how these relate to patient care. This is the basic information that will keep you out of trouble.
- Medical direction gives you the right and privilege to function as an EMT.
- EMTs must know their ethical responsibilities to their patient and to the patient's friends and family.
- EMTs must be knowledgeable about the different types of consent and how to apply them in various situations.

Learning Checklist

- ❏ The primary ethical responsibility of the EMT is to provide appropriate medical care with compassion and understanding.
- ❏ Your responsibilities may be initiated while on call or as a good Samaritan. Regardless, you should be aware of federal, state, and local laws and policies that define the standard of care and scope of your practice.
- ❏ Often your conscience will guide you.
- ❏ Certain principles are helpful in defining and then resolving an ethical dilemma. Autonomy requires you to honor a patient's rights. Always consider what is in the patient's best interest. "First, do no harm." You should be fair and objective in your patient care.
- ❏ It is very helpful to think about a previous or future dilemma and evaluate in your own mind the best way to resolve it.
- ❏ Quality of life is determined by the person whose life it is. Do not allow your own emotions or fears to interfere with your responsibilities.
- ❏ Decision-making capacity is a medical determination that is made on a case-by-case basis.
- ❏ Competency is a judicial determination and is not made at the time of patient care.
- ❏ Acceptance or refusal of medical treatment is based on decision-making capacity unless the patient has already been declared incompetent.

- ❏ Refusal of care requires the patient to understand fully what you want to do, the risks involved, and what could happen if you don't do it. The patient also must be free to decide whether he or she wants to refuse care. Such conversations should be clearly documented. Your convenience should never be a factor.
- ❏ The patient with decision-making capacity, a durable power of attorney for health care, or a legal guardian may sign refusals. If in doubt, "err on the side of life."
- ❏ An *advance directive* is a document that allows individuals to state in advance what they would or would not want done if their condition did not allow them to make such decisions. A patient must lack decision-making capacity for an advance directive to take effect.
- ❏ A living will usually requires that the patient have no hope for a meaningful recovery. It is somewhat restrictive. Usually it is not relevant in the prehospital emergency setting.
- ❏ A durable power of attorney for health care (agent) is a person appointed in advance by the patient to make all medical decisions on the patient's behalf. This agent is speaking "as the patient."
- ❏ Most states have a health care surrogate law that takes effect if no formal advance directive exists. The specific order of who is the decision maker is defined.
- ❏ Cardiopulmonary resuscitation is presumed to be performed on a patient unless it is specifically declined (DNR). A DNR patient may still receive aggressive treatment relative to the underlying condition up until the time of cardiopulmonary arrest. Comfort care is always indicated.
- ❏ Patient confidentiality should be honored. Always be vigilant in avoiding inadvertent comments that violate confidentiality. This confidentiality has been entrusted to you.
- ❏ Honest documentation is essential. *If you don't write it, you didn't do it.*
- ❏ All patients should be treated equally. However, the EMT should be aware of the need for donated organs as it applies to apparently futile situations.
- ❏ Your calling is to be an ethical human being. When confronted with an unethical situa-

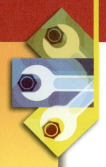

NUTS AND BOLTS

tion, you have an obligation to react with decency and conscience. Political and religious beliefs should be clarified in advance; patient care is not the time for debate or action. A mechanism for reporting an unethical situation should be in place, confidential, and supported.

Key Terms

Advance directive A legal document that allows individuals to provide directions regarding their health care in the event they cannot communicate. The usual examples are a living will or a durable power of attorney for health care.

Assault To create the fear of injury.

Autonomy Self-rule; patients have the right to determine for themselves what medical treatment they do or do not want.

Battery Touching a person without permission.

Coercion Forcing or pressuring a patient to make a decision that may not be of the individual's own choice.

Competency A judicial determination as to an individual's ability to care and make decisions for himself or herself. A guardian is appointed if the person is ruled incompetent.

Decision-making capacity A medical determination as to a patient's ability to understand and to accept or refuse treatment.

Do not resuscitate (DNR) A physician's order indicating that cardiopulmonary resuscitation is not to be performed in the event of cardiopulmonary arrest. It may not apply to medical treatment up until this event.

Durable power of attorney for health care A legal, signed document in which a person designates who will be empowered to make medical decisions on the individual's behalf if he or she cannot.

Good Samaritan A person who offers help when not specifically on call or obligated to do so.

Informed refusal The process of informing a patient of risks versus benefits in refusing medical treatment. The patient should clearly understand the risks and benefits, and the process should be well documented.

Living will A legal document prepared by a patient that gives direction to the person's physicians regarding end-of-life care. Usually not relevant to the prehospital setting.

Quality of life An individual belief as to what constitutes a meaningful existence.

Ration To specifically or arbitrarily determine which patients will receive the treatment or resources available.

Standing orders A document that describes the patient care to be performed when medical control is not contacted or is unavailable.

Surrogate An individual placed in the position of making decisions for another person; an advocate or alternate.

National Standard Curriculum Objectives

Cognitive Objectives

After completing this lesson, the EMT student will be able to do the following:

- Define the EMT scope of practice.
- Discuss the importance of DNR orders, advance directives, and local or state provisions governing their EMS application.
- Define consent and discuss the methods of obtaining consent.
- Differentiate between expressed and implied consent.
- Explain the role of consent of minors in providing care.
- Discuss the implications for the EMT of patient refusal of transport.
- Discuss the issues of abandonment, negligence, and battery and their implications for the EMT.
- State the conditions necessary for the EMT to have a duty to act.
- Explain the importance, necessity, and legality of patient confidentiality.
- Discuss the considerations of the EMT in organ retrieval.
- Explain the actions an EMT should take to assist in the preservation of a crime scene.
- State the conditions designated for mandated reporting by an EMT to local law enforcement officials.

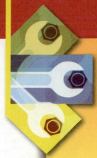

Affective Objectives

After completing this lesson, the EMT student will be able to do the following:

■ Explain the role of EMS and the EMT regarding patients with DNR orders.

■ Explain the need for and the benefits and use of advance directives.

■ Explain the rationale for having varying degrees of DNR.

Psychomotor Objectives

No objectives identified.

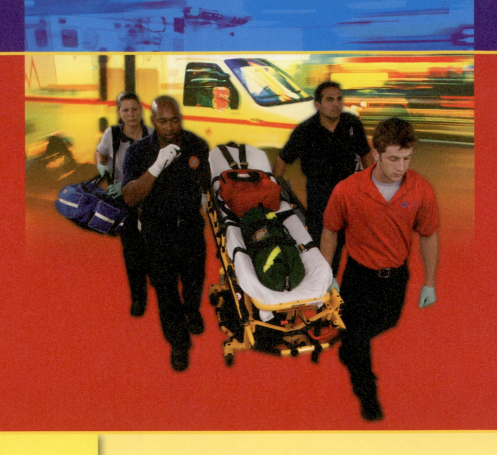

CHAPTER

4

CHAPTER OUTLINE

Body Directional Terms

Regions of the Body

Body Systems

LESSON GOAL

This chapter builds on the emergency medical technician's (EMT's) knowledge of the human body. It provides a brief overview of body systems, anatomy, physiology, and topographic anatomy. ■

OUTLINE

GOAL

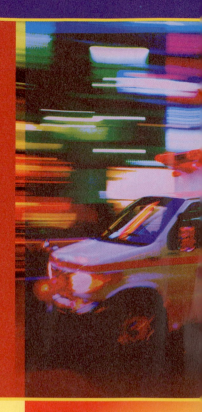

The Human Body

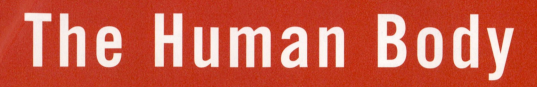

CHAPTER OBJECTIVES

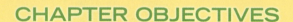

After completing this chapter, the EMT student will be able to do the following:

1 Explain the following directional terms:

- Medial
- Lateral
- Proximal
- Distal
- Superior
- Inferior
- Anterior
- Posterior
- Midline
- Right
- Left
- Midclavicular
- Bilateral
- Midaxillary

2 Describe the anatomy and function of the following major body systems: respiratory system, circulatory system, musculoskeletal system, nervous system, and endocrine system.

4

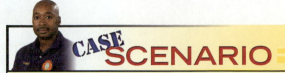

Jack is working with his classmates, trying to complete an in-class assignment from the instructor. Spread before them on the table are pieces of paper. On each piece of paper is written a word from the following list: right ventricle, left atrium, aorta, pulmonary vein, left ventricle, cardiac valve, vena cava, right atrium, pulmonary artery.

The assignment for Jack and his classmates is to arrange the pieces of paper in an order that would make sense of the cardiac system.

Question: *How should the papers be arranged so that they form a "picture" of the heart?*

E MTs are better able to identify life-threatening problems and communicate with other health care professionals if they have a thorough understanding of the basics of anatomy and physiology and are familiar with medical terminology. **Anatomy** is the structure and position of the body, and **physiology** is the function of the body. The use of a common medical language is essential for describing a patient's condition. With a common language, all members of the health care team can understand the location and extent of a patient's injuries. Knowledge of the human body is the cornerstone of the many skills you need to become an excellent EMT.

■ BODY DIRECTIONAL TERMS

Medical professionals always refer to the body in the **normal anatomical position.** In this position, the human body (the patient) is standing upright, facing you, with the arms at the sides and the palms turned forward. An imaginary vertical line drawn down the middle of the body is called the **midline.** All references to *right* and *left* refer to the *patient's* right or left. All of the following directional terms are based on the normal anatomical position of the patient (Fig. 4-1).

Anterior is toward the front of the body, and **posterior** is toward the back of the body. For example, during cardiopulmonary resuscitation (CPR), you perform compressions on the breastbone, in the anterior (front) chest. With each press downward, the heart is squeezed against the backbone, which is in the posterior (back) chest. When the body is in the normal anatomical position, you see the anterior (front) side.

Lateral means away from the patient's midline, and **medial** means toward the patient's midline. If you assess a runner who complains of pain on the outside

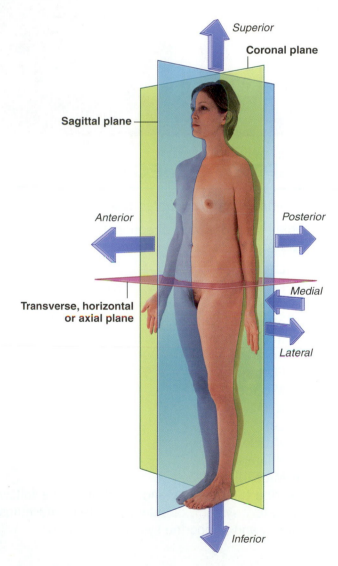

Fig. 4-1 The normal anatomical position, planes, and terms of location and orientation.

of the knee, you report this as pain to the *lateral knee.* If your patient has a cut on the inside of the knee, you report the injury as a laceration to the *medial knee.*

Superior is toward the patient's head, or top, and **inferior** is toward the patient's feet, or below. For example, the eyes are superior (above) to the mouth, and the chin is inferior (below) to the mouth. To describe injuries to the extremities, the term **proximal** is used to indicate injuries toward the trunk of the body, and the term **distal** is used to indicate injuries away from the trunk. For example, the elbow is at the distal end of the upper arm, whereas the shoulder is at the proximal end of the upper arm. As an EMT, you should always try to use directional terms to explain your assessment. For example, if you are assessing a child who fell from a swing, you may describe an injury such as "a deformity to the distal left forearm." This description is an accurate assessment and helps other health care providers prepare to receive the patient and select the appropriate equipment for treatment.

Specific terms also can be used to describe a patient's body position. **Supine** describes the position of a patient lying on the back, face up. This term would be used to describe a patient secured to a long backboard. **Prone** describes the position of a patient lying on the stomach. **Trendelenburg position** describes a patient lying in the supine position with the head lower than the feet. **Semi-Fowler position** describes a patient who is sitting in a semireclined position with or without the knees bent. This position traditionally is used to describe the way a conscious patient sitting on a cot is transported.

TABLE 4-1

Body directional and positional terms

Term	Meaning
Anterior	Toward the patient's front
Cephalic	Toward the patient's head
Distal	Away from the patient's trunk
Inferior	Toward the patient's feet/below
Lateral	Away from the patient's midline
Medial	Toward the patient's midline
Posterior	Toward the patient's back
Prone	Patient lying on the stomach
Proximal	Toward the patient's trunk
Semi-Fowler position	Semisitting position
Superior	Toward the patient's head/above/top
Supine	Patient lying on the back, face up
Trendelenburg position	Patient supine on an incline with the head lower than the feet

As an EMT, you may not be dealing with emergencies on a regular basis. Therefore you may not get the chance to practice regularly with medical and directional terms. If you are unsure which term to use, it is better to use common terms (e.g., *back* or *front*) to avoid confusion and inaccuracies. Table 4-1 presents a list of directional and positional terms.

■ REGIONS OF THE BODY

The body is also described in terms of regions. The three regions of the body are the *head* and *neck*, the *trunk*, and the *upper* and *lower extremities* (Fig. 4-2). The head is composed of the cranium, which houses the brain, and the face. The head is supported by the neck, which also connects the head to the trunk (also called the *torso*).

The trunk has three parts: the **thorax** (or chest), which contains the heart, lungs, and great vessels (which originate from the heart); the **abdomen;** and the **pelvis.**

The extremities (upper and lower) are attached to the trunk at the shoulders and hips. The upper extremity begins at the shoulder. It includes the arm, elbow, forearm, wrist, and hand. The hip, thigh, knee, leg, ankle, and foot make up the lower extremity.

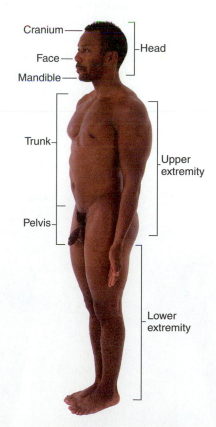

Fig. 4-2 The regions of the body.

This knowledge of basic anatomical terms, body directions, and body regions is the starting point for understanding how the body works and for communicating assessment findings with other health care workers. For instance, once you know how to locate the radial pulse in the distal forearm (wrist area), you can count the heart rate in beats per minute. By monitoring changes in the pulse quality and rate, you can determine whether the body is functioning normally. This information is critical to the health care team. Your understanding of the basic anatomy and physiology of the major body systems, which are covered in the following sections of this chapter, will help you provide a detailed assessment to other health care providers.

The Abdominal Quadrants

The abdomen is divided into four equal parts, known as *quadrants*, for reference purposes (Fig. 4-3). The quadrants are determined by drawing one imaginary horizontal line (side to side) across the abdomen through the umbilicus (belly button) and another imaginary line vertically (up and down) through the umbilicus. These regions are described as the *left upper quadrant (LUQ)*, *right upper quadrant (RUQ)*, *left lower quadrant (LLQ)*, and *right lower quadrant (RLQ)*. As an EMT, you should have a basic knowledge of the location of organs in the abdominal quadrants (Fig. 4-4). The RUQ holds the gallbladder and the major portion of the liver. The LUQ holds a smaller portion of the liver, the stomach, and the spleen. The RLQ holds the appendix. The small and large intestines wind through all four quadrants. Pelvic organs, such

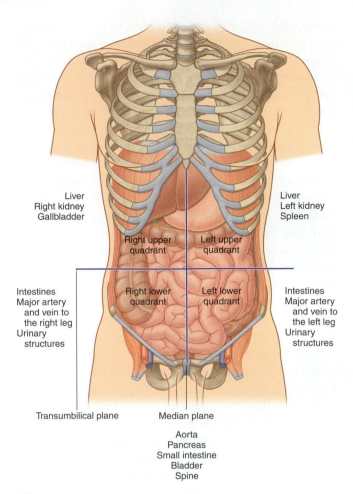

Fig. 4-4 The location of organs in the abdominal quadrants.

as the bladder and female reproductive organs, are also found in both of the lower quadrants (RLQ and LLQ). The kidneys are located behind the abdominal cavity, referred to as the *retroperitoneal area*. They are often described as being in the RUQ and LUQ as well as the right flank and left flank.

■ BODY SYSTEMS

It is important to know that the body is divided into separate yet interrelated systems. These are the respiratory, cardiovascular, nervous, musculoskeletal, integumentary, gastrointestinal, urinary, reproductive, endocrine, and lymphatic systems.

The Respiratory System

Our body tissues require a constant supply of oxygen to produce energy and to operate efficiently. Every function of the body, from muscle contraction to the

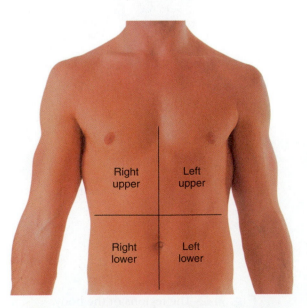

Fig. 4-3 The quadrants of the abdomen.

The Young and Not So Young

Pediatric and geriatric anatomy and physiology are sometimes different than that discussed here. Some differences are subtle, and some are significant. Anatomy and physiology changes as the newborn becomes an infant, then a child, and finally an adult. It begins to change again as adults become elderly and their body parts and systems begin to deteriorate. As an EMT, it is important that you understand these differences (which are discussed in later chapters of this textbook), because they will affect your assessments and interventions.

digestion of food, requires oxygen. During this process of *metabolism* (producing energy), body tissues give off waste products that need to be released. The respiratory system both delivers oxygen (O_2) to the blood and removes some waste products, primarily carbon dioxide (CO_2). A functional respiratory system is essential to survival. Irreversible damage to the brain and other organs can occur as early as 4 minutes without oxygen. Other body functions may deteriorate if CO_2 levels rise above normal. For these reasons, emergency care starts with assessment and management of the respiratory system. (Assessment and management of airway and breathing are discussed in more detail in Chapter 7.)

All the structures involved in the delivery of O_2 to the blood are components of the respiratory system (Fig. 4-5). Room air, which contains approximately 21% oxygen, enters the airway through the mouth and nose. Air (oxygen) entering the mouth passes through the oropharynx. Air that enters through the nose passes through the cavity above the roof of the mouth, called the *nasopharynx*. The cavities of the oropharynx and nasopharynx sometimes are referred to together as the *pharynx*. The epiglottis is located on top of the trachea in the posterior pharynx. This leaf-shaped flap prevents food and liquid from entering the lungs during swallowing. When the epiglottis opens, air enters the trachea (windpipe), which contains the larynx (voice box). You speak by passing air over the vocal cords in your voice box. Below the larynx, the trachea divides into two bronchi in the lungs. Each bronchus continues to divide into smaller and smaller branches. The air reaches the bronchioles, which finally connect to the alveoli (air sacs). Each alveolus is covered in a net of small blood vessels called *pulmonary capillaries*. When air enters the alveoli, molecules of oxygen freely cross through a thin membrane into the blood. CO_2 moves from the blood back into the alveoli, to be exhaled from the respiratory system through the lungs and out the mouth and nose.

The mechanical process of moving air into and out of the airways is called **ventilation.** Ventilation is accomplished through the movement of a dome-shaped muscle, the **diaphragm,** and other muscles in the chest wall. As the diaphragm contracts, it moves downward, expanding (enlarging) the lung and causing air to enter the lung (inspiration). The chest muscles assist by contracting to expand the thorax. When the diaphragm relaxes, the lung decreases in size and the air is pushed out (expiration).

The Cardiovascular System

The cardiovascular system consists of the heart (a pump), blood (fluid), and blood vessels (a container). The heart pushes blood through the blood vessels, transporting blood and nutrients to every re-

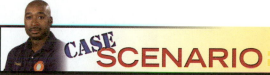

CASE SCENARIO
continued

After class Jack has a shift on the ambulance service. Their first call of the evening is for a female experiencing shortness of breath. Upon arrival at the patient's home Jack finds the patient sitting upright in a chair located in the living room.

Jack thinks that the patient, Marilyn Shorum, looks awfully pale. In fact, her skin appears to have almost a bluish tint. Mrs. Shorum is a 45-year-old female who had a sudden onset of shortness of breath that began almost without warning. She had had a short episode of sharp pain centered in the right side of her chest just before the respiratory distress began. Mrs. Shorum tried to ignore the problem, thinking it would go away on its own, but instead the discomfort worsened, and she feels as if she is going to pass out.

Question: What could be going on in the structures of the heart that could be causing Mrs. Shorum's condition?

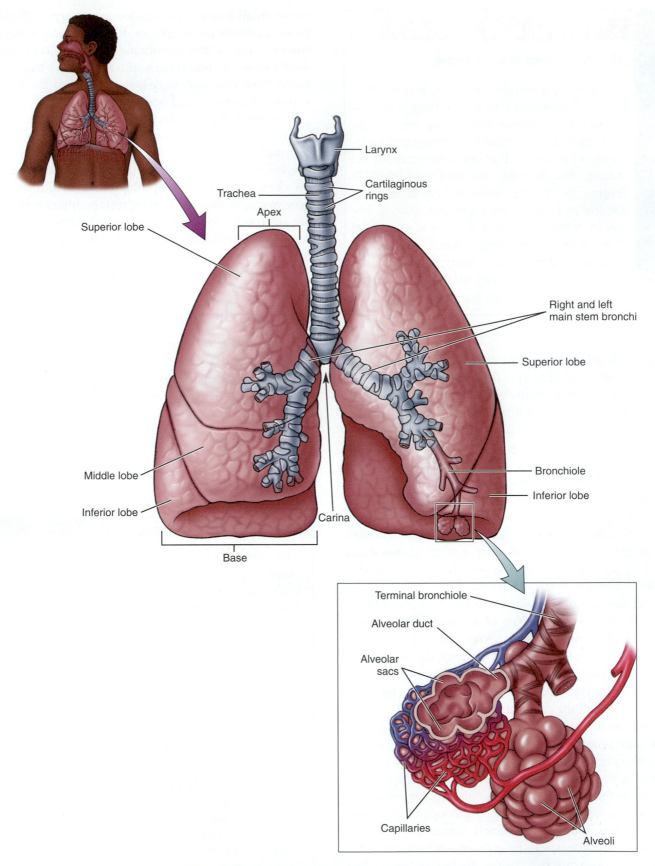

Larynx

Trachea

Cartilaginous rings

Apex

Superior lobe

Right and left main stem bronchi

Superior lobe

Middle lobe

Bronchiole

Inferior lobe

Inferior lobe

Carina

Base

Terminal bronchiole

Alveolar duct

Alveolar sacs

Capillaries

Alveoli

Fig. 4-5 The anatomy of the respiratory system.

gion of the body. In essence, the circulatory system is a transportation pipeline.

The Heart

The heart muscle is made up of four individual chambers (Fig. 4-6). One-way valves located between the four chambers allow blood to flow in one direction through the heart. The two top chambers are called the *left atrium* and the *right atrium;* the left and right atria receive blood from the rest of the body and direct it into the two lower chambers of the heart. The right atrium receives unoxygenated blood (blood that is low in O_2 and high in waste) from the veins (venae cavae). The left atrium receives oxygenated blood (blood that is high in O_2 and low in waste) from the lungs via the pulmonary veins. The lower chambers of the heart are called *ventricles.* The ventricles are bigger than the atria and have a larger muscle mass because they are responsible for pumping the blood throughout the body. The right ventricle has a smaller muscle mass and pumps unoxygenated blood to the lungs. The left ventricle has the largest muscle mass in the heart and pumps oxygenated blood to the rest of the body (excluding the lungs) through the arterial system. Each time the left ventricle contracts, it sends a pulse wave of blood into the arteries. You can palpate these pulse waves wherever an artery passes near the skin's surface over a bone. You will often use the carotid, femoral, radial, and brachial artery pulses to determine a patient's heart rate.

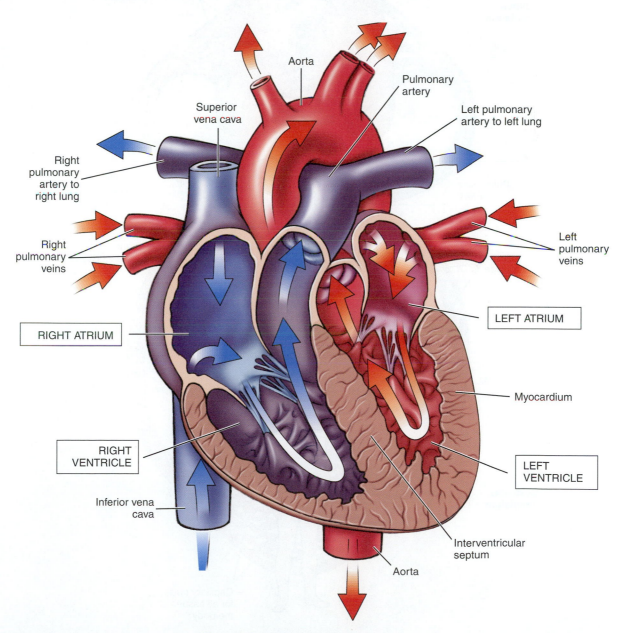

Fig. 4-6 The anatomy of the heart.

The heart has also been described as two independent pumps that work together to pump blood through the circulatory system (Fig. 4-7). The right side of the heart receives deoxygenated blood from the venae cavae. It pumps the waste-laden blood to the lungs, where CO_2 is removed and O_2 is added, as previously described. Highly oxygenated blood then returns to the left side of the heart, where it is pumped into the aorta to begin its cycle through the body again.

The Blood Vessels

Blood carries oxygen and other nutrients (e.g., glucose) to the cells and CO_2 and other wastes away from the cells. Blood is pumped through a closed system made up of a highly organized network of blood vessels. These blood vessels include arteries, arterioles, capillaries, venules, and veins.

Oxygenated blood leaves the left side of the heart and enters a system of large vessels called **arteries** (Fig. 4-8), which carry the blood away from the heart.

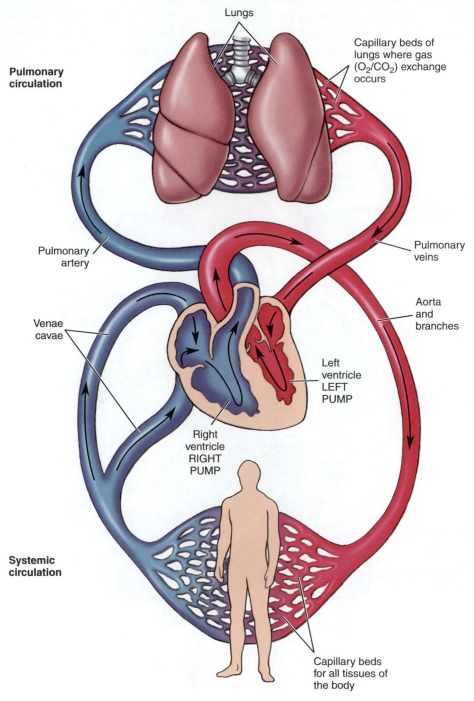

Lungs

Pulmonary circulation

Capillary beds of lungs where gas (O_2/CO_2) exchange occurs

Pulmonary artery

Pulmonary veins

Venae cavae

Aorta and branches

Left ventricle LEFT PUMP

Right ventricle RIGHT PUMP

Systemic circulation

Capillary beds for all tissues of the body

Fig. 4-7 The heart can be described as two independent pumps.

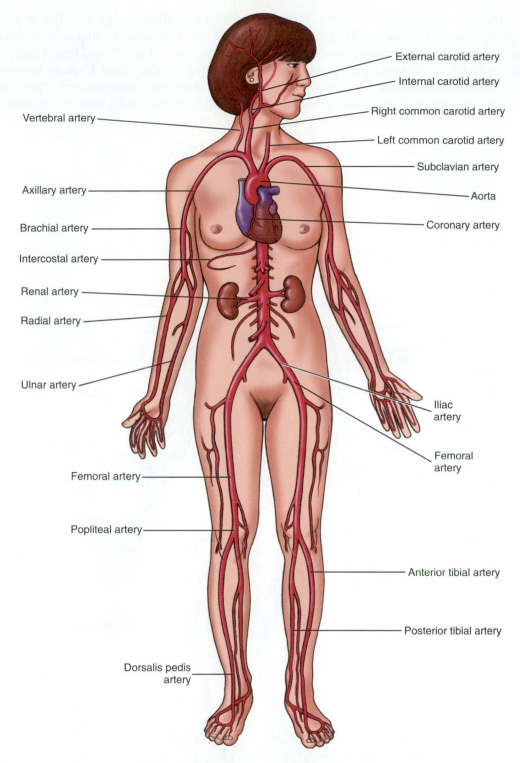

External carotid artery

Internal carotid artery

Right common carotid artery

Left common carotid artery

Subclavian artery

Aorta

Coronary artery

Vertebral artery

Axillary artery

Brachial artery

Intercostal artery

Renal artery

Radial artery

Ulnar artery

Iliac artery

Femoral artery

Femoral artery

Popliteal artery

Anterior tibial artery

Posterior tibial artery

Dorsalis pedis artery

Fig. 4-8 The major arteries of the body.

The aorta leaves the left ventricle of the heart, extending upward, and then arches downward (aortic arch) toward the chest, abdomen, and lower extremities. Several major arteries branch from the aorta to supply blood to the heart muscle (coronary arteries), the head (carotid arteries), the upper extremities, and the internal organs. The pulse of the carotid arteries is felt in the neck to the left and the right of the larynx. This pulse usually is stronger than that in other arteries because it is closer to the heart. Major arteries to the upper extremities also branch off the aorta to the brachial artery down each arm. To determine whether a pulse is present in an infant, you should check the brachial artery on the inside of the arm just above the elbow. This is a better site than the carotid artery in these patients because finding the carotid ar-tery in an infant is difficult. The brachial artery divides into two smaller arteries that deliver blood to the forearm and hand. You frequently palpate the radial artery in the distal forearm to count the pulse rate in conscious adult patients. This artery is located on the lateral (thumb) side of the wrist.

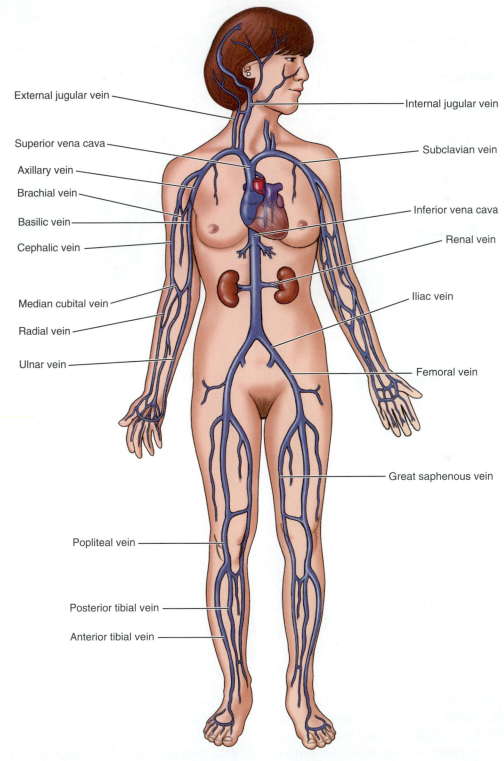

External jugular vein

Superior vena cava

Axillary vein

Brachial vein

Basilic vein

Cephalic vein

Median cubital vein

Radial vein

Ulnar vein

Popliteal vein

Posterior tibial vein

Anterior tibial vein

Internal jugular vein

Subclavian vein

Inferior vena cava

Renal vein

Iliac vein

Femoral vein

Great saphenous vein

Fig. 4-9 The major veins of the body.

The aorta continues downward through the chest and into the lower abdomen. There, it splits into two large arteries that pass through the pelvis to the lower extremities. Each femoral artery is the major artery for the thigh. The femoral artery can be palpated in the groin area near the crease between the abdomen and thigh. The femoral artery then divides into the smaller arteries of the leg and foot.

As blood is pumped through the arterial system, the vessels become smaller and are called *arterioles* (which still carry oxygenated blood). The arterioles connect to tiny capillaries, which are found in all tissues of the body. Capillaries supply the cells of the body with oxygen and nourishment. The capillaries also carry away CO_2 and other waste products from the cells of the body.

As blood leaves tissue capillaries, it enters small vessels called *venules*. Venules empty into **veins** (Fig. 4-9), which carry unoxygenated blood toward the heart. These small vessels join others to form larger veins as they carry away blood with waste. The largest vein in the body, the vena cava, empties directly into the right side of the heart.

The Nervous System

The nervous system controls the body's voluntary activities (movement that involves thought) and involuntary activities (movement that does not involve thought). It also provides for higher mental functions such as thought, emotion, and memory. The two main components of the nervous system are the central nervous system (CNS) and the peripheral nervous system (PNS) (Fig. 4-10).

The CNS is composed of the brain and spinal cord. The brain is the master control center of the body. It controls everything from muscle movements to emotional response. As you study this chapter, your brain is at work thinking and problem solving. In addition, your brain controls your finger muscles, which turn the pages (voluntarily) as you read. The brain also controls basic life functions, such as breathing and maintaining body temperature (involuntarily).

The spinal cord, a continuation of the brain, extends downward from the brain through the center of the spinal column. The spinal cord is like a high-speed information highway. It carries messages between the brain and the rest of the body. Proper functioning of the CNS is vital for the well-being and survival of the whole body.

The PNS is the system of nerves that carry messages between the body and the CNS. Two types of

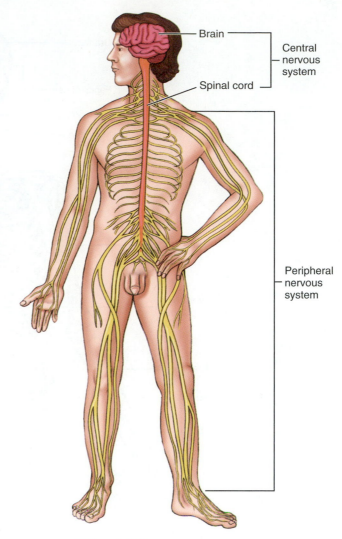

Fig. 4-10 The nervous system.

nerves make up the PNS: motor nerves, which carry information from the brain to the muscles of the body, and sensory nerves, which carry information from the body back to the brain. For example, when you decide to take a patient's pulse, your brain sends a "take the radial pulse" message down your spinal cord and motor nerves to your fingers to feel for the patient's pulse. The nerves in your fingers feel the patient's pulse waves. Your sensory nerves then collect the information about the pulse and deliver that information to your spinal cord and finally back to your brain. Your brain receives this message and then calculates the number of beats per minute.

The Musculoskeletal System

The musculoskeletal system consists of the bones, joints, connective tissues, and muscles. These compo-

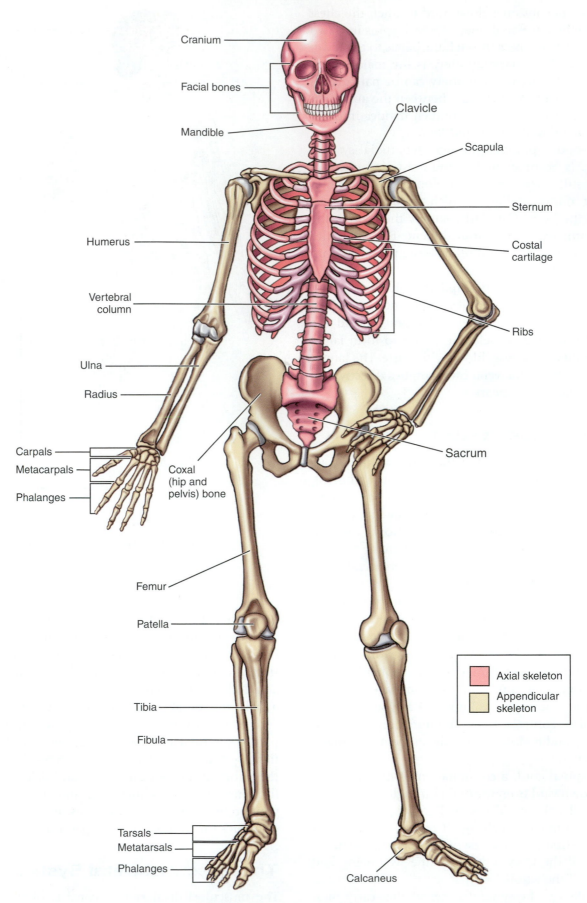

Fig. 4-11 The skeletal system.

nents work together to give the body form and allow it to move. The bones of the skeletal system provide body shape and protect vital internal organs. The muscular system provides movement to the skeletal system and is a part of every body system and container. The musculoskeletal system also is used as a reference for describing other body systems and anatomic parts. For example, the radial artery and radial nerve lie next to the radius bone in the forearm.

The Skeletal System

The skeletal system consists of the skull, spinal column, thorax, upper extremities, pelvis, and lower extremities (Fig. 4-11). The skull is divided into two parts, the cranium and the facial bones (Fig. 4-12). The cranium houses and protects the brain. The face is made up of several bones, including the mandible (jawbone). The mandible is an important landmark for learning how to open a patient's airway properly, as you will discover in Chapter 7

The spinal column is connected to the skull and extends the entire length of the back. Slightly S-shaped, it holds the body upright and allows for bending and twisting. The spinal column surrounds and therefore protects the spinal cord.

The spinal column is a collection of 33 individual bones, called *vertebrae*, which are stacked on top of one another (Fig. 4-13). Between the individual vertebrae is a round structure of cartilage called a *disk*. The disk helps give movement to the spinal column and plays a limited role as a shock absorber. The spinal column can be further defined by division of the vertebrae into five areas. Starting at the base of the skull, the first seven vertebrae make up the cervical spine. The next 12 vertebrae make up the thoracic spine. The next five vertebrae, which are the largest vertebrae of the spinal column, constitute the lumbar spine. The next area of the spinal column is the sacrum, which is made up of five fused vertebrae. The lowest section of the spinal column is the coccyx, which is composed of four fused vertebrae.

The thorax is comprised of 12 pairs of ribs (Fig. 4-14). The ribs are connected to the spinal column on the posterior side, and some are connected to the sternum (breastbone) on the anterior side. The **xiphoid process** is the lower portion of the sternum. The xiphoid process is an important landmark to know when delivering chest compressions during CPR. The clavicle (collarbone) connects the upper sternum to the scapula (shoulder blade), located in the posterior chest. The clavicle and scapula, along with the upper arm, form the shoulder joint.

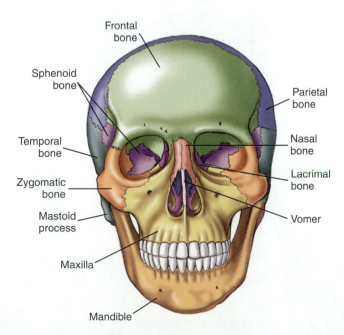

Fig. 4-12 The skull.

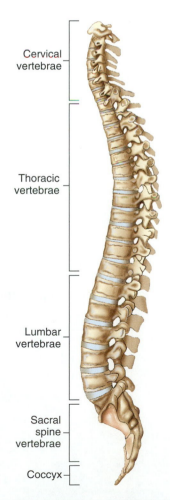

Fig. 4-13 The spinal column.

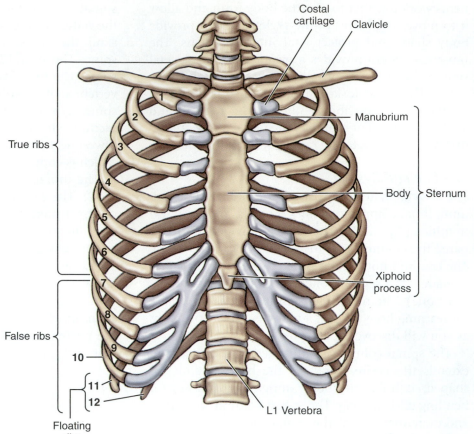

Fig. 4-14 The thorax.

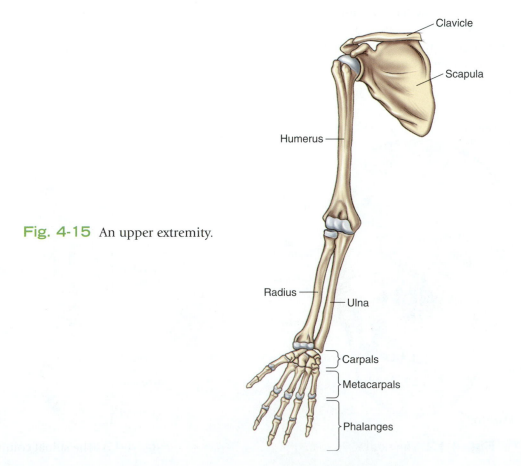

Fig. 4-15 An upper extremity.

Pelvis

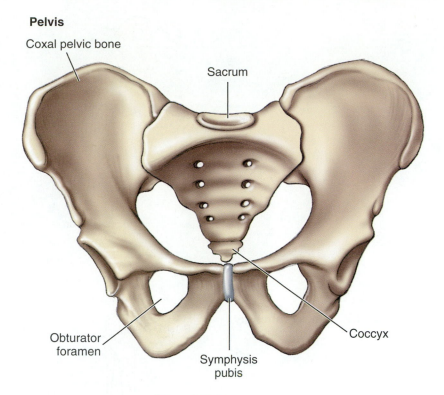

Coxal pelvic bone

Sacrum

Obturator foramen

Coccyx

Symphysis pubis

Fig. 4-16 The pelvis.

The upper extremity includes the humerus (upper arm). The proximal end of the humerus connects with the clavicle and scapula to complete the shoulder joint (Fig. 4-15). The distal end of the humerus meets the radius and ulna at the elbow joint. The radius is located on the lateral side of the forearm, and the ulna is on the medial side. The wrist is composed of many small bones, called *carpals.* The carpals join with the bones of the hand, the metacarpals, to allow movement. The many small bones of the fingers are called *phalanges.*

The pelvis is composed of two large bones that are attached to the lower portion of the spinal column. The pelvis is a large, bony ring that forms a cradle in the lower abdomen (Fig. 4-16). It is important to note that this cradle can collect a large amount of blood from internal bleeding.

The lower extremities connect to the pelvis. The head of the femur joins the pelvis to create the hip joint (Fig. 4-17). The femur is the longest, strongest single bone in the body. The distal end of the femur, along with the proximal end of the tibia, forms the knee joint. The patella (kneecap) covers the anterior knee and helps protect the joint. Distal to the knee are two bones that compose the lower leg. The larger tibia, or shinbone, is on the anterior, medial side of the lower leg. The smaller fibula lies posterior and lateral to the tibia. The distal ends of these two

bones are connected to the foot at the ankle joint. Bones of the ankle are called *tarsals.* A similar name, *metatarsals,* is given to the bones of the foot. Multiple smaller bones, called *phalanges,* form the toes.

The bones of the human skeleton are held together by connective tissues called *cartilage* and *ligaments.* When two or more bones come together to form a moveable joint, the bones are said to *articulate* (move) with each other.

The Muscular System

The human skeleton is much like a locomotive engine sitting at the train station. All the structures and joints are in place to allow movement, but it cannot move unless force is applied. The muscular system provides the force needed to get the work done through stimulation from the nervous system. It also helps define the body shape and gives limited protection to the internal organs (Fig. 4-18). The muscular system is composed of three types of muscle: voluntary muscles, involuntary muscles, and cardiac muscle.

- *Voluntary muscles* (also called *skeletal muscles*) are attached to bones by tendons. The contraction and relaxation of skeletal muscles creates and allows for movement. For example, as you take notes during your class, you are using this type of

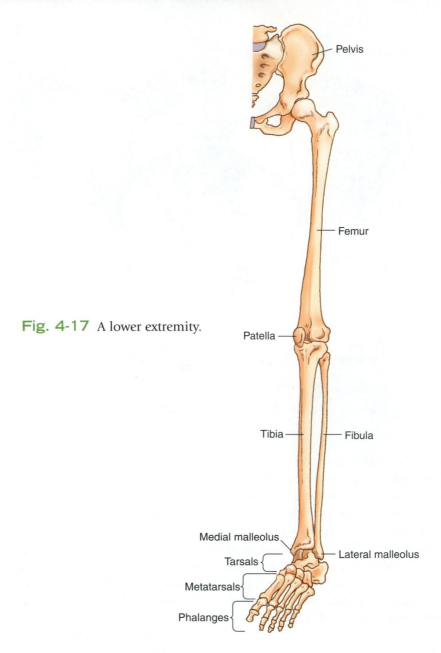

Fig. 4-17 A lower extremity.

muscle in your hand, through the voluntary control of your brain.

- *Involuntary muscles* (also called *smooth muscle*) are found in the walls of tubular structures such as blood vessels, the small airways of the lungs called *bronchioles*, the gastrointestinal tract, and the urinary system. As the name suggests, these muscles work involuntarily (without an active thought process). While you read this page, your stomach and intestines are moving to digest your

last meal, and your blood vessels are expanding and contracting to the size needed to keep blood flowing to all body tissues.

- *Cardiac muscle* is found only in the heart. It works constantly and automatically and requires a continual supply of oxygen-rich blood as fuel. Cardiac muscle can survive only a very short interruption of required blood flow. If cardiac muscle goes too long without oxygen, it dies (infarct).

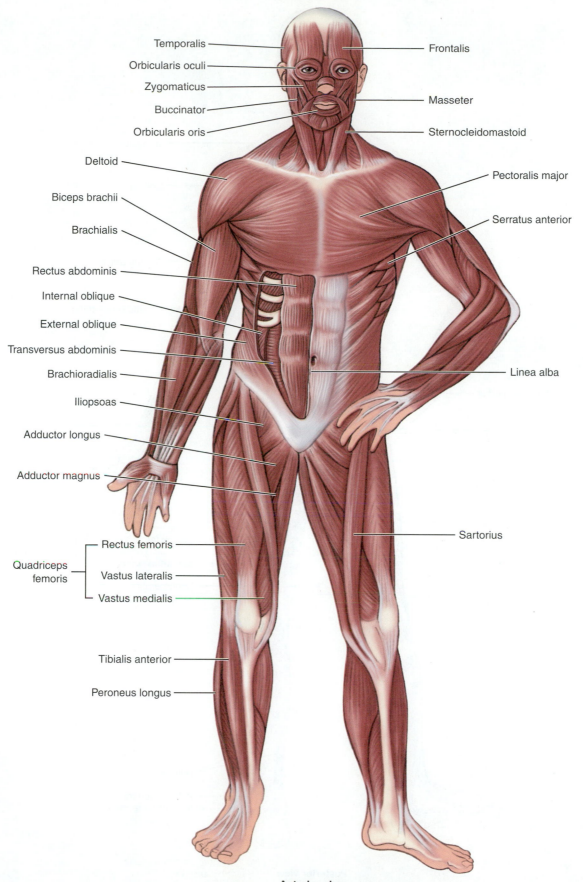

Temporalis

Orbicularis oculi

Zygomaticus

Buccinator

Orbicularis oris

Deltoid

Biceps brachii

Brachialis

Rectus abdominis

Internal oblique

External oblique

Transversus abdominis

Brachioradialis

Iliopsoas

Adductor longus

Adductor magnus

Rectus femoris

Quadriceps femoris

Vastus lateralis

Vastus medialis

Tibialis anterior

Peroneus longus

Frontalis

Masseter

Sternocleidomastoid

Pectoralis major

Serratus anterior

Linea alba

Sartorius

Anterior view
Fig. 4-18 The muscular system.

Continued

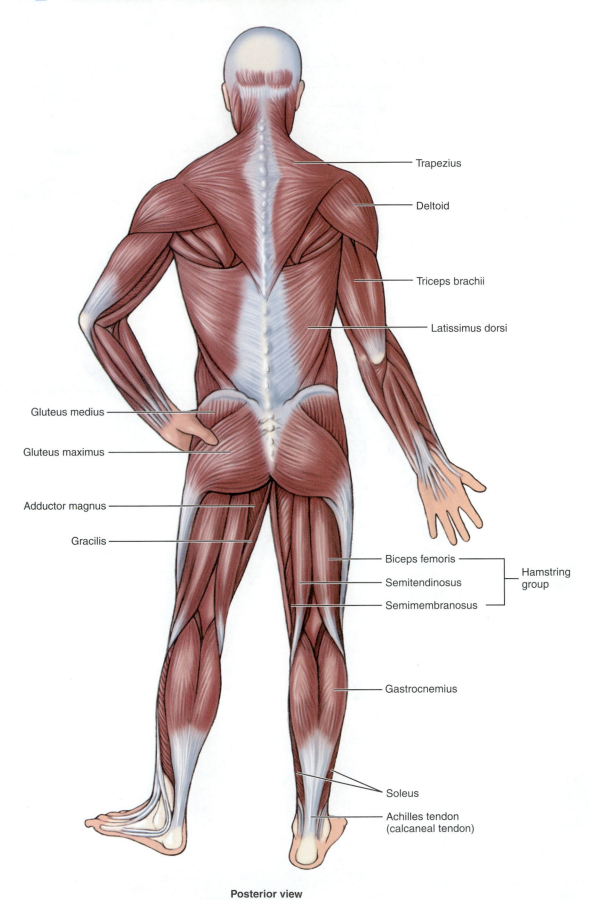

Trapezius

Deltoid

Triceps brachii

Latissimus dorsi

Gluteus medius

Gluteus maximus

Adductor magnus

Gracilis

Biceps femoris

Semitendinosus

Semimembranosus

Hamstring group

Gastrocnemius

Soleus

Achilles tendon (calcaneal tendon)

Posterior view

Fig. 4-18, cont'd　The muscular system.

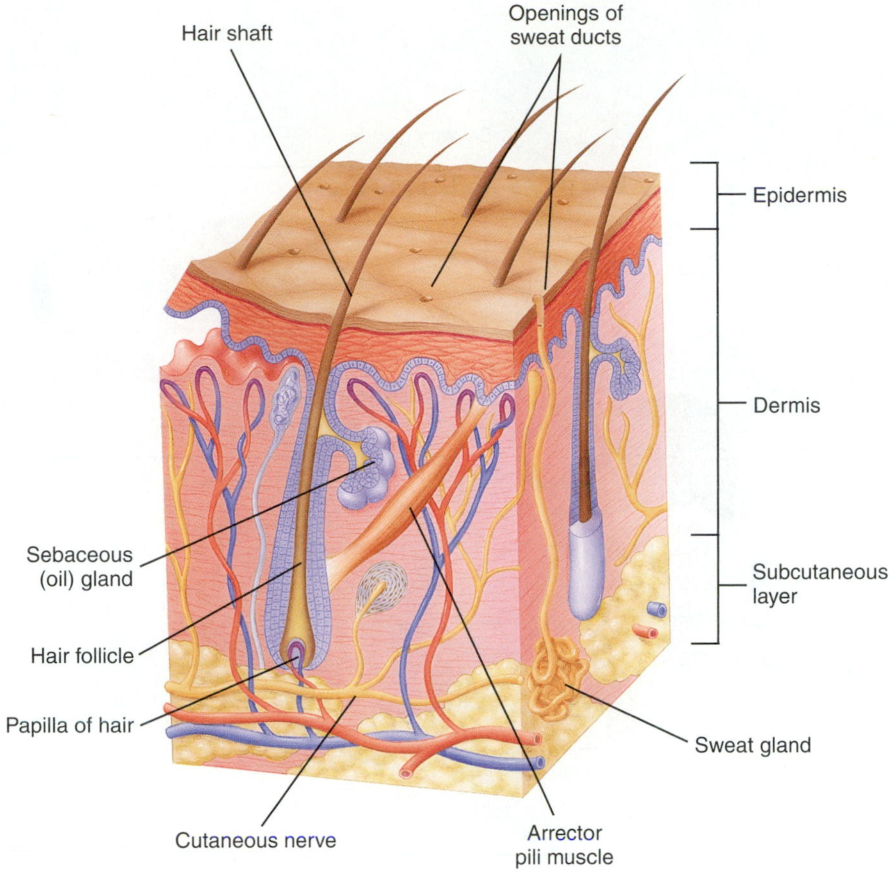

Hair shaft

Openings of
sweat ducts

Epidermis

Dermis

Subcutaneous
layer

Sebaceous
(oil) gland

Hair follicle

Papilla of hair

Cutaneous nerve

Arrector
pili muscle

Sweat gland

Fig. 4-19 The skin.

The Integumentary System

The integumentary system (the skin) protects the body from the environment and harmful substances. In addition, it helps regulate body temperature and provides sensory input to the brain. The skin also keeps the body from becoming dehydrated. The body is approximately 60% water and must maintain a specific balance of solutions to support normal body functions. The skin also provides a barrier against the elements, bacteria, and other sources of infection.

The skin plays a major role in the regulation of body temperature. It helps rid the body of excess heat and retains heat as needed. When a patient has a severe burn on a large surface area of skin, the damaged skin can no longer retain body heat, and the patient's body temperature drops.

Sensory nerves that gather information about temperature, touch, pressure, and pain are located in the skin. These nerves constantly relay information to the brain via the spinal cord.

The skin is divided into three layers (Fig. 4-19). The outermost layer is the *epidermis*. Cells that give the skin its color are located in the epidermis. The epidermis adheres to the second layer of the skin, the *dermis*. These two layers are so thin and so adherent they appear to be one layer. The dermis contains blood vessels, hair follicles, sweat glands, oil glands, and nerves. Below the dermis lies the *subcutaneous tissue*. This is a layer of fatty tissue that holds water and nutrients and provides insulation and cushioning to the body. The thickness of this tissue varies from body part to body part and from person to person.

The Gastrointestinal and Urinary Systems

The gastrointestinal and urinary systems are responsible for processing food and eliminating solid and liquid waste from the body. The digestive tract begins in the mouth and continues through the esophagus (located posterior to the trachea) to the stomach and into the small and large intestines, exiting the body at the rectal (anal) opening. As food moves through the digestive tract, mechanical and chemical processes promote absorption of nutrients and water. The leftover waste is eliminated as fecal material (Fig. 4-20).

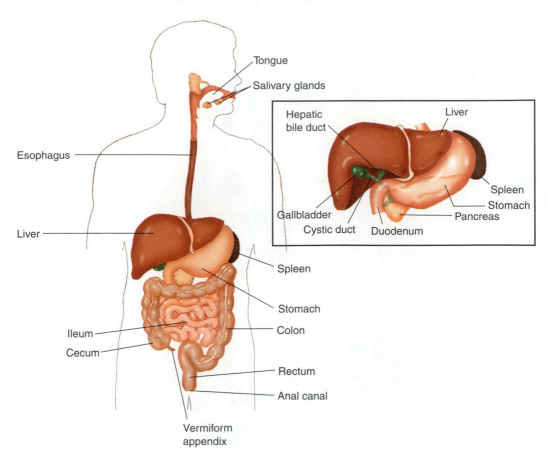

Fig. 4-20 The gastrointestinal system.

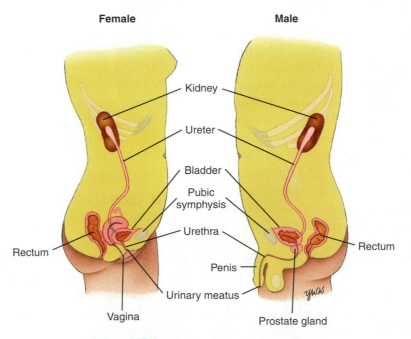

Fig. 4-21 The genitourinary system.

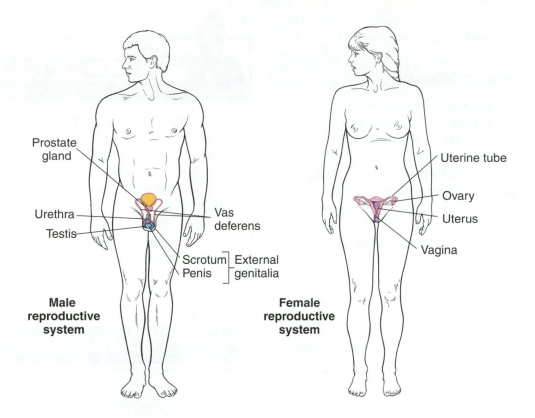

Fig. 4-22 A cutaway drawing of the male and female reproductive systems.

Blood carrying nutrients and water from the digestive tract also filters through the liver and kidneys, where the nutrients and water are absorbed and any extra water or any waste travels through ureters to the bladder and is eliminated as urine (Fig. 4-21).

The Reproductive System

The reproductive system is the system of structures and hormones required for reproduction. This system is closely associated with the urinary system, and together they sometimes are referred to as the *genitourinary system*. The reproductive system consists of the ducts, glands, and penis in the male and the ovaries, fallopian tubes, uterus, and vagina in the female (Fig. 4-22). The male testes produce semen, which combines with an egg released from the female ovaries to create a fetus.

The Endocrine System

The endocrine system is composed of glands that produce chemicals known as *hormones*. Endocrine glands include the pituitary, thyroid, parathyroid, and adrenal glands and the ovaries, testes, and pancreas (Fig. 4-23). Hormones provide strength, en-

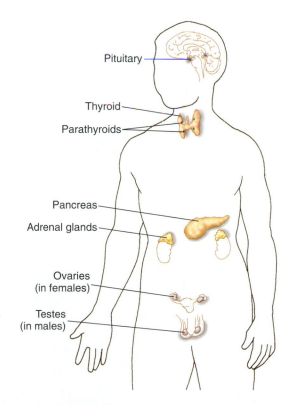

Fig. 4-23 The endocrine system.

durance, and the ability to move fuel into cells to create energy and to participate in reproduction.

The Lymphatic System

The lymphatic system links the digestive and circulatory systems by transporting vitamins and nutrients from the digestive tract into the blood. It also works as a bridge from tissues to the circulatory system by removing fluid and waste from tissues and transporting them into the circulatory system. Fluid and waste can then be transported to the liver and kidneys to be filtered out and eliminated. In addition, the lymphatic system participates in the immune response. It transports special substances to attack foreign bodies and fight infection.

Resources

Drake R, Vogl W, Mitchell A: *Gray's anatomy for students,* St Louis, 2005, Elsevier.

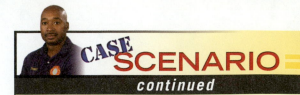

CASE SCENARIO *continued*

Mrs. Shorum is quickly loaded into the ambulance. Jack checks to make sure the oxygen mask he had put on her is still snugly in place. Her color has returned, but she is still pale and her heart rate is fast. Jack and his crew can see that their intervention has helped by ensuring that all the patient's blood is fully saturated with oxygen, but they know that this improvement is temporary at best and that Mrs. Shorum needs further care at the hospital. ■

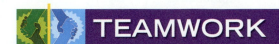

TEAMWORK

As discussed in this chapter, the EMT must have a basic knowledge of the human body and its many systems. As a member of the health care team, you will be working daily with a variety of professionals, including nurses, firefighters, physicians, and other EMS providers. A thorough knowledge of this basic information will better prepare you to communicate your findings effectively and professionally to all those involved in patient care.

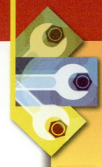

NUTS AND BOLTS

Critical Points

A knowledge of anatomy and physiology provides a solid foundation for learning patient care skills. A common language is essential for communicating effectively with other health care professionals. To identify a patient's needs, you must know how major body systems function and work together. EMTs must be able to recognize the structure and function of the respiratory, cardiovascular, nervous, and musculoskeletal systems and must understand the workings of other body systems.

Learning Checklist

❑ Normal anatomic position refers to the human body standing upright, facing forward, with the arms at the side and the palms of the hands turned forward.

❑ The directional terms *medial* and *lateral* are based on an imaginary vertical line, called the *midline*, that is drawn through the middle of the body. Lateral is away from the midline, and medial is toward the midline.

❑ Proximal is toward the trunk of the body, and distal is away from the trunk of the body.

❑ Anterior is toward the front of the body, and posterior is toward the back of the body.

❑ Superior is toward the head of the body, and inferior is toward the feet.

❑ The supine position refers to the body lying on its back, face up.

❑ The prone position refers to the body lying on its stomach.

❑ In Trendelenburg position, the patient is supine with the feet elevated higher than the head.

❑ In semi-Fowler position, the patient is in a semisitting position, bent at the waist.

❑ Body areas include the cranium, thorax, abdomen, pelvis, and extremities.

❑ The respiratory system is responsible for taking in oxygen and delivering it to the blood, eliminating waste, producing speech, and creating movements of ventilation.

❑ The respiratory system includes the oropharynx, nasopharynx, epiglottis, trachea, larynx, lungs, bronchi, and alveoli.

❑ The circulatory system is the transportation pipeline for moving blood throughout the body. Blood carries oxygen and nutrients to the cells and carbon dioxide and other wastes away from the cells.

❑ The cardiovascular system includes the arteries, veins, capillaries, and the heart.

❑ The nervous system controls the voluntary and involuntary activities of the body and provides higher mental functions, such as thought, emotion, and memory.

❑ The CNS includes the brain and spinal cord, and the PNS includes the motor and sensory nerves.

❑ The musculoskeletal system consists of the bones, joints, connective tissues, and muscles that work together to give the body form and allow it to move.

❑ The muscular system involves voluntary, involuntary, and cardiac muscle.

❑ The skeletal system includes the skull, facial bones, vertebrae, thorax, ribs, bones in the extremities, and pelvis.

❑ The spinal column (33 vertebrae) is made up of five sections: cervical, thoracic, lumbar, sacral, and coccyx.

❑ The integumentary system is the skin. The skin protects the body from the environment and harmful substances, helps regulate body temperature, and provides sensory input to the brain.

❑ The gastrointestinal system is responsible for processing food into nutrients.

❑ The urinary system is responsible for eliminating waste from the body in the form of urine.

❑ The reproductive systems of the male and female are closely associated with the urinary systems.

❑ Endocrine glands secrete hormones. These glands include the pituitary, thyroid, parathyroid, and adrenal glands and the ovaries, testes, and pancreas.

❑ The lymphatic system links the digestive and circulatory systems by transporting vitamins and nutrients from the digestive tract into the blood. This system also carries waste and fluid back from the tissues to the circulatory system and participates in the immune response of the body.

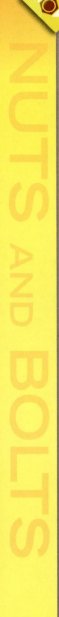

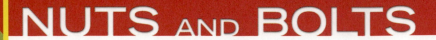
Key Terms

Abdomen The part of the body between the hips and chest.

Anatomy The structure of the body.

Anterior Toward the front of the body.

Arteries Blood vessels that carry oxygenated blood out to the body.

Axillary Pertaining to the armpit.

Bilateral Having or occurring on two sides.

Diaphragm Thin, dome-shaped muscle that forms the inferior border of the thoracic cavity and separates the contents of the chest from those of the abdomen. Flattening of the diaphragm with contraction expands the intrathoracic volume and draws air into the lungs. Relaxation of the diaphragm lessens intrathoracic volume and allows for exhalation.

Distal Away from the trunk of the body.

Inferior Toward the feet or bottom of the body.

Lateral Away from the midline of the body.

Medial Toward the midline of the body.

Midline An imaginary vertical line drawn through the middle of the body.

Normal anatomical position The position of a human body standing upright, facing forward, with arms at the side and the palms turned forward.

Pelvis The lower part of the trunk of the body.

Physiology The function of the body.

Posterior Toward the back of the body.

Prone The body lying face down.

Proximal Toward the trunk of the body.

Semi-Fowler position An inclined position in which the upper half of the body is raised by elevating the head about 30 degrees.

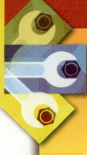

Superior Toward the head or top of the body.

Supine The body lying on its back.

Thorax The chest.

Trendelenburg position A position in which the body is supine with the feet elevated and the head down.

Veins Vessels that carry deoxygenated blood back to the heart.

Ventilation The mechanical process of inspiration and exhalation by which air rich in oxygen is breathed into the lungs and an equal volume of gas is expired, eliminating carbon dioxide from the body.

Xiphoid process Cartilaginous tissue at the distal end of the sternum.

National Standard Curriculum Objectives

Cognitive Objectives

After completing this lesson, the EMT student will be able to do the following:

- Explain the following topographic terms: medial, lateral, proximal, distal, superior, inferior, anterior, posterior, midline, right and left, midclavicular, bilateral, and midaxillary.
- Describe the anatomy and function of the following major body systems: respiratory system, circulatory system, musculoskeletal system, nervous system, and endocrine system.

Affective Objectives

No objectives identified.

Psychomotor Objectives

No objectives identified.

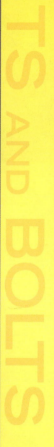

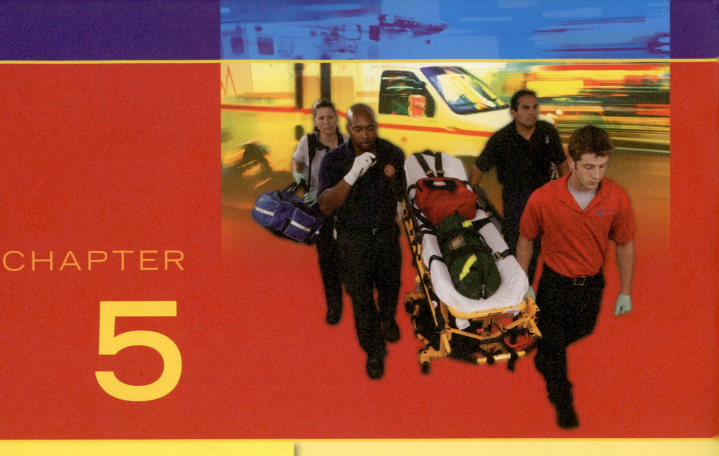

CHAPTER

5

LESSON GOAL

The goal of this lesson is to prepare the emergency medical technician (EMT) to obtain and interpret a patient's vital signs and SAMPLE history. The vital signs and history are the foundation on which many interventions in patient care are based. In addition, the vital signs demonstrate patient improvement or deterioration, so the EMT must be prepared to assess and interpret these basic patient findings accurately. ■

OUTLINE

GOAL

Baseline Vital Signs and SAMPLE History

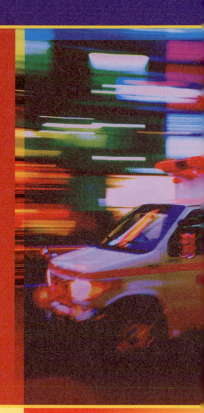

5

CHAPTER OBJECTIVES

After completing this chapter, the EMT student will be able to do the following:

1 Identify the components of vital signs.
2 Describe the methods to obtain a breathing rate.
3 Identify the attributes that should be obtained when assessing a patient's breathing.
4 Differentiate among shallow, labored, and noisy breathing.
5 Describe the methods to obtain a pulse rate.
6 List the information you should obtain when assessing a patient's pulse rate.
7 Differentiate between a strong and weak pulse and a regular and irregular pulse.
8 Describe the methods to assess the skin color, temperature, and condition (capillary refill in infants and children).
9 Identify the normal and abnormal skin colors.
10 Differentiate among pale, blue, red, and yellow skin.
11 Identify the normal and abnormal skin temperature.
12 Differentiate among hot, cool, and cold skin.
13 Identify normal and abnormal skin conditions.
14 Identify normal and abnormal capillary refill in infants and children.
15 Describe the methods to assess the pupils.
16 Identify normal and abnormal pupil size.

Continued

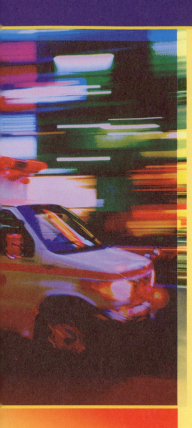

Chapter Objectives—cont'd

17 Differentiate between dilated (big) and constricted (small) pupil size.

18 Differentiate between reactive and nonreactive pupils and equal and unequal pupils.

19 Describe the methods to assess blood pressure.

20 Define systolic pressure.

21 Define diastolic pressure.

22 Explain the difference between auscultation and palpation for obtaining a blood pressure.

23 Identify the components of the SAMPLE history.

24 Differentiate between a sign and a symptom.

25 State the importance of accurately reporting and recording the baseline vital signs.

26 Discuss the need to search for additional medical identification.

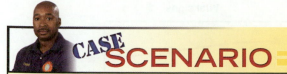

CASE SCENARIO

Jack was puzzled. A few hours earlier, he had been taking the vital signs of the ambulance crew members while back in the station. Although he had practiced counting a pulse and blood pressure on his fellow classmates, Jack had felt a little nervous when he took those vital signs on Elizabeth and the crew. To Jack's relief, Elizabeth complimented him on his skills and offered a couple of minor hints to help refine his technique. Now, they were in the back of an ambulance with Jonathon Parker, a 70-year-old man who had been complaining of mild shortness of breath for about 2 hours. At Eliza-beth's urging, Jack knelt down beside the patient and wrapped the blood pressure cuff around the patient's left arm. With the ambulance rumbling down the road, Jack tried to auscultate Jonathon's blood pressure using Elizabeth's stethoscope. However, he could not hear anything other than the noises around him as the ambulance was moving.

Question: *What can Jack do to obtain an accurate blood pressure in this situation? What alternative method could he try?*

When caring for patients, you will need to make several determinations. For example, you will need to know who your patients are, what happened, when the incident occurred, where your patients are, how the incident happened, and whether the scene is safe (Fig. 5-1). Once you have evaluated the scene, you will make contact with the patients and you will assess them to determine whether they are critical or not critical. You will do this by assessing how they respond to you and the scene, how they are breathing, and whether their circulation is adequate. If you find life-threatening issues during this time, you will begin treating these problems. After addressing the patient's airway, breathing, and circulation life threats, you will begin to collect more information about the patient. You will collect **vital signs** (specific measurements or assessments of a patient's skin, breathing, **pulse, blood pressure,** and **pupil** size and response). In addition, you will need to obtain a patient **history** (information about the patient's medical problems), and finally you will complete a more thorough assessment of the patient's body to determine whether there are injuries or complaints that you have not addressed to this point.

In this situation, you were able to determine the obvious. This was a motor vehicle crash, the two patients were out of the vehicles and sitting on the ground, and you will need to control traffic and continue to monitor for safety conditions. Both patients are alert and are talking to you, so each has a patent airway, is breathing, and has circulation. Your next steps would be to protect their cervical spines and be-

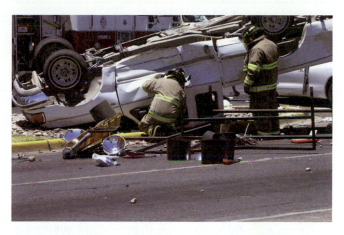

Fig. 5-1 Rollover motor vehicle crash.

gin collecting vital signs, take a history, and perform a physical exam.

■ BASELINE VITAL SIGNS

Vital signs consist of respirations; pulse; skin color, temperature, and condition; pupil size and response; and blood pressure. These components represent the status of the patient's vital functions: the patient's airway, breathing, and circulatory status. Because these are the patient's vital functions, it is essential that you learn to assess, report, and interpret them with skill and accuracy. Not only will you be using the vital signs, but also the ALS (advanced life support) crew will use them to continue care, as will the hospital emergency room staff and physicians.

Important Points
Vital signs represent the vital functions of the body and must be assessed accurately.

BOX 5-1

Vital Signs Provide a Clue to Patient Conditions

Current status of the patient
Patient improvement
Patient deterioration
Presence of illnesses or disease
Development of conditions

TABLE 5-1

Multiple sets of vital signs*

Pulse (per minute)	Respirations (per minute)	Blood Pressure (mm Hg)
88	16	126/72
90	16	124/74
94	20	118/82
98	22	114/86

*When you assess vital signs, you want to assess for trends.

Assessing vital signs is key to providing quality patient care because vital signs provide a *baseline* (standard or starting point) for you to compare future vital signs. This is important because vital signs can help you predict stability of the patient, improvement or deterioration, presence of diseases, and development of conditions (Box 5-1). Many times a single set of vital signs will help you determine a problem, but often you will need to obtain multiple sets (Table 5-1). These sets of vital signs then can be compared, and you will see a pattern develop (Fig. 5-2). The **trend** (or pattern) will give you the clues you need to recognize changes in the patient's condition and care appropriately for patients. In this set of vital signs, the patient's heart rate and breathing are increasing slowly, and the systolic blood pressure is decreasing slowly. Even though these changes are small and subtle, they may be key in identifying the early signs and symptoms of shock. It is your job to monitor these trends and to correlate them with the patient signs and symptoms to determine patient problems and treatment.

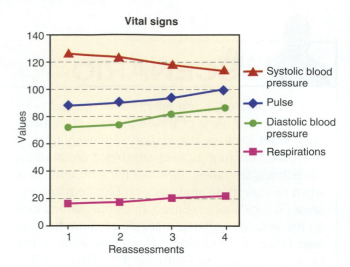

Fig. 5-2 When you graph these vital signs, you can see the pulse, respirations, and diastolic blood pressure are increasing while the systolic blood pressure is decreasing.

Important Points
Trends in vital signs help predict patient conditions.

SPECIAL Considerations

If the patient and the vital signs do not seem to match—your patient looks sick, but the vital signs seem to be within normal ranges—remember that it is the patient you were called to treat, not the patient's vital signs. If you think there is something wrong with the patient, always err on the side of caution and treat the patient.

■ RESPIRATIONS

When you assess a patient's **respiration,** you are assessing the act of breathing, or the process of moving air in and out of the lungs. At the same time, you are assessing the patient's airway. If a patient is breathing (moving air in and out of the lungs), the airway is open. Respirations can be assessed by finding the answers to the following questions:

- What is the respiratory rate?
- What is the quality?
- What is the pattern?

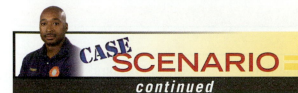

CASE **SCENARIO**
continued

Jack looked at Mr. Parker. Although he seemed to be improving with the oxygen therapy, he still looked anxious about what was happening to him. He was contemplating saying something when Elizabeth leaned over and said, "Why don't you try to determine his SAMPLE history?"

Question: Given the conditions of the noisy moving ambulance, what actions could Jack take to better establish a good rapport with Mr. Parker?

Rate

To evaluate the first question (What is the **respiratory rate?**), you will need to understand how to determine rate. You measure respiratory rate by the number of breaths a person takes in 1 minute. So a patient who breathes 16 times in 1 minute would have a respiratory rate of 16 breaths per minute. This often is documented as R 16 or Resp. 16. Because it takes what seems to be a long time to count respirations for a minute, respirations often are counted for 15 or 30 seconds and then are multiplied by 4 or 2 to determine a rate. For example, if a patient breathes 4 times in 15 seconds, you multiply 4 by 4 (because there are four 15-second time frames in a minute) to obtain 16 breaths per minute. If the patient breathes 8 times in

30 seconds, you would multiply 8 by 2 and have 16 breaths per minute. The process you use is not as important as the accuracy in counting the respirations.

Because it is sometimes difficult to see each individual respiration, you may want to look closely at the upper abdomen or rest your hand on the upper abdomen to feel the chest rise and fall with each breath. Because patients can change their breathing pattern when they know it is being assessed, you can place your hand on their pulse point and monitor their breathing before or after you take the pulse. You still can lay your hand across the upper abdomen while taking the pulse if their breathing is shallow and difficult for you to see (Fig. 5-3).

To know the normal respiratory rate for your patient is crucial. Table 5-2 outlines normal vital signs for each age group. Because pediatric vital signs are different for each age group and EMTs do not care for pediatric patients often, many departments post a chart such as this in their ambulances or in their pediatric kits. This serves as a reference for the crews when they are caring for pediatric patients.

The normal respiratory rate for an adult is 12 to 20 breaths per minute. If a patient is breathing more slowly than normal, you should consider assisting his or her breathing with positive pressure ventilation. Slow respirations suggest problems such as drug overdose, neurologic damage, or impending respiratory arrest. Oxygen administration without positive pressure ventilation is usually not adequate for these patients. If the patient is breathing more rapidly than normal, you should administer oxygen and assess the patient's response. If the breathing does not improve, once again you should consider positive pressure

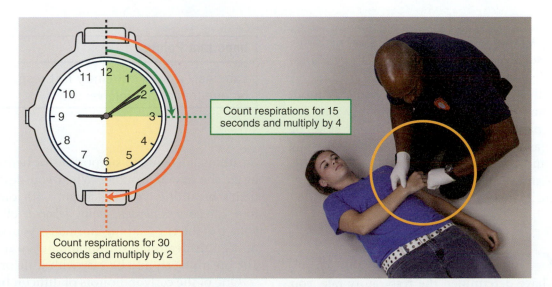

Count respirations for 15 seconds and multiply by 4

Count respirations for 30 seconds and multiply by 2

Fig. 5-3 Assess respirations by looking at or placing a hand on the upper abdomen while taking the pulse and by counting the number of breaths the patient takes.

TABLE 5-2

Normal vital signs by age group

Patient	Age	Respiratory Rate (breaths/min)	Pulse Rate (beats/min)	Blood Pressure* (systolic/diastolic, mm Hg)
Newborn	Birth-6 wk	30-50	120-160	(74-100)/(50-68)
Infant	7 wk-1 yr	20-30	80-140	(84-106)/(56-70)
Toddler	1-2 yr	20-30	90-130	(98-106)/(50-70)
Preschool	2-6 yr	20-30	80-120	(98-112)/(64-70)
School age	6-13 yr	18-30	(60-80)-100	(104-124)/(64-80)
Adolescent	13-16 yr	(12-20)-30	60-100	(118-132)/(70-82)
Adult	>16 yr	12-20	60-100	(100-150)/(60-90)

From Chapleau W: *Emergency first responder,* St Louis, 2004, Mosby.
*The normal systolic pressure in children aged 1 to 10 years can be calculated as 90 mm Hg + (child's age in years × 2) mm Hg. The lower systolic pressure in children aged 1 to 10 years can be calculated as 70 mm Hg + (child's age in years × 2) mm Hg.

TABLE 5-3

Breathing problems, causes, and interventions

Problem	Cause (Think)	Intervention
Stridor	Swelling of the airway	Humidified oxygen, ALS* intercept
Crowing	Airway obstruction or swelling	Humidified oxygen, ALS intercept
Gurgling	Fluids in the airway	Suction
Wheezing	Constriction of the lower airways (bronchioles)	Oxygen and a bronchodilator, ALS intercept
Grunting	Respiratory distress	Oxygen, ALS intercept
Snoring	Tongue obstructing the airway	Reposition the airway, oral or nasal airway
Labored respirations	Respiratory compromise	Oxygen, ALS intercept

*ALS, Advanced life support.

ventilation. A rapid respiratory rate is associated with problems such as stress, elevated temperatures, shock, inadequate breathing, and toxic exposure. A patient with an increased respiratory rate is more common than one with a slow respiratory rate. For the most part, patients with extremely slow or extremely fast respiratory rates have more serious problems and need rapid intervention (Table 5-3). Chapters 7 and 17 provide an in-depth discussion regarding the management of airway and breathing problems.

Quality

Once you have determined the respiratory rate, you should ask, "What is the quality?" Is this patient's

> **Important Points**
>
> Extremely slow or extremely fast respiratory rates require immediate intervention.

breathing adequate to support his or her needs, or is he or she having trouble? When you describe a patient's breathing, you will begin with one of these four categories: *normal, noisy, labored,* or *shallow.* If your patient is breathing normally, you should not notice the breathing. You should not hear any noise. The breathing should be easy with little or no effort.

One of the early indicators of difficult breathing is noisy respirations. *Noisy respirations* are present when

Important Points
Noisy respirations indicate some type of airway compromise.

you hear sounds as the patient breathes and are indicators of some type of obstruction. Noisy respirations are classified as **snoring, stridor, crowing, gurgling, wheezing,** or **grunting.** Snoring respirations are caused by the tongue falling back over the airway and partially obstructing it. Snoring is heard in patients with decreased levels of consciousness who are not awake enough to control their tongue and airway. Snoring is corrected by repositioning the patient, by performing a jaw thrust or head tilt–chin lift, or by stimulating the patient to wake up. You also may use oral and nasal airways to keep the tongue from obstructing the airway.

Stridor is a high-pitched sound heard during inspiration when the upper airway is partially obstructed by swelling. Stridor often occurs in children with croup. Any condition that causes the airway to swell may cause stridor and should be treated immediately with high-flow humidified oxygen. Rapid transport and ALS care should be considered because the airway may swell shut.

Crowing is a loud, shrill sound heard on expiration and indicates swelling or an obstruction of the upper airway. Crowing respirations may be associated with whooping cough and airway burns. This patient will need advanced care and should be transported as soon as possible and receive high-flow humidified oxygen.

Gurgling is a bubbling or gargling sound that occurs when blood or fluids are present in the airway. Gurgling is usually present in a patient with a decreased level of consciousness. The patient may have trauma to the face and upper airway, causing blood, vomit, or saliva to collect in the airway, thereby causing the gurgling. Regardless of the cause, suctioning, patient positioning, and airway management are indicated immediately. A patient with gurgling present has an increased chance of aspirating, or inhaling, the blood or fluids into the lungs and developing pneumonia or dying.

Wheezing is a whistling sound heard when the lower airways are obstructed by swelling, foreign bodies, or bronchospasm. Wheezing suggests problems such as asthma, chronic obstructive pulmonary disease, anaphylaxis, and other problems associated with lower airway obstruction and swelling. These patients will need oxygen and medications such as bronchodilators to manage the wheezing. You may hear the wheezing with just your ears, but more often you will need a stethoscope to listen to the chest to hear wheezes.

Grunting respirations are heard in newborns who have difficulty breathing. You will hear grunting sound each time they exhale. Infants do this to help keep their airways open at the end of each exhalation. Infants with grunting respirations should be treated as critical and should receive high-flow oxygen and rapid transport to ALS care or an appropriate facility.

Labored respirations are present when the patient is working to breathe. When you see a patient working to breathe, you should consider oxygen administration or assisting respirations with a bag-valve-mask device. A patient with labored breathing will be using the **accessory muscles** to breathe. The patient will be using the neck muscles and the intercostal muscles. You may see retractions (sucking in of the tissue) between the ribs, in the neck, and beneath the sternum (Fig. 5-4). Another way to identify labored respirations is to listen to the patient's ability to speak. A patient who is breathing normally can carry on a conversation without noticeable respiratory effort. A patient with difficulty breathing may be able to speak only one to two words without taking a breath.

Pattern

You may identify *respiratory patterns* when you assess breathing. These patterns often are associated with brain injuries or metabolic states (Fig. 5-5). **Apneustic respirations** are deep respirations associated with periods of apnea and commonly occur in stroke patients. **Ataxic respirations,** or Biot's respirations, are irregular respirations usually seen in stroke patients or patients with severe brain impairment. **Cheyne-Stokes respirations** are represented by a slow, shallow pattern that gradually increases in rate

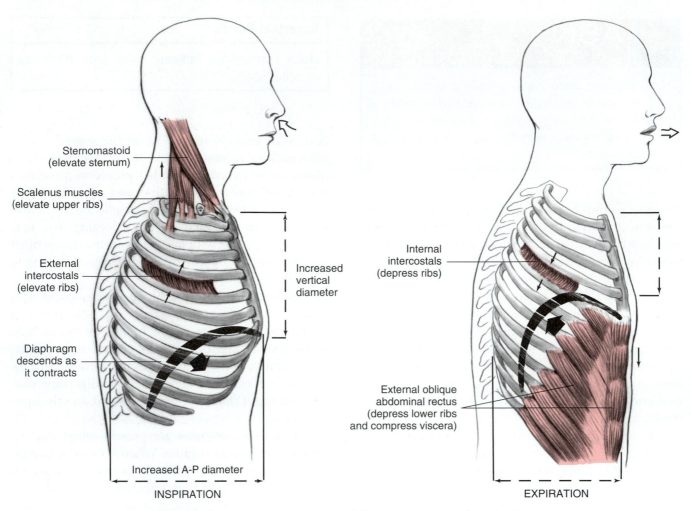

Fig. 5-4 Accessory muscles used for inspiration and expiration.

Apneustic	Long, deep breaths with periods of apnea between	Stroke, severe brain damage or disease
Ataxic or Biot's	Irregular, shallow and deep, no pattern	Stroke
Cheyne-Stokes	Respirations start slow and shallow and increase in rate and depth and then decrease with periods of apnea between	Stroke, metabolic problems
Central neurogenic hyperventilation	Continuous deep breaths; rate may be slow or fast	Acidosis, brain trauma
Kussmaul's	Regular deep breaths; visually rapid	Acidosis, commonly associated with diabetic ketoacidosis

Fig. 5-5 Common respiratory patterns and their causes.

and depth and then decreases again. This crescendo-decrescendo pattern is followed by a period of apnea before it begins again. Cheyne-Stokes respirations are associated with problems such as stroke or metabolic conditions. **Central neurogenic hyperventilation** and **Kussmaul's respirations** look alike, but the terms are associated with different conditions. Kussmaul's respirations are associated with diabetic ketoacidosis, whereas central neurogenic hyperventilation is associated more commonly with patients with head trauma. If you are unable to recall the exact name of the pattern, it is important to describe the breathing pattern and when you observed it. This may help advanced providers better identify the problem and care for the patient.

■ PULSE

When you take a pulse, you are feeling for the blood being pushed through the arteries with each heart-

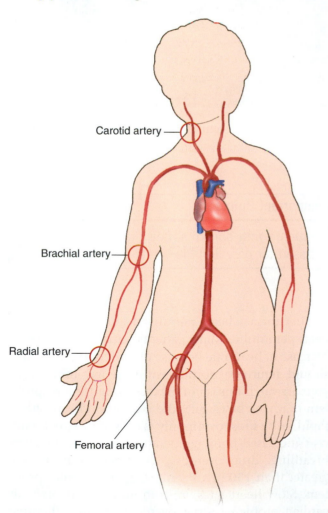

Fig. 5-6 Assess the carotid, brachial, radial, or femoral pulses.

Carotid artery

Brachial artery

Radial artery

Femoral artery

SPECIAL Considerations

Pediatric Consideration: Vital Signs
Measuring vital signs in pediatric patients is not as important in determining their status as it is in adults because compensatory mechanisms will mask physiologic damage. Instead, focus your attention more on the overall appearance of the "wellness" or "sickness" of the child.

SPECIAL Considerations

Pediatric Consideration: Pulse Oximeter
The use of an adult pulse oximeter finger clip on an infant or young child, even for a short time, can cause a burn. Always use a pediatric pulse oximeter clip.

beat. The pulse is a reflection of heart function and circulation. You can feel a pulse at points where the artery is near the surface of the skin. Fig. 5-6 illustrates common pulse points. As you assess the pulse, you will be asking yourself a series of questions, including the following:
- What is the rate?
- What is the quality?
- What is the rhythm?

In addition, you will be asking yourself whether there is anything significant to these findings (Table 5-4). Based on these findings, does my patient require intervention or assessment?

Rate

To take the pulse, you will use the same method described in the respiratory section. You will count the number of beats in 15 seconds and multiply by 4. So if you counted 22 beats in 15 seconds, the **pulse rate** would be 88. You also can count the number of beats in 30 seconds and multiply by 2. To locate the pulse, you may use many areas. The most common place to feel for a pulse is radial artery. This artery is in the wrist just above the thumb (Fig. 5-7). Use your index finger and apply gentle pressure to feel for a pulse. You also may find a pulse at the carotid artery in the neck (Fig. 5-8) and the **brachial artery** in the arm. The **carotid pulse** is used most often for unresponsive adults and larger children or patients with decreased circulation. The **brachial pulse** (Fig. 5-9) is used most commonly in infants and small chil-

TABLE 5-4

Pulse problems, causes, and interventions

Problem	Cause (Think)	Intervention
Rapid pulse	Shock, hypoxia, drugs, exertion, dehydration, cardiac problems	Oxygen, cooling, ALS* intercept
Slow pulse	Drugs, cardiac problems	Oxygen, ALS intercept
Irregular pulse	Cardiac problems	Oxygen, apply cardiac monitor, ALS intercept
Weak pulse	Shock, vascular compromise	Oxygen, treat for shock, reassess splinting if present, ALS intercept

*ALS, Advanced life support.

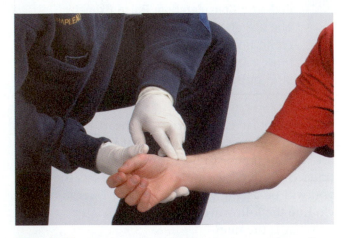

Fig. 5-7 Gently use your index finger to palpate for a radial pulse.

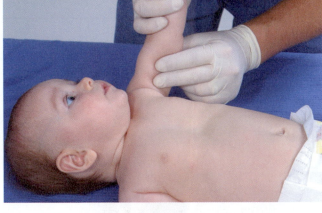

Fig. 5-9 The brachial artery usually is palpated in infants and small children.

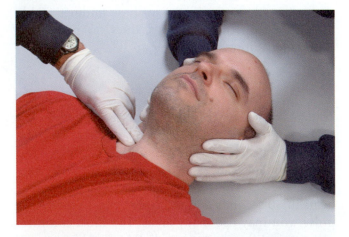

Fig. 5-8 When palpating for a carotid pulse, use one side of the neck.

dren whose necks are too small to palpate a carotid pulse easily. The pulse from the femoral artery is located in the groin and is palpated when a **radial pulse** cannot be obtained or a carotid pulse is not indicated.

Important Points

Patients with abnormal heart rates should be assessed for potential life threats.

The normal heart rate in an adult is 60 to 100 beats per minute. Many patients initially may have an increase in heart rate because of anxiety, but their rate should return to normal within a few minutes of your arrival. If this is not the case, monitor for a problem that may be causing the increase in heart rate. A rapid pulse most commonly is caused by stress, exercise, increased body temperature, hypoxia, difficulty breathing, drug overdose, or shock. A heart rate greater than 150 in an adult suggests a cardiac problem. Slow heart rates are common in patients with cardiac problems, drug overdose, or hypothermia. Sleeping patients and athletes also have slower heart rates.

Quality

When assessing the pulse, you also will be noting quality. Quality is the strength of the pulse. The pulse usually is described as strong or weak. A strong pulse that is easy to feel when you palpate is normal. If a patient has a weak pulse, it will be difficult to feel it on **palpation.** A weak pulse represents compromised circulation from vascular disease, vascular trauma, or shock. If a distal pulse such as a radial pulse is too difficult to feel, palpate a more central pulse such as the carotid or femoral. A weak pulse often is associated with a low blood pressure.

Rhythm

In addition to assessing for strength, you also will be assessing for rhythm. A pulse that is regular from beat to beat is normal. An irregular pulse may have many etiologies, but the primary cause is from the heart. If you feel an irregular pulse and can apply a cardiac monitor to obtain a recording of the rhythm, it is important to do so. Once again, describe what you feel and relay it to the receiving crew or facility, for changes in cardiac rhythm may be transient, so it is important to report your findings and the patient's response to the rhythm and rate.

■ SKIN

Even though the skin is discussed third, it is probably the first thing you will assess, and it rapidly will give you an indication of the patient's status. To assess the skin, you will look at and feel the skin to determine color, temperature, condition, and **capillary refill.** You see patients every day, so an internal alarm often goes off when you see a patient whose skin does not look normal. You should listen to this internal alarm because it is a valid indicator of patient status. You should ask yourself the following questions about the skin (Table 5-5):

- What is the color?
- What is the temperature
- What is the condition
- Is the capillary refill normal?

Color

Skin color will provide you with information regarding patient condition. Skin color may be difficult to assess on patients with dark skin. Use the lips or palms of the hands to assess for color. The skin usually is classified as normal, pale, flushed (red), cyanotic (blue), jaundiced (yellow), or **mottled** (splotched). Pale skin represents a decrease in blood flow to the skin. Pale skin is common with patients who are in shock, hypothermic, or anemic. Flushed or red skin usually represents an increase in blood flow to the skin. You will see this in patients who are hypertensive, are hot, have first-degree burns, or have poisoning such as from carbon monoxide. Cyanotic skin commonly is associated with decreased oxygen content in the blood. Many patients with respiratory disease show **cyanosis. Jaundice** is caused by liver disease and presents as a yel-

TABLE 5-5

Skin problems, causes, and interventions

Problem	Cause (Think)	Intervention
Pale	Shock (hypoperfusion)	Oxygen, treat for shock, ALS* transport
Flushed	Heat emergency, allergic reaction	Oxygen, cool if hot, monitor for anaphylaxis as needed
Cyanotic	Hypoxia	Oxygen, ALS intercept
Jaundiced	Liver problems	Oxygen, assess for gastrointestinal bleeding
Mottled	Shock (hypoperfusion)	Oxygen, treat for shock, ALS intercept
Moist	Shock (hypoperfusion), heat emergency	Oxygen, treat for shock, ALS intercept
Dry	Dehydration	Oxygen, treat for shock, ALS intercept
Cold	Cold emergencies	Oxygen, warm, ALS intercept
Cool	Shock (hypoperfusion)	Oxygen, treat for shock, ALS intercept

*ALS, Advanced life support.

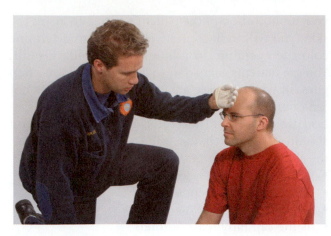

Fig. 5-10 Assess temperature by placing the back of your ungloved hand on the patient's skin.

lowish color to the skin. You initially may see the jaundiced color in the sclera or white portion of the eye. Mottled skin appears as a pale bluish splotched color to the skin. Mottled skin usually is present in shock and hypothermia.

Temperature

Feel the skin to assess the temperature. When you feel the skin, you should be assessing the skin with your hand—skin to skin. You can touch the skin with an ungloved hand or fold your glove down and touch the skin (Fig. 5-10). Normal skin temperature is warm. Cold skin suggests hypothermia. Cool skin is common in states of hypoperfusion. Hot skin is present in hyperthermia or in patients with fevers.

Condition

You also will be assessing the condition of the skin. Normal skin is dry. Moist, sweaty (diaphoretic) skin is present when the patient is sweating from exertion or an elevated temperature. Shock, or hypoperfusion, is another cause of moist skin. Patients who are dehydrated may have extremely dry skin that tents, or stays "pinched up," when the skin is pinched gently. You also may note edematous, or swollen, skin from too much fluid being present.

Capillary Refill

Capillary refill is assessed by pressing on the skin until the color leaves the area and then letting the pressure off and counting how many seconds it takes for the skin color to return to normal. Normal capillary refill

is less than 2 seconds. Hypothermia and shock may cause delayed capillary refill. A delayed capillary refill is a **sign** of decreased circulation to the area caused by vascular disease. Because adults are at risk for vascular disease, capillary refill may not be as accurate in determining systemic perfusion. Capillary refill is an accurate predictor of hypoperfusion in infants and children and is included in their assessment.

■ PUPILS

The pupil is the dark opening surrounded by the colored iris of the eye. The pupils are assessed for shape, equality, and response to light. To assess the pupils, look at the patient's eyes. The pupils should be round and equal. To assess response to light, shine a bright light into the pupils and monitor for response. In a darker area, the pupils **dilate** or become larger, and they normally **constrict** (get smaller) when exposed to light. Both pupils should be the same size and should constrict equally when you shine a light into them. Both pupils normally get smaller when a light is shined into one of them. To assess the reaction of each eye, cover one eye and shine a light into it and then cover the other eye and do the same. Watch for the pupils to constrict. If pupils do not react to light, you should suspect drug use or inadequate oxygena-

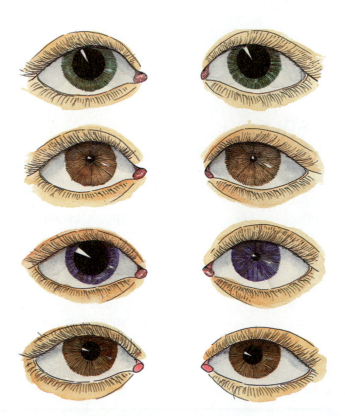

Fig. 5-11 Pupil assessment.

tion of the brain. If both pupils are dilated, suspect brain injury, drug use, or eye drop use. If both pupils are constricted, suspect a drug overdose (specifically narcotics) or eye drop use. If the pupils are unequal, you should suspect a stroke, brain trauma, or an artificial eye. Documentation of which pupil is larger than the other and the response is important to help the physician diagnose the patient problem (Fig. 5-11). Pupils that are not round suggest prior surgery of the eye or trauma with possible rupture of the globe (eyeball).

■ BLOOD PRESSURE

The blood pressure represents the pressure the blood produces in the arteries of the vascular system as it perfuses the body. The blood pressure is assessed using a **sphygmomanometer** (blood pressure cuff) and stethoscope. When you assess the blood pressure, you will obtain two numbers: a systolic blood pressure and a **diastolic pressure.** The systolic pressure is the higher number and represents the pressure in the vessels when the heart beats, and the diastolic pressure is the lower number and represents the pressure when the heart relaxes. The blood pressure is documented as the **systolic pressure** written over the diastolic pressure; for example, 122/76.

Table 5-2 lists normal blood pressure findings for adults and children. Overall, adults have higher blood pressures than children and infants. Proper measurement of the blood pressure is dependent on using the right sized cuff for the patient. You will need to carry smaller blood pressure cuffs for infants and children and larger cuffs for adults with large upper arms. High blood pressure or hypertension is associated with strokes. The other problem with high blood pressure is that it causes damage to the organs of the body from the continuous exposure to high pressures. Low blood pressure is caused by one of the forms of shock: septic, cardiogenic, hypovolemic, and neurogenic. Shock is discussed in detail in Chap-

ter 25. Just as high blood pressure can damage the organs, so can a low blood pressure. Each case must be addressed and managed immediately. Both cases often require ALS intervention for care (Table 5-6).

To obtain the blood pressure, you will use one of the following methods: **auscultation** or **palpation.** Auscultation is taking a blood pressure using a stethoscope and listening for a systolic and diastolic pressure (Skill 5-1). Palpation is taking the blood pressure by feeling or palpating for a blood pressure (Skill 5-2). When you palpate a blood pressure, you will obtain only a systolic pressure. It is best to obtain a pressure by auscultation because it provides the systolic and diastolic pressures, which are useful in identifying problems such as increased intracranial pressure, tension pneumothorax, or cardiac tamponade. Palpation is used when the surrounding environment is too loud to hear an auscultated pressure. Both auscultated and palpated blood pressures may be time consuming to obtain. If a patient is unstable with a life-threatening problem, use your other tools to aid in assessing the patient. A blood pressure can be obtained when the patient is more stable and the life threat is managed or you have additional assistance to obtain the blood pressure.

Auscultated Blood Pressure

To auscultate a blood pressure, you will need a properly fitting blood pressure cuff and a stethoscope. To ensure the cuff fits properly, the cuff size should be approximately two thirds the length of the upper arm and should encircle the arm to fit snugly. If the cuff is too large or too loose, you may obtain a false low reading. If the cuff is too small or too tight, you may obtain a false high reading.

Important Points
Do not delay care for life-threatening injuries to obtain a blood pressure.

TABLE 5-6

Blood pressure problems, causes, and interventions

Problem	Cause (Think)	Intervention
Low blood pressure (hypotension)	Shock (hypoperfusion)	Oxygen, treat for shock, ALS* intercept
High blood pressure (hypertension)	Stroke, drug use	Oxygen, ALS intercept

*ALS, Advanced life support.

SKILL 5-1
Auscultation of the Blood Pressure

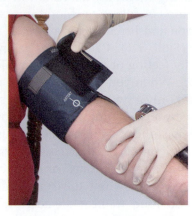

1. Place the blood pressure cuff on the patient and then place the stethoscope earpieces in your ears.

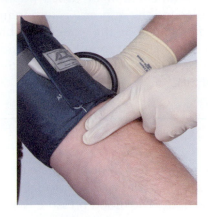

2. Palpate for the brachial artery.

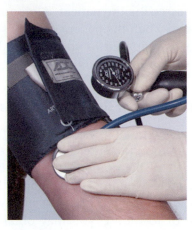

3. Place the diaphragm of the stethoscope over the brachial artery.

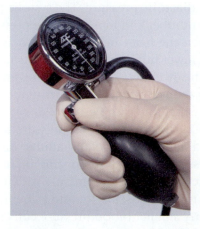

4. Ensure that the valve is closed and then inflate the cuff by squeezing on the bulb.

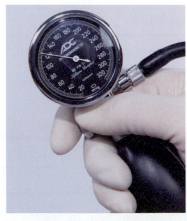

5. Slowly release the air from the cuff and listen for the first sound. The first sound is the systolic pressure.

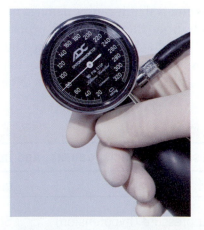

6. Continue to release the pressure slowly and listen for the last sound. The last sound heard is the diastolic pressure.

SKILLS

SKILL 5-2
Palpating a Blood Pressure

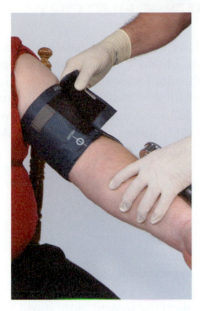

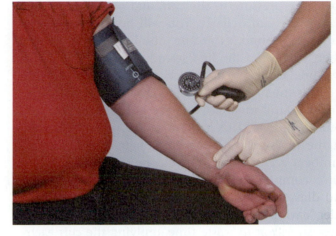

1. Place the blood pressure cuff on the patient's arm.

2. Palpate for a radial pulse.

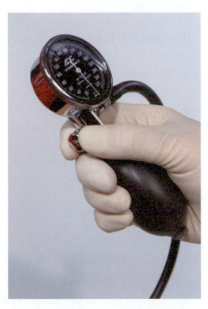

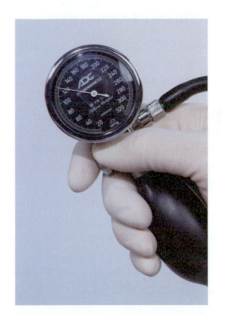

3. Ensure that the valve is closed and then inflate the cuff by squeezing on the bulb. This will obliterate the radial pulse.

4. Slowly release the air from the cuff and feel for the pulse. The first beat you feel is the systolic pressure.

SKILLS

Place the cuff 1 inch above the crease of the elbow with the bladder over the artery. Wrap the cuff snugly around the arm and secure the Velcro. Palpate the brachial pulse, and place the diaphragm of the stethoscope over the artery. Do not place the diaphragm under the cuff. Place the earpieces of the stethoscope in your ears. Ensure that the valve on the bulb of the cuff is closed and gently squeeze and release the bulb until the cuff is inflated and the pressure reads approximately 200 mm Hg. Gently let down the pressure in the cuff, and watch the numbers as the cuff deflates. You will be listening for a thumping sound. Note the number on the gauge when you heard the first sound. This is the systolic pressure. Continue to watch the numbers on the gauge as the pressure decreases. You will be listening for the sound to stop. Note the number for the last sound you hear. This is the diastolic pressure. If you let the pressure out too fast, you may not see the numbers accurately, so let the pressure out slowly. Once complete, you should document the systolic and diastolic numbers (for example, 138/66). Consider leaving the cuff in place for repeat blood pressures so as not to waste time applying the cuff each time.

Palpated Blood Pressure

To obtain a palpated blood pressure, you will need to place the cuff on the arm in the same manner. This time instead of listening for a thumping sound, you will be feeling for the pulse to return. To do this, feel for a radial pulse with your index and middle fingers. Inflate the cuff as described before. You will not be able to feel the pulse as you inflate the cuff. Once the cuff is inflated, slowly deflate the cuff, watch the gauge, and feel for the pulse to return. Note the number on the gauge when the pulse returns. This is the systolic palpated pressure. You will not get a diastolic pressure. Palpated pressures are documented as 132/P.

■ REASSESSMENT

You will need to reassess the patient's vital signs. In patients in critical condition, vital signs assessments are repeated at least every 5 minutes. In stable patients, vital signs assessments are repeated every 10 to 15 minutes or longer based on your protocols. As discussed before, you will want to monitor for trends and response to the care you have initiated. If vital signs are abnormal, your goal is to administer care that will help stabilize the patient and return the vi-

tal signs to the normal range. The transporting crew and receiving facility will want a current set of vital signs, so be prepared to provide updated vital signs as requested.

■ SAMPLE HISTORY

Once you have obtained the patient's vital signs, it is important to obtain a baseline history about the patient. The history focuses on information about the patient's medical condition and current medical problem or injury. At minimum, you will want to obtain a SAMPLE history (Table 5-7). **SAMPLE** is a mnemonic that stands for the following:

- **S**—*Signs* and *symptoms*
- **A**—*Allergies*
- **M**—*Medications*
- **P**—*Past medical history*
- **L**—*Last oral intake*
- **E**—*Events preceding*

As you collect the information, it will be necessary to use good listening and interviewing techniques. Some of the actions you can take to obtain a history include the following:

- Treating the person being interviewed with respect
- Listening to the answer as it is given
- Physically getting down on the person's level—face to face when possible
- Using words the person can understand
- Confirming answers as they are given
- Giving the person time to answer the question
- Asking open-ended questions as opposed to yes-or-no questions
- Getting an interpreter as needed

S—Signs and Symptoms

When you assess signs and symptoms, you are trying to identify the patient's problem. A sign is something you can see, hear, smell, or measure. For example, you can see a fractured arm or a bleeding laceration. You can hear problems such as snoring or wheezing. You can smell urine, feces, or bleeding from a gastrointestinal bleed. You can measure the vital signs. A **symptom** is something the patient feels. They can assign a severity or description to it, but you cannot measure it. Symptoms require more exploration so that you can ensure you understand the patient com-

TABLE 5-7

SAMPLE history

SAMPLE	Description	Emergency Medical Technician Activities
S Signs and Symptoms	Signs are problems you see, hear, feel, smell, or measure.	Ask about or Look for bleeding Listen for wheezing Smell for gastrointestinal bleeding Take the pulse
A Allergies	Symptoms are what the patient tells you. Materials, foods, or medications to which the patient is allergic	Ask the patient to describe how he feels Ask: Do you have any allergies to medications, food, or other material? Look: MedicAlert tags, vial of life, and old charts
M Medications	List of current medications the patient takes	Ask: Do you take any medications, herbs, vitamins, over-the-counter medications, or "recreational" drugs? Look: MedicAlert tags, vial of life, old charts, counter or cabinet for medications and dietary supplements, and paraphernalia for recreational drugs
P Past medical history	Pertinent medical history	Ask: Do you have any medical problems or see a doctor for any medical problems? You may use medication use to question about medical history as well. Look: For any medical assist devices such as oxygen, walkers, and nebulizers
L Last oral intake	Anything the patient last ate or drank	Ask: When did you last eat or drink anything? What and how much did you eat or drink? Look: Empty containers and dirty dishes
E Events preceding	What the patient did before the incident	Ask: What happened right before you called us? What caused your accident or illness? Describe the events before the incident. Look: Mechanism of injury and nature of illness

plaint. Assessment of symptoms is discussed more thoroughly in the medical assessment chapter (Chapter 11).

A—Allergies

Allergies are the reaction to something to which the patient is exposed. Allergens can range from dust and grass to medications to food items. Your major concern is medication allergies, but food allergies can be important because some medications originate from food items. For example, a shellfish allergy may coincide with an iodine allergy.

M—Medications

You will need to confirm whether your patient is taking medications. Medications include prescribed medications, over-the-counter medications, herbs, or any "recreational" or "street" drugs the patient may be taking. You need to confirm when the patient took the medication and how much the patient took.

Medications also may give you a clue to the patient's medical problems. For example, a "water pill" or furosemide (Lasix), which is a diuretic, may be taken for congestive heart failure. It is important that you see the name of the medication and write it down correctly because many names sound alike but are for different problems. Xanax (alprazolam) is a sedative for anxiety, and Zantac (ranitidine) is used to treat ulcers. Documenting or bringing a list with you of all the medications the patient takes is important because some medications may have interactions with currently taken drugs or drugs the patient may receive at the hospital.

P—Past Medical History

The patient's medical history is important to obtain because it may give you insight into problems to anticipate as you care for the patient. When you ask the patient for a history, be sure to ask about pertinent history. Information should be pertinent to the current problem. Knowing a patient had an appendectomy 10 years ago is important if he is complaining of abdominal pain but probably not important if the patient is complaining of a broken arm after a bicycle accident. You can identify pertinent history by asking if the patient is seeing a doctor for a medical condition, has had any recent medical problems, or has been hospitalized recently.

L—Last Oral Intake

Identifying what the patient last ate or drank is an important factor in the history. In diabetic patients, last oral intake may give you a clue to their blood sugar and level of response. If the patient requires surgery, the surgeon and anesthesiologist need to know this information. Last oral intake also may alert you to the potential for vomiting in your patient. Oral intake is also important in identifying dehydration in elderly and pediatric patients.

E—Events Preceding

Finding out what happened to the patient before you arrived can provide insightful clues as to the patient's condition. For example, knowing that an unconscious patient found on the ground outside fell off the roof would alter your assessment and treatment, just as finding that an ill child had been vomiting and had diarrhea for 2 days would influence how seriously you consider the child's illness. You should ask about mechanism of injury, nature of illness, and what happened before your arrival. If the patient is unable to communicate, look for anything that may provide a clue, such as damage to the vehicle, medication use, or poisoning exposure. You will be the eyes of the receiving crew or facility, so it will be important that you relay your findings to them.

■ BYSTANDER INFORMATION

Also important is to include family, friends, or bystanders in the collection of patient history. Patients may have a condition that alters their level of consciousness, so they may not be a reliable source of information. In children, parents may need to provide the information, so including them in the questioning process is important. As you collect the information, focus on the SAMPLE history and expand it as time allows.

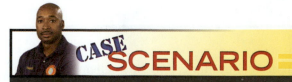

CASE SCENARIO
conclusion

The crew was finishing up the transfer of the patient at the hospital. The nurse who received the transfer came over to Jack and said, "The vital signs you took were accurate. We got the same information from the automated BP cuff, and more important, it was great to see the trending information about his blood pressure getting better as you transported him. I have no doubt that he was hypotensive when you first started with him." Jack thanked the nurse for the encouragement and feedback. He was also happy to see that the hospital took his information so seriously. ■

SPECIAL Populations

Cultural Consideration

Census data indicate that people of color (i.e., black, Asian or Pacific Islander, American Indian, Eskimo or Aleut, and Hispanic origin) are expected to compose a majority of the American population by the year 2020. Assessing skin color in the dark-skinned patient can be challenging. Assessing pallor, cyanosis, jaundice, and petechiae is best done in natural light. The emergency medical technician also can make use of the lips, oral mucosa, conjunctiva, palmar (palm) and plantar (sole of the foot) surfaces where the skin is lighter, and the nail beds.

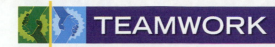

TEAMWORK

As discussed in this chapter, EMTs should be confident in obtaining and assessing the information obtained in baseline vital signs and history. Initially, this information may be received from family, friends, or first responders, and the clock will be ticking. How you interpret this information and establish subsequent care will make the difference in patient care.

Collecting vital signs and a history is one of the most important things you will do as part of a team process. The care providers will base their interventions and data collection on your initial findings. They will be using your baseline to determine whether the patient's condition is improving or deteriorating. They will expand their history-collecting information based on the history you collect. So, it is important for you not only to collect accurate information but also to relay that information. Documenting the information can be essential because a provider receiving the information may forget some of the information you provided, so it is important to write it down to prevent loss of information and loss of continuity of care. As you turn care over to another crew, they may ask you to continue to monitor vital signs as they initiate care. It is important that you do so accurately because processes such as medication administration or intubation may change the vital signs, so the ALS team will need to know immediately.

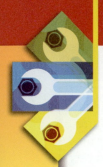

Critical Points

Vital signs represent the vital functions of the body and must be assessed accurately. Trends in vital signs help predict patient conditions. Extremely slow or extremely fast respiratory rates require immediate intervention. Noisy respirations indicate some type of airway compromise. Do not delay care for life-threatening injuries to obtain a blood pressure.

Learning Checklist

❏ After checking the patient's airway, breathing, and circulation, begin to collect more information about the patient. Vital signs consist of respirations; pulse; skin color, temperature, and condition; pupil size and response; and blood pressure.

❏ The trend or pattern in a patient's vital signs will provide clues about the care he or she needs. The first set of vital signs provides a baseline to compare with future vital signs.

❏ Assess respirations with regard to their rate, quality, and pattern. The normal respiratory rate for adults is 12 to 20 breaths per minute. Slow respirations suggest problems such as drug overdose, neurologic damage, or impending respiratory arrest. A rapid respiratory rate may be associated with stress, elevated temperatures, inadequate breathing, or toxic exposure.

❏ The four categories to describe the quality of respirations are normal, noisy, labored, or shallow. If a patient is breathing normally, you should not notice the breathing.

❏ Snoring is caused by the tongue falling back over the airway and partially obstructing it.

❏ Stridor is a high-pitched sound heard during inspiration when the upper airway is partially obstructed by swelling. Stridor often occurs in children with croup. Patients with stridor should receive high-flow humidified oxygen. Rapid transport and ALS should be considered because the airway may swell shut.

❏ Crowing is a loud, shrill sound heard on expiration and indicates swelling or obstruction of the upper airway. Crowing respirations may be associated with whooping cough and airway burns. Patients will need advanced care and should be transported as soon as possible and receive high-flow humidified oxygen.

❏ Gurgling is a bubbling or gargling that occurs when blood or fluids are present in the airway. Gurgling is usually present in a patient with a decreased level of consciousness. The patient may have trauma to the face and upper airway, causing blood, vomit, or saliva to collect in the airway, thereby causing the gurgling. Regardless of the cause, immediate suctioning, patient positioning, and airway management are indicated. A patient with gurgling has an increased risk of aspirating, or inhaling, the blood or fluids into the lungs and developing pneumonia or dying.

❏ Wheezing is a whistling sound heard when the lower airways are obstructed by swelling, foreign bodies, or bronchospasm. Wheezing suggests such problems as asthma, chronic obstructive pulmonary disease, anaphylaxis, and other problems associated with lower airway obstruction and swelling. These patients will need oxygen and medications, such as bronchodilators, to manage the wheezing. You may hear the wheezing without any equipment, but more often you will need a stethoscope to listen to the chest to detect wheezes.

❏ Grunting respirations are heard in infants who have difficulty breathing. You will hear a grunting sound each time they exhale. Infants do this to help keep their airways open at the end of each exhalation. Infants with grunting respirations should be considered in critical condition. They should receive high-flow oxygen and rapid transport to ALS care or an appropriate facility.

❏ Labored respirations occur when a patient is working hard to breathe. Oxygen administration or assisted respiration with a bag-valve-mask device should be considered for patients with labored breathing. Patients with difficulty breathing may be able to speak only one or two words without taking a breath.

❏ Respiratory patterns often are associated with brain injuries or metabolic states.

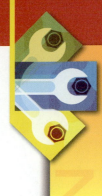

Apneustic respirations are deep respirations and periods of apnea; they are common in stroke patients. Ataxic (Biot's) respirations are irregular respirations commonly seen in stroke patients or patients with severe brain impairment. Cheyne-Stokes respirations follow a slow, shallow pattern that gradually increases in rate and depth and then decreases (a crescendo-decrescendo pattern), followed by apnea. Cheyne-Stokes respirations may be seen in stroke patients or metabolic conditions. Kussmaul's respirations are associated with diabetic ketoacidosis. Central neurogenic hyperventilation is associated most commonly with head trauma.

❑ The pulse is a reflection of heart function and circulation. When assessing the pulse, determine the rate, quality, and rhythm.

❑ The normal adult heart rate is 60 to 100 beats per minute. A heart rate greater than 150 in an adult suggests a cardiac problem.

❑ Quality is the strength of the pulse; it usually is described as strong or weak. A weak pulse represents compromised circulation from vascular disease, vascular trauma, or shock.

❑ Rhythm refers to the regularity of the pulse from beat to beat. A normal pulse is regular from beat to beat. An irregular pulse is one in which the beats occur at irregular intervals.

❑ The skin can provide a quick indication of the patient's status. Assess the skin by looking at and feeling the skin to determine color, temperature, condition, and capillary refill.

❑ The skin normally is classified as normal, pale, flushed (red), cyanotic (blue), jaundiced (yellow), or mottled (splotched). Skin color can be difficult to assess on patients with dark skin. Use the lips or palms of the hands to assess for color.

❑ Normal skin temperature is warm. Cold skin suggests hypothermia. Hot skin is present in hyperthermia or in patients with fever.

❑ Normal skin is dry. Moist, sweaty skin is present in patients who are sweating from exertion or have an elevated temperature. Shock also can cause moist skin. Dehydrated patients may have very dry skin that "tents" or stays pinched up when the skin is pinched gently. Edematous (swollen) skin is caused by too much fluid.

❑ Capillary refill is assessed by pressing on the skin until the color leaves the area and then releasing the pressure and counting how many seconds until the normal skin color returns. Delayed capillary refill is a sign of decreased circulation to the area caused by vascular disease.

❑ The pupils are assessed for shape, equality, and response/reaction to light. Both pupils should be the same size and should constrict equally when you shine a light into them.

❑ The systolic blood pressure is the higher number; it represents the pressure in the vessels when the heart beats. The diastolic pressure is the lower number and represents the pressure when the heart relaxes.

❑ Blood pressure is determined by auscultation (listening with a stethoscope when the blood pressure cuff is applied) or palpation (feeling for the pulse when the blood pressure cuff is applied. Only systolic pressure can be palpated. Palpated pressure is documented as X/P, where X is the systolic pressure).

❑ The SAMPLE history is useful for determining a patient history: S, signs and symptoms; A, allergies; M, medications; P, past medical history; L, last oral intake; E, events preceding.

❑ Family, friends, or bystanders can be helpful in the collection of a patient's history. Parents may need to provide history information for children.

❑ Assessing pallor, cyanosis, jaundice, and petechiae is best done in natural light, particularly in people of color. The EMT also can use the lips, oral mucosa, conjunctiva, palmar (palm) and plantar (sole of the foot) surfaces, and nail beds, where the skin is lighter.

Key Terms

Auscultation To listen with a stethoscope.

Accessory muscles Muscles of the anterior neck and intercostal spaces that pull the anterior portion of the rib cage upward and outward, expanding intrathoracic volume. Use of these muscles often signifies respiratory distress.

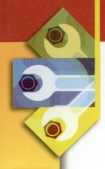

NUTS AND BOLTS

Apneustic respirations Respiratory pattern represented by long, deep breaths with periods of apnea between each breath.

Ataxic respirations Respiratory pattern represented by irregularly shallow and deep respirations with no pattern. Also known as Biot's respirations.

Blood pressure The pressure the blood exerts against the walls of the blood vessels.

Brachial artery The major artery of the upper arm.

Brachial pulse The pulse felt over the brachial artery in the upper arm.

Capillary refill The time it takes for the capillary bed to refill after it is compressed and the pressure is released.

Carotid pulse The pulse felt on either side of the neck.

Central neurogenic hyperventilation Respiratory pattern represented by continuous deep breaths; the rate may be slow or fast.

Cheyne-Stokes respirations Respiratory pattern represented by respirations that start slow and shallow and increase in rate and depth and then decrease in rate and depth with periods of apnea between.

Constrict To decrease in size or get smaller.

Crowing High, shrill sound heard during breathing.

Cyanosis Blue discoloration of the skin signifying poor oxygen delivery to the tissues. The oxygen-carrying molecule in red blood cells, hemoglobin, takes on a bluish color when not bound to oxygen. Thus when a high proportion of hemoglobin in the blood delivered to the tissues is not bound to oxygen, the tissues appear blue.

Diastolic pressure The pressure applied to the blood vessels during the relaxation phase of cardiac contractions. Represented as the bottom number of a blood pressure reading.

Dilate To increase in size or get larger.

Grunting A gruntlike sound heard at the end of respirations. Common in infants with respiratory distress.

Gurgling When a patient attempts to breathe, a sound made from the accumulation of fluids in the airway.

History Information gathered about a patient's medical condition.

Jaundice A yellowish color to the skin caused by liver disease.

Kussmaul's respirations Respiratory pattern represented by continuous deep breaths; the rate may be slow or fast. Associated with diabetic ketoacidosis.

Labored respirations Difficulty breathing represented by the use of accessory muscles and an increase in the work of breathing.

Mottled Having a blotchy skin appearance caused by decreased circulation.

Palpation To feel for injuries during patient assessment.

Pulse Measurement of the heart's contractions; can be felt anywhere an artery is close to the skin surface, overlying a bony structure.

Pulse rate The number of times the heart beats in 1 minute.

Pupil The black center or opening into the eye.

Radial pulse The pulse felt on the thumb side of the wrist.

Respiration The physiologic process by which oxygen that is drawn into the lungs is delivered to tissues and cells throughout the body and is exchanged for the waste products of cell metabolism.

Respiratory rate The number of times a patient breathes in 1 minute.

SAMPLE The mnemonic used to assist in collecting a patient history (S, signs and symptoms; A, allergies; M, medications; P, past medical history; L, last oral intake; E, events preceding).

Sign A patient finding you can see, feel, hear, smell, or measure.

Snoring The noise made during breathing as the tongue partially obstructs the airway.

Sphygmomanometer The cuff and gauge used to measure the blood pressure.

Stridor A high-pitched, harsh respiratory sound during inspiration that is a sign of upper airway obstruction.

Symptom A patient finding that the patient describes, such as pain. It cannot be observed or measured by another person.

Systolic pressure The pressure applied to the blood vessels during the contraction phase of the cardiac cycle. Represented as the top number of a blood pressure reading.

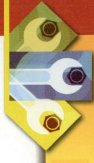

Trend The collection of several vital signs readings and comparing of the values for patterns.

Vital signs The specific measurements or assessments of a patient's skin, breathing, pulse, blood pressure, and pupil size and response

Wheezing High-pitched expiratory breath sounds caused by narrowing of the small air passages (bronchioles) in the lungs that most commonly is a result of an acute asthmatic episode.

National Standard Curriculum Objectives

Cognitive Objectives

After completing this lesson, the EMT student will be able to do the following:

- Identify the components of vital signs.
- Describe the methods to obtain a breathing rate.
- Identify the attributes that should be obtained when assessing breathing.
- Differentiate among shallow, labored, and noisy breathing.
- Describe the methods to obtain a pulse rate.
- Identify the information obtained when assessing a patient's pulse.
- Differentiate among strong, weak, regular, and irregular pulses.
- Describe the methods to assess the skin color, temperature, and condition (capillary refill in infants and children).
- Identify the normal and abnormal skin colors.
- Differentiate among pale, blue, red, and yellow skin.
- Identify the normal and abnormal skin temperature.
- Differentiate among hot, cool, and cold skin.
- Identify normal and abnormal skin conditions.
- Identify normal and abnormal capillary refill in infants and children.
- Describe the methods to assess the pupils.
- Identify normal and abnormal pupil size.
- Differentiate between dilated (big) and constricted (small) pupil size.

- Differentiate between reactive and nonreactive pupils and equal and unequal pupils.
- Describe the methods to assess blood pressure.
- Define systolic pressure.
- Define diastolic pressure.
- Explain the difference between auscultation and palpation for obtaining a blood pressure.
- Identify the components of the SAMPLE history.
- Differentiate between a sign and a symptom.
- State the importance of accurately reporting and recording the baseline vital signs.
- Discuss the need to search for additional medical identification.

Affective Objectives

After completing this lesson, the EMT student will be able to do the following:

- Explain the value of performing the baseline vital signs.
- Recognize and respond to the feelings patients experience during assessment.
- Defend the need for obtaining and recording an accurate set of vital signs.
- Explain the rationale of recording additional sets of vital signs.
- Explain the importance of obtaining a SAMPLE history.

Psychomotor Objectives

After completing this lesson, the EMT student will be able to do the following:

- Demonstrate the skills involved in assessment of breathing.
- Demonstrate the skills associated with obtaining a pulse.
- Demonstrate the skills associated with assessing the skin color, temperature, condition, and capillary refill time in infants and children.
- Demonstrate the skills associated with assessing the pupils.
- Demonstrate the skills associated with obtaining blood pressure.
- Demonstrate the skills that should be used to obtain information from the patient, family, or bystanders at the scene.

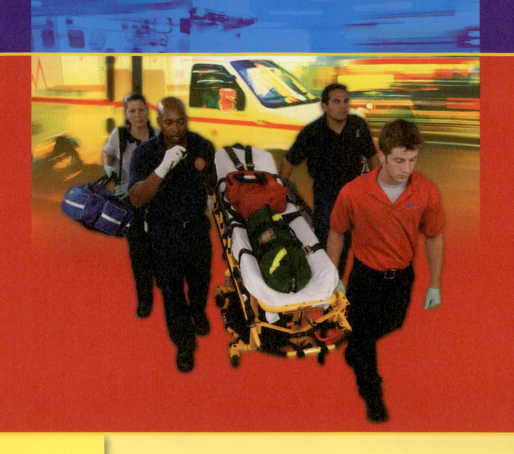

CHAPTER

6

OUTLINE

LESSON GOAL

This chapter focuses on the correct techniques, equipment, and positioning for moving a patient safely and effectively in a variety of situations and locations. ■

GOAL

Lifting and Moving Patients

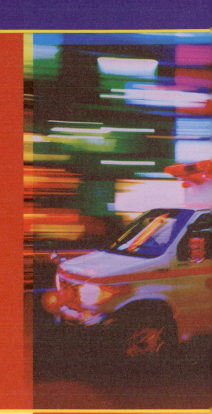

CHAPTER OBJECTIVES

After completing this chapter, the EMT student will be able to do the following:

1 Define body mechanics.
2 Discuss the importance of safety in lifting or moving a patient.
3 Identify the situations in which an emergency move is indicated.
4 Identify the situations in which a nonemergency move is indicated.
5 Understand the importance of patient positioning, the various types of patient positioning, and the indications for each type.
6 Discuss the importance of patient safety restraints.
7 Discuss the various types of transportation devices used in moving patients in the prehospital environment.
8 Demonstrate the various emergency moves.
9 Demonstrate the various nonemergency moves.
10 Demonstrate patient positioning based on the patient's condition.
11 Discuss the importance of patient safety restraints.
12 Select and demonstrate the use of the various types of equipment used to move patients in the prehospital environment.

6

OBJECTIVES

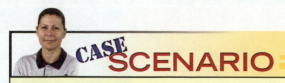

CASE SCENARIO

"How will you get me down those stairs?" Louise asked Elizabeth, her voice filled with fear and pain.

Elizabeth smiled and patted Louise's hand. "You let us worry about that, Mrs. Greenbaum. We have equipment that will help us get you down those stairs safely."

Louise had fallen earlier in the day, stumbling over a loose rug in the hallway. Landing on her right side, she could feel her hip pop and a sudden searing pain that went down her right leg. She tried to sit up, but the pain only got worse. The downstairs neighbor heard her calling out for help

and called 911 and then helped the ambulance crew enter the apartment by using a key. Once inside, Elizabeth quickly determined that Mrs. Greenbaum apparently has dislocated her right hip during her fall. They would need to extricate the patient down two flights of narrow stairs while the patient had to remain lying flat.

Question: Will Mrs. Greenbaum need to be moved urgently? Given the situation, what would you consider using to bring Mrs. Greenbaum safely down the stairs as comfortably as possible?

THE ROLE OF THE EMERGENCY MEDICAL TECHNICIAN

The goal of emergency medical services intervention is the delivery of the patient to definitive care. Therefore the emergency medical technician (EMT) must possess the knowledge and ability to perform the lifts, moves, carries, and drags necessary to meet this goal. This chapter focuses specifically on **emergency moves, nonemergency moves,** patient positioning, and the equipment used by the EMT in lifting and moving patients. Understanding, practicing, and mastering this miniarsenal of skills will go a long way in protecting the patient and the rescuers from unnecessary additional injuries or worse.

LIFTING AND MOVING PATIENTS SAFELY

Body Mechanics

One of the most common injuries incurred by emergency medical services responders while on the job is back strain. Often such injuries are the result of improper lifting and moving techniques. The safest and most effective way to use your body while lifting or moving a patient is referred to as using **body mechanics**. Using proper body mechanics and considering a few simple questions can help protect you and your partner when you attempt to move a patient:

- Is the patient accessible?
- Can my partner and I lift or move the weight of the patient?
- Can my partner and I safely overcome the obstacles or terrain while we are moving the patient?

If the answer to any of these questions is "no," or if the EMT feels unsure, it is always best to get additional help for moving a patient.

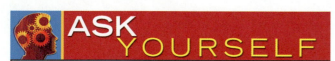

ASK YOURSELF

You and your partner are dispatched to a home for a patient with difficulty breathing. You find the patient, a 60-year-old man who weighs approximately 240 lb (110 kg), sitting on a chair in the tripod position and complaining of shortness of breath that started about 15 minutes ago. You complete your patient's medical history, assessment, and treatment and wish to move the patient to your collapsed wheeled stretcher, which you have placed next to the patient. What technique would you use to move this patient? In what position would you place the patient? Why is patient positioning important?

Principles of Lifting and Moving

To protect himself or herself and safely move a patient, the EMT should always follow these guidelines while lifting or moving patients:

- Avoid reaching more than 20 inches in front of you.
- Avoid reaching for a prolonged amount of time.
- When possible, push something, rather than pull it.
- Use your legs and *not* your back to lift. Bend at the knees and use the stronger muscles of the legs instead of the weaker back muscles (Fig. 6-1).
- Keep the weight of what you are lifting as close to your body as possible (Fig. 6-2).
- Move your body as a single unit.
- When carrying a patient up a flight of stairs, carry the patient head first. While going down stairs, carry the patient feet first.

- If possible, have backup help available to maneuver a patient through difficult terrain, past obstacles, or up or down stairways.

■ LIFTS, DRAGS, TAKEDOWNS, AND CARRIES

Wheeled Stretcher Operations

The wheeled stretcher (Fig. 6-3) is the most common means of transporting the patient to definitive care.

Hand position plays an important role in controlling the stretcher while hoisting or lowering. The **power grip** is the most effective way to accomplish this control. To hoist or lower the stretcher, place the hands approximately 10 inches apart, with the palms up and the fingers completely wrapped around the lift bar (Fig. 6-4).

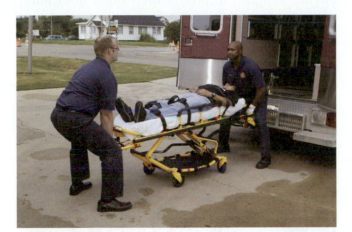

Fig. 6-1 Bend at the knees and remember to lift with the leg muscles and *not* the back muscles.

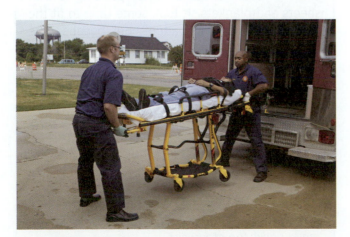

Fig. 6-2 Keep the weight of what you are lifting as close to your body as possible.

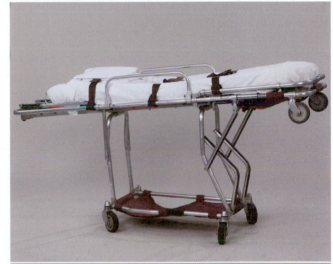

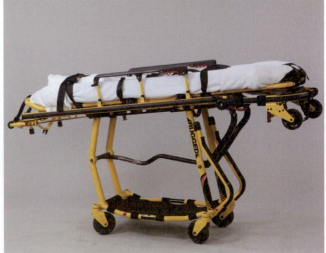

Fig. 6-3 Wheeled stretchers.

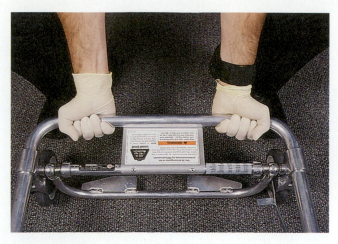

Fig. 6-4 Power grip for hoisting a stretcher.

The **power lift** is the safest and most effective way to lift a heavy object using proper body mechanics. While performing the power lift, it is important to remember to do the following:

- Keep your back locked and tighten your abdominal muscles.
- Feet should be shoulder-width apart and comfortably secure.
- Keep the lift as vertical as possible to avoid bending at the waist.

Skill 6-1 details the step-by-step process of the **head and foot method** using the power grip and power lift to hoist the stretcher from its down position. Skill 6-2 shows the **side-to-side method** for lifting a stretcher using the power grip and power lift. This same technique can be used while lifting or lowering a backboard or other similar device. These tools will be discussed later in this chapter.

Emergency Moves

Just as the name implies, emergency moves are techniques designed to move a patient from an unsafe environment in which additional injury to the patient, or injury to the EMTs, could result. Situations that merit an emergency move include the following:

- Fire or threat of fire
- Violence or threat of violence
- Explosives or the danger of explosion
- Imminent collapse of a structure
- Other hazards such as traffic, electrical, or chemical

The EMT also could encounter situations that are not immediately dangerous to the patient or himself or herself but still require an emergency move to provide adequate care:

- A patient in critical condition in a confined space in which there is not enough room to work.
- A patient in critical condition positioned in such a way as to prevent effective care. For example, a patient in cardiac arrest sitting in a chair needs to be moved to a hard, flat surface in a supine position.
- A patient in noncritical condition who must be moved in order to gain access to a patient who is in critical condition. This usually occurs at the scene of a motor vehicle collision.

These situations, and possibly others, require the EMT to make quick decisions regarding moving the patient. The EMT must remember that these moves are not designed to protect the patient from injury and may cause additional pain to the patient. Rather, these moves are designed only for situations in which there is a threat to life unless the patient is moved to a safer environment.

Drags

Emergency drags can be modified for one- or two-rescuer use depending on the circumstances. For ex-

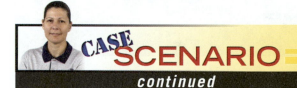

CASE SCENARIO
continued

The crew carefully moved Mrs. Greenbaum on the orthopedic stretcher, after padding it with sheets and blankets. It took some time to fit the stretcher around the patient, but because she had stable vital signs and no other major injury that required rapid transport, Elizabeth decided that it was critical to minimize the patient's pain and fears before and during the extrication process.

With the final straps in place, the crew prepared to lift Mrs. Greenbaum and maneuver themselves down the stairway.

Question: _If you were part of the crew, what are some lifting techniques to keep in mind as you move down the stairway?_

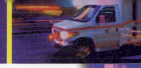

SKILL 6-1
◎ *Power Lift: Head and Foot Method*

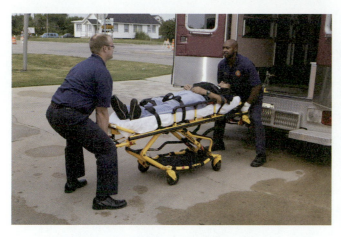

1. Emergency medical technicians using proper body mechanics and power grip to hoist stretcher. Remember to lift with your LEGS and *not* your BACK.

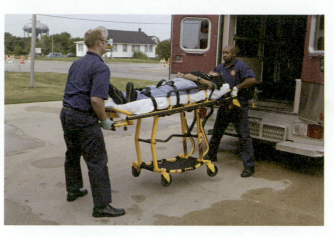

2. Simultaneously lift the stretcher until you hear it lock into place.

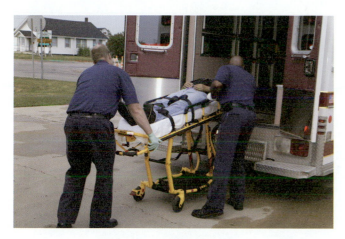

3. One emergency medical technician pushes the stretcher into the ambulance while the other guides it to the locking mechanism.

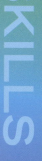

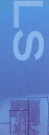

SKILL 6-2
Power Lift: Side-to-Side Method

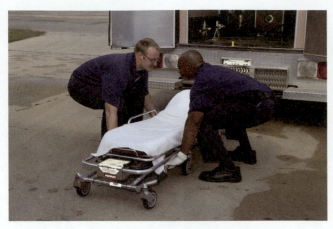

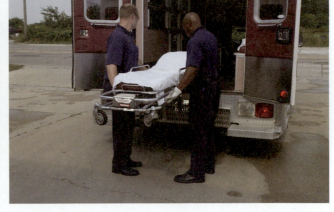

1. Some stretchers require the emergency medical technicians to be positioned on the sides of the stretcher instead of the head and foot.
2. Remember to lift with your legs and *not* your back.

3. While loading the stretcher into the ambulance, use a "shuffle step" and do not cross one leg over the other because this will cause twisting of the back.

ample, in the event of multiple patients, each EMT may be required to move a patient on his or her own, whereas a single patient could be moved by two EMTs. In either case, it is important to stabilize the head and neck of the patient as much as possible during the drag. Time may prohibit the use of a cervical collar and long backboard. Thus the EMT must remember to move the body as a single unit as much as possible. While moving the patient, the EMT also must remember to move along the long axis (length) of the patient. Skill 6-3 demonstrates several emergency drags one or two EMTs could use.

Carries

A **carry**, as the name implies, involves supporting part or all of the patient's weight while moving him or her. For this reason, it is recommended that two rescuers carry the patient. Granted, a patient could be carried by a single rescuer, provided that rescuer could support the weight of the patient adequately and safely while moving. Skill 6-4 demonstrates a variety of one- and two-person carries.

Standing Backboard Techniques

The **standing backboard techniques** can be qualified as emergency moves and as nonemergency moves, depending on the presenting situation. For example, a patient found standing in the middle of an area that just sustained an explosion needs to be removed quickly while protecting the patient's spine. This qualifies as an emergency move. However, the patient found out of his or her vehicle, walking around the scene of a motor vehicle collision but complaining of head and neck pain, would not fall necessarily into the category of a true emergency move. In this instance, the patient may have sustained a spinal injury. To have the patient sit or lie on the wheeled stretcher when he or she is found standing is inappropriate. Asking a patient to sit or lie changes the patient's center of gravity and could transform a minor injury into a major one. For this reason, *any* patient found standing after a motor vehicle collision *and* complaining of head, neck, or back pain or with signs of a position mechanism of injury should be placed on a backboard while standing.

The concept and skills of complete spinal immobilization will be covered later in this text. In the context of this chapter, however, when simply moving the patient from one point to another, the EMT must remember that his or her primary consideration is to remove the patient from the dangerous environment first and *then* to immobilize the patient completely once he or she is in a safe area. The EMT must realize that the skills shown in this chapter only minimally protect the integrity of the spine. The technique for applying a backboard to a patient who is standing is demonstrated in Chapter 29.

Rapid Extrication

Occasionally, the EMT is faced with having to care for a patient in critical condition in a confined space (e.g., inside a vehicle). The extrication devices, shown later in this chapter, are time-consuming to apply and should be used only on a stable patient. When faced with an unstable patient when time is critical, when a safe scene is becoming unsafe, or when a stable patient must be moved to attend to a more seriously injured patient, the EMT should rely on **rapid extrication.** Rapid extrication is the quick but safe manner to remove a patient from an area to provide meaningful intervention. Rapid extrication can be performed with two or more rescuers. The technique for three-person rapid extrication is shown in Chapter 29.

Nonemergency Moves

Nonemergency moves are performed when there is no immediate threat to the patient's life or the safety of the patient and the rescuers. Nonemergency moves are those used most often by EMTs in the course of their work. These moves include transferring a patient from his or her own bed to the stretcher, from the ground to the stretcher or backboard, and from the wheeled stretcher to the hospital gurney. The decision of which move to use, once again, depends on the presenting situation. If the EMTs feel that the patient's spine has not been compromised, then the direct ground lift or logroll without spinal precautions should be used, depending on whether the patient is prone or supine. Skills 6-5, 6-6, 6-7, and 6-8 demonstrate the various nonemergency moves. If the potential for spinal involvement exists, then the logroll using spinal precautions should be used. See Chapter 29 for additional skills involving spinal precautions.

■ TRANSPORTING PATIENTS SAFELY

Once definitive prehospital care has been given, the next goal of emergency medical services is the safe delivery of the patient to an appropriate facility. Not only should the EMT be aware of the medical needs

SKILL 6-3
One- and Two-Rescuer Emergency Drags

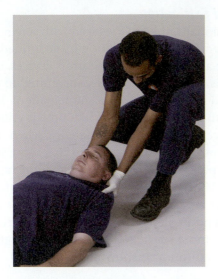

One-person clothing drag.

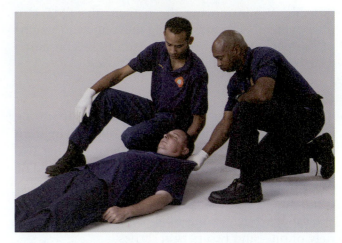

Two-person clothing drag.

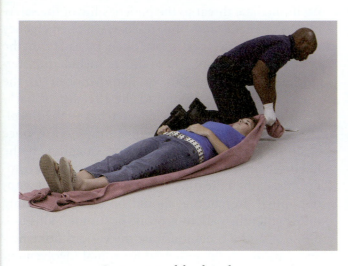

One-person blanket drag.

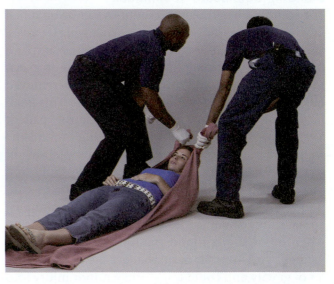

Two-person blanket drag.

SKILL 6-3
One- and Two-Rescuer Emergency Drags—continued

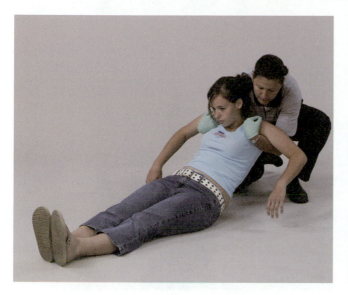

One-person upper extremity drag.

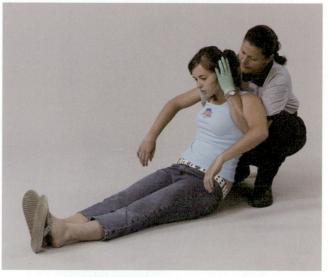

One-person modified upper extremity drag.

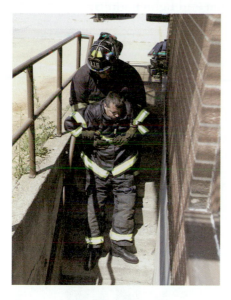

Incline drag.

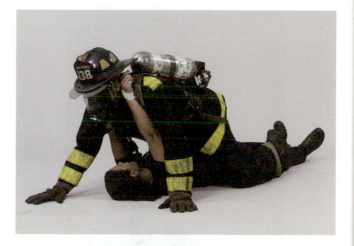

Firefighter's drag.

SKILLS

SKILL 6-4
One- and Two-Person Carries

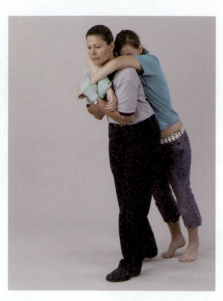

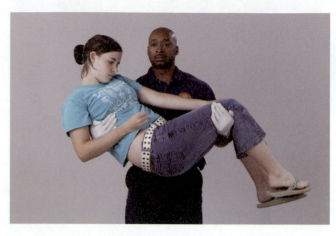

Pack strap carry. The emergency medical technician grasps the patient's arms around his or her neck and pulls the patient onto his or her back.

One-person cradle carry. This carry should be used on children and lighter adults.

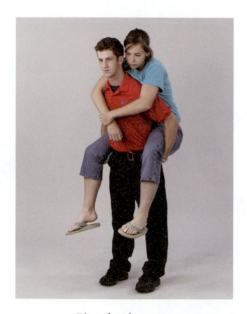

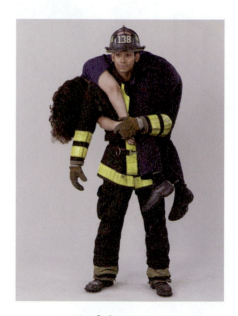

Piggyback carry.

Firefighter carry.

SKILL 6-4
One- and Two-Person Carries—continued

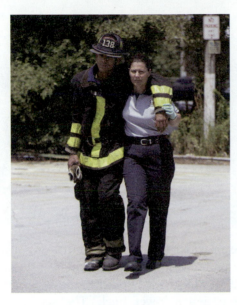

One-person assist. Support and steady the patient by grasping the patient's hand and supporting the patient with the emergency medical technician's other arm.

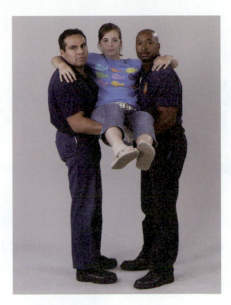

Two-person cradle carry. Not only can this carry be used to move a patient to safety, but also it can be used to move a patient from a sitting position.

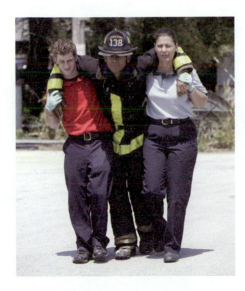

Two-person assist. Each emergency medical technician must have a firm grasp of the patient's wrist.

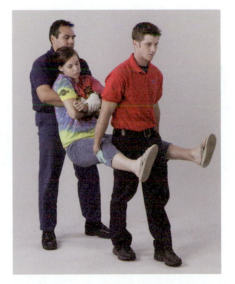

Two-person extremity carry. In an emergency situation, a patient can be carried down a flight of stairs or an incline. Remember to carry the patient feet first.

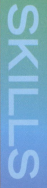

SKILL 6-5
◉ Direct Ground Lift*

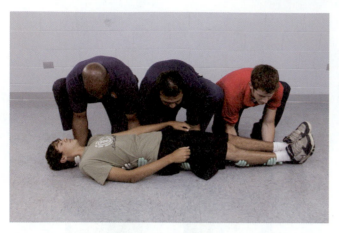

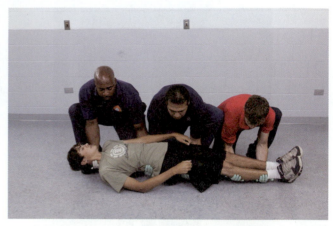

1. Two or three providers line up on one side of the patient. Providers kneel on one knee (preferably the same for all providers).

2. The provider at the head places one arm under the patient's neck and shoulder and cradles the patient's head while placing the other arm under the patient's lower back. The second provider places one arm under the patient's knees and the other under the patient's lower legs. The third provider places arms above and below the waist.

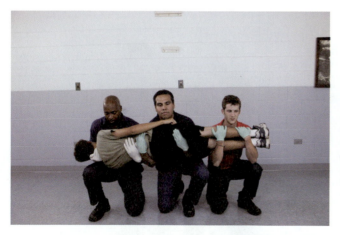

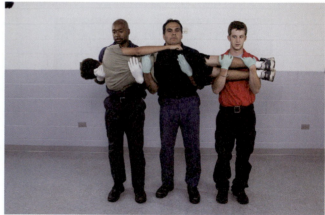

3. On signal, the rescuers lift the patient to their knees and roll the patient in toward their chests.

4. On signal the rescuers stand and move the patient.

5. To lower the patient, the steps are reversed.

---

*NOTE: The direct ground lift should be used only on lighter patients who have no suspected spinal injury. A minimum of three providers is necessary.

SKILLS

SKILL 6-6
Extremity Lift

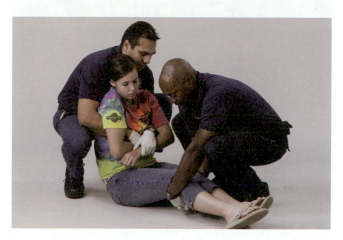

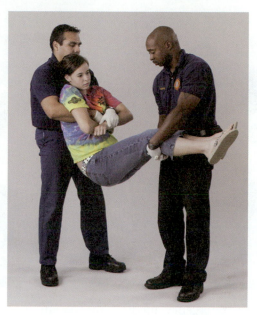

1. One provider kneels at the patient's head and another kneels at the patient's side by the knees. The provider at the head places one hand under each of the patient's shoulders and grasps the patient's wrists. The provider at the foot slips his or her hands under the patient's knees. Both providers move up to a crouching position.

2. The providers stand up simultaneously and move with the patient.

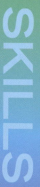

SKILLS

SKILL 6-7
● Draw Sheet Transfer

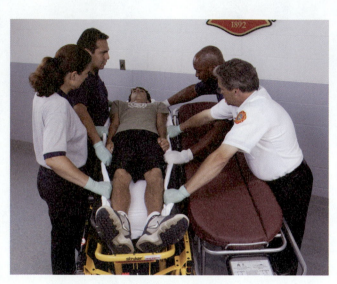

1. Two emergency medical technicians positioned on each side of the patient roll the edges of the sheet.

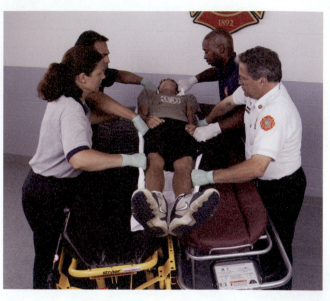

2. Lifting together on a three count, the technicians lift and move the patient to the adjacent bed or stretcher.

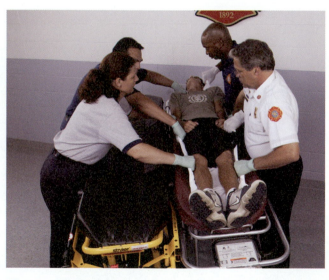

3. The patient is lowered gently onto the adjacent bed or stretcher.

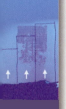

SKILLS

SKILL 6-8

◎ *Logroll with No Suspected Spine Injury*

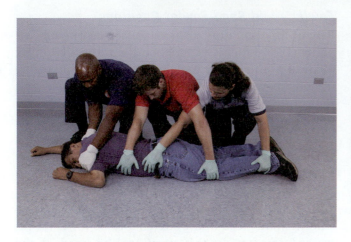

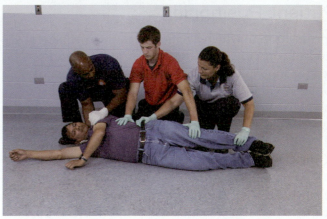

1. The three providers line up on the same side of the patient and are down on one or two knees. The provider at the head grasps the patient's arms and shoulders. The middle provider grasps the patient's torso and upper leg while the provider at the feet grasps the patient's feet and hips.

2. On the count of the person at the head, the providers roll the patient as a single unit toward themselves. From this position the patient's anterior can be assessed or the patient can be rolled completely over to a supine position.

of the patient, but also he or she should be aware of the patient's need for comfort and safety during the transport phase of the call. Patient positioning, depending on the patient's particular needs, and the use of safety restraint devices fulfill those needs.

Patient Positioning

The position in which a patient is found, the patient's level of consciousness, the type of mechanism of illness or injury, and how the patient feels most comfortable will determine how the EMTs will transport the patient. The EMT must know how to position a patient for transport because it is an important part of the documentation record on the narrative portion of the patient run sheet. For example, "Transported the patient in the position of comfort," tells the nurse or physician that the patient not only was cared for properly but also was made as comfortable as possible during transport.

Position of Comfort

Unless a patient has a specific condition that warrants transporting in a particular way (e.g., an immobilized patient), the best way to transport a conscious patient is in the **position of comfort.** The EMT must possess effective communication skills in order to assist the patient in finding that most comfortable position. Fig. 6-5 shows a patient with an isolated wrist injury that has been splinted, and the patient is being transported in the position of comfort.

Recovery Position

When treating an unconscious patient, protecting the patient's airway is of primary concern because the patient is not capable of protecting it. The **recovery po-** sition (Fig. 6-6) is the best method for the EMT to accomplish this protection. The recovery position allows the EMT access to the patient's airway and will assist in removing possible obstructions, such as blood or vomit.

Fowler's and Semi-Fowler Positions

Patients in respiratory distress, nauseated or vomiting patients, or patients experiencing dizziness or other medical problems are most often comfortable sitting upright in varying degrees while being treated and transported. For patients being treated and transported in the **Fowler's position**, the head of the wheeled stretcher is elevated to 45 to 60 degrees. This is the most common position for transporting patients in respiratory distress. Fig. 6-7 shows a patient being transported in the Fowler's position.

The **semi-Fowler position** is for those patients who wish the head of the stretcher to be lower for increased comfort. In this position, the head of the wheeled stretcher is raised to 30 degrees. Fig. 6-8 shows a patient in the semi-Fowler position.

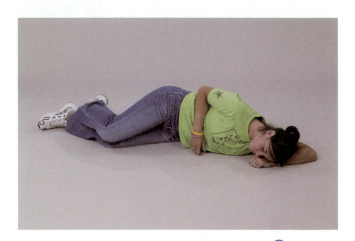

Fig. 6-6 Recovery position.

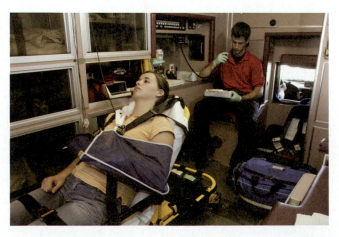

Fig. 6-5 Placing a patient in the position of comfort may make an unpleasant situation more tolerable and less painful.

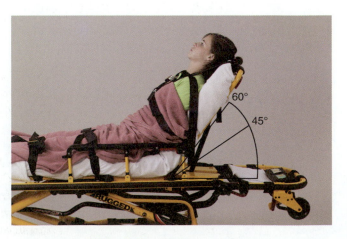

Fig. 6-7 Fowler's position.

Laterally Recumbent Position

Certain medical conditions, discussed later in this text, require a patient to be transported on his or her side, with the head of the stretcher flat. Often patients also will feel more comfortable while lying on their side, often with their knees bent upward. This position of transport is called the **laterally recumbent position**. This position is documented by the side on which a patient is lying: left laterally recumbent or right laterally recumbent. Fig. 6-9 shows a patient being transported in the left laterally recumbent position.

Patient Safety Restraints

Most states require some form of safety restraint device while transporting adult and pediatric patients, whether they are on the wheeled stretcher or the bench seat of the ambulance. Wheeled stretchers should have three restraint straps: one for the chest that should be secure but not so tight as to prevent adequate expansion of the patient's chest, one at the waist, and one at the legs (Fig. 6-10).

Pediatric patients should be transported in an approved child restraint seat (Fig. 6-11). If a child is found in a restraint seat (e.g., at the scene of a motor vehicle collision), it is appropriate for the EMT to remove the seat from the vehicle with the child in it to transport him or her, provided the seat is not damaged.

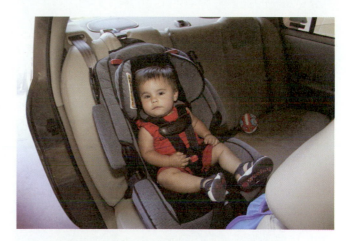

Fig. 6-10 A patient safely secured for transport.

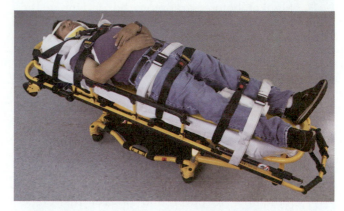

Fig. 6-11 Approved child restraint seat.

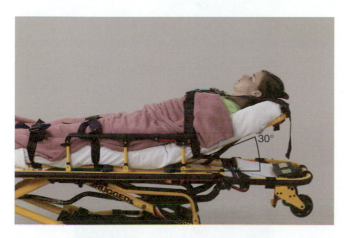

Fig. 6-8 Semi-Fowler position.

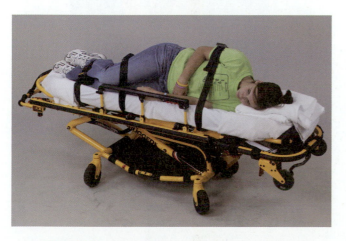

Fig. 6-9 Left laterally recumbent position.

SPECIAL Populations

Pediatric Consideration

In most states, child restraint laws do not exclude ambulances. When transporting a child who falls within the scope of the law, the child must be in an approved car seat unless the child cannot be seated because of treatment or immobilization issues. A car seat can be belted onto the stretcher or the attendant seat. Many ambulances carry an inflatable car seat for this purpose, or you also can use a car seat the child's family may have in their car.

SPECIAL Considerations

Whenever possible, first place an open blanket in the stair chair, and then place the patient onto the chair. Wrap the blanket around the patient with the patient's arms under the blanket before strapping the patient in the chair. This will prevent the patient from "helping you" by grabbing the railing and also will help you lift the patient from the chair to your stretcher.

SPECIAL Considerations

When moving patients who are immobilized, remember to cover and protect their face from rain, snow, and bright sun.

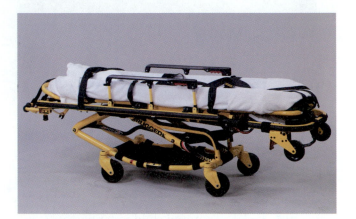

Fig. 6-12 Wheeled stretcher.

■ TRANSPORTATION DEVICES

Emergency medical technicians have a variety of equipment available to them to assist in lifting and moving patients. Local protocol generally dictates what equipment is available and in what situations the equipment can be used. The EMT should become familiar with the operation and use of all the

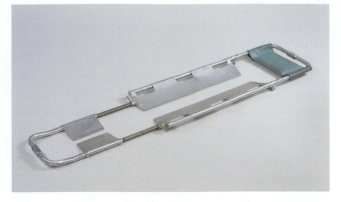

Fig. 6-13 Scoop stretcher.

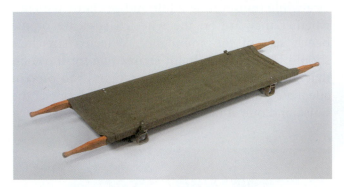

Fig. 6-14 Portable stretcher.

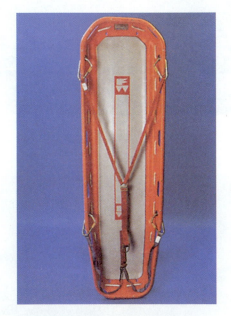

Fig. 6-15 Basket stretcher.

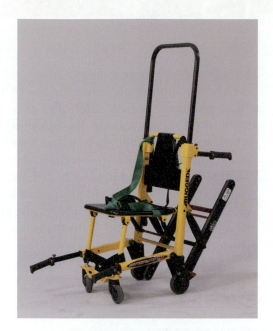

Fig. 6-16 Stair chair.

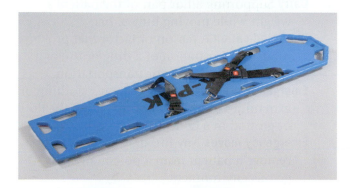

Fig. 6-17 Long backboard and straps.

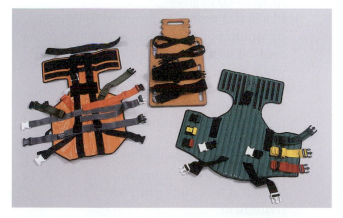

Fig. 6-18 Short backboard and straps and vest-type extrication devices.

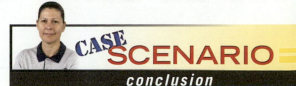

CASE SCENARIO

conclusion

Inside the ambulance, Mrs. Greenbaum relaxed noticeably. Although her hip still hurt, it was better than before and she realized that the crew worked hard at making her feel as comfortable and safe as possible while being carried down the stairs. The crew even made sure that the apartment was locked and let the neighbor know to which hospital she was being transported. ■

TEAMWORK

Teamwork is essential in the lifting and moving of patients. Whether a single patient is being transported by two EMTs or multiple patients are being transported by several ambulances, even from different agencies, working together is critical in maintaining the safety of the rescuers and the patients. Assistance from fire or police personnel, or even bystanders on the street, could greatly aid the EMTs responding to a situation. The responding EMTs must remember, though, that *they* are responsible for the patient's care. Therefore they should exercise due caution in assigning roles to anyone who is not trained to their level.

equipment available, not only during the initial training but also once the EMT has been in the field for a time. Frequent review and training with equipment will increase the confidence of the EMT in using the equipment. Review and training also will ensure that the patient receives the best possible care during transport in times of need. Figs. 6-12 to 6-18 show common equipment. During the skills labs associated with the EMT training, the instructor will demonstrate the use of each piece of equipment.

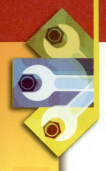

NUTS AND BOLTS

Critical Points

Think before you move! Ask yourself, "Is the scene safe?" "What is the patient's condition? Critical? Noncritical?" "Can my partner and I safely and effectively move this patient by ourselves? If so, how should we move the patient?" The ultimate goal of emergency medical services is to deliver the patient safely, stabilized to the best of the EMTs' abilities, to an appropriate facility. As such, the EMT has many responsibilities in caring for patients. Knowing *if, when,* and *how* to move a patient and deliver him or her to appropriate care is an integral part of the overall outcome of the patient. The EMT *must* be able to answer these questions *and* use the appropriate methods and equipment to accomplish this goal.

Learning Checklist

❑ The EMT must be able to identify whether a scene is safe for entry.

❑ An accurate initial assessment is crucial in determining whether the patient is critical or noncritical. A patient in critical condition must be moved in a more expeditious manner than one in a noncritical condition.

❑ Knowledge of proper body mechanics is essential in order to protect the EMT from injuring himself or herself while on a call.

❑ The most frequently used piece of transportation equipment is the wheeled stretcher. The EMT must be familiar with whatever product he or she is using. The EMT must know how to raise and lower the stretcher. In addition to the operation of the stretcher, the EMT must know how to use proper body mechanics in operating it.

❑ The EMT can choose from a variety of lifts, carries, and drags. The EMT must be able to determine which one to use and how to execute each one effectively and safely. The decision of which one to use is based on the situation. The EMT must decide whether an emergency move is indicated, or if there is no imminent danger, whether a nonemergency move should be used. The EMT also must decide whether the patient should be extricated rapidly from the vehicle. The EMT must

be able to make those determinations and execute the appropriate corresponding actions.

❑ To transport the patient safely and effectively, the EMT must know the position in which to transport the patient and how to secure the patient safely before transport.

❑ The EMT must be familiar with and proficiently use *all* the transportation equipment available to him or her. The EMT must know which device to use and its **indications** and **contraindications**.

Key Terms

Body mechanics The most effective way to use your body to lift or move a patient.

Carry Supporting all or part of the patient's weight while moving him or her.

Contraindication A reason or factor that prohibits administration of a drug or use of a method of treatment or transportation.

Emergency drags Using the patient's clothing or extremities to pull him or her along the floor or ground in a critical situation.

Emergency moves Any lift, drag, or carry to remove a patient from a potentially dangerous environment.

Fowler's position Placing a patient on a wheeled stretcher with the head of the stretcher raised to 45 to 60 degrees.

Head and foot method Hoisting or lowering a transportation device where one emergency medical technician is at the patient's head while the other is at the patient's feet.

Indication Conditions in which administering a specific drug or using a specific treatment or mode of transportation may benefit the patient.

Laterally recumbent position Placing the patient on his or her side. A patient lying on his or her left side is said to be "left laterally recumbent."

Nonemergency moves Any lift, drag, or carry used when the scene is safe or the patient is not in critical condition.

Position of comfort Placing the patient in his or her most comfortable position when there is no need for emergency procedures such as immobilization.

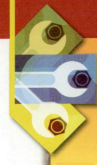

Power grip The correct hand placement for hoisting or lowering a transportation device. For hoisting, the hands should be spaced approximately 10 inches apart, with the fingers facing up. For lowering, the hands should be spaced the same distance apart, with the fingers facing down.

Power lift The most effective way to lift a heavy object.

Rapid extrication The rapid removal of a patient in critical condition from a vehicle.

Recovery position Placing an unresponsive, breathing, nontrauma victim on his or her side to allow access to the airway to keep it open.

Semi-Fowler position An inclined position with the upper half of the body raised by elevating the head or the stretcher about 30 degrees.

Side-to-side method Hoisting or lowering a transportation device where the emergency medical technicians are on either side of the device.

Standing backboard techniques Placing a standing patient with a suspected neck or spinal injury onto a long backboard, while the patient remains standing. These are two- or three-person techniques.

Transportation device Any equipment, such as stretchers, stair chair, long backboards, or vacuum backboards, used to move a patient from one location to another.

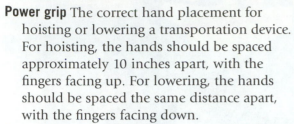

National Standard Curriculum Objectives

Cognitive Objectives

After completing this lesson, the EMT student will be able to do the following:

- Define body mechanics.
- Discuss the guidelines and safety precautions that need to be followed when lifting a patient.
- Describe the safe manner to lift a cot or stretcher.
- Describe the guidelines and safety precautions for carrying patients or equipment.
- Discuss one-handed carrying techniques.
- Describe the safe carrying procedure on stairs.
- Discuss the guidelines and applications for reaching.
- Describe correct procedures and reaching for logrolls.
- State the guidelines for pushing and pulling.
- Discuss the general considerations for moving patients.
- State three situations that may require an emergency move.
- Identify the following transportation devices:
  - Wheeled ambulance stretcher
  - Portable ambulance stretcher
  - Stair chair
  - Scoop stretcher
  - Long backboard
  - Basket stretcher
  - Flexible stretcher

Affective Objective

After completing this lesson, the EMT student will be able to do the following:

- Explain the rationale for properly lifting and moving patients.

Psychomotor Objectives

After completing this lesson, the EMT student will be able to do the following:

- Working with a partner, prepare each of the following devices for use, transfer a patient to the device, position and secure the patient for transport, and load the patient into the ambulance:
  - Wheeled stretcher
  - Portable stretcher
  - Stair chair
  - Scoop stretcher
  - Long backboard
  - Basket stretcher
  - Flexible stretcher
- Working with a partner, demonstrate proper techniques to move a patient from the wheeled stretcher to the hospital bed.

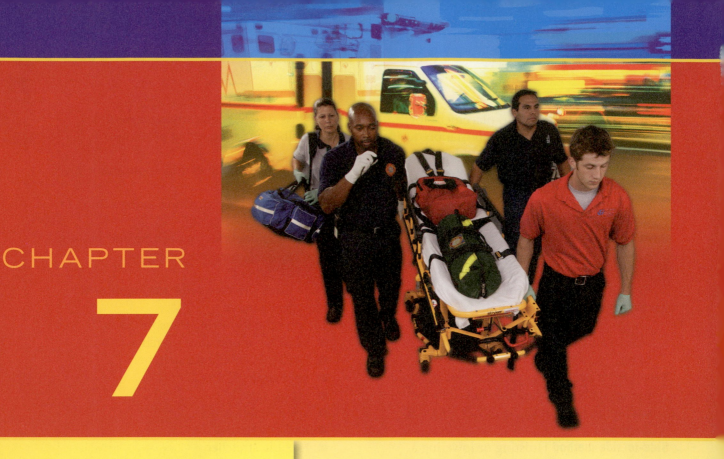

CHAPTER

7

OUTLINE

LESSON GOAL

GOAL

The purpose of this chapter is to instruct the emergency medical technician student in the fundamental principles of airway management. With this goal in mind, the basic anatomy and physiology of the human respiratory system are reviewed. The review is followed by a discussion of the signs and symptoms of normal and abnormal breathing in patients of varying ages. Specific interventions to open and maintain a patent airway, assist ventilation, and provide supplemental oxygen then are covered in detail. In this manner, this chapter allows readers to take the first steps toward becoming skilled in quickly recognizing and decisively managing the patient whose breathing is threatened. ■

Airway Management

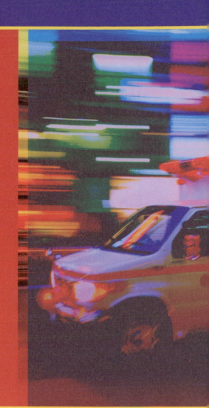

CHAPTER OBJECTIVES

After completing this chapter, the EMT student should be able to do the following:

1 Identify the major structures of the respiratory system, and explain the basic mechanics and physiology of breathing.

2 Recognize and explain the signs of adequate and inadequate breathing in pediatric and adult patients.

3 Perform proper airway opening maneuvers, such as the head tilt–chin lift and the jaw thrust techniques.

4 Define the indications for airway adjuncts and their correct insertion.

5 Deliver assisted ventilation effectively to the patient with compromised breathing by the mouth-to-mask, bag-mask, and flow-restricted ventilator techniques.

6 Explain different oxygen delivery systems along with the advantages and disadvantages of each.

7 List the special anatomic and physiologic considerations in evaluating and treating special populations such as infants and children with airway compromise.

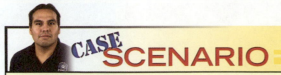

CASE SCENARIO

"Engine Twenty-seven, respond to Two Seven Four Four Five Wilshire Boulevard West, the Winton Hotel, room twenty-two seventeen, for a male short of breath. Timeout, One Zero Five." Rafael already has swung his feet out of the bed, quickly donning his boots and bunker gear. As he heads toward the apparatus bay, he can already hear the engine firing up its powerful diesel motor. Red and white flashes of light bounce off the walls as the engine rumbles out of the station and heads downtown. Within minutes, Rafael and his crew arrive in front of the hotel, where the security guard escorts them up the elevator to the twenty-second floor.

Upon entering the hotel room, Rafael finds an older man sitting on the edge of the bed. Although the lighting is poor, he can see that the patient is having some trouble breathing. His respiratory rate is quick, and his breaths appear shallow. His skin is pale, although he is warm and dry. As Rafael begins his assessment, Captain Alvarez opens up the airway bag.

Question: *Based upon the presentation of the patient, what should the captain pull out of the airway bag?*

Breathing is essential to life. The patient who is unable to breathe or who is for any other reason significantly deprived of oxygen will die within minutes. Ensuring adequate breathing and oxygenation is therefore the fundamental and most important responsibility of every emergency medical technician (EMT) during the care of a patient, regardless of the situation. Fulfilling this responsibility demands three things. First, it demands an understanding of the basic mechanics and physiology of breathing. Second, it demands an ability to recognize even the subtlest signs of actual or impending respiratory distress. Third, it demands an expertise with the variety of techniques and equipment available to assist any patient whose ability to breathe is threatened. Moreover, because time is so critical whenever a patient's breathing is endangered, the EMT must be rapid and decisive in identifying respiratory difficulty and intervening effectively to support breathing.

■ RESPIRATORY ANATOMY AND PHYSIOLOGY

The seemingly simple act of breathing is in actuality a complex and intricately coordinated process. This process serves a vital purpose: continually supplying the body with adequate oxygen while at the same time eliminating carbon dioxide, one of the major by-products of normal metabolism. Understanding the basic anatomic and physiologic principles of breathing is essential to the proper evaluation and management of any patient whose ability to breathe is compromised.

Respiration and Ventilation

Respiration is the physiologic process by which oxygen that is drawn into the lungs is delivered via specialized cells called **erythrocytes** in the bloodstream to tissues and cells throughout the body and is exchanged for the waste products of cell metabolism. Oxygen is essential to the survival and proper function of every living cell. At the same time, the constant removal of the by-products of cell metabolism from the body must take place. This removal maintains a carefully balanced chemical environment that allows cells to function normally and thrive. The most important of those waste products, hydrogen ion, is converted to water and carbon dioxide by the buffering system of the body. Carbon dioxide dissolves readily in blood. This allows it to be delivered to the lungs to be exhaled and thus eliminated from the body entirely.

Ventilation is the mechanical process by which oxygen is inspired deep into the lungs and carbon dioxide is exhaled. Continuous and adequate ventilation is essential if the physiologic process of respiration and thereby the health and survival of the body and its cells is to continue. Ventilation is the main function of the structures and organs that make up the human respiratory system.

Normal Anatomy of the Respiratory Tract

The **upper respiratory tract,** or airway, consists of the nose and mouth, the **pharynx,** the **larynx,** and the **trachea.** The upper respiratory tract channels air into and out of the passages of the **lower respiratory tract** and the lungs with each breath (Fig. 7-1). Air drawn in through the nose passes first through numerous convoluted passages formed by the nasal turbinates. Hairs and the moist mucosal surfaces that line these passages filter small particles inspired with the air. Air also is heated and humidified as it passes through the turbinates. Air also may be inspired through the mouth. However, the process of filtration, warming, and humidification is much less effective by this route.

Air taken in by either pathway passes next into the pharynx. The pharynx is a cavity situated immediately posterior to the nose and mouth (Fig. 7-2). The pharynx is divided into the **nasopharynx,** that portion directly behind the nasal passages, and the **oropharynx,** the open space lying at the back of the mouth. The larynx, or voice box, is a cartilaginous structure situated in the anterior neck, just below the pharynx (Fig. 7-3). The anterior aspect of the larynx is formed by the **thyroid cartilage** (known commonly as the Adam's apple). The Adam's apple usually is palpated easily on the front surface of the neck as a hard, somewhat mobile structure with a fluted notch at its superior aspect. As air courses through the larynx, finely controlled movement of small muscles and the **vocal cords** within this structure allow for phonation and speech. The superior opening of the larynx is protected by the **epiglottis.** The epiglottis is a flap of soft tissue that folds over to seal the larynx during the mechanical act of swallowing. It prevents food and liquid from passing deeper into the respiratory tract.

Beneath the larynx lies the trachea, or windpipe. This tubular structure is supported by numerous cartilaginous rings throughout its length as it descends into the chest. Only the uppermost of these rings, the **cricoid cartilage,** forms a complete circle around the trachea. The remaining tracheal rings are incomplete, C-shaped structures encircling only the anterior (front) two thirds of the windpipe at each level. The space between the lower aspect of the thyroid cartilage and the cricoid cartilage is spanned by a thin tissue known as the **cricothyroid membrane.** This membrane is another important anatomic landmark of the upper airway.

The trachea forms the transition between the upper and lower respiratory tracts (Fig. 7-4). At its lowermost end within the chest, the trachea forks into the right and left **bronchi.** These are the central conduits for air passage into and out of the lung on each corresponding side of the thoracic cavity. This branch point within the lower respiratory tract is known as the **carina,** and it is important to note that the division is not symmetric. The right bronchus descends into the right lung at less of an acute angle than does the left bronchus. For this reason, foreign bodies (including an endotracheal tube inserted too deeply into the airway) that pass into the lower respiratory tract tend to fall into and lodge within the right bronchus more often than the left.

As each bronchus enters the lung, it subdivides multiple times into smaller **bronchioles** before terminating in clusters of tiny air sacs. These air sacs are called the **alveoli.** Each alveolus is formed by a thin, elastic, and highly blood-enriched membrane. This membrane serves as the interface between the air spaces of the lungs and the blood as it passes through small capillaries coursing through each alveolus. Oxygen in the air drawn into the alveoli with each breath diffuses (transfers) across this membrane into the bloodstream. In the bloodstream, oxygen is taken up by erythrocytes for delivery to tissues throughout the body. Simultaneously, carbon dioxide that has accumulated in the blood as the result of cell metabolism diffuses in the opposite direction into the alveoli. Once in the alveoli, the carbon dioxide then can be exhaled.

Breathing

The mechanical act of breathing depends on the patency of the major structures of the upper and lower respiratory tracts described previously, as well as on changes in pressure within the thoracic cavity so that air can be inspired or exhaled. The floor of the thoracic cavity is composed of the **diaphragm.** This dome-shaped muscle separates the contents of the chest from the abdominal cavity. The bony frame formed by spinal column, ribs, and sternum and the intercostal muscles spanning the space between each of the ribs define the rest of the thoracic cavity.

During normal inspiration, contraction of the diaphragm draws it downward, increasing the volume (size) of the thoracic cavity. This creates a lower pressure within the chest relative to the outside atmosphere, and as as result of this pressure gradient, air is drawn through the respiratory tract and into the

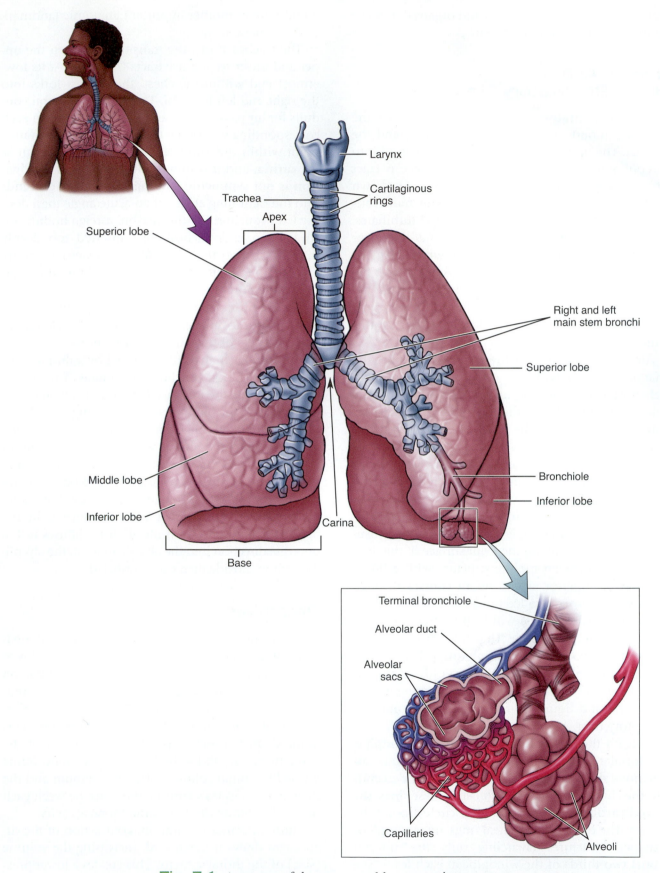

Fig. 7-1 Anatomy of the upper and lower respiratory tracts.

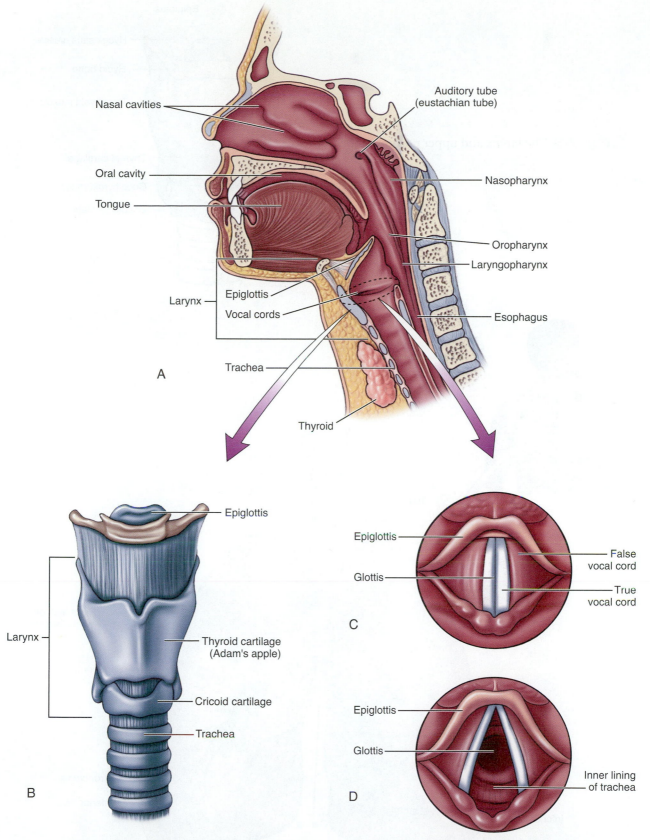

Fig. 7-2 Anatomy of the upper airway. **A,** Upper respiratory tract. **B,** Larynx showing thyroid cartilage. **C,** Vocal cords and glottis (closed). **D,** Vocal cords and glottis (open).

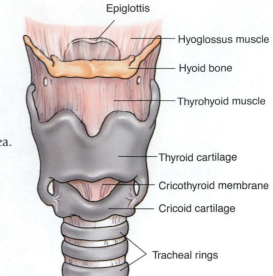

Fig. 7-3 The larynx and upper portion of the trachea.

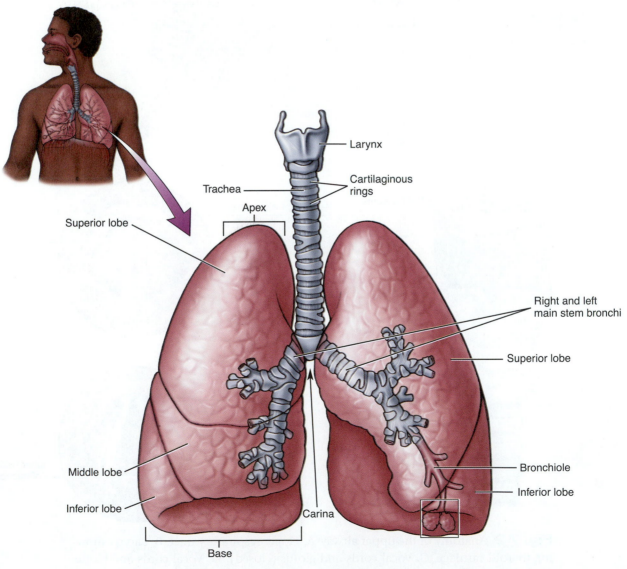

Fig. 7-4 Anatomy of the lower airway.

lungs. When greater volumes of air are required for breathing, as during heavy exercise or when some degree of obstruction of the respiratory tract is limiting the amount of air entering the lungs by diaphragmatic contraction alone, additional expansion of the thoracic cavity is necessary. Contraction of the external intercostal muscles and muscles connecting the upper portion of the anterior rib cage to the neck (referred to collectively as **accessory muscles** of breathing) further expands the rib cage upward and outward. This generates added intrathoracic volume and thereby the needed extra inspiratory pressure gradient and airflow (Fig. 7-5).

Reducing the volume of the thoracic cavity generates positive intrathoracic pressure, reversing airflow and thus causing exhalation. Simple, passive relaxation of the diaphragm and the accessory muscles aided by the retraction of elastic lung tissue to its preinhalation size usually increases the pressure within the chest sufficiently to expel a volume of air equivalent to that taken in with the preceding inspiration (Figs. 7-6 and 7-7).

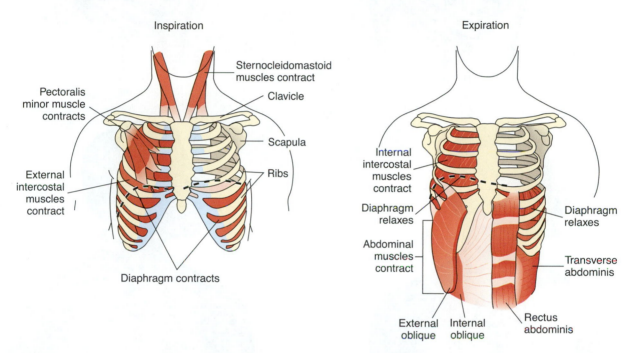

Fig. 7-5 The muscles of breathing.

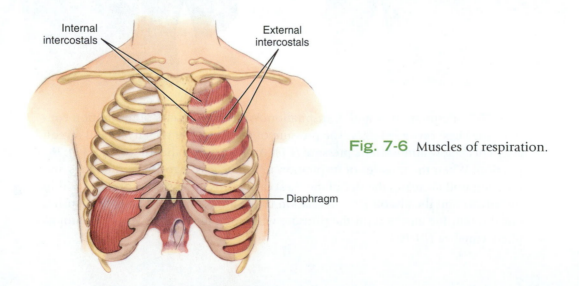

Fig. 7-6 Muscles of respiration.

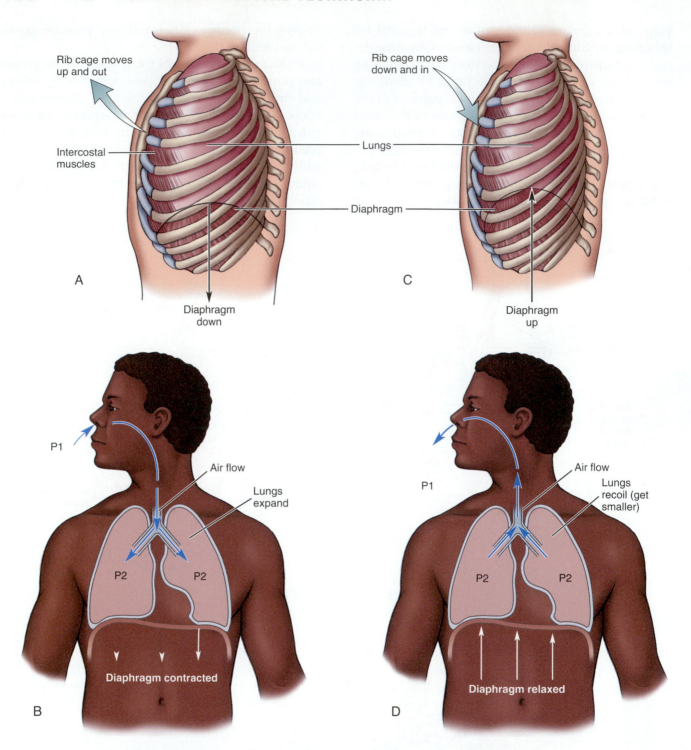

Rib cage moves up and out

Intercostal muscles

Lungs

Diaphragm

Diaphragm down

A

Rib cage moves down and in

Lungs

Diaphragm

Diaphragm up

C

P1

Air flow

Lungs expand

P2   P2

Diaphragm contracted

B

P1

Air flow

Lungs recoil (get smaller)

P2   P2

Diaphragm relaxed

D

Fig. 7-7 Respiration. **A** and **B,** Inspiration. When the muscles of inspiration contract, the chest cavity enlarges. The pressure of the air within the airway and alveoli *(P2)* falls below atmospheric pressure *(P1)*. Air rushes into the lungs. **C** and **D,** Expiration. When the muscles of inspiration relax, the elastic rocoil of the lungs and the chest wall decreases the size of the chest cavity. This increases the pressure within the airway and the alveoli *(P2)* in relation to the atmosphere *(P1)*. Air then rushes out through the airway until the pressure within the lungs and that of the atmosphere equalize *(P1-P2)*.

SPECIAL Considerations

Infants, Children, and the Elderly

The emergency medical technician must keep a number of anatomic considerations in mind with respect to the act of breathing for infants, small children, and older individuals. The passages of the nose and mouth are smaller in infants and children and thus are obstructed more easily. Moreover, in young individuals the tongue is proportionally larger and therefore occupies a greater proportion of the oropharynx compared with adults. The potential of the tongue to fall backward in a child lying supine and obstruct air passage though the pharynx is therefore significantly greater. The trachea is less rigid and narrower in infants and children, rendering it more susceptible to distortion or closure with swelling. Accessory musculature is less developed in younger individuals, leaving them more dependent on the diaphragm for breathing and with less of an ability to augment inspiratory effort when necessary.

Elderly individuals likewise deserve special attention when discussing the normal mechanics of breathing. Older persons are more likely to suffer from any number of chronic health problems that may limit their tolerance of an acute insult to the respiratory system. Illness and poor conditioning may diminish their ability to use accessory muscles of breathing to increase minute ventilation when needed. Those with chronic lung ailments such as emphysema may have suffered long-term damage to the lung tissue that not only impairs the gas exchange that takes place across the alveolar membrane but also destroys the elastic properties of the lung that allow for the normal, passive exhalation. As a result, the simple act of breathing for these individuals requires added work under the best of circumstances and may greatly limit the degree to which they can tolerate any added respiratory stress. Such persons are therefore at greater risk for sudden respiratory decompensation and failure when their breathing is impaired even minimally.

The amount of oxygen delivered to the tissues and, conversely, the amount of carbon dioxide eliminated from the body depend on the volume of the gas inspired and exhaled by the lungs over a given time. The **tidal volume** is the amount of air taken into the lungs with a single inspiration and subsequently exhaled. This averages about 500 mL in the average healthy adult. **Minute ventilation** refers to the tidal volume of an average breath multiplied by the number of times the individual breathes over 1 minute. Thus a normal adult with a tidal volume of 500 mL who is breathing at a rate of 12 times per minute has a minute ventilation of 6000 mL/min. Minute ventilation can be increased by increasing the depth, or volume, of breathing, or by quickening the rate of breathing. When either occurs, it may signify that the body has a greater need for oxygen or an increased amount of carbon dioxide to be eliminated.

■ ASSESSMENT

Every patient encounter must begin with a rapid but focused evaluation for the adequacy of breathing and ventilation. The first symptom of respiratory difficulty is **dyspnea**. This is the sensation on the part of the patient of being unable to breathe adequately. Dyspneic patients are often anxious and breathe at an abnormally high rate. The vital components of properly assessing the dyspneic patient include determining the patency of the airway and determining the effectiveness of breathing. Although the evaluations of the airway and adequacy of breathing often are discussed separately, in real-time patient assessments the two occur in tandem. Obstruction of the upper airway, for example, at first may draw attention because of obvious signs of labored breathing. Any sign of respiratory difficulty on the part of a patient therefore demands rapid, close, and repeated scrutiny of both elements of the evaluation.

Airway

Looking and listening are key to evaluating the airway for signs of actual or impending obstruction. A patient who is speaking in a normal voice, conversing in full sentences without difficulty, and showing no sign of respiratory distress is maintaining a patent airway for the moment.

However, the patient with major or total airway obstruction initially may show obvious signs of panic and agitation before progressing to lethargy and unconsciousness because of decreased oxygen delivery to the brain. Respirations may be rapid and labored, with significant accessory muscle use, or later they may be absent entirely. The entire absence of respirations is a condition known as apnea. The skin may exhibit **cyanosis,** a dusky blue appearance that reflects inadequate oxygen delivery to the tissues, and it may be cool and diaphoretic. However, cyanosis is a late sign of decreased oxygen in the conscious patient; speech may be distorted and shortened to one- or two-word gasps, or it may be impossible altogether. If able, the patient will try to maintain a position that maximizes the patency of the airway. This position often entails sitting upright and forward with the neck slightly extended. In the unconscious patient who is supine, a high likelihood exists for the tongue to fall backward into the oropharynx. The tongue would block the passage of air and cause sonorous, snoring respirations and, potentially, apnea (Fig. 7-8). Without quick recognition of these signs and intervention on the part of the EMT, the patient's death is imminent.

More subtle clues to upper airway compromise reflect the partial narrowing of one or more portions of the upper respiratory tract. Early appreciation of these signs is essential if progression to severe airway obstruction is to be prevented. **Stridor** is a high-pitched sound caused by air passing through an abnormally narrowed portion of the upper respiratory tract. Often stridor is heard easily with each inspiration of the patient. However, less dramatic stridor may be appreciated only by listening over the patient's anterior neck with a stethoscope. Changes in the pitch or volume of the patient's voice, drooling, and mild increases in respiratory rate and work of

BOX 7-1	
Normal Respiratory Rates Based on Age	
Infants	25 to 50 breaths per minute
Children	15 to 30 breaths per minute
Adults	12 to 20 breaths per minute

breathing are further signs that a threat to the airway may be present.

Breathing

Assessing the adequacy of a patient's breathing requires looking and listening to determine the rate, depth, quality, and rhythm of respirations. Normal respiratory rates vary by age (Box 7-1). An increased respiratory rate is one of the first signs of dyspnea as patients strive to maintain adequate minute ventilation.

Similarly, the depth of each respiration is important to note, not only because tidal volume is the other determinant of adequate minute ventilation but also because of the phenomenon of physiologic **dead space** within the respiratory tract. Dead space refers to the volume of gas—usually about 150 mL in a normal adult—that occupies the upper airway, bronchi, and bronchioles at the end of inspiration and does not reach the alveoli to participate in gas exchange. With each breath, the inhaled volume must exceed that of the dead space if fresh air is to reach the alveoli. By the same token, exhalation must expel a volume greater than the size of the dead space if the carbon dioxide accumulating in the alveoli is to be eliminated from the body entirely. Failure to exchange a sufficient amount of air with each respiration is known as **hypoventilation.** Thus a patient with shallow respirations of less than 150 mL of tidal volume is incapable of delivering oxygen to the tissues and eliminating carbon dioxide effectively, regardless of the number of times he or she is breathing per minute.

The quality of breathing may be appreciated first by inspecting the chest wall for symmetric (equal) expansion. Failure of one side of the chest to rise with inspiration may signify collapse of the underlying lung. The EMT should note signs of increased work of breathing, such as accessory muscle use. Infants and small children may show little evidence of accessory muscle use, however, despite significant respiratory distress. Flaring of the nostrils and **paradoxical breathing,** a "seesaw"

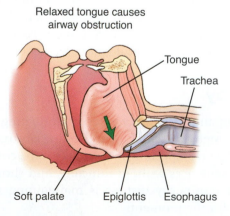

Relaxed tongue causes airway obstruction

Tongue

Trachea

Soft palate   Epiglottis   Esophagus

Fig. 7-8 Blockage of the airway by the tongue falling backward in the supine, unconscious patient.

movement of the chest and abdominal muscles to enhance movement of the diaphragm, may be more telling signs of labored breathing among these patients.

The EMT further assesses breathing quality by listening across the right and the left lung fields with a stethoscope. Normal breath sounds are sharp and brisk as air moves into and then out of the alveoli. **Wheezing** is a high-pitched sound that signifies air passing through bronchioles in the lower respiratory tract that have constricted, most often because of an acute asthmatic attack. Wheezing usually is heard diffusely. Wheezing is loudest during expiration because collapsing lung tissue narrows the bronchioles to the greatest degree during this phase of breathing. That narrowing makes it difficult for asthmatic patients to exhale effectively. This results in air trapping within the lungs at the end of exhalation. When this happens, the lungs are expanded abnormally as the next inspiration begins, and only a reduced tidal volume can be taken in with the next respiratory cycle. This is why patients with a severe asthmatic attack take rapid, shallow, and labored breaths, with significant accessory muscle use in an attempt to maximize chest wall expansion and inhale as great a volume of air as possible. **Rales** (pronounced *rawls*) are fine crackling sounds generated when fluid-filled or collapsed alveoli suddenly reexpand with inspiration. Fluid may accumulate within the alveoli because of infection, hemorrhage, or cardiac decompensation. Entirely absent breath sounds over one portion of the chest may signify collapse of the lung, severe bronchoconstriction to the point that no air is able to pass, or the accumulation of a large volume of fluid such as blood within that portion of the thoracic cavity.

Lastly, the EMT should note the rhythm of breathing. Normal ventilation is regular. Irregular breathing may signify impending respiratory failure, as the muscles of breathing reach the point of extreme fatigue, or damage to the portions of the central nervous system responsible for coordinating the normal cycle of inspiration and exhalation. **Agonal respirations** are infrequent, asynchronous gasps heard immediately before the total collapse of breathing and death.

■ MANAGEMENT

Proper support of the patient's airway and breathing is the fundamental and most important responsibility of the EMT. Providing such support demands proficiency in opening and maintaining a patent upper airway, assisting patient ventilation effectively, and

delivering supplemental oxygen efficiently to the patient with respiratory compromise. Additional interventions such as suctioning or inserting an airway adjunct may be required at any time during the patient's management and transport. Familiarity with these techniques is therefore also mandatory.

Opening of the Airway

The unconscious patient is vulnerable to upper airway obstruction because of the tendency for the tongue to fall backward into the posterior oropharynx, blocking all airflow. This is the most common cause for airway compromise in the unresponsive patient. Because the base of the tongue tightly adheres to the mandible, careful repositioning of the jaw often will pull the tongue away from the posterior pharynx and thus open the airway.

The unconscious, nonbreathing patient should be placed in the supine position (on the back). If the patient has not sustained significant trauma and no reason to suspect injury to the cervical spine exists, the **head tilt–chin lift** maneuver is a simple and effective method to open the airway (Skill 7-1). With one hand placed on the patient's forehead, the EMT positions two or three fingers of the other hand beneath the chin. The EMT should take care to put pressure only on the bony portion of the underside of the chin. The chin is then gently lifted upward as the head is tilted backward. Flexing the neck and pulling the mandible forward in this manner will pull the tongue out of the posterior pharynx. Compressing the soft tissues beneath the chin and along the anterior surface of the neck could potentially obstruct the airway further and must therefore be avoided.

If the potential for cervical spine injury is present, the head tilt–chin lift maneuver is contraindicated. The **jaw thrust** maneuver should be performed instead (Skill 7-2). With the patient supine, the EMT places one hand on either side of the patient's head to provide neutral, in-line cervical spine stabilization. The EMT then positions the fingertips of each hand behind the angle of the mandible. Forward pressure thrusts the jaw outward, thus lifting the tongue off the wall of the posterior pharynx.

Suctioning of the Airway

Proper suctioning is the next step in ensuring the patency of the upper airway in an unresponsive patient. Oral secretions, blood, food particles, loose teeth, or other solid objects may partially or fully block the

SKILL 7-1

◉ *Head Tilt–Chin Lift*

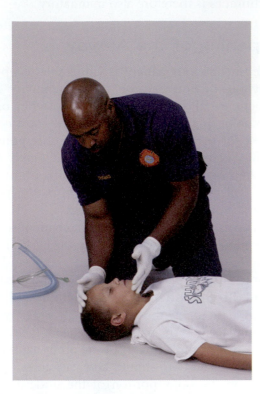

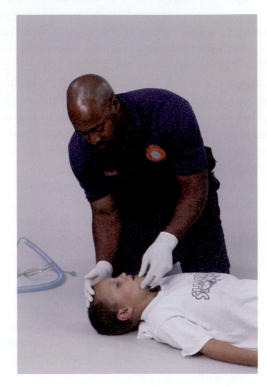

1. Place the patient in the supine position.
2. Stand or kneel at the patient's side.
3. Place the palm of one hand on the patient's forehead and the fingers of the other hand on the bony underside of the patient's chin. (Do not apply pressure to the soft tissues beneath the chin and along the anterior neck. This may occlude the airway further.)

4. Gently tilt the head backward and lift the chin to pull the tongue forward and open the airway.

SKILLS

154

SKILL 7-2
◎ *Jaw Thrust*

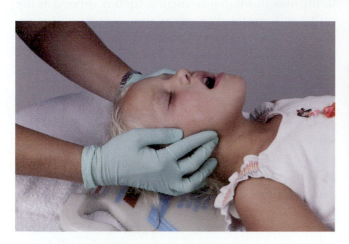 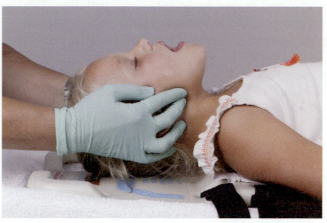

1. Place the patient in the supine position while maintaining in-line cervical spine stabilization.
2. Stand or kneel behind the patient's head.
3. Place hands on either side of the patient's head.
4. With the thumbs of each hand positioned on the patient's cheeks, place the ring fingers of each hand behind the angle of the mandible.

5. While maintaining in-line cervical spine stabilization, push the mandible forward to pull the tongue forward and open the airway.

SKILLS

movement of air through the oropharynx. These objects therefore must be suctioned out when present. Suctioning is indicated whenever repositioning maneuvers have failed to clear the airway, when gurgling or stridorous upper airway noises are audible, or when liquid or solid material is visible in the oropharynx. Proper body substance isolation measures are essential to the safety of the EMT performing suctioning of fluids from the oropharynx because of the high likelihood of contact with oral and respiratory secretions.

A variety of suction units and catheter attachments commonly are used in the prehospital setting (Fig. 7-9). Every ambulance should have a mounted suction unit using an electric pump as part of its standard operating equipment. Portable suction units consisting of a battery- or hand-powered pump are also available and useful when suctioning is needed before the patient can be transferred to the ambulance. All units should be mounted with a pressure gauge and should be capable of generating a vacuum pressure of at least 300 mm Hg. Suction devices should be inspected regularly to ensure proper function and, if applicable, adequate battery charge.

The catheter attachments used for suctioning may be rigid (the "tonsil tip" catheter) or soft (the French suction catheter). Rigid catheters are appropriate for suctioning fluids from the oropharynx of unresponsive adults, children, and infants. A rigid catheter should never be inserted blindly; its tip should be visible at all times during suctioning. Soft catheters are useful for suctioning fluids from the nasopharynx and other areas not reachable with a rigid catheter. A soft catheter should never be inserted farther than the base of the tongue, however. That distance is best estimated by measuring the distance from the tip of the patient's nose to the top of the ear.

Once the proper equipment is assembled, suctioning is performed by first inserting the chosen catheter as far as the base of the tongue (Skill 7-3). Ideally, this should be done before the suction unit is activated. When the catheter tip has been advanced to the maximum depth, suction then is applied as the catheter is removed slowly with a sweeping, side-to-side motion in the oropharynx. Suctioning of the posterior pharynx temporarily may obstruct the upper airway. Therefore the time to complete this maneuver should never exceed 15 seconds for adult patients. For infants and small children, an even shorter period of suctioning is preferred. If the initial suctioning attempt does not clear copious secretions or vomitus, the patient should be logrolled to the side as the oropharynx is cleared manually. Suctioning can be repeated after 2 minutes of adequate ventilation. This pattern of suctioning for 15 seconds, breathing or ventilation for 2 minutes, and suctioning again for 15 seconds may be continued during patient transport. Rinsing the catheter and tubing with water as needed will prevent clogging from dried secretions.

Airway Adjuncts

Airway adjuncts are simple devices that can aid greatly in maintaining an open passage between the tongue and the posterior wall of the pharynx in the supine patient. The use of an airway adjunct is thus an essential part of providing **assisted ventilation** to any patient who is unconscious or whose level of alertness is decreased to the point that he or she is unable to maintain airway patency without assistance.

The **oropharyngeal (oral) airway** is a rigid, curved device used for the patient who is unresponsive and without an intact gag reflex (Fig. 7-10). Several stan-

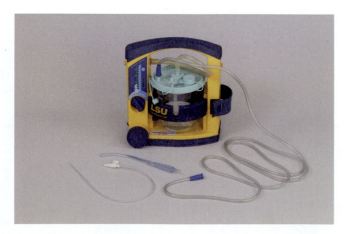

Fig. 7-9 Suction unit with tubing and catheter attachments.

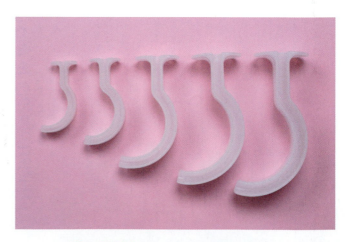

Fig. 7-10 Oropharyngeal airways.

SKILL 7-3

◎ *Suctioning*

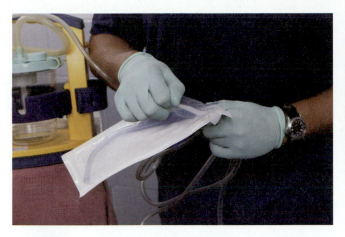

1. Assemble proper equipment based on the age of the patient and area to be suctioned, including the suction device, suction tubing, and a suction catheter (rigid versus soft tip).

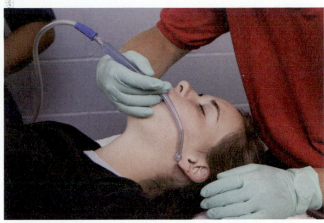

2. If a rigid suction catheter is chosen, measure a length equal to the distance from the tip of the patient's nose to the top of the ear.

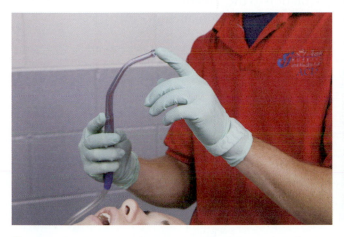

3. Test the assembly by turning on the suction device. Suctioning may be tested by sealing the side port on the selected catheter with one finger. Removing the finger from the port will discontinue suctioning. Once proper function is confirmed, remove the finger from the port or turn off the device.

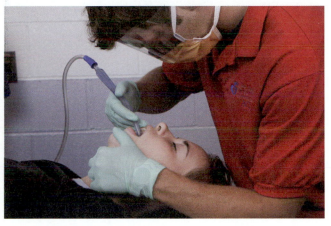

4. Insert the suction catheter into the patient's mouth or nose to maximal depth (as far as direct visualization allows for the tip of a rigid catheter or as far as the base of the tongue for a soft catheter).

Continued

SKILLS

SKILL 7-3
◉ *Suctioning—cont'd*

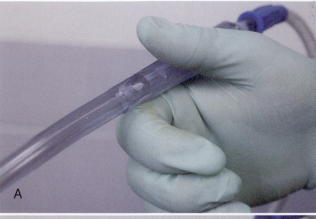

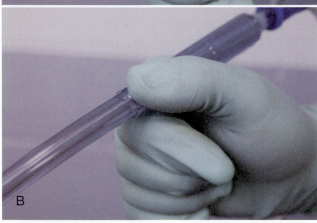

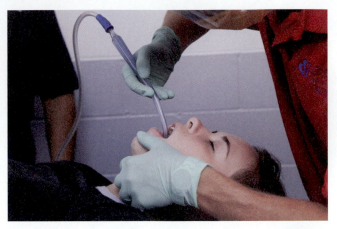

6. Slowly withdraw the catheter while sweeping from side to side to clear the airway. Do not suction for more than 15 seconds (less if suctioning fluids from an infant or small child). Provide ventilation to the patient for at least 2 minutes before any repeat suction attempt.

5. Turn on the suction device or cover the catheter side port with one finger to initiate suctioning.

dard sizes of oral airways exist. The proper size for each individual patient is determined best by measuring the distance from the corner of the patient's mouth to the angle of the mandible and choosing the airway that most closely approximates that length. In the adult patient, the oral airway is inserted properly into the mouth initially in an upside-down orientation. The curve of the airway should be directly opposite that of the tongue (Skill 7-4). Once the entire length of the airway has been inserted, it then is rotated 180 degrees, now parallel with the curvature of the tongue, and with the flange of the device resting at the patient's front teeth. This method is preferred because it minimizes the degree to which insertion pushes the tongue farther into the posterior pharynx. Alternatively, the EMT may use a tongue depressor to pull the tongue downward and forward while inserting the airway in a parallel orientation. This is the preferred technique in infants and small children. Because the tip of the properly placed oral airway rests against the posterior wall of the pharynx, this device should never be used for the patient with an intact gag response because vomiting likely will ensue.

A **nasopharyngeal (nasal) airway** is best for the patient with an intact gag reflex or who is otherwise unable to tolerate an oral airway. The nasal airway is a pliable tube inserted through the nose to rest with its tip in the posterior pharynx (Figs. 7-11 and 7-12). The proper size is chosen by matching the length of the nasal airway to the distance from the end of the patient's nose to the tip of the ear (Skill 7-5). Before insertion, the EMT should coat the tip of the nasal airway with a water-soluble lubricant. The EMT then places the device into the larger of the nasal passages with the bevel at the top of the airway oriented toward the base of the nostril or the nasal septum. The EMT should advance the nasal airway steadily but gently to avoid causing epistaxis (nosebleed). If significant resistance is met, the EMT may attempt insertion via the other nostril.

Assisted Ventilation

Assisted ventilation is the means by which adequate tidal volume is provided to the patient who has an insufficient respiratory depth or rate. The most important types of assisted ventilation include the

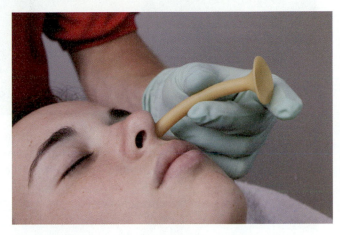

Fig. 7-12 Proper positioning of the nasopharyngeal airway.

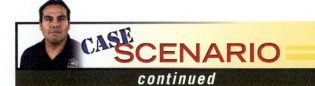

CASE SCENARIO
continued

"Mr. Wilson, is the oxygen mask helping you?" asked Rafael, leaning close to the patient's face.

Mr. Wilson could only nod his head because the breathing effort was so difficult. Rafael quickly continued his assessment of the patient, noting his vital signs and respiratory effort. He listened to Mr. Wilson's chest with his stethoscope; he could hear the odd popping sounds associated with fluid, also known as congestive heart failure. Rafael was concerned that because Mr. Wilson really could not speak to him that perhaps the oxygen mask was not enough to help his condition.

Question: *What could Rafael consider doing now to help Mr. Wilson breathe? What airway device could he use?*

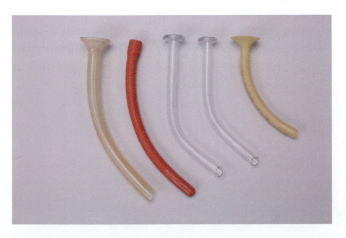

Fig. 7-11 Nasopharyngeal airways.

SKILL 7-4

◎ Oropharyngeal Airway Insertion

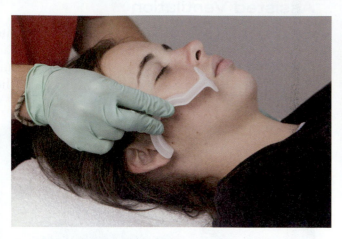

1. Select a properly sized oropharyngeal airway. (Length should match the distance from the corner of the patient's mouth to the angle of the mandible.)

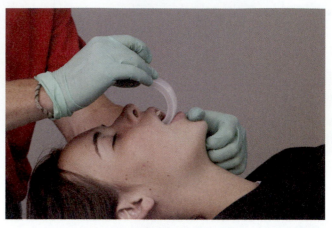

2. Open the patient's mouth and insert the airway with its curve opposite to the curve of the patient's tongue.

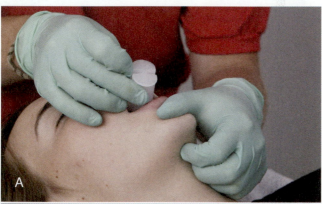

A

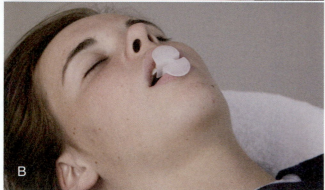

B

3. When the tip of the device is positioned in the posterior pharynx, rotate the oropharyngeal airway 180 degrees so that the curve of the device is parallel to that of the patient's tongue and the phalange is resting at the patient's front teeth.

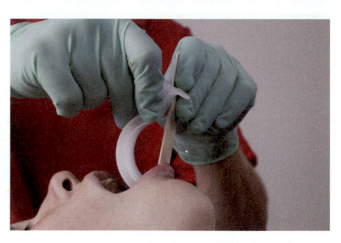

4. Alternatively, use a tongue depressor to pull the tongue forward and downward. Insert the oropharyngeal airway, with its curve parallel to that of the patient's tongue, until the tip of the device rests in the posterior pharynx and the phalange is situated against the patient's front teeth. Suction fluids as necessary and initiate assisted ventilation.

SKILLS

SKILL 7-5
◎ *Nasopharyngeal Airway Insertion*

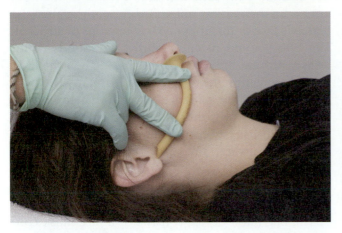

1. Select a properly sized nasopharyngeal airway. (Length should match the distance from the end of the patient's nose to the tip of the ear.)

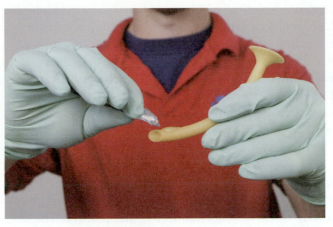

2. Apply a water-soluble lubricant to the tip of the nasopharyngeal airway.

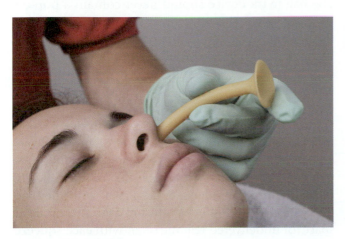

3. Select the larger of the patient's two nares as the place of insertion. Insert the tip of the nasopharyngeal airway with its bevel oriented toward the nasal septum or the base of the nose.

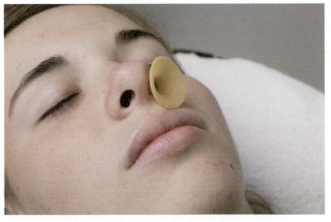

4. Apply gentle, steady pressure until the device is inserted to its full length with the phalange resting at the opening of the naris. Suction fluids and begin assisted ventilation as necessary.

mouth-to-mask technique, the **bag-valve-mask** technique performed by one person or two persons, and the use of a flow-restricted, oxygen-powered ventilator. One must recognize that assisted ventilation exposes the EMT to potential contact with respiratory secretions. Proper attention to and practice of body substance isolation measures is therefore mandatory. Moreover, no attempt at assisted ventilation will succeed unless an open airway is maintained at all times. Providing assisted ventilation therefore demands not only familiarity and skill with each described technique but also a careful, second-by-second coordination with the maneuvers for maintaining a patent airway discussed previously.

Protective barrier devices can be easily carried in a pocket or handbag. They are designed for placing over the mouth of a nonbreathing patient and include a one-way device so that air expired by the patient does not contaminate the rescuer. These devices allow safe mouth to barrier ventilation (Skill 7-6).

Mouth-to-mask ventilation is an effective technique that can be implemented by a single EMT. This is the preferred method of assisted ventilation for the EMT (Skill 7-7). The mask used fits over the patient's nose and mouth. At its apex is a mouthpiece with a one-way valve through which a rescuer can deliver breaths. A port allowing connection to supplemental oxygen tubing is also present. To use the device properly, the EMT should take a position above the supine patient's head and place the mask over the mouth and nose. Using both hands, the EMT obtains a firm seal of the mask on the face by applying pressure to the upper, nasal portion of the mask with both thumbs and to the lower segment of the device with each forefinger. The EMT then places the remaining fingers of each hand along the length of the jaw until the small fingers rest behind each angle of the mandible. With the fingers in these positions, the EMT then may initiate a head tilt–chin lift maneuver if no risk of cervical spine injury is felt to be present. Alternatively, a jaw thrust maneuver may be performed using the ring and small fingers of each hand. If the patient has dentures, the EMT should leave them in place in most cases while providing assisted ventilation. Dentures rarely obstruct the airway. Moreover, leaving them in place can help maintain the normal contour of the mouth to provide an adequate seal with the mask.

Once the mask is positioned with an adequate seal and the proper airway opening maneuver has been performed, the EMT delivers breaths at a depth and rate appropriate for the patient's age through the one-way valve. Supplemental oxygen should be connected and delivered through the appropriate port. The EMT should auscultate the chest wall for breath sounds and should observe for a smooth, symmetric rise and fall with each delivered breath. If this does not occur, the mask is not sealed properly against the patient's face or the upper airway remains obstructed. The EMT should listen carefully for sounds of air leaking around the edges of the mask. Then the EMT should reposition the device as appropriate. The EMT should return the patient's head and mandible to their neutral positions and then repeat the head tilt–chin lift or jaw thrust maneuver. If this fails to open the airway, the EMT should inspect the oropharynx and provide suction as needed and should insert an airway adjunct before repeating the mouth-to-mask ventilations.

The bag-mask device consists of a face mask connected by a one-way valve to a self-inflating bag and an oxygen reservoir (Fig. 7-13). Mask and bag sizes vary to accommodate infants, children, and adults. The bag-mask device should never contain a pop-off pressure valve. This may limit the force with which breaths can be delivered to a patient, rendering them inadequate. When connected to high-flow (15 L/min) supplemental oxygen and fitted with a true nonrebreather valve, the bag-mask device can deliver oxygen concentrations as high as 80% to 100%. The volume of a standard adult bag-mask device is 1600 mL. However, the mouth-to-valve ventilation delivers an actual tidal volume that is greater than that provided by bag-mask device. This is due to the difficulty in maintaining an adequate facial seal with the bag-mask device and the significant amount of dead space, or undelivered volume of air with each squeeze of the bag.

Proper bag-mask device ventilation can be performed by a single EMT. However, two EMTs working in tandem to deliver bag-mask device ventilations is greatly preferred because of the difficulty of adequately sealing the mask against a patient's face while simultaneously squeezing the bag with sufficient force to deliver useful breaths (Skill 7-8). An appropriately sized mask is placed over the face of the supine patient. Prior placement of an oral or a nasal airway will greatly aid in opening the airway and is highly recommended. If two persons are operating the bag-mask device, the first EMT positions the mask exactly as described previously for mouth-to-mask ventilation. Depending on the concern for cervical spine trauma and the need for head and neck immo-

SKILL 7-6
◎ *Mouth-to-Barrier Ventilation*

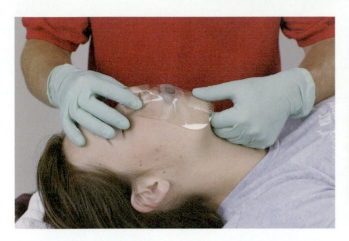
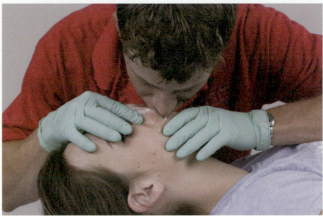

1. Put on appropriate personal protective equipment. Position yourself at the patient's head, and maintain an open airway through the use of the manual or mechanical techniques.
2. Place the barrier device over the patient's mouth.
3. Place your mouth over the mouthpiece, pinch the nostrils, and breathe slowly into the patient's mouth over $1\frac{1}{2}$ to 2 seconds for an adult and 1 to 2 seconds for an infant or child. The delivery of your breath should cause the patient's chest to rise visibly.

4. Remove your mouth from the mouthpiece and release the patient's nose to allow the patient to exhale. Continue rescue breathing for the patient at a rate of one breath every 4 to 5 seconds for an adult or one breath every 3 seconds for a child.
5. Continue to maintain an open airway and watch for any signs that the patient has vomited or has started breathing on his or her own.

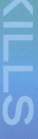

SKILLS

SKILL 7-7
◉ *Mouth-to-Mask Ventilation*

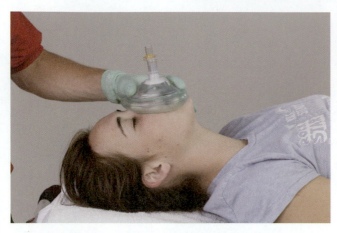

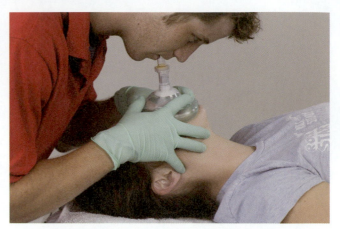

1. Assemble face mask with one-way breathing valve, supplemental oxygen tank, oxygen tubing.
2. Stand or kneel behind the supine patient.
3. If trauma is suspected, immobilize the head and neck.
4. Apply the mask to the patient's face with the apex over the nose and the base over the mouth. Obtain an airtight seal by applying pressure to the upper, nasal portion of the mask with both thumbs and to the lower segment of the device with each forefinger. Place the remaining fingers of each hand along the length of the jaw until the small fingers rest behind each angle of the mandible.

5. With the fingers in these positions, open the airway by tilting the head and lifting the chin upward or, if a potential for cervical spine injury exists, by performing a jaw thrust maneuver using the ring and/or small fingers of each hand.
6. Deliver breaths to the patient through the one-way valve at a rate and depth appropriate for the patient's age.

SKILL 7-8
◉ Bag-Mask Ventilation (Two Persons)

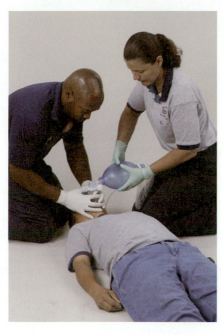

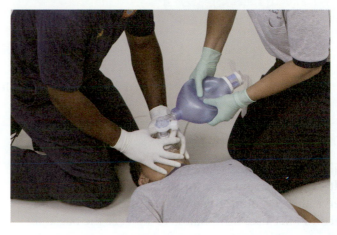

1. Assemble the bag-mask apparatus (face mask with one-way, self-inflating bag, oxygen reservoir, and supplemental oxygen tank with regulator and oxygen tubing).
2. Designate one emergency medical technician to stand or kneel behind the supine patient.
3. If trauma is suspected, immobilize the head and neck.
4. Insert an oral or nasal airway.
5. The emergency medical technician positioned at the patient's head applies the mask to the patient's face with the apex over the nose and the base over the mouth. Obtain an airtight seal by applying pressure to the upper, nasal portion of the mask with both thumbs and to the lower segment of the device with each forefinger. The remaining fingers of each hand are placed along the length of the jaw until the small fingers rest behind each angle of the mandible.
6. Perform a head tilt–chin lift (if no trauma is suspected) or jaw thrust maneuver (if trauma is suspected) as needed.
7. The second emergency medical technician delivers breaths by squeezing the bag with both hands at a rate and depth appropriate for age.

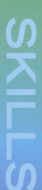

SKILLS

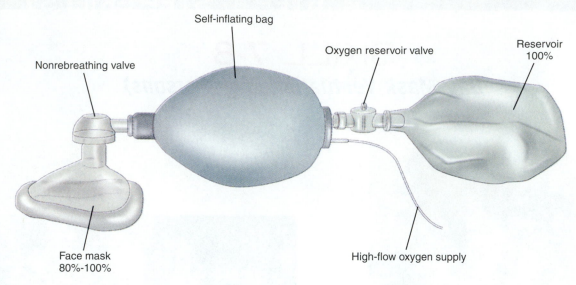

Nonrebreathing valve

Self-inflating bag

Oxygen reservoir valve

Reservoir 100%

Face mask 80%-100%

High-flow oxygen supply

Fig. 7-13 Assembled bag-mask device.

bilization, the first EMT then performs the head tilt–chin lift or the jaw thrust maneuver with in-line cervical spine immobilization. At the same time, the second EMT uses both hands to squeeze the bag at an age-appropriate rate with sufficient force to raise the chest wall.

Chest wall rise and audible breath sounds signify an adequate delivery of breaths. Absence of either should prompt inspection for a proper seal between the mask and the patient's face and reevaluation of the airway for persistent obstruction as described previously. If the breaths are too forceful with an airtight seal of the mask, however, air may be forced down the esophagus and into the stomach. Therefore the EMT must watch for signs of gastric distention and moderate the force with which breaths are delivered if vomiting and aspiration are to be avoided.

If a single EMT must perform BVM ventilation, an airtight seal of the mask against the patient's face is maintained with one hand while the other squeezes the bag to deliver breaths (Skill 7-9). This is done by using one hand to form a C around the delivery port of the mask, with the thumb at the apex of the mask and the forefinger at its base (Fig. 7-14). The middle, ring, and little fingers are positioned along the mandible to complete the seal of the mask while simultaneously performing a head tilt–chin lift or jaw thrust maneuver. Prior placement of an oral or a nasal airway greatly aids in maintaining a patent air-

way. When an adequate seal has been achieved and an appropriate airway opening maneuver performed, the EMT delivers breaths by squeezing the bag with the other hand.

A **flow-restricted, oxygen-powered ventilation device** is designed for use by a single EMT. These devices deliver 100% oxygen at rates as high as 40 L/min. An inspiratory pressure relief valve opens when airway pressures exceed 60 cm H_2O. This prevents excessive flow that can cause gastric distention and potential aspiration. When the relief valve opens, delivery of the breath to the patient ceases or is vented to the outside atmosphere. When this occurs, an alarm sounds to notify the EMT that the inspiratory flow has halted. Infants and children are more susceptible to lung injury in the setting of excessive airway pressures. Thus flow-restricted ventilators are used for adult patients only.

As with the other forms of assisted ventilation, an airway adjunct device is inserted and a mask is placed over the patient's face (Skill 7-11). Two hands form a seal between the mask and the patient's face. Then a head tilt–chin lift or a jaw thrust maneuver is performed in the same manner and with the same attention to the potential need for cervical spine immobilization as described previously. The flow-restricted ventilator attached to the mask has a trigger that can be activated easily with one of the fingers gripping the mask. When this is activated, inspiratory flow begins. As the chest wall rises, the EMT then releases the trigger to allow for

SKILL 7-9
◉ *Bag-Mask Ventilation (One Person)*

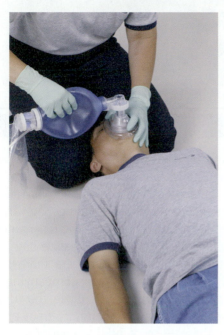
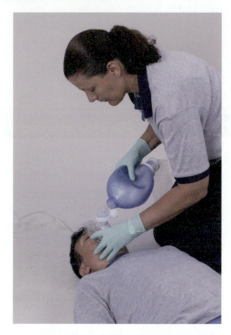

1. Assemble the bag-mask apparatus (face mask with one-way, self-inflating bag, oxygen reservoir, and supplemental oxygen tank with regulator and oxygen tubing).
2. Stand or kneel behind the supine patient.
3. If trauma is suspected, immobilize the head and neck.
4. Insert an oral or nasal airway.
5. Apply the mask to the patient's face with the apex over the nose and the base over the mouth. Obtain an airtight seal using one hand by applying pressure to the upper, nasal portion of the mask with the thumb and to the lower segment of the mask with the forefinger while the remaining fingers grip the length and the angle of the jaw.

6. Perform a head tilt–chin lift (if no trauma is suspected) or jaw thrust maneuver (if trauma is suspected) as needed.
7. Use the other hand to squeeze the bag and ventilate the patient at a rate and depth appropriate for age.

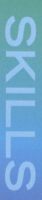

SKILLS

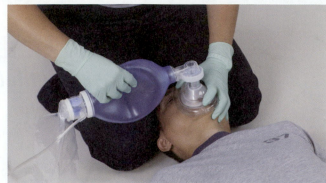

Fig. 7-14 Proper face mask application using one hand. Note the "C" formed by the thumb and index finger around the delivery port of the mask.

SPECIAL Considerations

Because of the smaller size and special anatomic considerations of infants and children, providing assisted ventilation to them demands special attention. Maneuvers to open the airway in these patients must take into account the fact that the trachea is much less rigid than in an adult and actually may kink if the neck is flexed or extended to an excessive degree. When an infant or small child is supine, the fact that the head is proportionately larger relative to the body means that the head tilts forward, flexing the neck and potentially closing the airway. Maximal airway patency is attained by positioning the infant's head in a neutral position, with the face parallel to the ground. For children, the neck may be extended slightly beyond the neutral position. Tilting the head too far back, though, will hyperextend the neck and cause narrowing of the trachea.

The emergency medical technician also must use special care when providing bag-valve-mask ventilations to these patients. The emergency medical technician must avoid excessive bag pressure because infants and children are more prone to gastric distention with the accompanying risk of vomiting and aspiration. Because the lungs and passages of the lower respiratory tract are much smaller than those of adults, overinflation of the lungs also is possible, causing tissue damage and potentially a pneumothorax. Use only enough bag pressure to cause the chest wall to rise visibly and to generate audible breath sounds when listening to the chest with a stethoscope.

SPECIAL Populations

Certain patients who require long-term assisted ventilation or who suffer from cancers of the head and neck undergo tracheostomy. This is a surgical procedure to provide an opening in the anterior neck that connects the trachea to the outside air. The opening is called a stoma. If the patient is alert and able to breathe spontaneously, he or she does so through this orifice. If the patient normally requires assisted ventilation, a tracheostomy tube is inserted and maintained in the stoma.

Emergency medical technicians frequently are called upon to provide assisted ventilation to tracheostomy patients. If a tracheostomy tube is present, this will attach to a bag-valve-mask device in place of the mask, and simple squeezing of the bag is sufficient (Fig. 7-15). Often, secretions will accumulate and obstruct the tracheostomy tube. This makes it difficult to provide ventilation to the patient. When this occurs, suctioning with a soft catheter often will clear the obstruction.

When only a stoma is present, the patient may be ventilated by placing an infant or child face mask over the opening and connecting the mask to a bag-valve or a flow-restricted ventilator. If neither of these is available, breaths may be delivered directly by placing the mouth over the stoma (Skill 7-10). Ideally, a plastic barrier device should be placed between the emergency medical technician's mouth and the stoma if this method is attempted. One must remember to seal the mouth and nose before delivering breaths through the stoma by any of these methods in cases where the upper airway remains patent. This will prevent air from escaping above instead of expanding the lungs.

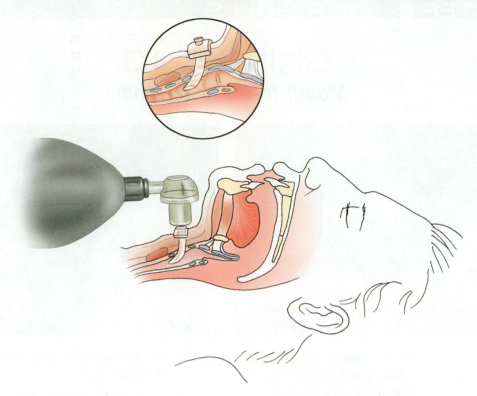

Fig. 7-15 Attachment of bag-valve to an indwelling tracheostomy tube.

exhalation. Active chest wall rise and audible breath sounds are the only reliable indicators that adequate ventilation is being achieved with the flow-restricted ventilator. If these are not present, the EMT must verify proper mask seal and airway patency.

Supplemental Oxygen

Any patient who complains of dyspnea or who manifests the signs of respiratory compromise described in this chapter should be provided with supplemental oxygen during prehospital evaluation and transport. This is essential in order to maximize the delivery of oxygen to tissues throughout the body. Although a theoretical concern exists over providing patients with chronic obstructive lung disease with too much oxygen and thereby suppressing their respiratory drive, this phenomenon rarely is encountered in the prehospital setting. Like all others, patients with chronic obstructive pulmonary disease depend first and foremost upon an adequate oxygen supply for survival.

Oxygen is stored in metal cylinders that vary in size. The U.S. Department of Transportation has des-

ignated each size with a corresponding letter that must be stamped on each cylinder (Box 7-2). When in use, every cylinder should be attached to a pressure regulator and flowmeter. The flowmeter indicates the current pressure of the oxygen contained within the cylinder and the rate at which oxygen is flowing through the regulator (Fig. 7-16). Regardless of the size, each cylinder when full should contain a sufficient amount of oxygen to generate 2000 psi of pressure. That pressure may increase or decrease depending on ambient temperature. The metal lining

---

BOX 7-2

U.S. Department of Transportation Letter Coding of Oxygen Cylinders

D Cylinder	350 L
E Cylinder	625 L
M Cylinder	3000 L
G Cylinder	5300 L
H Cylinder	6900 L

SKILL 7-10
Mouth-to-Mask-to-Stoma

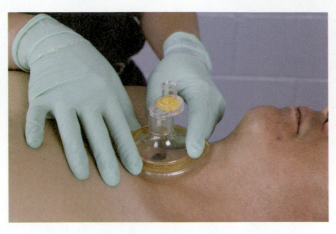 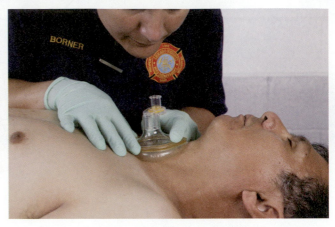

1. Place one hand under the patient's neck and use the other hand to obtain a seal using a pediatric mask over the opening in the patient's neck.

2. Provide ventilation as you would in mouth-to-mask ventilation.

SKILL 7-11
Flow-Restricted, Oxygen-Powered Ventilation Device

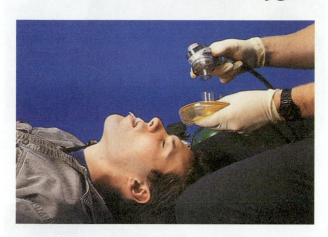
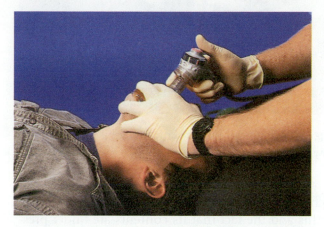

1. Position yourself at the top of the patient's head. Manually open the patient's airway. Size and insert an oral or nasal airway. Attach a flow-restricted, oxygen-powered ventilation device to the mask.

2. Apply the mask to the patient's face with the apex over the nose and the base over the mouth. Obtain an airtight seal using one hand by applying pressure to the upper, nasal portion of the mask with the thumb and to the lower segment of the mask with the forefinger while the remaining fingers grip the length and the angle of the jaw. Trigger the flow-restricted, oxygen-powered ventilation device until the chest rises. Release the trigger to allow passive exhalation. An adult patient should be ventilated at least once every 5 seconds.

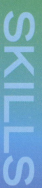

SKILLS

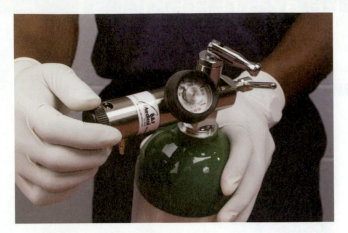

Fig. 7-16 Oxygen tank with attached regulator and flowmeter.

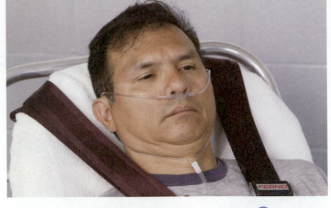

Fig. 7-17 Nasal cannula.

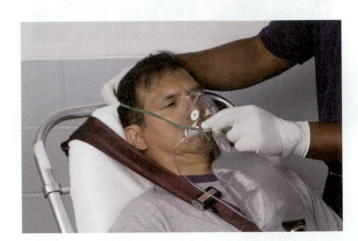

Fig. 7-18 Non-rebreather mask.

each cylinder is only a few millimeters thick. Because of this and the fact that its contents are under pressure, an oxygen cylinder should be transported and stored carefully to prevent falling and protected from blows to the regulator assembly.

Each fully pressurized oxygen cylinder should be fitted with a protective seal. The seal must be removed before use. Once this is done, the flow valve should be opened briefly and then closed. This will purge the valve of any particles that may have accumulated beneath the seal. The regulator and flowmeter then are attached to the cylinder. Tubing from a selected oxygen delivery device in turn is connected to the flowmeter, and the device itself is applied to the patient. Opening the flowmeter to an appropriate setting initiates the flow of oxygen to the patient. When use is complete, the delivery device is removed from the patient and is detached from the flowmeter. The valve on the oxygen cylinder then is closed while the flowmeter is left open. This releases pressure within the regulator, after which the flowmeter can be closed and the cylinder can be stored for future use (Skill 7-12).

Nasal cannula is a term commonly used to describe oxygen tubing with two small prongs that are inserted into the nostrils (Fig. 7-17). This is a relatively inefficient oxygen delivery device for several reasons. The maximal rate at which oxygen can be delivered via nasal cannula is 6 L/min. Flow at higher rates is irritating to the nasal mucosa. Oxygen delivered by the nasal prongs also mixes immediately with ambient air entering the nostrils and thus is diluted quickly. Consequently, the concentration of oxygen actually delivered to the alveoli by this method averages approximately 24%.

The **non-rebreather mask** (partial rebreather) is the best device for providing supplemental oxygen to a spontaneously breathing patient. The non-rebreather mask consists of a face mask, a bag reservoir, and a one-way flow valve that allows oxygen to flow from the reservoir into the mask without letting exhaled air into the reservoir (Fig. 7-18). A high concentration of oxygen therefore is maintained within the reservoir at all times, and the concentration of oxygen inhaled with each breath from the reservoir often exceeds 90%. Different mask sizes are available for children and adults. The mask should fit the patient snugly, but an airtight seal is not necessary (Skill 7-13). The reservoir bag should be inflated with oxygen before the mask is applied, and the flow rate should be sufficient (15 L/min) to prevent the bag from collapsing when the patient inhales.

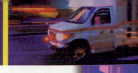

SKILL 7-12

Oxygen Tank/Regulator/Tubing Assembly

1. Ensure the protective seal has been removed from the valve on the tank. Do not lose the washer attached to the seal because it provides an airtight seal between the regulator and the tank.

2. Turn the valve away from yourself or anyone else. Quickly open and close the valve to blow any dirt or contaminants out of the tank opening.

3. Place the washer over the inlet port on the regulator.

4. Line up the regulator port and pins with the tank opening and holes in the tank valve.

5. Check the flowmeter to ensure it is turned off.

6. Tighten the screw by hand.

7. Open the tank to test for an airtight seal. If there is leakage, tighten the screw until the leak stops. Once you have made sure there are no leaks, the tank valve must be completely open or completely closed.

8. Adjust the flowmeter to the desired setting. When finished, turn off the flowmeter and close the tank valve.

9. Open the flowmeter momentarily to release the pressure from the regulator.

SKILL 7-13

Application of Non-rebreather Mask

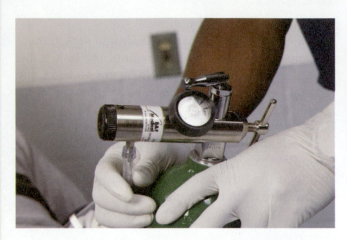

1. Attach non-rebreather mask to oxygen tank with regulator using connective tubing.

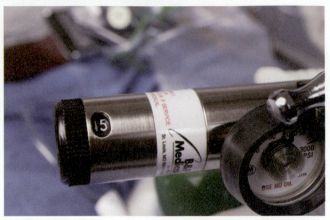

2. Adjust the regulator to deliver oxygen at 15 L/min.

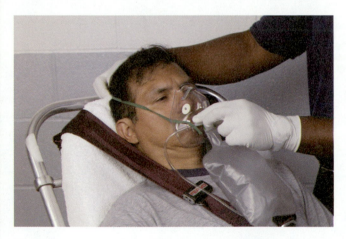

3. Insert a finger into the face mask and occlude the port connecting the face mask with the oxygen reservoir. Maintain the occlusion long enough (3 to 5 seconds, usually) for the reservoir bag to inflate fully.

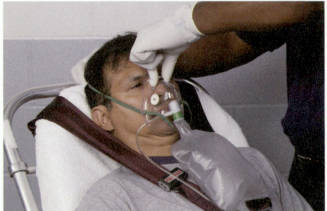

4. Place the mask over the patient's nose and mouth, and then secure it behind the patient's head with the attached elastic strap.

SKILLS

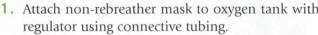

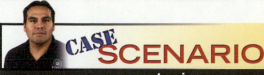

CASE SCENARIO
conclusion

With the assistance of his crew, Rafael worked to move Mr. Wilson to a semi-Fowler position, using pillows and blankets under Mr. Wilson's back as support. Using the bag-mask, he began to assist the patient's respiratory effort, squeezing the bag when Mr. Wilson tried to breathe in. He also encouraged Mr. Wilson to breathe as deeply as he could and to not fight the pressure feeling of the bag-valve-mask as it was being used. Mr. Wilson was frightened, but the young firefighter's reassuring words helped him to relax a little. Soon Rafael found he could provide ventilation to Mr. Wilson with the bag fairly easily. The medics arrived to take over care. ■

Resources

American Heart Association: *2000 Handbook of emergency cardiovascular care for healthcare providers*, Dallas, 2000, American Heart Association.

Ossmann EW: Pre-hospital pearls, pitfalls, and updates, *Emerg Med Clin North Am* 15(2):283-301, 1997.

Stapleton ER: Basic life support cardiopulmonary resuscitation, *Cardiol Clin* 20(1):1, 2002.

Wenzel V, Idris AH, Montgomery WH, et al: Rescue breathing and bag-mask ventilation, *Ann Emerg Med* 37(suppl):S36-S40, 2001.

Young KD: Pediatric cardiopulmonary resuscitation: state of the art, *Clin Pediatr Emerg Med* 2:80-84, 2001.

Young KD, Seidel JS: Pediatric cardiopulmonary resuscitation: a collective review, *Ann Emerg Med* 33:195-205, 1999.

TEAMWORK

The emergency medical technician (EMT) must be skilled in assessing and managing airway emergencies as they arise. However, the EMT also must be skilled in working and communicating effectively with other first responders and emergency medical personnel to ensure the best patient care possible. The EMT must be able and prepared to instruct other scene personnel on how best to assist with airway-opening maneuvers, assisted ventilation, and the provision of supplemental oxygen. Such instruction demands expertise on the part of the EMT with each of the interventions described in this chapter. Moreover, during base contact en route and upon arrival at the receiving medical facility, the EMT must list concisely and explain the reasoning for each action taken to secure the patient's airway and breathing. This information is vital to the emergency medical personnel who will assume care of the patient so that further support and intervention may be planned and carried out as needed.

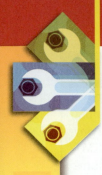

NUTS AND BOLTS

Critical Points

The emergency medical technician must begin every patient evaluation with an assessment for signs of an obstructed airway or compromised breathing. The quick recognition of these life threats requires understanding the fundamental anatomic and physiologic principles of breathing and the clinical symptoms exhibited by patients whose respiration is impaired. Upon identification, the emergency medical technician must meet any such threat with decisive and skillful action if the patient is to survive. Close familiarity with the equipment and techniques used to open the airway, provide assisted ventilation, and provide supplemental oxygen is therefore mandatory.

Learning Checklist

❑ Name the basic anatomic structures of the respiratory system, and explain the mechanics and physiology of breathing.

❑ Describe the signs of adequate and inadequate breathing in pediatric and adult patients, and explain them in the context of the mechanics and physiology of breathing.

❑ Describe the principles and proper performance of airway-opening maneuvers, such as the head tilt–chin lift and the jaw thrust techniques.

❑ Define the different types of airway adjuncts, the indications for their use, and the correct methods of inserting them.

❑ Describe in detail the equipment necessary and the proper means of delivering assisted ventilation using the mouth-to-mask, bag-valve-mask, and flow-restricted ventilator techniques.

❑ Explain different oxygen delivery systems along with the advantages and disadvantages of each.

❑ List the special anatomic and physiologic considerations in evaluating and treating special populations such as infants and children, the elderly, and patients with a tracheostomy and airway compromise.

Key Terms

Accessory muscles Muscles of the anterior neck and intercostal spaces that pull the anterior portion of the rib cage upward and outward, expanding intrathoracic volume. Use of these muscles often signifies respiratory distress.

Agonal respirations Short, irregular, and gasping breaths interspersed with long periods of apnea, usually signifying imminent death.

Alveoli Small air sacs within the lungs formed by elastic, highly vascularized membrane. Oxygen delivered to the alveoli during inspiration diffuses across the membrane and into the bloodstream. In the bloodstream oxygen is taken up by red blood cells, bound to hemoglobin, and transported to tissues throughout the body. At the same time, carbon dioxide dissolved in the blood diffuses in the opposite direction, crossing the membrane and accumulating within the alveoli to be exhaled.

Apnea The absence of spontaneous respiration.

Assisted ventilation Provision of breaths to a patient with inadequate or absent ventilatory effort.

Bag-mask Device used to provide assisted ventilation, consisting of a face mask connected by a one-way valve to a self-inflating bag and an oxygen reservoir.

Bronchi Large air passages that divide off of the trachea in the lower respiratory tract.

Bronchioles Smaller air passages within the lungs that divide off of the main bronchi and ultimately terminate in clusters of alveoli.

Carina The point at which the trachea divides into the left and right mainstem bronchi.

Cricoid cartilage Ring-shaped cartilaginous structure at the junction of the larynx with the trachea.

Cricothyroid membrane Thin sheet of connective tissue spanning the space between the anterior portions of the thyroid cartilage and the cricoid cartilage.

Cyanosis Blue discoloration of the skin signifying poor oxygen delivery to the tissues. The oxygen-carrying molecule in red blood cells, hemoglobin, takes on a bluish color when

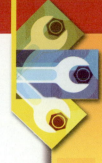

not bound to oxygen. Thus when a high proportion of hemoglobin in the blood delivered to the tissues is not bound to oxygen, the tissues appear blue.

Dead space Volume of gas that remains stagnant in the respiratory tract with each ventilation, usually about 150 mL in a normal-sized adult.

Diaphragm Thin, dome-shaped muscle that forms the inferior border of the thoracic cavity and separates the contents of the chest from those of the abdomen. Flattening of the diaphragm with contraction expands the intrathoracic volume and draws air into the lungs. Relaxation of the diaphragm lessens intrathoracic volume and allows for exhalation.

Dyspnea The sensation of difficulty breathing.

Epiglottis A curved flap of tissue that covers the opening of the trachea when swallowing occurs to prevent food or liquid from entering the lower respiratory tract.

Erythrocytes Red blood cells. These cells contain molecules of hemoglobin that bind oxygen diffusing into the bloodstream across the alveolar membranes in the lung for delivery to the tissues throughout the body.

Flow-restricted, oxygen-powered ventilation device Ventilator that, when triggered, delivers airflow through a face mask at a maximum flow rate of 40 L/min and a maximum inspiratory pressure of 60 cm H_2O.

Head tilt–chin lift Simple airway-opening maneuver accomplished with one hand placed on the patient's forehead and two or three fingers of the other hand positioned beneath the chin. The chin then is lifted gently upward as the head is tilted backward. Flexing the neck and pulling the mandible forward in this manner will pull the tongue out of the posterior pharynx. This technique is contraindicated if the potential for a cervical spine injury exists.

Hypoventilation Inadequate volume of gas exchange in the lungs.

Jaw thrust Airway-opening technique best suited for the supine patient with a possible cervical spine injury. One hand is placed on either side of the patient's head to provide neutral, in-line cervical spine stabilization, while fingers of each hand are positioned behind the angle of the mandible. Forward pressure thrusts the jaw outward, lifting the tongue off of the wall of the posterior pharynx.

Larynx Cartilaginous structure in the anterior neck connecting the posterior pharynx with the trachea in the upper airway. Also known as the voice box.

Lower respiratory tract Air passages formed by the trachea, bronchi, and bronchioles, and terminating in the alveoli.

Minute ventilation The tidal volume of an average breath multiplied by the number of times the individual breathes over 1 minute.

Mouth-to-mask ventilation Form of assisted ventilation in which the rescuer places a mask over the face of the victim, maintains an airtight seal against the face, and delivers breaths directly to the patient by blowing directly through a port in the mask.

Nasal cannula Oxygen tubing with two small prongs that are inserted into the nostrils. A relatively inefficient means of delivering supplemental oxygen.

Nasopharyngeal (nasal) airway Flexible tube inserted through one nostril into the posterior pharynx as a means of preserving the passage of air through the posterior pharynx.

Nasopharynx The cavity or air passage that lies immediately posterior to the nose and forms the upper portion of the pharynx.

Non-rebreather mask Combination of a face mask, a bag reservoir, and a one-way flow valve that allows oxygen to flow from the reservoir into the mask without letting exhaled air into the reservoir. This ensures that a high concentration of oxygen is contained within the reservoir at all times, in turn delivering a high concentration of oxygen with each inhalation.

Oropharyngeal (oral) airway Rigid, curved instrument that, when properly placed, maintains an open conduit for air passage between the tongue and the posterior wall of the oropharynx in the supine patient.

Oropharynx The air cavity/passageway situated at the back of the mouth.

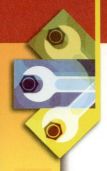

NUTS AND BOLTS

Paradoxical breathing "See-saw" movement of the chest and abdominal wall muscles with breathing in an effort to augment expansion of the thoracic cavity with inspiration. Often a sign of respiratory distress, particularly among infants and children.

Pharynx The cavity or open space above the larynx and posterior to the nose and mouth. May be subdivided further into the nasopharynx and the oropharynx.

Rales Fine crackling sounds generated when fluid-filled or collapsed alveoli suddenly reexpand with inspiration.

Respiration The physiologic process by which oxygen that is drawn into the lungs is delivered to tissues and cells throughout the body and is exchanged for the waste products of cell metabolism.

Stoma Opening on the anterior surface of the neck that connects the trachea directly to the outside air.

Stridor A high-pitched, harsh respiratory sound that is a sign of upper airway obstruction.

Thyroid cartilage Cartilaginous structure of the larynx, commonly known as the Adam's apple.

Tidal volume Volume of air inspired and exhaled with each breath, usually about 500 mL in an average-sized adult.

Trachea The air conduit that extends from the lower portion of the larynx into the chest, where it then divides into the right and left mainstem bronchi.

Tracheostomy Surgical procedure by which a channel is created in the anterior neck connecting the upper portion of the trachea to the outside air.

Upper respiratory tract A system of air passages formed by the nose and mouth, the pharynx, and the larynx.

Ventilation Mechanical process of inspiration and exhalation by which air rich in oxygen is breathed into the lungs and an equal volume of gas is expired, eliminating carbon dioxide from the body.

Vocal cords Thin strips of connective tissue attached to the muscles of phonation within the upper portion of the larynx. Variations in the vibration of the vocal cords caused by air passing through the upper airway generate the sounds necessary for speech.

Wheezing High-pitched expiratory breath sounds caused by narrowing of the small air passages (bronchioles) in the lungs that most commonly is a result of an acute asthmatic episode.

National Standards Curriculum Objectives

Cognitive Objectives

After completing this lesson, the EMT student will be able to do the following:

- Name and label the major structures of the respiratory system on a diagram.
- List the signs of adequate breathing.
- List the signs of inadequate breathing.
- Describe the steps in performing the head tilt–chin lift.
- Relate mechanism of injury to opening of the airway.
- Describe the steps in performing the jaw thrust.
- State the importance of having a suction unit ready for immediate use when providing emergency care.
- Describe the techniques of suctioning.
- Describe how to provide ventilation to a patient artificially with a pocket mask.
- Describe the steps in performing the skill of giving a patient artificial ventilation with a bag-valve-mask while using the jaw thrust.
- List the parts of a bag-valve-mask system.
- Describe the steps in performing the skill of giving a patient artificial ventilation with a bag-valve-mask for one and two rescuers.
- Describe the signs of adequate artificial ventilation using the bag-valve-mask.
- Describe the signs of inadequate artificial ventilation using the bag-valve-mask.
- Describe the steps in artificially ventilating a patient with a flow-restricted, oxygen-powered ventilation device.
- List the steps in performing the actions taken when providing mouth-to-mask and mouth-to-stoma artificial ventilation.

178

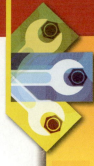

- Describe how to measure and insert an oropharyngeal (oral) airway.
- Describe how to measure and insert a nasopharyngeal (nasal) airway.
- Define the components of an oxygen delivery system.
- Identify a non-rebreather face mask, and state the oxygen flow requirements needed for its use.
- Describe the indications for using a nasal cannula versus a non-rebreather face mask.
- Identify a nasal cannula and state the flow requirements needed for its use.

Affective Objectives

After completing this lesson, the EMT student will be able to do the following:

- Explain the rationale for basic life support artificial ventilation and airway protective skills taking priority over most other basic life support skills.
- Explain the rationale for providing adequate oxygenation through high inspired oxygen concentrations to patients who in the past may have received low concentrations.

Psychomotor Objectives

After completing this lesson, the EMT student will be able to do the following:

- Demonstrate the steps in performing the head tilt–chin lift.
- Demonstrate the steps in performing the jaw thrust.
- Demonstrate the techniques of suctioning.

- Demonstrate the steps in providing mouth-to-mask artificial ventilation with body substance isolation (barrier shields).
- Demonstrate how to use a pocket mask to give a patient artificial ventilation.
- Demonstrate the assembly of a bag-valve-mask unit.
- Demonstrate the steps in performing the skill of giving a patient artificial ventilation with a bag-mask device for one and two rescuers.
- Demonstrate the steps in performing the skill of giving a patient artificial ventilation with a bag-mask device while using the jaw thrust.
- Demonstrate artificial ventilation of a patient with a flow-restricted, oxygen-powered ventilation device.
- Demonstrate how to give artificial ventilation to a patient with a stoma.
- Demonstrate how to insert an oropharyngeal (oral) airway.
- Demonstrate how to insert a nasopharyngeal (nasal) airway.
- Demonstrate the correct operation of oxygen tanks and regulators.
- Demonstrate the use of a non-rebreather face mask, and state the oxygen flow requirements needed for its use.
- Demonstrate the use of a nasal cannula, and state the flow requirements needed for its use.
- Demonstrate how to give artificial ventilation to the infant and child patient.
- Demonstrate oxygen administration for the infant and child patient.

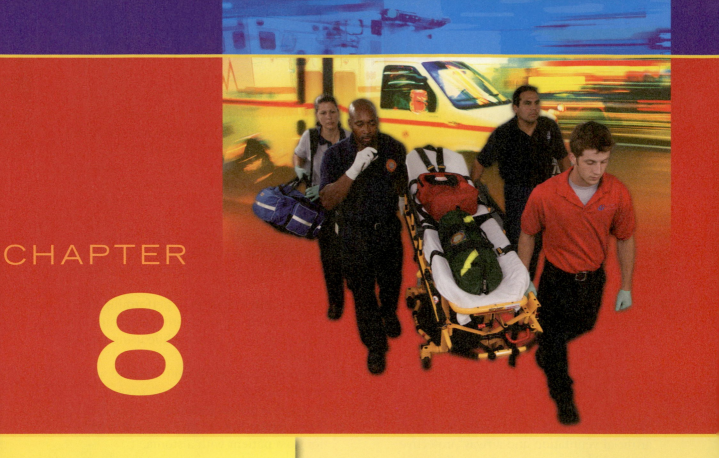

CHAPTER

8

OUTLINE

GOAL

LESSON GOAL

This chapter provides the emergency medical technician student with the information necessary to evaluate a scene during the initial stages of response. It emphasizes hazard awareness, mechanism of injury, nature of illness, patient numbers, and the need for additional assistance. ■

Scene Size-up

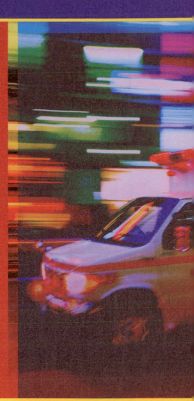

CHAPTER OBJECTIVES

After completing this chapter, the EMT student should be able to do the following:

1 Discuss the different hazards that the emergency medical technician may face at the scene.

2 Describe common hazards found at the scene of a trauma situation and a medical situation.

3 Determine whether the scene is safe to enter.

4 Discuss common mechanisms of injury and nature of illness.

5 Explain why it is important to know the number of patients at the scene.

6 Discuss why it is important to know when you need more help or assistance.

7 Discuss the reasons crew members should make sure the scene is safe before entering.

8 Explain the rationale for crew members to evaluate scene safety before entering a scene.

9 Serve as an example for others by explaining how patient situations affect your evaluation of mechanism of injury or nature of illness.

10 Observe various scenarios and identify potential hazards.

8

OBJECTIVES

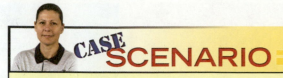

CASE SCENARIO

Elizabeth scans the scene in front of her as the unit nears the scene of the motor vehicle crash. The intersection is the busiest one in town, where two four-lane roadways cross each other. Over the years, traffic engineers have adjusted the timing of the intersection lights to reduce the number of incidents, but crashes occur when drivers try to "beat the red." Tonight appears to be no exception. Elizabeth and her crew observe that a late-model four-door sedan has struck the driver side of an older compact car just behind the door. Deformity to the side of the car is obvious; from a distance, Elizabeth estimates that there is at least a foot of intrusion into the passenger compartment of the small car. Broken window glass litters the street, and brown and green fluids are coming from under the vehicles.

One police cruiser is on the scene, parked across the two center lanes to block traffic. One of the officers is waving off oncoming vehicles. The other is speaking to what appears to be the driver of the larger car. Elizabeth notes that the driver of the compact car is still in the driver's seat.

The ambulance comes to a stop just beyond the crash scene, blocking another two lanes of traffic. Elizabeth and her crew carefully exit the rig, making sure no vehicles are passing by them. As Elizabeth grabs the first-in bag, her crew members put on latex gloves and safety glasses and gather various immobilization equipment and place it on the gurney. They begin to move toward the crash scene.

Question: *What are a few of the hazards that face Elizabeth and her crew? What actions can be performed to help minimize the risk to the rescuers on scene?*

■ SCENE SIZE-UP FACTORS

The emergency medical technician (EMT) should consider a number of factors when conducting the scene size-up:

- Scene safety
- **Mechanism of injury**
- **Nature of illness**
- Number of patients
- Need for additional assistance

■ SCENE SAFETY

Your first responsibility is to evaluate the scene for safety. You should assess for your ability to handle this situation safely by yourself. Do you need help? Should you just back out and wait? You can use the *Who, What, Where, When, Why,* and *How* method to establish safety (Fig. 8-1; Table 8-1):

Who: When you arrive on the scene, look around at all the individuals who are present. Then ask yourself, "Who at this scene could make things unsafe for the patient, my partner, or myself?" If you identify a person or group that may be a haz-

SPECIAL Considerations

Are There Hazardous People on the Scene?
"During a 12-year employment period, paramedics received an average of nine assaults per paramedic. Assault injuries resulted in 170 cases of blunt trauma, 73 lacerations, 2 gunshot wounds, 10 stabbings, 1 burn, 8 fractures, 9 dislocations, 1 choking, and 56 cases of miscellaneous body injuries."[1]

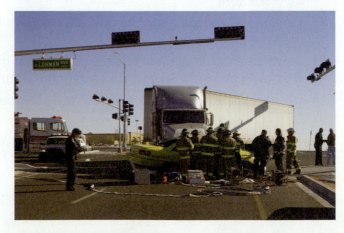

Fig. 8-1 Assess the situation for hazards: *Who, What, Where, When,* and *How?*

TABLE 8-1

Who, What, Where, When, Why, and **How** of scene safety

Factor	Question	Examples
Who	Who at this scene could make this situation unsafe for you?	• A violent patient or bystander • An unruly crowd • Alcohol- or drug-impaired person on scene • An exposure patient (blood or body fluids present) • A large patient • Unaccounted for persons at the scene (Who is missing?)
What	What is present at this scene to make it unsafe?	• Gunshots • Family altercation • Traffic • Smoke • Fumes • Fluid leaks • Placards (indicating hazards) • Low oxygen area • Weather
Where	Where are safety issues at this scene?	• Unstable vehicle • Uncontrolled traffic • Dark house • Dog present • Unsafe footing
When	When is this scene most likely to be unsafe?	• During initial contact • When a patient is suicidal • As traffic begins to move • As extrication begins • During patient movement
Why	Why is this scene unsafe?	• Lack of lighting • Lack of crowd control • Tempers • Presence of body fluids
How	How could this scene become unsafe?	• Additional personnel on scene creating safety issues • A glove is punctured • It begins to rain • An argument begins

ard, determine whether it is safe to continue. If it is safe to continue, stay alert to changes in this person's or group's behavior, and be prepared to change your plans or leave the scene as indicated. Perhaps someone who should be at the scene is not present. For example, the family member who abused your patient may be absent; however, he or she may return suddenly. Be sure to assess the need for law enforcement. In addition, keep your partner informed of your concerns.

> **Important Points**
>
> Keep your partner informed of any scene safety concerns you have.

You also may be required to care for a person who is bleeding, vomiting, or presenting some other type of exposure concern. You should wear gloves, eye protection, a gown, and a mask as the scene dictates. To treat all patients as potential exposure hazards and to wear your **personal protective equipment** upon arrival at the scene for every patient encounter is the best practice. That way, if a safe scene suddenly becomes unsafe—for example, a patient vomits—you are protected.

Another type of patient who may be a hazard to emergency medical services personnel is a very large patient or a patient who may have to be moved a long distance. Because of the weight or distance, you may be putting your back, knees, and ankles at risk for injury. When encountering such a patient, protect yourself with good body mechanics and additional assistance as needed.

What: What is present at this scene to make it unsafe? Have you been dispatched to the scene of "shots fired," "family fight," "altercation," or "possible suicide"? If you have been dispatched to one of these or any other potentially violent scene, it is best to wait until law enforcement arrives to secure the scene before you enter.

SPECIAL Considerations

Following several publicized incidents where gang members shot the patient the emergency medical technicians were treating, many emergency medical services agencies believe it may be safer to leave the scene with the patient before performing a complete assessment when responding to calls that may be related to gang violence to avoid further injury to their patient and injury to themselves.

Important Points

Treat all patients as if they pose an exposure risk. Wear your personal protection equipment.

Important Points

Use good body mechanics and additional resources to move large patients.

Important Points

Do not enter a violent scene until it is controlled by law enforcement.

With motor vehicle incidents, you should be assessing for traffic control. Consider whether other vehicles can see you, you are off the road, and the traffic has been controlled. Look for smoke, fumes, fluid leaks, and placards when appropriate. If any of these are present, take the appropriate hazardous materials or fire precautions. If you respond to a scene with unconscious victims, consider that you may have entered an environment with inadequate oxygen and the potential effect on your crew and yourself.

You should consider the weather to be a hazard as well. Fog, rain, sleet, and snow can alter the environment significantly and put you at risk. These elements may impair vision or make surfaces slick or unstable. In addition, extremes in temperature may affect your crew and patients and put them at risk for heat and cold emergencies, such as hypothermia, frostbite, heat stroke, or heat exhaustion.

Where: You also should be asking yourself, "Where are the safety issues at this scene?" Look around and evaluate the scene for safety hazards. For example, at a motor vehicle crash the most common hazards are an unstable vehicle and traffic. Thus you will need to focus on each of these, ensuring that traffic is diverted around your work zone and that vehicles are stabilized. At a home the potential risks to safety include body fluid exposure, violence, and protective dogs. Responding to a dark house should alert you to a possible problem, as well. Usually if you have been called to help, a light will be on and someone will greet you at the door.

Injuries are one of the biggest problems for EMTs. Therefore it should be a priority to monitor your footing for slick areas, materials to trip over, and

Important Points

Use resources to control traffic, fire, and hazardous materials incidents.

Important Points

Weather may make the scene unsafe.

Important Points

Awareness of your surroundings is key to scene safety.

SPECIAL Considerations

The following are some tips related to scene safety:

- Do not get lulled into a false sense of security: just because you have been here 10 times before does not mean it will be safe this time.
- Do not ignore risks of violence during travel to and from the call and trips back and forth to the apparatus while on the scene.
- Do not be confrontational or abusive to anyone or any group.
- Do not become an easy target: call for law enforcement early, and be prepared to bail out when the need arises. Do not become a dead hero.
- Do not ignore your gut feeling: when it does not feel right, it probably is not right.

Important Points

A change in the scene usually indicates a change in safety.

Important Points

Anticipating potential hazards will decrease your chances of injury.

holes into which to fall. You could injure an ankle, a knee, or your back from unstable footing.

When: In addition, you should be considering when a scene is unsafe. You can do this by asking yourself, "When is this scene most likely to be unsafe?" Even though you should always be aware of scene safety, with most scenes there are predictable times that a scene becomes unsafe or unstable. For instance, as you enter and leave a scene, you change the dynamics of the situation. Therefore you need to be aware of changing safety points. For example, you may be focused on finding an address on a house at night and may not be aware of a car pulling out of a driveway ahead of you. Or, for example, as metal begins to give under pressure, a previously safe extrication can become unsafe. The tool can break loose the metal it is supporting or change the balance of a vehicle on the cribbing or jacks. Continuously

reevaluating the scene will keep you aware of when safety aspects change.

How: "How might this scene become unsafe?" As you evaluate the scene, anticipation is important. You should always be thinking ahead about how a scene could deteriorate. For instance, the more persons present at a scene, the greater the potential for human error, which is one of the major contributors to injuries in the prehospital setting. You should anticipate the potential for harm from something as simple as a punctured glove causing a possible exposure to a change in behavior of a patient, which may cause major harm to you or your crew.

■ ENTERING THE SCENE

Once you have established the potential hazards of a scene, take precautions to control the hazards. If the scene cannot be made safe, do not enter (Fig. 8-2). If you anticipate a violent scene, wait for law enforcement. When a scene involves hazards such as fire or chemical exposure, notify the fire department or hazardous materials team.

Your service should have policies or protocols to address unsafe scenes. Following the protocols and notifying the appropriate authorities are important. If you do not have training to manage the hazard or do not have the appropriate resources, call for help as necessary. A two-way radio or other form of communication may be essential to maintaining your safety. If you have entered a scene and the safety conditions have deteriorated, you should exit the scene as soon as possible. The priority at all scenes is to maintain your safety and the safety of your partner.

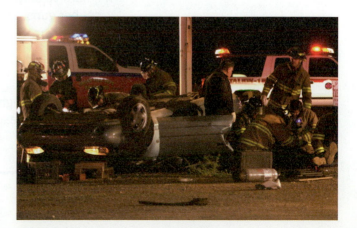

Fig. 8-2 As you enter the scene, control the hazards and be aware of changes.

TABLE 8-2

Common mechanisms of injury and patterns of injury

Mechanism of Injury	Predictors	Associated Patterns of Injury
Motor vehicle crash (type of impact and damage to the interior of the car may help predict the injuries)	Unrestrained	Multiple trauma, head, and neck injuries, scalp and facial lacerations
	Air bag	Head and neck, facial, and eye injuries
Motor vehicle/pedestrian crash (children are more commonly struck head-on, whereas adults are struck from the side)	Low speed	Lower extremity fractures
	High speed	Chest and abdominal injuries
Fall from a height	Low height	Upper or lower extremity fractures
	Medium height	Head and neck injuries, upper and lower extremity fractures
	Great height (3 times the patient's height = critical injuries)	Chest and abdominal injuries, head and neck injuries, upper and lower extremity fractures
Fall from a bicycle	Without a helmet	Head and neck injuries, scalp and facial lacerations, upper extremity fractures
	With a helmet	Upper extremity fractures
	Hitting the handlebar	Internal abdominal injuries
Motorcycle crash	Low speed	Lower extremity fractures and burns
	Medium speed	Head and neck injuries, upper and lower extremity fractures
	High speed	Chest and abdominal injuries, pelvic and femur fractures, head and neck injuries, upper and lower extremity fractures
Penetrating trauma	Low velocity (knives, ice picks)	Isolated to the area of penetration, severe blood loss possible
	Medium velocity (handguns, .22-caliber guns, shotguns)	Usually isolated to the area of penetration, but a wider area of damage should be suspected; also may have ricocheting of bullet through body Severe injury more likely
	High velocity (high-powered rifles and assault weapons)	Area of damage much larger than area of penetration Critical life-threatening injuries more likely

From Chapleau W: *Emergency first responder: making the difference,* St Louis, 2004, Mosby.

DETERMINING WHAT HAPPENED

As you enter a scene and establish safety, you also will be trying to determine what happened. You will look at a traumatic event and assess the forces and damage that occurred. This is referred to as the mechanism of injury. In a medical situation, you will try to identify the patient's medical condition and the resulting signs and symptoms. This is referred to as the nature of illness. Too often, emergency medical services providers assume that a patient has only a medical complaint or a traumatic injury. However, many patients can present a confusing picture. They may have a combination of medical and traumatic complaints. Provision of appropriate care will be based on identifying patient problems. Therefore it is essential that you understand and evaluate for both situations.

COMMON MECHANISMS OF INJURY

One of the clues you will use to determine patient injury is mechanism of injury (Table 8-2; Fig. 8-3). The mechanism of injury is the process of evaluating the forces involved in the incident and applying them to the injuries a patient has received. To understand the mechanism of injury, you must understand some basic laws of physics. These include **Newton's law of motion** and the law of kinetic energy. Newton's law of motion states, "A body in motion will stay in motion and a body at rest will stay at rest until acted on by an outside force." These principles can be applied to all trauma situations.

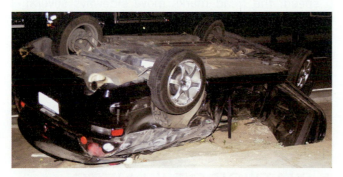

Fig. 8-3 Use the mechanism of injury to help predict patient injuries.

For example, in motor vehicle crashes the vehicle stays in motion until it comes into contact with another car, a tree, or any other object. Once that object is struck, the motion of the car will stop. Because the energy generated by the car cannot be destroyed, it must be used up in some way. The typical way the energy is used up is in destruction and damage to the car. The same principles apply to the persons inside the car (Fig. 8-4). The type of impact should help the EMT predict the types of injuries that may be present (Table 8-3). When motor vehicle crash victims are restrained, injuries tend to be less severe. However, the injuries may involve bruising from seat belts and burns and abrasions from air bag deployment.

As with any of these traumatic situations, speed is the deciding factor. The greater the speed, the greater the amount of damage. This is true of blunt and penetrating trauma. In blunt trauma, damage is caused by forces crushing and tearing the tissue internally, usually without an open wound (Fig. 8-5). These types of injuries are common in most sporting, car versus pedestrian, and motor vehicle incidents. Penetrating trauma is characterized by an open wound. Damage is caused by an object passing through the

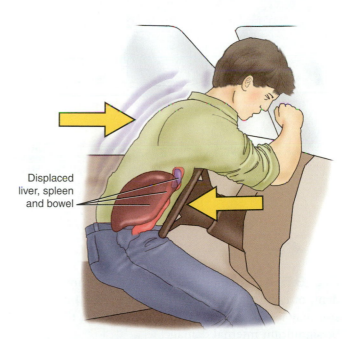

Displaced liver, spleen and bowel

Fig. 8-4 A frontal impact can cause potential injuries to the head, neck, chest, and pelvis.

Important Points

Mechanism of injury is key to patient assessment.

Important Points

Types of impact help predict injuries.

TABLE 8-3

Injuries in unrestrained motor vehicle crashes

Motor Vehicle Crashes	Indicator	Type of Injury
Frontal impact	Severity of damage to front of vehicle Starring of the windshield Damage to the steering wheel or dash	Head, neck, chest, and abdominal injuries from impact on dash, steering wheel, and windshield. Suspect lower extremity fractures from impact on dash
Lateral impact	Severity of damage to the side of the vehicle Broken side window Damage to door and panels	Head, neck, shoulder, upper arm injuries, lateral rib fractures, pelvic and hip injuries
Rear impact	Appropriate use of head rests Front and rear impact	Neck injuries and possible anterior chest damage

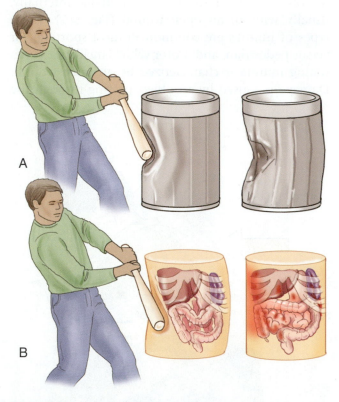

Fig. 8-5 **A**, Swinging a bat into a steel drum leaves a dent, or cavity, in its side. **B**, Swinging a bat into a person may leave no visible cavity even though there may be significant internal damage.

tissue and damaging it directly or by the cavity that is formed around the object as it forces its way through the tissue. The cavity damages the tissue by tearing and stretching the tissue. External bruising and wounds provide clues to the internal structures or organs damaged.

Important Points

The greater the speed at the time of impact, the greater the damage.

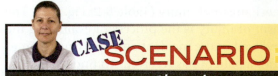

CASE SCENARIO continued

The police officers arriving on the scene quickly secure the intersection with traffic cones and flare patterns. Elizabeth moves toward the driver who is still in her car. From the tire skid marks on the ground, Elizabeth realizes that the car must have been struck at a fairly high rate of speed: the tread marks move sideways several feet. The driver appears to be awake as Elizabeth approaches the door, although she is not moving.

Question: *Based on the presentation of the vehicles, what injuries might Elizabeth expect of the driver?*

■ NATURE OF ILLNESS

If your patient has a medical condition, then your primary concern will be the nature of his or her illness. The best way to determine the nature of illness is to ask the patient or family members why they called you. The patient's **chief complaint,** or prob-

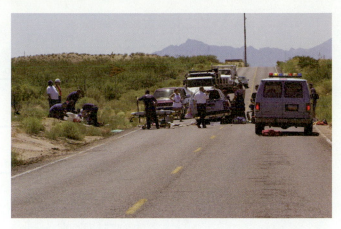

Fig. 8-6 Carefully assess the scene to locate patients.

lem, usually will give you a clue to the patient's illness. Your goal is to determine whether the patient has any condition that may be immediately life threatening or a safety risk to you or your crew. Life-threatening conditions are usually respiratory or cardiac or involve major bleeding or an alteration in the patient's mental status. Safety conditions may include exposure to a communicable disease. Therefore taking personal protective precautions is crucial.

Other sources that may assist you in determining the patient's medical problems are the presence of medical equipment, such as oxygen or a walker, and the presence of medications. Oxygen may indicate a respiratory problem, and a walker may indicate arthritis or recent hip or knee surgeries. Medications also can provide clues to a patient's problem. Medications are discussed in depth in Chapter 16. The information provided in that chapter will guide your assessment and history-gathering activities.

PATIENT NUMBERS

As you approach the scene, another factor you will need to consider is the number of patients involved. The more patients you have, the more resources you will need and use. Therefore it is essential to identify patient numbers as soon as possible. Ideally, you can do this by counting the number of patients present. On occasion, however, this may not be so simple. As crowds gather to view an incident, the patients can be difficult to identify. Thus when in doubt, simply ask. Moreover, patients can walk away from scenes or can be thrown clear of a crash site. Locating the child or passenger ejected during a motor vehicle crash may involve searching the site and asking bystanders and other victims what they saw and remember. You may even find yourself combing a scene for extended periods as you try to locate all the victims involved (Fig. 8-6).

ADDITIONAL ASSISTANCE

You should request additional assistance as soon as you think the potential need exists (Fig. 8-7). The assistance can always be cancelled. However, if you wait to call for assistance, you may be overwhelmed by the situation before help can arrive. The situation will dictate the assistance you need. For instance, the assistance you need may be as simple as extra personnel or as specific as a farm implement dealer who can assist you in disassembling a bailer to remove a patient. Regardless, the key is anticipation and early notification.

In summary, scene size-up requires you to be able to complete a rapid assessment of safety, mechanism of injury, nature of illness, number of patients, and the need for additional resources (Fig. 8-8). The scenes may be simple and easy to manage or over-

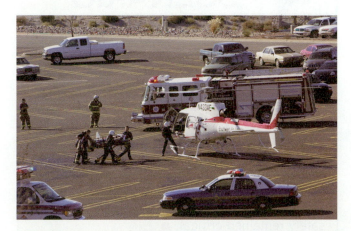

Fig. 8-7 Call for additional resources as needed: consider additional transport units, law enforcement, rotorcraft, and fire department.

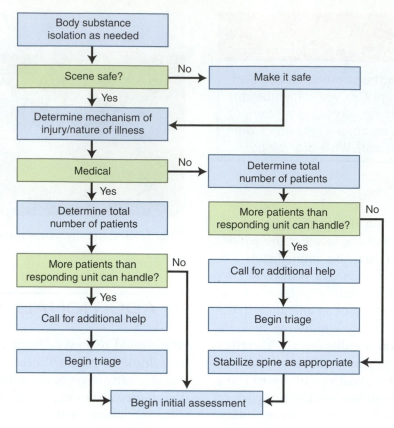

Fig. 8-8 Scene size-up algorithm.

whelming and full of complexities. The key is to be flexible and constantly aware of the changing dynamics and needs of the setting and to adjust your priorities accordingly.

Reference

1. Walsh DW: An analysis of paramedic-encountered violence in a large urban EMS system. *JEMS Prehospital Care Research Forum* p S-10, March 1996.

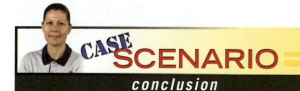

CASE SCENARIO
conclusion

Although it took some effort, the ambulance crew quickly extricated the driver out of the ambulance and secured her to a backboard. Someone had moved the ambulance closer to the scene, and they were able to load the patient right into the back. The driver maneuvered the unit out of the intersection, being careful not to run over the cones and flares that police had set up to secure the scene. The officers were going to be on the scene for a while still, so scene safety remained critical. ■

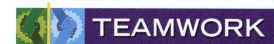

TEAMWORK

As previously discussed in this chapter, emergency medical technicians often are the first to arrive on the scene. Whether the scene is a traffic accident, hazardous materials incident, or crime scene, working together safely with law enforcement, firefighters, and other responders will contribute positively to the rescue. Understanding clues, signs, and symptoms will help emergency medical technicians determine the mechanism of injury or nature of illness when no other information is available. Remember at the end of the shift, we all want to go home to our loved ones safe and uninjured.

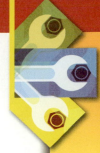

Critical Points

Keep your partner informed of any scene safety concerns you have. Treat all patients as if they pose an exposure risk. Wear your personal protection equipment. Use good body mechanics and additional resources to move large patients. Do not enter a violent scene until it is controlled by law enforcement. Use resources to control traffic, fire, and hazardous material incidents. Weather may make the scene unsafe. Awareness of your surroundings is key to scene safety. A change in the scene usually indicates a change in safety. Anticipation of potential hazards will decrease your chances of injury. Mechanism of injury is key to patient assessment. Types of impact help predict injuries. The greater the speed at the time of impact, the greater the damage.

Learning Checklist

❏ Your first responsibility is to evaluate the scene for safety.
❏ You can use the *Who, What, Where, When, Why,* and *How* method to establish safety.
❏ *Who:* Who at this scene could make things unsafe for the patient, your partner, or yourself?
❏ *What:* What is present at this scene to make it unsafe?
❏ *Where:* Where are the safety issues at this scene?
❏ *When:* When is this scene most likely to be unsafe?
❏ *How:* How might this scene become unsafe?
❏ Once you have established the potential hazards of a scene, take precautions to control the hazards. If you anticipate a violent scene, wait for law enforcement. When a scene involves hazards such as fire or chemical exposure, notify the fire department or hazardous materials team.
❏ If the scene cannot be made safe, *do not enter.*
❏ Following the protocols and notifying the appropriate authorities are important.
❏ If you do not have training to manage the hazard or do not have the appropriate resources, call for help as necessary.

❏ A two-way radio or other form of communication may be essential to maintaining your safety.
❏ If you have entered a scene and the safety conditions have deteriorated, you should exit the scene as soon as possible. The priority of a scene is to maintain your safety and the safety of your partner.
❏ As you enter a scene and establish safety, you will be looking at a traumatic event and assessing the forces and damage that occurred. Patients may have a combination of medical and traumatic complaints, and it is essential that you understand and evaluate for both situations.
❏ The mechanism of injury will help to determine patient injury. The mechanism of injury is the process of evaluating the forces involved in the incident and applying them to the injuries a patient has received.
❏ If your patient has a medical condition, then your primary concern will be the nature of his or her illness. The patient's chief complaint, or problem, usually will give you a clue to the patient's illness.
❏ Your goal is to determine whether the patient has any condition that may be immediately life threatening or a safety risk to you or your crew. If you should identify any such condition, take steps to deal with it immediately.
❏ As you approach the scene, another factor you will need to consider is the number of patients involved. The more patients you have, the more resources you will use and need. Therefore it is essential to identify patient numbers as soon as possible.
❏ You should request additional assistance as soon as you think the potential need exists. If you wait to call for assistance, you may be overwhelmed by the situation before help can arrive.

Key Terms

Chief complaint The patient's initial or primary statement of what the problem is.
Mechanism of injury The cause of the injuries or damage to the patient.

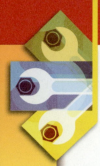

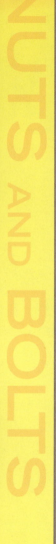

Nature of illness A determination of the patient's illness from findings.

Newton's law of motion A body in motion will stay in motion and a body at rest will stay at rest until acted on by an outside force

Personal protective equipment Equipment used to isolate a health care worker from a patient's body substances. Also refers to specialty equipment used by emergency providers during the course of a rescue or a fire.

National Standard Curriculum Objectives

Cognitive Objectives

After completing this lesson, the EMT student will be able to do the following:

- Recognize hazards/potential hazards.
- Describe common hazards found at the scene of a trauma and a medical patient.
- Determine whether the scene is safe to enter.

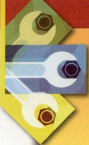

- Discuss common mechanisms of injury and nature of illness.
- Discuss the reason for identifying the number of patients at the scene.
- Explain the reason for identifying the need for additional help or assistance.

Affective Objectives
After completing this lesson, the EMT student will be able to do the following:

- Explain the rationale for crew members to evaluate scene safety before entering.

- Serve as a model for others by explaining how patient situations affect your evaluation of mechanism of injury or illness.

Psychomotor Objective
After completing this lesson, the EMT student will be able to do the following:

- Observe various scenarios and identify potential hazards.

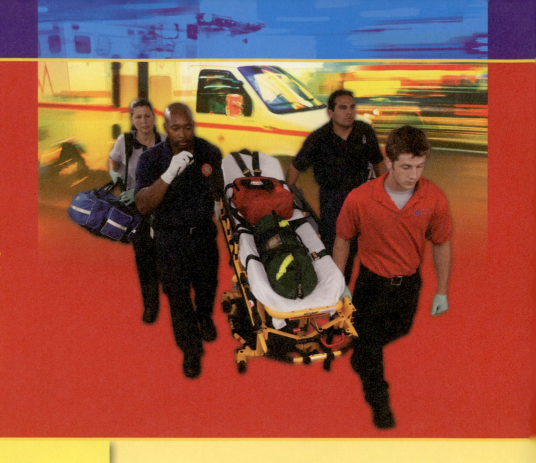

CHAPTER

9

LESSON GOAL

GOAL

This chapter provides the emergency medical technician (EMT) with the knowledge and skills to perform an initial assessment of a medical or trauma patient. This assessment involves forming a general impression of the patient and determining whether the patient is in critical condition. In addition, you will learn to determine the adequacy of the patient's airway, breathing, and circulation, and initial measures for supporting each of these functions. ■

Initial Patient Assessment

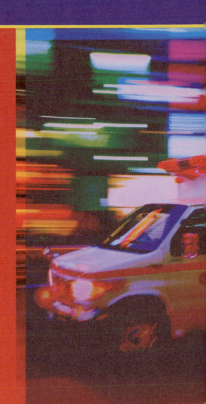

CHAPTER OBJECTIVES

9

After completing this chapter, the EMT student will be able to do the following:

1 Discuss why it is important to form a general impression of the patient.
2 Discuss the ways to assess a patient with altered mental status.
3 Discuss the differences in assessing altered mental status.
4 Discuss methods of assessing the airway.
5 Discuss why it is important to manage the cervical spine of a trauma patient.
6 Describe methods of assessing whether a patient is breathing.
7 State the care that should be provided to a patient with adequate breathing.
8 State the care that should be provided to a patient without adequate breathing.
9 Discuss the difference between a patient with adequate breathing and one with inadequate breathing.
10 Describe the methods used to obtain a pulse.
11 Discuss the need for assessing the patient for external bleeding.
12 Describe normal and abnormal findings when assessing skin color.
13 Describe normal and abnormal findings when assessing skin temperature.
14 Describe normal and abnormal findings when assessing skin condition.
15 Explain the reason for prioritizing a patient for care and transport.
16 Explain the importance of forming a general impression of the patient.

Continued

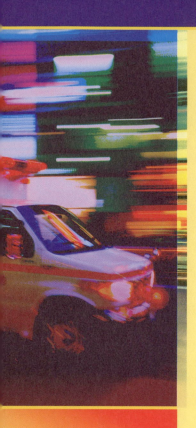

Chapter Objectives—cont'd

17 Explain the value of performing an initial assessment.

18 Describe and perform the techniques for assessing mental status.

19 Describe and perform the techniques for assessing the airway.

20 Describe and perform the techniques for assessing whether the patient is breathing.

21 Describe and perform the techniques for assessing whether the patient has a pulse.

22 Describe and perform the techniques for assessing the patient for external bleeding.

23 Describe and perform the techniques for assessing the patient's skin color, temperature, and condition and capillary refill.

24 Demonstrate the ability to prioritize patients.

CASE SCENARIO

"Fire Department! Did someone call for help?" Captain Alvarez pounds on the door to the small, single-family home not far from the station. Behind the door, the captain and his crew can hear the muffled cry of a woman, "The door's unlocked! Please come in!"

Cautiously Captain Alvarez opens the door and steps into a dim living room. He immediately hears sounds coming down the hallway from the back of the building. "Fire Department!" he calls out again. "Where are you?"

"Back here in the kitchen! Hurry!" the woman cries.

Looking over the captain's shoulder, Rafael sees the legs of a person lying on the kitchen floor. As the crew makes its way down the hall, they hear a woman counting, "One and two and three and..."

Coming into the kitchen, Rafael sees a woman in her twenties frantically performing chest compressions on a man lying supine on the floor. A cordless phone lies nearby. He hears the voice of one of the county's telecommunicators coming from the phone, encouraging the woman to continue cardiopulmonary resuscitation (CPR). The crew members quickly begin their assignments. While one of the firefighters opens the silver pouch containing the automatic external defibrillator (AED) patches, Rafael kneels at the patient's head to begin his initial assessment.

Question: What should Rafael's first steps be in beginning his assessment? Why is it important to perform these steps before continuing with care?

Patient assessment is the process by which the EMT systematically evaluates a patient for injuries or illness (Fig. 9-1). In this assessment, you focus on any injury or medical problem that immediately threatens the patient's life **(life threat).** If a life threat is identified, you combine your assessment skills with your treatment skills to correct the life threat. If you are certain no life threat is present or after you have treated the life threat, you can move on to assessing for less serious problems.

■ GENERAL IMPRESSION

To become an expert at patient assessment, you must be a good investigator and a good problem manager. You must be able to assess your patient and the scene systematically and to interview patients and bystanders. Once you have collected the information, you must form an impression about the situation and anticipate how the patient may respond. This first impression of the situation is referred to as a **general impression.** It guides your next actions. In addition, you must be able to communicate your findings to many other providers.

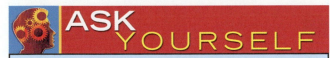

ASK YOURSELF

Have you asked yourself yet, "I wonder what my first call will be like? What kind of injuries or illness will my patient have? Will the problems be life-threatening or minor? What will I do? Can I provide good patient care for my first patient?"

SPECIAL Populations

Pediatric Perspectives

Assessing for orientation can be challenging in pediatric patients. Infants are unable to provide answers for you. Children who are just starting to talk generally can tell you their name but little else. Children who are a little older may be able to answer some basic questions about where they are. With very young children, the most important part of your assessment is observing the child's interaction with you (or, in many cases, the child's unwillingness to interact with you), the surroundings, and the parent or caregiver.

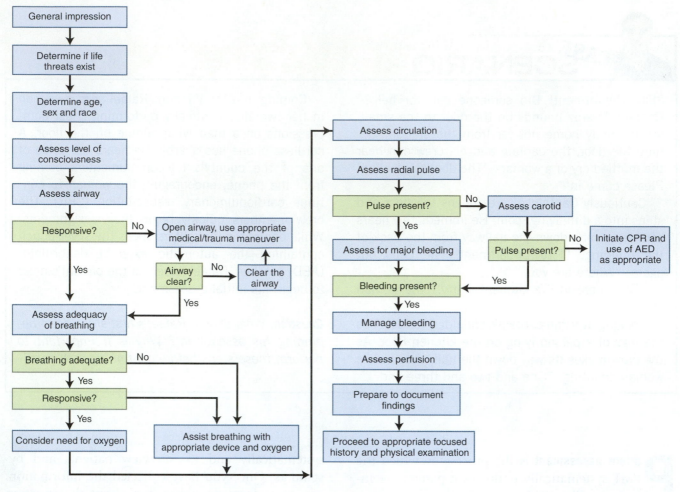

Fig. 9-1 Initial patient assessment flow chart.

The general impression includes assessing the nature of the illness or the mechanism of injury. The term **nature of the illness** typically is used for patients with medical conditions. It helps determine the type of medical problem these patients have. For example, a patient with slurred speech and weakness on one side may be having a stroke. The nature of this illness would be a neurologic emergency. The nature of the illness for a patient with difficulty breathing and a history of asthma is respiratory distress. The nature of the illness usually correlates with the affected body system.

When a patient is involved in a traumatic event, the situation is assessed for the mechanism of injury. Determining the **mechanism of injury** involves assessing the scene for the events that caused the patient's injuries. Examples of mechanisms of injury include motor vehicle crashes, motor vehicle–pedestrian crashes, falls, motorcycle and bicycle crashes, and gunshots or stabbings (see Table 8-2).

Even though the nature of the illness and the mechanism of injury are considered separate entities,

SPECIAL Considerations

Cultural Perspectives

First impressions are important. Although European Americans typically are encouraged to look people in the eye when speaking to them, some Asian and Native American groups may consider this disrespectful or impolite. Many people of Middle Eastern descent see direct eye contact between a man and a woman as a sexual invitation. Observe your patients when talking and listening to them for clues regarding appropriate eye contact.

it is important to recognize that both may be present. A patient involved in a motor vehicle crash may drive himself home and call for emergency medical services (EMS) several hours later, complaining of shortness of breath resulting from injuries received during the crash. If you do not collect a thorough history and maintain an index of suspicion, you might assume that the patient has a medical problem. An elderly patient with a cardiac history may call EMS with a complaint of hip pain after a fall. You may find the hip pain but miss the cause, which was a fainting spell caused by an irregular heartbeat.

A patient's age, gender, and race may be useful information when you are forming a general impression and identifying the patient's problem. For example, if you are dispatched on a call for a 2-year-old child with difficulty breathing, you should make a mental list of common respiratory problems associated with that age group. These problems may include croup, pneumonia, and foreign body aspiration. A 60-year-old male with difficulty breathing may have chronic obstructive pulmonary disease (COPD), a myocardial infarction (heart attack), or pneumonia. A 23-year-old female with abdominal pain may be assessed for appendicitis, kidney stones, or an ectopic pregnancy. A 16-year-old African American male with leg pain may be assessed for trauma, insect bites, or sickle cell disease. Even though the patient may not have any of the problems you think up, each problem is an area of assessment that should be

Important Points
Age, gender, and race are a few factors that can help you begin to mentally list possible injuries or illness.

considered when preparing to care for these types of patients.

The key factors for forming a general impression include the following:

- Life threats
- Nature of the illness
- Mechanism of injury
- Age, gender, and race (some diseases predominantly affect one race, such as sickle cell anemia, which primarily affects African Americans)

As you investigate and determine whether life threats exist, you must be prepared to solve the problems you find. Such problems may include an unsafe scene, a patient who is not breathing, or an equipment problem. You must know when to act quickly and when you have time to continue your investigation. In addition, you must select and apply the appropriate intervention or solution for the patient or situation. Once you have taken an action, you must evaluate the effect of that action on the patient or problem. You have many resources at your disposal, and you must determine which ones to call for and use and when. As you perform all these activities, you must plan which interventions to complete immediately and which to complete in the future. You also must develop a sense of flexibility, because each situation is unique and will change as you go along.

Excellent assessment skills are the most important skills an EMT can develop. It takes time, commitment, knowledge, and flexibility to develop such skills. When each of these factors is invested in learning these skills, the results save lives.

Once you have formed a general impression, you can start to focus on mental status and airway, breathing, and circulation. While these things are traditionally taught sequentially, usually beginning with the airway, in most situations you can and will assess these elements at the same time. For example, if you enter a patient's home and the patient is talking to you, you know the person is awake, has an open airway, is breathing, and has a pulse or circulation. Your job then is to determine whether each component is adequate. On the other hand, if you

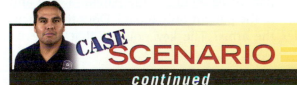

CASE SCENARIO continued

With the AED pads in place, Rafael presses the "Analyze" button on the machine and directs everyone to break contact with the patient. Within a few seconds the machine indicates that an electrical shock needs to be delivered to the patient. Rafael looks around the patient to make sure no one is touching the man. He then presses the button to deliver the charge. The man's body twitches for a moment as the electrical shock runs through it, trying to correct the electrical abnormality in the cardiac conduction system. Five seconds later, the AED provides a warning: "No shock indicated. Check pulse. Check breathing."

Question: Why is it important for Rafael to perform the initial assessment again? What might happen if he does not check the patient's pulse and breathing?

enter a home and the patient does not move or acknowledge you, you must systematically determine the patient's mental status and airway, breathing, and circulatory status. Establishing a systematic review process that covers each of these components is an important part of your EMT training.

■ ASSESSING THE PATIENT'S MENTAL STATUS

Once you arrive on scene, you determine the patient's **mental status,** which means how the person is responding to the current situation. To do this, you must determine whether the patient is awake and able to respond normally to the situation or to questions you ask. As you begin this process, you must take steps to protect the patient's spine if you suspect any type of trauma. This is done by stabilizing the patient's head and neck manually (see Chapter 29). Once the head and neck have been stabilized, you can continue assessing the patient's mental status.

To assess mental status, first ask, "Is the patient responsive or not?" You can assess this by speaking to the patient and evaluating the person's response to you. In many situations the patient will be awake and talking to you as you enter the scene. If so, the patient is responsive, and you can move to the next level of assessment. This also provides you immediate information about the patient's airway, breathing and circulation. If the patient is talking to you, you know

the patient has a pulse and you can obtain information about the airway based upon the quality of the speech, visible drooling, and whether or not there is any respiratory distress. If the patient does not respond to you, you must evaluate the responsiveness element in more detail. A tool you may find useful for evaluating a patient's responsiveness uses the mnemonic **AVPU** (Table 9-1).

The *A* represents the alert and talking patient. This is the responsive patient just described. To make sure that patients are alert, confirm that they are *oriented;* that is, they know their name, where they are, what day it is, and what happened to them. Patients who are oriented are able to provide all this information. This often is referred to as "alert and oriented to person (who), place (where), time (date), and situation (what)." Patients who are disoriented may be able to recall their name but none of the other information. These patients are described as alert and oriented to name but disoriented to place, time, and situation. A disoriented patient is considered a higher priority for a potential life threat than a patient who is oriented.

The *V* component of AVPU is used when the patient does not immediately respond to you when you enter the scene. It means that you have to speak to or shout at the patient, or use verbal stimuli, to get the person to respond to you. It also is important to note how the patient responds. Is the patient awake and alert? Does the patient only moan? Does the patient just flex the arms? The key point is that a greater

---

Important Points

If you suspect trauma, manually stabilize the patient's head and neck before continuing with treatment.

Important Points

Disorientation or an abnormal response to the alert, verbal, painful, and unresponsive (AVPU) assessment should produce a high index of suspicion for a potential life-threatening problem.

TABLE 9-1

Assessment tool: AVPU (alert, verbal, painful, unresponsive)

Responsive	Alert	Awake	Awake and oriented; responds to surroundings without being prompted or stimulated
	Verbal	Responds to verbal stimuli	Responds to verbal commands or to questions
	Painful	Responds to painful stimuli	Responds when a painful stimulus (e.g., a pinch) is administered
Non-responsive	Unresponsive	No response to stimuli	Does not move or respond verbally when questioned or when a painful stimulus is administered

SKILL 9-1
Initial Assessment: Unresponsive Patient

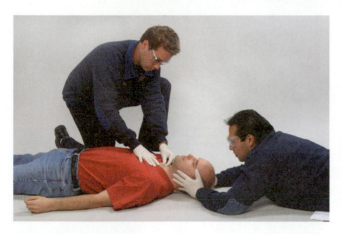

1. Evaluate general impression; assess degree of unresponsiveness.

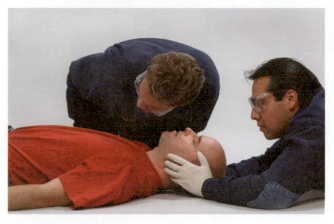

2. Assess airway and breathing.

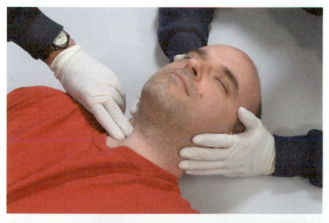

3. Assess for a pulse.

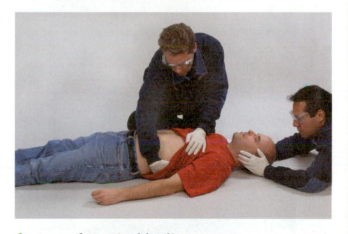

4. Assess for major bleeding.

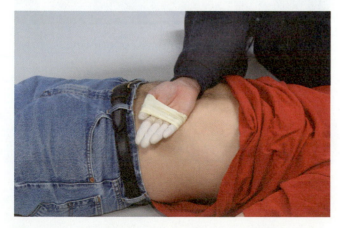

5. Assess the skin.
6. Determine disability and assess priority.

SKILL 9-2
Initial Assessment: Responsive Patient

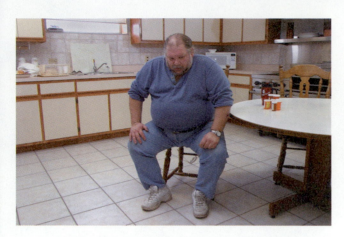

1. Evaluate general impression.

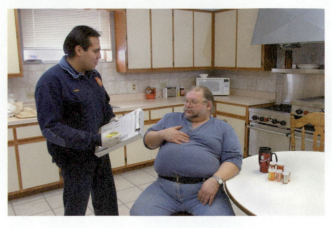

2. Assess responsiveness, airway, and breathing.

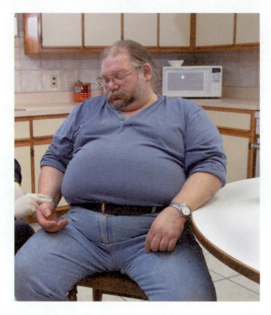

3. Assess circulation.

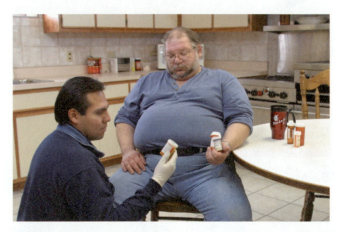

4. Determine disability and assess priority.

stimulus is required to get this patient to respond. If the response is anything but normal, the patient may have a serious or even critical condition.

The *P*, or painful, component is used when the patient is not alert and does not respond to verbal commands. When using painful stimuli, you do not want to injure the patient. You apply just enough uncomfortable stimuli to see whether the patient can be roused. Such stimuli can include pinching the shoulder or rubbing the sternum. As with the verbal component, your patient may respond normally or abnormally. Because this is a more aggressive stimulus, an abnormal response suggests that the patient should be monitored for more serious problems.

A patient who does not respond to voice or pain is considered unresponsive (the *U* component). You should treat this individual as a patient in critical condition and immediately focus on assessing the airway, breathing, and circulatory status. You also should consider rapid transport and, when possible, advanced life support (ALS) intercept (meeting up with an ALS unit while transporting the patient to the hospital).

The **Glasgow Coma Scale** is a tool for obtaining a more detailed evaluation of the patient's neurologic status. This technique not only assesses the patient's responsiveness but also motor functions and eye-opening response (see Chapter 10). (See the Special Populations box for assessing orientation in pediatric patients.)

■ ASSESSING THE PATIENT'S AIRWAY

After the patient's mental status has been established, the next priority is the airway. Airway assessment and management are discussed in detail in Chapter 7, therefore this section focuses on *initial* assessment and management.

In assessing the airway, you are determining whether the patient has an open, an obstructed, or a partly obstructed airway. A patient who is awake and talking to you has an open airway. Therefore you may begin assessing breathing adequacy. If your patient is not awake, you can assess the airway by performing a head-tilt/chin-lift (medical maneuver) or jaw thrust (trauma maneuver) and begin to look, listen, and feel for breathing. If the patient is breathing, the airway is open. If you do not hear breathing, ventilate the patient and clear any obstruction as soon as possible. You also may encounter a noisy airway. A noisy airway is a partly obstructed airway. You must clear it immediately by means of positioning or suctioning

as indicated. Consider using the recovery position to help maintain the patient's airway after you have it cleared. Once you have cleared and established an airway, it is essential that you continuously monitor its adequacy the entire time you are with the patient.

■ ASSESSING THE PATIENT'S BREATHING

After the airway has been assessed and managed, the next step is to evaluate breathing (see Chapter 5 for a detailed description of this process). Your focus in this step is to determine whether breathing is adequate. If the patient is not breathing, begin rescue breathing immediately. If the patient's breathing is adequate, move on to assessing the circulation. If the patient's breathing is not adequate (i.e., a respiratory rate of fewer than 8 or more than 24 breaths per minute), administer oxygen or assist respiration with a bag-mask device as indicated. A respiratory rate below 8 breaths per minute requires BVM assistance with 100% oxygen. A respiratory rate above 24 breaths per minute requires oxygen administration through a nonrebreather mask. Patients with inadequate respirations may need positive-pressure ventilation if they do not improve with administration of supplemental oxygen. Patients whose respiratory rate falls between 8 and 24 breaths per minute may also need oxygen, depending on their presentation and your assessment findings. If you have any question as to whether a patient needs oxygen, it is best to administer it in an appropriate manner.

■ ASSESSING THE PATIENT'S CIRCULATION

After the airway has been controlled and breathing supported, the next step is to determine circulation adequacy. (Circulation assessment and management are covered in detail in Chapters 5, 18, and 25.) The initial assessment of circulation is a three-step process.

1. **Is the pulse present?** You can assume your patient has a pulse if the person is awake and talking or trying to communicate with you in some way. If the patient is not responding or breathing, check the pulse immediately. If no pulse is present, initiate CPR. If the patient has a pulse, you must determine whether it is adequate. If the heart rate is below 60 or above 100 beats per minute, the patient may be showing

signs of a life-threatening condition that requires early intervention and rapid transport.

2. **Is major bleeding present?** Check for major bleeding. To do this, you may need to remove the patient's clothing and turn the person to assess for concealed injuries. Control any severe bleeding by using direct pressure, elevation, pressure points, and tourniquets as indicated. Major blood loss can lead to shock and death in a very short time. Therefore it is essential that you find any severe bleeding and control it. Keep in mind that not all bleeding occurs externally. If you think the patient may have major internal bleeding as a result of trauma or a medical cause (e.g., a ruptured aorta), immediately begin transport and attempt an ALS intercept.

3. **Is perfusion adequate?** Patients with warm, dry, normal-colored skin who are alert and oriented have good perfusion. Inadequate perfusion usually manifests as a change in responsiveness and changes in skin condition. Cool, moist, pale, or mottled skin is a sign of inadequate perfusion. You also will often find a weak and rapid or weak and slow pulse, delayed capillary refill, and decreased blood pressure. If perfusion is inadequate, you must begin oxygen therapy and assess and treat the patient for causes of shock. These patients need early transport and ALS care as soon as possible.

■ PRIORITIZING PATIENTS FOR CARE AND TRANSPORT

The goal of the initial assessment is to begin sorting patients and assign priorities for treatment and transport. Through the initial assessment, you can identify patients who are in critical condition or who have life threats (Table 9-2). These patients need immediate correction of the life threat, early and timely transport, and ALS care as soon as possible. Your job is to initiate the care as you assess and begin to plan transport. Once you have assessed a patient and determined that no life threats are present, or if you have stabilized the conditions you identified, you can move on to the next step, a focused history and physical examination.

TABLE 9-2

Indicators of a patient in critical condition

Assessment Factor	Indicators
General impression	Poor general impression
	Severe mechanism of injury
	Patient not moving
Mental status	Patient unresponsive
	Patient confused or disoriented
	Abnormal response to alert, verbal, painful, unresponsive (AVPU) assessment
	Pediatric patient: glassy stare, does not acknowledge caregiver
	Changing level of consciousness
Airway	Compromised airway
	Noisy respirations (e.g., stridor, snoring, or gurgling); grunting possibly present in infants
Breathing	Absence of breathing
	Inadequate rate and quality of breathing
	Difficulty breathing
	Use of accessory muscles
Circulation	Absence of pulse
	Weak, irregular pulse
	Extremely slow or fast pulse
	Cool, moist, pale, or cyanotic skin (shock)
	Delayed capillary refill, especially in children

Modified from Chapleau W: *Emergency first responder: making the difference*, St Louis, 2004, Mosby.

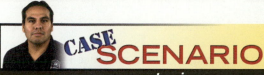

CASE SCENARIO

conclusion

The paramedics from Rescue 15 arrive on scene. Rafael quickly provides a report to the lead paramedic: "Upon our arrival, we found the patient's wife performing CPR. When we had her stop, I checked the man's airway, breathing, and circulation status. He wasn't breathing and had no pulse. We defibrillated him with the AED twice. When I checked his status again, he had a pulse, but he wasn't breathing. We continued to ventilate him with the BVM and oxygen." Rafael looks down at the patient for a moment. "And now he's beginning to breathe on his own."

The paramedic thanks Rafael for his report and kneels next to the patient to begin her care. Rafael and the other rescuers prepare to move the resuscitated patient to the ambulance. ■

TEAMWORK

As discussed in this chapter, EMTs must be confident in their assessment skills. How you interpret the information given to you by family, friends, bystanders, or first responders can greatly improve the patient's outcome. Continual patient assessment by the EMT, followed by proper treatment and transfer to an appropriate facility, certainly benefits everyone involved. Always remember that you are part of the health care community.

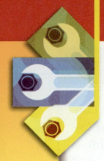

NUTS AND BOLTS

Critical Points

- Use age, gender, and race as factors that can help you begin to make a mental list of possible patient injuries or illnesses.
- If you suspect trauma, manually stabilize the patient's head and neck before continuing treatment.
- Disorientation or an abnormal response to AVPU should produce a high index of suspicion for a life-threatening problem.

Learning Checklist

- ❑ *Patient assessment* is the process of systematically evaluating a patient for injuries or illness. Priority is given first to life-threatening conditions and then to minor conditions after any life threats have been managed.
- ❑ You must systematically assess your patient and the scene and interview patients and bystanders. You must form an impression about the situation and anticipate how the patient may respond. This first impression is called the *general impression.*
- ❑ Young patients may not be able to express themselves well enough to aid you in your evaluation. With very young children, observing their interaction with you (or in many cases their unwillingness to interact with you), their surroundings, and the parent or caregiver can give you valuable insight to the child's condition.
- ❑ The general impression includes assessing the nature of the illness or the mechanism of injury.
- ❑ The term *nature of the illness* typically is used for patients with medical conditions. It aids in determining the type of medical problem these patients have.
- ❑ Determining the mechanism of injury involves assessing the scene for the events that caused the patient's injuries.
- ❑ Even though the nature of the illness and the mechanism of injury are considered separate entities, it is important to recognize that both may be present.

- ❑ A patient's age, gender, and race may be useful information when establishing a general impression and identifying a patient's problem. For example, when dispatched on a call for a 2-year-old child with difficulty breathing, you should make a mental list of common respiratory problems associated with that age group.
- ❑ As you investigate, you must also be prepared to solve the problems you find. Such problems may include an unsafe scene, a patient who is not breathing, or an equipment problem.
- ❑ You need to know when to act quickly and when you have time to continue your investigation. In addition, you must select and apply the appropriate intervention or solution for the patient or situation.
- ❑ Once you have taken an action, you must evaluate the effect of that action on the patient or problem.
- ❑ You have many resources at your disposal as you make your assessment, and you must determine which ones to call for and use and when.
- ❑ As you perform all your assessment activities, you also must plan which interventions to complete immediately and which to complete later.
- ❑ Once you have formed a general impression, you can start to focus on mental status and airway, breathing, and circulation.
- ❑ When you arrive on scene, you must determine the patient's *mental status,* or how the person is responding to the current situation. To do this, you must determine whether the patient is awake and able to respond normally to the situation or to questions you ask.
- ❑ A tool you may find useful for evaluating a patient's responsiveness is the mnemonic AVPU, which stands for alert, verbal, painful, and unresponsive.
  - ❑ *Alert* refers to patients who are oriented and responsive to their environment. This is often referred to as "alert and oriented to person (who), place (where), time (date), and situation (what)." *Verbal* refers to patients who require verbal stimulation

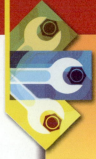

before they respond. *Painful* refers to patients who require a painful physical stimulus before they respond. A patient who does not respond to verbal or painful stimuli is considered *unresponsive*.

❑ The Glasgow Coma Scale provides a more detailed evaluation of a patient's neurologic status.

❑ Once a patient's mental status has been established, the next priority is to assess the airway.

❑ After the airway has been assessed and managed, the next step is to evaluate breathing.

❑ After the airway has been controlled and breathing supported, the next step is to determine circulation adequacy.

❑ The goal of the initial assessment is to begin to prioritize patients and to identify those who are in critical condition or who have life threats. These patients require immediate correction of the life threat, early and timely transport, and ALS care as soon as possible. If you have assessed a patient and determined that no life threats are present, or if you have stabilized the conditions you identified, you can move on to the next step, a focused history and physical examination.

Key Terms

AVPU A mnemonic assessment tool used to determine a person's mental status: *a*lert (the person is alert, awake, and oriented); *v*erbal (the person responds to voice); *p*ainful stimuli (the person responds only to a painful stimulus); *u*nresponsive (the person is not awake and is completely unresponsive to any type of stimulation).

General impression The first impression formed by the EMT on arrival at the scene.

Glasgow Coma Scale A quick, practical, standardized system for assessing the degree of conscious impairment in critically ill patients; it is also used to predict the duration and ultimate outcome of coma. This scale is used primarily for patients with head injuries.

Life threat Injuries or medical problems that threaten the patient's life.

Mechanism of injury The cause of a patient's injuries.

Mental status An assessment of how the patient responds mentally to the situation around him or her.

Nature of the illness A determination of the patient's illness from findings.

Patient assessment The process of systematically evaluating a patient for injuries or illness.

Perfusion The circulation of blood to the tissues of the body.

National Standard Curriculum Objectives

Cognitive Objectives
After completing this lesson, the EMT student will be able to do the following:

■ Summarize the reasons for forming a general impression of the patient.

■ Discuss methods of assessing altered mental status.

■ Differentiate the methods of assessing altered mental status in an adult, a child, and an infant.

■ Discuss methods of assessing the airway in an adult, a child, and an infant.

■ State the reasons for managing the cervical spine once a patient has been categorized as a trauma patient.

■ Describe methods of assessing whether a patient is breathing.

■ State the care that should be provided to an adult, a child and an infant with adequate breathing.

■ State the care that should be provided to an adult, a child, and an infant without adequate breathing.

■ Differentiate between a patient with adequate breathing and one with inadequate breathing.

■ Distinguish between methods of assessing breathing in an adult, a child, and an infant.

■ Compare the methods of providing airway care to an adult, a child, and an infant.

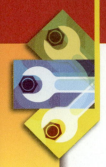

- Describe the methods used to obtain a pulse.
- Differentiate the methods used to obtain a pulse in an adult, a child, and an infant.
- Discuss the need for assessing a patient for external bleeding.
- Describe normal and abnormal findings when assessing skin color.
- Describe normal and abnormal findings when assessing skin temperature.
- Describe normal and abnormal findings when assessing skin condition.

- Describe normal and abnormal findings when assessing skin capillary refill in a child and in an infant.
- Explain the reason for prioritizing a patient for care and transport.

Affective Objectives
After completing this lesson, the EMT student will be able to do the following:

- Explain the importance of forming a general impression of the patient.
- Explain the value of performing an initial assessment.

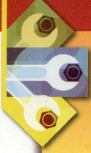

Psychomotor Objectives

After completing this lesson, the EMT student will be able to do the following:

- Demonstrate the techniques for assessing mental status.
- Demonstrate the techniques for assessing the airway.
- Demonstrate the techniques for assessing whether the patient is breathing.
- Demonstrate the techniques for assessing whether the patient has a pulse.
- Demonstrate the techniques for assessing the patient for external bleeding.
- Demonstrate the techniques for assessing the patient's skin color, temperature, and condition and capillary refill (infants and children only).
- Demonstrate the ability to prioritize patients for care and transport.

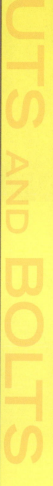

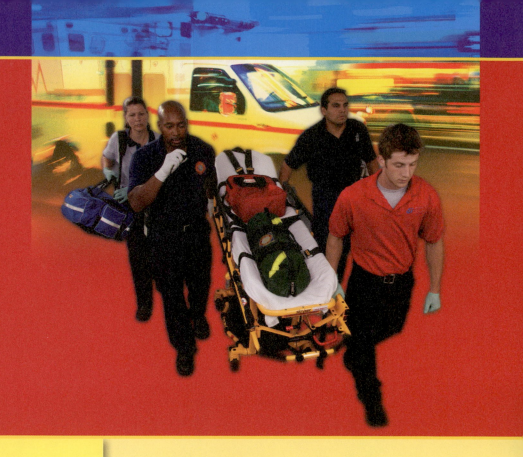

CHAPTER

10

OUTLINE

LESSON GOAL

GOAL

This chapter provides the emergency medical technician (EMT) with the knowledge and skills to recognize the **mechanism of injury** and how it relates to the prediction of injuries in the trauma patient. In addition, you will learn to identify trauma patients with life-threatening and non-life-threatening injuries and to prioritize and differentiate those injuries. You also will learn to determine the appropriate assessment for critical and noncritical patients. ■

Focused History and Physical Examination of Trauma Patients

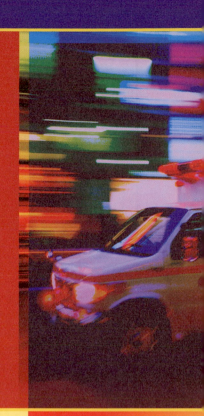

CHAPTER OBJECTIVES

After completing this chapter, the EMT student will be able to do the following:

1 Discuss why it is important always to consider the mechanism of injury.

2 State the reasons for performing a rapid trauma assessment.

3 Give examples of situations calling for a rapid trauma assessment and explain why it is appropriate in each case.

4 Explain the elements of a rapid trauma assessment.

5 Discuss when it is appropriate to change the rapid assessment to allow for patient care.

6 Discuss the reason for performing a focused history and physical exam.

7 Discuss the feelings patients might experience during assessment.

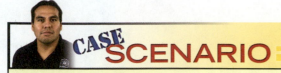

CASE SCENARIO

The crackle of police radios fills the air as Rafael steps off the engine. Taking the jumpkit out of the side cabinet, he swings it over his shoulder and heads into the dimly lit bar. Inside he finds several officers gathered around a young male lying on the littered floor. One of the officers turns to Rafael and says, "He's been shot in the stomach." Rafael notes that the man's shirt seems to be soaked with blood. He appears very anxious and is breathing rapidly.

Question: *Which should Rafael address first, the breathing problem or the bleeding? What are some of the steps Rafael should take to manage this patient?*

The case scenario highlights many of the important measures you have already learned. The first is scene safety. Police officers are already on the scene, therefore, as an EMT, you should know that they can provide some background information and can assure you that it is safe for you to proceed with assisting the patient.

The injured man has a wound that requires you to remove his shirt to examine him better. It is important to consider the patient's privacy as much as possible, especially if a crowd is present, as in this case. With the information from the police and the obvious gunshot wound, you have already formed a general impression of the patient. Now is the time to consider whether the wound is life threatening and whether you need additional backup. For example, are there any other patients? Once you have completed the initial assessment, you can perform the **focused history** and physical examination of this trauma patient. You will be looking for any other injuries and medical conditions this patient may have. You may have to ask personal questions, therefore it is important to maintain a professional and respectful attitude.

For your focused exam, you should always keep airway, breathing, and circulation (known as the *ABCs*) in mind. These are the factors most likely to cause life-threatening problems. If you identify a compromise in one of these factors, stop your physical exam and refocus on the initial assessment, correcting any life-threatening problems. If a life threat is identified, consider advanced life support (ALS) intercept and rapid transport. Once the life threat has been managed, you can return to the focused history and physical exam.

As you perform your focused history and exam, make sure you take steps to maintain spinal stabi-

ASK YOURSELF

Have you asked yourself, "What am I going to do when I arrive on that first trauma call, no one is on the scene, and the patient is unconscious? How am I going to determine what happened and, more important, what injuries has the patient sustained?"

SPECIAL Considerations

Cultural Perspectives
Touching during the physical exam is viewed differently by people of different cultures. With Muslim women, the clothing should be left in place and the patient should be examined by a female EMT whenever possible. This is a matter of religious upbringing for Muslims. With patients of Southeast Asian heritage, the head should be touched only after asking permission whenever possible. These patients consider the head to be sacred, and improper touching can be seen as an insult to the patient.

Important Points

Be respectful and professional as you assess the patient.

Important Points

Assessing for and treating life threats always takes precedence over a focused history and physical exam.

Important Points
Maintain spinal stabilization throughout the assessment.

Important Points
Just because a patient involved in a motor vehicle accident was restrained does not mean that the person was not injured.

lization. Many trauma patients have been exposed to violent forces, therefore damage to the spinal cord or its supportive structures is possible. Manual protective measures must be maintained throughout the assessment until stabilization equipment such as cervical collars and backboards can be applied.

■ SIGNIFICANT MECHANISMS OF INJURY

Use the mechanism of injury to guide your focused history and physical exam. Injuries may not be obvious, and the mechanism of injury can help you identify hidden problems so that you do not miss them. Injuries should be suspected when significant forces or mechanisms are encountered or certain patient conditions are seen, such as those in the following list:

- Ejection from a vehicle
- Death that has occurred in the same passenger compartment
- Falls greater than 20 feet (or two times the patient's height)
- Vehicle rollover
- High-speed vehicular collision
- Vehicle-pedestrian collision
- Motorcycle crash
- Unresponsive patient or patient with altered mental status
- Penetration of the head, chest, or abdomen

■ RESTRAINT SYSTEM INJURIES

Unrestrained patients in motor vehicle crashes are at greatest risk for critical injures. Restrained patients involved in motor vehicle collisions may suffer injuries from the restraint systems. Patients who are protected only by seat belts may have bruising to the abdomen and crushing injuries to the abdominal contents and the spine. These patients also may rotate forward and strike the dashboard or steering wheel.

SPECIAL Populations

Geriatric Considerations

Older patients are at greater risk for fractures and underlying tissue damage if their bones are brittle as a result of osteoporosis. They often have multiple medical conditions and a diminished ability to respond to the stress of trauma, factors that increase the potential for more severe injuries.

Shoulder harnesses often cause neck abrasions and bruising over the shoulder area. Clavicle fractures also may occur. Victims who wear only the shoulder harness may slide down under the strap and have significant neck injuries. Also, the lower body may slide under and strike the dashboard, causing femur, knee, and hip fractures.

Air bags offer additional protection but are designed to be used with shoulder harness and seat belt systems. When air bags are used with these systems, the most common injuries are facial abrasions, burns, and eye damage. As lateral air bags become more common, similar injuries will be found to the side struck by the lateral air bag. Suspect critical injuries if a child or small adult is struck by an air bag. Air bags are good only for the initial impact, and additional injuries may occur with a second impact. One way to determine whether a patient struck the steering wheel after the air bag deployed is to lift the air bag and check the steering wheel for damage.

Young patients may suffer critical injuries from the mechanisms of injury listed previously. Their injury patterns are similar to those seen in adults. In addition, young patients may suffer critical injuries with the following mechanisms of injury:

- Falls greater than 10 feet
- Bicycle collisions
- Medium-speed vehicular collisions

■ CONSIDERATIONS AFTER SCENE SIZE-UP AND INITIAL ASSESSMENT

You have completed the scene size-up and the initial assessment and you have reassessed the mechanism of injury. At this point, you should ask yourself, "Is the patient stable enough for me to continue my assessment on scene?" If the answer is no or if you suspect, based on the mechanism of injury, that this patient may become unstable, you should package the patient and initiate transport before you continue your assessment. It is always better to be en route to an appropriate facility with a patient who begins to deteriorate than to be sitting on scene with limited resources. You can continue your assessment during transport as time allows.

As you begin your assessment of the trauma patient, you have three routes to follow (Fig. 10-1). If your patient has a significant mechanism of injury, a life threat you have stabilized, or an altered level of consciousness, start with a **rapid trauma assessment.** This means that you start at the head and rapidly assess the patient in an orderly manner all the way to the toes. If the patient is stable and has an isolated injury, such as a fractured arm, you can focus your assessment on the arm and then expand the assessment as needed. With a critical patient whom you are unable to stabilize, you should stay in the initial assessment, focusing on the ABCs until the patient is stable. You may then move on either to the rapid trauma assessment or the focused trauma assessment.

■ WHO NEEDS A RAPID TRAUMA ASSESSMENT?

EMTs must be able to recognize when a patient needs a rapid trauma assessment. This assessment is indicated for patients with life-threatening or potentially life-threatening injuries. Such injuries usually involve the head, neck, chest, or abdomen. If any of the following are factors in the case, you should consider a rapid trauma assessment:

- Significant mechanism of injury
- Altered level of consciousness
- Actual or suspected head trauma
- Actual or suspected chest trauma
- Actual or suspected abdominal trauma
- Altered respiratory or pulse rates that have not responded to care started in the initial assessment
- Signs and symptoms of shock

■ WHY DO A RAPID TRAUMA ASSESSMENT?

The rapid trauma assessment is done to provide a more detailed evaluation of the areas that may involve potential life threats. This helps the EMT to assess injuries more specifically, to treat the injuries, and to identify patients who need advanced care and rapid transport.

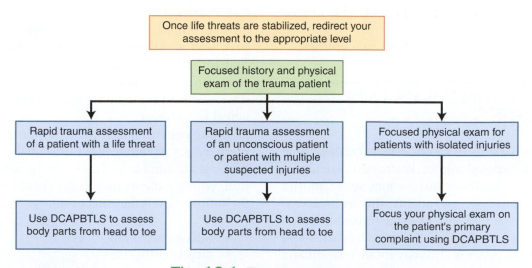

Fig. 10-1 Trauma assessment.

Elements of a Rapid Trauma Assessment

The rapid assessment should include a quick, efficient evaluation of the body to assess for injuries and to reassess problems that may have been identified in the initial exam. The rapid assessment should begin at the head and move in an orderly fashion to the toes. Assessment tools such as **inspection, palpation,** and **auscultation** are used in this assessment. You actually will have started the rapid assessment during the initial exam, but you will take it to the next level during this stage.

Reassessing Mental Status

During the initial assessment (see Chapter 9), you used the **AVPU** assessment tool to evaluate your patient. This provided you with information about the amount of stimuli necessary to get the patient to respond. Now it is time to take the mental status assessment to the next step. In this step you want to know the type of response to the stimuli. The Glasgow Coma Scale (GCS) is a tool often used to assess mental status (Table 10-1). The GCS has been modified slightly for children (Table 10-2). The GCS assesses eye opening, verbal response, and motor response and assigns a number to the level of patient response. The numbers from each section are added to obtain a score. For example, a patient who does not open the eyes, who moans to pain, and who extends the left arm and flexes the right arm would be rated as follows: eye opening—1, verbal response—2, and motor response—3, for a GCS total score of 6. Because this patient's motor response has two levels (3 and 2), it is important to assign the best score the patient achieves. Documentation of the GCS score helps care providers determine the patient's baseline neurologic status and continued progress, just as vital signs serve as a baseline for documenting patient response.

Inspection and Palpation

Now you can begin your physical exam of the patient. You do this by inspecting (looking at) and palpating (feeling) each body part for injuries. The mnemonic **DCAPBTLS** can be used as a guide in identifying injuries (Table 10-3). Using the letters of the acronym, you should look for *d*eformities, *c*ontusions, *a*brasions, *p*unctures, *b*urns, *t*enderness (T), *l*acerations, and *s*welling. To assess for pain and/or tenderness, you must ask the patient if he or she hurts anywhere. You may also elicit pain or tender-

TABLE 10-1

Glasgow Coma Scale for adults

Criteria	Patient Response	Score
Eye opening	Spontaneously	4
	To speech	3
	To pain	2
	None	1
Verbal response	Oriented	5
	Confused	4
	Inappropriate words	3
	Incomprehensible words	2
	None	1
Motor response	Obeys commands	6
	Localizes pain	5
	Withdraws to pain	4
	Flexion to pain	3
	Extension to pain	2
	None	1

ness when you palpate an injured area. Deformity may not be visible initially but may be identified as you palpate an injury. Rapid assessment findings that should be considered priorities are presented in Table 10-4.

Assessing the Head

As your partner maintains cervical spine stabilization, you should begin with the head and inspect for injuries or bleeding. Lacerations of the head can bleed severely and must be controlled quickly (see Chapter 25). Palpate the head for irregularities that may indicate skull fractures or swelling caused by bleeding under the skin or scalp (Fig. 10-2). External injuries, such as bruising behind the ears and around the eyes, suggest the possibility of injury to the brain

SPECIAL Populations

Pediatric Considerations

When a physical assessment must be performed on a conscious infant or toddler, doing a "toe to head" assessment is less frightening for the child, allows the child to start trusting you, and generally is more productive.

TABLE 10-2

Modified Glasgow Coma Scale for children and infants

Criteria	Child	Infant	Score
Eye opening	Spontaneous	Spontaneous	5
	To verbal stimuli	To verbal stimuli	4
	To pain only	To pain only	3
	No response	No response	2
Verbal response	Oriented, appropriate	Coos and babbles	5
	Confused	Irritable, cries	4
	Inappropriate words	Cries to pain	3
	Incomprehensible sounds	Moans to pain	2
	No response	No response	1
Motor response*	Obeys commands	Moves spontaneously and purposefully	6
	Localizes painful stimuli	Withdraws to touch	5
	Withdraws in response to pain	Withdraws in response to pain	4
	Flexion in response to pain	Abnormal flexion posture to pain	3
	Extension in response to pain	Abnormal extension posture to pain	2
	No response	No response	1

From Aehlert B: *Pediatric advanced life support study guide,* ed 2, St Louis, 2005, Mosby.
*If the patient is intubated, unconscious, or preverbal, the most important part of this scale is motor response. Motor response should be evaluated carefully.

TABLE 10-3

DCAPBTLS assessment for injuries

D	Deformities	Abnormal shape to a body part, often from a broken bone
C	Contusions	Bruising or bleeding under the skin
A	Abrasions	Scrapes to the skin that rub off the top layers of the skin
P	Punctures or penetrations	Open wounds, gunshot or stablike wounds to the skin
B	Burns	Burning or blistering of the skin from heat, electrical current, or chemical exposure
T	Tenderness	Complaints of pain caused by an injury; tenderness cannot be seen, it is indicated by the patient
L	Lacerations	Cuts or open wounds into the skin
S	Swelling	Increase in size as a result of bleeding or fluids under or into the skin

itself. Patients with external injuries should be monitored for signs of brain injury or increased intracranial pressure (see Chapter 29). Fluid leaking from the nose, mouth, or ears may be cerebrospinal fluid and may indicate an open skull fracture. If you have not yet assessed the patient using the GCS, you should do

that now. In a patient with an altered level of consciousness, you should also assess the pupils for size, equality, and responsiveness to light (see Chapter 5). Evaluate the mouth and nose for bleeding and a patent airway. Suction or intervene as needed if problems are identified.

TABLE 10-4

Priority findings in a rapid trauma assessment

Assessment	DCAPBTLS	Injuries/Concerns
Head	Deformities	Skull fractures
	Contusions	Bruising behind the ears (Battle's sign) and beneath the eyes (raccoon's eyes) suggests basilar skull fractures and possible brain injury.
	Burns	Monitor for airway burns.
Neck	Deformities	Deviated trachea Cervical spine injuries
	Contusions	Swelling from the contusion may obstruct the airway.
	Punctures or lacerations	May affect a major vessel; treat with an occlusive dressing.
	Swelling	Distended neck veins suggest possible tension pneumothorax or cardiac tamponade.
	Tenderness	Possible cervical spine damage
Chest	Deformities	Rib fractures or flail chest
	Contusions and abrasions	Underlying heart and lung damage
	Punctures and lacerations	May cause sucking chest wounds and should be managed with an occlusive dressing
	Burns	May restrict breathing as a result of pain or severity
	Tenderness and swelling	May indicate rib fractures
Abdomen	Contusions and abrasions	Suspect injuries to the organs that lie below the external wounds.
	Punctures and lacerations	Consider applying an occlusive dressing; protect bowel if exposed
	Tenderness	May be represented by guarding (tensing of the abdominal muscles)
Pelvis	Contusions and abrasions	Suspect injuries to the bladder or pelvic fractures.
	Tenderness or crepitus	Suspect pelvic fracture and internal bleeding.
Extremities	Swelling	Suspect internal bleeding that may contribute to shock.
	Distal pulses, sensation and movement	Compare side to side to assess for extremity injury or head injury.
Back	Tenderness or deformity	Assess for spinal injury.
	Contusions	Monitor for bleeding from retroperitoneal organs (kidneys and aorta).

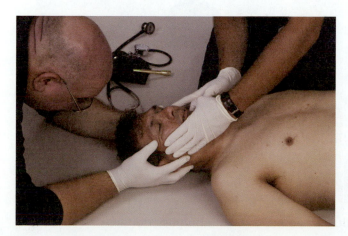

Fig. 10-2 Inspect and palpate the head and face.

Assessing the Neck

Assess the neck for open wounds or deformities. If open wounds are identified, apply an occlusive dressing and control the bleeding. Palpate to see whether the trachea is in the midline. Also, inspect for **jugular vein distention (JVD),** which may be a sign of tension pneumothorax or cardiac tamponade. Both of these are life-threatening conditions. Look for neck muscle use during breathing, which may indicate severe respiratory distress. Palpate the posterior aspect of the neck for deformities of the spine. Once the neck has been evaluated, you may apply a cervical immobilization collar (Skill 10-1).

Assessing the Chest

Now you can move to the chest. You will need to expose the patient by removing the person's clothing. When removing clothing by cutting, make sure to avoid disturbing any stab or gunshot wound holes. Inspect and palpate the chest As you inspect the chest, assess for open wounds, bruising, unequal movement, or deformity. Open wounds should be covered with an occlusive dressing to prevent abnormal air movement into and out of the chest. With bruising or abrasions of the chest wall, you should consider the possibility of damage to the heart or lungs. Unequal movement or **paradoxical movement** of the chest wall may indicate rib fractures or a flail chest and may make breathing difficult for the patient. If you find a chest injury, consider auscultating the chest at this time. You should auscultate both for normal and abnormal lung sounds (see Fig. 10-3). Absent or decreased lung sounds on one side may suggest a pneumothorax, hemothorax, or tension pneumothorax. All these conditions require ALS

care and immediate transport. The patient may complain of pain or tenderness as you palpate the chest, or you may feel **crepitus** (a crackling feeling produced when broken bone ends rub together), which suggests broken ribs. Subcutaneous emphysema (crepitus or a crackling feeling under the skin caused by air leakage) may also be felt, which suggests a pneumothorax.

Assessing the Abdomen

The abdomen is the next focus of the DCAPBTLS assessment. As you assess the abdomen, it is important to remember that bleeding into the abdomen frequently is a cause of shock in the trauma patient. Inspect the abdomen for bruises or open wounds. Open wounds to the upper quadrants of the abdomen should be managed with an occlusive dressing. With an evisceration (bowel or other abdominal contents protruding from the abdomen), manage the condition as described in Chapter 27. Bruising and abrasions may represent damage to internal organs. If you find bruising over the upper left quadrant, suspect spleen damage. Contusions to the upper right quadrant should make you suspect liver damage. Because both of these organs can bleed severely, monitor for signs and symptoms of shock when these injuries are found. You also should suspect intraabdominal bleeding with bruising around the umbilicus. Seat belt abrasions or bruising across the abdomen should raise suspicion of internal organ damage or lumbar spine fractures. Abdominal distention (enlargement of the abdomen) may also be noted. Be sure to palpate the abdomen gently so as not to increase bleeding. **Guarding** (tensing of the abdominal muscles) and tenderness are also indicators of possible internal

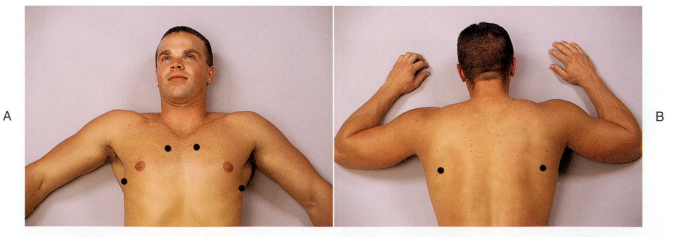

Fig. 10-3 A, Common anterior auscultation points. B, Common posterior auscultation points.

SKILL 10-1
Cervical Spine Immobilization

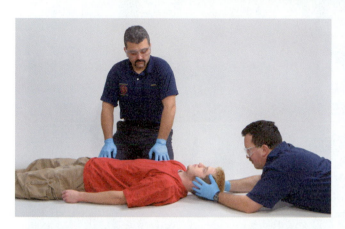

1. Apply and maintain manual stabilization of the head and neck in a neutral, inline position.

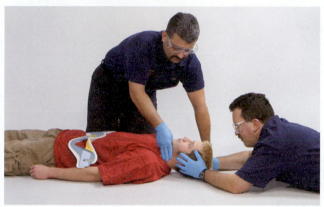

2. Using your fingers, measure the distance between the patient's lower jaw and shoulder (make sure your fingers are placed parallel to the patient's jaw.)

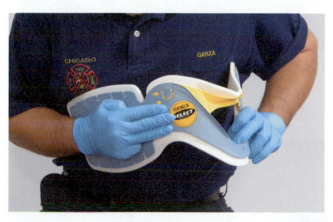

3. Find a cervical collar that matches the patient's measurements or adjust the collar size to fit the measurement.

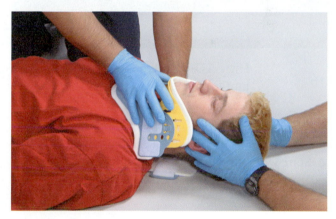

4. Apply the cervical collar and secure it.

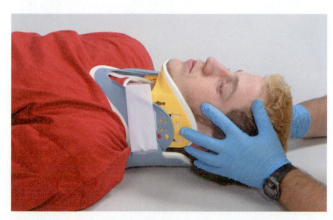

5. Maintain manual stabilization until the patient is fully immobilized on a long backboard.

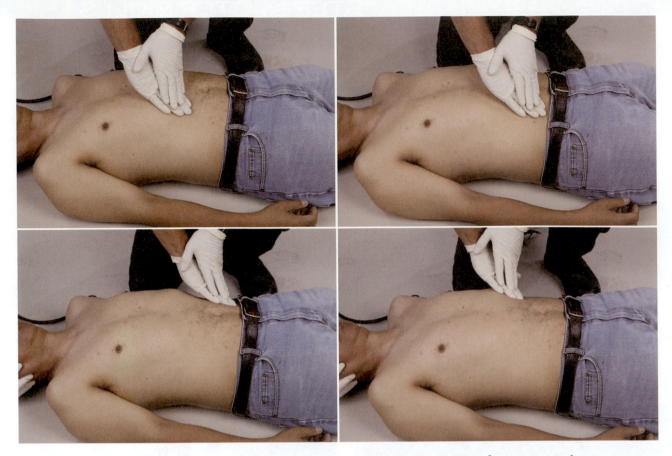

Fig. 10-4 Palpate the abdomen in an orderly manner, moving from one quadrant to the next.

damage. It is important to be systematic as you palpate. Start with the upper right or left quadrant and move progressively to each of the other quadrants (Fig. 10-4).

Assessing the Pelvis

The next step is assessment of the pelvis. Look for contusions or abrasions caused by seat belts. As you expose the pelvic area in male patients, it is important to assess for bleeding from the urethral meatus (the opening of the penis) and to communicate this finding to the receiving emergency department or ALS crew, because it represents possible damage to the urethra. Palpate the pelvis by applying gentle inward and downward pressure to the iliac crests (Fig. 10-5). Pain or crepitus in this area indicates a pelvic fracture, and severe bleeding may be present. If you identify a pelvic fracture, you should consider applying a pneumatic antishock garment (PASG) for patients in shock or with pelvic fractures that are unstable. Burns to the perineal area are considered critical, and transport to a burn center is recommended.

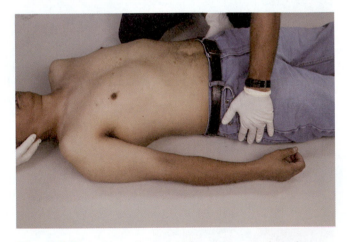

Fig. 10-5 Palpate the pelvis for crepitus and tenderness.

Assessing the Extremities

Each extremity should be assessed using the DCAPBTLS assessment tool. In addition to this assessment, evaluate each extremity for **distal pulses, sensation,** and **motor function** (Fig. 10-6). Compare

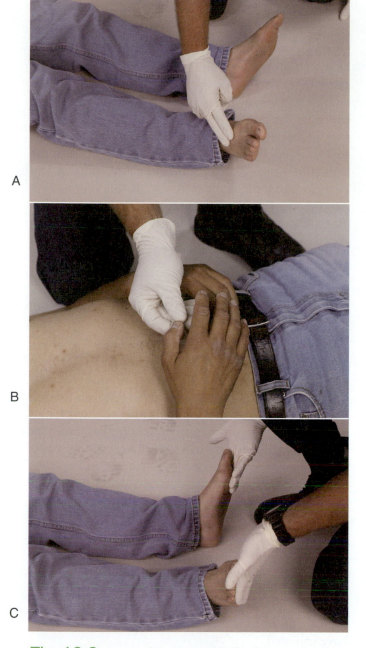

Fig. 10-6 Assess the extremities for **(A)** distal pulses, **(B)** sensation, and **(C)** motor response.

the extremities to detect injury. Injury should be suspected if an extremity does not appear or feel the same as the corresponding one. If injuries are found, consider splinting or caring for them at this point if the patient is stable.

Assessing the Back

Gently roll the patient onto the left or right side, keeping the spine in alignment, so that you can inspect and palpate the back (Fig. 10-7). If the patient

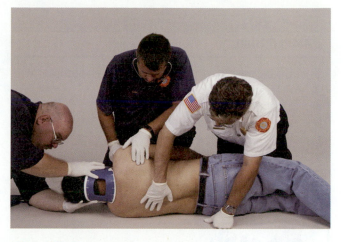

Fig. 10-7 Assess the back before placing the patient on a backboard.

is lying on either side or on the abdomen, you may do this assessment before you roll the person onto the back. You may assess the back before placing a patient on a backboard, because often the back is not assessed until the patient is removed from the backboard. Inspect and palpate for deformities to the spine area which may have caused cord damage. Open wounds should be managed with occlusive dressings. Contusions may represent damage to the kidneys or leaking of the aorta or vena cava.

SAMPLE History

After completing the rapid assessment, assess the vital signs if they were not obtained previously (see Chapter 5) and collect a SAMPLE history (Box 10-1). The acronym *SAMPLE* stands for the elements included in this history: *s*igns and *s*ymptoms of the chief complaint, *a*llergies, *m*edications, *p*ast pertinent medical history, *l*ast oral intake, and *e*vents preceding the incident (see Chapter 5). It is important to obtain a medical history for the trauma patient. The signs and symptoms can direct you to the patient's injuries. Allergies are important information to relay to the hospital. The patient may not be able to give this information to the hospital staff later and thus would be at risk for receiving a medication to which the person is allergic. Patient medications may alert you to a problem or may change the way a patient responds. For example, a patient may be taking a beta blocker to control the heart rate or blood pressure; however, this drug may limit the body's ability to increase the heart rate if the patient is bleeding and in shock. That is, because of the medication, the patient's body may not be able to compensate as well. The past medical

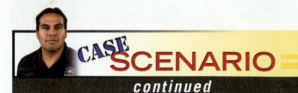

CASE SCENARIO continued

With the patient's shirt cut off, Rafael can see the wound in the right chest. Bright red blood is running out of it and dribbling down the side of the patient's chest. Palpating around the area, Rafael can't feel any broken ribs, but he detects a sensation of popping and crackling under the skin around the wound, which indicates that air is entering under the skin (subcutaneous emphysema) which suggests a collapsed lung (pneumothorax).

Question: *What could Rafael do right now to correct the problem? Should he focus on this issue or continue his assessment?*

history may alert you to a respiratory problem, such as chronic obstructive pulmonary disease (COPD), which may make breathing more difficult for the patient. If the patient requires surgery, the last oral intake is important information for the surgeons. The events preceding the incident may be useful for identifying the cause of the problem. For example, the patient may have had a seizure and then fell or had an accident.

Although the rapid trauma assessment requires a fairly long discussion, it can be performed in a relatively short time. It is essential to be orderly and thorough as you perform this assessment, because this helps reduce the chance that injuries will be missed. Depending on the patient's stability and the transport times, you should treat any injuries and package the patient for transport if this has not yet been done. For injuries that have been treated, reassess the areas as needed to check the patient's response to treatment.

■ FOCUSED TRAUMA ASSESSMENT

The focused trauma assessment is used when a patient has an isolated injury and the person has not shown an alteration in mental status or experienced a significant mechanism of injury. DCAPBTLS is also used in these cases to assess the injury. It often is used for an isolated extremity injury, such as a burn, laceration, or fracture. Once you have assessed the extremity, assess the vital signs, collect a SAMPLE history, and reassess as needed. You also must document and relay your findings to the receiving facility or transporting emergency medical services (EMS) crew.

Caring for the trauma patient requires you to be detailed, comprehensive, and efficient. You must designate your patient as critical, potentially critical, or noncritical. As you assess, correlate your findings with potential patient problems. In addition, constantly monitor the patient's response to the care you have initiated.

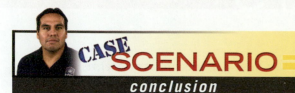

CASE SCENARIO conclusion

With the occlusive dressing in place, the fire crew works to get the patient prepared for rapid transport to the trauma center. The rest of the patient's clothes are removed, and he is placed on a backboard. The patient is covered with blankets to reduce any further heat loss. Rafael continues to monitor the oxygen flow rate to the mask and reassesses the patient's airway, breathing and circulatory status. ■

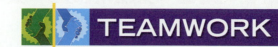

TEAMWORK

You may receive a patient from first responders. Therefore you must listen to their report and continue your assessment based on that report. In turn, you may deliver the patient to a transporting crew. In such cases you must report your findings to them and assist with the care and packaging of the patient. These crews may want to do their own assessment to confirm your findings and establish their own baseline for the patient. If you transport the patient, you continue your care, reassess the patient, and then document your findings and report them to the receiving facility. Whatever the circumstances, your report should include five primary elements: (1) the initial assessment, (2) the mechanism of injury, (3) any injuries found, (4) the care you initiated, and (5) the patient's response to that care.

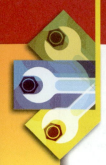

Critical Points

- EMTs must understand the mechanism of injury and the associated injuries the patient may sustain.
- Understanding the differences between the rapid trauma assessment and the focused assessment saves valuable time and ensures that you prioritize your patient's injuries correctly.
- EMTs must make sure that proper spinal immobilization is initiated and maintained until the patient has been properly secured.
- EMTs must understand passenger restraint systems and the injuries that may result even when restraints are used properly.

Learning Checklist

- ❑ The focused exam should always be conducted with the ABCs in mind. If a compromise is identified in one of these factors, stop the physical exam, refocus on the initial assessment, and correct any life-threatening problems. Consider ALS intercept and rapid transport.
- ❑ The mechanism of injury can serve as a guide for the focused history and physical exam. Injuries may not be obvious, therefore the mechanism of injury may help identify hidden problems.
- ❑ Although unrestrained passengers in motor vehicle crashes are at greatest risk for critical injuries, restrained passengers may also suffer injuries from the restraint systems. Shoulder harnesses can cause neck abrasions, bruising over the shoulder area, and clavicle fractures. If passengers wear only a shoulder harness, they may slide down in the vehicle and strike the dashboard, possibly suffering femur, knee, and hip fractures.
  - ❑ The most common air bag injuries are facial abrasions, burns, and eye damage. Children or small adults can sustain critical injuries if struck by an air bag. To determine whether the patient struck the steering wheel, lift the air bag and check the steering wheel for damage.

- ❑ Older patients are at greater risk for fractures and underlying tissue damage because of osteoporosis (brittle bones).
- ❑ The rapid trauma assessment starts at the head and progresses in an orderly manner to the toes. If the patient is in stable condition and has an isolated injury, focus the assessment on the injured area and expand the assessment as needed. A rapid trauma assessment is indicated for patients with life-threatening injuries or potentially life-threatening injuries. Such injuries usually involve the head, neck, chest, or abdomen. Use assessment tools such as inspection, palpation, and auscultation.
- ❑ The Glasgow Coma Scale is used to assess mental status. A modified version of the scale is used for children. Document the GCS score in the patient care report.
- ❑ The assessment mnemonic DCAPBTLS is used to identify injuries. Inspect for *d*eformities, *c*ontusions, *a*brasions, *p*unctures, *b*urns, *t*enderness, *l*acerations, and *s*welling.
- ❑ The rapid trauma assessment proceeds in the following order: assessment of the head, neck, chest, abdomen, pelvis, extremities, and back. Be mindful of the possible need for spinal immobilization.
- ❑ After completing the rapid assessment, assess the vital signs (if not previously obtained) and collect a SAMPLE history.
- ❑ The focused trauma assessment is used when the patient has an isolated injury and has no alteration in mental status, and no significant mechanism of injury was involved. Designate the patient as critical, potentially critical, or noncritical. Correlate your findings with potential problems. Constantly monitor the patient's response to the care you have initiated.

Key Terms

Auscultation An assessment technique that involves listening to sounds inside the body with a stethoscope.

AVPU A mnemonic assessment tool used to determine a person's mental status. The

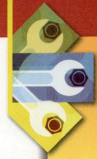

acronym stands for *a*lert (the person is alert, awake, and oriented); *v*erbal (the person responds to voice); *p*ainful stimuli (the person responds only to a painful stimulus); *u*nresponsive (the person is not awake and is completely unresponsive to any type of stimulation).

Crepitus A crunching or grating sound heard when broken bone ends rub together.

DCAPBTLS A mnemonic used to identify injury to the body. The acronym stands for *d*eformity, *c*ontusions, *a*brasions, *p*uncture, *b*urns, *t*enderness, *l*aceration, and *s*welling.

Distal pulses Pulses taken at a point farther from the midline of the body, such as the pedal or radial pulse.

Focused history Information obtained from a patient regarding the person's medical history.

Guarding Tensing of the muscles or other body parts to protect an area.

Inspection An assessment technique that involves looking for injuries or problems.

Jugular vein distention (JVD) Enlargement of the jugular veins on the sides of the neck.

Mechanism of injury The cause of a patient's injuries.

Motor function The ability to move.

Palpation An assessment technique that involves feeling for injuries during the patient assessment.

Paradoxical movement Movement associated with a flail chest in which the chest wall moves in on inspiration and out on expiration.

Rapid trauma assessment A rapid, orderly, head to toe assessment of a trauma patient.

Sensation The ability to feel.

National Standard Curriculum Objectives

Cognitive Objectives

After completing this lesson, the EMT student will be able to do the following:

- Discuss the reasons for reconsideration concerning the mechanism of injury.
- State the reasons for performing a rapid trauma assessment.
- Give examples of situations calling for a rapid trauma assessment and explain why it is appropriate in each case.
- Describe the areas included in the rapid trauma assessment and discuss what should be evaluated.
- Explain when the rapid assessment may be altered to allow patient care.
- Discuss the reason for performing a focused history and physical exam.

Affective Objective

After completing this lesson, the EMT student will be able to do the following:

- Recognize and respect the feelings patients might experience during the assessment.

Psychomotor Objective

After completing this lesson, the EMT student will be able to do the following:

- Demonstrate the rapid trauma assessment that should be used to assess a patient based on the mechanism of injury.

CHAPTER

11

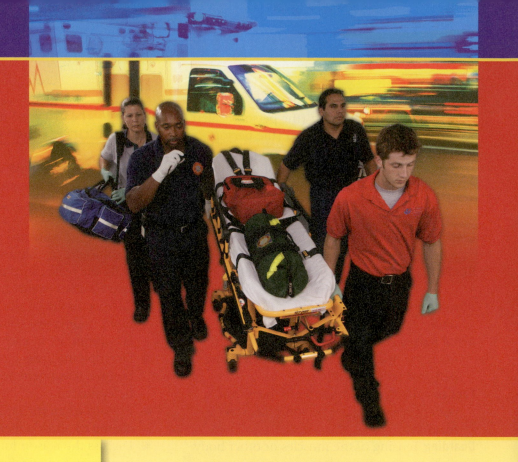

CHAPTER OUTLINE

Scene Size-Up

Initial Assessment

Focused History and Physical Exam: Medical

Providing Emergency Medical Care

OUTLINE

LESSON GOAL

The goal of this chapter is to prepare the emergency medical technician (EMT) to assess a medical patient properly. As an EMT, you must understand the priorities in taking a patient's history and must be able to complete a focused exam based on the patient's chief complaint and history. Ultimately, you must be able to connect information obtained through the history and physical exam findings to disease processes to provide the appropriate interventions. ■

GOAL

Focused History and Physical Examination of Medical Patients

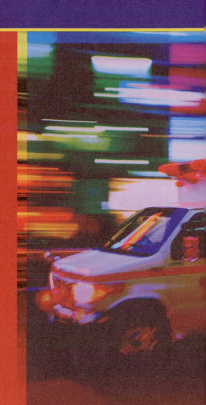

CHAPTER OBJECTIVES

After completing this chapter, the EMT student will be able to do the following:

1 Discuss factors the EMT should consider when assessing a patient with a specific chief complaint and no known history.

2 Explain the difference between assessment of a responsive patient with no known history and assessment of a responsive patient with a known history.

3 Discuss factors the EMT should consider when assessing a patient who is unresponsive or who has an altered mental status.

4 Explain the difference between assessment of a patient who is unresponsive or who has an altered mental status and assessment of other medical patients.

5 Understand the need to be sensitive to the feelings patients might experience during assessment.

6 Demonstrate the assessment skills used to assist a responsive patient with no known history.

7 Demonstrate the assessment skills used to assist a patient who is unresponsive or who has an altered mental status.

11

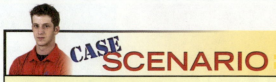

"Oh, Ray, thank goodness it's you!" Mrs. Jameson exclaims. "I don't know what's wrong with me, but it hurts real bad." Ray smiles and puts his hand reassuringly on Mrs. Jameson's shoulder as he kneels beside her. "No worries," he says simply and clearly. "Tell me where it hurts."

Mrs. Jameson holds the lower half of her abdominal region. "Right here," she says stiffly, grimacing.

"What does it feel like?" Ray asks as he takes the stethoscope and blood pressure cuff out of the medical kit.

"Like a really bad cramp, but worse than I've ever had," Mrs. Jameson replies.

Question: *Ray's questions are an example of what technique? What other questions should he ask the patient?*

A medical emergency is one of the most frequent calls you will receive as an EMT. On these calls you will use some of the skills discussed in previous chapters, as well as additional skills:

- Scene size-up
- Initial assessment
- Focused history and physical exam (with a medical emphasis)
- Rapid assessment
- Vital signs
- Ongoing assessment

A crucial skill for EMTs is the ability to differentiate between critical and noncritical patients. You must be able to gather a thorough history and choose an appropriate assessment. When you care for medical patients, the history is your main emphasis. You will use the SAMPLE history (signs, allergies, medications, past medical history, last oral intake, and events preceding) discussed in previous chapters, but you will expand this history in medical patients to understand the problem more completely. Your patient may know what is wrong, or this may be a new problem that you will have to identify and treat. Not only will you gather a history, you also will perform a physical exam to confirm the patient's signs and symptoms. With unresponsive patients or patients with multiple complaints, you may include a rapid assessment that moves from head to toe. For patients with isolated complaints, your assessment focuses on the patient's chief complaint and expands as needed.

■ SCENE SIZE-UP

When you arrive at the site of the call, you perform a scene size-up to make sure the area is safe. You also evaluate the mechanism of injury and the nature of the illness. With medical patients, you generally will not find a mechanism of injury, but you should always be conscious of the possibility of trauma. For example, when you respond to the scene of a female patient with abdominal pain, it would be reasonable to assume a medical cause for her pain. As you complete your physical exam of her abdomen, you note contusions. On further questioning, she tells you that her boyfriend beat her, but she was afraid and did not want anyone to know. Therefore a perceived medical condition is now a traumatic condition. The nature of the illness plays a larger part with medical patients. Environmental clues can help you determine the nature of the illness (Table 11-1). If possible, you also should question the patient about the illness or the reason you were called. You should take body substance isolation (BSI) precautions at this time.

■ INITIAL ASSESSMENT

Once you have completed the scene size-up, you can move on to the initial assessment. Form an initial impression of the patient; assess the patient's mental status and airway, breathing, and circulation; and assign a priority to the patient. At this point, you must determine whether the patient is stable enough for you to continue to a medical assessment or whether the

TABLE 11-1

Nature of the illness

Clue	Patient Problem
Oxygen tank, tubing, nebulizer	Respiratory emergency
Wheelchair, walker, crutches	Arthritis, neurologic problem
Smell of old blood	Gastrointestinal bleeding
Foley catheter, strong urine smell	Neurologic problem, sepsis, kidney or bladder problem, possible abuse or neglect
Chemical smell	Poisoning, respiratory distress, safety issue
Unclean house or food preparation area	Food poisoning, sepsis, abuse or neglect
Amputation, prosthetic device	Vascular disease, diabetes
Medication	Disease associated with medication
Alcohol or drug paraphernalia, odor	Overdose, gastrointestinal bleeding, safety issue

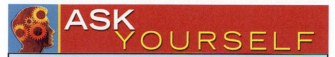

ASK YOURSELF

Consider this scenario: You arrive on the scene of a medical emergency. Your patient is a middle-aged man who is confused and unaware that you are in the room. No one else is home. What should you do next? Where do you begin?

person is critical and needs immediate intervention. If your patient is unstable, treat the problems found in the initial exam until the patient's condition has stabilized. Once the patient is stable, move on to the focused history and physical exam for medical patients.

■ **FOCUSED HISTORY AND PHYSICAL EXAM: MEDICAL**

The focused history and physical exam: medical is the process for assessing a medical patient. All components of the process should be completed, but the order in which they are performed may change, depending on whether the patient is conscious or unconscious. The components are as follows:

- Assessing the history of the present illness
- Assessing complaints and signs and symptoms (OPQRST)
- Assessing the SAMPLE history
- Performing a rapid assessment

- Assessing baseline vital signs
- Providing emergency medical care

Assessing the History of the Present Illness

To assess the history of the present illness, it is easiest to start with the chief complaint. The *chief complaint* is the problem the patient is complaining about when you arrive. One way to determine the chief complaint is to ask the patient the following questions:

- "Why did you call us?"
- "What problem made you call for an ambulance today?"

The chief complaint should be recorded in the patient's own words. If the patient says to you, "My head hurts," then the chief complaint is "Head hurts," not "Headache" or "Possible stroke." "Headache" or "Stroke" would be your interpretation of the chief

SPECIAL Considerations

Cultural Perspectives

Using family members, especially young children, as interpreters can be problematic. The person may not have adequate language skills in one or both languages. Also, culturally based modesty barriers may exist regarding discussion of certain topics, especially across genders and age groups, leading to difficulty discussing medical problems.

complaint and that should be determined after you have completed your assessment. Once you have established a chief complaint, you should explore it for more information. One technique for exploring the chief complaint or the patient's signs and symptoms uses the mnemonic **OPQRST,** which stands for the following criteria:

O	Onset
P	Provocation
Q	Quality
R	Radiation
S	Severity
T	Time

The answers to the questions you ask using the OPQRST technique (Table 11-2) can provide you with information on what the patient was doing when the problem began (onset), what makes the problem better or worse (provocation), what the problem feels like (quality), whether it moves to another part of the body (radiation), how bad it is (severity), and when the problem began and how it has changed since then (time). The OPQRST technique helps you to clarify a problem so that it can be identified and treated. As you ask these questions, you not only are collecting the data but also looking for clues as to what is causing the patient's problem and what treatment may be required. In most cases the OPQRST questions serve as a starting point for further questioning and information gathering.

Onset

Onset addresses the patient's activities before the problem began. You are trying to identify an event that may have caused the problem. For example, in a patient with shortness of breath, the onset could have happened while the patient was eating. This should make you think of possible aspiration or an allergic reaction. You could go on to explore these two possibilities by confirming that the patient did not choke or eat anything that would trigger any known food allergies. If the patient ate strawberries and is allergic to them, you may focus your care on an allergic reaction and monitor for anaphylaxis. In such cases, you continue the history collection as the patient's condition allows.

Important Points

OPQRST is a beginning point, not an ending point, for history gathering.

SPECIAL Considerations

Talking and Breathing
Quantifying the degree of dyspnea in a patient with severe shortness of breath can be difficult. A useful technique is to count the number of words the patient can speak between breaths. Thus three words and then a breath is three-word dyspnea.

TABLE 11-2

OPQRST questions

OPQRST Component	Possible Questions
Onset	"What were you doing when the problem started?" "What happened that may have caused the problem?"
Provocation	"What makes the problem better or worse?" "What do you think is causing the problem?"
Quality	"Can you describe the problem?"
Radiation	"Does the pain move anywhere? If so, where?" "Do you feel pain or discomfort anywhere else? If so, where?" "Can you show me where the pain is and how it moves?"
Severity	"On a scale of 1 to 10, with 10 being the worst pain you've ever had, what is the severity of this pain?" "What type of pain have you had before? How bad is this pain compared with your other pain?"
Time	"What time did this problem start?" "How long have you had this problem?" "How has the problem changed since it began?"

Provocation

Provocation relates to any action that either brings the problem on or changes the problem, making it either better or worse. For example, if a patient is dizzy, the person may feel better when lying down but get dizzier when sitting up. This is important, because dizziness or lightheadedness in a patient when sitting up is one of the signs of hypoperfusion. You therefore would assess for any other signs and symptoms of shock. Provocation may be assessed by asking the patient whether anything provokes the problem, or this may be determined during the physical examination, such as when performing palpation. For example, the patient may tell you, "It hurts more in my lower chest when you push on it."

Quality

Quality pertains to the description of the problem. The best way to obtain information on the quality of the problem is to ask the patient to describe it. This way, you are not describing the problem for the patient and are more likely to get a better description of it from the patient's point of view. If the patient has trouble describing the problem and you decide to ask more specific questions, give several choices and allow time for the patient's own description. For example, you might ask, "Is the pain stabbing, sharp, dull, cramping, constant...?" The quality of the pain is important, because different types of pain are associated with different problems. For example, a cramping pain in the abdomen is more common with hollow organs, whereas a constant pain is more common with solid organs. Therefore the better description you can get of the pain and any changes that have occurred is helpful in determining the overall cause of the patient's problem.

Radiation

Radiation refers to pain or discomfort that is associated with or that moves into another area of the body. For example, in a patient experiencing chest pain, the pain may radiate into the arm, neck, or jaw. These symptoms are commonly associated with a heart attack or an acute myocardial infarction. Patients also may have *referred pain*, which is pain that manifests in another body part when the original site is irritated. For example, a patient with gallbladder disease may complain of pain in the back between the right shoulder blade and the spine. For patients who do not have pain, you can use the *R* element to assess for related symptoms, such as nausea and vomiting.

Severity

Severity describes the intensity or strength of a pain. Pain usually is rated on a scale of 1 to 10, with 1 being the least pain and 10 being the most severe pain. Pain is difficult to assess, because it is a subjective sensation. One patient with a pain severity of 8 may be yelling, screaming, and writhing, whereas another patient with the same pain level may be stoic and not moving. Therefore comparing the present pain with other types of pain the patient has had may help you with the assessment. For example, you can ask the patient to compare this pain with other pain previously experienced and to rate this pain according to that incident. Pain levels of 9 to 10 often represent potentially critical patients, and rapid transport is indicated, regardless of how ill you think the patient may be at this time. It also is important to note how the pain has changed and whether any factors affect it. For example, if you give medications, such as nitroglycerin for chest pain, you should note the pain severity before and after administration of the medication. The FLAC (*f*ace, *l*egs, *a*ctivity, *c*onsolability) pain scale can be a useful tool for qualifying a patient's pain (Table 11-3).

Time

Time is assessed by asking the patient how long the problem has existed, when it started, and how it has changed over time. This gives you information on the progression of the problem. For example, you may be caring for a patient with breathing difficulty. The patient may tell you the trouble started several hours ago and has gotten worse in the past 15 minutes, so that chest tightness is preventing the patient from breathing. This patient is progressing and becoming more critical, therefore rapid transport should be considered with advanced life support (ALS) intercept. If the patient tells you that the trouble started several hours ago but has not worsened, you should continue with your assessment and determine the appropriate care and transport. A rapidly deteriorating patient indicates a critical patient, therefore the progression of symptoms over time is a vital factor to assess.

Medical Patient Assessments

As you have noted, the OPQRST history is important for qualifying patient conditions. In addition to individuals with pain, OPQRST can be applied to and expanded for many other types of patients, such as those with respiratory difficulties (Table 11-4), cardiac problems (Table 11-5), altered mental status (Table 11-6), an allergic reaction (Table 11-7),

TABLE 11-3

FLAC pain scale

FLAC Component	Score 0	1	2
Face	No particular expression or smile	Occasional grimace or frown; withdrawn, disinterested, or worried look; lowered eyebrows; partly closed eyes; pursed mouth	Frequent to constant frown, clenched jaw, quivering chin, deeply furrowed forehead, closed eyes, open mouth, deeply lined nose/lip area
Legs	Positioned normally or relaxed	Uneasy, restless, tense, increased in tone, rigid, intermittently flexed/extended	Kicking or drawn up, hypertonic, extremely flexed/extended, trembling
Activity	Lying quietly, assuming normal position, moving easily and freely	Squirming, shifting back and forth, tensing up, hesitating to move, guarding	Arching, becoming rigid or jerking, assuming fixed position, rocking, moving head side to side, rubbing body part
Cry	No cries/moans (awake or asleep)	Moans or whimpers, occasional cries, sighs, occasional complaint	Steady cries, screams, sobs, moans, grunts, frequent complaints
Consolability	Calm, content, relaxed, does not require consoling	Reassured by occasional touching, hugging, or being talked to; distractible	Difficult to console or comfort

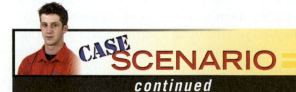

CASE SCENARIO
continued

Ray begins to assess Mrs. Jameson's abdominal region. On inspection, the area does not appear overly swollen, bruised, or otherwise injured. He asks Mrs. Jameson, "Is it okay for me to gently feel around your abdomen? I'd like to make sure there aren't any unusual findings."

Question: *Where should Ray palpate the abdomen first? What are some of the unusual findings he might detect?*

poisoning/overdose (Table 11-8), an environmental emergency (Table 11-9), obstetric conditions (Table 11-10), and behavioral emergencies (Table 11-11). (Each type of patient assessment, presentation, and care is discussed in greater detail in later chapters.)

SAMPLE History

To evaluate your medical patient, you also must collect a SAMPLE history (the acronym *SAMPLE* stands for *s*igns and symptoms, *a*llergies, *m*edications, *p*ast medical history, *l*ast oral intake, and *e*vents preceding the incident problem). The SAMPLE history commonly proceeds as follows:

- Assess any signs and symptoms the patient has. If the signs and symptoms identified are different from the chief complaint, you can use the OPQRST method to explore them.
- Assess for allergies. This is important in assessing for possible allergic reactions or anaphylaxis and for alerting the medical staff to allergies as they begin drug administration.
- Determine whether the patient has been taking any medications. This includes herbs, prescribed medications, over-the-counter medications, homeopathic medications, or recreational (street) drugs or alcohol. The medications may give you a clue as to medical problems. If the patient is unsure which

Text continued on p. 236

TABLE 11-4

Respiratory assessment considerations

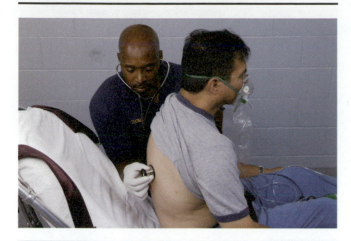

Assessment Component	Considerations
Onset	What caused the patient's respiratory problem?
Provocation	What makes it easier or harder for the patient to breathe?
Quality	Describe how the patient feels when breathing.
Related symptoms	Does the patient have any other problems when breathing?
Severity	On a scale of 1 to 10, with 10 being the hardest to breathe, how hard is it for the patient to breathe?
Time	How long has the patient had trouble breathing?
	How has the patient's breathing changed since the difficulty started?
Other	Has this ever happened to the patient before? If yes, what happened?
	What was done to correct the patient's breathing problem?
Focused physical exam	Assess the chest for accessory muscle use.
	Listen to breath sounds.

Modified from National Registry of Emergency Medical Technicians: *Patient assessment/management: medical* (skill sheet), Columbus, OH, 2000, NREMT.

TABLE 11-5

Cardiac assessment considerations

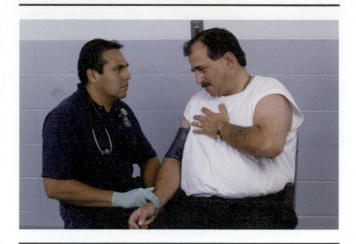

Assessment Component	Considerations
Onset	What was the patient doing when the chest pain started?
Provocation	What makes the pain better or worse?
Quality	Describe the pain.
Radiation	Does the pain go anywhere? Does the patient have any other pain?
Severity	On a scale of 1 to 10, with 10 being the worst pain the patient has ever had, how does this pain rate?
Time	How long has the patient had the pain?
	How has the pain changed since it started?
Other	Has this ever happened to the patient before? If yes, what happened?
	What was done to treat the patient's chest pain before?
Focused physical exam	Apply a cardiac monitor.
	Palpate the chest for pain.
	Inspect the neck for jugular vein distention (JVD).
	Inspect the feet for edema.
	Assess the chest for accessory muscle use.
	Auscultate breath sounds.

Modified from National Registry of Emergency Medical Technicians: *Patient assessment/management: medical* (skill sheet), Columbus, OH, 2000, NREMT.

TABLE 11-6
Altered mental status assessment considerations

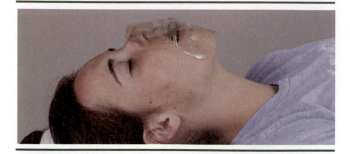

Assessment Component	Considerations*
Onset	What was the patient doing before losing consciousness?
Provocation	Has anything seemed to wake the patient up?
Quality	Describe the episode.
Related symptoms	Did the patient have any associated symptoms?
Severity	To what does the patient respond (AVPU, GCS)?
Time	How long has the change of consciousness been present?
Other	Has this ever happened to the patient before? If yes, what happened?
	What was done to treat the altered level of consciousness before?
	Did the patient have a seizure? If so, describe it.
	Has the patient had a fever?
	Does the patient have diabetes or take any drugs such as narcotics?
	Is there any chance the patient fell or hit his or her head?
	Has the patient had any previous trauma?
	Has anything been done to treat this patient?
Focused physical exam	Determine responsiveness
	Evaluate and ensure patent airway
	Look for signs of external trauma
	Check pupils
	Evaluate for possible spine injury
	Assess the blood glucose

Modified from National Registry of Emergency Medical Technicians: *Patient assessment/management: medical* (skill sheet), Columbus, OH, 2000, NREMT.
AVPU, An assessment mnemonic for *a*lert, *v*erbal, *p*ainful, *u*nresponsive; *GCS*, Glasgow Coma Scale.
*These questions may be addressed to family members or bystanders.

TABLE 11-7
Allergic reaction assessment considerations

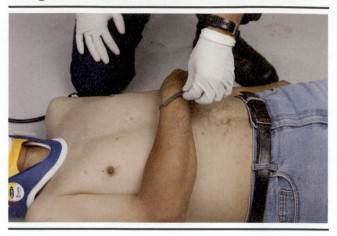

Assessment Component	Considerations
Onset	What was the patient doing when the episode started?
Provocation	Has anything happened to make the patient better or worse?
Quality	Describe the allergic reaction.
Related symptoms	Is the patient having any other problems?
Severity	On a scale of 1 to 10, with 10 being the worst reaction the patient has ever had, how does this reaction rate?
Time	When did the reaction start?
	How has the reaction changed since it started?
Other	Has this ever happened to the patient before? If yes, what happened?
	What was done to treat the patient's allergic reaction before?
	How was the patient exposed to the allergen (substance)?
	To what was the patient exposed?
	Has the patient ever had an anaphylactic reaction?
Focused physical exam	Apply a cardiac monitor.
	Assess the chest for accessory muscle use.
	Auscultate breath sounds.
	Assess for rash.
	Assess for stingers.
	Assess for signs of shock.

Modified from National Registry of Emergency Medical Technicians: *Patient assessment/management: medical* (skill sheet), Columbus, OH, 2000, NREMT.

TABLE 11-8

Poisoning/overdose assessment considerations

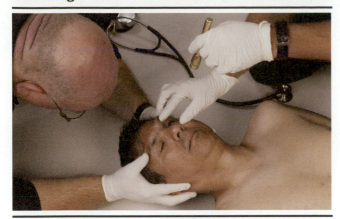

Assessment Component	Considerations
Onset	What caused the overdose/poisoning?
Provocation	Has anything been done to make the patient better or worse? If so, what?
Quality	Describe what the patient has been like since the overdose/poisoning occurred.
Related symptoms	Does the patient have any other symptoms?
Severity	How severe/critical does the patient appear?
Time	How long ago did the poisoning/overdose happen?
	How has the patient changed since the overdose/poisoning occurred?
Other	What substance caused the problem?
	How did the exposure occur?
	How much was ingested?
	Over how much time did the ingestion occur?
	What is the patient's estimated weight?
	What interventions were attempted?
Focused physical exam	Ensure scene safety.
	Apply a cardiac monitor.
	Auscultate breath sounds.
	Look for signs of poisoning/overdose (e.g., burns to the mouth, vomit, drug paraphernalia, empty medication bottles)
	Sniff for signs of exposure.
	Assess for track marks.
	Check pupils.

From National Registry of Emergency Medical Technicians: *Patient assessment/management: medical* (skill sheet), Columbus, OH, 2000, NREMT.

TABLE 11-9

Environmental emergency assessment considerations

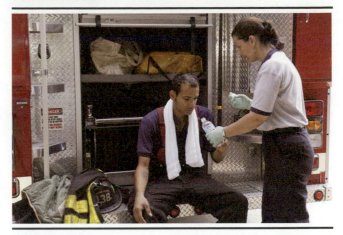

Assessment Component	Considerations
Onset	What was the patient doing when the incident happened?
Provocation	Has anything been done to heat or cool the patient?
Quality	Describe how the patient looks.
Related symptoms	Does the patient have any other problems?
Severity	What is the patient's temperature? How hot or cold is the person?
Time	How long has the patient been exposed to the heat or cold?
	How has the patient's presentation changed during the exposure?
Other	What is the source of the exposure?
	Has the patient lost consciousness?
	Is the patient having local or systemic effects?
Focused physical exam	Apply a cardiac monitor.
	Auscultate breath sounds.
	Assess for tissue damage.

From National Registry of Emergency Medical Technicians: *Patient assessment/management: medical* (skill sheet), Columbus, OH, 2000, NREMT.

TABLE 11-10
Obstetric assessment considerations

Assessment Component	Considerations
Onset	What was the patient doing when the contractions or pain started?
Provocation	What makes the pain better or worse?
Quality	Describe the pain or contractions.
Radiation/ related symptoms	Does the pain go anywhere? Does the patient have any other pain? Does the patient feel the need to push?
Severity	On a scale of 1 to 10, with 10 being the worst pain the patient has ever had, how does this pain or contraction rate?
Time	How long has the patient had the pain or contractions? What changes have occurred in the pain or contractions since the beginning?
Other	When was the patient's last menstrual period? Is the patient pregnant? Has the patient had any vaginal bleeding or discharge? If yes, how did it look? How far along is the patient's pregnancy? Has the patient had prenatal care? Does the patient anticipate problems with this pregnancy? Is the patient expecting more than one baby?
Focused physical exam	Palpate the abdomen. Monitor the contractions. Inspect for crowning as appropriate.

From National Registry of Emergency Medical Technicians: *Patient assessment/management: medical* (skill sheet), Columbus, OH, 2000, NREMT.

medications are being taken, ask what the medications are for and try to find the original bottle when possible. If you cannot find the container, bring in the medications for identification. Find out how much medication is being taken, when the last dose was taken, and whether the medication is being taken as prescribed.

• The past medical history is important in caring for the medical patient, because the patient may be manifesting a known problem and may be able to

TABLE 11-11
Behavioral emergency assessment considerations

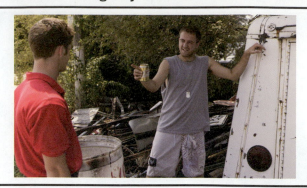

Assessment Component	Considerations*
Onset	What was the patient doing when this behavior/problem started?
Provocation	Does anything make the behavior/problem better or worse?
Quality	Describe the behavior/problem.
Related symptoms	Is the patient seeing, hearing, or feeling anything else?
Severity	On a scale of 1 to 10, with 10 being the worst episode the patient has ever had, how does this episode rate?
Time	When did this behavior/problem start? How has the behavior/problem changed since it started?
Other	Is the scene safe? Is the patient suicidal? Is the patient a threat to self or others? Does the patient have medical problems that could contribute to the behavior/problem or that need to be managed? Have any interventions been tried so far? Has this ever happened to the patient before? If yes, what happened? What was done to treat this problem before? Does the patient have adequate resources available?
Focused physical exam	Assess the areas the patient will let you assess, as reasonable, given the patient's condition. Consider a neurologic exam. Assess the blood glucose level.

From National Registry of Emergency Medical Technicians: *Patient assessment/management: medical* (skill sheet), Columbus, OH, 2000, NREMT.
*These questions may be directed to the patient or to family members or bystanders, depending on the patient's response.

TABLE 11-12

Rapid assessment for medical patients

Assessment Component	Consideration
Equality	Compare the two sides of the body; they should be equal in function and appearance.
Function	Assess to see whether each body part is working or moving normally.
Guarding	Assess for protecting of a body part (i.e., holding the muscles tense or protecting the area with another part of the body, such as holding the hands over the abdomen).
Masses	Inspect and gently palpate for masses, feeling the consistency or any unusual details (e.g., a pulsating mass).
Pain	Does the patient inform you that a body part hurts?
Tenderness	Determine whether the patient experiences any pain when the body is moved or palpated.

provide you with more information about needs and treatment. Sometimes the patient has an unknown or a new problem. You must assess the medical history for possible causes of the signs and symptoms in order to eliminate or establish one of the previous problems as the cause.

- The last oral intake may be useful in guiding you to such problems as low blood sugar or food poisoning. It is important that you document what was ingested, how much, and when. This also is important information for the physicians should surgery be required.
- The events preceding the incident can be evaluated by asking the patient what happened before the incident. This information gives you insight into the mechanism of injury, the nature of the illness, or factors that may contribute to the patient's progression.

You may opt to collect the SAMPLE history in a different order, but it is important that all components be explored so that no significant information is missed.

Rapid Assessment

The rapid assessment may be performed before, during, or after collection of the history. With a conscious patient, you usually will collect the focused history first and then move on to the physical exam. This provides you with information to focus your assessment, and it allows time for the patient to become more comfortable with you before you begin palpating the patient's body. Taking your time often increases the patient's trust and results in a more thorough history and a more accurate physical exam. With a patient who is in serious condition but still conscious, you may find yourself beginning your assessment as you question the patient about his or her history. Another way to

collect a history and complete a physical exam at the same time is to have your partner question the family or bystanders about the patient's history as you perform the assessment. With unconscious patients, you usually will perform a rapid assessment and then collect the history. Regardless of the method selected, you should be systematic and consistent in the process so that you do not leave out important information.

Rapid assessment of a medical patient proceeds from the head to the toes. It includes the head, neck, chest, abdomen, pelvis, extremities, and posterior body. You may want to keep the mnemonic *DCAPBTLS* (*d*eformities, *c*ontusions, *a*brasions, *p*unctures or *p*enetrations, *b*urns, *t*enderness, *l*acerations, *s*welling) in the back of your mind as you do the assessment, because the patient may have trauma injuries. However, with a medical patient, the assessment focuses on **equality, function, guarding, masses, pain, and tenderness** (Table 11-12). You may include the entire body if the patient is unconscious or unable to communicate a specific problem.

If the patient is conscious, assess the area where the person has a specific complaint (detailed assessment of each body part is discussed in Chapter 12). You can use the specific component of this assessment for the focused exam, but you usually will not assess the entire body.

Vital Signs

Vital signs must be obtained with all medical patients (see Chapter 5). The EMT monitors the various components of the vital signs for trending in medical patients. This requires obtaining multiple sets of vital signs to determine the patient's response to treatment and how the patient has changed over the time that you are with the patient. This is important information to provide to medical control as decisions are made about medical care.

PROVIDING EMERGENCY MEDICAL CARE

As you complete your assessment, you will be initiating or planning to initiate patient care. This care focuses on the symptoms you identified and on the patient's condition. In some cases you must differentiate between problems and at times relay that information to medical control to obtain orders to administer medications. In other cases you must match the patient's signs and symptoms to your protocols and select the protocol that best fits the patient's condition; treatment then is initiated based on the protocol.

Specific Chief Complaint: Known History

Some patients have a specific chief complaint or a known medical problem. With these patients, you still complete the scene size-up and initial assessment. As you begin collecting a history, you may find that the patient's chief complaint and medical history coincide. For example, a patient who complains of chest pain may have a cardiac history. In this case, you continue your assessment to include assessment of the chest and the vital signs. Once all this information has been gathered, you select the chest pain protocol or guidelines to follow. In all likelihood, your protocol will include administration of oxygen and preparation for transport.

The protocol may include additional steps, such as assisting the patient with his or her own nitroglycerin after contacting medical control (this process is discussed in detail in Chapter 16). You must describe your patient so that medical control can see that you have effectively assessed the patient, formed the correct impression, and collected the proper informa-

tion to assist with the nitroglycerin. An example of such a report is as follows:

> Unit 22 to Heart Hospital; we are en route to your facility with a conscious, 52-year-old male with crushing midsternal chest pain. He describes the pain as an 8 in severity. The pain began 15 minutes ago and is continuous. It radiates to his left arm. He has oxygen at 10 via non-rebreather (NRB) mask, with no relief to the pain. His vital signs are P 88 and regular, R 16 and regular with clear bilateral breath sounds, BP 142/84, skin cool and pale, pupils equal, round, reactive to light (PERRL). He has a history of a previous heart attack and does have his own nitroglycerin but has not taken it. The nitro is current and prescribed for this patient. We are requesting permission to assist the patient with one of his nitroglycerin tablets sublingual per protocol.

By outlining the pertinent patient history, assessment, and vital signs, the report suggests a patient with a cardiac problem, therefore the EMT chose to follow the service's cardiac protocol. The protocol required that vital signs be taken and be adequate and that the medication be the patient's own and current. This was all confirmed and relayed to medical control, along with a request for an order to administer nitroglycerin. When you are this thorough, the physicians are more likely to trust your assessment and judgment and issue you the order you request.

Specific Chief Complaint: No Known History

Other emergency medical services (EMS) patients may have a specific chief complaint but no known medical problem. These patients can be a challenge, because the cause is more likely to be unknown. You do not have a previous diagnosis to help you with the patient. In this case, complete a scene size-up, initial exam, and focused history and physical exam and obtain vital signs. Try to identify a cause of the chief complaint, but if you are unable to do so, treat the patient's signs and symptoms and transport the person. For example, you may care for a patient with abdominal pain. The patient denies any allergies, medications, or medical problems and tells you that the pain came on suddenly while the patient was watching TV. The pain is cramping, does not radiate, and is a 6 on the pain scale. The pain started 30 minutes ago and has not changed. The patient had a sandwich for lunch about 3 hours ago. The lower left abdomen is soft and tender to palpation. The patient indicates feeling slightly nauseated. You decide to treat the patient for an acute abdomen. The vital signs are pulse (P) 92 and regular, respirations (R) 16 and regular, blood pressure (BP) 114/68, skin warm and moist, and pupils PERRL. You administer oxygen and place the patient in the position of comfort for transport. You arrive at the hospital without incident. Because this patient did not have a problem that you could treat in the field, oxygen and transport are the best options for management.

Unresponsive Medical Patient

With an unresponsive patient, the EMT must rely on the patient's presentation and on bystanders or family members for information. With this type of patient, perform a scene size-up as usual, but pay even more attention to the environment for clues to the patient's problem. Next, perform the initial assessment. Because the patient is unconscious, the person must be treated as critical. Therefore you should anticipate ALS intercept. If ALS intercept is not possible and the patient's airway, breathing, or circulation (ABCs) has been compromised, make sure you can manage the airway, oxygenate the patient, support circulation, and initiate transport. The recovery position (Fig. 11-1) allows the patient to better protect the airway and should be considered unless contraindicated by the patient's condition. (You can complete your rapid exam and history and obtain vital signs en route, if necessary.) If the patient's ABCs are stable, move directly to the rapid assessment and then obtain vital signs. While you perform these tasks, your partner can check the bathroom, kitchen, or refrigerator for medications or a **Vial of Life,** which may provide clues to the patient's problem. In addition, you should question bystanders and family members about the patient's history. If no one is available to answer questions, initiate transport and continue the assessment. Consider asking other EMS care providers present whether they know the patient from previous calls.

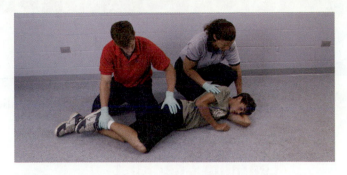

Fig. 11-1 Place the patient in the recovery position.

Medical patients can have many presentations. It is important to adjust your assessment and management to the presentation. However, in adjusting the assessment, you must make sure you do not omit necessary information. You also must relate your findings to medical control in an orderly, understandable manner to complete a radio or oral report on a patient and to obtain orders to initiate treatment. Medical patients can have complex conditions involving multiple factors, and you often will feel challenged as you care for them. Working to solve the puzzles they present can be a satisfying and enlightening experience.

TEAMWORK

As previously discussed, EMTs arrive on a scene to find various types of patients in distress. Often the patient's chief complaint is not obvious. Working together with other responders and looking for clues or evidence of what has transpired may lead you to the underlying problem. You may find yourself directing others to look for medications or other information sources. Working together and understanding how to find information when the patient is unable to assist you greatly benefits everyone involved.

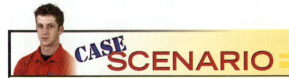

CASE SCENARIO

"Do you really think I should go to the hospital?" Mrs. Jameson asks as Ray gets the stretcher ready.

"Yes, ma'am, I do," Rays responds. "Your abdomen is very tender to the touch. I'm not sure what's going on, but the fact that you have so much pain worries me. On the other hand, your vital signs are pretty good, and that makes me a little less worried."

"Okay, Ray," Mrs. Jameson replies. "Thanks for being so concerned about me." ■

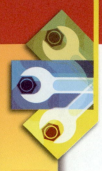

NUTS AND BOLTS

Critical Point

- OPQRST is a beginning point, not an ending point, in history gathering.

Learning Checklist

❏ The EMT needs to differentiate between critical and noncritical patients. A thorough history helps in choosing appropriate assessment tools. For unresponsive patients or those with multiple complaints, a rapid assessment moves from head to toe. For patients with isolated complaints, the assessment is focused on the patient's chief complaint and is expanded as needed.

❏ After ensuring that the scene is safe, the EMT can also evaluate the mechanism of injury and nature of illness. Use environmental clues to help determine the nature of the illness.

❏ The initial assessment helps to determine whether the patient is stable enough to continue to a medical assessment or the patient is in critical condition and needs immediate intervention.

❏ The focused history and physical exam: medical is the process of assessing a medical patient.

❏ Start with the chief complaint to assess the history of the present illness. The chief complaint should be noted in the patient's words. Use OPQRST to obtain more information about the patient's problem.

❏ Onset refers to what the patient was doing before the problem began.

❏ Provocation relates to any action that changes the nature of the problem—makes it better or worse.

❏ Quality refers to the description of the problem, including the quality of pain the patient is feeling.

❏ Radiation refers to movement or association of pain or discomfort into another part of the body. Referred pain may be present in a different part of the body from the original site of the problem.

❏ Severity correlates to the strength or intensity of the pain. Pain rated as 9 or 10 on a 10-

point scale often indicates the potential for critical patients, and rapid transport is indicated.

❏ Time is assessed in reference to how long the problem has existed, when it started, and how it has changed over time since it first began.

❏ The SAMPLE history is used to collect a history for medical patients. S = Signs and symptoms; A = allergies; M = medications; P = past medical history; L = the last oral intake; E = events preceding the call for help.

❏ For unconscious patients, the rapid assessment is usually performed before obtaining the history. The rapid assessment is conducted from head to toe and includes the head, neck, chest, abdomen, pelvis, extremities, and posterior body.

❏ The mnemonic DCAPBTLS is useful in patient assessment. D = Deformities; C = contusions; A = abrasions; P = punctures/penetrations; B = burns; T = tenderness; L = lacerations; S = swelling.

❏ Vital signs are monitored for tending in medical patients as multiple sets of vital signs are obtained to assess the patient's response to emergency care.

❏ Bystanders, family, and friends may provide information for unresponsive patients.

❏ All necessary information is included in the patient care report. Findings should be related in an orderly, understandable manner to complete radio or oral reports and to obtain orders to initiate treatment.

Key Terms

Equality A term used for comparing the body side to side to determine sameness.

Function The assessment factor that pertains to normal movement and operation.

Guarding Tensing the muscles or using other body parts to protect an area.

Onset An event that causes a symptom to occur.

OPQRST An acronym used in collecting a patient history about a specific sign or symptom. The letters stand for *o*nset, *p*rovocation, *q*uality, *r*adiation, *s*everity, and *t*ime.

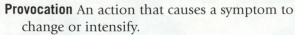
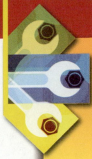
Provocation An action that causes a symptom to change or intensify.

Quality The assessment factor that pertains to the description of a symptom.

Radiation Movement to another area; the term often is used to describe pain that moves from one location to another.

Severity The assessment factor that pertains to qualification of a symptom's intensity.

Vial of Life A container that holds medical information about a patient.

National Standard Curriculum Objectives

Cognitive Objectives

After completing this lesson, the EMT student will be able to do the following:

- Describe the unique requirements for assessing a patient with a specific chief complaint and no known history.
- Differentiate between the history and physical exam for responsive patients with no known history and the history and physical exam for responsive patients with a known history.
- Describe the requirements for assessing an unresponsive patient.
- Differentiate between the assessment for a patient who is unresponsive or has an altered mental status and the assessment for other medical patients.

Affective Objective

After completing this lesson, the EMT student will be able to do the following:

- Attend to the feelings patients might experience during the assessment.

Psychomotor Objectives

After completing this lesson, the EMT student will be able to do the following:

- Demonstrate the patient assessment skills for assisting a responsive patient with no known history.
- Demonstrate the patient assessment skills for assisting a patient who is unresponsive or has an altered mental status.

CHAPTER

12

LESSON GOAL

This chapter focuses on the skills the emergency medical technician (EMT) must acquire to complete a detailed physical exam, to understand the findings, and to use the findings to provide appropriate patient care. Assessment related skills form the foundation of the EMT's ability to practice. ■

The Detailed Physical Examination

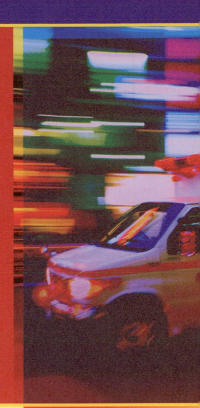

CHAPTER OBJECTIVES

After completing this chapter, the EMT student will be able to do the following:

1 Discuss the components of the detailed physical exam.

2 State the areas of the body that are evaluated during the detailed physical exam.

3 Explain what additional care should be provided while the detailed physical exam is performed.

4 Distinguish between the detailed physical exam performed on a trauma patient and that performed on a medical patient.

5 Explain the rationale for emotional feelings patients may experience during the detailed physical exam.

6 Demonstrate the skills required to perform the detailed physical exam.

OBJECTIVES

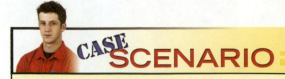

CASE SCENARIO

The mountain bike rider looks a bit embarrassed as Ray walks up to him. Ray and his partner had responded to a report of a "cyclist down" on one of the many trails in the vast park. They had to hike in a few hundred yards to reach the scene.

"Hey there, we're from the hospital ambulance service," Ray says to the young man. "What's your name?"

"Josh," the bike rider replies.

"How are you doing, sir?" Ray asks as he reaches to check Josh's radial pulse. It is strong and regular.

"Oh, I'm okay," Josh answers. "My wrist hurts, but I don't think it's broken."

"Did you fall off the bike?" Ray asks.

"Yep," says Josh. "Hit the rock over there at the wrong angle, flipped right over."

Ray's partner reaches behind Josh to manually stabilize the young man's neck and head.

"Don't move for a moment, okay?" Ray tells Josh. "Let me just check you over quickly to make sure you're not hurt anywhere else."

Question: *Why did the fire crew establish manual stabilization of the spine? Is this a "load and go" situation, or is the patient stable?*

The **detailed physical exam** is performed to assess each body part individually to determine whether injury or a medical problem is present. It is the process of starting at the patient's head and moving to the toes in order to systematically evaluate the body. The detailed physical exam is more thorough and time-consuming than the rapid assessment completed on trauma and medical patients. The detailed physical exam is used for trauma patients with a significant mechanism of injury to ensure that the whole body is completely reassessed for injuries. It also may be used for unconscious medical patients when the EMT is trying to detect problems. For conscious medical patients, you may select the components of the detailed physical exam that correlate with the patient's problem. For example, for a patient with abdominal pain, you may use only the abdominal component of the detailed physical exam.

A detailed exam is not performed on every patient. For example, a patient who steps in a hole and twists an ankle but does not fall and has no other problems would not need a detailed physical exam. A patient who falls, twists an ankle, hits the head, and has a history of diabetes and cardiac problems may require a detailed physical exam.

Because this is a detailed exam, you must **expose** the patient and then **inspect** and **palpate** the body thoroughly as well as auscultate when appropriate. This can make your patient feel very uncomfortable or embarrassed, therefore you need to make every reasonable effort to protect the patient's privacy and to be professional in your actions. You can do this by moving the patient to a private area, such as the back of the ambulance, to do the assessment or by shielding the patient with a blanket. Also, you should keep exposure time to a minimum and then cover the patient. This not only protects the patient's privacy, but also keeps the person warm.

You most often will start the detailed exam at the patient's head and work toward the toes. Infants and children are the exception to this rule. Many young children do not like having their head touched, so you may find the assessment easier if you start at the toes and move toward the head in a conscious child.

The detailed physical exam should be started only after the initial exam has been completed and any life-threatening conditions have been stabilized. If

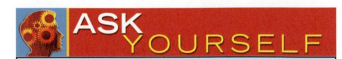

ASK YOURSELF

You may be asking yourself, "Detailed physical exam? I thought we already learned how to conduct an exam. What's the difference between the detailed exam, the rapid trauma exam, and the medical assessment? Will the detailed physical exam really make a difference? Are we wasting time by conducting this exam?"

Important Points
Consider toe to head assessment in pediatric patients.

Important Points
Do not start your detailed assessment until all life threats have been stabilized.

your patient is not stable, the detailed physical exam should not be completed. The goal of the detailed physical exam is to identify any problems you may have missed or any changes that may have occurred since your previous exam. Because many of your patients will be trauma patients, you should continue to provide spinal stabilization throughout the assessment.

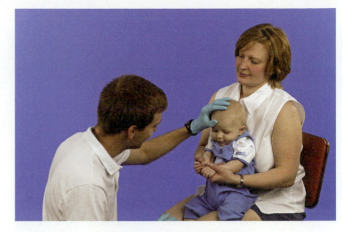

Fig. 12-1 Gently palpate the fontanels to determine whether they are bulging or sunken.

■ THE DCAPBTLS METHOD

As you assess the patient's body, use the mnemonic **DCAPBTLS** again. Following the letters of the acronym, you should assess for *d*eformities, *c*ontusions, *a*brasions, *p*uncture wounds, *b*urns, *t*enderness, *l*acerations and *s*welling. You also should assess for crepitus, distention, equality, function, guarding, and masses. Individual body parts or systems may require assessment of additional points (these points are addressed in the following sections on specific areas). The order of this assessment may be adjusted as needed. The flow described is for discussion purposes only and is not the only way an assessment can be completed.

Head

Your assessment of the patient's head should involve a breakdown into the individual components: head, face, eyes, ears, nose, and mouth. Inspect and palpate for DCAPBTLS. The hair can hide injuries, therefore it is important to take your time as you assess patients with a lot of hair or very thick hair. Gently palpate the scalp, and check your hands frequently for blood. If you find bleeding, consider controlling it, depending on the severity, because scalp wounds can bleed profusely. You may note a spongy feeling as you palpate the scalp. This is common in patients who have had their hair pulled and is a frequent finding with abuse, especially in the elderly. In infants, you should palpate the **fontanels** (Fig. 12-1). A bulging fontanel sug-

gests bleeding or **meningitis,** whereas a sunken fontanel most often is associated with **dehydration.**

Face

Assess the patient's face, again checking for DCAPBTLS. Also assess **equality,** or *symmetry.* Ask yourself whether the two sides of the patient's face look equal. To assess function, have the patient smile and lift the eyebrows. This tells you whether the facial muscles and nerves are intact. If you note drooping on one side, the patient may have suffered a stroke or may have nerve damage. Palpate the face gently. Begin at the forehead and slowly move to the orbits and then to the cheekbones, **maxilla** (upper jaw bone) and **mandible** (lower jaw bone). If you note trauma to the face, reevaluate the airway, because it can become obstructed by blood, secretions, or swelling. Brain trauma also should be a consideration, therefore continue monitoring neurologic function using the AVPU assessment tool (i.e., *a*lert, *v*erbal, *p*ainful, *un*-responsive) and the Glasgow Coma Scale.

Eyes

Look at the patient's eyes. What do they look like? Are they open and looking at you? Is the sclera of the eye white, red, or yellow? White is normal, red (bloodshot) occurs with irritation, and yellow suggests liver damage. Do you see blood in the anterior chamber of the eye (in front of the pupil and behind the cornea)? This is a sign of trauma and requires transport to an appropriate facility for evaluation. Look for contact lenses. Are the eyes clear or glazed over? If you note bilateral bruising, or **raccoon's eyes**

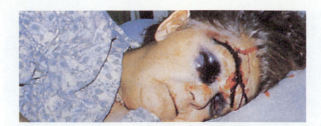

Fig. 12-2 Assess for raccoon's eyes.

(Fig. 12-2), without direct trauma to the facial area, suspect a possible **basilar skull fracture.**

Do the patient's eyes look straight at you or do they **deviate** to one side? Are they still or continuously moving or shaking back and forth **(nystagmus)?** Look at the pupils. Are they round and of equal size? Shine a bright light into each pupil. Do they both constrict? (Pupil reaction is discussed in Chapter 5.) If the patient is awake, check the visual acuity (ability to see). Hold up a certain number of fingers and confirm that the patient can tell you the number, or have the patient identify an object close by. Make sure the eyes have normal movement. You can do this by moving your finger to the left, right, up, down, and to each corner and observing whether the patient's eyes follow. If the patient's eye movement cannot follow that of your finger, damage to the nerves or entrapment of the eye from a fracture may be present. Other problems associated with eye movement are described in Table 12-1.

Ears

Look in and behind the patient's ears. If you see fluid or blood flowing from the ear, cover it with a light dressing but do not occlude the flow. Occluding the flow may lead to increased intracranial pressure and worsening of the patient's head injury. Note the color of the fluid. Fluid leaking from the ear may be cerebrospinal fluid (CSF). One way to identify CSF is to get a small amount of the fluid on a piece of gauze. If a halo forms around the fluid, it most likely is CSF. This is called a **halo test.** Another way to assess for CSF is to test the fluid with a **glucometer.** If the sample tests positive for sugar, it probably is CSF. This is important, because it means that the skull has been fractured and CSF is leaking through the fracture site to the outside of the body. In most cases, however, CSF will also be mixed with blood, making field diagnosis extremely difficult. Also check behind the ears for bruising. If bruising is noted, this is called **Battle's sign** (Fig. 12-3). Battle's sign is a late sign of a basilar skull fracture.

Nose

Assess the patient's nose for leaking fluids or blood. If blood or fluids are present, assess for CSF leakage as previously described. Accumulated fluid or blood may affect breathing, particularly in infants, and should be cleared immediately. Singed nasal hairs in burn patients suggest airway burns. If drug use is sus-

TABLE 12-1

Examination of the eyes

Eye Movement	Possible Problems
Eyes move in different directions (disconjugate gaze).	Head injury, direct trauma to the eye
Eye is paralyzed (unable to move from the upward gaze).	Fracture of the orbit
Eyes are deviated to the right or left.	Stroke, meningitis, tumor
Nystagmus (involuntary jerking of the eyes) is present.	Stroke, head trauma, inner ear problems, tumors, multiple sclerosis, drug or alcohol ingestion; *or* may be normal

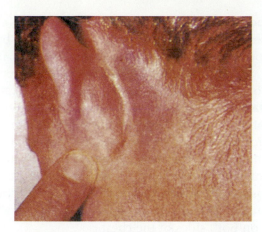

Fig. 12-3 Look behind the ears for Battle's sign.

pected, residual drug may be noted in the nostrils of patients who "snort" or inhale drugs.

Mouth

Look in the patient's mouth for blood, fluids, or vomit and make sure the airway is clear. Assess to see that the teeth are intact. Consider removing dentures if they jeopardize the airway. Have the patient open the mouth and clench the teeth. Look for lacerations or swelling of the tongue. If the patient is unable to open the mouth or if the teeth do not line up properly, the person may have a broken jaw. Check for odors, such as alcohol, vomit, gasoline, paint, or a sweet smell (which may suggest acidosis, typically related to complications of diabetes).

Neck

Continue your DCAPBTLS assessment. Remove the clothing from the patient's upper body and gently palpate the neck for tenderness and deformity while maintaining inline spinal stabilization, when trauma is a consideration. If the patient is wearing a cervical collar and you feel reassessment is necessary, maintain stabilization and gently open the collar to progress with your assessment of the neck and then reapply the collar. Assess the anterior neck for jugular vein distention. Any open wounds should be managed with an occlusive dressing. Assess for neck muscle (accessory muscle) use with breathing, which indicates respiratory distress. Swelling, foreign bodies, or masses in the neck area may lead to airway obstruction, therefore reassess the airway frequently if any of these is present. Listen for stridor during inspiration indicating airway obstruction. Palpate the trachea to assess its position. A shift in the trachea

away from the midline is a late sign of tension pneumothorax. A cervical collar should be applied when the neck assessment is completed if one had not been applied previously whenever spine trauma is a possibility. If bruising or abrasions are noted and are hidden by the collar, make sure to tell the receiving facility about them. This is important, because underlying damage to the large vessels of the neck may be present, but the signs and symptoms of damage may not develop until later.

Chest

As you inspect the patient's chest using DCAPBTLS, look for open wounds. If open wounds are found, apply an occlusive dressing and secure it on three sides. Note any scars on the chest. For example, a midline scar over the sternum suggests cardiac surgery. An incision in the lateral aspect of the chest suggests cardiac or pulmonary surgery. The patient may have had a portion of the lung removed, and breath sounds may be absent in that area. When a scar is found, therefore, it is important to ask why the patient has the scar or what surgery was performed. This provides insight into possible medical problems. The

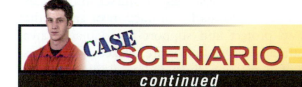

CASE SCENARIO *continued*

Ray continues his detailed physical examination. He finds that Josh has abrasions and contusions along both lower legs and on the palms of both hands. A bruise is forming on the upper left thigh. Josh can move all his extremities, although his thigh hurts when he pushes with his left foot against Ray's extended palm. He also feels pain in his left wrist when he tries to squeeze Ray's finger. That wrist has a spoonlike shape and is painful to mild palpation.

"Josh, you look okay, considering the fall you took," Ray says. "Even though you were wearing a helmet, I'd like to place a cervical collar around your neck and have my partner help keep your head still until the medics arrive."

"My neck doesn't hurt," Josh protests. "Why do I need a cervical collar?"

Question: *Why should Josh's head and neck be immobilized, at least for now?*

shape of the chest may also provide clues to a patient's medical problem. For example, a barrel-shaped chest is found in patients with emphysema.

Palpate the chest for tenderness and crepitus. **Point tenderness** may occur with rib fractures, bruising of the chest wall, or pleurisy. Point tenderness is present when the patient can point to the location of the pain. **Crepitus** is a crunching feeling that may be noted with rib fractures as the broken bones rub against each other. A crackling feeling **(subcutaneous emphysema)** that is detected as air leaks into the skin may also be noted. This commonly occurs with a pneumothorax,.

Also assess for equality of chest movement. To do this, place your hands on the lower chest wall with your thumbs meeting at the xiphoid process. Then ask the patient to take a deep breath. Observe the distance the thumbs move away from each other. If one side of the chest expands or moves more than the other, consider the presence of a pneumothorax, hemothorax, or tension pneumothorax. **Paradoxical movement** (in which a portion of the chest bulges on expiration and sinks in on inspiration) occurs when consecutive ribs are broken, causing that portion of the chest to float and to move in the opposite direction from the rest of the rib cage. This is known as a **flail chest.** A flail chest may be missed initially because of adjacent muscle contraction or spasm that occurs to protect and support the damaged area. When these muscles tire or are relaxed by administration of medication, the paradoxical movement becomes more apparent.

Once you have inspected and palpated the chest, you should **auscultate** the lungs. This is done by using your stethoscope to listen to the lungs. At minimum, you should listen at the apices (the upper portion of the lungs, just under the clavicles, at the midclavicular line) and at the bases (the lower portion of the lungs, at the midaxillary line). Listening at additional sites may be beneficial for noting changes. Auscultation of the posterior chest also should be part of your assessment. As you listen, move your stethoscope from side to side, comparing the sounds you hear. Normal breath sounds are clear and the same on both sides of the chest.

In some cases, you will hear abnormal breath sounds, which include rales, or *crackles,* and wheezes. In other cases, you may hear breath sounds on one side but not on the other (Table 12-2). That is why it is so important to compare one side of the chest to the other. **Rales (crackles)** are heard when fluid accumulates in the lungs. As the patient inhales or exhales, air moving through the wet alveoli makes a crackling sound that can be heard when you auscultate the lungs. Rales (crackles) are commonly associated with congestive heart failure, pulmonary edema, pneumonia, and bronchitis. **Wheezes** are whistling sounds made as air passes through narrowed airways, usually during expiration. Wheezes are commonly heard with conditions such as bronchitis, emphysema, asthma, and anaphylaxis. Breath sounds may be decreased in one area of the lungs or completely absent. This is common in conditions such as a hemothorax, a pneumothorax, or atelectasis (collapse of a portion of the lungs).

TABLE 12-2

Auscultation of the lungs

Sound	Description	Possible Cause
Rales (crackles)	Crackling noise caused by air moving through fluid in the lungs	Congestive heart failure Pulmonary edema Bronchitis Pneumonia
Wheezes	Whistling noise caused by air moving through narrowed airways	Asthma Bronchitis Emphysema Anaphylaxis Pneumonia
Absent	No breath sounds heard over an area of the lung	Hemothorax Pneumothorax Tension pneumothorax Atelectasis

In some situations you may also apply a cardiac monitor. If you do so, noting the rhythm or printing a copy for advanced life support (ALS) providers may be appropriate at this time. You can listen to heart tones and relay any abnormal sounds heard. Murmurs or other sounds that may be heard when you listen to the heart are beyond the discussion in this text but are important to relay to other providers.

Whenever abnormal findings are identified, you should begin appropriate treatment, whether that involves giving oxygen, applying an occlusive dressing, or administering medications. You also should reassess the patient's respiratory status frequently for response to the treatment. This is true for both medical patients and trauma patients. Assessment and reassessment of the respiratory status are crucial to quality patient care.

Abdomen

As you complete your DCAPBTLS assessment, you should evaluate the patient's abdomen for disten-

tion, rigidity, and softness. Unexplained signs and symptoms of shock may be caused by abdominal bleeding, therefore it is important to keep this fact in mind as you assess the abdomen. Any external injuries or complaints of pain should be correlated with a possible internal injury or medical problem with the organs listed in Table 12-3.

Distention is swelling of the abdomen. If you are assisting a patient's ventilation and note distention in the **epigastric** (upper abdominal) area, consider repositioning the airway or reassessing the device you are using. You may be filling the stomach with air as a result of improper airway positioning or because of an improperly positioned airway device (and sometimes distention with air is not avoidable). In pediatric patients, distention may be caused by the swallowing of air when the patient cries. Distention may also be caused by intestinal obstruction as gas accumulates in the blocked bowel. Finally, distention may also be caused by blood accumulating in the abdomen. A large amount of blood is required to cause

TABLE 12-3

Abdominal assessment

Location	Organs and Possible Problems
Upper right quadrant	Liver: Hepatitis, trauma, abscess Gallbladder: Cholecystitis, gallstones Pancreas: Pancreatitis Lung: Pneumonia, pulmonary emboli Bowel: Ulcer
Upper left quadrant	Spleen: Ruptured spleen Stomach: Ulcer, gastritis Bowel: Ulcer, diverticulitis Pancreas: Pancreatitis Lung: Pneumonia, pulmonary emboli
Lower right quadrant	Appendix: Appendicitis Ovary, fallopian tubes: Cysts, ectopic pregnancy, infection Bowel: Diverticulitis, obstruction Kidney: Kidney stone
Lower left quadrant	Ovary, fallopian tubes: Cysts, ectopic pregnancy, infection Bowel: Diverticulitis, obstruction Kidney: Kidney stone
Referred pain	Shoulder: Ruptured ovary or fallopian tube (female), swollen or ruptured spleen (left shoulder), swollen or ruptured liver (right shoulder) Right scapula: Gallbladder pain Epigastric area: Pneumonia, pleurisy, acute myocardial infarction, early appendicitis Midback: Pancreatitis, aortic aneurysm Umbilicus: Appendicitis, colon obstruction, diverticulitis Groin: Kidney stone

the abdomen to distend. Bruising may also be noted. You may see it in the flank area or around the umbilicus. Unless trauma has caused **superficial** damage, bruising usually is a late sign. You should note the presence of scars or any devices, such as a drain, **colostomy bag,** or tubes placed in the abdomen.

After you inspect the abdomen, you should begin palpation. Palpate the unaffected **abdominal quadrants** first. For example, if a patient complains of pain in the upper right quadrant, you should begin palpating in the upper left quadrant, move to the lower left quadrant, then to the lower right quadrant, and finally up to the upper right quadrant. By assessing the non-painful quadrants first, you will usually find that the patient is less likely to be **guarding** the area that hurts and will allow you to complete a more accurate assessment. To palpate the abdomen, place your hand on the area you wish to assess. Place the other hand on top and gently press your hand into the abdomen, rolling down from your palm to your fingers. As you palpate, feel for guarding, firmness, or softness. Normally the abdomen is soft to palpation in all quadrants. Watch the patient's face for grimaces or other indications of pain. If you note firmness or a mass, feel for **pulsation.** If that is noted, inform the receiving caregivers, because an aortic aneurysm may be present.

Pelvis

Remove the clothing from the patient's lower body and inspect the pelvis for bruising. You may also note **incontinence** (involuntary loss of urine or stool). In trauma patients, attention should be paid as to whether or not there is blood at the urethral meatus, suggesting injury to that structure. When assessing the pelvis, you may find a **urinary catheter** (a tube placed in the bladder to drain urine) in place. If so, note the amount and color of the urine. If a bag is present, keep the bag lower than the patient's pelvic area to prevent backflow of urine into the bladder. If indicated, expose the perineal area and note bleeding, drainage, or wounds. In cases of pregnancy, assess for **crowning** (the baby's head bulging from the vaginal opening). In some male patients you may note a condition called **priapism** (persistent erection of the penis). This is a sign of spinal cord injury or other medical problems.

Palpation of the pelvis is done when the patient complains of pain. You may also palpate the pelvis to see whether you can identify tenderness. To palpate the pelvis, place both hands on the iliac crest and gently press down. If the patient complains of pain or if you feel crepitus, note the location. If crepitus is identified, do not repeat the procedure.

Extremities

As you complete your DCAPBTLS assessment of the patient's extremities, compare each extremity with the corresponding one to check for symmetry. Inspect the extremities. They should be mirror images of each other. Note and report any differences. As you inspect, look at length and positioning. For example, a shortened and externally rotated leg suggests a fractured hip. Also look at the color of the extremities, and check for swelling. A **mottled** or **cyanotic** extremity indicates inadequate blood flow to the area. Redness and warmth in an area may suggest a venous **embolus.** Swelling in an area suggests injury or decreased venous return. **Pedal edema** (swelling of the feet and ankles) commonly is associated with right-sided heart failure.

Palpate the extremities for pain, crepitus, or deformity. When you have completed the palpation, assess for distal pulses, sensation, and movement. Again, you should assess for equality of the two sides of the body. To do this, palpate the radial or pedal pulses. These pulses should be equal and easily palpated. If an extremity is injured or has decreased circulation and repeated assessment of the pulse will be required, you can mark the pulse by drawing an X over the site with a pen to make locating it easier. To assess sensation, touch the patient's toes on each foot and ask the patient to tell you which toe is being touched. Assess movement by asking the patient to push their feet against your hands and then to pull their feet back as you grip them with your hands. The two legs should have equal strength as they push and pull. The arms are assessed similarly. Palpate for a radial pulse. Touch the fingers and ask the patient to identify the one touched. To test strength, have the patient squeeze your hands and assess for equality and strength.

Back

The final step in the detailed physical assessment is to assess the patient's back. As with the other areas of the body, inspect and palpate for DCAPBTLS. If the patient already is immobilized on a backboard, this step should have been performed. You do not need to remove the patient from the backboard to complete this assessment. If the patient is not secured to a backboard, perform the back assessment and consider auscultating the lungs posteriorly. Breath sounds often are easier to hear through the back. Auscultate from side to side and compare sounds as described in the section on chest assessment. Breath sounds will be best heard if you listen between the spine and the scapula.

Vital Signs

Take the patient's vital signs again and compare the results with previous findings to determine the patent's response to treatment. Report the vital signs to the receiving crew or facility and reassess any abnormal findings as needed.

■ OTHER ASSESSMENT TOOLS

In addition to the physical exam, you may want to consider using a pulse oximeter, a cardiac monitor, and a glucometer to assist you with your assessment. A **pulse oximeter** (Fig. 12-4) provides information about the patient's oxygenation status. A **cardiac monitor** provides information on the patient's heart rhythm. A **glucometer** (Fig. 12-5) is used to determine the patient's blood glucose level and can be useful with patients who are unconscious or who have diabetes.

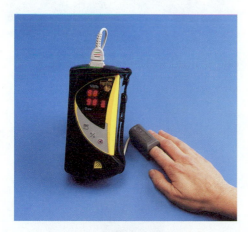

Fig. 12-4 Consider using a pulse oximeter to assess oxygenation.

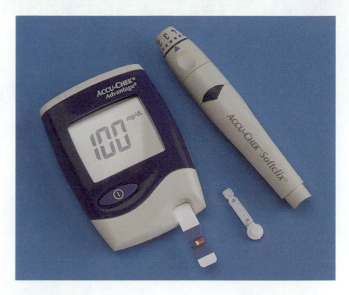

Fig. 12-5 Consider using a glucometer to check the patient's capillary blood glucose level.

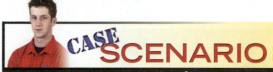
CASE SCENARIO
conclusion

Although Josh did not appear to have any injury to the head or neck, immobilizing his spine to a long backboard after application of a cervical collar would be prudent because of the mechanism of the injury. In addition, the crew splints Josh's left wrist and places some activated cold packs around the injury site on the wrist, which helps ease Josh's pain. ■

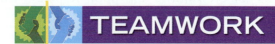
TEAMWORK

As discussed in this chapter, EMTs may be called to a residence, an athletic event, or some other scene. Regardless of the locale, EMTs and responders must provide the best possible care to the patient. Conducting a detailed physical exam that is complete and thorough ensures that your patient will receive the best possible care. It is important to keep in mind that, as you conduct the detailed physical exam, other tasks can be performed, equipment can be prepared for use, vehicles can be moved for a prompt departure, and information can be retrieved or relayed. Having confidence in your assessment skills always benefits the patient.

SKILL 12-1
The Detailed Physical Examination

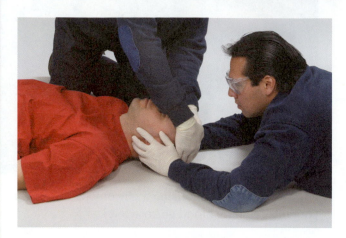

1. Inspect and palpate the scalp.

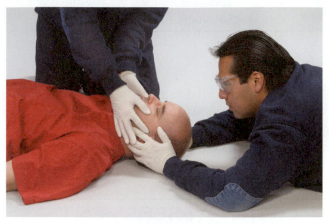

2. Inspect and palpate the face.

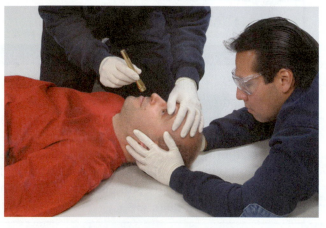

3. Look for eye injuries and pupil response. Do not palpate eye injuries.

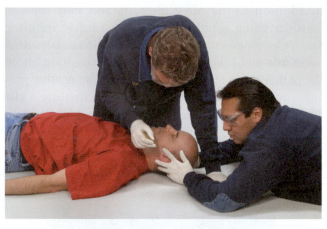

4. Look for fluid leaking from the ears.

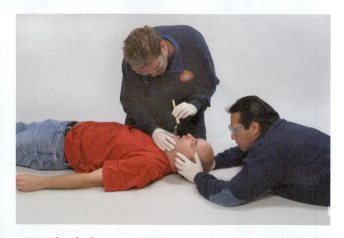

5. Check the mouth for any bleeding or injuries.

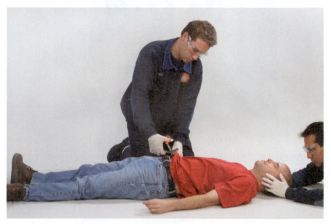

6. Remove the clothing from the patient's upper body.

SKILLS

SKILL 12-1
The Detailed Physical Examination—cont'd

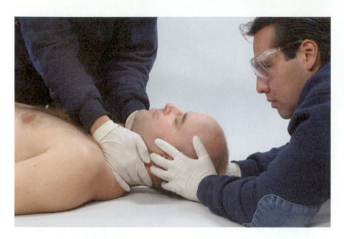

7. Inspect and palpate the front and the back of the neck.

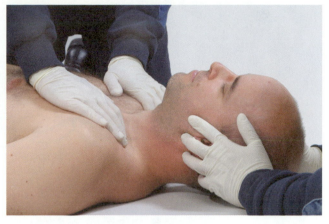

8. Inspect and palpate the chest.

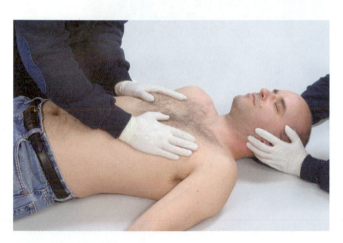

9. Compare the two sides of the chest to check for any abnormality.

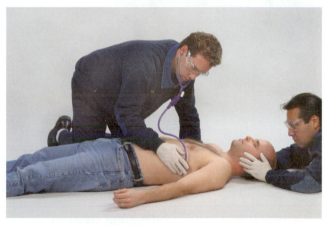

10. Auscultate the chest.

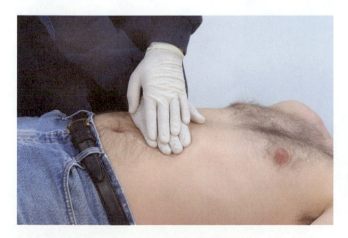

11. Inspect and palpate the abdomen.

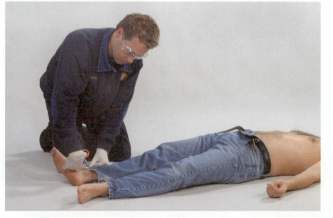

12. Remove the clothing from the patient's lower body.

Continued

SKILL 12-1
The Detailed Physical Examination—cont'd

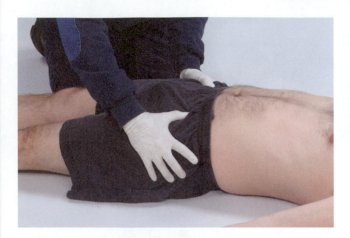

13. Palpate the pelvis.

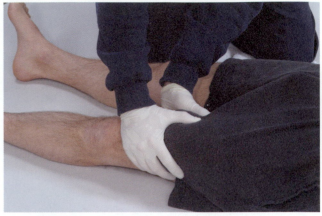

14. Inspect and palpate each upper leg.

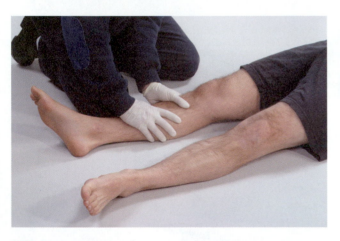

15. Inspect and palpate each lower leg.

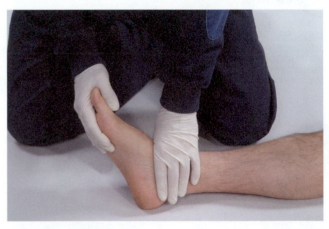

16. Assess movement and sensation in each foot.

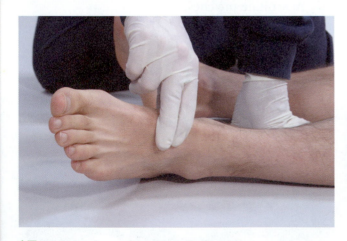

17. Assess the pulses in each foot.

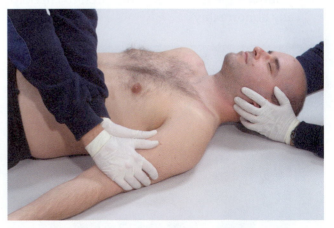

18. Inspect and palpate each upper arm.

SKILLS

SKILL 12-1
The Detailed Physical Examination—cont'd

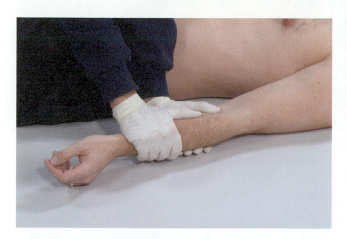

19. Inspect and palpate each lower arm.

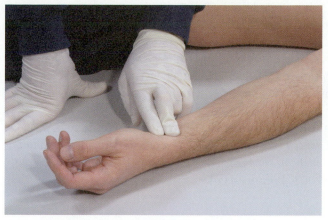

20. Assess the radial pulse in each arm.

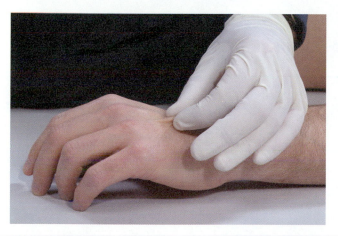

21. Assess movement and sensation in each hand.

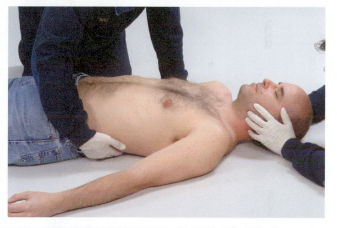

22. If possible, log roll the patient and assess the back.

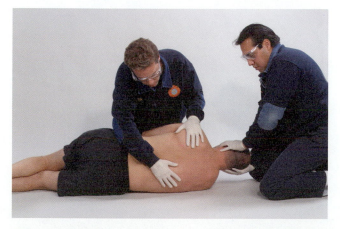

23. Palpate the back and inspect for signs of bleeding.

SKILLS

Resources

American College of Surgeons: *Advanced trauma life support for doctors*, ed 6, Chicago, 1997, First Impressions.

Bates B: *A guide to physical examination and history taking*, ed 4, Philadelphia, 1987, JB Lippincott.

Butman AM, Martin SW, Vomacka RW, McSwain NE: *Comprehensive guide to pre-hospital skills: a skills manual for EMT-Basic, EMT-Intermediate, EMT-Paramedic*, Akron, OH, 1995, Emergency Training.

Caroline N: *Emergency care in the streets*, ed 5, Boston, 1995, Little, Brown.

Dalton AL, Limmer D, Mistovich JJ, Werman HA: *Advanced medical life support: a practical approach to adult medical emergencies*, ed 2, Upper Saddle River, NJ, 2003, Prentice-Hall.

Emergency Nurses Association: *Emergency nursing pediatric course*, Park Ridge, IL, 1993, The Association.

Emergency Nurses Association: *TNCC: trauma nursing core course*, ed 4, Des Plaines, IL, 1995, The Association.

Nursing 86 Books: *Nurses reference library: assessment*, Springhouse, PA, 1986, Springhouse Corp.

Nursing 86 Books: *Nurses reference library: signs and symptoms*, Springhouse, PA, 1986, Springhouse Corp.

Prehospital Life Support Committee, National Association of Emergency Medical Technicians, and the Committee on Trauma, American College of Surgeons: *Basic and advanced prehospital trauma life support*, ed 5, St Louis, 2003, Mosby.

Stoy WA: *Mosby's EMT-Basic textbook*, St Louis, 1996, Mosby.

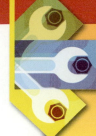

Critical Points

- The detailed physical exam is a thorough, meticulous process that forces the EMT to focus on hidden injuries or problems.
- To perform the detailed physical exam correctly, the EMT must know how to delegate. As you find problems, allow one of your teammates to address the problem while you continue your exam.
- EMTs must be completely familiar with their equipment (e.g., pulse oximeters, glucometers) and how it works.

Learning Checklist

- ❏ The detailed physical exam is more thorough and time-consuming than the rapid assessment. It is used for trauma patients with a significant mechanism of injury to make sure the entire body is completely reassessed for injuries. In unconscious patients, the detailed exam may be used to help detect problems.
- ❏ During the detailed physical exam, the patient's body is exposed as you inspect and palpate the body. Make every effort to protect the patient's privacy and be professional in your actions.
- ❏ Infants and children are the exception to the head to toe approach to the detailed exam. With a conscious child, the assessment may go more easily if you start at the toes and move toward the head.
- ❏ Start the detailed exam only after the initial exam has been completed and life-threatening conditions have been stabilized.
- ❏ Assessment of the patient's head includes inspecting and palpating for DCAPBTLS. Check the individual components: head, face, eyes, ears, nose, and mouth. In infants, palpate the fontanels.
- ❏ Assess the face for symmetry and function. If trauma to the face is noted, reevaluate the airway. Blood, secretions, or swelling may cause the airway to become obstructed. Monitor neurologic function using the AVPU assessment tool and the Glasgow Coma Scale.

- ❏ Fluid or blood flowing from the ear should be covered with a light dressing that does not occlude the flow. CSF may leak from the ear. Battle's sign is a late sign of a basilar skull fracture.
- ❏ Examine the eyes for color and note the presence of any blood in the anterior chamber of the eye. Blood is a sign of trauma and requires transport to an appropriate facility. The pupils should be round and of equal size. In awake patients, check the visual acuity. Raccoon's eyes indicate a basilar skull fracture.
- ❏ Fluid or blood accumulation in the nose may affect breathing, particularly in infants, and should be cleared immediately.
- ❏ Assess the patient's mouth for blood, fluids, or vomit and make sure the airway is clear. The teeth should be intact. Lacerations or swelling of the tongue should be noted. Also, check for odors (e.g., alcohol, vomit, paint, gasoline, or a sweet smell).
- ❏ Palpate the neck for tenderness and deformity while maintaining inline spinal stabilization. Assess the neck for jugular vein distention. Treat any open wounds with an occlusive dressing. Use of accessory muscles may indicate respiratory distress. Apply a cervical collar once the neck has been assessed if a collar had not been applied previously.
- ❏ Assess the chest for open wounds, which should be covered with an occlusive dressing and secured on three sides. Scars on the chest may suggest previous cardiac or lung surgery. Also assess the chest on each side for equality of movement of the two sides. Check for tenderness and crepitus.
- ❏ As you auscultate the lungs, compare the sounds from side to side. Rales (crackles) are heard with fluid accumulation in the lungs. A cardiac monitor may be used in some cases.
- ❏ Assessment of the abdomen includes checking for distention, rigidity, and softness. Assess the abdomen quadrant by quadrant.
- ❏ Bruising or incontinence of urine or stool may be noted during the assessment of the pelvis. In pregnant women, the baby's head may bulge from the vaginal opening

(crowning). The pelvis is palpated when the patient complains of pain or to identify tenderness.

❑ Compare each extremity with the opposite side to ensure symmetry. Also check for coloring and swelling. Palpate for pain, crepitus, or deformity. Check for a radial pulse, and assess movement, sensation, and strength.

❑ The detailed physical exam concludes with assessment of the patient's back. Inspect and monitor for DCAPBTLS.

❑ Check vital signs frequently to determine the patient's response to treatment. Report vital signs to the receiving crew or facility.

❑ Other assessment tools may include a pulse oximeter, a cardiac monitor, and a glucometer.

Key Terms

Abdominal quadrants The four sections into which the abdomen is divided to aid assessment.

Auscultate To examine by listening to the body with a stethoscope.

Basilar skull fracture A fracture of the base of the skull.

Battle's sign Bruising or bluish discoloration of the bone behind the ear, indicating a basilar skull fracture.

Cardiac monitor A machine that reads the electrical activity of the heart.

Colostomy bag A bag placed over the opening of a colostomy (an opening made into the abdomen where the bowel is brought to the surface, allowing bowel contents to empty into the bag).

Crackles Crackling sounds heard in the lungs that are caused by the alveoli popping open; usually the result of fluid accumulation in the lungs.

Crepitus A crunching or grating sound heard when broken bone ends rub together.

Crowning The appearance of the head of the infant at the vaginal opening during delivery.

Cyanotic Characterized by bluish skin discoloration caused by low oxygen saturation of the blood.

DCAPBTLS A mnemonic used to identify injury to the body. The acronym stands for *d*eformity, *c*ontusions, *a*brasions, *p*uncture, *b*urns, *t*enderness, *l*aceration, and *s*welling.

Dehydration The decrease of fluid in the body caused by problems such as vomiting, diarrhea, or excessive sweating.

Detailed physical exam The process of systematically evaluating the body, starting at the head and progressing to the toes.

Deviate To move to one side.

Distention A state of swelling or enlargement; the term usually is used to describe the abdomen.

Embolus A mass (liquid, solid, or gas) that occludes a blood vessel.

Epigastric A term that refers to the upper midabdomen, just below the sternum.

Equality A term used for comparing the body side to side to determine sameness.

Expose To remove the clothing to assess a patient.

Flail chest A condition in which several ribs are broken in two places, causing a floating segment; it may also occur if the sternum breaks free from the rib cage.

Fontanels Openings or spaces between the bones of the skull in infants and small children. The openings close as the child grows.

Glucometer A device for measuring the amount of glucose in blood.

Guarding Tensing of muscles or use of other body parts to protect an area.

Halo test A test in which a small amount of fluid is placed on a piece of gauze to determine whether cerebrospinal fluid is present.

Incontinence Involuntary loss of urine or stool.

Inspect To look for injuries or problems.

Mandible The lower jawbone.

Maxilla The upper jawbone.

Meningitis Inflammation of the membranes surrounding the brain.

Mottled Blotchy appearance of the skin caused by a decrease in circulation.

Nystagmus Continuous movement or shaking back and forth of the eye.

Palpate To feel for injuries during the patient assessment.

Paradoxical movement Movement associated with a flail chest in which the chest wall

NUTS AND BOLTS

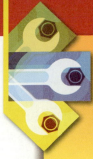

moves in on inspiration and out on expiration.

Pedal edema Swelling of the ankles and feet.

Point tenderness Pain in a specific location to which a patient usually can point.

Priapism Persistent erection of the penis associated with spinal cord injury or other medical conditions.

Pulsation A rhythmic beating or pulsing.

Pulse oximeter A device for measuring the oxygen saturation of hemoglobin.

Raccoon's eyes Bilateral bruising around the eyes; often associated with a basilar skull fracture.

Rales (crackles) Fine crackling sounds produced when fluid-filled or collapsed alveoli suddenly re-expand on inspiration.

Subcutaneous emphysema A condition characterized by leakage of air into the chest wall, which produces a crackling feeling under the skin on palpation; it often is caused by an injury to the lung.

Superficial On the surface of the body.

Urinary catheter A tube placed in the bladder to drain urine; also referred to as a Foley catheter.

Wheezes A whistling sound heard in the lungs that is caused by air moving through narrowed bronchioles.

National Standard Curriculum Objectives

Cognitive Objectives

After completing this lesson, the EMT student will be able to do the following:

■ Discuss the components of the detailed physical exam.
■ State the areas of the body evaluated during the detailed physical exam.
■ Explain what additional care should be provided during the detailed physical exam.
■ Distinguish between the detailed physical exam performed on a trauma patient and that performed on a medical patient.

Affective Objective

After completing this lesson, the EMT student will be able to do the following:

■ Explain the rationale for the emotional feelings patients might experience during the detailed physical exam.

Psychomotor Objective

After completing this lesson, the EMT student will be able to do the following:

■ Demonstrate the skills required to perform the detailed physical exam.

CHAPTER

13

OUTLINE

LESSON GOAL

The goal of this lesson is to prepare the emergency medical technician to perform an ongoing assessment. This chapter focuses on reassessment and confirmation of the patient status, review of the assessment, and checking of interventions for adequacy and patient response. ■

GOAL

Ongoing
Assessment

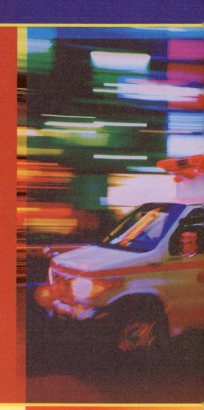

CHAPTER OBJECTIVES

After completing this chapter, the EMT student will be able to do the following:

1 Discuss the reasons for repeating the initial assessment as part of the ongoing assessment.

2 Describe the components of the ongoing assessment.

3 Describe the trending of assessment components.

4 Explain the value of performing an ongoing assessment.

5 Recognize and respect the feelings that patients might experience during assessment.

6 Explain the value of trending assessment components to other health professionals who assume care of the patient.

7 Demonstrate the skills involved in performing the ongoing assessment.

13

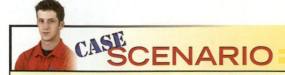

CASE SCENARIO

"How does that ice feel, Josh?" Ray asked as he reached for the on-board blood pressure cuff.

"Good. My wrist is numb."

"It will be. That's good, it will keep the swelling down. I am going to recheck your blood pressure and pulse, just to make sure everything is okay." Ray began his ongoing assessment of the patient by performing another initial assessment. Josh remained alert, oriented, and cooperative. He was answering questions easily, speaking in full sentences, indicating that his airway was open and that he was breathing normally. His pulse rate was strong, although it was a bit faster than before.

Question: *Why is ongoing assessment of the patient important, even though there appeared to be no changes in the vital signs?*

This chapter can be summed up in three words: *reassess, reassess, reassess.* This may seem simplistic, but it is crucial to the process of providing excellent patient care. You want to ensure that your initial impression of the patient is correct, that you have found and treated all life threats, that you have not missed any reasonably identifiable problems, that you are aware of the patient's current condition, and that the patient is responding as expected to the treatment you initiated. The only way to do this is to reassess. Ideally, you would perform a detailed physical exam before you begin your **ongoing assessment,** but a patient in critical condition may require that you reassess, treat, reassess, and treat life threats over and over again. If that is the case, focus your ongoing assessment on life threats and move on only when the patient is stable enough for you to do so.

How often should you reassess? Continuously. You should always reassess your patients each time you look at or interact with them. If something does not seem right, then you should be formal and systematic in your reevaluation. For patients in stable condition, an ongoing assessment should be completed every 15 minutes. For patients in critical condition, an ongoing assessment should be repeated every 5 minutes. Regardless of these recommendations, you should reassess the patient as frequently as needed.

■ REPEAT THE INITIAL ASSESSMENT

Begin your reassessment with the initial exam (Fig. 13-1). The ongoing assessment includes the following:

- Reassessing the mental status
- Reassessing and maintaining an open airway

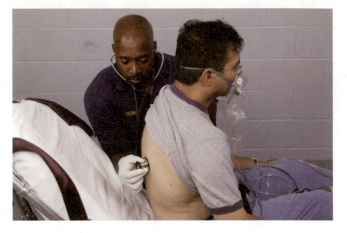

Fig. 13-1 Repeat the initial exam.

- Monitoring breathing for rate and quality
- Reassessing the pulse for rate and quality
- Monitoring the skin color and temperature
- Assessing the patient's response to your interventions
- Reestablishing patient priorities

Reassess the patient's responsiveness using the AVPU (alert, verbal, painful, unresponsive) scale. Patients who responded only to pain earlier but who are now responding to voice or are alert are much more reassuring than patients who were alert and are now only responding to pain or not all. Reassess the airway for patency, and correct any problems identified. If the patient had snoring respirations earlier, ensure that the airway is open and that the snoring is no longer present. Your job is to focus on the problems, ensure that they are corrected, and document the changes. Next, monitor the breathing for rate and quality. Now that you have opened the airway, ask yourself whether the breathing is adequate. Did you apply oxygen? Has the respiratory rate slowed? Does the patient need you to assist the breathing? Once again, take action based on your assessment of the patient status.

After you have reassessed and managed the airway and breathing, you can move on to circulation. Is the pulse rate returning to normal? What is the quality? If the circulation is returning to normal and of good quality, you can move on. If not, consider actions to support the circulation or rapid transport if you cannot do anything more for the patient with the resources you have. Reevaluate the skin color and temperature. If you find that the patient is showing signs and symptoms of hypoperfusion, apply oxygen and treat the patient for shock. You should expect the skin color to return to normal from pale or cyanotic. As the shock and hypoxia reverse, you should feel the skin start to become dry and warm. To know what to expect, you will need to understand what happens to the body during different medical conditions. This will allow you to determine whether the patient is improving or deteriorating based on your treatment. If a patient is not responding as expected, you may have missed an injury or initiated the wrong treatment or inadequate treatment for the patient's problem. Do not hesitate to reassess when the patient is not responding to a treatment in the way you anticipated. The patient's response may be a clue that you need to refocus your assessment and add treatment modalities or change the ones you have initiated.

After you have reevaluated the initial exam and the patient's response to care, you should reestablish your priorities. For example, initially the priority may have been to open and stabilize the airway, but on reassessment the skin is cool and moist, the heart rate has increased, and the pulse has become weaker. Now the priority has shifted from an airway problem to a circulatory problem. Now the focus should be treating for shock and reassessing the patient's response to this intervention. Patient assessment and priorities are dynamic and constantly changing, so it is essential to maintain an ongoing assessment and to be flexible to adjust to patient needs.

■ REASSESS AND RECORD VITAL SIGNS

Just as reevaluating the initial assessment is important to patient care, so too is reassessing the vital signs (Fig. 13-2). You will need to reassess the following:

• Respiratory rate, quality, and pattern
• Pulse rate, quality, and rhythm

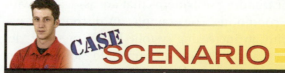

CASE SCENARIO continued

Ray compared Josh's current vital signs with the first set he had taken on scene. They were as follows:

Time	Pulse Rate	Respirations	Blood Pressure
1007	86	16	130/76
1030	96	20	132/74

Ray looked at Josh's skin. Shining a penlight onto the patient's face, Ray could see that Josh looked a little pale around his eyes and over his mouth. Although Josh had stopped sweating earlier, beaded sweat was beginning to appear over his lip.

Ray reached over to begin another hands-on assessment.

Question: *What about the vital signs might be concerning Ray?*

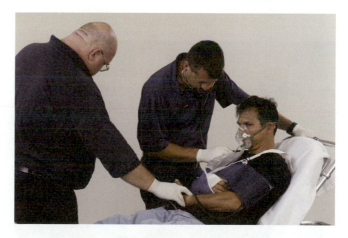
Fig. 13-2 Repeat the vital signs.

• Skin color and condition
• Pupil response
• Blood pressure

As discussed before, it is important to obtain and document an initial set of vital signs to serve as a baseline. Also important is that you obtain and document additional sets of vital signs. This will allow you to monitor patient conditions in measurable terms and look for **trending** or patterns that are associated with certain conditions. For example, an unconscious patient with an increasing systolic blood pressure, decreasing diastolic blood pressure, and slowing heart rate would be showing signs of increased intracranial pressure (referred to as Cushing's triad) and a worsening of the head injury. You would not find this deterioration if you did not repeatedly obtain vital signs and document them. So it is important to reassess the vital signs, to document them, and also to be aware of the implications of the changes and trends.

REPEAT THE FOCUSED ASSESSMENT

Repeat the focused assessment regarding the patient's complaint or injuries. You should assess for improvement in the condition. For example, if a patient had abdominal pain, you should reassess the area for location of the pain and changes in the pain or any associated conditions, such as nausea. You should use the same tools identified previously: DCAPBTLS and OPQRST. You may expand these areas as needed. You also may expand the assessment of the patient history at this time (Fig. 13-3). Patients may add to the information they have provided initially as they become more comfortable with the provider and recover from

the stress of the initial contact. Patients can tire of repeated assessments, so it is important to explain the importance of the ongoing assessment and to be respectful of patients' needs and frustrations.

■ CHECK INTERVENTIONS

The final focus of the ongoing assessment is to check interventions. You should make sure bleeding is controlled, oxygenation is maintained, and respirations are supported. You should also ensure that the interventions you have initiated are not causing harm to a patient (Fig. 13-4). For example, you should evaluate distal circulation, sensation, and motor response of an extremity before and after it has been splinted. If any of these is diminished, you may need to loosen or readjust the splint to allow for normal return of these functions.

As you can see, the ongoing assessment is crucial to quality patient care. Your documentation of these assessments is just as essential and will be reviewed by your medical director or quality improvement personnel to ensure that your assessment and care are of high quality. Accurate and honest reporting of patient findings, responses, and interventions is important,

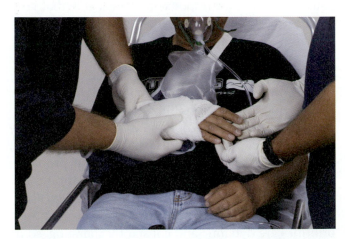

Fig. 13-4 Reassess adequacy of interventions.

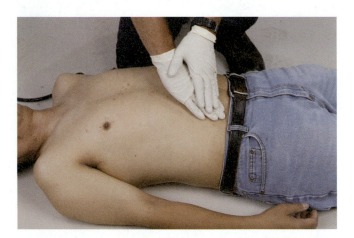

Fig. 13-3 Repeat the focused physical exam.

SPECIAL Populations

When treating a patient who is partially fluent in English, speak slowly; use short, simple sentences; and avoid technical terms, professional jargon, and American idioms.

SPECIAL Considerations

EMT Training – Not just for ambulances
The body moves blood from the surface to the core in a cold environment and increases blood flow to the surface when in a hot environment. The emergency medical technician should take into account that a patient will have skin color changes based on the move from the outside temperature to the ambulance.

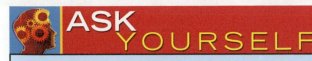

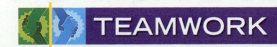

ASK YOURSELF

Now that you have learned the first five components of the patient assessment, you must be wondering, are we done yet? What else could there be? What else can I do for the patient? Have I forgotten anything?

for this may be the only information that travels with the patient from the scene once you turn over care of that patient. You need to tell the story of what happened to this patient, what you found, what treatments you administered, and how the patient responded. This story will represent your insight into this patient's problems and priorities and your ability to provide the necessary care.

TEAMWORK

The ongoing assessment is vital to determine patient response to your care. Your job is to communicate your assessment and the trends you saw during care. The relay of all your findings is important if you transfer the patient's care to another provider before you reassess interventions you have started. The next provider may take your baseline data and provide the ongoing assessment, so you will need to relay your concerns and priorities in written and oral format. Because a patient receiving prehospital patient care may see a number of providers (first responder, EMT, EMT-Paramedic, nurse, emergency room physician, and specialty physician), maintaining continuity of care and ongoing assessments may be a challenge. Do all you can to help maintain continuity and quality of care.

CASE SCENARIO

Josh winced as Ray palpated along his left flank. "Ouch, that hurts," he said.

"Sorry about that," Ray replied. He looked in the area where he had just palpated. Although most of the area was covered by the backboard, Ray thought he saw that the area was reddened, and was just beginning to show a hematoma. He reached over Josh and pulled an oxygen mask out of the cabinet. Filling it with oxygen, he placed it over Josh's mouth and nose. "I'd like you to breath some oxygen right now, Josh. It might smell a little funny, but I want to be safe rather than sorry." ■

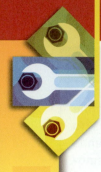

NUTS AND BOLTS

Critical Points

- The ongoing assessment is a critical part of the overall patient management that allows the EMT to evaluate whether or not the patient is improving or deteriorating and what the response to treatment has been.

Learning Checklist

❑ An ongoing assessment should be repeated every 15 minutes for patients in stable condition. For patients in critical condition, an ongoing assessment should be repeated every 5 minutes. Regardless of these general recommendations, you should reassess your patient as frequently as needed.

❑ The ongoing assessment includes the following: reassessing the mental status, reassessing and maintaining an open airway, monitoring breathing for rate and quality, reassessing the pulse for rate and quality, monitoring the skin color and temperature, assessing patient response to interventions, and reestablishing patient priorities.

❑ If a patient does not respond as expected, check to see whether you may have missed an injury. You may have initiated the wrong

or inadequate treatment for the patient's problem. The lack of response may indicate that you need to refocus your assessment and add or change treatment modalities.

❑ Repeat the focused reassessment regarding the patient's complaint or injuries. You should assess for improvement in the patient's condition.

❑ Use the same tools you used in the initial assessment: DCAPBTLS (Deformities, Contusions, Abrasions, Punctures or Penetrations, Burns, Tenderness, Lacerations, Swelling) and OPQRST (Onset, Provocation, Quality, Related symptoms, Severity, Time). Expand these areas as needed. You also may expand your assessment of the patient history.

❑ Explain the importance of the ongoing assessment to the patient and be respectful of the patient's needs and frustrations with repeated assessments.

❑ The final focus of the ongoing assessment is to check interventions. Ensure that bleeding is controlled, oxygenation is maintained, and respirations are supported.

❑ Documentation of your ongoing assessment is just as essential as the care you provide. Accurate reporting of findings, responses, and interventions are important for the patient's continuing care.

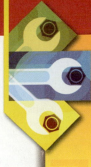

Key Terms

Ongoing assessment The process of monitoring a patient over time. It includes repeating the initial assessment, reassessing and recording vital signs, repeating the focused assessment, and checking interventions.

Trending The process of monitoring findings over time to identify patterns.

National Standard Curriculum Objectives

Cognitive Objectives

After completing this lesson, the EMT student will be able to do the following:

- Discuss the reasons for repeating the initial assessment as part of the ongoing assessment.
- Describe the components of the ongoing assessment.
- Describe trending of assessment components.

Affective Objectives

After completing this lesson, the EMT student will be able to do the following:

- Explain the value of performing an ongoing assessment.
- Recognize and respect the feelings that patients might experience during assessment.
- Explain the value of trending assessment components to other health professionals who assume care of the patient.

Psychomotor Objective

After completing this lesson, the EMT student will be able to do the following:

- Demonstrate the skills involved in performing the ongoing assessment.

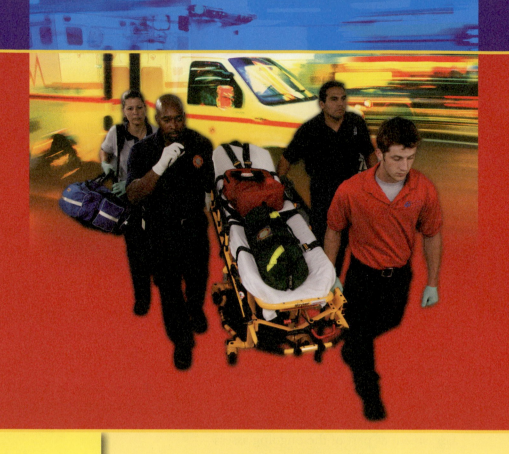

CHAPTER

14

CHAPTER OUTLINE

Communication Model

Patient Communication

Remote Communications

Hospital Communications

Verbal Reports

OUTLINE

LESSON GOAL

A critical component of being an effective emergency medical technician is knowing how to communicate with patients, dispatchers, other emergency service providers, and the hospital. This chapter introduces the communication model. It also identifies the elements, techniques, and common pitfalls of effective communication. Communication technology, such as two-way radios and other devices used by the emergency medical technician, is introduced as well. In addition, the chapter addresses the appropriate use of this equipment when one is communicating with other providers, the dispatch center, and online medical control. ■

GOAL

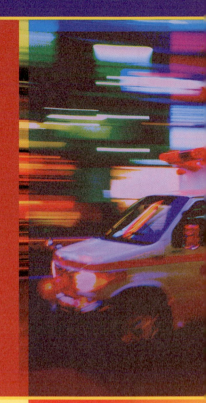

Communications

14

OBJECTIVES

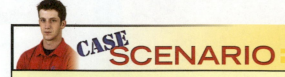

Ray looked through the opening separating the patient compartment from the front of the ambulance to get his bearings on their current location. Consulting with his partner, they decided to divert the transport from the local community hospital to a landing zone nearby. Turning back to the patient, Ray said, "Josh, I am a bit concerned by the pain you're having in your side. For your safety, we are going to rendezvous with a medical helicopter in about ten minutes. We are going to transfer you to the helicopter crew, and they will take you to the county trauma center. It will be faster than taking you there by ambulance. Are you okay with that?" Josh simply nodded yes. He was not feeling well now at all, and for the first time he felt a bit nervous about what was happening. Ray reached for the radio microphone and switched the channel to the hailing frequency for the county communication center. In a few minutes he and the crew of the responding medical evacuation helicopter were speaking to each other.

Question: *What information should Ray provide to the helicopter crew?*

Communication is an integral part of your career as an emergency medical technician (EMT). During a typical call, you will communicate with several persons face-to-face and over the radio or telephone. You will have to communicate with your patient and his or her family to obtain an adequate history and physical so that you can treat effectively. You will have to communicate with your partner and other personnel on the scene to work efficiently as a team. Plus, communication with dispatch is essential. Dispatch needs to know where you are, if you are safe, and what your status is. Finally, you will have to transfer all the information you have gained during your time with your patient to the hospital staff. This allows for the continuation of the treatment you have initiated.

As an EMT, you must understand the process and principles of interpersonal communications with your patients, their families, and other providers. This understanding will ensure that you do not lose or overlook valuable information. You also must have a basic understanding of radio systems and their components, as well as how to use them appropriately. The two-way radio remains the mainstay of remote communication in the prehospital setting. However, several other technologies also are being used. Wireless computer connections, data transmission, and cellular phones are common components of prehospital communications. You may use these systems daily. The overall goal of communication is that information is exchanged and understood by all parties involved, whether information is related to patient care or communications with your dispatch center.

■ COMMUNICATION MODEL

Although a common topic of conversation, communication is not very well understood. Consider all of the seminars that are offered on effective communication. Also consider the number of incidents that occur as a result of a misunderstanding during a conversation. Regardless of the method of communication, all communication follows the same model (Fig. 14-1).

Encoding and Decoding

When two persons communicate, one person is the communicator (who does the **encoding**) and the other is the receiver (who does the **decoding**). The communicator has a message to convey to the receiver. These roles will change as the dialog progresses and information flows back and forth between the individuals. However, the process remains the same. The communicator will encode the message in a medium that the receiver can understand. This medium may be verbal, nonverbal (e.g., gestures), or written. Basically, communication may involve any medium that the communicator and the receiver understand.

This book is an example of the communication process. Certain information has to be delivered. In this case, the information is encoded in writing. In reading the text, you (the receiver/reader) decode the message and receive the intended information. In the classroom, your instructor will encode information verbally. Then you will decode the message being delivered. Regardless

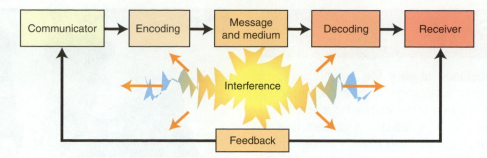

Fig. 14-1 Basic communication model.

of the medium being used, once the message is encoded to a medium, the receiver can decode the message. This results in communication.

Feedback

A key component of effective communication is **feedback.** Feedback is given to the communicator. Feedback ensures the message that was intended to be given was actually the message that was received. If it becomes evident that the message intended was not the message received, the process starts all over until the correct message is exchanged. As an EMT, you will use this process in all of your communications. You may need to initiate the feedback phase with your patient if you are not certain he or she has understood your questions or instructions. You can initiate feedback by asking questions to clarify a patient's response. You also can ask the patient to explain his or her understanding of your questions or instructions. An example in which you use feedback involves the patient who refuses care or transport. As you have learned, in this situation you must receive an *informed refusal.* Through feedback, you will ensure that your patient truly understands the benefits of treatment and the risks of refusal.

Interference

Interference in the communication process may lead to miscommunication and misunderstanding. Interference takes many forms. It can occur during any phase of the communication process. Moreover, interference is the most common cause of miscommunication among individuals. Therefore you should use feedback to help eliminate interference. Interference may occur if the message has been encoded in a manner or medium that the receiver does not understand. For example, your emergency medical service (EMS) system may use

codes for communication between dispatch and other units. However, the hospital to which you are transporting may not understand these codes. If you use the codes during your radio report, the receiver may not decode them accurately.

A language barrier is another classic form of interference. With this type of interference a medium that both parties understand will have to be found. A noisy environment also can interfere with communication. Similarly, interference can occur with a patient who is uncomfortable answering certain questions in a public area.

Interference to effective communication even can be internal. This is interference that is present within the patient's or the provider's mind. This type of interference has a great impact on effective communication. When in need of medical care, patients often are focused on several things other than the questions you are asking. They may be thinking about their quality of life after the incident, their survival, the financial impact of medical care, whether they trust you and your care, and many other things. All of these thoughts are distracting. They interfere with the patient's ability to decode accurately the questions you are asking. The EMT also may experience internal interference. While you are formulating your questions and interpreting the answers, you also will be determining what is wrong with the patient, planning your treatment, conducting your treatment, and making a transport decision. You also may be distracted by the type of day you have had. If you are still thinking about your last call, wondering if you turned the stove off at the station before you left, or thinking about anything other than your patient, your ability to communicate effectively will be diminished greatly. As an EMT, your responsibility is to make every effort to reduce interference in communication. You also have the responsibility to use feedback to ensure that effective communication takes place.

ASK YOURSELF

Think of an instance in your life in which miscommunication or a misunderstanding occurred. Maybe you were given instructions for a specific task, and after you completed it, you were told, "That is not what I asked you to do." What happened? Why did you think you were asked one thing, but the person who asked you felt he or she asked you something completely different? How can these situations be avoided?

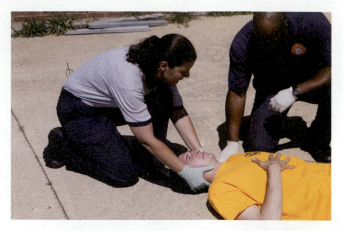

Fig. 14-2 Patient care in a public setting can affect the answers your patient may give or not give.

■ PATIENT COMMUNICATION

Nothing is more essential to appropriate patient care than obtaining a good history. The ability to obtain a good history requires effective communication skills. In your career as an EMT, you may hear "Patients will lie to you." When you hear this statement, evaluate it carefully and do not allow yourself to fall into this way of thinking. Rarely will patients intentionally deceive you. More often, the perceived deception is the result of how or where the questions were asked or how the EMT conducted the interview. In addition to aiding you in gathering information, communication with the patient allows you to establish rapport and build your relationship. This relationship determines the patient's comfort level in answering questions. One tenet of emergency medicine you must never forget is that you arrive at one of the worst times in someone's life—as a complete stranger. Then you immediately begin to ask personal questions, things the patient may not want even his or her own family to know. Without a good relationship and the patient's complete trust, you are more likely to get superficial answers to your questions than all of the information you need. Later, when the patient gives the whole story to another practitioner, you may be left with the feeling you were deceived. If this happens, it is imperative that you evaluate what you may have done to cause the patient to withhold information or to give incomplete information.

Setting

The setting in which you communicate with your patient can have a dramatic impact on its effectiveness. The setting can help establish or can destroy a trusting relationship between you and your patient. Al-

though the prehospital setting is not always the best setting for talking with your patient, the EMT should be aware of several factors that affect communication and how to mitigate them.

Privacy

Ideally, any communication should take place in a private setting. This is a setting in which the patient can feel comfortable that the conversation will not be overheard by others. However, this is not always possible. Often you will find yourself responding to a call in a public area with little or no **privacy** (Fig. 14-2).

When this happens, the EMT needs to be aware of how this may affect the patient and his or her answers. Whenever possible, questions about sensitive topics should be deferred until you are in a more private setting. If you must ask such questions in a public setting, it is advisable to ask them again once you are in a private setting, such as inside the ambulance. When re-asking questions in a private setting, to receive an answer such as "Now that we are alone, I can tell you. ..." is not uncommon. Often the information gained will affect your thoughts significantly regarding the patient's condition and subsequent treatment.

Interruptions

Think of a situation in which you were trying to tell a story and were interrupted constantly. How did it make you feel? Most likely, you felt as though the other person was not truly interested in what you had to say. You probably abbreviated the story or stopped telling it altogether. Communicating with patients is no different. Patients are telling you the story of their illness or injury. Although occasionally you may need to ask questions to help guide the interview, you want to ensure that you do not interrupt constantly. Common interruptions at a typical scene include the EMT taking over the conversation, allowing the family or bystanders to take the role of the patient in answering questions, or the EMT having a conversation with his or her partner while the patient is talking. Any of these can cause the patient to abbreviate or stop telling his or her story. He or she may feel you have all the information you need, or that he or she cannot add anything significant. The end result is an incomplete story. Thus you will not receive all of the available information to make your treatment decision.

Physical environment

As an EMT, you will provide emergency care in a variety of environmental conditions. When a patient is concerned about his or her physiologic well-being, higher-level cognitive functioning is difficult. For example, a patient who is lying on the highway on a cold and rainy night is focused primarily on getting warm and dry. In such a case, his or her ability to decode questions accurately is diminished severely and may result in superficial answers to your questions. Much like with privacy, if you have to ask a patient questions when he or she is uncomfortable, be sure to ask them again when the patient is comfortable and feels safe. Then the patient will be able to give more thoughtful and complete answers to the questions you are asking.

Lighting

The EMT must be aware of lighting conditions, particularly the sun and lights on emergency vehicles. Whenever possible, any bright lights should be positioned to the side of the patient and the EMT. That way, neither person will be looking directly into the lights. If this is not possible, consider what effect the light will have on communication. If the patient is staring into the light, you become a shadowy figure in silhouette. This may make it hard for the patient to identify you or establish a relationship with you. As a result, the patient interview turns into an interrogation, which seldom provides in-depth, personal responses. A good practice is to ensure the patient is never looking into a bright light during an interview.

Distance

Your **distance** from the patient should be comfortable for you and the patient. Speaking with the patient from across the room may imply that you are not interested in what is being said. However, being too close can cause discomfort. Either of these actions may damage the relationship you are trying to forge with the patient. Your distance also may affect

SPECIAL Considerations

To avoid distracting a patient from communicating clearly, it is always preferable that the patient not have to look into a bright light. The bright light may make the patient feel as if he or she is being interrogated instead of interviewed. However, if the emergency medical technician is looking into the light, the patient becomes a silhouette. This can affect the assessment, which normally is performed by visualizing the patient. Bright light also can create scene safety issues because the emergency medical technician cannot clearly see the patient and his or her actions. As an emergency medical technician, you must weigh the variables of each scene carefully. Moreover, you must determine the best option when it comes to lighting.

the amount of information the patient provides. Take cultural considerations into account with the amount of distance that you place between you and your patient. In the United States, "personal space" is typically anywhere from 2 to 5 feet. Other cultures, however, may define personal space as closer or farther. If you are constantly "chasing" your patient while conducting the interview, he or she may be trying to tell you something. Most likely, increasing the amount of space between you and your patient will often result in more effective communication.

Eye contact

"The eyes tell all": You have probably heard this phrase numerous times, but have you ever stopped to consider what it really means? A significant emphasis is placed on the eyes during communication. The eyes send strong nonverbal messages. Many questions often are answered with only the eyes. For example, "Is he or she sincere?" "Is he or she interested?" "Is he or she being deceptive?" These and many other questions often are answered with the eyes. In the United States and most Western cultures, eye contact during communication is expected and should be maintained. Eye contact expresses interest and sincerity. Furthermore, it can help to develop a trusting relationship with the patient. This is not the case in all cultures, however. If you notice the patient is uncomfortable and constantly looking away from you, reduce the amount of eye contact you use. Then evaluate the effect on his or her comfort level. Avoid

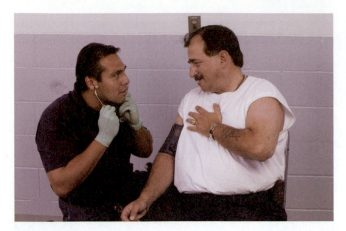

Fig. 14-3 Remain at eye level with your patient, and maintain eye contact.

wearing sunglasses. They not only interfere with eye contact but also can give the impression that you are hiding something. They hide strong nonverbal clues for which your patient will be looking.

In addition to maintaining eye contact with the patient, the EMT should make every effort to place himself or herself at eye level with or lower than the patient (Fig. 14-3).

Standing above or "looming over" your patient may seem authoritarian. Most persons are not comfortable with this. Patients should have a feeling of equality during the interview and during subsequent care decisions. At times, the configuration of your equipment automatically will place you above the patient. This occurs, for example, when you are sitting on the bench seat while the patient is supine on the stretcher. If this becomes an obstacle to effective communication, consider kneeling between the stretcher and bench seat to place yourself closer to the patient's level.

Approach

Once you have considered the setting and made it as comfortable as possible for the patient, you need to determine how to approach the conversation. Just as with the setting, how you initiate and conduct the conversation will have a large impact on the relationship that is developed, the patient's trust, and the completeness of the information you gain. The key to effective communication is to be open and honest with your patient.

Introduce yourself to the patient with your name and level of certification. Let your patient know you genuinely are interested in what he or she has to say. If the patient appears uncomfortable answering ques-

---

BOX 14-1

When You Really Do Not Know the Answer

You may be asked a question to which you do not know the answer. Responding with "I don't know" is often the first reaction of the emergency medical technician. This makes sense, because you are answering the question honestly. However, be cautious with this reply. Consider the position of the patient or family member who asks this question. To them, you are the expert, educated in emergency medicine, and they are looking to you for answers. Answering with "I don't know" and no further explanation can cause your knowledge to be brought into question. It may leave them wondering whether they or their loved one was cared for in the best possible manner. Consider the following scenario. You are treating a patient in cardiac arrest when a family member asks whether she will survive. You answer, "I do not know, but we are breathing for her, circulating her blood with chest compressions, and analyzing her heart rhythm." This is not only an honest answer but also one that informs the family of what is being done. It also does not leave them questioning the care that was provided.

---

tions, explain why the information is important to his or her care. Also assure the patient that his or her answers will be held in confidence. The EMT should always be friendly to patients in all situations. However, the EMT also should maintain the high professional standards patients expect from a medical professional. Additionally, the EMT must always be honest with his or her patients. You may be asked questions for which you do not know the answer (Box 14-1). For example, a patient with chest pain may ask, "Am I having a heart attack?" In this situation, be honest with the patient and explain what you suspect. If you think it is a possibility, tell the patient so. However, if the same patient asks, "Should I go to the hospital?" the answer becomes much easier. This is a new experience for the patient. Therefore your honest answer of "Yes" followed by why you think he or she should go can provide the guidance for which patients often are looking. Whereas, an answer such as "That is your decision" may leave the patient unsure of the correct course of action. When speaking with a patient, always consider the following guidelines.

Address the patient by name

After introducing yourself to the patient, be sure to ask his or her name and use it. Unless the patient is a child, always use his or her title and last name. This is especially relevant in the older population. The EMT must recognize that cultural standards change over time. In the past, respect for elders was emphasized much more than it is today. In fact, it was never acceptable to call someone older than you by his or her first name. Therefore, calling anyone, other than a child, by his or her first name upon first meeting may be considered offensive and may harm the relationship you are trying to build. As a result, you may get simple and superficial answers to the questions you are asking. This in turn degrades the quality of your history. If, once you address the patient by his or her title and last name, the patient asks you to call him or her something different, respect those wishes as well. However, do not assume such familiarity upon your initial introduction.

Questioning

When initiating a conversation, the EMT should begin with broad, general questions. "Mr. (or Mrs.) Smith, how can I help you today?" provides the patient an opportunity to begin telling you the story of his or her illness in his or her own words. Such a general question will help guide the history and assessment. You already may have received information regarding the patient complaint from dispatch. However, be sure not to accept this at face value. Instead, determine what the patient's complaint truly is. For example, if you are dispatched for chest pain, you may want to start with "Mrs. Smith, our dispatcher told us you were experiencing chest pain today. Is this true?" Be sure to avoid opening questions that could have negative connotations. Asking "Mr. Jones, what is your

problem today?" or "What is your complaint?" immediately can place the patient on the defensive. This can affect any further communication. The remainder of the conversation is guided by the response to these broad questions, and the questions generally will be one of the following types.

Open-ended questions

Open-ended questions are those that cannot be answered with a "yes" or "no" response. These questions provide the most information. They allow the patient a good deal of liberty in his or her response as he or she tells you what he or she is experiencing. This will allow the EMT the most insight into the patient's condition. Examples of open-ended questions are "Tell me about your chest pain" or "What did you mean when you said you are having trouble breathing?" Open-ended questioning is the preferred method of communicating with your patient.

Closed or direct questions

At times, patients may not respond well to open-ended questions. When asking a patient to describe his or her abdominal pain, the response may be as simple as "It hurts." The patient may give no further explanation. This can be frustrating for the EMT, and an alternative line of questioning must be found. The classic **closed or direct questions** are ones that can be answered with a "yes" or "no" response. Closed questions should be phrased carefully so the patient provides as much information as possible. If the EMT asks, "Is your chest pain dull?" and receives an answer of "Yes," the EMT is forced to wonder if that is his or her own description of the pain or the patient's description.

Regardless of the type of question, the EMT should speak clearly, in a normal tone, at a normal rate. Furthermore, the EMT should be sure to ask only one question at a time and give the patient adequate time to answer. Appearing rushed or interrupting a patient as he or she is answering will give the impression that you are not interested in what the patient has to say. Plus, it may cause the patient to abbreviate further answers.

When asking closed questions, give the patient as many options as possible for his or her response. Ask if the chest pain is dull, sharp, stabbing, burning, or tingling. Determine the effect the condition has had on the patient. If the call is for respiratory distress, ask the patient how far he or she can walk before becoming short of breath. Also ask how this compares with how far he or she normally can walk. This type of questioning provides more guidance than open

---

SPECIAL Populations

Terms of Endearment

During your career as an emergency medical technician, you may see many providers using terms of endearment when speaking to elderly patients. Addressing a patient as "sweetie," "honey," "dear," or worse yet "granny" or "pops" is not only disrespectful but also not acceptable for a medical professional. Do not allow yourself to use these terms, even though you may hear your co-workers and others doing so.

questioning. However, it provides more information than a "yes" or "no."

Closed questioning should be used only when open questioning does not work. Moreover, how you ask the question often dictates how it will be answered. Consider the following two questions: "How would you rate your chest pain?" and "Your chest pain is not too bad, is it?" Although both questions are seeking the same information, they give different messages to the patient. The first is asking for the patient's opinion or evaluation of the pain. With the second, the patient is forced to evaluate the pain on what the EMT considers bad. Most likely the patient is unsure of the definitions of good and bad the EMT is using; thus the patient is forced to speculate. Often the answer to this type of question will be "Well, I guess it is not too bad."

Communication Techniques

Regardless of the type of questioning you use, you must allow the patient to tell the story of his or her illness as he or she perceives it. Interrupting too soon or interjecting questions inappropriately can result in the patient abbreviating his or her story. Moreover, you may not get the information you were seeking originally. However, you must take an active role in communication to keep the interview focused on the current complaint. The EMT can use several techniques to guide the conversation (Box 14-2).

Each technique is not appropriate for all interviews. Therefore you must choose the one that matches the current situation.

Facilitation

Facilitation is the process by which you encourage the patient to provide more information or to continue with his or her response. This can be done verbally and nonverbally. Verbal responses may include phrases such as "Go on," "I'm listening," and other similar responses. These facilitate the continuation of the conversation. Nonverbal responses may include

---

BOX 14-2
Communication Techniques

Facilitation
Reflection
Clarification
Empathetic responses
Confrontation
Interpretation

---

leaning forward or nodding your head. These also indicate that you are interested in what the patient is saying and would like for him or her to continue or expand upon the current answer or description.

Reflection

Reflection is a powerful communication technique in which you repeat the patient's answers back to him or her for further description or explanation. Saying to your patient, "You said your chest hurts whenever you take a deep breath. Can you tell me more about that?" informs the patient that you are interested in what he or she said and would like more information about it. You also gain the complete description from the patient and do not risk stopping him or her from giving further information by taking over the conversation.

Clarification

Clarification is similar to reflection in that you will repeat part of what the patient said. This technique can be used when the EMT is not sure what the patient means in his or her description of the condition. An example of clarification would be "You said you have felt strange every time you stood up over the last few hours. Can you tell me what you mean when you say 'strange'?" Perhaps the EMT believes the patient means he or she feels dizzy, when in actuality the patient means he or she feels light-headed but not dizzy. Often the cause of miscommunication is that the receiving party does not receive the actual message intended by the receiver. Clarification ensures that the message intended is the message received. Clarification also is an excellent example of feedback.

Empathetic responses

Empathetic responses are those that acknowledge the patient's feelings and let him or her know that those feelings are acceptable. These responses are important in building a trusting relationship. When you recognize and accept a patient's feelings, this not only builds the patient's trust in you but also allows him or her to provide more in-depth and sometimes personal information without fear of being judged. For example, a patient involved in a motor vehicle accident may be visibly upset while telling you how she saw the tree coming at her and there was nothing she could do. A response of "That must have been very scary for you" lets her know it is okay to feel that way. It also allows her to continue her description.

When replying empathetically, however, avoid the response "I understand." This response may sound as if it expresses acceptance and forges a connection with the patient. However, it often can have the reverse effect. Telling a patient who is having a stroke that you understand how he or she feels or what he or she is going through may cause the patient to ask you when *you* had a stroke. When you tell the patient that you have not had one, he or she may feel as if you are being patronizing. Then the relationship you are trying to forge may weaken. Any further communication from the patient most likely will be superficial at best and will not provide the information you need to treat the patient adequately. You even may have experienced a similar situation, such as a stroke, as the patient. However, avoid using "I understand" as an empathetic response because individuals respond to the same situation in different ways. If your patient is having a myocardial infarction and you also have had a myocardial infarction, your response, outlook, and feelings may be completely different. In short, there is no way someone truly can understand what another person is feeling. If a patient expresses concern about his or her particular condition, a better response would be "I can imagine this must be very difficult for you." This response expresses the same concern and empathy without damaging the patient relationship and further communication.

Confrontation

Confrontation is used to point out something about the patient's actions or behavior that is not consistent with what he or she is telling you. Possibly, the patient is not providing the whole story. Possibly, the patient also is denying that he or she is ill or injured. Confronting the patient with inconsistencies may allow him or her to accept the situation and provide further information. A patient who denies abdominal pain yet winces every time you palpate the abdomen may provide further information if you say, "You told me your abdomen did not hurt, yet every time I touch it, you wince in pain. Can you tell me what you are feeling?"

Interpretation

A correct interpretation of what the patient tells you shows you are interested in what has been said. It also shows that you have been truly listening. This technique can forge strong patient relationships and greatly enhance further communication. However, use of this technique has risks as well. If you are incorrect in your interpretation, the patient may feel as though you have not been listening and that you do not care what he or she has to say. The patient also may feel that there is no value in providing more in-

formation. Rather than providing further information and initiating conversation, the patient may resort to giving superficial and incomplete answers to the questions you initiate.

Nonverbal Communication

Whenever two persons interact, a constant stream of **nonverbal communication** is being exchanged. The patient will make decisions about you based on the way you present yourself. Do you appear professional? Is your uniform neat and clean? Are you well groomed, neat, and clean? A patient may assume that if you are not concerned about your appearance, you may not be concerned about the quality of care you provide. As a result, the patient may be less likely to have complete trust in you. The patient also may not give complete answers to your questions. Your stance should be open and friendly, and you should maintain eye contact. In addition, your facial expressions and gestures should indicate that you truly are interested in what your patient has to say. An example of poor nonverbal communication would include an EMT standing with arms crossed and staring into space when someone is talking to him or her. If your body language says you are not interested in what a patient has to say, you will not get the complete story, regardless of what you may say verbally.

As an EMT, you will receive as much nonverbal information from your patient as he or she receives from you. This information is valuable in determining how forthcoming your patient is in answering the questions you ask. In addition, the nonverbal information makes up a large part of your physical exam. How is the patient dressed? Is the clothing appropriate for the weather and situation? Is the clothing worn together appropriately? Someone who is wearing a heavy winter coat with shorts on or plaids and stripes together simply may have an alternative fashion style. However, he or she may have an underlying psychiatric disorder or organic brain syndrome that you need to consider for treatment and the manner in which you conduct the conversation. Look at the patient's body language. Does the patient look at you when he or she speaks with you or stare blankly at you? Is the patient sulking in the corner with his or her arms crossed, or is the patient open in his or her posture? What types of gestures and facial expressions does the patient make during the conversation? All of these are important clues to the quality and completeness of the information you receive from the patient. This information must be complete because it ultimately guides your treatment of the patient.

Pitfalls of Communication

Despite all efforts to ensure the most effective communication possible, the EMT can do other things to cause the patient to provide limited information. Although easily avoidable, the following items are common ways EMTs unknowingly encourage their patients not to communicate openly (Box 14-3).

False reassurance

Patients are often able to comprehend the severity of their illness or injury. When the EMT falsely assures a patient that there is nothing wrong or that things will be fine, the patient may well know better. This calls into question the honesty and the competency of the EMT. If the patient has doubts in either of these areas, he or she is unlikely to provide complete information or answers to the questions the EMT asks.

Avoidance

As an EMT, you often will respond to calls during which you must discuss subjects with which you are uncomfortable. In this situation, it is human nature to avoid the topic. This often occurs subconsciously through word choice, body language, or facial expressions. Doing so expresses disinterest in what the patient has to say and discourages him or her from providing what may be the information you need to treat the condition correctly. Through experience, you will become more comfortable discussing a variety of topics. However, if you are ever in a situation where you are uncomfortable, but the information is relevant to patient care, you must make sure you do not avoid the topic.

Sensitive topics

Although similar to avoidance, sensitive topics are those with which the patient or the patient and EMT are uncomfortable, such as alcohol use/abuse or sexual history. When asking questions about subjects that may be considered sensitive, you should work your questions into the conversation, as you would with any other question. Remember, the patient may be accustomed to answering these questions from prior visits to medical personnel. Thus the more comfortable you appear when asking the question, the more comfortable the patient will be in answering it.

Medical terms

Throughout your EMT course, you will become familiar with medical terms and medical terminology. This is the language of medical professionals. You should use it when speaking with others in the medical profession. When communicating with patients, however, you must make sure you are speaking to them in a language they can understand. To tell a patient his or her rhinitis and rhinorrhea is most likely the result of exposure to an allergen that caused immunoglobulin E–mediated degranulation of the mast cells is probably pointless. As you talk with your patient, you will determine how questions and statements need to be phrased. You may be able to ask one person about his or her dyspnea, whereas you will have to ask another about his or her respiratory distress and a third about his or her smothering spells. In short, the medium in which the sender encodes the message must be one the receiver can decode.

Leading questions

Often associated with closed questions, **leading questions** lead the patient to an answer that may not be his or her own answer. An example of a leading question is "Your chest pain is dull, right?" If the patient answers "Yes," is it because he or she thinks the pain is supposed to be dull or because it truly is dull? If the patient answers "No," is it because the pain truly is not dull or because he or she is denying the possibility of cardiac problems and does not want to admit pain that may be from the heart? When questioning your patients, pay close attention to how you phrase questions. Make sure your questions do not lead patients to a specific answer.

Dominating the conversation

Allow the patient to provide as much of the information as possible. Often the EMT will take over the conversation after only a few seconds. This often occurs because once the patient states that he or she has, for example, abdominal pain, the EMT has a series of questions he or she wants to ask specifically about the abdominal pain. As a result, the patient may feel the EMT has all the information he or she needs. The patient may not feel compelled to offer any more information other than cursory responses

---

BOX 14-3

Pitfalls of Communication

False reassurance
Avoidance
Sensitive topics
Medical terms
Leading questions
Dominating the conversation
"Why" questions

to questions he or she is asked directly. By allowing the patient time to tell his or her story, the EMT often will gain the same information while affirming that what the patient has to say is important and valuable. Another common scenario in which someone other than the patient dominates the conversation involves the family and bystanders. The family and bystanders may answer every question for the patient. These individuals can provide important information. However, the EMT must ensure the patient is allowed to provide answers whenever he or she is capable. After all, no one knows better how the patient feels than the patient.

"Why" questions

Although valuable, "why" questions also tend to make patients feel challenged. These questions may make patients feel as if they have to justify what they are feeling or what they have done to try and treat their illness or injury. Asking several "why" questions in a row may make the conversation feel more like an interrogation. In response, patients often become defensive. Persons who are defensive often will not provide in-depth information because they fear having to provide further justification for their statements. Use these types of questions sparingly. In addition, space them well apart from each other.

Family and Friends

Often EMTs find themselves in situations where the patient is unable to provide a history or to answer questions. When faced with this, you may have to turn to a family member or friend to gain certain information. You even may find yourself speaking with a third party to gain further information from what the patient already has told you or valuable information the patient did not supply (Box 14-4).

The same basic principles for speaking with a patient apply when speaking with a third party. However, there are also disadvantages to speaking with

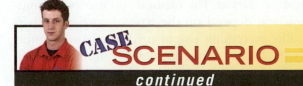

CASE SCENARIO
continued

"Repeat the landing zone you are heading to, County Ambulance Seven."

"LifeFlight, County Seven is heading to the high school sports field, LZ-Two. Do you receive?"

Ray could hear the helicopter blades in the background as the pilot responded. "We copy you are heading to LZ-Two. Thanks for the report, and we'll see you in five minutes."

Ray hung up the microphone and turned his attention back to Josh. The patient looked very worried now and uncomfortable. As Ray reached for the blood pressure cuff again, he updated Josh as to what was happening.

Question: *What communication techniques could Ray use to calm and support Josh?*

someone other than the patient. Only the patient truly can describe what he or she is feeling or experiencing. Information gained from others will be based on their thoughts, experiences, biases, and needs, not the patient's. Family and friends will provide information based on what they think is wrong with the patient. For example, if you are speaking with the parents of a patient with abdominal pain and the patient's sister had appendicitis at the same age, the parents are likely to give information that leads you toward appendicitis. This is often done unknowingly by the family member. Therefore the EMT must understand this tendency of third parties to frame the information they provide. When interviewing others, the EMT also must look for clues as to the quality of the relationship between the patient and the individual giving the information. Indications of a good relationship will lend credibility to the information being given. However, clues to a bad relationship may bring the information into question.

Communication Barriers

Nothing emphasizes the importance of being able to communicate with your patient more than when you are not able to do so. In such a case the EMT must be resourceful and attempt to find a way around the **com-**

BOX 14-4

Communication with Third Parties

When speaking with someone other than the patient, you should gain the patient's permission whenever possible. If the patient has the mental ability to give consent or deny consent, you would be violating his or her confidentiality by speaking to anyone else about his or her condition without approval.

munication barrier. The method you use for communication will depend on the type of barrier. Furthermore, like everything else in medicine, your comfort level with alternative methods of communication will grow as you gain more experience using them.

Language barriers

One of the most frustrating situations in medicine can result from a patient and provider who speak different languages. Your ability to gain information in order to treat your patient effectively is gone until you can find a way to exchange information. Several bilingual questionnaires are available that can be used for this purpose. In these questionnaires, the questions are written in the languages of the EMT and the patient. Responses to the questions are written in the same manner. The EMT simply can point to the question, and the patient then can point to the appropriate response. Whenever possible, however, you should use a trained medical interpreter who is familiar with the terms and general process used in patient-practitioner communications. One imperative is that the EMT remember that a few broken words spoken by each person is inadequate communication on which to base treatment. The EMT must find a better method of communication.

Hearing-impaired patients

Much like a language barrier, communicating with a deaf or hearing-impaired patient can prove to be a challenge. The one advantage over a language barrier is that usually the EMT and the patient will have the same language base and the only difference will be the method of expression.

Depending on the degree of hearing loss and the age at which the hearing loss occurred, each individual will have a preferred method of communication. The EMT should ascertain what this method is early on and use it whenever possible. One common misconception regarding deaf individuals is that they cannot use their voice. The ability to hear and the ability to use the vocal cords are in no way related. Unless there is a separate issue with the vocal cords, deaf patients indeed can use their voice. As a general rule, those patients whose deafness is prelingual regularly will choose not to use their voice. Those patients whose deafness is postlingual may use their voice regularly. However, during the stress of an emergency, do not be surprised if a deaf patient is using his or her voice.

Although many ways of communicating with the deaf or hearing-impaired patient are available, the following general concepts apply to all interactions.

Do not raise your voice unless the patient requests this of you. Depending on the severity of the hearing loss, the patient will not hear you anyway or will hear only incomprehensible noise. Visual contact is important in deaf culture and should be maintained at all times. A hearing patient will hear someone call you and understand why you suddenly turn away from him or her, whereas the deaf patient will respond differently to the same situation, wondering if you suddenly have lost interest or if a major incident has just occurred. Many events the hearing population associate with sound, such as a telephone ringing, an alarm clock buzzing, or a doorbell ringing, are associated with lights in the deaf population. As a result, most deaf individuals are sensitive to light. Therefore the EMT must be aware of lighting, including the distraction and visual disturbance emergency vehicles can create.

The following methods generally are used in communication with a deaf or hearing-impaired patient:

Sign language

Not all deaf and hearing-impaired patients use sign language. However, if the patient uses it, it most likely will be his or her preferred method of communication. If you know sign language, no matter how little, you should attempt to use it if the patient prefers. Even if you are unable to complete the entire conversation with sign language, you can supplement it with one of the other methods. One fact about sign language that generally is not known among the hearing population is that it is not universal. Each country has its own sign language. Therefore if you happen to know American Sign Language and your patient is from another country, there is a good chance you will not be able to use this method of communication. You will have to choose another method.

Gestures

Gestures can be an effective form of communication if the EMT does not know sign language. The EMT can "act out" the message he or she is trying to send to the patient. Although gestures are not an element of sign language, you often will find that the gesture you use is the correct sign for what you are trying to say. The other factor that makes gestures so effective is that deaf individuals are much more accustomed to communicating with hearing individuals than hearing individuals are with deaf individuals. As a result, you often will find that the patient will understand what you are trying to say much more easily than you will understand him or her.

Writing

If the EMT does not know sign language or the patient is from another country with a different sign language, but there is a common written and spoken language, then writing will be the best option for communication. Although this method may take more time, it will eliminate any error or miscommunication that may result from poorly understood gestures or sign language.

Lip reading

Lip reading is the most ineffective method of communication. It should be the last choice when you are speaking with a deaf or hearing-impaired patient. Lip reading is an acquired skill that takes considerable practice to develop. Contrary to popular belief, many deaf individuals do not use lip reading regularly. This may be because they primarily interact with the deaf community. Therefore do not assume that because a patient is deaf, he or she is a skilled lip reader. Also consider the fact that there are approximately 44 sounds in the English language used to create an extraordinary number of words. Without the benefit of sound, many words, such as "pregnant" and "brain dead," look exactly the same for lip readers. Because of these factors, lip reading is roughly 33% accurate at best and often is much less effective.

If you are faced with a situation where lip reading is your only option for communication, be sure both parties are looking directly at each other and neither person is looking directly into a bright light. Remove any objects from your mouth, and be sure there is nothing covering your mouth. Speak at a normal rate and tone, distinctly and clearly. Shouting or overexaggerating your words will distort your lip movements and make lip reading even more difficult (Box 14-5).

Interpreters

When dealing with a language barrier or a deaf or hearing-impaired patient, the best course of action is to use a medical interpreter. These interpreters are trained specifically for medical interpretation. They are familiar with medical terms and the patient interview process. Moreover, they will remain neutral and will not interject their own thoughts or feelings into the conversation between the patient and provider. Check for medical interpreters at the local hospital, public health agency, or local civic organizations.

Regardless of who is used to help interpret, remember that the interpreter is simply a conduit for communication. He or she is not a participant in the conversation. Observe the following guidelines whenever you are using anyone as an interpreter:

- Speak directly to the patient, not the interpreter. Ask, "Where is your pain?" rather than, "Can you ask him where the pain is located?"
- Maintain eye contact with the patient, not the interpreter.
- Do not "think out loud." Patients will wonder what is not being interpreted.
- Speak at a pace that allows time for interpretation.
- Clarify with your interpreter if you want him or her to interpret simultaneously (interpreting what is said at the time it is said) or consecutively

---

BOX 14-5

Challenge Yourself

Sit across from someone and read a phrase to him or her without making any sound. Be sure to look directly at the person and use the techniques for lip reading mentioned in the chapter. Can the person figure out what you said? How many words did he or she get, and how many did he or she miss? What was your percentage of effectiveness? Try watching television without the sound on. Can you keep up with the dialog?

SPECIAL Considerations

Unfortunately, in the prehospital setting a medical interpreter is rarely available. The emergency medical technician often is forced to use the patient's family members or friends as an interpreter. In this situation, you must appreciate the fact that the person you use as an interpreter has a vested interest in the patient's condition and outcome. In addition, just as any other time you use a family member for information, he or she is likely to interject his or her own thoughts and opinions. Inform the person acting as the interpreter to interpret exactly what you say and exactly what the patient says. The interpreter should not paraphrase or add his or her own opinions to the conversation. Medical interpreters will not need these instructions, for they will remain neutral to the situation. This is strongly emphasized in their training.

(waiting until the person is done speaking and then interpreting everything at that time).

- Avoid medical terms that may make interpretation more difficult. Although a medical interpreter may be familiar with medical terms, family and friends who are acting as interpreters will find them difficult.

Elderly Patients

As you will learn, the body goes through numerous physiologic changes as a person ages. After the age of 30, all systems start to lose some function. By the age of 60, as much as a 30% decline has occurred. Through this process, the visual field narrows and hearing loss occurs, starting in the higher-frequency ranges. Visual acuity also diminishes because of the growth of the lens, loss of accommodation, decreased ability to focus, and development of cataracts.

Always be sure to place yourself at eye level in front of the patient so you can be sure you are within his or her visual field. In addition, speak slowly and distinctly in a low voice. If the patient wears glasses or has a hearing aid, make every effort to find it for him or her.

In addition to visual and auditory deficits, you must consider other challenges to communication when speaking with the elderly patient. As patients age, their response time to questions will be slower. To receive accurate information, the EMT must be patient and allow the patient to answer questions fully. If you interrupt prematurely, you may stop the patient from giving you the information you were seeking. Elderly patients may downplay or deny symptoms they are experiencing for several reasons. They simply may attribute the symptoms to the aging process and not consider them relevant. Also, they may be taking multiple medications, which may mask symptoms. Moreover, they may be concerned about the financial impact of medical care or may be worried that they may lose their independence. Finally, many elderly patients believe that patients go to hospitals to die. They may know of many friends and family members who were transported to a hospital and never returned home. This can result in the

patient denying symptoms to avoid transport. Any indication that the patient is not completely forthcoming with his or her entire history should prompt further exploration by the EMT. Facilitation and confrontation are especially useful in these situations.

Other important considerations are the age of the patient and the time in which he or she grew up. Most patients who are currently in their fifth decade or beyond grew up in a time when persons did not seek medical attention for "every little thing." Determine the patient's perception of medical care and how often he or she uses the health care system. The patient who rarely saw a physician as a child or young adult because such issues were dealt with at home has made a significant decision when requesting an ambulance. The chest pain he or she describes as "a little twinge" and rates as 2/10 might be described as debilitating 10/10 pain by the majority of the other patients for whom you care.

■ REMOTE COMMUNICATION

Much of the communication performed by an EMT will be done remotely. In other words, you will communicate with someone in another location. The two-way radio remains the mainstay of remote communications in EMS. However, cellular phones, facsimiles, wireless computer connections, and wireless handheld computers are becoming more common.

Communication Systems

A **communication system** in EMS can range from simple to complex. This usually depends on the needs of the particular department. These systems contain some, if not all, of the following components:

NOTE

If the patient is having difficulty hearing you and does not have a hearing aid, you can place a stethoscope in his or her ears and speak into the diaphragm.

///CAUTION!

Most radio frequencies used by emergency medical services are considered public domain. Although the Federal Communications Commission regulates who can *transmit* on them, there is no regulation regarding who can *receive* them. Whenever you speak on the radio, you must assume someone other than the person to whom you are talking also is listening. Personally identifiable patient information should *never* be transmitted over the radio.

Base stations

The **base station** is a radio at a fixed location, such as a dispatch center, EMS station, or hospital (Fig. 14-4).

These radios are generally high powered. They have the longest transmission range of all the radios used in EMS. Two types of base stations are common to EMS. With one type, the control head (for selecting the frequency and adjusting the volume), the transceiver (a piece of equipment that transmits and receives), and the antenna are in the same location. The control head and transceiver may be integrated into one unit, or they may be separate pieces of equipment. In either case, the transceiver is connected directly to the antenna, which may be on top of the building or on a tower just outside (Fig. 14-5).

The transmission distance is limited by the power of the radio (measured in watts) and the height of the antenna.

Another base station configuration is the remote console. With this type, the control head is in one location and is connected by telephone lines to the transceiver. The antenna is in another location. This allows the antenna to be placed on the highest geographical point, which greatly increases transmission range. Another advantage of the remote console configuration is that it is possible to have control heads in multiple locations (i.e., dispatch, the hospital, and each station) connected to one transmitter. In this situation, the control heads also are connected by telephone lines and often have an intercom function. This allows communication between base stations without transmitting on the frequency (Fig. 14-6).

Mobile radios

Mobile radios are radios that are mounted permanently in your vehicle (e.g., ambulance, fire truck, or police car; Fig. 14-7).

The power of mobile radios is generally lower than that of base stations. Power generally ranges from 20 to 50 W, although it can also be as high as 100 to 175 W (Box 14-6). The average transmission range of a **mobile radio** is 10 to 15 miles. However, this varies widely depending on its power, and the terrain the radio waves must cross. Flat terrain will in-

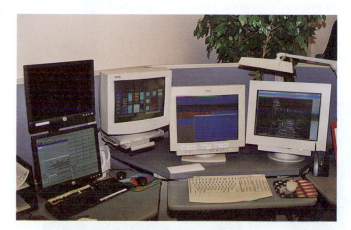

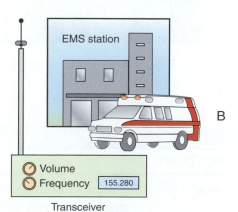

Fig. 14-4 Base stations have the greatest transmission distance of all radios. The transmitters of most modern dispatch centers are controlled by computer.

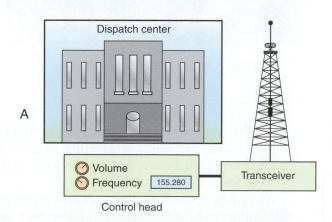

Fig. 14-5 Base station configuration with all components at the same location. **A,** Control head and transceivers are separate pieces of equipment. **B,** Control head and transceiver are integrated into the same piece of equipment.

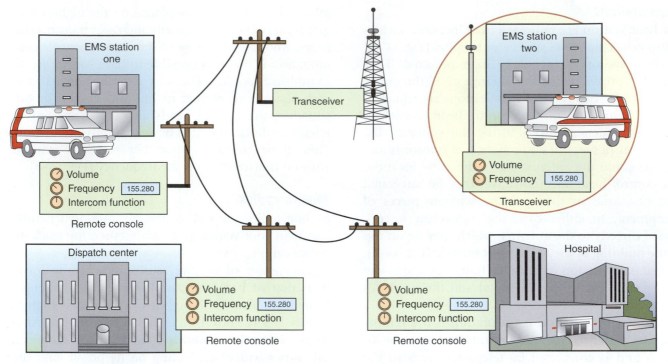

Fig. 14-6 Base station configuration using remote consoles. Each remote console is connected to a common transceiver and the other consoles via telephone lines, which allows intercom communications between each console. Emergency medical services station two is not connected to the remote console network and has its own transceiver. Therefore transmissions from this location are done over the radio frequency and cannot be done over the intercom.

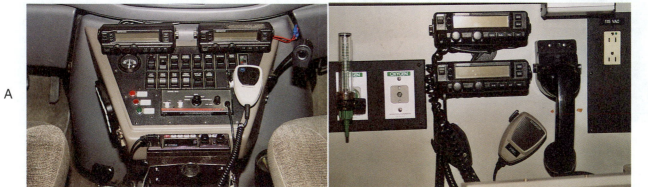

Fig. 14-7 **A,** Mobile radio in the cab. **B,** Mobile radio in the patient care compartment.

BOX 14-6	
Important Terms	
Frequency	The number of cycles a radio wave makes in 1 second
Hertz (Hz)	1 cycle per second
Kilohertz (KHz)	1,000 cycles per second
Megahertz (MHz)	1,000,000 cycles per second

crease the range, whereas obstructions such as buildings or mountains will decrease the range. Certain frequencies work better than others over different types of terrain.

As with base stations, there are two types of mobile radios. The control head and transceiver may be contained in the same unit, or multiple control heads may be connected to a transceiver, which is mounted elsewhere in the vehicle. The latter is the more com-

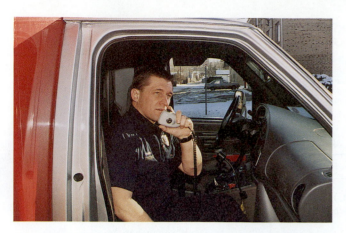

Fig. 14-8 The passenger should use the radio when possible to allow the driver to focus on driving.

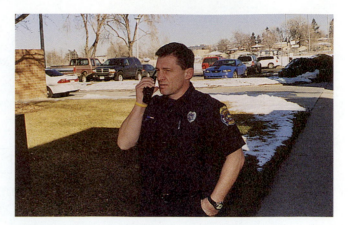

Fig. 14-9 Handheld radios are low power with limited transmission distance.

mon configuration in an ambulance. This allows a control head to be in the cab and one to be in the patient care compartment. Generally, only one control head can be used at a time. Thus you will have a method to activate the control head you want to use. *Whenever possible, the passenger should coordinate all vehicular radio communications to allow the driver to concentrate on driving* (Fig. 14-8).

Portable radios

As the name implies, the **portable radio** is a transceiver that is handheld (Fig. 14-9).

The **Federal Communications Commission** limits the power of this type of radio to 5 W. This results in transmission ranges of only a few miles. Portable radios are a key component of EMS communications. They allow you to talk with the dispatcher, hospital, or other providers while still on the scene of an emergency without having to return to the vehicle radio.

Pagers

A pager is a radio that only receives. It has no capability to transmit. In EMS, pagers are used to alert crews that they have a call. The dispatcher activates a set of tones, which "opens" the pager. This allows for reception of the radio frequency. The pager remains "open" and all transmissions on the frequency will be heard until it is reset, usually by pushing a button. After resetting, nothing will be heard over the pager until it is "opened" manually or is reactivated by the tones.

Repeaters

Repeaters are transceivers that may be combined with a base station or may stand alone. A radio signal received by a **repeater** on one frequency is rebroadcast

at the power of the repeater on another frequency. This dramatically increases its range. For example, you are on a scene on your 5-W handheld radio. You need to communicate with someone who is 30 miles away. Normally this would not be possible because of the low power of the handheld. In a repeated system, the low-power transmission from the handheld goes to the repeater. The transmission then is rebroadcast by the repeater at 100 W (Fig. 14-10).

Essentially, in a repeated system, you have the full power of the repeater transceiver at your disposal no matter what type of radio you are using.

Repeaters also can be mounted in the ambulance and turned on with a switch when arriving on scene. Once turned on, the mobile repeater functions the same as a stationary repeater. If a situation requires the response of multiple ambulances, generally only the first ambulance on scene activates its vehicle-mounted repeater.

Cellular phones

As cellular phones have become more common and less expensive, many EMS systems use them as primary or backup methods of communication. The cellular phone adds a slight amount of security over standard radio frequencies. However, the EMT must remember that it is still a radio and it is possible for the conversation to be overheard. When using a cellular phone, you should not dicuss patient-identifiable information. Advantages of the cellular phone are that it allows the EMT to carry on a conversation with medical control and for medical control to speak directly with the patient if needed. Disadvantages of cellular phones are the lack of coverage in certain areas and the possibility of system outages and overloads, such as those that occur during a major disaster.

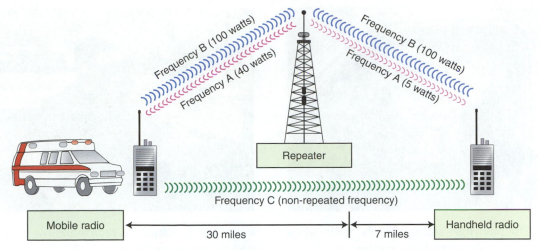

Fig. 14-10 Repeaters greatly increase the transmission range of low-powered radios. The repeater receives on one frequency and rebroadcasts the transmission at high power on another frequency. Although the radios transmit and receive on different frequencies, you cannot transmit and receive simultaneously in most systems. Most repeater systems also have a nonrepeated or direct frequency. This frequency does not activate the repeater, and transmission distance is limited by the power of the original radio.

Other communication methods

Advances in computer and wireless technology have created a variety of other devices that are becoming more common in EMS communications.

Computers

Many ambulances now are being equipped with computers that are connected directly to the dispatch center (Fig. 14-11). This allows direct access to the computer-aided dispatch system, as well as text-based communication with the dispatcher and other emergency vehicles. Printers also are being installed in ambulances. This allows the crews to complete and print written documentation, regardless of their location.

Facsimiles

Facsimiles may be sent from a variety of computer equipment and EMS equipment while still in the field.

Digital equipment

Unlike analog radio equipment, which transmits voice by changing its fluctuation on an electromagnetic wave, digital equipment converts information into a binary language (a language comprised of 0s and 1s). This technology is much more secure than analog devices. Plus, it allows for the transmission of voice or data. In addition, digital technology is not subject to the signal degradation of analog equipment. You must understand that all computer systems use binary language and that digital communi-

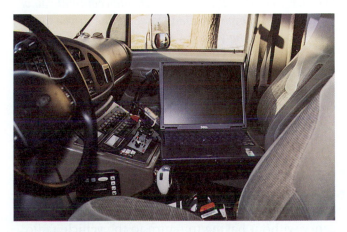

Fig. 14-11 A laptop computer mounted in the cab can enhance communications greatly by providing the same information the dispatcher has: Global Positioning System moving map displays, hospital status, and text messaging between emergency vehicles.

cation equipment can interfere with medical equipment. If you notice any abnormal function of your medical equipment while using digital communication devices, you immediately should change to an analog device.

System maintenance

Regardless of the type of equipment used in a communications system, the equipment must have regular maintenance to operate effectively. The EMT

should always care for radio equipment according to the recommendations of the manufacturer. Radios should not be dropped, mishandled, or abused. They also should not be immersed in liquids or exposed to unusually low or high temperatures, unless designed to do so. A common component of your daily ambulance check will be to call the dispatcher to ensure your radio is transmitting and receiving correctly. This may be done daily or weekly. Radios also should be evaluated periodically by a qualified technician. This will ensure that there are no problems that would not be identified through normal use. Because radio communications are so critical to the provision of EMS, there should be backup systems in place in the event the primary communication system fails.

Federal Communications Commission

The Federal Communications Commission (FCC) is responsible for regulating all radio communications within the United States. Organizations that use radio transmissions must receive a license from the FCC authorizing them to do so. The license will specify the frequency or frequencies the organization may use. It also will specify the number of base stations, mobile radios, handheld radios, and pagers that may be used. Frequencies used by EMS agencies fall within the public safety radio pool. Anyone granted a license within this pool of frequencies must meet certain criteria regarding frequency use and the service provided. Through this process, the FCC can ensure maximum use of available bandwidth. In addition, it can prevent multiple departments in the same geographic area from using the same frequencies and interfering with each other's communications.

The FCC also monitors radio transmissions for appropriate use, the intentional disruption of radio communications, or profanity and obscene language. Fines for inappropriate use or language can be large. All frequencies used by EMS agencies must be used for EMS-related communication. This includes "talk around" channels, which are frequencies other than the primary dispatch frequency. These frequencies may or may not be received and heard by the dispatch center.

Typical communications

During an EMS response, several events will occur that require communication with the dispatcher, other emergency service providers, or the hospital. Most EMS systems use **plain English** when speaking on the radio. In this method of communication, the message to be conveyed is stated clearly and exactly. This prevents confusion between individuals. In the past, codes commonly were used on the radio. The most common were 10-Codes (Box 14-7).

These codes were thought to reduce transmission time and add some level of privacy to radio communication. However, if all departments involved in a call do not use the same codes, communication actually is disrupted. In addition, most persons monitoring emergency frequencies know the codes as well if not better than emergency responders. Thus privacy can become an issue. As a result, the use of codes in emergency medicine is rare in modern EMS. During an EMS response, the following communications typically take place.

Dispatch

The dispatch center or **public safety dispatch point** receives notification that an emergency response is needed (Fig. 14-12).

In most areas of the country, the system is activated by the 911 system. This system was established

---

BOX 14-7

Sample Associated Public Safety Communications Officers 10-Codes

10-1 Signal weak
10-2 Signal strong
10-3 Stop transmitting/Clear the frequency
10-4 Message received/Affirmative
10-5 Relay information
10-6 Busy
10-7 Out of service
10-8 In service
10-9 Repeat
10-10 Negative
10-12 Stand by
10-17 En route
10-18 Urgent
10-20 Location
10-21 Call by phone
10-22 Disregard
10-23 On scene
10-24 Assignment complete
10-25 Meet
10-33 Emergency
10-41 On duty
10-42 Off duty
10-50 Motor vehicle collision
10-52 Ambulance

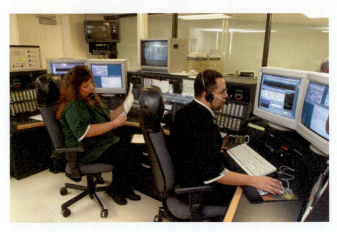

Fig. 14-12 Dispatchers gain information from callers and determine the needed resources.

by AT&T in 1968. Depending on the capability of the public safety dispatch point, the dispatcher may have only the information provided by the caller, or the caller's location may be displayed on a computer map along with the phone number, address, and information about any prior calls to that location.

Some dispatch centers use emergency medical dispatchers. These dispatchers are trained to provide pre-arrival medical instructions to the caller and gain additional information for the responding ambulance. Once the nature of the call is determined, the appropriate resources are dispatched to the call. An ambulance may be dispatched because the call is in its response district. However, an ambulance may be selected because it is closest. The dispatcher may have a computerized map that shows the current location of all ambulances. This automated vehicle locating system often allows the dispatcher to track the progression of the ambulance to the call and assist with directions as needed. The initial dispatch simply may advise the particular ambulance that they have an emergency call or may provide all available information about the call and will include the time (Box 14-8).

For example, a call might be "Medic Ten, C-Med, emergency traffic reference abdominal pain, Fourteen Sixty-Three Garrison Road, map three-four-six-two-eight-four, time twelve fifty-seven."

Call acknowledgment

Once the call is received, the crew must acknowledge the call "C-Med, Medic Ten, copy emergency traffic."

En route

You must understand that the unit is not en route until the crew is in the ambulance and ready to respond: "C-Med, Medic Ten, we are en route."

BOX 14-8

24-Hour Clock

In emergency services, all times are given according to the 24-hour clock, as an hour followed by the appropriate minutes. For example, 12:34 AM would be 0034. This eliminates any confusion between AM and PM times.

0100 = 1 AM
0200 = 2 AM
0300 = 3 AM
0400 = 4 AM
0500 = 5 AM
0600 = 6 AM
0700 = 7 AM
0800 = 8 AM
0900 = 9 AM
1000 = 10 AM
1100 = 11 AM
1200 = 12 PM
1300 = 1 PM
1400 = 2 PM
1500 = 3 PM
1600 = 4 PM
1700 = 5 PM
1800 = 6 PM
1900 = 7 PM
2000 = 8 PM
2100 = 9 PM
2200 = 10 PM
2300 = 11 PM
0000 = 12 AM

All times associated with an EMS response are tracked in order to make the system more efficient. This includes the time the dispatch center received the call, the time it was dispatched, and the time the crew was actually en route. The difference between the time the call is dispatched and when the crew is en route often is referred to as "chute time." Standard acceptable chute times are between 30 and 60 seconds. Incorrectly stating you are en route when you are actually acknowledging the call limits the ability to find system weaknesses.

Call information

Once the crew is in the ambulance and ready to receive the information, the dispatcher will provide all available information about the call. "Medic Ten, C-Med, emergency traffic Fourteen Sixty-Three Garrison Road, map three-four-six-two-eight-four, reference a seventy-three-year-old female who is conscious and alert complaining of chest pain. Card Ten—Delta Three, time now twelve fifty-eight." After receiving the complete dispatch information, the crew members should confirm they have the information. This keeps the dispatcher from having to wonder if the transmission actually was received: "C-Med, Medic Ten, copy information."

Scene arrival

When the crew members arrive on scene, they notify the dispatcher. That way, your location is known at all times, and response time can be tracked: "C-Med, Medic Ten, we're on scene." The dispatcher then will confirm your arrival: "Medic Ten, C-Med, copy on scene at thirteen-o-five."

Status check

Some systems will check on a crew after a predetermined amount of time on scene. This ensures the safety of the crew and helps to determine whether additional resources are needed: "Medic Ten, C-Med, status check." The response is generally a short description of the call: "C-Med, Medic Ten, we are ten-four, female patient chest pain."

En route to the hospital

You need to notify the dispatcher when the crew leaves the scene for the hospital and what the transport mode is. This keeps the dispatcher notified of the progress of the call and allows for the tracking of scene times: "C-Med, Medic Ten, en route to Memorial Hospital with one patient, nonemergency." The dispatcher then will acknowledge this with an associated time: "Medic Ten, C-Med, copy en route to Memorial, thirteen twenty-two."

Arrival at the hospital

The crew members inform the dispatcher when they arrive at the hospital: "C-Med, Medic Ten, we are out at Memorial." The dispatcher then acknowledges this: "Medic Ten, C-Med, copy out at Memorial, thirteen thirty-five."

Call complete/ready for service

For the dispatcher to know the ambulances that are available for calls at all times, the crew members should notify the dispatcher as soon as they are ready for service. In addition to clearing a call, the crew members also should state their intentions. These could include remaining at the hospital to complete paperwork or returning to their district, station, or some other location. This helps the dispatcher better

track the location of each ambulance. It also allows for the dispatch of the closest available unit for additional calls: "C-Med, Medic Ten, we are clear and back in service, remaining at Memorial to complete paperwork." A typical response to this would be "Medic Ten, C-Med, copy clear and back in service, time now thirteen fifty-five. Advise when you are en route back to your district."

Radio Procedures

Radio use is a fairly simple and straightforward skill to master. To ensure clear radio transmissions, always speak at a normal rate and in a normal voice without wide fluctuations in tone. Clearly state your request or intentions in a professional manner, without slang, ambiguous terms, or profanity. Adhere to the following principles whenever you are using the radio:

- Ensure the radio is on and the volume is adjusted properly.
- Make sure the frequency is clear before beginning your transmission.
- Press the microphone key or "push to talk" key and wait 1 or 2 seconds before speaking. This allows the circuitry of the radio to engage and ensures that the beginning of your transmission is heard.
- Speak in a normal tone of voice, at a normal rate, with the microphone 2 to 3 inches from your mouth.
- Identify who you are calling, followed by who you are.
- Wait for a response from whom you are calling that indicates you can "go ahead" with your transmission.
- Unless codes are standard for the system, use plain English or clear text.
- Keep transmissions brief, avoiding meaningless phrases. However, ensure that your complete message is received and understood.
- Clarify sound-alike phrases to avoid confusion. Names such as "Brandy Wine Road" and "Branding Iron Road" may not be distinguishable on the radio. Numbers also often sound similar. The receiving facility may not be sure if your estimated time of arrival (ETA) is 4 to 5 minutes, or 45 minutes. When needed, state the individual digits of the number.
- An EMT rarely acts alone. The term *we* generally should be used rather than *I*.
- Use words that are easy to hear, such as *affirmative* and *negative* rather than *yes* or *no*.

NOTE

Always make it a habit to turn your portable radio off when you are in the ambulance. This eliminates any feedback that may occur when using the mobile radio. In addition, it prevents the possibility of your sitting in a way that presses the key of the portable radio. More than one "private" conversation in an ambulance has been overheard because someone was leaning on the key of his or her radio. Not only can this lead to an embarrassing situation, but also it makes the frequency unavailable for use by others.

■ HOSPITAL COMMUNICATIONS

Communicating with hospitals is an integral part of most EMS responses. These communications fall within one of two categories: consulting with medical direction for advice on patient care issues or medication orders, and notifying the receiving hospital of your ETA and the patient's condition.

Communication with Medical Direction

Depending on the structure of the EMS system, the hospital the EMT contacts for medical direction may or may not be the hospital to which the patient is being transported. Regardless, the procedure remains the same. Most often the EMT will contact medical direction for orders to administer medication or to assist the patient with his or her own medication. In this situation, the physician will make the determination to grant or deny your order based on the information you provide (Box 14-9).

The goal of the EMT is to provide a clear, accurate description of the patient and current illness, or to "paint a picture" of the patient. The more clearly the physician is able to see what you are seeing, the more accurate the patient care decisions will be. The physician also must be comfortable with the skill level of the EMT and the accuracy of the assessment that was done. These competencies are conveyed through the verbal interaction that takes place. As you gain experience as an EMT, your skill at accomplishing these two goals will increase.

Hospital Notification

When en route to the hospital with a patient, the EMT must notify the receiving facility to allow time

BOX 14-9
Medication Orders

When requesting medication orders, it is best to notify the physician of your request and then follow this with your report of the patient condition and complaints. This allows the physician to listen to your report with the ultimate goal in mind and to ask appropriate questions as needed. Also, correctly stating the treatment you want to provide shows your competence and greatly increases the physician's confidence in your assessment of the patient. If you receive an order that is unclear, beyond your scope of practice, or inappropriate, your duty is to question the physician and clarify the order. Repeat all orders back to the physician to reduce any misunderstanding. As an emergency medical technician, your responsibility is to know the proper indications, contraindications, and doses of the medications with which you can assist or administer. You are accountable for your actions and must know your limitations. Do not assume the physician is familiar with your scope of practice. Doing something "because the physician told me to" is not a defense for inappropriate treatment.

for any preparations that must be made before arrival (Fig. 14-13).

A room or equipment may need to be prepared, or specialists may need to be notified for certain types of patients. The amount of time the hospital needs will vary from system to system. However, a minimum notification time of 10 to 15 minutes generally is expected. Always ensure that your reports are objective and nonjudgmental. False information about a patient could lead to charges of slander. The information given and format of the radio report is as follows:

- Identify whom you are calling and who you are. If you need to speak with a physician, provide that information on your initial contact. Wait for a response before continuing your report. This avoids tying up the frequency when no one may be listening.
- When you receive a response, reidentify your unit and identify yourself and your level of provider. If you requested a physician and are unsure who has answered the radio, restate your request.
- State the purpose of your call, ETA (if applicable), and the age and sex of your patient.
  - "We are on scene requesting nitroglycerin orders for a seventy-three-year-old female patient."

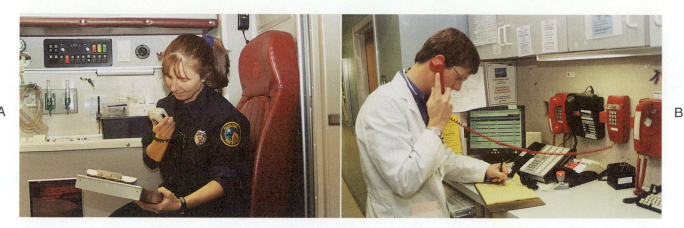

Fig. 14-13 **A,** Notify the hospital you are en route as soon as possible. **B,** Medical direction should be used as a resource when needed.

- "We have an ETA of fifteen minutes to your facility with a seventy-three-year-old female patient."
- Provide the patient's chief complaint, any significant associated complaints, and a brief pertinent history of the present illness.
- If the patient has a medical history that includes any major illnesses or conditions, include these.
- State the patient's current mental status and baseline vital signs.
- Provide the findings of your physical exam, your treatment, and the patient's response to treatment.
- Repeat any instructions you are given.
- Recontact the hospital if there are any significant changes in the patient's condition after your initial contact, particularly if the patient deteriorates.

The radio report for the example call given before would be as follows:

Ambulance: "Memorial Hospital, this is Medic Ten (I need a physician to the radio please)."
Hospital: "Medic Ten, this is Memorial, go ahead."
Ambulance: "Memorial this is Medic Ten, EMT Smith, we have an ETA of fifteen minutes to your facility with a seventy-three-year-old female patient with a chief complaint of chest pain associated with respiratory distress and diaphoresis. The patient describes the pain as eight out of ten, substernal, dull and crushing, radiating to the left arm, with an onset of thirty minutes ago while at rest. The patient had a myocardial infarction three years ago and states this pain is similar to that episode. She is conscious and alert, responding to all questions appropriately. Her initial vitals were blood pressure one thirty-two over eighty-eight, respirations twenty-two, and pulse eighty-four. Her airway is clear, respirations are labored without use of accessory muscles, and breath sounds are clear and equal. Her pulse is weak and regular, and the skin is pale, cool, and diaphoretic. She took three, zero-point-four–milligram nitroglycerin pills before our arrival without relief. We currently have her on fifteen liters per minute of oxygen by non-rebreather and have administered three hundred twenty-four milligrams of aspirin with no change in condition or complaints. We will advise you of any changes en route, go ahead."
Hospital: "Medic Ten, affirmative, we will see you in fifteen minutes, room one on arrival. Memorial clear."
Ambulance: "Copy room one on arrival, Medic Ten clear."

■ VERBAL REPORTS

When you arrive at the hospital, the proper transfer of care from the ambulance staff to the receiving staff at the hospital must include a **verbal report.** During this report, you will have the opportunity to give a more comprehensive description of the patient's complaint and conditions. You also will have the chance to provide any assessment and treatment information not included in the initial verbal report or any findings or changes after you made initial radio contact.

If you are giving the report to a person to whom you did not give your radio report, you will have to include all the information from your radio report and this additional information. If you are giving the report to the same person with whom you spoke on the radio, the verbal report will include only additional information not transmitted or information found after transmission. Always include the following information in the verbal report:

- The patient's name
- Description of the patient's complaint(s) and condition
- History that was not provided over the radio
- Treatment and response to treatment administered after radio contact
- Vital signs taken after radio contact

Resources

Bates B: *A guide to physical examination and history taking*, ed 5, Philadelphia, 1991, JB Lippincott.

Department of Transportation, National Highway Traffic Safety Administration: *EMT-Basic National Standard Curriculum*, Washington, DC, 1994, Department of Transportation.

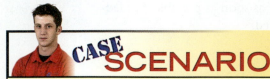

CASE SCENARIO

As the ambulance pulled onto the edge of the field, Ray could hear the distant sound of the medical evacuation helicopter. Their timing was pretty good. In a few minutes, the helicopter was circling the field as the pilot surveyed the site before landing. As the unit landed, Ray took one last set of vital signs before opening the back doors of the ambulance. He spoke with the helicopter medic, providing the information he knew about the patient and his findings during the assessment. The paramedic agreed with Ray that Josh needed to be transported to the trauma center as soon as possible. ■

NUTS AND BOLTS

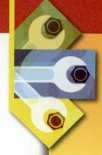

Critical Points

Communication is critical to your ability to be an effective EMT. You must understand the common barriers and pitfalls of the communication process that lead to misunderstanding. You also must understand how to overcome these. Your entire course of treatment will be based on the information you gain from the patient. Moreover, effective care is the result of an accurate history. This information has to be passed along to other medical professionals who will be caring for the patient after your care is complete. If you cannot effectively pass along the patient's complaints, history, progression, your treatment, and its effects, valuable information will be lost, as well as the time it takes to repeat everything you have done. Radio communication equipment is one of the most commonly used tools in an EMS system. You must be able to use the radios adequately and have backup plans in the event of equipment failure. Your personal safety could depend on the dispatcher's knowledge of your location and situation. The dispatchers are an integral part of the EMS system and must be informed during all phases of a call.

Learning Checklist

❑ Understanding how communication is achieved and understanding the principles of encoding, decoding, feedback, and interference is critical to effective communication.

❑ Patient communication is the key to effective treatment. You have to consider many factors when obtaining a patient history to ensure it is complete and accurate. The first of these factors is the setting. The ideal setting for interviewing a patient is one that is private, free of interruptions, and comfortable for the patient and the emergency medical technician.

❑ When speaking with a patient, always use his or her title and last name. Using terms of endearment with the elderly population can be considered insulting.

❑ Questions should be open-ended. This allows the patient the freedom to respond completely. If you use closed questions, be sure they are not leading, and give several options as answers.

❑ Communication techniques used with patients include facilitation, reflection, clarification, empathetic responses, confrontation, and interpretation.

❑ Nonverbal communication is a critical component of communication. It often provides as much information as what actually is said.

❑ There are several common pitfalls of communication. Avoid these at all times. They include false reassurance, avoidance, mishandling of sensitive topics, use of medical terms that are not understood, leading questions, overuse of "why" questions, and the emergency medical technician's dominating the conversation.

❑ Family and friends can be valuable sources of information. However, because of their tendency to present information based on their own needs and experiences, this information is not always entirely accurate. You should always receive permission from the patient before speaking about his or her condition with anyone else.

❑ Dealing with patients who speak another language or hearing-impaired and deaf patients can present a formidable communication barrier. Gaining information from the patient is essential to proper care and treatment. Make every effort to find a common medium of communication. This may include the use of interpreters, sign language, gestures, writing, and lip reading.

❑ Elderly patients often have visual and auditory impairments that can hinder communication. Use methods to overcome these barriers. Pay special attention to their views and use of health care, as well as to their fears. These can provide valuable insight into the completeness of the information provided.

❑ Communication systems used in emergency medical services can range from simple to complex. As an emergency medical technician, you will use these systems daily and must understand their capabilities and limitations. You are likely to use base stations, mobile radios, portable radios, pagers, repeaters, cellular phones, and computers daily. Your responsibility is to know how to use the equipment appropriately and how to keep it in good working order.

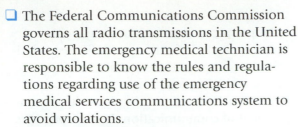

❑ The Federal Communications Commission governs all radio transmissions in the United States. The emergency medical technician is responsible to know the rules and regulations regarding use of the emergency medical services communications system to avoid violations.

❑ A typical emergency medical services response involves several methods of communications with several persons. You must keep the dispatcher informed of your location and status at all times. This ensures your personal safety and efficient use of resources. You must inform the dispatcher when you are en route to a call, when you are on scene, when you transport and arrive at the hospital, and when you are clear. You also must contact the hospital for medical direction and notification that you are en route with a patient.

❑ The verbal report to hospital personnel is a required component of the patient transfer. When transferring a patient, you should always use the patient's name and inform the receiving medical professional of the chief complaint, pertinent history, patient condition, details of the physical assessment, your treatment, and the response to treatment.

Key Terms

Base station Radio at a fixed location, such as a dispatch center, hospital, or emergency medical services station that cannot be moved from place to place. This type of radio is the most powerful radio in the emergency medical services communication system.

Closed or direct questions Closed questions are those that can be answered with a "yes" or "no" response. If used, options should be provided for the patient, and the question should not be phrased in a manner that leads him or her to a specific answer.

Communication barrier A condition that interferes with standard communication, such as a language barrier or a patient who cannot hear you. When faced with these situations, the emergency medical technician must do whatever is necessary to overcome the barrier.

Communication system A system composed of radios, computers, and other equipment that allows the emergency medical technician to communicate with others from remote sites.

Confrontation A communication technique used to point out something about the patient's actions or behavior that is not consistent with what he or she is telling you.

Decoding The process by which the intended receiver interprets the meaning of the message sent by another individual.

Distance When one is speaking with a patient, a distance of 2 to 5 feet should be maintained for patient comfort.

Empathetic responses A communication technique that acknowledges the patient's feelings and lets him or her know those feelings are acceptable.

Encoding The process by which the sender of a message places the message into a format that the receiver can understand.

Facilitation A communication technique that encourages the patient to provide more information or to continue with his or her response.

Federal Communications Commission An agency of the federal government that is responsible for governing all radio transmissions in the United States.

Feedback An integral part of the communications process that determines whether the message intended was actually the message received.

Interference A component of the communication model that is responsible for most instances of miscommunication.

Leading questions Questions that are phrased in such a way that they lead the patient to an answer that may not necessarily be the most correct answer.

Mobile radio A radio that is mounted in a vehicle.

Nonverbal communication An important element of communication in which messages are relayed through movements, posture, gestures, and the eyes.

Open-ended questions Questions that cannot be answered with a "yes" or "no" response. These questions provide the most information because they allow the patient free rein in response as the patient tells you what he or she is experiencing. They also allow the emergency medical technician the most insight into the patient's condition.

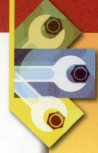

Plain English The preferred method of emergency medical services radio communication in which information is stated directly and not coded in any manner.

Portable radio A radio that can be taken wherever the emergency medical technician goes. These are generally low-power handheld radios with limited transmission distance.

Privacy An environment that protects the patient from exposing themselves or their conversation to individuals not involved with their medical care. In a private setting, patients are more comfortable and more likely to provide complete answers to questions asked. If your initial interview was conducted in a public setting, ask questions again when privacy may allow more open responses.

Public safety dispatch point Commonly referred to as a dispatch center, these points receive calls for service from the public and assign resources to each incident. Public safety dispatch points also track the movement of emergency equipment and may provide pre-arrival instructions to callers.

Repeater A piece of radio equipment that receives low-power radio transmissions and rebroadcasts them at a higher power. Repeaters may be vehicle mounted, free-standing, or associated with a base station.

Verbal report An essential component of the patient transfer to the hospital. The verbal report should contain the patient's name. It also should inform the receiving medical professional of the chief complaint, pertinent history, patient condition, details of the physical assessment, your treatment, and the response to treatment.

National Standard Curriculum Objectives

Cognitive Objectives

After completing this lesson, the EMT student will be able to do the following:

- List the proper methods of initiating and terminating a radio call.
- State the proper sequence for delivery of patient information.

- Explain the importance of effective communication of patient information in the verbal report.
- Identify the essential components of the verbal report.
- Describe the attributes for increasing effectiveness and efficiency of verbal communications.
- State legal aspects to consider in verbal communication.
- Discuss the communication skills that should be used to interact with the patient.
- Discuss the communication skills that should be used to interact with the family, bystanders, and individuals from other agencies while providing patient care, and the difference between skills used to interact with the patient and those used to interact with others.
- List the correct radio procedures in the following phases of a typical call:
  - To the scene
  - At the scene
  - To the facility
  - At the facility
  - To the station
  - At the station

Affective Objective

After completing this lesson, the EMT student will be able to do the following:

- Explain the rationale for providing efficient and effective radio communications and patient reports.

Psychomotor Objectives

After completing this lesson, the EMT student will be able to do the following:

- Perform a simulated, organized, concise radio transmission.
- Perform an organized, concise patient report that would be given to the staff at a receiving facility.
- Perform a brief, organized report that would be given to an advanced life support provider arriving at an incident scene at which the EMT already was providing care.

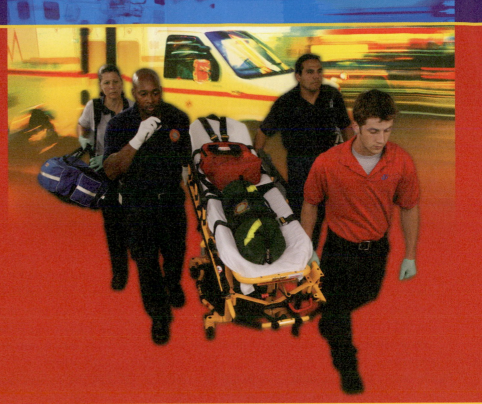

CHAPTER

15

LESSON GOAL

GOAL

A valuable aspect of patient care and the emergency medical services system is documentation. This chapter explains the importance of documentation as it relates to the patient, the prehospital care provider, and the health care system. It also examines the various methods and tools used to complete the prehospital care report properly. ■

Documentation

CHAPTER OBJECTIVES

After completing this chapter, the EMT student will be able to do the following:

1 Explain the components of the written report and list the information that should be included in it.

2 Identify the various sections of the written report.

3 Describe the information required in each section of the prehospital care report and the way in which it should be entered.

4 Define the special considerations concerning patient refusal.

5 Describe the legal implications associated with the written report.

6 Discuss state and/or local record and reporting requirements.

7 Explain the rationale for patient care documentation.

8 Explain the rationale for using medical terminology correctly.

9 Explain the rationale for using an accurate and synchronous clock to aid in trending observations.

10 Complete a patient care report.

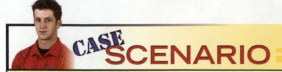

Just as a picture paints a story, the **prehospital care report** (also called a patient care report or PCR) should paint a picture of what occurred during a call. When any person reviews a PCR, it should give that person a clear understanding of what occurred. The PCR should paint a picture in the mind of the person reading it. This picture should provide an accurate image and understanding of what transpired during that particular event with that particular patient.

This chapter examines the purpose and design of accurate report writing. It identifies the content and structure of the PCR. In addition, it identifies a variety of methods to create a well-written patient narrative. This chapter also considers the legal implications of documentation and the importance documentation has in relation to quality patient care and system development.

■ COMPONENTS OF THE WRITTEN REPORT

Prehospital care reports come in a variety of formats (e.g., handwritten, typed, or electronic) and styles (e.g., narrative and checkboxes). However, all contain basic elements regarding call information.

Minimum Data Set

Minimum data set refers to information documented on the PCR that is gathered for statistical purposes. This information is used in a variety of ways. Minimum data often are used to validate the systematic need for prehospital care. Minimum data are used to improve patient care, **patient trends,** and system **quality assurance.** Minimum data can be required by and submitted to local, regional, state, and national organizations. Most states have minimum requirements for data collection and reporting.

Minimum data are collected in two areas: **patient information** and **administrative information.**

Patient information includes information about the call that relates specifically to the patient. (Box 15-1). Administrative information includes run information that relates specifically to the system response (Box 15-2).

Synchronous Clocks

Accurate and **synchronized time recording** is important. Synchronizing your own personal time device (wristwatch) with that of your partner and that of

BOX 15-1
Minimum Data Set: Patient Information

Age and gender
Chief complaint
Mechanism of injury or nature of illness
Level of consciousness (AVPU [alert, verbal, painful, unresponsive]/Glasgow Coma Scale)
Pertinent medical history
Signs and symptoms
Vital signs
Blood pressure (in patients over 3 years of age)
Pulse
Respirations
Skin perfusion
Treatment provided
Patient response to treatment provided

BOX 15-2

Minimum Data Set: Administrative Information

Date of call
Times
Time dispatched
Time responded
Time arrived at the scene
Time departed from the scene
Time arrived at destination (health care facility)
Location of call
Call type
Medical or trauma
Emergent or nonemergent to and from the scene
Use of lights and sirens
Crew information
Names of personnel responding
License or certification number

your service (ambulance wall clock) at beginning of each shift is imperative. This helps to ensure accurate recording of the treatment of the patient, documentation of events, and submission of data for system evaluation.

Frequently, time factors are considered to aid in observing patient trends and determining appropriate treatment. Patient trends are the changes in a patient's condition during a given period. Recording of accurate times of vital signs and reassessment findings can help in determining how a patient is responding to treatment and whether adjustments in care are needed.

■ FUNCTIONS OF THE WRITTEN REPORT

Continuity of Care

The PCR provides **continuity of care** for the patient. Often patient care occurring before arrival at the emergency department has an effect on the care that is rendered once the patient arrives. Certain elements are important in determining the appropriate continuing care of the patient. These elements include the history of the present complaint (often only available from witnesses at the scene), care given to the patient, and patient response to care given at the scene and during transport. Transfer of care and ongoing treatment decisions in the emergency department or other health care facility frequently depend on the patient documentation that the prehospital care provider leaves behind with the patient.

Legal Implications

The PCR is a legal document. As such, it should be respected as a valuable part of patient care and as an integral component of the patient medical record. The PCR should provide information that explains the entire call and should include the following:

• Accurate times
• Environment and surroundings in which the patient was found
• General impression of the patient
• Chief complaint
• Assessment and treatment provided
• Patient's response to the treatment provided
• Where patient was transferred and who assumed patient care
• Status of the patient when care was transferred

Objective and subjective information

Information documented about a call should be objective. **Objective information** is factual information that is based on observations by the emergency medical technician (EMT). Personal bias and judgment should not be included during the call or within the documentation. **Subjective information** is information that is perceived by the patient or bystander and not by the EMT. Documentation should explain what the EMT observed in an objective manner. An example of such includes "The patient appeared to have difficulty with speech and motor coordination." However, "The patient seemed intoxicated" is not considered objective. Without the definitive results of a lab test, determining whether a patient is intoxicated or chemically altered is impossible. Even if the patient tells you that he or she has used alcohol or drugs, you still should document it as "The patient states [blank]," which is objective.

The EMT simply should document his or her observations and treat the patient according to signs and symptoms. Many illnesses can mimic the signs and symptoms of chemical- or alcohol-induced characteristics. Moreover, even patients who are under the influence of alcohol or drugs still have the right to receive good patient care. Your documentation should reflect that.

As an EMT, you may be asked to testify in a court of law regarding care rendered during a call, the patient's condition upon your arrival, or your observations. Your first defense as an EMT is good patient care. However, years after an incident, if you are in court and have to testify, your best, and likely only, resource will be the accurate, clear, and legible documentation of that patient care and event on the PCR. An unorganized, sloppy, incomplete, and inaccurate

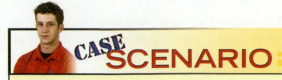

CASE SCENARIO

Ray looked up from the patient care report he had been filling in. He wanted to be sure that the information was especially accurate because there had been a change in the patient's condition that necessitated a dramatic change in Josh's care and transport. The form contained the following information.

Ray spent a few more seconds organizing his thoughts and then began to fill out the narrative section.

Question: *Think back to the patient scenario. Is the information that Ray documented accurate? What would you change? Now, think about what you would write down for the narrative sections.*

APALA CTY PATIENT CARE REPORT

00069729

DISPATCH DATE 05-12-05	CASE NUMBER 0 0 0 0 7 6 4 2	PT NUMBER 1 of 1	PAGE NUMBER 1 of 2	Service Type	Scene Transfer

INCIDENT LOCATION BEAR PARK, SW ENTRANCE	Location Type L R E C	Estimated Incident Date & Time SAME

PATIENT NAME (Last, First) PADUI, JOSHUA	PATIENT ADDRESS 1080 BENTON AV, BROWNSVILLE MN	TELEPHONE NUMBER 270-555-1234

BIRTHDATE 10-10-78	SSN 123-45-6789	INSURANCE INFORMATION ☐ MediCare/Cal ☑ Kaiser ☐ Work Comp. ☑ Pvt	POLICY NUMBER

AGE 27 ☑Y ☐M ☐D	GENDER ☑M ☐F ☐UNK	WEIGHT (kg) 85	MEDICATIONS DENIES ☑Denies	ALLERGIES NKA ☑NKDA

PAST MEDICAL HISTORY ☑Denies
☐MI ☐CHF ☐HTN ☐Other Cardiac ☐Asthma ☐COPD
☐Pneumonia ☐Other Respiratory ☐Immunocompromised
☐Diabetes ☐Kidney Failure ☐Cancer ☐Psychiatric ☐Seizures
☐CVA / TIA ☐Neurological ☐Pregnancy ☐Recent Surgery
☐Alcohol/Substance Abuse ☐History of Current Complaint
☐Other: _____

PRIMARY M.D. NONE

NATURE OF DISPATCH FALL	CHIEF COMPLAINT (L) WRIST PAIN

PRIMARY IMPRESSION WRIST INJURY	CODE 2	SECONDARY IMPRESSION INTERNAL BLEEDING	CODE 3	SUSPECTED ETOH/DRUG USE Y (N)

FIRST RESPONDER UNITS	DISPATCH CODE	DISPATCH TIME	ON SCENE TIME	AT PATIENT TIME	ASSISTED TRANSPORT	EMT NAME	CARE PROVIDERS ID #	EMT-P NAME	ID #
BLS	2 (3)				Y N				
ALS	2 3				Y N				

FIRST RESPONDER NOTES N/A

TREATMENT: O₂ _____ l/m NC NRB BVM NPA OPA Suction C-Spine Bandage Splint Oral Glucose Other: _____

BYSTANDER CARDIAC ARREST INFORMATION	FIRE DEPARTMENT CARDIAC ARREST INFORMATION
Witnessed: ☐Y ☐N Time of Arrest ___:___ N/A	Time CPR Started: ___:___ N/A
Bystander CPR: ☐Y ☐N Time CPR Started ___:___	Fire Department AED Placed: ☐Y ☐N Shock Advised: ☐Y ☐N
Public Access Defibrillator Available: ☐Y ☐N Placed: ☐Y ☐N	Time of 1st Shock ___:___ Number of AED Shocks Delivered: ___
Shock Advised: ☐Y ☐N Number of Shocks Delivered: ___	Pulse Return (ROSC) ☐Y ☐N

TIME	BP	PULSE	RESP	SpO₂	BGL	CARDIAC RHYTHM		GCS	GLASGOW COMA SCALE
1007	130/76	86	16	/	/	/	/	15	
1030	132/74	96	20	/	/	/	/	15	

GLASGOW COMA SCALE

EYE OPENING	VERBAL	MOTOR
4 Spont.	5 Oriented	6 Obeys
3 Voice	4 Confused	5 Purpose
2 Pain	3 Inapprop.	4 Withdraw
1 None	2 Garbled	3 Flexion
	1 None	2 Extension
		1 None

FR SIGNATURE

TRANSPORT UNIT ID A705	DISPATCH TIME 0928	ON SCENE TIME 0955	AT PATIENT TIME 1002	DEPART SCENE TIME 1030	START MILEAGE 072.5	ARRIVE DESTINATION TIME 1042	END MILEAGE 084.1	DISPATCH CODE 2 (3) U D

TRANSPORT CODE 2 3 U D

ATTENDANT I / ID# R. BARNES/171 EMT	ATTENDANT II / ID# J. Smith/272 EMT	INTERN / OBSERVER N/A	RESCUE CAPTAIN / ID# N/A

ASSISTING UNITS	SFFD	RC	SFPD	PRIVATE AMBULANCE	OTHER ANGEL AIR 295

DISPOSITION: ☐SFFD Transport ☐AMA ☐PDT ☐SFPD ☐UTL ☐NOM ☐MAP ☐Medical Examiner ☐Pvt Amb Transport ☑Other: _____

DESTINATION MUH	REASON DDTT	CONDITION AT DESTINATION: ☐Unchanged ☐Improved ☑Deteriorated	EKG: N/A

PCR-1103 (Rev. 11/04)

CASE SCENARIO

NARRATIVE / HISTORY OF CHIEF COMPLAINT:

HEAD	⊖ EENT
NECK	non-tender
CHEST	⊖ Breath sounds, nontender on palpation
ABDOMEN	soft, nontender
BACK	Ⓛ Flank bruising, tenderness on palpation
PELVIS	Nontender
ARMS	Ⓛ wrist deformity, tenderness ⊕ ROM, Ⓡ thigh
LEGS	abrasions Ⓛ knee bruise

LUNG SOUNDS

L	Normal	R
L	Rales	R
L	Rhonchi	R
L	Wheezes	R
L	Diminished	R
L	Absent	R

PUPILS

L	Normal	R
L	Constricted	R
L	Dilated	R
L	Pinpoint	R
L	Unreactive	R

RESPIRATORY EFFORT
☒ Normal ☐ Labored
☐ Depressed ☐ Absent

PERFUSION
☒ Normal
☐ Decreased

SKIN SIGNS:
☐ Pink ☐ Flushed ☒ Pale
☐ Blue
☒ Warm ☐ Hot ☐ Cool
☐ Cold
☐ Dry ☒ Moist
☐ Diaphoretic

TIME	MEDICATION / PROCEDURE	PATIENT RESPONSE	BY
	Assess, exam, hx, vital signs	A/ox 3, Ⓛ wrist pain	
	C/spine precautions		
	splint Ⓛ wrist/apply cold	⊕ ROM before/after	
	Begin transport		
	Reassess vital signs	↑ pulse rate, diaphoresis	
	Reexamine patient	Consult, reevaluate Destination	
	Rendevous air ambulance	Divert to MOSS playground	
	Transfer to angel air ambulance	without incident	

Revised Trauma Score: 12

ADVANCED AIRWAY MANAGEMENT PROCEDURES

RESPIRATIONS	SYSTOLIC BP	GCS
4- 10-29/min	4- ≥ 90 mm Hg	4- 13-15
3- ≥ 30/min	3- 76-89 mm Hg	3- 9-12
2- 6-9/min	2- 50-75 mm Hg	2- 6-8
1- 1-5/min	1- 1-49 mm Hg	1- 4-5
0- No Spont	0- No Pulse	0- 3

PROCEDURE	# ATTEMPTS	SUCCESSFUL	BY
ETT NTT NC CBT		Y N	
ETT NTT NC CBT		Y N	
ETT NTT NC CBT		Y N	
ETT NTT NC CBT		Y N	
Pleural Decomp R		Y N	

COMPLICATIONS:
☐ Difficult Anatomy ☐ Combative Patient
☐ Equip. Failure ☐ Vomit/Blood ☐ FBAO
☐ ⊕ Gag ☐ Trismus ☐ Other:

Vocal cords clearly visualized ☐ Y ☐ N
Bilat LS confirmed by both paramedics ☐ Y ☐ N
EDD bulb reinflated < 5 sec. ☐ Y ☐ N
Capnometer Reading: ☐ Purple ☐ Yellow ☐ Beige
End tidal CO₂ reading _____ mm Hg

	MECHANISM OF INJURY	INJURY CONTRIB. FACTORS	SAFETY FACTORS	FACTORS AFFECT EMS CARE
1				
2				
3				
4				

BASE CONTACT ☐ Radio ☐ Landline **Time:** **Base MD:**

RECEIVING HOSPITAL NOTIFICATION ☒ RH Notified ☐ Attempted/Failed ☐ ECD Relay ☐ No Notification

REPORT GIVEN TO: ANGEL AIR - EMTP DONOHUE

REPORT AUTHOR SIGNATURE / ID#

---

patient care record often leads the reader to assume the care provided also was unorganized, sloppy, incomplete, and inaccurate. You may provide the best patient care possible, provide the most accurate and diligent treatment to a patient, but if your documentation does not reflect that, no one will know.

Ordinarily, the person completing the PCR is the person who also will go to court to testify, if needed.

The primary care provider on the call is usually the person who completes and attests to the PCR.

Educational Tool

Many prehospital care services use the written PCR as an educational tool. The report is used to **critique** a call. The report can be examined to evaluate what was done correctly or what could have been differently or better. Quality assurance activities monitor and improve the care provided through review of the documentation of patient care. Some calls that involve difficult or infrequently occurring circumstances may be examined through the documentation to evaluate the situation for future strategies.

Often, the critique is performed by focusing on the documentation itself. Medical directors or administrators may look at different aspects of the PCR to see whether the documentation of the report was complete and concise. Accuracy in documentation includes not only spelling but also fluency, organization, and completion.

Administrative Uses

Other functions of the PCR include administrative uses. Billing and statistical information are obtained from the documentation. The patient's insurance information and subsequent payment for the service provided often depends on the medical documentation. This documentation helps to determine reimbursement. Accuracy is needed to ensure appropriate handling of fiscal responsibility. Many prehospital care providers may feel that this aspect of the job is neither their responsibility nor their focus. However, because documentation often is a concern for the patient, the EMT should give it serious consideration. Moreover, documentation can have an impact on the sustainability of the prehospital medical care system as a whole.

Documentation of prehospital care commonly is used to gather operational statistics for individual ambulance services. Common statistical data gathered for analysis include the number of calls made in a year, the type of calls (medical or trauma), and the frequency and criticality of call types. Statistics are used to assess the needs of the patient population served. They also are necessary to build and support the system so that it best meets the needs of the community. Statistics also can be used to assess needs for education, training, and staffing.

Research

Research in emergency medical services (EMS) is critical for growth and system building. Collected data are valuable for assessing current treatment trends and scope of practice. The data also are valuable for evaluating the need to adjust treatment modalities based on needs and historic patient outcomes. Accurate and complete data reports are essential to researchers. These reports aid researchers in having an appropriate analysis of **patient data** in any given focus of study.

Evaluation and Continuous Quality Improvement

Once an area of research and statistical gathering is complete, the data can be analyzed and evaluated for changes that may be appropriate. Research and evaluation can help determine areas of concern. These processes also validate the need for modification. Any change in the treatment standards should be research based and should be validated by evaluation and data analysis, including patient outcomes.

Continuous quality improvement is just as it implies, continuous. It should be ongoing. In addition, continuous quality improvement should consider all aspects of prehospital care: the patient, the service, the financial charges, and the system. Emergency medical services is ever evolving and changing, just as health care is ever evolving and changing. Quality improvement should not be focused solely on a single aspect but should look at the system as a whole and continually strive to evaluate and improve it.

■ FORM TYPES

The traditional PCR is in paper form (Fig. 15-1). Generally, these reports will have a check box, circle, or fill-in-the-box format, with a section for a patient narrative.

As technology has advanced, more and more prehospital services are using reports that are electronic (Fig. 15-2). Several computerized versions of run reports are on the market today. Computerized run reports have the added benefit of electronic data retrieval for statistical information, as discussed previously in this chapter. They also can decrease the time it takes to complete the report. In addition, they can store patient demographics and medical history if the patient has been seen before.

■ SECTIONS OF THE REPORT

Regardless of whether the report is handwritten or electronically entered, all have similar information requirements. Common sections include **run data**, patient data, check boxes, patient narrative, and others, depending on state or local requirements.

RUN # _____

PATIENT INFORMATION

Date of Run |__|__|__|__|__|__|
mo.   day   yr.

VEHICLE # _____

LOCATION
_____

DISPOSITION
_____

Last Name   First   MI

Home Address   Street/RFD

City   State   ZIP

Age ____ DOB |__|__|__|__|__|__| Sex: M F
mo.   day   yr.

Physician(s)

Insurance

	TIME	
Serv Noti	_____	
Time Out	_____	
At Scene	_____	
Dep Scene	_____	
At Dest	_____	
In Serv	_____	

VHF ☐   Emer. ☐
S.O.P. ☐   Non. Emer. ☐
Phone to ☐
Cellular Phone ☐

MILEAGE
Ending |__|__|__|__|__|
Beginning |__|__|__|__|__|
Run Total |__|__|__|__|__|

CAUSE OF INJURY
01 Assault/Batt
02 Bicycle
03 Chemical
04 Electrical
05 Fall
06 Fire/Explos
07 Gun/Knife
08 Moped
09 Motor Veh
10 Motorcycle
11 Rail/Air
12 Sports/Rec
13 Veh/Ped
14 Water Acc
99 Other

ASSESSED CONDITION
01 Allergic Reaction
02 Behavioral/OD
03 Cancer
04 Cardiac
05 Cardio/Resp
06 Diabetes
07 Exposure - Cold
08 Exposure - Heat
09 GI/GU
10 Neonate
11 Neuro/Seizure
12 OB/GYN
13 Poison
14 Respiratory
15 Trauma
16 Vascular/Stroke
99 Other

VITAL SIGNS

Time	Respiratory Rate	Effort	Pulse Rate	Quai	B/P	Cap Ref	Glasgow Scale ④ Eye	⑤ Ver	⑥ Mot	⑮ Tot	Pulse - OX Reading
		1 Nor 0 Abn 0 Abs		0 Reg 0 Irr		2 Nor 1 Del 0 Abs					
		1 Nor 0 Abn 0 Abs		0 Reg 0 Irr		2 Nor 1 Del 0 Abs					
		1 Nor 0 Abn 0 Abs		0 Reg 0 Irr		2 Nor 1 Del 0 Abs					

Lung Sounds _____
Skin Color/Temp/Moist _____
Pupils _____

PAST MED HISTORY   ALLERGIES

CURRENT MEDS

IV SOLUTIONS   Number attempted _____   Number successful _____

TIME	BAG SIZE/TYPE	RATE

AID PROVIDED BY OTHERS?
Y   N   TX Number
01 Citizen _____
02 Fire _____
03 FR _____
04 Law Enf. _____
05 Med Pers _____

TREATMENT (TX)
01 Airway Cleared
02 Airway Adjunct _____ type
03 Bleed Control _____ method
04 Cervical Collar
05 Cold/Heat Applied
06 CPR (time began) _____
07 Dressing Applied
08 Elevation
09 MAST Applied
10 MAST Inflated _____ time
11 OB Assist
12 O2 _____ LPM via _____
13 Psychological Support
14 Restraints Used
15 Scoop
16 Spineboard-Long
17 K.E.D.
18 Heart Monitor
19 Defibrilation
20 Bashaw
21 Splint _____ type
22 Doppler
23 I.V. Maintenance
24 I.V. Therapy
25 Other

DEFINITIVE THERAPY

TIME	ECG RHYTHM/RATE	DRUG/DOSE/ROUTE	DEFIB/JOULES

INTUBATION
TIME   ATTEMPTS
CT _____   _____
ET _____   _____

NARRATIVE

_____

PERSONNEL   Title / Cert #
Driver _____
Attendant _____
Attendant _____

Fig. 15-1 Traditional prehospital care report in written format.

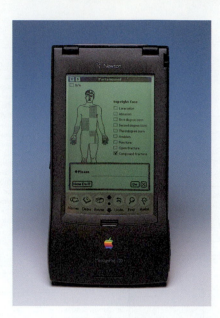

Fig. 15-2 A computer-based prehospital report system.

Run Data

Run data are data regarding the operational aspects of the call, without the patient element. Run data include the following elements:

• Date
• Times (notification, en route, at the scene, depart the scene, arrive at hospital, back in service)
• Service name
• Unit number
• Crew members' names
• EMS call identifier (usually a number)

Patient Data

Patient data are just as the name implies. Patient data are information specific to the patient. Patient data include the following elements:

• Name
• Address
• Date of birth
• Insurance information
• Gender
• Age
• Nature of illness/mechanism of injury
• Location of patient
• Treatment rendered before the EMT's arrival (if applicable)
• Signs (objective), symptoms (subjective)
• Emergency care administered by the EMT or others
• Vital signs

• SAMPLE history (*S*igns and symptoms, *A*llergies, *M*edications, *P*ast medical history, *L*ast oral intake, *E*vents preceding)
• Changes in the patient's condition
• To whom the patient care was turned over and where

Check Boxes

Many forms have a check box, circle, or fill-in-the-blank area for ease of use. These features aid in the efficiency of documentation. These areas may include information such as male/female, medical/trauma, assessed condition, and other information common to all patients. Check boxes also may appear for common treatment information, such as oxygen administered, splinting, and patient refusal of transport. In addition, some forms may have a fill-in-the-box area for vital signs or other information that frequently is gathered in the patient assessment. With any check box, be sure to fill in the box completely. Be careful not to leave unintentional marks on the form.

Patient Narrative

Run report forms generally have a section for the patient narrative. The patient narrative is a description in the writer's own words of the events of the call. Complete and accurate documentation is important when one is writing this section of the PCR. Correct spelling, accurate use of medical terms, and a conscientious attention to detail are paramount. Information in the patient narrative section should not conflict with information in other parts of the run report. Vital signs and treatments listed in the check box area should not conflict with what is described in the patient narrative section. For example, in the vital signs section, if you note that the patient's initial breathing rate is 20 breaths per minute and your narrative states the patient's breathing rate is 36, then there is a conflict. Your narrative should explain why the rate is different from that documented in the "boxed" area.

In the patient narrative, the EMT should describe the call without making conclusions. You can determine what to include for complete and accurate documentation by what you learn in assessment and intervention for patients, including the following:

• Scene size-up
• Initial assessment
• Focused history and physical exam/rapid assessment
• SAMPLE history
• Treatment provided

- Ongoing assessment
- Transfer of care

Subjective information can be included in the narrative; this information may be helpful and relevant. However, you should make a distinction between the information that is subjective by using quotation marks around what the patient stated or what bystanders stated.

As mentioned previously, a common phrase in health care is "If it wasn't written down, it wasn't done." Keep this in mind when completing any PCR.

Pertinent negatives

Pertinent negatives are important to document in the patient narrative. Pertinent negatives are signs or symptoms that are not present but that you would expect to see given a specific scenario. An example of a pertinent negative is a patient with a chief complaint of headache but who has no history of recent or past head trauma.

Scene information

Include important information regarding the scene. In a motor vehicle collision, information such as the position of the vehicles, path of impact (e.g., head-on, side, rear-end), location of the patients, use of seat belts, environment (weather), and surroundings can be important in determining the mechanism of injury. Some EMS services use Polaroid or digital photography at the scene of a crash to help visually describe the vehicle damage. Record any unusual circumstances about the scene as well. You may be the only person who has access to that information, information that could be essential in determining a patient's needed treatment. Unusual odors in the home, such as gas, can be a key factor in assessing a patient's condition and determining appropriate treatment. Documentation for suspected suicide or crime scenes should also include pertinent information regarding the scene.

Several methods can be used for writing the patient narrative. Some EMS providers prefer to write their patient care narrative sequentially, in the order the events occurred. Some providers prefer a more structured method. Box 15-3 shows examples of charting methods that can be helpful when writing a patient narrative.

Medical abbreviations

Use of medical abbreviations is common in documentation. You must be certain, however, that the abbreviations you use are universal and will be understood easily by other health care providers

---

BOX 15-3

Report Writing Methods

CHART Method

C: Chief complaint—What the patient tells you

H: History—The history of the present illness, including any precipitating events and medications the patient currently is taking

A: Assessment—The full assessment, including initial and focused

R: (Rx) Treatment—Treatment to the patient at the scene, including any treatment provided before emergency medical services arrival. Include patient response to interventions.

T: Transport—Treatment provided to the patient en route to the medical facility and patient response to interventions. To whom care was transferred at the medical facility and the condition of the patient at that time

SOAP Method

S: Subjective—Information that the patient or bystanders tell you

O: Objective—Observations made from your physical examination of the patient and observations of the scene

A: Assessment—Your physical assessment of the patient and your field impression

P: Plan—Treatment you provided to the patient

(Table 15-1). Approved medical abbreviations may be used. Your service should have a list of approved standard abbreviations that may be used in documentation. Avoid radio codes altogether in the written report. Other health care providers may not be familiar with radio codes or may have a different system for radio codes than the organization for which you work.

Sensitive and protected information

When documenting sensitive information, such as a potential crime or a communicable disease, you should be sure to document the source of the information. The source of the information may include, for example, law enforcement, the patient, or bystanders. These should be clearly identified in your documentation as the source of the information provided.

State reporting requirements

You should be familiar with and comply with any reporting requirements of your state. Certain types of patient calls have attached reporting requirements.

TABLE 15-1

Common abbreviations and symbols used in prehospital care documentation

Abbreviation or Symbol	Definition
♂	Male
♀	Female
$\bar{a}$	Before
BP	Blood pressure
BVM	Bag-valve-mask
$\bar{c}$	With
c/o	Complaining of
CPR	Cardiopulmonary resuscitation
DOB	Date of birth
Hx	History
LLQ	Left lower quadrant (of abdomen)
LUQ	Left upper quadrant (of abdomen)
NTG	Nitroglycerin
O_2	Oxygen
po	By mouth
Pt	Patient
Px	Physical examination
RLQ	Right lower quadrant (of abdomen)
RUQ	Right upper quadrant (of abdomen)
SL	Sublingual
SOB	Shortness of breath
Tx	Treatment
y/o	Years old

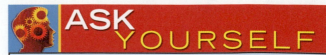

ASK YOURSELF

You and your partner respond to a 911 call requesting assistance for a motor vehicle collision involving a single vehicle. Upon arrival, you survey the scene and see a compact vehicle sitting upright in the roadway. Law enforcement has secured the scene and is directing traffic. First responders are on scene assisting the patient. First responders report that this adult patient is alert and conscious with airway, breathing, and circulation intact. They direct you to the patient, who is still in the vehicle, with vehicle restraints in place.

What about the scene survey is important to document?

What is the significance in documenting the position and condition in which the vehicle was found?

Is it important to document what the first responders reported to you?

Is it important to document how this patient is removed from the vehicle? Why?

Other than questions relating to your physical assessment, what other questions are important to ask the patient?

Is it important to obtain the names of first responders who assisted this patient?

When you approach this patient, she states she feels fine and does not feel she needs treatment or transport.

What is your appropriate action at this point?

What would you tell your patient to convince her to agree to treatment and transport?

What is important to document on the patient refusal form about this scenario?

For instance, there are mandatory reporting laws for child and dependent adult abuse and for criminal activity or communicable diseases. Become familiar with local and state requirements and the methods your organization has for reporting these situations.

Accurate, thorough, and legible documentation

Be sure you spell words correctly. Correct spelling of all medical terms and simple words is critical for clarity, accuracy, and credibility in your report. If you are not sure how to spell a word correctly, do not guess. Find out, or use a different word with the same meaning.

For the ongoing assessment, record times and findings. Even if vital signs have not changed or the patient's condition has not changed, this information still should be documented with a time. That way, it is clear that the patient's condition was the same at that specific time. If your service uses a handwritten report, be sure to write or print legibly. When others, or even you, cannot read and interpret what has been written in the report because of poor handwriting, it is not only embarrassing but also unacceptable.

■ CONFIDENTIALITY

As with all other medical records, the PCR is confidential. The PCR is patient information; thus it is protected by laws of **patient confidentiality.** Be aware of state laws that address how and what information can be released and to whom. Release and distribution of the completed form should comply with local and state protocol and law.

HEALTH INSURANCE PORTABILITY AND ACCOUNTABILITY ACT

The Health Insurance Portability and Accountability Act (HIPAA) created national standards to protect individual's medical records and other personal health-related information while also giving patients more control over their health information. The act sets limitations on the use and release of health records and establishes safeguards that health care providers must implement to protect the privacy of a patient's health information.

Because HIPAA has different levels of standards based on the health care provider and/or services provided, each EMT should check with his or her employer to learn how HIPAA requirements are to be applied and met.

FALSIFICATION

Falsification of any type of medical report is a crime. Inclusion of false information or omission of information about the call is illegal. Not only is it illegal, but also it puts the patient at risk. The continuum of medical care for the patient can be affected significantly by what is in your documentation. This is particularly relevant if you make an error in your patient care. Make it clear in your documentation what you did, what steps you took to remedy the situation, and what the results to the patient were. In the best interest to you and your patient, document honestly what occurred. Falsifying patient documents subjects you to possible revocation or suspension of your EMT certification or license. It also puts you and your ambulance service at risk of legal action.

PATIENT REFUSAL

Any competent adult has the right to refuse treatment. If you encounter this situation, you should treat the patient with respect regarding his or her wishes. However, you also should make every effort to ensure the patient is informed of and understands the potential consequences of his or her refusal of treatment. You can do this by explaining the potential risks of not receiving medical care in simple terms that can be understood easily. You also should be certain the patient is able to make a rational decision and is not influenced by drugs, alcohol, injury, or illness, which may affect his or her judgment.

You should attempt to persuade the patient to seek medical treatment. Enlist the aid of the patient's family or friends at the scene. If the patient continues to refuse transport or treatment, ask the patient if you can take vital signs as well as complete any other assessment that you feel is needed at the scene. Conducting a brief assessment will enable you to document the patient's condition while you are at the scene. Contact medical direction as indicated by local protocol.

Any patient who has refused treatment or transport should sign a **patient refusal form** (Fig. 15-3). Read the form to the patient and explain its content and purpose. The form should be signed by the patient and by a witness. If the patient refuses to sign the form, have a family member or bystander sign it.

You also should assure the patient that it is acceptable to contact you for help again, if he or she changes his or her mind, his or her medical condition worsens, or to seek alternative medical care if he or she wishes.

Even in the case of a patient refusal, you should complete the PCR and attach the completed and signed patient refusal form. The PCR should include as much information as possible. It also should follow the same documentation guidelines used for patients who are treated and transported. Include patient assessment findings, vital signs, recommendations for care, treatment provided if any, and information to inform the patient and persuade him or her to approve of transport and treatment. The documentation of patient refusal is just as crucial as the documentation for patients to whom treatment is provided.

SPECIAL SITUATIONS/ INCIDENT REPORTING

Error Corrections

Correct errors made while writing the PCR. This can be accomplished by drawing a single line through the error, initialing it, and writing the correct information beside it. Do not try to obliterate the error. This act could be interpreted as trying to mask an error in patient care.

Errors discovered after the PCR has been submitted also should be corrected by drawing a single line through the error. However, use a different color of ink. Initial and date it and add a note with the correct information. Information that was omitted erroneously should be added with an additional note. The EMT also should initial and date this. (Follow local protocol.)

GCH EMS RELEASE FORM

I, THE UNDERSIGNED, DO AGREE THAT THE GREATER COMMUNITY HOSPITAL AMBULANCE SERVICE ANSWERED MY CALL FOR ASSISTANCE TO MY SATISFACTION. THROUGH MY OWN FREE WILL, (OR SOMEONE RESPONSIBLE), I AT THIS TIME REFUSE THE SERVICE OF THE AFOREMENTIONED ORGANIZATION AND RELEASE GCH EMS AND ANYONE AFFILIATED WITH IT OF ANY RESPONSIBILITY FOR MY HEALTH AND WELL BEING.

THE POSSIBLE CONSEQUENCES OF MY REFUSING MEDICAL TREATMENT AND NECESSARY PRECAUTIONS LISTED BELOW, WERE EXPLAINED TO ME AND I UNDERSTAND COMPLETELY:

HEAD INJURY

_____ Hard to wake up
_____ Change in usual behavior
_____ Can't walk or talk right
_____ Vomits more than once
_____ Headache that worsens over 24 hours
_____ Blurred vision, double vision, or unequal pupils

SPRAIN INJURY

_____ Elevate injured part above the level of chest
_____ Use cold packs while swollen, for 20 min., several times/day.

INFECTIONS/LACERATIONS

_____ Keep area clean and dry
_____ Call your Dr. if you have any of the following:
Pus, red streaking, worse pain, fever, or chills.

SPECIAL INSTRUCTIONS

_____
_____
_____
_____
_____
_____

VITAL SIGNS

BP_____ PULSE _____ RESP. _____

_____ Pt. refuses to allow vital signs to be taken.

_____ Pt. refuses the recommended immobilization, but does agree to be transported.

I was advised to, and will seek further medical care as needed, if any of the above or other symptoms develop or worsen.

_____   _____
Witness   Name (Print)

_____   _____
Witness   Address

_____   _____
Driver   Date of Birth   Age

_____   _____
Attendant   Signature

_____   _____
Date   Time   Relationship to Patient

Fig. 15-3 Patient refusal form.

Multiple-Casualty Incidents

In some situations a call cannot be documented immediately. It may be necessary to complete a detailed prehospital report at a later time if, for instance, there are multiple patients or there is a high call volume. Generally, reports should be completed as soon as possible. However, if it is physically impossible to do so, the EMT should take notes about the patient and use these notes to aid in completing the report later. Often in this situation, triage tags, patient summary sheets, or abbreviated patient report forms are used. Your local multiple-casualty plan should have guidelines regarding the appropriate methods for documentation in these instances.

Special Situation Reports

Certain events in the prehospital management of patient care may warrant special reporting guidelines in addition to the PCR. Common occurrences that may have special reporting requirements are the following:

- Child abuse
- Dependent adult abuse
- Suspected criminal activity
- Hazardous materials incidents
- Employee injury
- Exposure of the patient or care provider to bloodborne pathogens
- Certain communicable diseases
- Documentation of restraint usage

These reports, just as any other medical report, should be documented and submitted to the appropriate authorities in a timely manner. They should be accurate and complete as well. Moreover, the EMT should attach a copy to the PCR and keep a copy for his or her own records. Local protocol should explain what type of documentation format to use and to whom the documentation should be submitted. In some cases, local protocol also may specify a time line requirement for submission of special documentation or reporting.

RESOURCES

Stanford TM: *EMS report writing: a pocket reference*, Englewood Cliffs, NJ, 1992, Prentice Hall.

Birmingham J: *Medical terminology*, ed 3, St Louis, 1999, Mosby.

Gurchiek D, Maggiore WA: How to document the unthinkable, *JEMS*, 29(10):78-85, 2004.

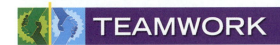

TEAMWORK

In many calls for prehospital medical care, other providers are also aiding the patient. Documentation should always include other resources that have been assisting with the call. Law enforcement on scene, medical first responders, and others are an important element and integral part of patient management in the prehospital setting.

Other resources may provide you with their documentation to aid in the continuity of care for the patient. A first responder may give you a written handoff report of the patient condition and assessment he or she performed before your arrival. As the emergency medical technician providing continued care for the patient, you also should provide written documentation to the care providers to whom you transfer the patient care. This written documentation is an important part of the overall patient care and management of the call. It provides a written sequence of events from the initial patient contact to the disposition of the patient for definitive medical care.

CASE SCENARIO

Ray and his partner already were heading back to the hospital as he was finishing the narrative section of the patient care report. It took longer than normal for Ray to complete the form; there was a lot of information and detail that he wanted to document. He also realized that he had made a mistake on the form and crossed it out. After initialing the cross-out, he filled in the correct information next to it. ■

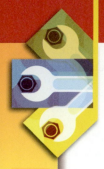

Critical Points

The importance of documentation cannot be overstated. Documentation should encompass the entire call, from initial notification of the transport EMS service to disposition of the patient at the medical facility. Documentation offers legal protection for the provider and the EMS organization. Moreover, documentation provides vital information to other health care professionals in providing continued care for the patient.

Learning Checklist

❑ Components of the prehospital care report include the minimum data set. Minimum data set includes patient information and administrative information. Documentation should be completed using synchronized time. Synchronous time recording assists in evaluating patient trends and appropriate treatments.

❑ Continuity of care for the patient is a critical aspect of patient care. Continuity of care often depends on documentation from the previous health care provider.

❑ The prehospital care report is a legal document. As such, the prehospital care report can offer protection to the emergency medical technician in defending his or her actions in case legal litigation should occur. Generally, the person completing the prehospital care report is also the person who testifies in court.

❑ Documentation should be objective. Objective documentation states factually what the prehospital care provider observed or assessed. Subjective information, what the patient perceives and expresses to you, should be identified clearly in the documentation as such.

❑ The prehospital care report has many educational uses. It can be used to evaluate a call, assess quality improvement, and build on documentation skills.

❑ Administration uses the prehospital care report for billing and statistical information.

Accurate documentation can aid in evaluating system needs and improvement. In addition, documentation can be an important source of determining appropriate reimbursement benefits for the patient.

❑ Research is an important part of health care. Growth of emergency medical services and improved patient care and outcomes are based on the analysis of research. Research often is conducted using prehospital care report documentation. Accuracy and data are essential to researchers in any given study.

❑ Evaluation and continuous quality improvement are required in system response building and improved patient care. Change in system response and changes in patient treatment standards should be evaluated continually and improved upon where needed.

❑ Prehospital care reports come in traditional and handwritten formats and, more recently, electronic formats. Regardless of the format, prehospital care reports have common sections: run data and patient data. Run data are operational information about the run exclusive of patient information. Patient data are information about the specific patient. Most prehospital care reports have a check box, circle, or fill-in-the-box area, as well as an area to write the patient narrative. The check box areas aid in ease of documentation and contain information that may be common to all patients. The patient narrative section should describe the call in the writer's own words.

❑ The ambulance agency should have a list of common, approved medical abbreviations that may be used. Avoid the use of radio codes when completing documentation.

❑ Always identify information that comes from sources other than the patient. Sensitive information provided about crime scenes or certain communicable diseases should have the source clearly identified in your documentation.

❑ Falsifying documentation is a criminal act that is subject to legal action. Falsifying a

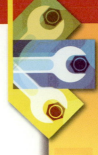

document puts your certification or licensure at risk, and most importantly, it can put your patient at risk for inappropriate medical care.

❑ Special forms should be available to document a patient refusal. The patient and a witness should sign the forms. Attempts to persuade the patient to accept transport and treatment should be well documented. In addition, the emergency medical technician should document the discussion of consequences of refusing patient care. Moreover, the emergency medical technician should assure the patient that he or she may call for assistance again, if needed. Prehospital care providers should complete a prehospital care report and attach documentation of the completed patient refusal form.

❑ Errors made while documenting should be corrected by drawing a line through the error, not by obscuring the error. This correction should be initialed. The correction should be written beside the error or clearly defined on an attached note.

❑ Multiple-casualty incidents have unique documentation requirements. These documents take into consideration the situation and volume of patients. Know your local protocol for documentation requirements during these incidents.

❑ Special situations can arise in which the emergency medical technician may need to complete documentation in addition to the prehospital care report. Examples of such incidents include injury to the prehospital care providers, exposure to blood-borne pathogens, suspected dependent adult or child abuse, and criminal acts. Know your local protocol for documentation requirements in these situations.

Key Terms

Administrative information Information that relates to the call but not specifically to the patient, such as date and time of dispatch.

Continuity of care Care that is continued by other health care providers after the patient has been released from your care.

Continuous quality improvement Continual evaluation of system response and patient care with the purpose of maintaining or obtaining the highest standard of care possible.

Critique Evaluation of an emergency medical services call through documentation.

Minimum data set Data that include patient information and administrative information documented on the prehospital care report. This information is used for statistical purposes.

Objective information Factual information that is based on observations of the emergency medical technician.

Patient confidentiality The legal right of patients to have their medical information protected and not shared.

Patient data Data about the call that are specific to the patient.

Patient information Information that relates specifically to the patient, such as age and gender.

Patient refusal form Specific form to document a patient's refusal of treatment and transport.

Patient trends Evaluation of a sequence of patient vital signs and assessments that indicate improvement or deterioration of the patient's condition.

Pertinent negatives Findings that are not present that may be expected given the scenario.

Prehospital care report The standard form used for documenting patient care in emergency medical services systems; also referred to as a patient care report or PCR.

Quality assurance Method of ensuring quality patient care and system response.

Run data Data about the call that do not include the patient element.

Subjective information Information that is perceived by the patient or bystanders and not by the emergency medical technician.

Synchronized time recording The act of matching your time device (wristwatch) with that of other time devices (wall clock).

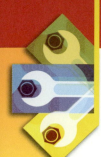

NUTS AND BOLTS

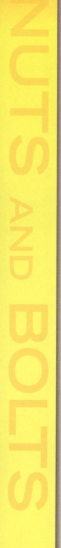

National Standard Curriculum Objectives

Cognitive Objectives

After completing this lesson, the EMT student will be able to do the following:

- Explain the components of the written report and list information that should be included in the written report.
- Identify the various sections of the written report.

- Describe the required information in each section of the prehospital care report and the way in which it should be entered.
- Define the special considerations concerning patient refusal.
- Describe the legal implications associated with the written report.
- Discuss state and/or local record and reporting requirements.

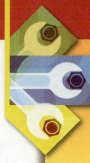

Affective Objectives

After completing this lesson, the EMT student will be able to do the following:

- Explain the rationale for patient care documentation.
- Explain the rationale for using medical terminology correctly.
- Explain the rationale for using an accurate and synchronous clock to aid in trending observations.

Psychomotor Objective

After completing this lesson, the EMT student will be able to do the following:

- Complete a patient care report.

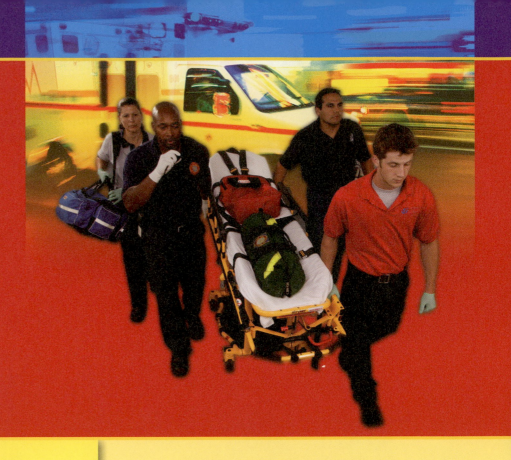

CHAPTER

16

OUTLINE

LESSON GOAL

This lesson introduces the emergency medical technician student to an overview of pharmacology as it relates to emergency medical services. Students will learn drug names, forms, indications for usage, and how to assist patients in self-administering medications. They also will become familiar with prescription labels to obtain vital information about medications. ∎

GOAL

Pharmacology

CHAPTER OBJECTIVES

After completing this chapter, the EMT student will be able to do the following:

1 Using the generic name, identify the medications that are carried on the unit.

2 Name the types of medications for which the emergency medical technician may assist the patient in administration.

3 Discuss the various forms of medications.

4 Discuss the purpose of the administration of medications to patients.

5 Be able to demonstrate the process for assisting a patient who is self-administering a medication.

6 Be familiar with prescription medication labels in order to obtain vital information about those medications.

OBJECTIVES

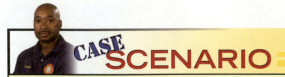

CASE SCENARIO

Auntie Janice looks awfully pale, Jack thought to himself. They were at a family picnic. The kids were off splashing in the lake, and the adults were kicking back in the shade of a few large oak trees. Jack knew that Janice had been to the doctor's office lately for some medical problems she had been experiencing. Touching her on the shoulder, Jack asked, "Auntie, are you feeling okay?"

"I'm not sure. I feel like I'm having some squeezing in my chest." She pointed to the center of her chest, clutching her fist.

"Have you had this before?"

"Yes. I had been seeing Dr. Trinh for it. He's not sure what it is exactly."

Jack felt his aunt's radial pulse. It felt strong, though a little fast. Her skin did not feel cool and was dry. "Did Dr. Trinh prescribe you any medication?"

"He did." She began to reach for her purse. "I think it's in here."

Jack motioned her to stop. "Is it okay if I got it for you? I just want you to relax for now and not exert yourself."

Janice nodded. Reaching in to the purse, Jack found a small spray bottle that looked like a breath freshener dispenser, only a little thicker. "Is this it? Nitroglycerin spray?"

"Yes, that's it."

Question: What does nitroglycerin do? What can Jack deduce about Janice's medical condition?

The topic of pharmacology can be rather intimidating, regardless of one's level of training or education. The percentage of individuals who are taking at least one form of medication continues to rise annually. However, the prehospital provider does not need to know the names of all of the potential medications patients may be taking, although knowledge of the most common medications is helpful. Nor does the prehospital provider need to understand the complex chemistry and mechanisms of action of the thousands of commonly used medications. What the emergency medical technician (EMT) does need to know about pharmacotherapy includes the following:

1. Names of the drugs. (Drugs have two names: a **trade name** and a **generic name.**)
2. How to use a pharmacopeia. Names of drugs are listed in a drug "phone book" called a pharmacopeia.
3. How to read a drug label. This will assist in documenting and communicating information about the patient's medications.
4. The critical types of medications that an EMT can help a patient to self-administer.
5. A handful of medications that are safe and easily administered can be life threatening.

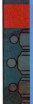

SPECIAL Populations

More than 80% of the elderly in the United States take at least one prescription medication, and one third of those take three or more drugs per day.

■ DRUGS AND THEIR EFFECTS

The first rule of pharmacology for health care providers at all levels is that there is no such thing as a "good (safe) drug." All drugs have adverse effects and risks; however, the beneficial effects of a particular medication typically outweigh the risks. In fact, before prescribing a medication, a physician must determine that the specific benefits of a medication outweigh the potential harmful effects. Upon deciding to start an individual on a particular medication, the physician educates the patient and monitors the patient for the development of potential complications from the administered medication.

The most well-known complication from a medication is an allergic reaction. Allergic reactions have a broad spectrum of clinical presentations (see Chapter 21). The most dramatic of these is **anaphylaxis.** Anaphylaxis is a life-threatening allergic reaction. This reaction may be characterized by rash, swelling, respiratory distress, and shock. Most commonly, a person's allergic response to a medication typically manifests itself as a rash. Such rashes slowly can progress to involve the whole body and, in the case of certain medications, eventually sloughing of the skin.

■ DRUG NAMES

The names of medications can be rather confusing. All drugs have at least two names. A generic name essentially can be viewed as the scientific or chemical name for a drug. The generic name is registered with the U.S. government in a large directory of drugs known as the **United States Pharmacopeia.** The *Pharmacopeia* is similar to a phone book and contains basic information on all medications that are available in the United States. Trade names are the names created for drugs by the drug companies for marketing purposes (Box 16-1). When developing pharmaceutical trade names, most drug companies look for memorable and descriptive names that will help with the marketing of that specific drug to physicians and patients.

■ FORMS OF MEDICATION

Different medications come in different forms. Sometimes a single medication can come in a variety of forms. Often the form of a medication is determined by the nature and urgency of the problem the drug is being used to treat.

If someone is having a severe asthmatic attack, he or she needs relief immediately. An **oral medication** (pill, liquid, suspension) that needs to be swallowed, digested, absorbed, and then circulated through the body may take 30 minutes to an hour to provide the patient with relief. Therefore in the case of asthma, for example, an oral medication is inappropriate, and an inhaled, and in some cases injected, medication is preferable. In contrast, an oral medication is appropriate for the treatment of a stable chronic condition such as hypertension or an acute non–life-threatening condition.

An **injectable medication** can be injected directly into a muscle (intramuscular) or into a vein (intravenous). Injectable medications are absorbed rapidly and circulate through the body, often in less than several minutes. The drawback of injectable medications is that special training is required to administer these, and in the case of **intravenous medications,** one needs special equipment as well. Intravenous routes are preferred for the **administration** of cardiac medications in advanced life support situations in order to deliver the medications to the heart in a matter of minutes. For a patient having an asthmatic attack, intravenous medications would provide the patient with immediate relief. However, an asthmatic patient may have several attacks a day. In addition, these attacks can occur at work or at home. Therefore starting an intravenous line or giving an **intramuscular medication** with each attack is impractical. Instead, **inhaled medications** often are used to deliver medication to patients with asthmatic attacks or other similar respiratory diseases.

Inhaled medications are rapidly active, easy to administer, and often convenient. Most persons with asthma will have prescribed inhalers. These inhalers contain fine powders of medications that will act virtually immediately on the lung when administered. Another form of inhaled medications is liquid medications. These are nebulized into small particles by a machine and then are delivered to the patient by inhalation. Nebulized medications require a small oxygen-powered machine to deliver the medication to the patient. However, not all medications can be administered in this fashion. You must know which medications can and cannot be given this way.

Some medications are delivered by absorption across mucous membranes (mucosa) or the skin. For example, glucose gels (Fig. 16-1) can be administered between the cheek and gums of a diabetic patient with low blood sugar. The glucose gel is absorbed and increases the patient's blood serum glucose level. Nitroglycerin is another medication that can be absorbed in a variety of forms. In one form, nitroglycerin is a compressed powder that is formed into tablets (Fig. 16-2). A nitroglycerin tablet can be placed

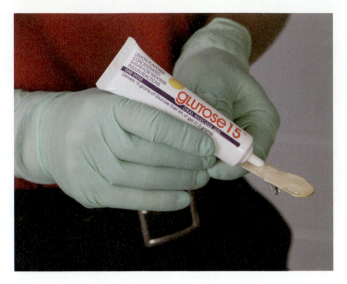

Fig. 16-1 Oral glucose gel.

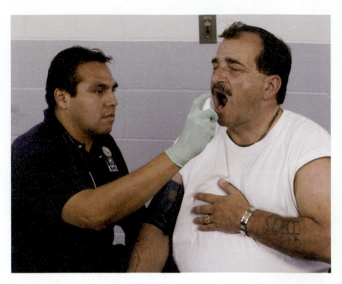

Fig. 16-3 Nitroglycerin spray administered sublingually.

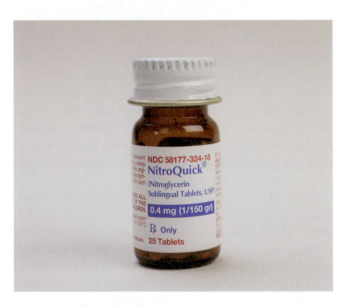

Fig. 16-2 Nitroglycerin tablets.

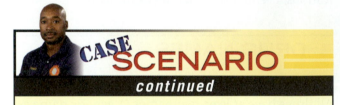

CASE SCENARIO *continued*

"Okay, Janice, Uncle Harold called for the ambulance, and they are on their way." Jack was helping Janice settle into a comfortable position, out of the sun.

"I'll be okay. He didn't have to do that."

"Are you still having that squeezing feeling in your chest?"

"Yes."

Looking at the bottle again, Jack confirmed that the medication was nitroglycerin and that it had not expired. "Okay, I am going to help you with your medication. Follow my directions."

Question: What directions should Jack provide? What are some possible side effects he should tell the patient about?

under a patient's tongue, where the tablet is absorbed rapidly. As an alternative to the tablet, one can spray nitroglycerin under a patient's tongue where it is absorbed rapidly through the mucous membrane (Fig 16-3). A third preparation of nitroglycerin is as a **transdermal medication,** a paste or an ointment that is absorbed through the skin.

Another form of delivering drugs includes the use of gases. The drug most commonly used by prehospital providers is oxygen, which is a **gas** form of a drug. Inhaled nitrous oxide is another drug in the gaseous form that sometimes is used in the prehospital setting.

Each drug is manufactured in one or more of the particular forms mentioned previously to allow the medication to be delivered through the bloodstream in a specific concentration to a target organ. Various forms of a medication exist to provide options for ease and rapidity of delivery based on the needs of the clinical scenario.

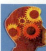

Have you realized the tremendous responsibility that comes with the administration of medications? Have you thought about the following questions: What if I give too much? Too little? Did I administer the medication via the correct route? Did I give the medication to the right patient? How do I ensure that I am administering the medication correctly?

■ VITAL DRUG INFORMATION

Six pieces of vital information exist for every medication: indication, **dosage,** administration, actions, **side effects,** and **contraindications.** Emergency medical technicians need to know the six pieces of vital information for each drug they will be assisting with or delivering to their patients (Box 16-2).

Indications are the reasons for giving a patient the medication. This could be, for example, to treat the respiratory distress of an asthmatic attack or for the relief of chest pain from angina.

Dosage is simply how much of the medication is given to the patient. For nitroglycerin, this could be one tablet. A bronchodilator for treating an asthmatic patient could be two puffs of a metered dose inhaler.

Administration refers to the route used to give the medication to the patient. The route of administration depends largely on the *form of the medication.* Routes of administration include oral, sublingual (under the tongue), mucosal, transdermal (across the skin), inhaled, subcutaneous, intramuscular, or intravenous. Nitroglycerin can be administered sublingually as a tablet or spray and transdermally as a

paste; glucose gel is administered to the oral mucosa at the gum line; activated charcoal (Fig. 16-4) is taken orally as a suspension; and epinephrine can be given as an intramuscular or intravenous injection to treat anaphylaxis.

The **drug actions** are the desired effects of the drug in the treatment of a particular problem. For example, nitroglycerin is given to dilate coronary arteries to provide relief of cardiac chest pain.

Every medication has side effects. Side effects are the nondesirable and sometimes dangerous actions of the administered drug. Some common side effects

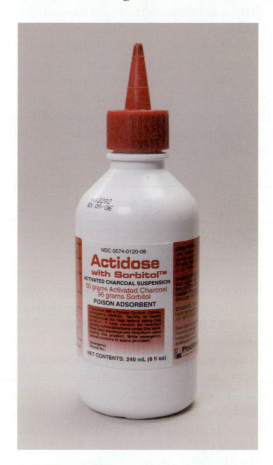

Fig. 16-4 Activated charcoal.

BOX 16-2

Prescription Drug Labeling

All prescription drugs are required to have a label affixed to their container that has, at a minimum, the following information:
Patient's name
Drug name (generic and/or trade name)
Strength of drug
Dosage
Prescribing physician

///CAUTION!

The Five Rights
Before administering any medications to a patient, the emergency medical technician should verify the following rights:
Right patient
Right time
Right drug
Right dose
Right route

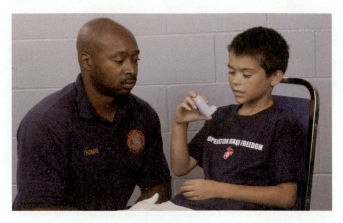

Fig. 16-6 Metered dose inhaler.

of many medications include nausea, emesis (vomiting), diarrhea, tachycardia, hypertension, hypotension, or altered level of consciousness.

Contraindications are those conditions in which the medication should *not* be given to a patient. A drug is contraindicated when a particular patient condition or situation will produce an undesirable effect, such as anaphylaxis, that may harm the patient. This undesirable effect negates any potential benefit of the drug.

■ ASSISTED PATIENT MEDICATION ADMINISTRATION

Emergency medical technicians are permitted to assist patients in taking certain classes of medications that previously have been prescribed by that patient's physician. Of course, this varies based on individual system protocols and medical direction. In the absence of a standing protocol, the EMT should seek approval from medical control before assisting the patient with his or her medication. Those medications with which the EMT can assist include autoinjected epinephrine (EpiPen) (Fig. 16-5), nitroglycerin, and metered dose inhalers (Fig. 16-6; Table 16-1). Details

TABLE 16-1	
Patient-assisted medications	
Generic Name	**Trade Name**
Nitroglycerin	Nitrostat (tablet)
	Nitrolingual (spray)
Autoinjectors	
Epinephrine	EpiPen
	EpiPen Jr
Metered dose inhalers	
Albuterol	Proventil
	Ventolin
Metaproterenol	Alupent

for administering these medications are covered in the chapters addressing specific medical problems. Before administering a patient's medication, the EMT must *read the label*. Also, the EMT must read the *name printed on the label*. Some patients may be taking prescription medications that were not prescribed to them. Only administer medications that are prescribed specifically for your patient. In addition, read the *dosage*; a patient may be taking a medication in a manner other than the way it was prescribed. Administer the medication as it was prescribed or as directed by your medical control.

■ EMERGENCY MEDICAL TECHNICIAN– ADMINISTERED MEDICATIONS

Emergency medical technicians are permitted to administer some medications in certain clinical circum-

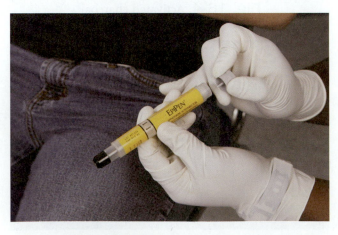

Fig. 16-5 EpiPen (epinephrine).

stances. These medications include activated charcoal, oral glucose gel, and oxygen. Each of these agents is discussed in detail in the respective clinical chapters.

■ DETERMINATION OF EFFECTIVENESS AND REASSESSMENT

Reevaluation of a patient following the administration of any medication is imperative for the provider. Ideally, one hopes to observe that a medication has its desired effect. For instance, one expects that a patient with angina pectoris will experience relief of his or her chest pain after assisting him or her in taking a nitroglycerin tablet. Similarly, a diabetic patient with a low blood sugar should report subjective improvement following application of a glucose gel to the mucous membranes of the mouth. On rare occasions, a patient may have an adverse or even allergic reaction to a medication administered, and the patient's condition actually may worsen following the intervention. Following administration of any medication, a provider needs to repeat taking the vital signs, conduct a repeat patient assessment, and document any observations or changes. As a result, the provider can determine whether the pharmacologic intervention was beneficial. If the patient's condition

does not improve, the prehospital provider will need to seek an alternative mode of therapy. A habit of early and repeated assessment will allow for early and almost immediate intervention to any adverse drug effect.

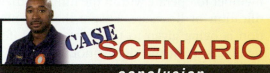

CASE SCENARIO conclusion

Jack noted that his aunt looked like she had less discomfort a few minutes after the administration of nitroglycerin. Janice had complained of a brief headache that also was going away as time went on. "Are you feeling dizzy at all?" he asked Janice.

"No. Do I still need to go to the hospital, Jack?"

"I think you should go, Auntie. I'm not absolutely sure, but it's possible that you might be having some problems with your heart, and I would really like for you to see a doctor right away."

"As long as you come along with me in the ambulance. I would be scared without you."

Jack smiled. "Of course! What is family for, after all?" ■

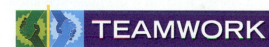

TEAMWORK

As discussed in this chapter, the emergency medical technician first must ensure that he or she is operating within the scope of practice. Although you will be working with other health care providers, remember to do only what is allowed by standing orders or is recommended by medical direction. The emergency medical technician should ensure that a proper report is relayed to those assuming patient care, complete with information relating to the medication given, dose, route, and time administered. Your patient will benefit from your ability to administer a medication.

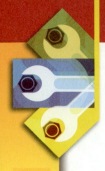

NUTS and BOLTS

Critical Points

Emergency medical technicians must always remember to operate within the limits of their certification or licensure. Ensure that the medication is being given to the right patient, for the right reason, at the right amount, via the right route. Understand the information on the medication label. Stay current on issues related to the medications that you are allowed to administer or with which you may assist.

Learning Checklist

❑ The emergency medical technician needs to know the following aspects of pharmacology: drug names, how to use a pharmacopeia, how to read drug labels, the types of medications an emergency medical technician can assist patients in self-administering, and the medications carried on the ambulance that the emergency medical technician can administer safely.

❑ There is no such thing as a "good (safe) drug"; all drugs have adverse effects and risks.

❑ An allergic reaction is the most well-known complication of medication usage.

❑ Anaphylaxis is a life-threatening allergic reaction. Anaphylaxis may cause rashes, swelling, respiratory distress, and shock.

❑ The generic name of a drug is the scientific or chemical name.

❑ The trade name of a drug is the name used by the drug company that manufactures and markets the drug.

❑ The form of medication is determined by the nature and urgency of the problem the drug is used to treat.

❑ Oral medications include pills, liquids, and suspensions that are taken by mouth.

❑ Injectable medications are injected directly into a muscle or vein.

❑ Inhaled medications are fine powder or liquid forms of medication that are inhaled by mouth or through the patient's nose.

❑ Absorbed medications include gels, pastes, and ointments. The medication is absorbed through the patient's skin.

❑ Indications are the reasons a patient is taking a given medication.

❑ The dosage of a drug is how much of a medication is given to the patient.

❑ Administration refers to the delivery route of the medication. Drugs can be delivered orally, sublingually (under the tongue), mucosally, transdermally (across the skin), intravenously, by inhalation, or intramuscularly.

❑ Drug actions are the desired effects of the medication in treatment of a particular problem.

❑ Side effects are the nondesirable and sometimes dangerous actions of the administered drug.

❑ Contraindications are the conditions in which a patient should *not* take a given medication.

❑ Emergency medical technicians are allowed to assist patients in taking epinephrine by means of an autoinjector (EpiPen), nitroglycerin, and metered dose inhalers.

❑ Emergency medical technicians may administer some medications in certain clinical situations. These include activated charcoal, oral glucose gel, and oxygen.

❑ The five "rights" for medication administration are right patient, right time, right drug, right dose, and right route.

Key Terms

Administration The route or how a drug is delivered.

Anaphylaxis A severe, life-threatening hypersensitivity reaction to a previously encountered antigen that results in vasodilation and subsequent hypotension.

Contraindications Reasons or factors that prohibit administration of a drug.

Dosage Amount of a medication that should be administered.

Drug actions The means by which a drug exerts a desired effect.

Gas The form of a drug or element that is neither liquid nor solid; a gas has no definite shape, and its volume is determined by its container and by temperature and pressure.

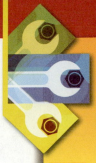
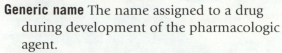
Generic name The name assigned to a drug during development of the pharmacologic agent.

Indications Conditions in which administering a specific drug may benefit the patient.

Inhaled medications Medications that are introduced into the body by breathing in by the mouth or nose.

Injectable medication A medication that is administered by injection beneath the skin or into a vein.

Intramuscular medication A medication that is administered by injection into a muscle.

Intravenous medication A medication that is delivered by injection directly into a vein.

Oral medication A medication that is delivered by mouth.

Side effects Any reactions to or consequences of a medication or therapy.

Trade name The name given to a drug by the manufacturer.

Transdermal medication A medication that is delivered by being applied to the skin; the drug is absorbed through the skin.

United States Pharmacopeia The official publication including all drugs officially recognized by the federal Food, Drug, and Cosmetic Act.

National Standard Curriculum Objectives

Cognitive Objectives

After completing this lesson, the EMT student will be able to do the following:

- Identify which medications will be carried on the unit.
- State the medications carried on the unit by the generic name.
- Identify the medications with which the EMT may assist the patient in administration.
- State the medications with which the EMT can assist the patient by the generic name.
- Discuss the forms in which the medications may be found.

Affective Objective

After completing this lesson, the EMT student will be able to do the following:

- Explain the rationale for the administration of medications.

Psychomotor Objectives

After completing this lesson, the EMT student will be able to do the following:

- Demonstrate general steps for assisting patients with self-administration of medications.
- Read the labels and inspect each type of medication.

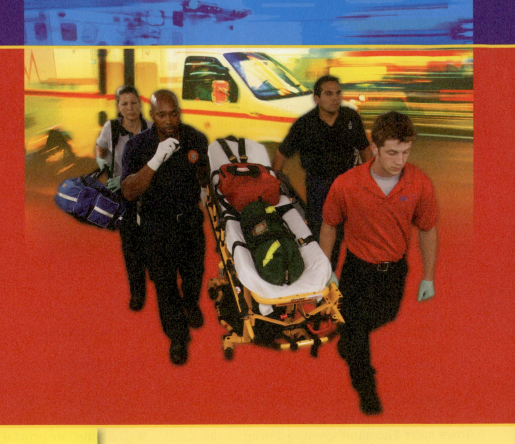

CHAPTER

17

OUTLINE

GOAL

LESSON GOAL

A patient who cannot breathe may deteriorate quickly. The emergency medical technician must be prepared to give a thorough assessment and provide timely treatment and transport to the appropriate medical facility as needed for adults, children, and infants. ■

Respiratory Emergencies

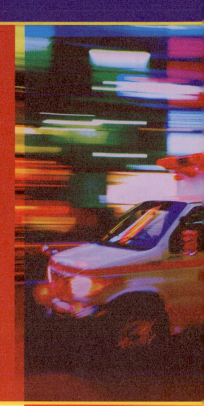

CHAPTER OBJECTIVES

After completing this chapter, the EMT student will be able to do the following:

1. List the parts of the respiratory system and how they work.
2. Discuss the way a patient having breathing problems might present.
3. Describe the emergency medical care of the patient with breathing difficulty.
4. Discuss the role of medical control in the treatment of a patient with breathing difficulty.
5. Describe the emergency medical care of the patient with breathing distress.
6. Discuss when the patient with breathing difficulty may need airway management.
7. List the signs of adequate air exchange.
8. Know and discuss the medications used in a prescribed inhaler.
9. Describe the differences in treating an infant, child, and adult patient with breathing difficulty.
10. Discuss the differences in upper airway obstruction and lower airway disease in the infant and child.
11. Explain the reasons for giving an inhaled treatment.
12. Demonstrate the emergency medical care for breathing difficulty.

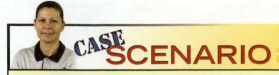

CASE SCENARIO

The nurse's office in the elementary school is typically a quiet, peaceful place—but not today. Sitting on one of the couches is a frightened 6-year-old boy who is having a difficult time taking a deep breath. His chest feels so tight, it is almost as if someone had him in a bear hug and was preventing him from expanding his chest. Usually when this happens his mom or dad takes care of him and it gets better, but he is at school and they were not there to comfort him. The school nurse is there, but she is trying to put a green mask on him and it makes him even more scared.

Elizabeth and her crew enter through the doorway. As she sizes up the scene, she notes that the school nurse is attempting to place a simple face mask on the face of a boy who wants nothing to do with it. The boy's face appears pale, and Elizabeth can hear wheezing even though the boy is several feet away.

Question: What can Elizabeth do to reassure this young boy? What signs and symptoms should she assess?

One of the most common complaints to which the emergency medical technician (EMT) will respond is difficulty breathing, or **dyspnea.** Patients who are having difficulty breathing may deteriorate rapidly. For the responding EMT, these patients need thorough assessment, timely treatment, and transport to the appropriate medical facility. Numerous conditions may cause difficulty breathing, and numerous factors often are involved. Chest pain, as well as the accompanying anxiety, may cause a patient to feel as if he or she cannot catch his or her breath, just as a broken leg may increase the respiratory rate. The job of the EMT is to provide the appropriate treatment, not necessarily to identify correctly the exact cause of the dyspnea.

This chapter focuses on the anatomy and physiology of the respiratory system, the pathophysiology of respiratory diseases and conditions, the assessment of respiratory status, the indicators of adequate and inadequate breathing, and the standard treatment for those patients experiencing respiratory difficulty.

From the perspective of patients, rarely is any situation as important and immediate as when they feel as though they cannot breathe. They need the EMT to be confident, calm, reassuring, and effective in managing their emergency. The information in this chapter provides the EMT with the necessary knowledge and tools to manage patients with respiratory distress effectively.

■ RESPIRATORY SYSTEM ANATOMY AND PHYSIOLOGY

You previously have covered the anatomy and physiology of the respiratory system. That information is reviewed in this section in an effort to enhance your ability to assess and treat the patient with respiratory distress.

Upper Airway

Under normal conditions, ambient air (room air contains roughly 21% oxygen) enters through the nose. The nasal passages are thickly lined and richly supplied with blood, allowing the inspired air to become warmed and slightly humidified. The air also is filtered by the hairs and cilia lining the nasal passages. When patients are short of breath, you may see open-mouth breathing in an attempt to pull in even more air. (Consider an athlete who has just finished a 400-m dash, or an EMT who has just run up three flights of stairs.) This open-mouth breathing is often a sign of respiratory distress. In these cases, the air then enters the pharynx, which passes the air to the larynx. The entrance to the esophagus is also located at this level. The larynx, or voice box, serves as the entrance to the trachea, or windpipe. Externally, the larynx can be identified by the Adam's apple. At the top of the larynx is the epiglottis. This leaf-shaped structure guards the entrance to the trachea. The epiglottis prevents food and liquid from entering the trachea during swallowing. You no doubt have experienced this airway protection firsthand when trying to drink and talk at the same time. The epiglottis is open to allow air out of the trachea and to allow speech, and the liquid runs right down "the wrong pipe." The resultant airway reaction involves forceful coughing in an attempt to rid the airway of the foreign substance. The reaction also can involve laryngospasm (the involuntary closing of the vocal cords in the larynx) to prevent further insult.

The trachea is approximately 11 cm long and approximately 2 cm in diameter.[1] (The trachea is usually the size of the patient's little finger.) Anatomically, the trachea is located in the neck and chest and runs from approximately the sixth cervical vertebra to the fifth thoracic vertebra and is supported by C-shaped rings of cartilage. The trachea bifurcates (divides) into the left and right mainstem bronchi. The right mainstem bronchus is shorter and more vertical than the left. The mainstem bronchi continue to divide, with the walls becoming thinner with each division (Fig. 17-1).

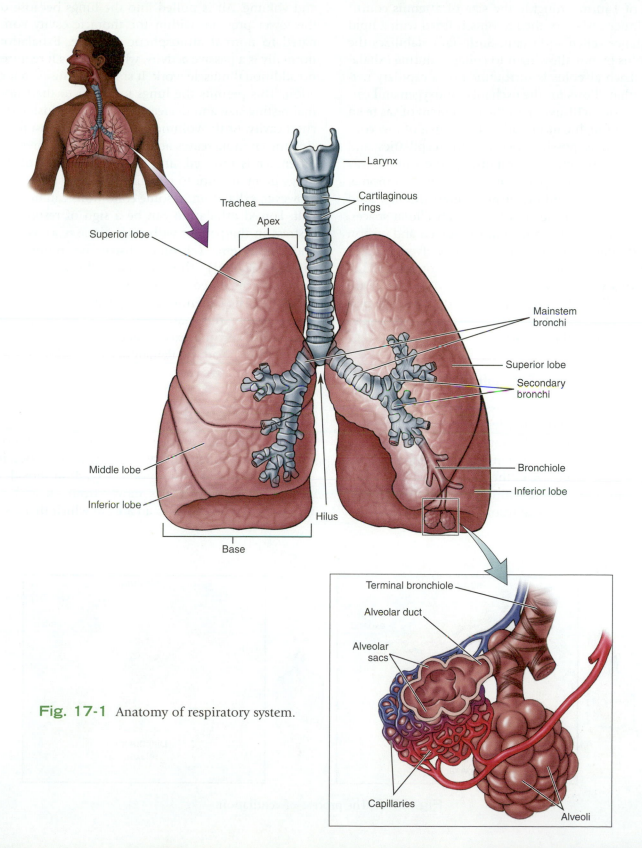

Fig. 17-1 Anatomy of respiratory system.

Lower Airway

The bronchi further divide into bronchial tubes, bronchioles, alveolar ducts, alveolar sacs, and ultimately into the functional unit of respiration: the alveolus. Alveoli are thin-walled sacs numbering about 300 million and provide an exchange surface area of 140 m^2, roughly the size of a tennis court.[1] The inner surface of the alveolus is lined with a lipid substance called surfactant. Surfactant stabilizes the alveolus by not allowing it to collapse during exhalation. Each alveolus is surrounded by a capillary network that allows for the exchange of oxygen and carbon dioxide. **Diffusion,** or the movement of gas from an area of high concentration to an area of low concentration, is possible because the capillaries and alveoli are in contact, with nothing to get in the way of the gas exchange. (In diseases such as pneumonia, congestive heart failure, or **pulmonary edema,** fluid or mucus can fill the alveolar or extracellular spaces, making it more difficult to move oxygen and carbon dioxide into and out of the patient's alveolar capillaries.) The pulmonary circulation consists of the pulmonary artery, which carries *deoxygenated* blood to the lungs, the capillary network, and the pulmonary vein, which carries *oxygenated* blood back to the left atrium of the heart.

Mechanics of Respiration

Inspiration is an active process requiring muscle contraction. The inferior border of the chest cavity is comprised by the diaphragm. The diaphragm is a thin sheet of muscle that upon inspiration flattens out, increasing the size of the thoracic cavity and thus decreasing the pressure within the lungs. In addition, the accessory muscles of respiration—namely, the intercostal muscles, muscles of the neck, and the abdominal muscles—also contract, increasing the volume of the chest cavity, which in turn further lowers the pressure within it. Air then enters the chest cavity in an attempt to equalize pressure.

An inverse relationship exists between pressure and volume. Air is pulled into the lungs because of the lower pressure within the thoracic cavity compared to normal atmospheric pressure. Exhalation normally is a passive activity, which means it requires no additional muscle work. It simply is muscle relaxation. This permits the lungs to return to their normal resting size and decreases the volume inside the chest cavity. As the volume decreases, the pressure inside the chest increases accordingly, and the pressure difference is reversed, and air is pushed out of the lungs in an attempt to equalize pressure (Fig. 17-2). However, exhalation in some conditions can be difficult. Forced exhalation can be a sign of respiratory distress in the patient with such diseases as **asthma** and **emphysema (chronic obstructive pulmonary disease [COPD]).** Those patients who are working hard to exhale require aggressive assessment and treatment. The patient is working hard to push the air out through the narrowed air passages (bronchospasm) and the excess mucus that is produced with an asthma attack. Remember, exhalation should occur with relative ease.

Gas Exchange

The alveoli contain air rich in oxygen, and the blood from the pulmonary artery contains blood poor in oxygen and full of waste products (carbon dioxide). As covered previously, gas moves from an area in which there is an excess to an area in which there is a

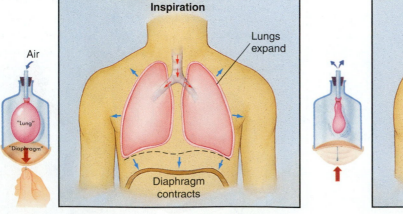
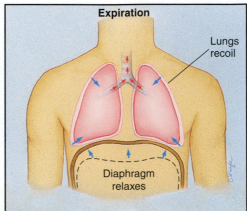

Fig. 17-2 The process of ventilation.

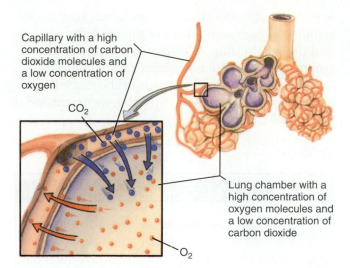

Capillary with a high concentration of carbon dioxide molecules and a low concentration of oxygen

CO_2

Lung chamber with a high concentration of oxygen molecules and a low concentration of carbon dioxide

O_2

Fig. 17-3 Diffusion of oxygen and carbon dioxide in the lungs.

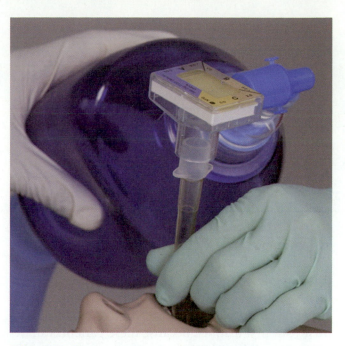

Fig. 17-4 Colorimetric end-tidal carbon dioxide detector.

deficiency. In the case of the alveoli, they are rich in oxygen and poor in carbon dioxide, so oxygen moves into the red blood cells of the capillaries and carbon dioxide moves from the capillaries where it was abundant into the alveoli for elimination. Fig. 17-3 illustrates the diffusion process. At the cellular level, the alveoli give up their oxygen to the red blood cells, while the cells release their carbon dioxide to the capillaries.

Any interference in this process, such as fluid, blood, mucus, or infectious processes, decreases the amount of oxygen and carbon dioxide being exchanged and therefore may cause a feeling of dyspnea. Think of the patient with pneumonia. He or she is tired, coughs up this pungent sputum, has absolutely no energy, and gets winded just getting off of the couch. The infection is inhibiting gas exchange.

Lung Volumes

From the moment a person takes his or her first breaths, the lungs will always contain air. In other words, no exhalation can completely empty the alveoli. The total lung capacity is 5400 to 5800 mL in the adult. The adult male forcibly can expel up to 4800 mL. This is called the *vital capacity*. The average amount of air taken in with each breath is 500 mL. This is called *tidal volume*. Of the 500-mL tidal volume, 150 mL stays in the airway (trachea, bronchi). This is referred to as *dead space air*. That leaves 350 mL for actual gas exchange and alveolar filling.[2] Taking the respiratory rate at 18 breaths/min, the lungs process more than 9000 L of air each day. Remembering that ambient air that is inhaled contains almost 20% oxygen, and the air you exhale contains

16% oxygen, this 4% difference is the amount retained by the body for use by the tissues, or almost 360 L. (This underscores the importance of maintaining a patent airway and adequate ventilation.)

Control of Respiration

The respiratory center is located in the brainstem, or more specifically the medulla oblongata. The respiratory center is sensitive to pH, blood pressure, and more importantly, carbon dioxide levels. When chemoreceptors detect a rise in the carbon dioxide levels, the respiratory center increases the rate of breathing in order to get rid of enough carbon dioxide to return it to normal levels. Conversely, when the carbon dioxide levels become too low, the rate of breathing slows to allow the necessary buildup of carbon dioxide in order to again return to normal levels. Capnography, or the measurement of carbon dioxide levels, is becoming the standard means of determining the effectiveness of the EMT's intervention, including cardiopulmonary resuscitation (Fig. 17-4). A carbon dioxide level within normal limits reveals that ventilation and perfusion (blood flow) are being achieved. Those two elements (ventilation and perfusion) must be present for adequate gas exchange in the lungs, which when done efficiently, will produce relatively normal carbon dioxide levels (35 to 45 mm Hg). Table 17-1 gives normal breathing rates.

TABLE 17-1

Normal respiratory rates

Age Group	Respiratory Rate (breaths/min)
Adult	12-20
Child	15-30
Infant	25-30

■ ASSESSMENT OF THE RESPIRATORY SYSTEM

It is imperative for the EMT to develop the ability to identify quickly and confidently those patients who are in respiratory distress. You will need to be able to trust your first instinct, because these patients can deteriorate rapidly. The information contained in this section will help you to develop these abilities.

Breathing provides the fuel that feeds the machinery of life. A person must take in enough oxygen to supply the energy required to perform vital body functions. Think of your body as an automobile. You may have the biggest and best engine, but if you cannot supply enough fuel to run that big motor, it does you absolutely no good. Your car may sputter, stall, or quit running altogether, leaving you stranded, all because of a fuel supply problem. Your vehicle gives you all sorts of signs and symptoms. A good mechanic can diagnose the problem of your car based on what you tell him or her about the performance (symptom) and what he or she observes during the exam (sign). For a timely repair, it is important to relay the correct symptoms. Whether the problem is a broken/clogged fuel line (airway), tainted fuel source (water in the fuel, improper fuel mixture, carbon monoxide, or any hypoxic environment), or that you are simply low on or even out of fuel, the result is the same: noticeably poor performance. Correct identification of symptoms gives you a starting point for further exam and efficient treatment.

Adequate Breathing

Going back to the mechanic analogy, what do all good mechanics have in common? One predominant factor is that they have a deep understanding of how your vehicle is supposed to work. They understand the relationships between systems and individual parts. They can tell you how one simple malfunction can lead to a total system failure. The EMT in many

ways is no different than the mechanic. Your understanding of each component of the respiratory system and the relationship of those parts to the entire system makes for easier assessment and treatment.

The following observations must be made in your assessment of the patient in order to determine if there is adequate breathing.

Rate

SPECIAL Considerations

You must take the scene and situation into consideration. An adult patient who was involved in a minor collision may breathe more than the 20 breaths/min because of his or her anxiety, not necessarily because of respiratory compromise.[3]

Rhythm

Patients who are not experiencing respiratory distress exhibit basically regular and rhythmic breathing. The next breath usually can be predicted in time and depth. Remember that talking will interrupt the rhythm, as will any discomfort found during the exam. When assessing the respiratory rate and rhythm, attempt to be subtle. If the patient knows his or her respirations are being counted, he or she may inadvertently alter their breathing, giving you an inaccurate result.

SPECIAL Considerations

An effective way of counting respirations is to hold your pulse check for an additional 30 seconds. While your patient thinks you are taking his or her pulse, you will be counting the respirations. This method redirects the patient's attention away from breathing, leading to a more accurate reading.

Quality

Your exam of the eupneic (normally breathing) patient should reveal clear and equal breath sounds across the chest. Upon auscultation with a stethoscope, you should hear air movement in all fields. Upon inspection, both sides of the chest should rise and fall equally. You also must assess the depth of respiratory effort to ensure adequate tidal volumes. Remember that normal adult tidal volume is 500 mL.

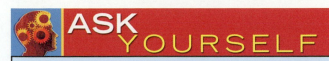

Breathing Status Assessment

Patients who cannot breathe may not be the most willing participants in a detailed physical exam. They are focused on one thing: breathing. They do not want to talk, move, or do anything that may require additional fuel. It will serve you well to assess all that you possibly can without causing the dyspneic patient to further exert. That may mean writing on a pad of paper instead of soliciting verbal responses or instructing the patient simply to nod *yes* or shake his or her head *no*. This only works if you use close-ended questions. Close-ended questions require yes or no answers. Open-ended questions require explanations and effort. Under these circumstances, you need to know what information is important for your assessment and appropriate treatment and what is unnecessary. This requires you to have a working knowledge of the respiratory system, common complaints, and the ability to discern what information is essential for appropriate treatment. *In other words, you have to know what information is necessary for appropriate and timely patient care.*

The following are pertinent items for respiratory assessment:

- *General appearance:* First impressions are usually correct. Take a second and assess the patient as a whole. What is his or her anxiety level? What is he or she telling you? At this point, you must begin to determine whether this patient can wait or whether he or she requires "right foot therapy" (rapid transport) to the medical center. Take what the patient tells you as true, especially if he or she relays that he or she has had similar episodes.
- *Environment/surroundings:* Observe the location for temperature, unusual odors, oxygen cylinders, and concentrators along with "miles" of tubing throughout the residence, a *No Smoking Oxygen in Use* warning on the front door, nebulizer machines, and any number of prescription medications. Look for these medications in the bathroom, in the kitchen cupboards, on the counter and table, on the nightstand, and even in the re-

frigerator. You may run across a *Vial of Life* on the front of the refrigerator. This contains a medical history, current medications, allergies, physicians, and family contacts. These can prove invaluable in assisting the unconscious or obtunded patient.

- *Patient position:* Patients experiencing dyspnea seldom will be supine or prone. Rather, they usually will be sitting upright or in the tripod position with their elbows on their knees and leaning forward. (Calloused elbows may indicate chronic respiratory problems.) Along with wishing to remain upright or forward, these patients will prefer their legs dangling from the chair or ambulance cot. With the help of gravity, this drains fluid away from the lungs in patients with congestive heart failure, making diffusion of oxygen into the red cells of the capillaries easier. The feet and ankles, of course, will become edematous. *(Pedal edema is a cardinal sign of fluid overload.)*
- *Speech:* Patients should be able to speak in full sentences without appearing short of breath. If the patient can say only a few words in between breaths, that is a sign of severe dyspnea. The severity of the dyspnea is categorized by the number of words the patient can speak in between taking a breath. For example, if the patient can only say two words before taking his or her next breath, he or she is said to have two-word dyspnea. As mentioned previously, use close-ended questions if possible. Your patients will appreciate the fuel they save by not having to relay their medical life story.
- *Mental status:* The brain is a greedy organ, using 20% of the oxygen taken into the body. Therefore the brain is one of the first organs to produce warning symptoms (warning lights on the dash). Lack of oxygen can cause confusion, anxiety, lethargy, aggressiveness, or other aberrant and bizarre behavior.
- *Skin color:* Any variance from the usual skin color may indicate poor respiratory status. Cyanosis, pallor, and mottling are common findings in those patients with significant respiratory distress.
- *Work of breathing:* Is your patient breathing easily, or is he or she using accessory muscles? (Children tire easily because of immature chest musculature.) Some patients when working hard to breathe flare their nostrils in an effort to pull in as much oxygen as possible. This is called nasal flaring. Patients also may exhibit open-mouth breathing. Again, this is an attempt to pull in as much oxygen as possible because the demand is exceeding the supply.

TABLE 17-2

Noisy breathing sounds and their significance

Respiratory Sound	Description	Possible Significance
Stridor	High-pitched sound, usually heard on inspiration	Obstruction of the *upper airway* from foreign body or swelling; swelling can be caused by allergic reactions or infections of the epiglottis, larynx, or trachea
Audible wheezing	High-pitched whistling noise from narrowed bronchioles; usually heard on expiration	Caused by constriction or partial obstruction of the *lower airways*
Gurgling	"Wet" sounds generated by air moving through fluid in the airway	Caused by fluid in the upper or lower airway from aspiration, near-drowning, or heart failure
Snoring	Low-pitched sounds, usually associated with partial closure of the airway by the tongue	Deep unconscious states or other cases of partial obstruction of the pharynx by the tongue

From Henry MC, Stapleton ER: *EMT prehospital care,* ed 3, St Louis, 2004, Mosby.

- *Breathing patterns:* Is your patient exhibiting any abnormal or irregular breathing patterns?
- *Noise of respiration:* Coughing, gurgling, snoring, **stridor,** and **wheezing** may indicate respiratory compromise. Remember, any process that interferes with gas exchange—whether it is water, mucus, blood, or any other substance—causes a decrease in the amount of oxygen available for general use. Table 17-2 reviews breath sounds.
- *Rate:* Adults usually breathe 12 to 20 times per minute. Breathing too slowly may cause a lack of oxygen in the system **(hypoxia)**, whereas breathing too quickly **(hyperventilation)** may result in getting rid of too much carbon dioxide (hypocarbia).
- *Respiratory quality:* Are lung sounds clear and equal? Does the chest rise and fall equally?

Pediatric Considerations

The primary medical cause of life-threatening emergencies in pediatric patients is difficulty breathing. Hypoxia is the leading cause of cardiac arrest in children. Children require twice the amount of energy as adults to do the same daily body work. The following are some of the important physiologic differences:

- Children have large tongues, small mouths, smaller-diameter airways (approximately the size of the child's smallest finger), and a large epiglottis compared with airway size.

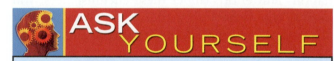

ASK YOURSELF

Without proper intervention, why do some of your hyperventilation patients pass out?

- They have less protection to the airway because of the cartilaginous structures of the airway are softer and can collapse with relative ease.
- Infants are obligate nose breathers and cannot breath through their mouths. Make sure the nasal passage is clear of mucus and obstruction.
- Immature chest musculature does not allow for prolonged accessory muscle use; therefore children fatigue quickly.
- The diaphragm is the main muscle of breathing, more so than in adults. Abdominal distention can interfere with diaphragmatic function and impair breathing.
- Smaller lung volumes and smaller blood volumes place a premium on having an adequate airway, ventilation, and circulation.[4]

Inadequate Breathing

One of the most crucial skills an EMT will learn is the rapid identification of respiratory distress. As part of the ABCs (airway, breathing, circulation), breathing carries great importance. Remember, as an EMT assessing the ABCs, you do not continue your assessment until you have addressed any life-threatening problems found during the primary assessment such as breathing. You previously have covered the findings of adequate breathing. The following are assessment findings associated with inadequate breathing:

- *Rate:* Less than 10 and greater than 30 per minute
- *Rhythm:* Irregular
- *Quality:* Shallow or very deep (tidal volume problems)
- *Effort:* Accessory muscle use (neck, intercostal, chest, and abdominal muscles), diaphoresis (sweating from the work of breathing), head-bobbing and fatigue (often seen in children), nasal flaring, and mouth breathing
- *Position:* Sitting upright or leaning over (tripod position) with forearms on legs, standing, or any other position in which the patient feels most able to breathe.

///CAUTION!

Do NOT attempt to place these patients supine. They will fight you all the way, making their hypoxia worse.

- *Appearance:* Poor skin color (pale; cyanosis is a late sign of hypoxia)
- *Sound:* Diminished or even absent breath sounds (Remember that pediatric patients have thinner chest walls, making the auscultation of breath sounds typically easier. Diminished sounds in children are pertinent findings.)
  - Snoring respirations indicate a partial airway obstruction.
  - Wheezing noises are a sign of airway constriction.
  - Coughing is a sign of airway irritation.
- *Agonal respirations,* or occasional gasping breaths, may be seen as a preterminal event. These are not considered functional respirations.

■ RESPIRATORY DISTRESS

During your career as an EMT, you may respond to more calls for difficulty breathing than any other single complaint. Remember that you are being called because someone feels that he or she cannot breathe adequately. You must respect the patient's complaint, for it is entirely subjective. Even if all exam findings are negative, the patient still may be experiencing

some degree of dyspnea. As an EMT, the exact cause of the dyspnea is not as important as your reaction and subsequent treatment. Is the dyspnea caused by respiratory disease, such as asthma or **chronic obstructive pulmonary disease** (COPD), cardiac dysfunction as in myocardial infarction and congestive heart failure, or traumatic injury? All of the previous conditions may cause the same sense of difficulty breathing, and it is up to you to administer the proper treatment.

Signs and Symptoms of Respiratory Distress

The following are signs and symptoms of respiratory distress:

- Restlessness, anxiety, and mental status changes
- Tachycardia (bradycardia in children)
- Tachypnea or bradypnea
- Skin color changes
- Noisy breathing
- Speaking difficulty because of breathing
- Accessory muscle use
- Abdominal breathing
- Tripod or forward-leaning position
- Pursed lips, nasal flaring, and open-mouth breathing
- Pulse oximeter reading of less than 95% (oxygen saturation) at sea level

Remember that obtaining a focused history from a patient with severe respiratory distress can be challenging. You may be dealing with altered mental status and the patient's inability to explain fully his or her situation because of dyspnea. Do not forget the alternate means of obtaining this important focused history, mainly pen and paper, medications, and yes/no questions. Fig. 17-5 reviews the pertinent history points in the assessment of the patient with respiratory difficulty.

Additional Assessment

You can use the OPQRST mnemonic to obtain additional information in the assessment of the patient's respiratory condition:

O—Onset: When did this episode begin? Is this the first episode?
P—Provocation: What were the circumstances when it began?
Q—Quality: Ask the patient to describe his or her situation.

SAMPLE History for Difficulty Breathing

S   **S***igns and Symptoms* of respiratory distress include the following:
Obvious distress
Signs of increased effort
Fast, slow, or labored breathing
Wheezing or other respiratory noises
For the complaint of breathing difficulty use OPQRST:
O*nset*—Ask the patient when the problem started.
P*rovocation*—Does anything make breathing better or worse (e.g., increased activity, sitting, standing, lying down)?
Q*uality*—How does the patient describe the distress? Tightness in the chest or shortness of breath? Is there any associated pain? Where is the pain? Is the pain worse with breathing? Sharp pain or dull?
R*adiation*—Does the pain go anywhere else (e.g., the arm, neck, or jaw)?
S*everity*—On a scale of 1-10, with 10 being the most difficult it has ever been to breathe, how severe is the difficulty breathing? If this has happened before, how does this episode compare to other episodes?
T*ime*—How long has the patient had difficulty breathing (e.g., it may have started a couple of days ago, but it has been getting much worse over the last half hour)?

A   **A***llergies.* A history of allergies may give important clues for a patient with shortness of breath. For example, an acute episode of asthma is often triggered by allergies to such things as dust, pollen, or animal dander. An anaphylactic (severe allergic) reaction may be the result of a bee sting to which the patient is allergic.

M   **M***edications.* The medications that a patient takes can give an indication of an underlying medical condition. For example, a patient may have an inhaler for asthma. If medications are readily available you should have them gathered for the responding EMS team. Patients with chronic lung disease may have oxygen at home. Oxygen is considered a medication and you should note the type of device and the dose (liters per minute).

P   **P***ertinent past medical history.* Common conditions that are associated with breathing difficulty include asthma, emphysema, chronic bronchitis, congestive heart failure, or pulmonary edema.

L   **L***ast oral intake.* The last oral intake (solid or liquid) may be important for medical attention that is received at the hospital.

E   **E***vents leading to the illness.* What was the patient doing before he or she began to have difficulty breathing? Has it been getting worse over time? Has he or she received treatment for this type of problem before? When and what happened? Try to establish a brief time sequence (e.g., the patient had fever and chills for 2 days before the breathing difficulty started).

Fig. 17-5 SAMPLE history for difficulty breathing.

R — Radiation: Do symptoms spread to other body regions?

S — Severity: Using the 10 scale, gather his or her distress level (1 least; 10 most).

T — Time: How long has the patient had these symptoms?

Has the patient done anything to attempt to relieve the symptoms? This may include over-the-counter remedies, prescription medicines (his or her own or someone else's), other personal remedies, and even cultural remedies.

■ **TREATMENT FOR RESPIRATORY DISTRESS**

Oxygen Therapy

Do not withhold oxygen from anyone who is short of breath. For anyone in respiratory distress, the nonrebreather mask at 12 to 15 L/min of oxygen is appropriate. Some patients will not be able to tolerate the mask on their face. They may feel like they are being smothered, and again this agitation requires more fuel, making their situation worse. Explain their need for oxygen, and apply a nasal cannula at 2 to 6 L/min of oxygen. If you have a pulse oximeter device available, the amount of oxygen given should be titrated to maintain an oxygen saturation as close to 100% as possible.

Position the patient in his or her position of comfort. As mentioned previously, do not place the patient supine unless you are going to provide ventilation for him or her. The truly dyspneic patient who allows supine positioning is usually in critical condition and will require aggressive airway and ventilatory management.

Ventilation

After a thorough assessment and focused history, it is time to formulate a treatment plan. Some steps, such as ensuring a patent airway and detecting respiratory effort, are obvious. If you feel that the patient is not breathing adequately via rate or depth, you will need to assist ventilation. Do not be afraid to use the bag-valve-mask (BVM). If you do need to assist ventilation with the BVM, be sure to connect it to supplemental oxygen in order to deliver close to 100% oxygen, as opposed to 21% without it. Remember to synchronize your assisted ventilations with your patient's inspiratory patterns. Ventilating against the patient's breathing efforts only worsens the hypoxia. Adequate ventilation is being achieved when the following occur:

- The chest rises and falls with each artificial ventilation.
- Proper rates are maintained: 12 breaths/min for adults, 20 breaths/min for children and infants.
- The heart rate returns to within normal limits.

///**CAUTION!**

Consider advanced life support assistance for any patient with significant difficulty breathing.

TABLE 17-3

Signs of adequate versus inadequate positive pressure ventilation

Adequate	Inadequate
Chest rises and falls with each breath.	No chest rise occurs with breaths.
Breathing rate is sufficient:	Breathing rate is too slow or too fast.
Approximately 12 breaths/min for adults	
Approximately 20 breaths/min for infants and children	
Heart rate returns to normal with positive pressure ventilation.	Heart rate does not return to normal.

From Henry MC, Stapleton ER: *EMT prehospital care,* ed 3, St Louis, 2004, Mosby.

Oxygenation versus Ventilation

You have just read of the importance and the use of supplemental oxygen. Although adequate oxygenation is important, the importance of adequate ventilation is covered now. Remember that ventilation is the process by which air is taken into the lungs for diffusion and distribution. You can place a nonrebreather mask with 15 L/min supplemental oxygen on a patient, but if the patient cannot breathe in the oxygen because of ventilatory compromise, it is of little help. Take the simple example of filling your car with fuel. You pull up to the pump, remove the gas cap, and place the nozzle into the tank. Is your car going to fill itself? Why not, if the fuel is there and the hose is there? What is the holdup? Of course, you know you have to squeeze the handle of the fuel nozzle to transport the fuel into your car. That is comparable to ventilation: mechanically transporting fuel to the proper destination. If your patient is not effectively pulling in the oxygen, he or she will require assistance. The role of the EMT is to "squeeze the handle," in effect, and assist the ventilation process.

The EMT also must understand that ventilation involves inhaling and exhaling. If your patient is breathing in poorly, he or she also is breathing out poorly. Retaining too much carbon dioxide because of poor ventilation can have a negative effect on patient outcome. By physically inflating the lungs, you effectively are exhaling also, for exhalation is a passive process dependent upon inspiratory tidal volumes. Table 17-3 reviews the signs of adequate and inadequate ventilation.

■ COMMON RESPIRATORY CONDITIONS

Asthma

Asthma is a member of the family of conditions known as chronic obstructive pulmonary disease. Asthma is an inflammatory disease causing air-

> ### ///CAUTION!
> Ventilation must be synchronized with the inhalation of a spontaneously breathing patient. Do not fight him or her and work in opposition to his or her efforts. Let the patient know what your intentions are so that he or she can help you.

flow restriction via bronchospasm and excess mucus production. Asthma is a chronic condition; however, prehospital providers will see it in a more acute setting. Asthma attacks have many triggers; including allergy, physical activity, stress, and some environmental components. The smaller airways, or bronchioles, experience swelling and muscle spasm which cause air passage narrowing, while the release of histamine in the body causes the capillaries to become leaky. As a result, the patient has to push the air out through the mucus, edema, and bronchospasm. Think of how difficult it would be to exhale a full breath through a small straw. This leads to the retention of carbon dioxide and the increasing inability to fill the alveoli with oxygen. Remember, if the alveolus cannot empty its carbon dioxide, it cannot efficiently fill with oxygen. Diffusion depends on efficient respiration and alveolar filling in a clean, barrier-free exchange environment.

Presentation

The most common symptoms of an asthma attack are dyspnea, coughing, increased respiration rate greater than 30 breaths/min, and wheezing. Signs of progressive worsening of the attack include exhaustion, cyanosis, bradycardia, altered mental status, and a silent chest. The silent chest is an ominous finding. It indicates no air movement within the lungs. In

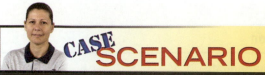

CASE SCENARIO
continued

The "care bear" was doing what it was intended to do—reassure the young boy while providing some much-needed blow-by oxygen. Elizabeth continued her assessment of the child's respiratory status. As the boy became calmer, the once-audible wheezes decreased until she could barely hear them. With her stethoscope she still can hear them in the lung fields. As Elizabeth stands up, the nurse comes over with the boy's metered dose inhaler. "This is his medication. I had a hard time finding it in the storeroom. Also, the child's parents are on the phone. They would like to know what's going on with their son."

Question: *Should Elizabeth talk to the parents over the phone? Or should she first help the patient take his medication?*

SPECIAL Considerations

If the patient is experiencing an anaphylactic reaction and has an available autoinjector EpiPen (epinephrine) prescribed for him or her, you will want to assist the patient with the administration of this medication to assist the patient's airway and ventilation efforts.

other words, coughing and some wheezing are not actually negative findings. They tell you that the airway is open, some air is moving in and out of the lungs, and diffusion is happening on some level.

Management

Treatment of the asthma attack by an EMT consists of ensuring a patent airway, oxygen administration (nonrebreather mask with 15 L/min), ventilatory assistance if necessary, and the use of the patient's prescribed inhaler. The medicine contained in these "puffers" reverses the bronchospasm and helps calm down the reaction, lessening mucus production, thus freeing the trapped air for exhalation.

Anaphylaxis

You will encounter patients who do not have a history of asthma or COPD but who may be coughing, wheezing, and having difficulty breathing. This could be due to an allergic reaction to food, medicine, or the environment. The most severe type of allergic reaction is anaphylaxis. This is a life-threatening reaction during which the airways swell and the blood vessels dilate. Patients with this reaction experience extreme dyspnea along with profound hypotension. Most anaphylactic reactions occur within 30 minutes of exposure, and all may progress into respiratory failure. A

bee sting is one of the most common causes of anaphylaxis. Persons who know they are severely allergic to bee stings may carry an EpiPen. This is an autoinjector pen containing epinephrine, a medicine that can reverse the bronchoconstriction and raise the blood pressure by vasoconstriction (see Chapter 16).

Presentation

Most patients present in serious respiratory distress, in the upright or tripod position, with an altered mental status. Other common findings include diaphoresis, cool and pale skin often with hives (urticaria), and inspiratory and expiratory wheezing.

Management

Aggressive airway management and ventilation are standard management goals. High-flow oxygen, upright positioning, and rapid transport to the hospital complete the anaphylaxis treatment. If local protocols permit, the EMT may help the patient administer his or her epinephrine via autoinjector. This is a grave emergency that requires immediate and decisive action.

Pulmonary Edema

Pulmonary edema is caused by the inability of the heart, mainly the left ventricle, to pump blood effectively. When the heart cannot handle the volume of fluid normally supplied, that fluid begins to back up. Using your knowledge of anatomy and physiology, you realize the blood will back up into the lungs from the left side of the heart. The fluid interferes with diffusion, and the resulting pulmonary edema can lead to respiratory failure.

Presentation

Patients with pulmonary edema complain of extreme dyspnea. They have wet lung sounds (crackles) and exhibit **orthopnea**, or difficulty breathing while supine (Box 17-1). These are the persons who sleep in the recliner or with four or five pillows to keep their head up so that gravity can draw some of the fluid

BOX 17-1
Signs and Symptoms of Pulmonary Edema

Extreme diaphoresis
Feeling of impending doom
Hypotension
Pedal edema
Pink, frothy sputum
Rales with all respiratory effort
Rhonchi
Severe dyspnea
Upright or tripod position
Wheezing (small airway protection)

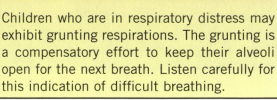

SPECIAL Populations

Children who are in respiratory distress may exhibit grunting respirations. The grunting is a compensatory effort to keep their alveoli open for the next breath. Listen carefully for this indication of difficult breathing.

away from their lungs. A late and ominous sign of pulmonary edema is frothy, pink sputum coming out of the patient's mouth. This indicates that blood has backed up into the lungs, turning the sputum pink.

Management

Management of these patients includes maintaining an airway, high-flow oxygen (15 L/min) via nonrebreather mask, possibly assisting ventilation, and sitting them upright, maybe even with their legs on either side of the cart to promote dependent fluid flow away from the lungs. You often can hear these patients breathing the moment you set foot in the house. These patients are easy to spot but require aggressive treatment. They are so exhausted from their work of breathing that they easily can progress into respiratory arrest. For this reason, these patients require rapid assessment, management, and transport to the nearest medical facility.

Emphysema

Emphysema is another member of the COPD family of diseases. It is characterized by destruction of the alveoli, which makes exchange gas much more difficult. The most common cause of emphysema is the repeated exposure to noxious substances in the air. This includes primary and secondhand smoke, dust, air pollution, and other caustic substances found in the air. With emphysema the alveoli lose some of their elasticity, further decreasing diffusion, and causing carbon dioxide retention. The loss of elasticity reduces the ability of the small airways to remain open during exhalation. This causes patients to trap air in their small airways. This air trapping is the reason for the "barrel chest" appearance. In an attempt to keep as many of the small airways open as possible during exhalation, these patients will breathe through pursed lips. This

forces some pressure into the small airways, helping to keep them open for the next inspiration. Over time, the body will compensate for the constant hypoxia and produce extra red blood cells. This enables the patient to carry more oxygen in the blood. Together, the pink appearance of the skin and the pursed lip puffing are the reason this patient may be called a "pink puffer." Another common finding in emphysema is a productive cough, caused by irritation of the bronchial lining. As discussed previously, any foreign substance in the alveolar/capillary matrix will decrease gas exchange, making it that much harder to breathe.

Presentation

These patients present usually upright or in the tripod position (watch for calloused elbows) and are often quite thin because of the constant extra work of breathing which causes weight loss. They may exhibit pursed lip breathing, a compensatory mechanism that places additional pressure in the alveoli in order to keep them open for the next breath. They are found upright with rapid and shallow respirations, and they experience distress with any sort of activity.

Because of the chronic gas exchange problems, these patients retain abnormally high amounts of carbon dioxide in their systems. This is important when you recall the normal stimulus the brain uses to regulate respiratory effort: carbon dioxide levels. Over time, the receptors become ineffective, and the body must look for a new respiratory stimulus. Many patients with COPD breathe based on **hypoxic drive.** Instead of carbon dioxide, the body now senses oxygen levels. Simply stated, when the brain thinks it needs more oxygen, the person breathes. When it is content, respiratory effort slows. This is important for the EMT to understand when administering supplemental oxygen to these patients.

Management

If the patient's distress is not substantial, begin oxygen therapy conservatively with a nasal cannula at 2 to 6 L/min. In theory, by giving these patients high-flow oxygen (15 L/min via nonrebreather mask), their brain might tell them they have enough oxygen, and their respiratory effort may decrease or stop altogether. If they do stop breathing or slow to an ineffective rate or depth, pull out your BVM with supplemental oxygen and ventilate them appropriately. However, this theoretical concern should never prevent the EMT from providing supplemental oxygen to a patient who is dyspneic, regardless of the cause.

Chronic Bronchitis

Presentation

Chronic **bronchitis** is a condition in which the lining of the airway becomes irritated and produces excessive mucus. This is normally due to prolonged exposure to harmful pollutants, such as with long-term smoking. The excess mucus production actually plugs the bronchioles and significantly reduces alveolar ventilation. These poorly ventilated alveoli in turn will cause cyanosis because of the lack of oxygen in the blood. These patients may also have noticeable edema, usually in the dependent areas such as the ankles or abdomen. This edema is caused by right ventricular failure, which is another condition precipitated by COPD. Because these patients present cyanotic and bloated, they sometimes are called "blue bloaters." They also may have wheezing, **rhonchi,** and a productive cough. As you would expect, they often are found sitting upright or in the tripod position.

Management

Oxygen therapy begins with a nasal cannula at 2 to 4 L/min. If the patient's condition warrants, go ahead and place him or her on a nonrebreather mask with 15 L/min of oxygen. These patients may require suction and ventilation. Sit these patients upright, and do not require them to expend great amounts of energy in the exam or history.

Pulmonary Embolism

A **pulmonary embolism** is a blood clot in the pulmonary circulation. These clots usually arise from the legs (lower extremities) and travel to the pulmonary circulation. As previously covered, for diffusion to occur, there must be a constant supply of blood coming to and going from the alveolar beds. If a section of the lung is cut off from the fresh blood, the alveolar beds cannot take on oxygen and release carbon dioxide. Patients with pulmonary embolus usually present with sudden onset of chest pain associated with severe respiratory distress. Persons at greater risk for pulmonary embolism include the following: young adults, smokers, females taking birth control pills, pregnant women, and patients after surgery. These are not the only patients who can have pulmonary emboli, but this is a significant risk group. A pulmonary embolism is a dire emergency requiring rapid recognition and transport.

Presentation

Your patient will be experiencing substantial dyspnea that has nothing to do with his or her ability to breathe in and out. The hypoxia occurs because of the impaired diffusion. Along with severe dyspnea, the patient may experience sudden, sharp, severe chest pain.

Management

These patients require rapid transport to the hospital, along with the standard dyspnea treatment: oxygen at 15 L/min via non-rebreather mask, airway management, upright positioning, and if necessary, assisted ventilation via BVM and supplemental oxygen.

Hyperventilation

Hyperventilation is the condition in which your patient is breathing too quickly, often due to a stressful or anxiety-producing event. This rapid breathing causes him or her to lose too much carbon dioxide. As you have learned, carbon dioxide levels are the stimulus to breathe. The only way for the body to keep more of its carbon dioxide and return to normal levels is to slow down the breathing process. These patients need the *Reset* button activated. That is why *syncope* is a common symptom of hyperventilation. Once patients pass out, they return to normal breathing rates, and the carbon dioxide levels again fall within normal limits.

Presentation

Along with an increased breathing rate and an increase in anxiety, these patients may complain of numbness to their hands and feet and actually may experience finger and toe cramping. These are called carpal and pedal spasms. When the respiratory rate slows down, these symptoms will dissipate. These patients also may develop chest pain with deep inhalation.

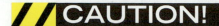

///CAUTION!

Hyperventilation and pulmonary embolism can have the same presentation and even may occur in the same risk group population. Always take the dyspneic patient seriously.

Management

The initial presentations of pulmonary embolism and hyperventilation are similar; therefore, hyperventilation should be considered only after all other causes have been excluded. Be careful. Do your best to coach the patient down to a manageable respiratory rate. Ask the patient to take a breath, hold it for a count of three, and then exhale. You need to remind the patient constantly of this pattern until the respiratory rate slows. Traditional methods of treating hyperventilation have included the use of a paper bag to allow patients to rebreathe their own carbon dioxide, replacing it as they go. You probably have seen this done. The big issue with this treatment lies in the possibility that the cause for the patient's rapid breathing is not simple hyperventilation. Therefore, the worst possible problem should be considered and all patients should be given oxygen (15 L/min) via a non-rebreather mask.

Airway Obstruction

The tongue is the most common cause of airway obstruction. Foreign bodies, including vomitus, foreign objects, dentures, and blood can all lead to airway obstruction. As you learned in cardiopulmonary resuscitation training, the first intervention in any unconscious patient is to open the airway. The head tilt–chin lift maneuver simply moves the flaccid tongue out of the airway space, allowing respiration to occur. You must identify the presence of an airway obstruction before the administration of oxygen. Remember, fuel does you no good if you cannot get it to the motor.

Presentation

An otherwise healthy child who has a sudden onset of difficulty breathing needs airway management above all else. Think about the field of vision of some of these children: it is floor level. As you know, everything they can grab goes right into their mouths. In situations like the one just mentioned, you must consider an upper airway obstruction and take the required steps to relieve the obstruction.

Airway obstructions in adults are less common, but no less lethal. Most often, these incidents occur while eating and consuming alcohol. Interestingly, you may find that these choking patients leave the public setting and go into the bathroom.

Management

In the unconscious patient who has no chest rise, open the airway and ventilate. If you still have no chest rise, initiate abdominal thrusts in an attempt to clear the airway. An unconscious adult, or any person with an altered mental status, may vomit and not be able to protect his or her airway, resulting in aspiration of vomitus into the lungs. This too is an airway obstruction and must be cleared before oxygen administration. Do not forget about the ABCs!

■ PRESCRIBED INHALERS

As an EMT, you will be presented with numerous situations in which your actions truly will make the difference in your patient's life. One such situation involves the administration of your patient's inhaler (Skill 17-1). Along with paramedics, you are able to assist those in need by facilitating the administration of their medicine.

Patients with chronic obstructive diseases often require the use of their prescribed medicine inhaler (Fig. 17-6). This is a device that delivers a metered dose of a bronchodilator, a medicine that relaxes the air passages and allows better airflow. You will find some of the following medicine names on these inhalers: albuterol (Proventil, Ventolin), metaproterenol (Alupent), ipratropium (Atrovent), terbutaline (Brethine), and isoetharine. These drugs have basically the same mechanism of action (beta-agonists) and side effects with the exception of ipratropium (parasympatholytic). These drugs, along with the desired bronchodilation, can cause increased heart rate, anxiety, and tremors. Remember, the positive effect of better breathing usually outweighs the potential side effects. As with any medicine, you must ask the patient whether he or she has any allergies to these types of medicines.

Indications for Inhaler Use

The following are indications for use of an inhaler:

1. The patient exhibits signs and symptoms of respiratory distress.
2. The patient has a physician-prescribed handheld inhaler.
3. You have specific authorization by medical direction to assist.

SKILL 17-1
◉ *Inhaler Administration*

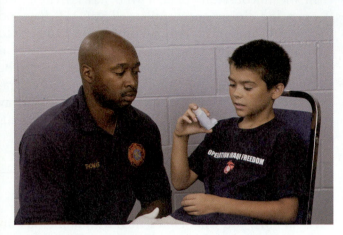 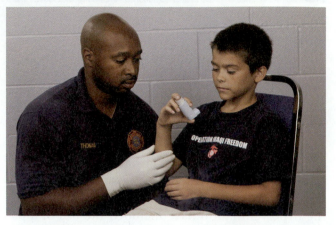

Follow these guidelines before assisting with a patient's inhaler administration:

1. Obtain an order from medical direction, either off-line or online.
2. Make sure the inhaler is at least room temperature.
3. Verify the right medication, right patient, and right route.
4. Be sure the patient is alert enough to use the inhaler.
5. Be sure the inhaler is not expired.
6. Confirm how many doses, if any, the patient has taken before your arrival.
7. Shake the inhaler vigorously several times.
8. Briefly remove supplemental oxygen.
9. Encourage the patient to exhale deeply and place his or her lips around the end of the device.
10. As the patient inhales, have him or her depress the inhaler.
11. Instruct the patient to inhale as deeply as he or she can and hold his or her breath for maximum medication absorption.
12. Replace supplemental oxygen device.
13. Reassess vital signs.
14. Allow the patient a few normal breaths, and repeat as needed per medical direction.
15. Be alert for anxiety, tremors, and increased heart rate.
16. If the patient has a spacer, a device placed between the inhaler and the patient, allow him or her to use it. Spacers provide a more effective administration of the medicine.

SKILLS

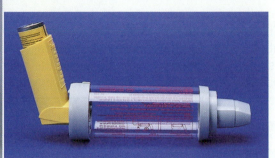

Fig. 17-6 **A,** A metered dose inhaler delivers a specific dose of medication to the lungs. **B,** A spacer device used with an inhaler increases the amount of medication going to the lungs.

Contraindications for Inhaler Use

The following are contraindications for use of an inhaler:

1. The patient is unable to use the device.
2. The inhaler is not prescribed for the patient.
3. You do not have permission from medical direction.
4. The patient already has met the maximum prescribed dose before EMT arrival.

Pediatric Concerns

Handheld inhalers are commonly used in treating asthma in children. The same guidelines for use hold true for this patient group. The patient must have an order and his or her own inhaler in order for the EMT to assist with administration. Remember, cyanosis is a late sign of respiratory distress in children. Often the pediatric patient with an asthma attack will have coughing and mucus problems, not necessarily the classic wheezing.

SPECIAL Populations

Two common childhood infections can have profound effects on the respiratory system. These conditions are discussed briefly[3]:

Croup, or laryngotracheobronchitis, is a viral infection involving the airway, mostly the upper airway. The tissue around the trachea becomes inflamed, narrowing the airway. Croup is seen primarily in the late fall and early winter months in children between 6 months and 3 years old. Children tend to develop symptoms after a mild fever and upper respiratory illness, and symptoms seem to intensify toward evening. Signs and symptoms of croup include the development of a harsh, barking cough, inspiratory stridor, and if allowed to progress, restlessness, cyanosis, and tachycardia. Patients experiencing croup will want to sit up and should be placed in the position of comfort. Additional treatment includes cool, moist air, such as from an open window, or humidified oxygen.

Epiglottitis is a potentially life-threatening bacterial infection in which the epiglottis becomes inflamed and can obstruct the airway. Epiglottitis affects children ages 3 to 7 years. These children usually awaken in the night with a high fever and drooling, caused by the painful act of swallowing with the enlarged epiglottis. These children are found upright with shallow respirations, dyspnea, and inspiratory stridor. Epiglottitis is a true emergency and requires proper management. DO NOT examine the airway or place anything into the airway; it may precipitate full airway obstruction. Position these patients upright and even tripod if they are comfortable. Use cool, humidified oxygen, and avoid any agitation. Keeping parents or caregivers near the patient will help keep your patient calm.

A dyspneic child often will display a tripod position with the head in the hands. Remember, as discussed, children fatigue easily, and this is a compensatory mechanism used to assist respiratory effort. Children with impending respiratory failure often exhibit head-bobbing in an attempt to maximize inspiratory effort, often at a cost of expending all their energy.

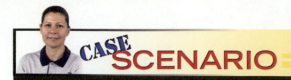

CASE SCENARIO

conclusion

"Yes, he's getting better. Yes, we will be transporting to Children's Hospital. You'll meet us there? Very good. See you soon." Elizabeth hung up the phone. Turning to the boy, she said, "Well, Mike, how are you feeling?" The boy was able to nod his head that he was feeling better. His skin color had returned to his cheeks, and he was not breathing nearly as fast as before. Holding onto the care bear, Mike got on the stretcher and was wheeled down the hallway back to the waiting ambulance. ■

TEAMWORK

As an emergency medical technician, you may be called upon to administer oxygen and provide assistance with inhalers or to assist other health care providers to do so. You must understand the principles behind these techniques to assist others more effectively.

References

1. Martini FH, Bartholomew EF, Bledsoe BE: *Anatomy and physiology for emergency care*, Englewood Cliffs, NJ, 2002, Prentice Hall.
2. Sanders MJ: *Mosby's paramedic textbook*, ed 2, St Louis, 2000, Mosby.
3. Pons P, Cason D: *Paramedic field care: a complaint based approach*, St Louis, 1997, Mosby-Year Book.
4. American Academy of Pediatrics: *APLS: the pediatric emergency medicine course*, ed 2, Dallas, 1993, American College of Emergency Physicians.

Resource

American College of Emergency Physicians: *Advanced pediatric life support (APLS)*, Dallas, 1993, American College of Emergency Physicians.

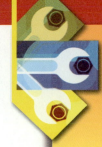
Critical Points

As an EMT, you will encounter countless patients with difficulty breathing. Your role will be to provide an accurate assessment and timely and sometimes lifesaving treatment. Few patients deteriorate more quickly than those who are experiencing difficulty breathing.

As stated previously in this text, scene safety is always priority No. 1. Patients who are having difficulty breathing may have mental status changes because of hypoxia and may make your situation unsafe. Always take the patient's mental status into consideration in your scene safety plan. Remember to talk to your patient and tell him or her what you are doing and why. A less anxious patient uses less fuel, possibly improving breathing status.

Patients who are experiencing difficulty breathing will need to conserve all the oxygen they can. Do not ask them to relay their entire medical history, for talking may worsen their condition. Get the basic information you need, and be resourceful in your search for any pertinent findings.

Talk to these patients. They likely will be frightened, whether or not this has happened to them before. Let them know you grasp the seriousness of their situation and are going to help them. Ask for their cooperation without requiring them to expend their much-needed energy.

Difficulty breathing can result from medical and traumatic conditions. Regardless of the origin, *never* withhold oxygen from a patient in respiratory distress.

Your treatment options for the patient in respiratory distress include oxygen administration, proper positioning (usually upright), an appropriate assessment, possibly the need for ventilation assistance using the bag-mask device, assistance with administration of the patient's own metered dose inhaler, and maybe even airway management with adjunct placement. No matter what treatments you decide on, every dyspneic patient will need your calm, reassuring, and confident attention. Treat the patient first. As mentioned previously, do not forget to treat the human component to your patient's problem. Connecting with him or her puts everyone more at ease, and that is in your patient's best interest.

Learning Checklist

❏ The assessment of the patient with respiratory distress includes scene size-up, initial assessment, SAMPLE history (*S*igns and symptoms, *A*llergies, *M*edications, *P*ast medical history, *L*ast oral intake, *E*vents preceding) and vital signs, and detailed physical examination as needed.

❏ To calm and reassure your patient is important. The human component of respiratory care cannot be stressed enough. These patients know that if they cannot breathe, they may die. Your confident and empathetic manner may improve your patient's condition. Remember that anxiety causes increased body functions, using more of the already depleted fuel supply.

❏ Listen closely to what your patient tells you and also look, listen, and smell to grasp what the scene is telling you. Do you see a nebulizer in the room, indicating chronic respiratory problems? Is there a haze of cigarette smoke in the room with the already dyspneic patient? Are there "miles" of oxygen tubing along the baseboards, again indicating chronic respiratory problems? Do you hear the gurgling and bubbling of a patient in pulmonary edema? Are there any unusual odors that may trigger respiratory problems?

❏ Look to see whether your patient is wearing any medical identification indicating an allergy, medical condition, or medication.

❏ Note the position of your patient upon your arrival. Remember that patients who are having difficulty breathing rarely are supine or prone; rather, they are bolt upright or even in the tripod position.

❏ Adequate oxygenation depends on ventilation rate and quality, actual lung condition (any fluid or mucus may hinder gas exchange), and the oxygen content of the environment. Emergency medical technicians have the ability to influence each of these components and improve respiratory status.

❏ Your patient's respiratory status can be determined by examining the following: general appearance, patient position, speech or lack thereof, mental status, skin color, work of breathing, and breathing rate and quality.

❑ Adults with breathing rates of less than 10 per minute and more than 30 per minute will likely have inadequate breathing. Again, take into consideration the scene, and account for any possible changes, such as anxiety, nervousness, or a physical struggle. The numbers are not absolute. Treat the patient, and not the breathing rate.

❑ Signs of respiratory distress include restlessness, mental status changes, tachycardia, skin color changes (e.g., pale and cyanotic), noisy respirations, difficulty speaking in sentences, accessory muscle use in breathing including the abdomen, tripod positioning and orthopnea, pursed lip breathing, nasal flaring, and mouth breathing.

❑ Signs and symptoms of an asthma attack include anxiety, coughing, wheezing, and altered mental status.

❑ Signs and symptoms of pulmonary edema include extreme difficulty breathing, wet lung sounds (rales), pink and frothy sputum, and hypotension.

❑ Signs and symptoms of emphysema include chronic dyspnea and productive cough, pursed lip breathing, and hypertension. These patients commonly are found upright and may be using oxygen at home.

❑ Signs and symptoms of a pulmonary embolism include a sudden onset of chest pain accompanied by significant difficulty breathing. Prehospital care involves high-flow oxygen, airway management and ventilation, and rapid transport to the nearest hospital.

❑ The dyspneic patient may use his or her handheld inhaler to minimize asthma symptoms. The emergency medical technician must be aware of these devices, how they work, and the need for medical direction.

Key Terms

Apnea The absence of spontaneous respiration.
Asthma A respiratory disorder characterized by recurring episodes of dyspnea and wheezing caused by constriction of the bronchi, coughing, and viscous mucus secretions.

Bronchitis Acute or chronic inflammation of the mucous membranes of the tracheobronchial tree.

Chronic obstructive pulmonary disease A progressive and irreversible condition characterized by diminished capacity of the lungs caused by airway constriction and mucous obstruction. Chronic bronchitis, emphysema, and asthma are forms of the disease.

Croup An acute viral infection of the upper and lower airway that may cause partial obstruction and a barking cough. Croup usually is seen in children 3 months to 3 years old.

Diffusion The process by which gases or particles in a fluid move from an area of higher concentration to an area of lower concentration in an effort to equalize distribution.

Dyspnea The sensation of difficulty breathing.

Emphysema A respiratory condition characterized by overinflation and destructive changes to alveolar walls, resulting in a loss of lung elasticity and decreased gas exchange.

Epiglottitis Inflammation of the epiglottis, usually bacterial, causing marked airway obstruction and requiring rapid definitive intervention.

Hyperventilation Rapid and deep breathing resulting in a decrease in carbon dioxide retention.

Hypoxia Inadequate cellular oxygenation.

Hypoxic drive The low arterial oxygen pressure stimulus to respiration.

Orthopnea Respiratory difficulty when supine. Breathing is much easier sitting upright or standing.

Pulmonary edema The accumulation of extravascular fluid in the lung tissues and alveoli, caused mostly by congestive heart failure.

Pulmonary embolism The blockage of a pulmonary artery by a blood clot .

Rales Fine crackling sounds generated when fluid-filled or collapsed alveoli suddenly reexpand with inspiration.

Rhonchi Abnormal, coarse sounds heard over the upper airways as air moves through thick mucus secretions. Rhonchi often clear with coughing.

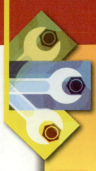

Stridor A high-pitched, harsh respiratory sound that is a sign of upper airway obstruction.

Wheezing High-pitched expiratory breath sounds caused by narrowing of the small air passages (bronchioles) in the lungs that most commonly is a result of an acute asthmatic episode.

National Standard Curriculum Objectives

Cognitive Objectives

After completing this lesson, the EMT student will be able to do the following:

- List the structure and function of the respiratory system.
- State the signs and symptoms of a patient with breathing difficulty.
- Describe the emergency medical care of the patient with breathing difficulty.
- Recognize the need for medical direction to assist in the emergency.
- Discuss the emergency medical care for the patient with breathing distress.
- Establish the relationship between airway management and the patient with breathing difficulty.

- List the signs of adequate air exchange.
- State the generic name, medication forms, dose, administration, action, and indications and contraindications for the prescribed inhaler.
- Distinguish between the emergency medical care of the infant, child, and adult patient with breathing difficulty.

Affective Objectives

After completing this lesson, the EMT student will be able to do the following:

- Defend treatment by the emergency medical technician for various respiratory emergencies.
- Explain the rationale for administering an inhaler.

Psychomotor Objectives

After completing this lesson, the EMT student will be able to do the following:

- Demonstrate the emergency medical care for breathing difficulty.
- Perform the steps necessary in facilitating the use of an inhaler.

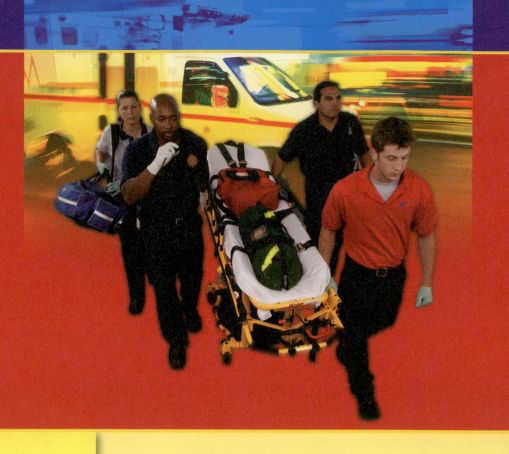

CHAPTER

18

OUTLINE

GOAL

LESSON GOAL

A cardiovascular event is a true medical emergency for a patient. The recognition and treatment of a cardiovascular event can mean the difference between life and death. This chapter reviews the circulatory system, discusses the anatomy and physiology of the cardiovascular system, and discusses the assessment and treatment of a patient experiencing a cardiac event. The chapter also covers the link between early recognition and treatment of a cardiovascular event and patient outcome. ■

Cardiovascular Emergencies

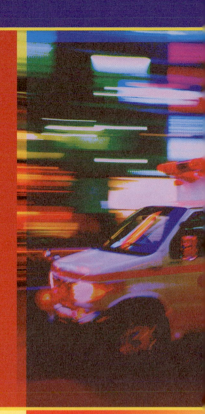

CHAPTER OBJECTIVES

After completing this chapter, the EMT student will be able to do the following:

1 List the parts of the cardiovascular system and how they work.
2 Describe the emergency medical care of the patient experiencing chest pain/discomfort.
3 List the indications and contraindications for automated external defibrillation.
4 Define the role of the emergency medical technician in the emergency cardiac care system.
5 Explain the impact of age and weight on defibrillation.
6 Discuss the position of comfort for patients with various cardiac emergencies.
7 Explain the importance of airway management in the patient with cardiovascular compromise.
8 Predict the relationship between the patient experiencing cardiovascular compromise and basic life support.
9 Discuss the fundamentals of and reasons for early defibrillation.
10 Explain the importance of prehospital advanced cardiac life support (ACLS).
11 Explain the importance of urgent transport to a facility with ACLS.
12 Discuss the various types of automated external defibrillators and the difference between the fully automated and the semiautomated external defibrillator.

Continued

18

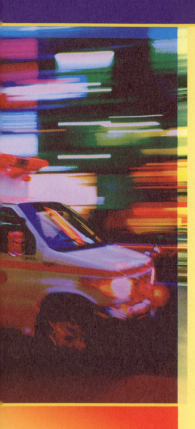

Chapter Objectives—cont'd

13 State the reasons for ensuring that the patient is pulseless and apneic before using the automated external defibrillator.

14 Discuss what might cause inappropriate shocks.

15 Explain when you would stop cardiopulmonary resuscitation to use the automated external defibrillator.

16 Discuss rhythm monitoring.

17 List the steps in the operation of the automated external defibrillator for one emergency medical technician and two emergency medical technicians.

18 Discuss the standard of care to use when treating a patient with constant ventricular fibrillation when ACLS is not available.

19 Discuss the standard of care to use when treating a patient with recurrent ventricular fibrillation when ACLS is not available.

20 Explain the reason for not checking a pulse between shocks with an automated external defibrillator.

21 Discuss the importance of and components for postresuscitation care.

22 Explain the role medical direction plays in the use of automated external defibrillation.

23 State the reasons for reviewing each call following the use of the automated external defibrillator.

24 Discuss the components that should be included in a case review.

25 Explain the role of medical direction and protocols in the emergency medical care of the patient with chest pain.

26 List the indications for the use of nitroglycerin.

27 State the contraindications for and side effects of the use of nitroglycerin.

28 Describe the controls on an automated external defibrillator and how they work.

29 Describe event documentation.

30 Explain why the maintenance of automated external defibrillators is important.

31 Explain the reasons for giving nitroglycerin to a patient with chest pain or discomfort.

32 Demonstrate the assessment and emergency medical care of a patient experiencing chest pain/discomfort.

33 Demonstrate the application and operation of the automated external defibrillator.

34 Demonstrate the maintenance of an automated external defibrillator.

35 Demonstrate the assessment and documentation of the patient's response to the automated external defibrillator.

36 Perform the steps in assisting the patient to use nitroglycerin for chest pain or discomfort.

37 Demonstrate the assessment and documentation of patient response to nitroglycerin.

38 Practice completing a prehospital care report for patients with cardiac emergencies.

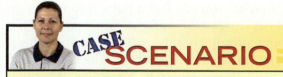

CASE SCENARIO

Dinner is almost done. Jack is cleaning up the remainder of the dishes while Elizabeth wipes down the table. Jane is using the broom, sweeping around the table. The ride-along, Jack, is already off to the common area, looking again at his emergency medical technology book, hoping that the tones go off soon. They already have had two runs earlier in the shift, causing dinner to run late. But it was so exciting to see the crew in action; they seemed to work so well together.

Jack's prayers are answered: The county tones begin to warble, and the house lights came on. "Rescue Six Thirty-six, Seventy-three Talbert Road, cross of Main, report of respiratory distress." Jack wipes his hands and heads to the garage to start up the ambulance.

They pull up to a single-story tract home in one of the older sections of town. An older woman greets them at the door, looking anxious. "My husband is in the back room. I think he fainted. Please hurry!"

"What is his name, ma'am?" asks Elizabeth, while walking down the narrow hallway toward the back bedroom.

"Jim Markham," replies the woman.

In the bedroom, Elizabeth leans over to the man, who is lying on the bed. "Mr. Markham, how are you doing?"

"I am . . . okay," the patient replied slowly, as if he were trying to convince himself that in fact he was. Although awake, Mr. Markham looked a bit confused as to where he was. He was pale, and sweating profusely. Following instructions he received from Elizabeth earlier in the shift, Jack opened the first-in bag to retrieve the penlight, stethoscope, and blood pressure cuff. Jane is busy opening the airway kit and cracking open the oxygen tank.

Question: *What are some of the procedures the emergency medical services crew should do immediately to help manage this patient?*

More than 600,000 persons die each year from various types of cardiovascular disease. Approximately half of those deaths result from sudden cardiac death. Sudden cardiac death is often the first warning sign a patient displays of cardiac disease. Up to 50% of sudden cardiac deaths occur before the patient reaches a hospital.

Cardiac events are true medical emergencies. In the prehospital setting, emergency medical care can make a significant difference in the patient's survival and outcome. This chapter discusses the assessment and treatment of cardiac emergencies and the management of **cardiac arrest.**

■ REVIEW OF THE CIRCULATORY SYSTEM

The circulatory system can be thought of as a transport system for the body, with various one-way streets and highways along the way. As discussed in Chapter 4, the circulatory system includes not only the heart but also an integrated arterial and venous system that serves specific functions to keep the body working.

The circulatory system transports oxygen and nutrients to the body and removes carbon dioxide and other wastes from the tissues.

Anatomy

Heart

The heart is more than a muscle. The heart is the "engine" of the circulatory system. The heart is composed of two sides, the right side and the left side. A wall called the **septum** divides the two sides. Each side of the heart has an **atrium** and a **ventricle,** separated by a one-way valve, meaning the valve only allows blood to flow in one direction.

The right atrium receives oxygen-depleted **blood** from the **veins** of the body and the heart and pumps it to the right ventricle. From the right ventricle the oxygen-poor blood is pumped to the lungs to be "refueled." Picking up oxygen in the lungs, the blood returns to the left atrium of the heart via the pulmonary veins. The left atrium pumps the now oxygen-rich blood to the left ventricle which then pumps the blood out to the body so that the blood can deliver oxygen and nutrients.

The one-way valve that separates the atria and ventricles prevents the backflow of blood and enables a one-way flow of blood through the heart (Fig. 18-1).

Blood Vessels

In addition to the heart, the circulatory system is composed of various vessels called **arteries** and veins in a network that is connected to the heart. Each of these arteries and veins has a specific route and a function to provide for the body.

Arteries carry blood away from the heart to the rest of the body. They carry oxygen-rich blood and deliver nutrients to the various organs of the body. With each contraction of the heart, you can feel it pumping blood through the body wherever you are able to palpate a **pulse.** You can feel a pulse through an artery that lies close to the surface of your skin and lies over a bony prominence. Fig. 18-2 shows peripheral and central pulse sites. Arteries become smaller and smaller until they connect to **arterioles.** Arterioles become smaller and smaller until they connect with **capillaries.** Capillaries are intertwined with all of the tissues in the body, allowing the exchange of oxygen for carbon dioxide. The capillaries then join with tiny vessels called **venules.** The venules join with veins, which become larger and larger in diameter returning to the right atrium. In the right atrium, the process begins all over again.

The largest artery (in diameter) of the body is the **aorta.** The aorta is a major artery that originates from

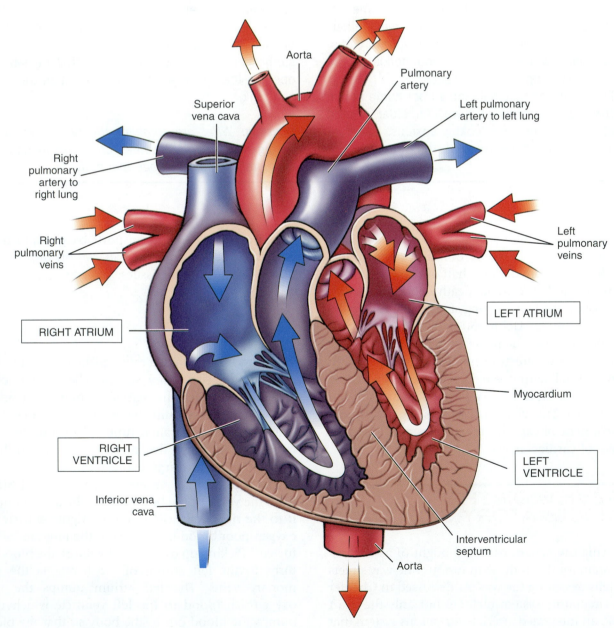

Fig. 18-1 Anatomy of the heart.

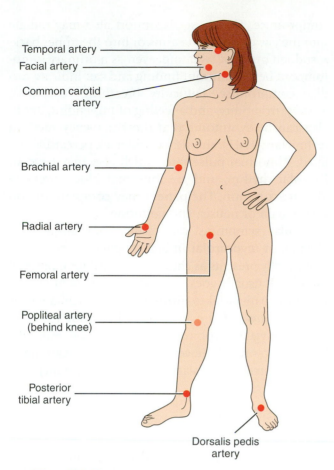

Temporal artery
Facial artery
Common carotid
artery
Brachial artery
Radial artery
Femoral artery
Popliteal artery
(behind knee)
Posterior
tibial artery
Dorsalis pedis
artery

Fig. 18-2 Peripheral and central pulse sites.

the heart and lies in front of the spine in the thoracic and abdominal cavity. At the level of the navel, the aorta divides to form the **iliac arteries.** These arteries supply the lower extremities with oxygen and nutrients.

The **pulmonary artery** originates in the right ventricle of the heart. It carries oxygen-poor blood and delivers it to the lungs to be replenished. The pulmonary artery is the only artery in the body that carries oxygen-poor blood instead of oxygen-rich blood.

The **carotid arteries** are the major arteries in the neck. They supply the head with oxygenated blood. The carotid pulse can be felt on either side of the neck next to the trachea.

The **femoral artery** is the major artery of the thigh and supplies the groin and lower extremities with oxygenated blood. Femoral pulses can be felt on either side of the groin area at the crease between the abdomen and thigh.

The **radial artery** supplies the lower arm and hand with oxygenated blood. Radial pulses can be felt in the distal anterior area of the wrist (near the base of the thumb on the palm side of the wrist).

The **brachial artery** can be felt in the upper arm and can be palpated on the inside of the arm be-

tween the elbow and the shoulder. The brachial artery most commonly is used to determine a **blood pressure** with a **sphygmomanometer** (blood pressure cuff) and a stethoscope. The sphygmomanometer is placed over the brachial artery and the blood pressure is auscultated at the distal end of the brachial artery in the antecubital fossa at the elbow.

Arteries that can be palpated in the lower extremities are the posterior **tibial artery** and the **dorsalis pedis artery.** The posterior tibial artery is located on the medial side of the malleolus (near the inside of the ankle). The dorsalis pedis artery is located on the anterior surface of the foot.

The primary function of the **venous system** (veins) is to carry blood back to the heart after the *arterial system* has delivered oxygen and nutrients. The **pulmonary vein** carries blood to the left atrium of the heart from the lungs after being replenished with oxygen. From there, the blood once again is pumped out into the body. Consequently, the pulmonary vein is the only vein in the body that carries oxygen-rich blood.

The **venae cavae** are major veins that consist of two branches: the **superior vena cava** and the **inferior vena cava.** The superior vena cava carries oxygen-poor blood from the head and arms. The inferior vena cava carries oxygen-poor blood from the lower extremities and torso. This oxygen-poor blood in both of these major veins is transported to the right atrium of the heart. As mentioned previously, the blood then is carried to the lungs from the right atrium via the right ventricle and pulmonary artery to be reoxygenated.

Blood Composition

What is blood? Blood is composed of numerous components including **red blood cells** (erythrocytes), **white blood cells** (leukocytes), **plasma,** and **platelets.** Red blood cells give blood its red color. They also carry oxygen to the organs of the body and carry carbon dioxide away from the organs. White blood cells help defend the body against infections. Plasma is the fluid that moves the red and white blood cells and nutrients throughout the body. It contains a variety of proteins, hormones and infection-fighting chemicals called antibodies. Platelets are special cells that make the blood form clots and help the body to stop bleeding.

Physiology

The left ventricle of the heart contracts, sending the oxygen-rich blood through the arteries of the body. As this occurs, you can simultaneously feel that push of blood by palpating any of the major arteries that are located over a bone near the surface of the skin. This is called a pulse.

To review, peripheral pulses are the following:

- Radial
- Brachial
- Posterior tibial
- Dorsalis pedis

Central pulses are the following:

- Carotid
- Femoral

Blood pressure is the pressure exerted against the walls of an artery when the left ventricle contracts. When one is using a sphygmomanometer, this reading is called the **systolic blood pressure.** This pressure is recorded as the top number of the blood pressure reading.

The pressure against the arteries when the left ventricle completes its contraction and is at rest is called the **diastolic blood pressure.** This pressure is recorded as the bottom number of the blood pressure reading, when assessed with a sphygmomanometer.

Inadequate circulation can cause a state of profound depression to the vital processes of the body called **shock** (hypoperfusion). A lack of blood volume or a lack of blood circulating in the body can cause shock. Shock can be recognized by specific signs and symptoms as the body reacts and attempts to compensate for its loss of perfusion. Signs and symptoms of shock include the following:

- Pale, cyanotic, cool, clammy skin
- Weak but rapid pulse
- Rapid and shallow breathing
- Restlessness, anxiety, or mental dullness
- Nausea and/or vomiting
- Low or decreased blood pressure
- Subnormal temperature

Chapter 25 further discusses the effects shock (hypoperfusion) has on the body.

■ CARDIAC COMPROMISE

As you perform your patient assessment, look for signs and symptoms that may indicate **cardiac compromise.** Chest pain that the patient describes as a dull pressure, a dull ache, or a squeezing or tightness can be a symptom of **myocardial** (cardiac muscle)

compromise. The chest discomfort also may radiate into the jaw or down the arms or into the upper back. A sudden onset of sweating, even as a primary symptom, can be a significant finding and can indicate cardiac compromise. Difficulty breathing (dyspnea), anxiety, irritability, and a feeling of impending doom also can be symptoms that the emergency medical technician (EMT) should consider to be cardiac related. Abnormal pulse rate, which also may have an irregular rhythm, and an abnormal blood pressure also are common. The patient may complain of epigastric pain or nausea and vomiting.

Similar symptoms can result from **angina, ischemia,** or **myocardial infarct.** Angina is a condition that usually presents as chest discomfort upon physical exertion. It usually goes away when the patient rests or when the patient takes **nitroglycerin.** Ischemia results when an area of the heart muscle is not receiving enough oxygen. Myocardial infarction is the result of a blockage to one of the vessels in the heart resulting in death (infarction) of heart muscle (myocardium).

Assessment

Well-developed assessment skills are essential in forming a field impression to determine an appropriate treatment plan for a patient with possible cardiac compromise. The initial assessment for any patient with suspected cardiac disease is the same as it is for any other type of patient. Once your scene is secure and you have your necessary personal protective gear in place, assessment can begin. Assessment should include forming a general impression and continuing with your evaluation of airway, breathing, and circulation and determining the priority status or criticality of your patient. Apply high-flow oxygen as soon as possible to any patient showing signs and symptoms of cardiac compromise.

If the patient is able to interact with you and has a known history of cardiac problems, move on to your focused assessment and physical examination after your initial assessment. Patients tend to place themselves in a position that provides the most comfort to them. Be sure to allow the patient to continue to assume his or her position of comfort as you are assessing, treating, and transporting him or her. Patients with *hypotension* (low blood pressure) or who complain of being light-headed or dizzy may feel best when lying down. Patients who are complaining of difficulty breathing may feel best when sitting up. Be sensitive to what feels the most comfortable to the patient. Patients with cardiac symptoms should not exert themselves. Any patient who is suspected of having cardiac-related signs and symptoms should not be allowed to get up and move about and should not be allowed to walk. For the patient to remain at rest during assessment and transport is crucial to avoid increasing cardiac workload.

Obtain baseline vital signs including skin assessment and mental status.

Important questions to ask your patient in assessing any chest pain are the *OPQRST* questions:

- *O*—Onset
- *P*—Provocation
- *Q*—Quality
- *R*—Radiation
- *S*—Severity
- *T*—Time

Box 18-1 gives further details of the OPQRST assessment for evaluating a patient with chest pain.

Any prior cardiac-related history is pertinent information. Included in your SAMPLE history (*S*igns and symptoms, *A*llergies, *M*edications, *P*ast medical history, *L*ast oral intake, *E*vents preceding), you should ask the patient about any prescribed cardiac medica-

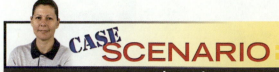

CASE SCENARIO
continued

Jack's first set of measured vital signs were:

Pulse	Respirations	Blood Pressure
110	20	86/64

From Elizabeth's SAMPLE history and OPQRST of the complaint, Jack suspected that Mr. Markham was experiencing a cardiac emergency. His history indicated that he had high risk: he was taking medications for high blood pressure and high cholesterol. Elizabeth held up one of the medications. "Jack, should we help him with his nitroglycerin?"

Question: Given Jack's findings, should Mr. Markham receive nitroglycerin? Why or why not?

tion. You also should ask whether he or she has been prescribed nitroglycerin.

Nitroglycerin

Nitroglycerin (generic name) most commonly is found in the form of **sublingual** (under the tongue) tablets or in sublingual spray (Fig. 18-3). Common trade names for nitroglycerin are Nitrostat or Nitrolingual (nitroglycerin translingual) Spray.

Action

Nitroglycerin dilates blood vessels, decreasing the workload of the heart, which in turn alleviates cardiac-related signs and symptoms. With dilation of the blood vessels, however, comes a risk that the patient's blood pressure may decrease. If the patient's systolic blood pressure decreases to less than 100 mm Hg, place the patient in the **Trendelenburg position** (supine with his or her feet elevated) and withhold further administration of nitroglycerin.

If the patient has a current prescription of nitroglycerin that has been issued to him or her, ask whether the patient has taken any before your arrival. For the conscious and alert patient showing signs and symptoms of a cardiac emergency, consider administration of nitroglycerin. The EMT should examine the patient's prescription of nitroglycerin to ensure that it is prescribed for the patient, is not expired, is the correct **dosage**, and is to be ad-

BOX 18-1
OPQRST Assessment for Chest Pain

*O*nset: When did the symptoms first occur? What were you doing when they first started?

*P*rovocation: Does anything make the pain worse or better? Does it hurt when inhaling or exhaling?

*Q*uality: Describe the pain. Is it sharp or dull? Is it constant, or does it subside and get worse?

*R*adiation: Does the pain go to anywhere else besides the chest? Is there pain in the jaw, arm, or back?

*S*everity: How bad is the pain? A tool that is useful for assessing the pain of a patient with cardiac disease is the 1-to-10 pain scale. Ask the patient to rate his or her chest pain or discomfort, with 1 being the least pain and 10 being the worst pain he or she can imagine. This initial rating makes it easier to evaluate the level of pain during your ongoing assessment of the patient. It also helps you to determine whether the interventions performed are benefiting the patient and easing his or her symptoms.

*T*ime: How long have you had the pain? When did it start and has it come and gone?

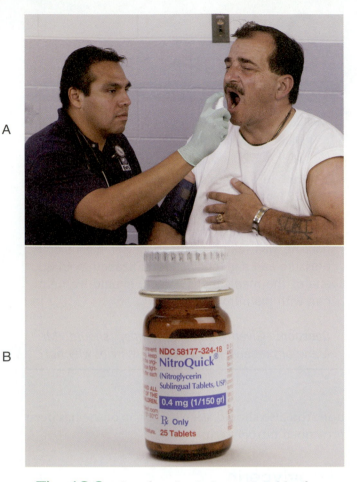

Fig. 18-3 Nitroglycerin. **A,** Spray. **B,** Tablet form.

ministered sublingually. The patient may take up to three consecutive doses of nitroglycerin, either by sublingual pill or spray. If the patient has not met the maximum dosage, the EMT should obtain orders (online or off-line) for authorization to assist the patient with nitroglycerin administration. Once orders are obtained from medical direction for the administration of nitroglycerin, the EMT must be sure the patient meets the following criteria:

- Signs and symptoms of cardiac-related chest pain
- Systolic blood pressure greater than 100 mm Hg
- Physician-prescribed nitroglycerin tablets or spray in the patient's name
- Specific authorization from medical direction

The EMT also must be certain that none of the following **contraindications** are present before administering nitroglycerin:

- Systolic blood pressure less than 100 mm Hg
- Head injury

- Use of sildenafil (Viagra), vardenafil (Levitra), tadalafil (Cialis), or similar types of drugs for erectile dysfunction within the previous 48 hours
- Infants and children
- Patient has met maximum dosage before arrival of emergency medical services (EMS)
- Patient does not have his or her own prescribed medication
- Medical direction has not authorized administration of nitroglycerin for this patient

The EMT should be knowledgeable about any drug for which he or she is responsible for administering or with which he or she can assist.

Dosage

The dosage for nitroglycerin is one tablet or one metered spray under the tongue (0.3 to 0.4 mg). This dosage may be repeated in 3 to 5 minutes if there is not sufficient relief of the patient's symptoms. A maximum of three doses may be given with approval from medical direction. The EMT should reassess the patient after each dose of nitroglycerin before assisting the patient with more doses. Be especially alert for blood pressure that drops less than 100 mm Hg after giving nitroglycerin.

Administration

Once medical direction has issued orders to administer nitroglycerin and the EMT has found no contraindications, the EMT should assist the patient with administering nitroglycerin. Be sure to follow the *four R's of medication administration:* the right medication, the right patient, the right dose, and the right route. The patient must be alert as well. Check the expiration date of the nitroglycerin. Ask the patient to lift his or her tongue and place or have the patient place the nitroglycerin tablet or one pump of spray under his or her tongue (Skill 18-1). Instruct the patient to keep his or her mouth closed and not to swallow until the tablet completely dissolves and is absorbed. Reassess the patient's blood pressure within 2 minutes of administration of the nitroglycerin. For a patient to complain of a headache or a burning sensation under the tongue is normal. Record administration of the nitroglycerin along with accurate times of the administration and any effects it has had in relieving the patient's signs and symptoms.

Reassessment

Ongoing assessment of the patient with cardiac disease is important. Vital signs, pain assessment, and assessment of the effects of interventions should be recurrent.

SKILL 18-1
Administration of Nitroglycerin

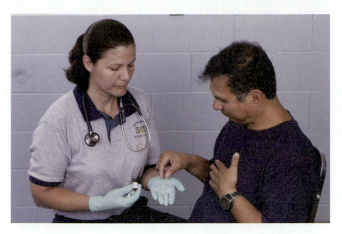

1. Follow appropriate body substance isolation precautions and assess the patient's vital signs. Consult medical direction regarding nitroglycerin administration.

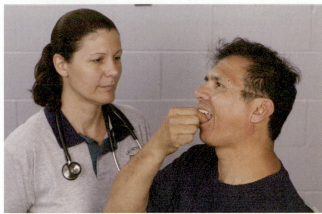

2. Instruct the patient to lift his or her tongue. Place one tablet under the tongue and ask the patient to close his or her mouth. Instruct the patient to leave the tablet under the tongue until it is completely dissolved and to not chew the tablet.

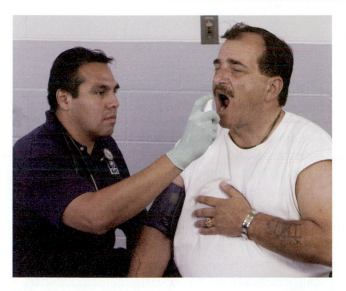

3. If the patient uses nitroglycerin spray, spray once under the tongue. Instruct the patient to close his or her mouth quickly.

4. Take the patient's blood pressure within 2 minutes of administration. Record the patient's name, the name of the medication, the dosage of the medication (listed on bottle), the time of administration, and the name of the ordering physician providing medical direction.

5. Reassess and record all vital signs. Also assess and document any effects the medication has had on the patient. Notify medical direction of any changes in the patient's condition or for requests for additional doses.

Transport

Do not allow the patient to move himself or herself, as exertion only serves to increase the workload of the heart. Moreover, transport the patient in a position that is most comfortable for him or her. Consider any patient with signs and symptoms of cardiac compromise as critical. If available, request a **tier** rendezvous with advanced life support. Consider methods of transportation that are best for the patient. For example, although a patient's situation may be urgent and critical and rapid transport may be necessary, lights and sirens may cause added fear and anxiety for the patient. Assess what is necessary and explain to the patient what will occur. If it is determined that lights and sirens are needed to help control traffic, explain this to the patient. Assure the patient that safety is the primary concern. A calm and careful transport for the patient is best, and safety is the most important consideration.

■ BASIC LIFE SUPPORT

Not all patients who experience cardiac compromise experience cardiac arrest. That possibility does exist, however, and the EMT must be prepared to manage such an event by being proficient in cardiopulmonary resuscitation (CPR). Any patient who is complaining of breathing difficulty or chest pain or discomfort should be considered a candidate for potential cardiac arrest. Therefore the EMT should be prepared and have the necessary equipment nearby in anticipation of such an event (Skill 18-2).

Good basic life support skills are essential. Emergency medical technicians rarely have a situation in the field that calls for performing one-person CPR (Skill 18-3). However, some situations may require it. For example, your partner may need to prepare or retrieve equipment. Similarly, he or she may be driving en route to the hospital while you are the only other EMS provider on the scene or in the back of the ambulance.

You should practice these techniques and enhance them during your EMT course. In addition, **defibrillation** should be integrated into your one- and two-rescuer CPR skills. The use of automated external defibrillation devices is discussed later in this chapter.

As a professional emergency medical provider, learning basic life support includes using body substance isolation techniques, airway adjuncts, and oxygenation and ventilation equipment such as oral or nasal airways, bag-valve-mask, and flow-restricted oxygen-powered ventilation devices. The use of these devices is discussed in Chapters 7 and 17. The EMT must practice and become proficient at using these devices along with the integration of CPR. The EMT also must assume responsibility for keeping informed of current trends in treatment standards and the latest developments in technology.

Obtaining a pertinent history by interviewing bystanders and/or family members is important. The history can aid in determining the nature of cardiac arrest and what may have led to it. Document this information. Also share this information with other health care providers to assist in determining further management of the patient's condition.

When available, request advanced cardiac life support (ACLS) to tier with any patient with cardiac arrest in order to continue the **chain of survival**. The American Heart Association defines the chain of survival as a series of actions that include early access to EMS, early CPR, early defibrillation, and early ACLS[1] (Box 18-2).

BOX 18-2
Chain of Survival

Early access: Early identification of a cardiac emergency and access to emergency medical services. Training the public to recognize signs of cardiac arrest and when to contact emergency medical services.

Early cardiopulmonary resuscitation: Lay public education and training in performing cardiopulmonary resuscitation until emergency medical personnel can arrive. Early cardiopulmonary resuscitation is an essential element in the patient's chance of survival.

Early defibrillation: Defibrillation is the most important element in reversing ventricular fibrillation and aiding the heart to resume functioning. Public access defibrillation is becoming more widespread.

Early advanced care: Access to advanced cardiac life support is needed to provide the necessary life support needed for a cardiac arrest victim.

SKILL 18-2
Two-Rescuer Cardiopulmonary Resuscitation

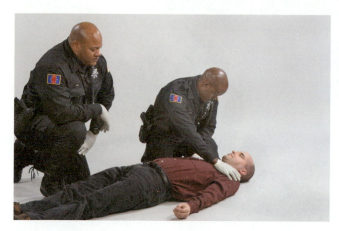

1. Establish responsiveness.

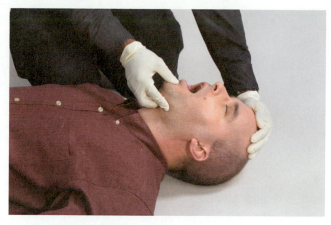

2. If patient is unresponsive, one rescuer should call for help or retrieve the AED if available, while the other opens the patient's airway with a head tilt–chin lift or jaw thrust.

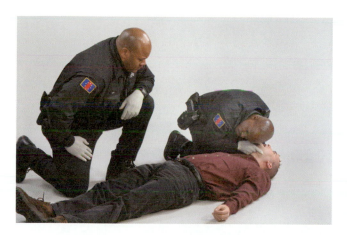

3. Look, listen, and feel for breathing.

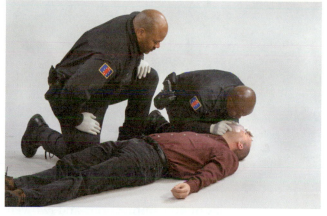

4. If there are no signs of breathing, provide two rescue breaths or retrieve the AED if available.

Continued

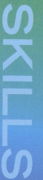

SKILLS

SKILL 18-2
Two-Rescuer Cardiopulmonary Resuscitation—cont'd

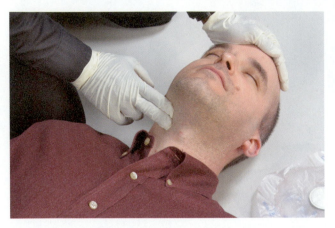

5. Check for signs of circulation, including carotid pulse, signs of normal breathing, coughing, or movement.

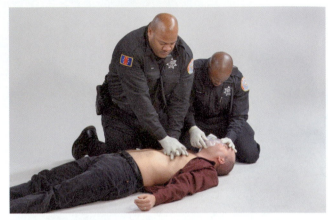

6. If no signs of circulation, one rescuer performs 30 chest compressions, followed by two ventilations given by the second rescuer.

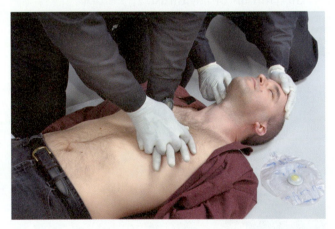

7. After five cycles of 30 compressions and two ventilations, the rescuer at the head should check for signs of circulation. If no signs of circulation, resume cardiopulmonary resuscitation. Check for signs of circulation after every five cycles (about 2 minutes). Rescuers should switch between providing compressions and ventilations as they tire and as convenient.

SKILL 18-3
One-Rescuer Cardiopulmonary Resuscitation

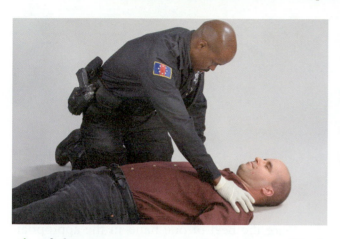

1. If the rescuer witnesses the patient suddenly collapse, the rescuer should establish unresponsiveness, then phone 911 or get the AED if available. If the lone rescuer is called to an asphyxial cause such as a drowning, the rescuer should perform five cycles of CPR (30 compressions to two ventilations each).

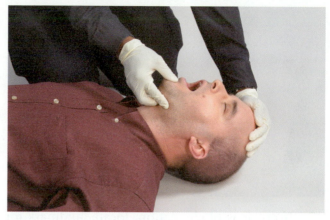

2. Open the airway with a head tilt–chin lift or jaw thrust.

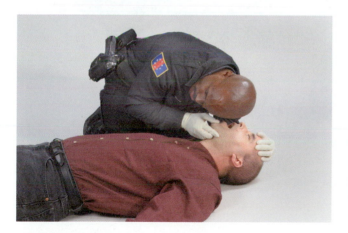

3. Look, listen, and feel for breathing.

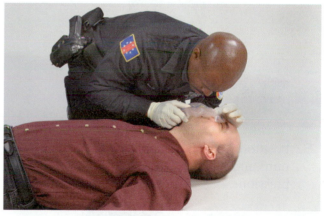

4. If no signs of breathing, provide two rescue breaths.

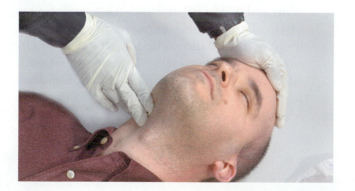

5. Check for signs of circulation including carotid pulse, signs of normal breathing, coughing, or movement.

Continued

SKILLS

SKILL 18-3
One-Rescuer Cardiopulmonary Resuscitation—cont'd

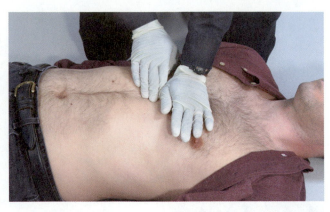

6. If no signs of circulation, locate landmark for compressions on the lower portion of the sternum.

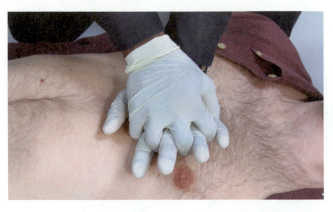

7. Place the heel of one hand in the appropriate spot and place your other hand on top. Use the force from the heels of your hands only.

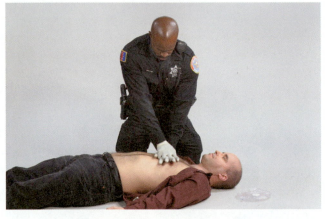

8. Position yourself directly over the patient's sternum and lock your elbows to deliver 30 compressions.

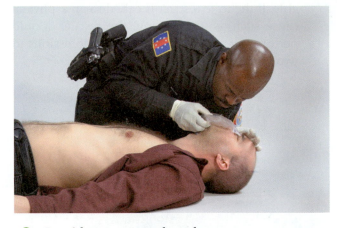

9. Provide two rescue breaths.

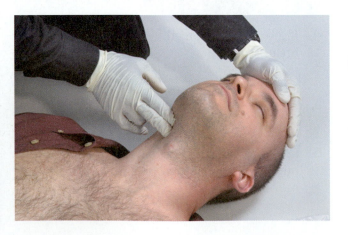

10. After approximately five cycles of 30 compressions and two ventilations, check again for signs of circulation. If no signs, resume cardiopulmonary resuscitation, checking for signs of circulation every five cycles. If there are signs of circulation but no signs of breathing, continue rescue breathing at a rate of one breath every 5 seconds.

■ AUTOMATED EXTERNAL DEFIBRILLATION

Cardiac arrest, sometimes referred to as sudden death, can be a sudden loss of heart function. Most sudden deaths from cardiac arrest occur when the electrical impulses in the heart become rapid and chaotic. Impulses in the heart that are rapid and chaotic do not allow the heart to pump blood out to the body as it is designed to do. This electrical activity is called **ventricular fibrillation** (Fig. 18-4) and sometimes can be reversed with the use of a cardiac **defibrillator.**

Early defibrillation, a continued link in the chain of survival, includes recognizing and treating ventricular fibrillation. The **automated external defibrillator** (AED; Fig. 18-5) is a machine designed to evaluate and recognize a patient's cardiac rhythm and deliver a shock if the patient displays a cardiac rhythm such as ventricular fibrillation.

Many EMS systems have demonstrated increased survival rates of patients with cardiac arrest when using AEDs as opposed to CPR alone. Early defibrillation programs are gaining popularity in the public and in traditional health care arenas. Automated external defibrillators are functional and simple to use. As **public access defibrillation** programs are gaining popularity, and access to AEDs is becoming more common, response time in the chain of survival is decreasing, and survival rates for victims of sudden cardiac arrest is increasing.

Overview of the Automated External Defibrillator

Health care providers have been using defibrillation for cardiac arrest for many years. With the advancement of computer technology, defibrillation has evolved into an easy-to-access, easy-to-learn, and easy-to-perform treatment.

Defibrillators deliver a shock to the patient's chest. The intent is to reverse the rapid, chaotic electric activity the heart experiences during ventricular fibrillation. Ventricular fibrillation sometimes is described as the heart "quivering" and not producing the organized impulses necessary to cause the heart to contract in an effective manner. Defibrillation can interrupt that chaotic electrical impulse and cause the heart to start contractions in a more orderly fashion. The more orderly fashion enables the heart to pump blood out to the body as designed.

Most commonly, AEDs come fully automated or semiautomated. Fully automated external defibrillators require the EMT simply to apply two electrode patches to the patient's chest, attach the electrodes to the AED, and turn on the machine. The AED then an-

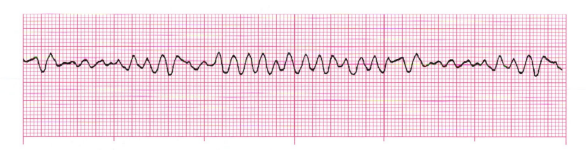

Fig. 18-4 Ventricular fibrillation.

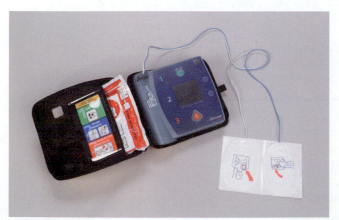

Fig. 18-5 Example of an automated external defibrillator.

alyzes the cardiac rhythm and delivers shocks to the patient when appropriate.

A **semiautomated external defibrillator** operates in much the same way. The EMT turns on the power to the AED, applies the electrodes (adhesive patches) to the patient's chest, and attaches the electrode wires to the AED. The EMT then must press a button telling the machine to analyze the cardiac rhythm. Once the cardiac rhythm is analyzed, the machine, through a computer-synthesized voice, will instruct the EMT on subsequent needed actions. If it is determined that a shock is needed, the voice on the AED will instruct the EMT to deliver a shock by pushing the shock button.

The AED is designed to deliver a shock only if the patient has a "shockable" rhythm. The AED has a microprocessor installed that evaluates the cardiac rhythm and determines whether it is a rhythm for which a shock is indicated. Ventricular fibrillation and **ventricular tachycardia** are rhythms that the AED will shock. Ventricular tachycardia is a rapid cardiac rhythm in which the heart beats so rapidly that it is not producing output to the rest of the body (Fig. 18-6). When the cardiac rhythm is ventricular tachycardia, the patient may or may not have a discernable pulse. The AED will advise to shock for ventricular tachycardia once the rate ex-

ceeds 180 beats per minute. The AED cannot determine whether the patient has a pulse. It can determine only what electrical rhythm the heart has. To avoid delivering a shock to a patient who has a pulse, attach the AED only to patients who are unresponsive, breathless, and pulseless. Patients with a pulse still have electrical impulses in the heart that are functioning. Shocking a patient with a pulse can cause the heart to convert into ventricular fibrillation or into **asystole.** Asystole (Fig. 18-7) also is known as flatline or cardiac standstill. Asystole indicates that the heart has stopped all function, including any electrical activity.

In very few instances has an AED delivered an inappropriate shock. These machines are accurate at interpreting cardiac activity and which rhythms require a shock and which rhythms do not. Often failure of the machine is due to human error. A priority at every shift check is making sure that batteries are working and that extra batteries are available. The AED should not be placed on patients who have a pulse. Moreover, it should never be operated when in a moving vehicle or while moving the patient. Stop CPR while the machine is analyzing the patient's heart rhythm and while shocks are being delivered. The person operating the device should ensure that no one is touching the patient while the AED is analyzing the cardiac

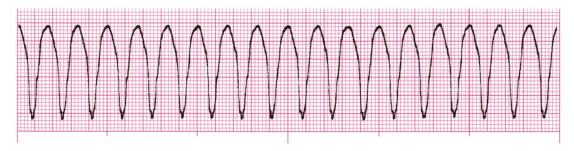

Fig. 18-6 Ventricular tachycardia.

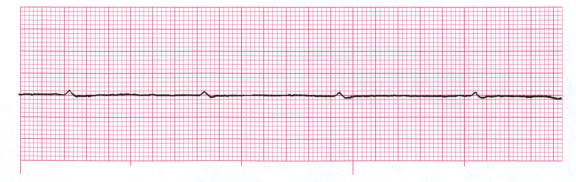

Fig. 18-7 P-wave asystole.

rhythm or while shocks are being delivered. Stop CPR and artificial ventilations while the machine is analyzing and while it is delivering shocks to the patient. Anyone touching the patient can be shocked as well. Although CPR is part of the chain of survival for patients with cardiac arrest, early defibrillation is more effective in terminating ventricular fibrillation. Because most patients with shockable rhythms are in ventricular fibrillation, stopping CPR to defibrillate is more beneficial to the patient. Cardiopulmonary resuscitation may be resumed after the initial shocks are delivered.

Advantages of the Automated External Defibrillator

The AED has many advantages. Operation is simple and quick. Learning to use a defibrillator is easier than learning the techniques of CPR. However, one must memorize the appropriate sequence for using the AED. After the initial training is completed, continuing education should be in place. Moreover, regular practice sessions using an AED trainer and various cardiac arrest scenarios should be in place. Skills should be evaluated periodically. Medical direction should be involved in ensuring a system of quality assurance and evaluation of cardiac arrest events.

The machine can be attached to the patient and the first shock delivered within 1 minute of arrival at the patient's side. Adhesive pads make using the AED a hands-off operation. Automated external defibrillation is safer than traditional ACLS defibrillation, which requires placing and holding paddles directly onto the patient's chest. Electrodes are large and easy to place on the patient. Some AEDs have an optional rhythm-monitoring system that can be beneficial when tiering with ACLS services.

Automated External Defibrillator Operation

Approaching a patient with cardiac arrest requires the same initial actions as any other call requires. Practice body substance isolation using personal protective gear. If possible, don your gear while en route to the scene. Once you arrive on scene, survey the scene and ensure safety. If additional resources have not been called for already, you should request resources such as ACLS.

Perform your initial assessment of patient responsiveness, airway, breathing, and circulation. If CPR is

in progress by bystanders, ask them to stop while you verify pulselessness and apnea. Once it is verified the patient is pulseless and breathless, have your partner resume CPR for 5 cycles (about 2 minutes) while you prepare the AED.

Skill 18-4 outlines the steps for using an AED as described in this section. Turn on the defibrillator power. Attach the adhesive pads to the patient's chest, and ensure the electrodes are attached to the AED. If the AED is a machine that has an event voice recorder, begin your narrative. Stop CPR and ask all bystanders to "clear" (stand away from and do not touch) the patient. Rescuers who are managing the patient's airway also must be clear of the patient. Initiate the analysis of the cardiac rhythm by pushing the analyze button.

Fig. 18-8 depicts a universal algorithm protocol for operation of an AED.

Shock Advised

If the AED advises to deliver a shock, again **clear the patient** by ensuring that no one is touching the patient. Once the machine charges and advises to deliver the shock, press the shock button. Allow the

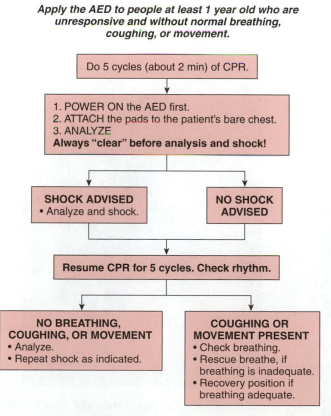

Fig. 18-8 Automated external defibrillator protocol.

SKILL 18-4
◎ *Use of the Automated External Defibrillator*

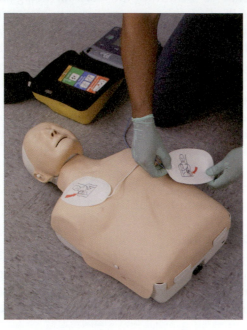

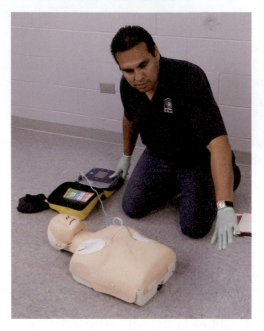

1. Place the automated external defibrillator (AED) next to the patient's left ear if possible. Turn the AED on.
2. Attach the AED pads to the patient's chest as directed on the pads.

3. Allow the AED to analyze the patient's rhythm. Do not touch the patient.
4. If the AED states that a shock is advised, ensure that everyone is clear of the patient.

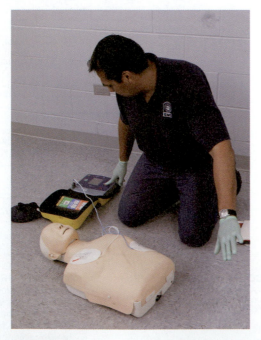

5. Press the shock button. Once the shock is delivered, immediately begin 5 cycles (about 2 minutes) of CPR beginning with chest compressions.

SKILLS

machine to shock the patient. Immediately resume CPR for 5 cycles. Check rhythm.

If the patient is not breathing, provide mechanical ventilations with supplemental oxygen and initiate transport.

If after any rhythm analysis, the machine advises *no shock,* check the patient's pulse. If the patient has a pulse, check the patient's breathing. If the patient is breathing adequately, apply high-flow oxygen by non-rebreather mask and initiate transport. If the patient is not breathing adequately, provide mechanical ventilation with supplemental oxygen and initiate transport.

Standard Operational Procedures

The EMT must be familiar with the operation of the device that is used in his or her EMS system. No AED can work without properly functioning batteries. Thus the EMT should check to see that the batteries are in working order at the beginning of each shift. Extra batteries also should be carried and should be accessible at all times.

Although rapid defibrillation is of utmost importance, airway and ventilation are prime concerns for the patient also. As emphasized in previous learning, the body and the brain cannot survive without oxygen. Therefore, manage airway and breathing concurrently while carrying out the AED protocol. Stay clear of patients when the AED is analyzing and delivering shocks, but provide airway support and ventilations when performing CPR.

If the patient has persistent ventricular fibrillation (the machine repeatedly advises to deliver a shock) and there is no ACLS available, transport as soon as possible. Additional shocks may be delivered to the patient in persistent ventricular fibrillation en route. Automated external defibrillators cannot analyze a rhythm accurately when an emergency vehicle is in motion. Thus you first must have the driver stop the vehicle before you have the AED analyze the patient's cardiac rhythm. Defibrillation in a moving vehicle is never safe because of the potential for the rescuer to be shocked.

If en route with an unconscious patient who has a pulse or a patient who has been resuscitated but is unresponsive, monitor the patient's pulse frequently (every 30 seconds). If you subsequently determine that a pulse is not present, do the following:

- Stop the vehicle.
- Start CPR if the defibrillator is not immediately available.

- Once the AED is attached, analyze the rhythm.
- Deliver one shock if indicated.
- Resume CPR for 5 cycles.
- Continue transport.

Single Rescuer with Automated External Defibrillator

As a professional provider, you likely will not find yourself in a position of being a lone rescuer on a call. However, in the event this should occur, follow this sequence for using the AED:

- Perform the initial assessment (airway, breathing, and circulation).
- Ensure the patient is pulseless and apneic.
- Turn on AED power.
- Attach the device to the patient.
- Initiate rhythm analysis.
- Deliver the shock if directed.
- Follow AED protocol.

Your protocols should have criteria in place for using ACLS tiers within your EMS system. Advanced cardiac life support is not required in order to use an AED; however, ACLS is a link in the chain of survival. Advanced cardiac life support can provide ongoing additional care for the patient in cardiac arrest. Implement ACLS as soon as possible. Protocols established by medical direction should explain what ac-

SPECIAL Considerations

The automated external defibrillator generally is not used for patients under the age of 1 year old. Most children experience cardiac arrest following respiratory arrest. Automated external defibrillators designed for adults may deliver a shock that has too much energy for a child less than 55 lb. This can cause additional damage to the myocardium. Many AED manufacturers now offer child pads that deliver less energy. Use these pads for children if available. If child pads are not available, use adult pads. Consult medical direction and become familiar with your local protocols and equipment for recommendations on using the automated external defibrillator for pediatric patients.

tions to carry out if you are waiting for ACLS to arrive on scene.

The AED is an electrical device and should be handled appropriately. Never operate the AED in or near water or in the rain. Water can transport an electric current from the device not only to the patient but also to the rescuer and bystanders if used in or near water. If necessary, move the patient to the ambulance and remove any wet clothing he or she may be wearing. When operating the AED, be sure the patient is not touching anything metal. Metal also has the ability to transmit the electric current. The possibility of electric current being transmitted when delivering a shock to the patient is an important consideration when clearing bystanders.

Postresuscitation Care

If the patient remains pulseless once the AED protocol has been completed, follow local protocol regarding transport with CPR, ACLS tier activation and rendezvous, and continued use of the AED. If the patient does regain a pulse after AED protocol has been followed, ensure a patent airway and maintain basic life support. Keep the AED attached to the patient while transporting to the receiving facility. Continue with a focused assessment and ongoing assessment en route. Be sure to reassess frequently any interventions you have initiated.

Documentation

Documentation is an important part of ongoing medical care for the patient. Document the initial and ongoing assessments and interventions performed. Also document any response or lack of response to interventions you have performed. Documentation should include shocks that have been delivered and analysis of *no shocks advised*. Also document the patient's vital signs and airway, breathing, and circulatory status during the AED protocol. Some systems use a standard documentation form for patients with cardiac arrest with AED use. This may be helpful in documenting the event.

Defibrillator Maintenance

Defibrillators require regular maintenance. The EMT should complete a maintenance checklist every shift (Fig. 18-9). Each unit the system has should be checked. Defibrillator failure is usually due to improper maintenance, most commonly battery failure.

A schedule for regular replacement of batteries should be established. The American Heart Association has published information regarding guidelines and additional information for the use of automated external defibrillation.

Skills Maintenance

Most systems require a 90-day rotation of skills verification for operation of the AED. To be well prepared during a cardiac event, you should practice your skills frequently, incorporating various cardiac arrest scenarios.

Training to use an AED as an EMT does not automatically allow you to use it legally. State laws and rules and local medical direction will determine whether your EMS system is allowed to use defibrillation during a cardiac arrest event. Every cardiac arrest call with an AED used should be reviewed by the medical director or his designee. Reviews can be written reports or, if used, voice recording or solid state or magnetic tape recordings that are stored in the AED. Reviewing AED calls helps to aid in quality improvement and assurance. The review process should involve review of operator performance and review of the EMS system as a whole. This will help to ensure that every link in the chain of survival has been established and is used.

■ VASCULAR EMERGENCIES

All chest pain is not cardiac. The great vessels share the chest cavity with the heart, and disorders of or injury to these structures can cause pain and dysfunction that may mimic cardiac problems.

Aneurysms

This is a weakening and dilation of the artery wall. The layers that make up the artery separate, and a hematoma or bulge develops. This bulge can impair circulation beyond the aneurysm and it can leak or rupture, creating complications in the chest cavity or shock and death.

Aortic Dissection

Over 85% of aortic dissections present as acute chest pain. Patients most frequently will describe abrupt severe chest pain. Often patients describe the pain as going to the back between the scapulas. Many patients describe a "ripping or tearing" sensation in their chest.

The condition is caused by a tear that causes the layers in the aorta to separate, and blood can then enter between the layers, further separating them. This can happen spontaneously, often in patients with hypertension, or it can be brought on by trauma or possibly medical procedures like catheterizations.

During assessment, vital signs may indicate extension of the developing dissection. As blood flow into the arteries branching off the aorta is compromised, the pulse in one or more extremity may be diminished or obliterated. This condition can cause further cardiac complications by involving the coronary arteries, and rupture of the dissection can cause bleeding into the pericardial space.

These patients require urgent medical or surgical intervention depending on the location of the aneurysm. Field care will include IV access and infusions, at least 95% oxygen by mask, and expeditious transport to an appropriate facility.

Vascular Occlusions

Vascular occlusions occur particularly in patients between the ages of 50 and 70. Narrowing of the vessels due to chronic atherosclerotic disease further complicated by emboli can narrow and obstruct arteries. Sudden occlusion of a vessel will cause hypoxia to the tissues counting on the vessel for its blood sup-

Medtronic

LIFEPAK® CR Plus
Defibrillator
User's Checklist

Year: ___   Unit Serial Number: ___   Location: ___

MONTH
DATE
INITIALS

Instruction and Recommended Corrective Action

Check defibrillator for damage or foreign substances.
If it appears that unit was tampered with, immediately notify: ___

OK is visible on readiness display.
If not, refer to Troubleshooting Table.

Note date electrode pads expire: ___
If date is passed notify: ___

Extra set of electrode pads stored with AED (optional).
If missing notify: ___

Infant/child electrode pads* stored with AED (optional).
Expiration date: ___
If missing notify: ___

Resuscitation Kit containing: disposable gloves, face mask, trauma scissors and razor stored with AED.
If kit or items missing notify: ___

Other resuscitation equipment stored with AED: ___
If missing notify: ___

NOTE: If corrective action is needed, leave box unchecked and complete troubleshooting log.

Troubleshooting Readiness Display

CHARGE-PAK™ charger and electrode pads need to be replaced **OR** CHARGE-PAK charger is not installed
Notify: ___ . Use AED if needed.

Service needed
Immediately notify: ___ . Attempt to use AED in an emergency. If AED is inoperable, retrieve another AED if possible and continue CPR until EMS arrives.

Internal battery not fully charged
Verify CHARGE-PAK charger is installed. If missing notify: ___
If CHARGE-PAK charger installed use unit if needed.

* The LIFEPAK CR Plus AED may be used on children up to 8 years old or 25kg (55 lbs) only with the Infant/Child Reduced Energy Defibrillation Electrodes.

Fig. 18-9 Automated external defibrillator operator checklist.

LIFEPAK® CR Plus Defibrillator

Troubleshooting Log

Date/Time	Action Taken	User's Checklist

Signature Log

Initials	Print Full Name	Initials	Print Full Name

©2004 Medtronic. LIFEPAK is a registered trademark of Medtronic.
CHARGE-PAK is a trademark of Medtronic Physio-Control Corp.
MIN 3204089-000 / CAT. 26500-001766

Fig. 18-9, cont'd Automated external defibrillator operator checklist.

ply. These patients present with sudden onset pain, paresthesia, paralysis, and pulselessness to the extremity deprived of circulation.

These patients require definitive care at the hospital, and management focuses on IVs, oxygen, and cardiac monitoring (possible movement of clots and cardiac complications).

Deep Vein Thrombosis

Trauma, prolonged immobility, advanced age, birth control pills, cancer, obesity, pregnancy, and other conditions can promote development of clots. Most commonly, older women are affected, and calves and thighs are most often the sites.

When red blood cells and platelets for thrombi attach to vessel walls, blood flow is occluded. These thrombi can break off and move, creating pulmonary emboli. Inflammation of venous walls where thrombi have attached is called *thrombophlebitis*.

Pain and swelling are common in patients with deep vein thrombosis due to partial or complete obstruction of blood flow. Redness and warmth and hardness to the extremity are common. The involved extremity should be immobilized, and the patient should be monitored for possible progression of clots into the lungs.

Emergency medical technicians can offer three of the links in the chain of survival: early EMS, early CPR, and early defibrillation. Once these are accom-

ASK YOURSELF

You and your emergency medical technician partner have just finished your shift checks, restocking and checking your ambulance equipment, when you are dispatched to a local public eating establishment for an adult patient who is complaining of chest pain.

- While en route to the scene, what can you do to prepare for this call?
- What essential equipment should you take with you to the patient's side?

The scene is safe, and as you approach the patient, you see an adult man, approximately 70 years of age who is sitting upright on a chair. The patient appears alert but pale and diaphoretic.

- What information is important to gather about this patient's history?
- What essential links in the chain of survival have been established up to this point?
- As an emergency medical technician, what can you do to continue the chain of survival for this patient?

The patient states he has a history of cardiac problems. He also explains that his chest pain started about an hour ago and has become increasingly worse.

- What questions should you ask this patient about his chest pain?
- What tool can you use to help gauge the severity of this patient's pain?

- What intervention can you provide to this patient at this time?

The patient states he takes nitroglycerin and has it with him.

- What factors are important in determining whether nitroglycerin should be given to this patient?

You have determined the patient has no contraindications for nitroglycerin use and have contacted medical control. Medical control directs you to proceed with assisting this patient in administering nitroglycerin.

- What things should you confirm before giving the nitroglycerin?
- What questions can you ask this patient to determine whether the nitroglycerin is helping?
- What is the maximum dose of nitroglycerin this patient can take?

With your assistance and instruction, your patient has taken one dose of nitroglycerin. He states he is afraid he is dying and suddenly slumps over. You and your partner lower him to the floor. Your partner confirms the patient is unresponsive, breathless, and pulseless.

What is the most important intervention you can provide for this patient at this time?

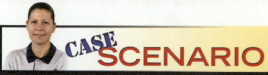

CASE SCENARIO

conclusion

Jack held onto Mr. Markham's hand. He was looking very sick; Jack had never seen someone so ashen. The ambulance moved swiftly toward the hospital, with Elizabeth providing an urgent report over the radio to the receiving hospital. "The patient's blood pressure has been decreasing over the past 20 minutes, but he remains alert. We have him on high-flow oxygen, and our ETA is less than 5 minutes." Hanging up the radio, Elizabeth looked at Jack. "Not giving him the nitro—does that make sense to you?"

Jack nodded. "His BP was too low to support a drug that tends to lower blood pressure by its mechanism of action."

"Unfortunately, that is true in this case. Even if it could help, it's too dangerous. We can only hope that we get him to a coronary care unit where they might be able to help." ■

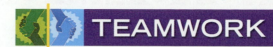

TEAMWORK

Every link in the chain of survival needs to be realized in order for the patient to have the best chance of survival and the best outcome from a cardiac event. Early access to emergency medical services involves the patient or bystanders recognizing a cardiac emergency. Early cardiopulmonary resuscitation from bystanders and emergency medical services is crucial in the fight against time in saving these patients.

EMTs cannot be understated. Without excellent basic life support techniques, advanced life support measures are futile. From the layperson to the advanced care provider, cardiac emergencies are conditions that truly do take a team effort to create the best outcome possible for the patient.

Reference

1. American Heart Association: *Circulation* 112(24)(suppl), December 13, 2005.

Resources

American Heart Association: *Circulation* 112(24)(suppl), December 13, 2005.
EMS Magazine: The Journal of Emergency Care, Rescue and Transportation
JEMS: A Journal of Emergency Medical Services

plished, the next link, early advanced care, needs to be activated. Advanced cardiac life support offers the patient further treatment in the fight against cardiac arrest. Specific advanced procedures and drug therapy work best for the patient when accessed as early as possible. Emergency medical technicians should activate and request ACLS services as soon as they are aware the patient is in a cardiac crisis.

Even with the recognized need for advanced life support, the value of basic life support offered by

Critical Points

Cardiac events can be considered true emergencies for the patient and the prehospital provider. An essential part of caring for a patient with cardiac disease is acting quickly to assess your patient and determine the nature of the chest pain. As an emergency medical technician, you must know your protocols and must be proficient at skills required in managing a cardiac emergency. Cardiac events are emergencies in which emergency medical services truly can make a difference in the patient's outcome.

Learning Checklist

❑ Sudden cardiac arrest accounts for more than 300,000 deaths per year, with up to half of those deaths occurring in the prehospital setting. Sudden cardiac arrest is often the first warning sign a person displays of cardiac disease.

❑ Cardiac events are true medical emergencies.

❑ The circulatory system is a transport system for the body. This system includes the heart and arterial and venous systems.

❑ The circulatory system transports oxygen and nutrients to the body and removes waste from the tissues.

❑ The heart is made up of two sides: the right side and the left side. Both sides have an atrium and a ventricle.

❑ The right atrium receives oxygen-poor blood from the body.

❑ The right ventricle pumps the oxygen-poor blood to the lungs to replenish oxygen.

❑ The left atrium receives oxygenated blood from the lungs. The left ventricle pumps the oxygenated blood out to the body.

❑ Arteries carry oxygenated blood away from the heart.

❑ Veins carry deoxygenated blood back to the heart.

❑ Capillaries are vessels in which the exchange of oxygen for carbon dioxide occurs.

❑ The largest artery in the body is the aorta.

❑ The aorta divides into the iliac arteries.

❑ The pulmonary artery originates in the right ventricle of the heart and delivers blood to the lungs to be oxygenated. The pulmonary artery is the only artery in the body that carries deoxygenated blood.

❑ Carotid arteries supply the head with blood.

❑ Femoral arteries supply the lower body with blood.

❑ Radial arteries supply the lower arm and hand with blood.

❑ Brachial arteries most commonly are used to obtain a patient's blood pressure reading.

❑ Tibial pulses are located near the inside of the ankle.

❑ Dorsalis pedis pulse can be felt on the top of the foot.

❑ Pulses are felt when an artery runs along a bony prominence.

❑ The primary function of the veins is to carry deoxygenated blood back to the heart.

❑ The pulmonary vein carries blood to the left atrium of the heart from the lungs.

❑ The pulmonary vein is the only vein in the body that carries oxygenated blood.

❑ The venae cavae are the major veins of the body and consist of two branches: the superior vena cava and the inferior vena cava. The superior vena cava carries oxygen-depleted blood from the head and arms. The inferior vena cava carries oxygen-depleted blood from the lower extremities and the torso.

❑ Blood consists of red blood cells, white blood cells, plasma, and platelets.

❑ Signs and symptoms of shock are pale, cyanotic, cool, clammy skin; weak, rapid pulse; rapid, shallow breathing; restlessness, anxiety, or mental dullness; nausea or vomiting; and decreased or low blood pressure.

❑ Cardiac chest pain may not be described as pain but as an ache, pressure, tightness, or squeezing sensation. The pain also may radiate into the jaw, arms, back, or epigastric region.

❑ Sudden onset of diaphoresis may be the only significant symptom of cardiac compromise. Anxiety, restlessness, and dyspnea also can be associated with cardiac emergencies.

❑ Angina, ischemia, or myocardial infarct can produce similar symptoms.

❑ Initial assessments for cardiac emergencies are the same as they are for any other type of emergency.

- Apply high-flow oxygen to patients with cardiac disease as soon as possible.
- Obtaining a patient's medical history is important in determining the nature of the chest pain.
- Allow the patient to remain in a position of comfort if at all possible.
- Never allow a patient with cardiac disease to move about or to walk.
- Transport patients with cardiac disease with caution, realizing that lights and sirens may cause additional anxiety to the patient and stress to the heart.
- Use the OPQRST acronym when assessing patients with chest pain.
- Use nitroglycerin for cardiac chest pain if the patient meets all of the criteria for it and shows no contraindications. Additionally, the patient must be alert.
- Up to three doses of nitroglycerin may be administered if approved by medical direction.
- Monitor patient vital signs before and after the administration of nitroglycerin.
- Do not give nitroglycerin to patients with a systolic blood pressure less than 100 mm Hg.
- Perform frequent reassessments for any patient with chest pain.
- Ventricular fibrillation is a heart condition. With this condition the heart produces electrical signals in a rapid and chaotic manner that does not allow the heart to pump blood to the body effectively. Defibrillation can reverse ventricular fibrillation of the heart.
- The emergency medical technician must become proficient with using the automated external defibrillator during a cardiac arrest. Time is crucial for the survival of victims of cardiac arrest.
- The rescuer is responsible for clearing bystanders when the automated external defibrillator is analyzing and shocking the patient.
- The emergency medical technician should never analyze or shock the heart while in a moving vehicle or while moving the patient.
- Apply the automated external defibrillator only to patients who are breathless and pulseless.
- Advanced cardiac life support is an important part of the chain of survival. Request it (if available) for all patients with cardiac disease.
- Most automated external defibrillator manufacturers now offer child pads that deliver less energy than adult pads, and should be used for all pediatric patients when available. If not available, use adult pads.
- The automated external defibrillator is an electric device and should not be handled in water. Remove wet clothing from the patient before applying the automated external defibrillator.
- Documentation of the events of any cardiac call, including events while using the automated external defibrillator, is important. Accurate documentation is needed for the continuum of patient care.
- Maintenance of the automated external defibrillator should be performed at every shift. Batteries should be checked, and spare batteries should be on hand and readily accessible. Mechanical failure of the automated external defibrillator is most commonly due to human error and batteries that are not working.
- Emergency medical technicians are responsible for maintaining their skills. Automated external defibrillator skills verification should be done at least every 90 days.
- Even though emergency medical technicians are trained to use an automated external defibrillator, they need to be familiar with their local laws and rules regarding the use of automated external defibrillators by emergency personnel.

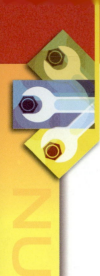

NUTS AND BOLTS

Key Terms

Angina Chest discomfort felt upon exertion and usually relieved when resting.

Aorta The largest artery in the body. It originates from the heart and lies in front of the spine in the thoracic and abdominal cavities.

Arteries Blood vessels that carry oxygenated blood out to the body.

Arterioles Smallest arteries of the body.

Asystole Event in which the heart has no rhythm and has ceased all electrical activity.

Atrium Upper chamber of the heart. The heart has a right atrium that receives oxygen-depleted blood from the body, and a left atrium that receives oxygen-enriched blood from the lungs.

Automated external defibrillator Machine that is designed to deliver a shock for defibrillation of a cardiac rhythm known as ventricular fibrillation.

Blood The fluid in the body that is made up of red blood cells, white blood cells, platelets, and plasma.

Blood pressure The pressure the blood exerts against the walls of the blood vessels.

Brachial artery The major artery of the upper arm.

Capillaries Tiny vessels that allow the exchange of oxygen and carbon dioxide and nutrients and waste to occur.

Cardiac arrest The halting of all functioning heart activity.

Cardiac compromise A term used for harmful cardiac conditions.

Carotid arteries Arteries that supply the head and neck with blood.

Chain of survival A term used by the American Heart Association to define a series of actions that include early access to emergency medical services, early cardiopulmonary resuscitation, early defibrillation, and early advanced cardiac life support.

Clear the patient A phrase used to describe the action an emergency medical technician must take to ensure that no bystander is touching the patient while the emergency medical technician is analyzing or shocking with an automated external defibrillator.

Contraindications Reasons or factors that prohibit administration of a drug.

Defibrillation Administering a shock to a patient in ventricular defibrillation in order to cause the heart to regain function.

Defibrillator Name for a machine that defibrillates specific cardiac arrhythmias.

Diastolic blood pressure The pressure applied to the blood vessels during the relaxation phase of cardiac contractions. Represented as the bottom number of a blood pressure reading.

Dorsalis pedis artery Artery that supplies the foot with blood.

Dosage Amount of a medication that should be administered.

Femoral artery Artery that supplies the upper and lower leg with blood.

Iliac arteries Arteries that supply the lower extremities with oxygen and nutrient-enriched blood.

Indications Conditions in which administering a specific drug may benefit the patient.

Inferior vena cava Large vein that carries oxygen-poor blood from the lower extremities and torso.

Ischemia When an area of the heart muscle is not receiving enough oxygen.

Myocardial Referring to cardiac muscle.

Myocardial infarct Heart attack; caused when an artery of the heart is blocked partially or completely, causing damage to the heart.

Nitroglycerin The generic name for a drug that acts to dilate the blood vessels, decreasing the workload of the heart.

Plasma Fluid in the blood that helps move the blood cells and platelets.

Platelets Cells that cause the blood to clot in order to stop bleeding.

Public access defibrillation Laypersons trained to use an automated external defibrillator in public areas.

Pulmonary artery Artery that carries deoxygenated blood from the right ventricle of the heart to the lungs.

Pulmonary vein Vein that carries oxygenated blood from the lungs to the left atrium of the heart.

Pulse Area where an artery can be felt over a bony prominence in the body when the heart contracts.

Radial artery Artery located on the thumb side of the wrist.

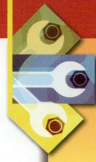

Red blood cells Cells that carry oxygen and are transported in the blood.

Semiautomated external defibrillator Type of automated external defibrillator that requires operator direction to analyze and shock.

Septum The wall that divides the right side of the heart and the left side of the heart.

Shock The inadequate delivery of oxygen and nutrients to cells, resulting in organ system malfunction. Eventually shock is detectable with abnormal vital signs. It can lead to death.

Sphygmomanometer The cuff and gauge used to measure the blood pressure.

Sublingual Under the tongue.

Superior vena cava Large vein that carries oxygen-poor blood from the head and arms.

Systolic blood pressure The pressure applied to the blood vessels during the contraction phase of the cardiac cycle. Represented as the top number of a blood pressure reading.

Tibial artery Artery located in the lower extremities.

Tier Action of continued care when a prehospital emergency medical services system continues care with an advanced prehospital emergency medical system.

Trendelenburg's position A position in which the body is supine with the feet elevated and head down.

Veins Vessels that carry deoxygenated blood back to the heart.

Venae cavae Major veins that carry blood back to the right atrium of the heart from the body.

Venous system System of veins in the body.

Ventricle Lower chamber of the heart. The heart has a right ventricle that pumps deoxygenated blood to the lungs and a left ventricleal that pumps oxygenated blood to the body.

Ventricular fibrillation A rapid, chaotic cardiac rhythm in which the heart "quivers" with electrical impulses but fails to contract.

Ventricular tachycardia Rapid heartbeat that does not allow the heart time to fill and pump blood properly.

Venules Smallest size of vein.

White blood cells Cells in the blood that help the body fight infection.

National Standard Curriculum Objectives

Cognitive Objectives

After completing this lesson, the EMT student will be able to do the following:

- Describe the structure and function of the cardiovascular system.
- Describe the emergency medical care of the patient experiencing chest pain/discomfort.
- List the indications for automated external defibrillation.
- List the contraindications for automated external defibrillation.
- Define the role of emergency medical technician in the emergency cardiac care system.
- Explain the impact of age and weight on defibrillation.
- Discuss the position of comfort for patients with various cardiac emergencies.
- Establish the relationship between airway management and the patient with cardiovascular compromise.
- Predict the relationship between the patient experiencing cardiovascular compromise and basic life support.
- Explain that not all patients with chest pain experience cardiac arrest and do not need to be attached to an automated external defibrillator.
- Explain the importance of prehospital advanced cardiac life support intervention if it is available.
- Explain the importance of urgent transport to a facility with advanced cardiac life support if it is not available in the prehospital setting.
- Discuss the various types of automated external defibrillators.
- Differentiate between the fully automated and the semiautomated defibrillator.
- Discuss the procedures to take into consideration for standard operations of the various types of automated external defibrillators.
- State the reasons for ensuring that the patient is pulseless and apneic when using the automated external defibrillator.
- Discuss the circumstances that may result in inappropriate shocks.

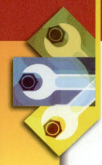

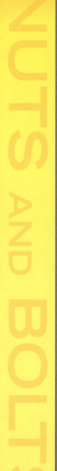

- Explain the considerations for interruption of cardiopulmonary resuscitation when using the automated external defibrillator.
- Discuss the advantages and disadvantages of automated external defibrillators.
- Summarize the speed of operation of automated external defibrillation.
- Discuss the use of remote defibrillation through adhesive pads.
- Discuss the special considerations for rhythm monitoring.
- List the steps in the operation of the automated external defibrillator.
- Discuss the standard of care to use to provide care to a patient with persistent ventricular fibrillation and no available advanced cardiac life support.
- Discuss the standard of care to use to provide care to a patient with recurrent ventricular fibrillation and no available advanced cardiac life support.
- Explain the reason for not checking pulses between shocks with an automated external defibrillator.

- Discuss the importance of coordinating providers trained in advanced cardiac life support with personnel using automated external defibrillators.
- Discuss the importance of postresuscitation care.
- List the components of postresuscitation care.
- Explain the importance of frequent practice with the automated external defibrillator.
- Discuss the need to complete the Automated Defibrillator: Operator's Shift Checklist.
- Discuss the role of the American Heart Association in the use of automated external defibrillation.
- Explain the role medical direction plays in the use of automated external defibrillation.
- State the reasons why a case review should be completed following the use of the automated external defibrillator.
- Discuss the components that should be included in a case review.

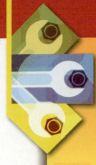

- Discuss the goal of quality improvement in automated external defibrillation.
- Recognize the need for medical direction of protocols to assist in the emergency medical care of the patient with chest pain.
- List the indications for the use of nitroglycerin.
- State the contraindications and side effects for the use of nitroglycerin.
- Define the function of all controls on an automated external defibrillator, and describe event documentation and battery defibrillator maintenance.

Affective Objectives

After completing this lesson, the EMT student will be able to do the following:

- Defend the reasons for obtaining initial training in automated external defibrillation and the importance of continuing education.
- Defend the reason for maintenance of automated external defibrillators.
- Explain the rationale for administering nitroglycerin to a patient with chest pain or discomfort.

Psychomotor Objectives

After completing this lesson, the EMT student will be able to do the following:

- Demonstrate the assessment and emergency medical care of a patient experiencing chest pain/discomfort.
- Demonstrate the application and operation of the automated external defibrillator.
- Demonstrate the maintenance of an automated external defibrillator.
- Demonstrate the assessment and documentation of patient response to the automated external defibrillator.
- Demonstrate the skills necessary to complete the Automated Defibrillator: Operator's Shift Checklist.
- Perform the steps in facilitating the use of nitroglycerin for chest pain or discomfort.
- Demonstrate the assessment and documentation of patient response to nitroglycerin.
- Practice completing a prehospital care report for patients with cardiac emergencies.

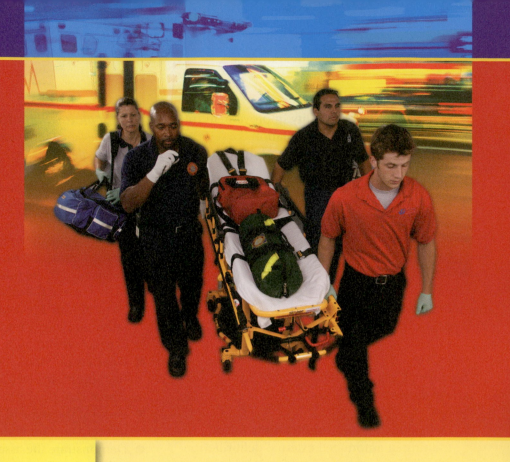

CHAPTER

19

LESSON GOAL

GOAL

This chapter focuses on emergencies involving the gastrointestinal and genitourinary systems. Although abdominal pain and injury can be painful to the patient, other than supportive care (e.g., control of pain or extensive hemorrhage), little definitive care can be given outside the hospital. The emergency medical technician will learn to recognize, assess, and treat injuries to provide that care for patients with injuries involving the abdominal cavity. ∎

Gastrointestinal/ Genitourinary Emergencies

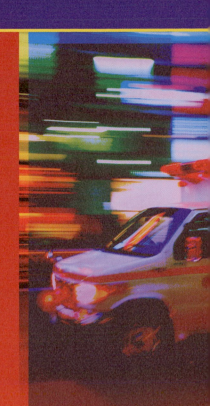

CHAPTER OBJECTIVES

After completing this chapter, the EMT student will be able to do the following:

1 Discuss the different causes of nontraumatic abdominal emergencies.
2 Discuss the signs and symptoms of nontraumatic abdominal emergencies.
3 Describe the proper way to perform an assessment on a patient with nontraumatic abdominal pain.
4 Identify the four quadrants of the abdomen.
5 Identify the hollow organs within the abdomen.
6 Identify the solid organs within the abdomen.
7 Discuss the function of the kidneys.
8 Discuss visceral pain as it relates to the gastrointestinal tract.
9 Discuss somatic pain as it relates to the gastrointestinal tract.
10 Describe the emergency care of a patient with nontraumatic abdominal pain.

OBJECTIVES

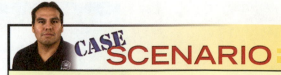

CASE SCENARIO

Firefighter Rafael Gonzales stepped off the engine and pulled the jump kit out of its compartment. The engine had just arrived in front of the largest senior citizen housing complex in their response district, a 10-floor apartment building, for a report of an "unknown medical." In addition, the mobile data terminal in the pumper included information that a forced entry may be required to gain access. However, the building superintendent met them at the main door and escorted the crew into the building.

Taking the elevator to the seventh floor, the crew stopped in front of apartment 728. As Rafael knocked briskly on the door, he called out, "Fire department! Did someone call for help?"

Distantly, they could hear a faint voice calling for help. The superintendent inserted the master key and opened the door into a dimly lit, small apartment. Even though it was midday, the shades were tightly drawn. No lights were on inside the apartment. The captain found a light switch and turned it on, illuminating the contents of the room.

Rafael could hear someone calling from the back bedroom at the end of the hall. Walking cautiously, the firefighters made their way past several piles of old newspapers and other belongings lining the hallway floor. Cigarette burns marred the carpet.

Looking into the bedroom, Rafael observed an elderly woman lying in the bed. Although it was dark in the room, she looked pale and was breathing a bit quickly. As the crew pulled open the shades and began to empty out the egress route, Rafael began to pull out his equipment. Kneeling down by the patient, he said, "Hi, my name is Rafael. I am an EMT. What is your name?"

She responded in a weak voice, "Monica Hostetler." Rafael could hear that even just those two words caused the patient to breathe a little harder.

As he reached over to feel the patient's radial pulse, Rafael replied, "May I call you Mrs. Hostetler?" Her skin felt cool to the touch and diaphoretic. Her radial pulse was present, although it was faint and fast.

Mrs. Hostetler nodded. Rafael made note of her respiratory rate: it was 24 times per minute. "Tell me what is bothering you today."

"My stomach really hurts." She rubbed her lower abdomen as she spoke.

"OK. Is there anything else that bothers you today?"

"I was just in the bathroom. Almost passed out while I was having a bowel movement. I think I saw blood in the toilet after I finished."

Questions: *Based upon Rafael's initial assessment, does Mrs. Hostetler's condition appear to be stable or unstable? Why? On what questions should Rafael focus? What physical assessment techniques should he use to gain additional information? What care should the crew provide at this point?*

■ GASTROINTESTINAL SYSTEM

General Anatomy, Physiology, and Pathophysiology

The abdomen is surrounded by the diaphragm at the top, the abdominal muscles in the front, the pelvis at the bottom, and the flank, back muscles, and spinal column in the back (Fig. 19-1). Historically, the abdomen has been divided into four equal **quadrants** (Fig. 19-2). One imaginary plane runs down the middle of the abdomen through the umbilicus (navel). A second imaginary plane runs perpendicular to the first, again through the umbilicus. The abdomen also can be divided from the front (abdominal cavity) to the back (retroperitoneal cavity).

As with other cavities in the body, the abdominal cavity is lined with several layers of tissue. These layers of tissue include skin, fatty tissue, muscle, and in the case of the abdomen, a tough layer of elastic tissue called the **peritoneum** (Fig. 19-3). The peritoneum can become irritated from blood or inflammation, causing discomfort and pain. These layers combine to protect, cushion, and provide blood flow to the internal organs that are primarily responsible for digestion of food products necessary for metabo-

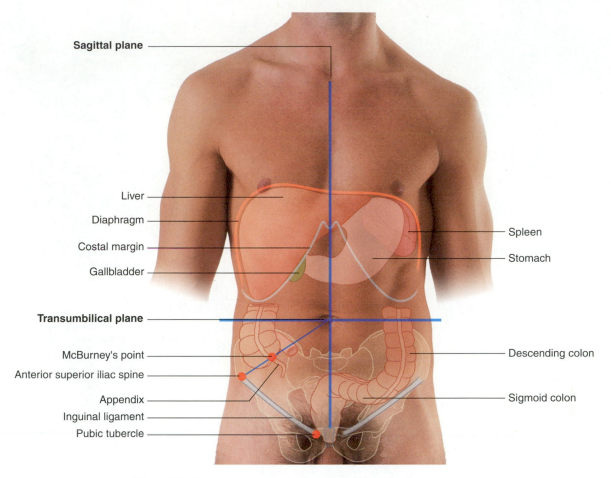

Fig. 19-1 Organ location within the abdominal quadrants.

lism. In addition, the layers protect, cushion, and provide blood flow to other critical organs and structures, such as the **kidneys, ovaries** in females, and major blood vessels.

Digestive System

The organs that are responsible for digestion generally are separated into two categories (Fig. 19-4). The **digestive or gastrointestinal tract** is the hollow tube in which most digestion takes place. The digestive tract really begins in the mouth and esophagus. However, in the abdominal cavity, the digestive system is made up of the stomach, small intestine, and large intestine. The mechanical and chemical breakdown of food occurs within the digestive tract. Nutrients and water also are absorbed through the intestinal walls. The intestinal organs, which are **hollow organs,** are prone to a variety of conditions, including blockage, hemorrhage, and perforation, resulting in spillage of gastric or intestinal contents into the abdominal cavity. Blood also can be contained within the cavity, most commonly after trauma, often without being readily apparent to the

patient or emergency medical technician examining the patient.

The **accessory organs** provide the chemicals necessary for the breakdown of food products as they pass through the digestive tract. These organs include the liver, gallbladder, and pancreas. The liver and the pancreas, as well as another abdominal organ called the spleen, are examples of **solid organs.** These solid organs require a great deal of blood flow to function correctly. These organs are reasonably well protected, as they are located mostly under the lower ribs. However, after trauma, they have a tendency to bleed significantly if they are injured. Additionally, they are prone to illnesses brought on by disease or toxic conditions, such as the overuse of alcohol.

Urinary System

The **urinary system** is primarily responsible for the collection and removal of waste buildup in the human body (Fig. 19-5). The major organ of the urinary system is the kidney. Two of these solid organs are located in the retroperitoneal space on either side of the spinal column in the flank area just beneath the

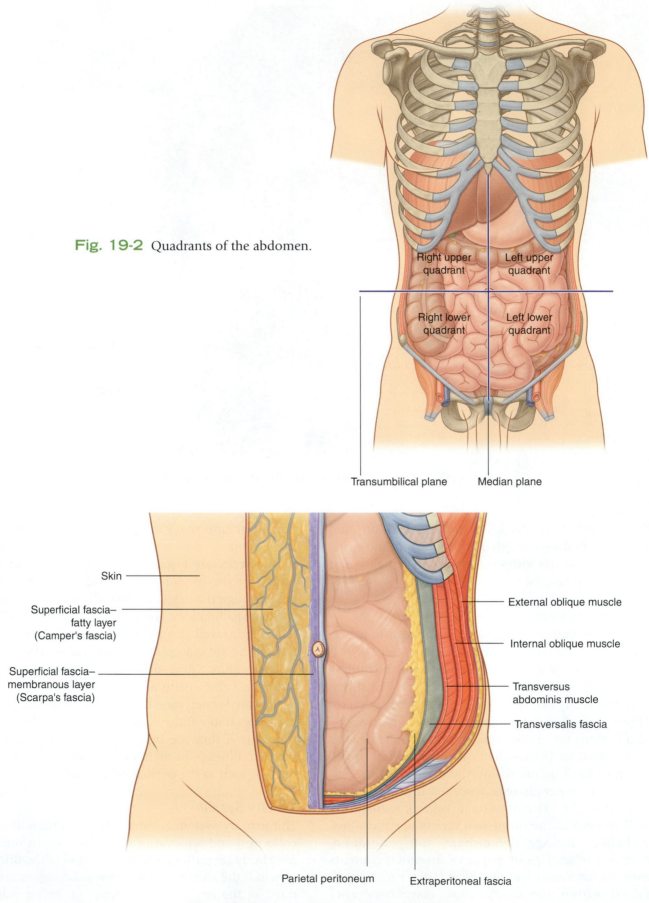

Fig. 19-2 Quadrants of the abdomen.

Right upper quadrant

Left upper quadrant

Right lower quadrant

Left lower quadrant

Transumbilical plane

Median plane

Skin

Superficial fascia–
fatty layer
(Camper's fascia)

Superficial fascia–
membranous layer
(Scarpa's fascia)

External oblique muscle

Internal oblique muscle

Transversus
abdominis muscle

Transversalis fascia

Parietal peritoneum

Extraperitoneal fascia

Fig. 19-3 Layers of the abdominal wall.

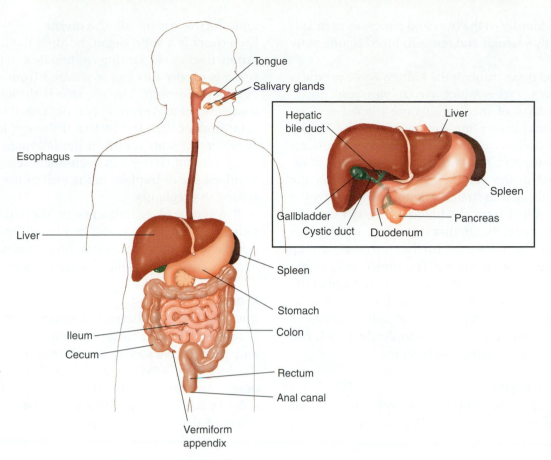

Fig. 19-4 The digestive tract.

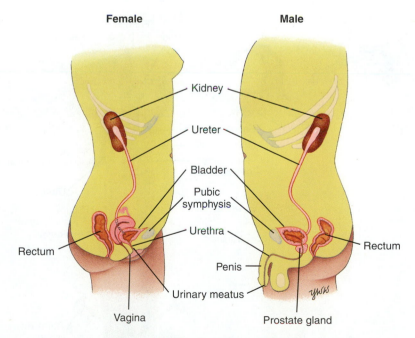

Fig. 19-5 The urinary system.

lower ribs. Similar to the liver and pancreas, each kidney is highly vascular and tends to bleed significantly if injured.

As blood flows through the kidney, waste products such as urea, excess water, electrolytes, and breakdown products of medications are filtered and removed. These wastes are drained from the kidney through a hollow tube called a **ureter.** The ureters carry the waste to a hollow organ known as the **bladder,** located in the pelvis. Urine is collected in the bladder, causing it to stretch over time. Eventually the urine is expelled from the bladder through the urethra. In the male, the urethra exits the body through the penis. In the female, the urethra is shorter, ending at the opening of the vagina. The ureter and urethra provide a convenient method for bacteria to enter the body, often causing infection and inflammation. In addition, excessive salts may cause kidney stones to block the urethra partially or completely, which can produce significant pain and bleeding.

Reproductive System

In the female the reproductive system is found within the abdominal cavity (Fig. 19-6). The main reproductive organs are the **uterus** and two ovaries. Each ovary is a solid organ, holding the female's reproductive eggs. During a female's reproductive years, generally one egg is released from one of the ovaries per month. The egg travels through the **fallopian tubes** and eventually is deposited into a muscular organ called the uterus. If the egg is fertilized after contact with sperm in the fallopian tube, several profound changes in hormone levels permit the fertilized egg to implant in the wall of the uterus, resulting in pregnancy.

If a fertilized egg attaches to the fallopian wall rather than the uterine wall in a condition known as ectopic pregnancy, significant, life-threatening bleeding may occur if the fallopian tube bursts.

Blood Vessels

Running close to the spinal column are the major blood vessels that bring oxygen and nutrients to and return wastes from the abdominal organs and the legs (Fig. 19-7). The descending aorta travels downward through the abdominal cavity and divides in half in the pelvic area. Composed of three layers of tissue, the aorta is flexible yet tough. Dis-

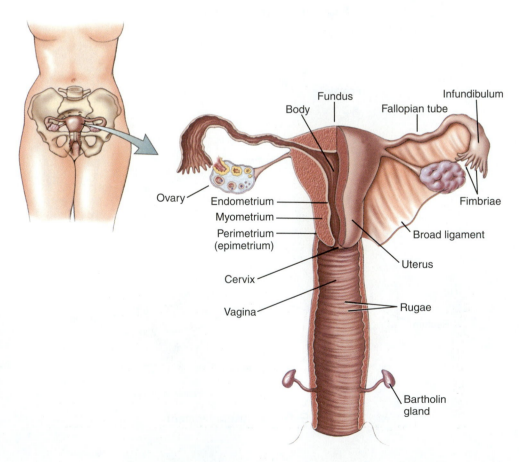

Fig. 19-6 The female reproductive system.

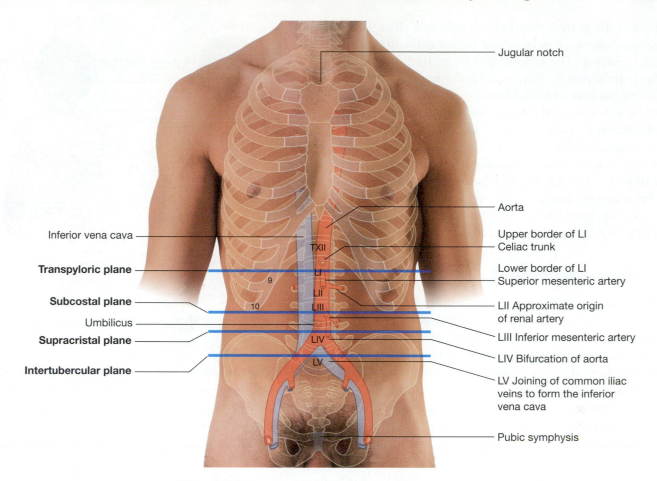

Fig. 19-7 Major blood vessels of the abdomen.

SPECIAL Populations

In the elderly, back pain and collapse with decreased level of consciousness should be considered a ruptured abdominal aortic aneurysm until proved otherwise. Assess for a pulsatile abdominal mass and signs and symptoms of hypoperfusion.

ease of the aorta may result in dilation and even rupture of the aorta with hemorrhage into the abdominal cavity.

The abdominal organs are supplied with blood through a network of vessels. This network of vessels is found in a "webbing" of connective tissue collectively known as the **mesentery.** Like the arteries that supply blood to the brain and heart, the mesenteric arteries can be blocked by emboli. This can result in death of the tissue (such as the small or large bowel) being supplied by that particular artery.

■ GENERAL ASSESSMENT

The general assessment of a patient complaining of an abdominal discomfort or pain is similar to the approach used in other medical patients. The emergency medical technician should pay attention to several physical and historical findings in these patients.

Scene Size-up

Your scene size-up for a patient with an abdominal complaint is the same as any other scene size-up: First check for hazards that may endanger you and your crew. Before entering the scene, establish body substance isolation and take universal precautions. As you evaluate the scene, check for signs that may be related to an abdominal complaint. Look for emesis (vomit) on the patient or around the environment. Check vomitus, if present, for the presence of blood. Check medications, prescribed and over-the-counter (such as large, empty bottles of antacids), that might point to a preexisting medical condition. The appearance of the patient may provide valuable clues. Is the patient supine, or is he or she having difficulty standing or sitting? The latter might be an initial sign that the patient may be having difficulty maintaining perfusion because of blood loss.

As you gather the scene information, determine whether your patient is ill or injured. A patient who has sustained an injury to the abdomen will need transport to and early assessment and intervention by a skilled surgical team at a trauma receiving facility. The minimal amount of time you spend on scene evaluating your patient with abdominal trauma may relate directly to a better outcome.

Initial Assessment

As you contact the patient, perform an initial assessment. Carefully evaluate the patient's airway. Is there vomit or are there secretions in the airway? Is there a need for suctioning or, in the case of a patient with altered mental status, a need to position the head to maintain a patent airway? If there is a trauma mechanism, do cervical spine precautions need to be performed while you manage the airway?

Once the airway has been established, look at the work of breathing. Is the patient's respiratory rate adequate? Is the depth of breathing appropriate? If the patient is in shock because of low blood volume, his or her breathing effort will increase to try to maintain adequate oxygen levels in the bloodstream.

Check for the presence of a radial pulse. Is it strong and regular? Is it fast? Again, if blood volume is low because of internal bleeding, the heart will attempt to speed up to try to compensate for the loss. In addition, the body will force blood flow back into the core circulation, causing the skin to be pale and become diaphoretic.

History and Physical Exam

After conducting the initial assessment and identifying and managing any life-threatening conditions, begin evaluating the patient's history and perform the focused physical exam on the conscious patient.

Pain

The classic sign for a patient with an abdominal complaint is pain. Pain that originates from deep inside the abdomen often can be vague and generalized. The patient often complains of an "aching," "twisting," or "crampy" type of sensation that can be difficult to pin-

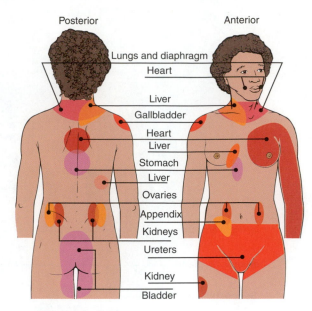

Fig. 19-8 Typical areas of referred pain.

point. This is known as **visceral pain.** Such pain can be caused by a variety of conditions that cause the affected organ or area to become inflamed (swollen), ischemic (low in oxygen), or distended (stretched). Hollow organs such as the large and small intestines tend to produce visceral pain responses.

Sometimes the abdominal pain is sharp and easily localized by the patient. The pain signals travel along well-defined nerve pathways that are interpreted easily by the brain. This is known as **somatic pain.** Solid organs such as the kidney and pancreas tend to produce somatic pain responses.

Occasionally, the pain or discomfort felt in the abdomen actually is coming from a location outside the cavity. This is known as **referred pain** (Fig. 19-8). Patients who are experiencing a cardiac emergency sometimes can feel discomfort in the upper abdominal (epigastric) region rather than in the chest itself.

SPECIAL Considerations

With patients having cognitive impairment or other inability to communicate, watch for the following "pain behaviors":

Frowning, frightened face
Rapid blinking
Grunting, groaning
Rigid, tense postures and movements
Increasing pacing or rocking movements
Mobility difficulty

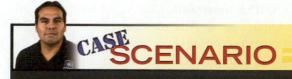

CASE SCENARIO

continued

Over the next few minutes, Rafael examined the patient and asked her more detailed questions about her complaints. In the meantime, one firefighter filled a non-rebreather mask with oxygen and placed it over the patient's face. The other crew members cleared a path from the bedroom to the front door and also looked for medication bottles and other indications of a medical history.

Soon, Rafael had the following information:

Chief complaint: "My stomach hurts."

Onset: 3 days ago

Provocation/palliation: She awoke with the discomfort, and it had been getting steadily worse since then. Nothing seems to help.

Quality: A dull ache in the lower abdomen

Radiation/related symptoms: The pain did not radiate. She complained of ongoing episodes of diarrhea and loss of appetite.

Severity: Pain was not bad originally, but today it was "pretty bad."

Time: The pain just continued to worsen steadily over time.

The oxygen seemed to help Mrs. Hostetler slow her breathing down a bit. She was able to speak longer sentences without becoming short of breath. Her SAMPLE history revealed that she had a long history of diabetes, which was controlled with an oral medication. She also experienced hypertension and was on a medication for that. She was not allergic to any medications. Her last meal was earlier that day, although it was not much—toast and coffee. No information was reported that indicated a fall or any other type of trauma mechanism.

Her vital signs were recorded as follows: respirations, 20 (24 originally); pulse, 100, blood pressure, 104/68. Her skin was still pale and cool but not as wet as before.

The physical exam revealed that Mrs. Hostetler was tender throughout her abdomen, but especially over the two lower quadrants. The abdomen was not distended, and there was no skin discoloration. She had pulses in both of her femoral arteries. She denied any chest pain. She had several bowel movements yesterday, all of them loose and progressively darker. A firefighter confirms that she saw what appeared to be dark red blood in the toilet.

Questions: *Based upon Rafael's findings, what do you suspect is happening with Mrs. Hostetler? The patient had complained also of almost "passing out" while she was having a bowel movement earlier. How can this be explained?*

The reverse also can occur. For example, the gallbladder is located just under the liver in the right upper quadrant. The gallbladder can become blocked, causing it to inflame and become ischemic. Patients with this condition, known as cholecystitis, often complain of a dull, achy discomfort under their left scapula that sometimes is confused with muscle pain.

History

The mnemonic for pain, *OPQRST*, can yield a great amount of information about the patient's abdominal complaint. Each question can provide valuable clues to the cause of the patient's complaint:

O—*Onset.* Sudden onset of pain or discomfort can indicate a rapid onset or change in the patient's condition. For example, the appendix that has become swollen from infection may burst suddenly, causing a rapid onset of sharp, right lower quadrant pain. A slower onset of discomfort may indicate an infection or a blockage condition that has taken some time to develop.

P—*Provocation* or *palliation.* Was there something that caused the pain to occur? For example, abdominal pain that begins shortly after a meal may point to a gastrointestinal problem. However, epigastric pain that occurs without provocation may be an indication of a cardiac emergency. For you to ascertain whether anything relieves or reduces the pain (palliation) is equally important. For example, a patient with a peritoneal condition will try to relax the peritoneum by lying on his or her side and bringing his or her knees toward his or her chest, assuming a fetal-like position. Reducing flank pain by standing up may indicate kidney stones.

Q—*Quality.* A dull, achy pain with a location that is difficult to pinpoint may point to a bowel obstruction or other hollow organ problems. A sharp, tearing pain may result from a solid organ disorder.

R—*Region, related* symptoms, and *radiation.* Remember that pain can refer from one location to another. Is the patient nauseated or experiencing vomiting? If there is vomiting, can the emesis be described? If the patient describes vomit that is reddish, there may be active bleeding in the upper part of the digestive tract, such as in the esophagus or stomach. If the vomit contains clots, is dark brown or black, and has a coffee-ground consistency, it may be blood that has been in the digestive tract long enough to be processed.

Ask about the patient's bowel movements or urine output. A patient who has not had a bowel movement for many days may be experiencing an intestinal blockage. However, diarrhea (loose, fluid-filled bowel movement) may indicate an infectious process or food poisoning. Dark, black, tarry-like feces or stool may indicate bleeding deep inside the intestine.

Determine whether any changes in the color or amount of urine output have occurred. Urine should be clear, with a light to moderate yellow or amber tint. Dark, cloudy urine may indicate infection. Concentrated urine may be a sign of dehydration. Pain or burning upon urination may be related to infection or the formation of kidney stones. Occasionally, blood may be seen in urine, indicating possible trauma or a serious condition involving the kidney or bladder.

Ask whether the patient feels feverish. A history of flulike symptoms or fever may indicate an infectious process.

S—*Severity.* Be aware that the level or intensity of the pain or discomfort being reported by the patient may not match the patient's actual level of discomfort. However, pain that continues to worsen over time is a significant finding that the condition is worsening.

T—*Time.* Determine how long the discomfort has been occurring. During that time, has the pain remained constant, intermittent, or steadily increasing or decreasing?

The SAMPLE mnemonic (Signs and symptoms, Allergies, Medications, Past medical history, Last oral intake, Events preceding) can provide insight into the patient's current medical condition by providing clues about the medical history. Currently prescribed medications may indicate a preexisting genitourinary/gastrointestinal condition. A patient with a history of peptic ulcers or kidney stones may be experiencing an exacerbation of those conditions.

Pay attention not only to when the last oral intake occurred but also to what was ingested. For example, a patient who eats a meal that is high in fat or oil followed a short time later with significant right upper quadrant pain, cramping, and referred pain to the shoulder may be experiencing a gallbladder attack. Another example would be abdominal pain or discomfort following the ingestion of alcohol, a possible sign of pancreatitis.

In females of childbearing age, ask about sexual activity. A woman who is experiencing an ectopic pregnancy may be in a critical condition if the fallopian tube bursts and uncontrolled bleeding into the abdomen occurs. Refer to the chapter on obstetrics and gynecology for more information on this life-threatening condition.

Look for other clues as well that might suggest an ongoing abdominal problem. Examination of the skin and eyes may reveal yellow or orange discoloration associated with liver diseases such as cirrhosis or hepatitis. Examination of the conjunctiva inside the eyelids may reveal a very pale pink color suggesting blood loss.

Vital Signs

Obtain a complete set of vital signs as the history is being elicited. Pay particular attention to signs of potential stress on the cardiovascular system, such as tachypnea, tachycardia, and skin signs. An important diagnostic test for patients with abdominal discomfort is determining whether the patient is exhibiting **postural vital signs.** Also known as a "tilt test," a patient's pulse rate and blood pressure are measured initially while the patient is lying supine. The patient then is moved to the seated position. Alternatively, the patient may begin in the seated position and then may be moved to a standing position. In either case, the pulse rate and blood pressure are measured again approximately 1 minute after changing positions. If the systolic blood pressure falls by more than 20 mm Hg or the pulse rate rises by 20 beats/min, the test is positive and may mean that the patient is hypovolemic. Be aware that a patient almost immediately may exhibit signs of hypovolemia—such as light-headedness, fainting, sudden blanching of the skin, or diaphoresis—when changing positions. In these situations, immediately place the patient back into his or her original position, without waiting to measure the pulse rate or blood pressure.

In addition, if the patient is tachycardic or hypotensive in whatever position the patient is first contacted or if the patient complains of symptoms—such as dizziness, light-headedness, or fainting when standing—that suggest that the patient is volume depleted, you do not need to check the postural vital signs.

Physical Exam

The physical exam should be brief and focused. Little can be gained by causing the patient additional discomfort or prolonging transport with a detailed physical exam. Several key findings to observe and document about the patient are relevant to an abdominal complaint:

Visualization. Observe the patient's condition. Is he or she sitting or lying still? A fetal position may indicate significant discomfort, and being curled up may be the most comfortable position the patient can find. Expose and look at the abdomen first. Is it of normal shape and size, or is it abnormally distended? Distention may be due to air, excessive fluid or blood, or bowel obstruction. Are there any marks, bruises, discoloration, or hematomas? These may be due to trauma or changes in circulatory patterns.

Palpation. Ask the patient to point to the site of the pain or discomfort. Using the flats of your fingers, first palpate the quadrant diagonally across from the quadrant with the pain. Palpate gently but with enough depth to check for masses. Note if there is any guarding (sudden tensing of the abdominal muscles) or any appearance of discomfort by the patient. Work your way around the nonaffected quadrants to see whether palpation worsens the pain. Finally, gently palpate the area to which the patient originally pointed, being careful not to cause significantly more discomfort or pain. Stop palpating immediately if you find an area that feels as if it may have a "pulse"—possibly a blood vessel that may be ready to burst.

In females of childbearing age, pain upon palpation of the lower quadrants may indicate possible ectopic pregnancy or infection in the pelvis.

Although a specific diagnosis is generally not possible in the field, the location of the patient's pain may suggest certain problems:

Right upper quadrant:	Gallbladder disease Hepatitis Pneumonia
Epigastrium:	Ulcers Pancreatitis Myocardial infarction
Left upper quadrant:	Splenic problems Stomach problems Pneumonia
Right lower quadrant:	Appendicitis Ovarian problems in women Ectopic pregnancy
Suprapubic:	Bladder infections Uterine problems such as miscarriage
Left lower quadrant:	Diverticulitis (large bowel) Ovarian problems in women Ectopic pregnancy
Flank and back pain:	Kidney problems (stones, infection) Abdominal aortic aneurysm

■ GENERAL TREATMENT

The treatment of abdominal discomfort is mainly supportive. Determining the patient's best position of comfort is essential. The drive to the hospital may be painful to the patient. Patients with peritoneal pain may not be able to lie in the semi-Fowler position or supine on the gurney. Placing the patient in a lateral recumbent position with knees bent may be most comfortable.

If any signs of shock exist, provide appropriate measures. Cover the patient to maintain body temperature. Apply high-flow oxygen and assist with respiration if the patient's breathing appears inadequate. Be vigilant for sudden vomiting that may compromise the airway.

Ensure that the patient does not ingest anything orally. Even water may cause vomiting to occur,

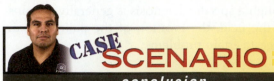

CASE SCENARIO
conclusion

The engine crew worked quickly to prepare Mrs. Hostetler for transport. Because she was already feeling faint, Rafael decided not to assess whether the patient had positive postural vital signs. He was concerned that she actually would faint if they tried to sit her up. He did note that there were additional blood stains on the bed, coming from her rectum. Rafael concluded that, based on the exam findings and the history provided by the patient, she was in shock and needed to be moved carefully but quickly to the hospital. A blanket was paced over Mrs. Hostetler's torso to help retain body heat, and her legs were elevated slightly to maintain blood return back to the heart. Oxygen was maintained at high flow. Within a few minutes of the engine crew's arrival, Rafael could hear the siren of the medic unit pulling up to the apartment complex. ■

which may compromise the airway. In addition, if the patient has a problem that ultimately requires surgical intervention, it is preferable to not have the patient have anything in the stomach when he or she is put under anesthesia.

Resources

Jarvis C: *Physical examination and health assessment*, ed 2, Philadelphia, 1996, WB Saunders.

Price SA, Wilson LM: *Pathophysiology: clinical concepts of disease processes*, ed 4, St Louis, 1992, Mosby-Year Book.

Sanders MJ, McKenna K: *Mosby's paramedic textbook*, rev ed 2, St Louis, 2002, Mosby-Year Book.

Tintinalli JE, Kelen GD, Stapczynski JS: *Emergency medicine: a comprehensive guide*, ed 6, Chicago, 2004, McGraw-Hill.

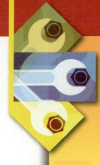

Critical Points

The specific cause of abdominal pain cannot be diagnosed in the field. Spending a minimal amount of time on the scene is important to the outcome of the patient. Transport the patient without delay in a position of comfort. Protect the patient's body temperature and airway, and administer high-flow oxygen.

Learning Checklist

❑ The abdomen generally is divided into four quadrants. The abdomen also can be divided from the front (abdominal cavity) to the back (retroperitoneal).

❑ The abdominal cavity is lined with several layers of tissue, including skin, fatty tissue, muscle, and the peritoneum.

❑ The peritoneum is a tough layer of elastic tissue. It combines with the other layers to protect, cushion, and provide blood flow to the critical organs and structures in the abdominal cavity.

❑ Most digestion takes place in the digestive tract, which begins in the mouth and esophagus.

❑ The intestinal organs are hollow organs, which are prone to a variety of conditions, including blockage and perforation.

❑ The accessory organs include the liver, gallbladder, and pancreas.

❑ The major organ of the urinary system is the kidney. The kidneys are solid organs located on either side of the spinal column, just beneath the lower ribs.

❑ Waste products such as urea, excess water, electrolytes, and breakdown products of medications are filtered and removed as blood flows through the kidney. The wastes are drained from the kidney through the ureter, a hollow tube that carries the waste products to the bladder. Urine eventually is expelled from the bladder through the urethra.

❑ The descending aorta travels downward through the abdominal cavity and divides in half in the pelvic area. The mesentery is the "web" or network of connective tissues that supplies the blood to the abdominal organs.

❑ Visceral pain is pain that is aching, twisting, or crampy. Hollow organs such as the large and small intestines produce visceral pain responses.

❑ Somatic pain is sharp and easily localized by the patient. Solid organs such as the kidneys and pancreas produce pain responses.

❑ Referred pain is pain that is felt in one area but originates in another part of the body.

❑ Postural vital signs refer to vital signs obtained when the patient is supine and then is moved to a sitting position or when the patient is sitting and then is moved to an erect or standing position.

❑ The location of the patient's pain within a certain abdominal quadrant can provide clues to certain problems.

Key Terms

Abdominal aortic aneurysm Dilation of the wall of the abdominal aorta caused by a weakness in the vessel that may be full of fluid or clotted blood.

Accessory organ An organ or other distinct collection of tissues that contributes to the function of another similar organ.

Bladder The membranous sac that serves as a receptacle for secretions; the urinary bladder collects urine.

Digestive tract The musculomembranous tube extending from the mouth to the anus; the tube is lined with mucous membrane and is part of the digestive system. The mouth, pharynx, esophagus, stomach, small intestine, and large intestine compose the digestive tract.

Fallopian tubes Paired structures extending from each side of the uterus to each ovary. The tubes provide a way for the egg to reach the uterus.

Hollow organs Intestinal organs through which materials pass, such as the stomach, small intestine, large intestine, ureters, and bladder.

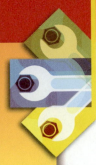

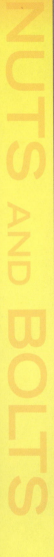

Kidneys The pair of bean-shaped organs that filter the blood and eliminate wastes in urine.

Mesentery A fold of tissue that attaches organs to the body wall. Mesentery usually refers to small bowel mesentery, which anchors the small intestine to the back of the abdominal wall. Blood vessels, nerves, and lymphatic vessels branch through the mesentery to supply the intestine.

Ovaries The paired female reproductive organs found on each side of the lower abdomen.

Peritoneum Membrane lining a body cavity.

Postural vital signs Vital signs obtained when the patient is supine and then is moved to a sitting position or when the patient is sitting and then is moved to an erect or standing position.

Quadrants The four quarters of an anatomic area.

Referred pain Pain that is felt at a site different from that of an injured or diseased organ or body part.

Solid organs Organs including the heart, lungs, kidneys, pancreas, and liver.

Somatic pain Pain that is sharp and easily localized.

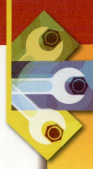

Ureter One of a pair of tubes that carries urine from the kidney into the bladder.

Urinary system All organs and ducts involved in the secretion and elimination of urine from the body.

Uterus The hollow, pear-shaped internal female reproductive organ in which the fertilized ovum is planted and develops.

Visceral pain Abdominal pain that is caused by any abnormal condition of the viscera; it is usually severe, diffuse, and difficult to localize.

National Standard Curriculum Objectives

Cognitive Objectives
No cognitive objectives identified.

Affective Objectives
No affective objectives identified.

Psychomotor Objectives
No psychomotor objectives identified.

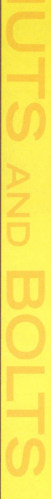

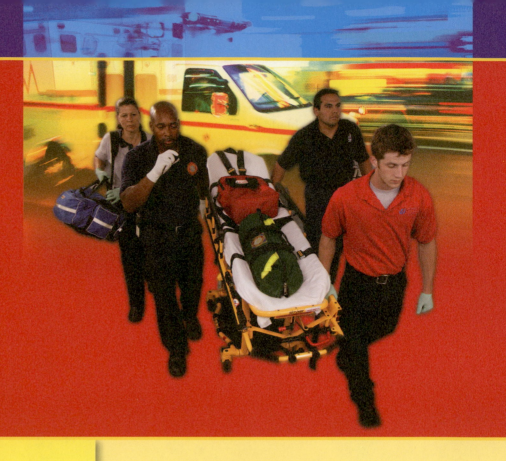

CHAPTER

20

CHAPTER OUTLINE

Altered Level of Consciousness

General Care of Patients with Altered Mental Status

Specific Causes of Altered Mental Status

LESSON GOAL

As an emergency medical technician (EMT), you will encounter patients with an altered mental status or changes in the level of consciousness. This chapter provides information on how to identify, approach, and care for these patients. ■

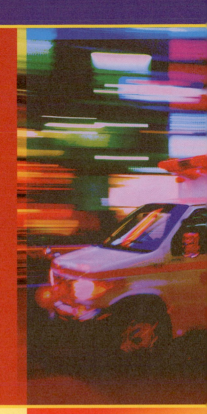

Altered Mental Status

CHAPTER OBJECTIVES

After completing this chapter, the EMT student will be able to do the following:

1 Discuss the importance of appropriate airway management in a patient with an altered mental status.
2 Discuss the general approach and care of the patient with an altered mental status.
3 Identify a patient with an altered mental status who has a history of diabetes.
4 Identify a patient with an altered mental status who is taking diabetic medications.
5 Outline the steps in caring for a patient with an altered mental status who has diabetes.
6 Outline the important pharmaceutical characteristics of oral glucose: generic name, trade name, dosage forms, dose, method of administration, action, and contraindications.
7 Discuss the assessment and treatment approach for a patient having a seizure.
8 Identify the patient who may be having a stroke.
9 Discuss the role of medical direction in the emergency care of a patient with an altered mental status.
10 Explain the rationale for administering oral glucose.
11 Demonstrate the steps in the assessment and treatment of a patient with an altered mental status who has diabetes.
12 Demonstrate the appropriate administration of oral glucose.
13 Demonstrate the appropriate reassessment and documentation of the response to oral glucose in a patient with an altered mental status who has diabetes.
14 Demonstrate completion of the patient care report for a patient with an altered mental status.

20

OBJECTIVES

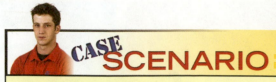

CASE SCENARIO

The police officer waves Ray and his partner over to his patrol car. "Hey Ray, how are things going?" he says.

"Same as always, overworked and underpaid," Ray replies. "What's going on?"

The officer points at the driver of the car he had pulled over a bit earlier for driving erratically. "I thought the driver was intoxicated. He failed a sobriety test, but I can't smell anything on his breath. Can you tell whether he is on drugs?"

Ray replies, "I probably can't, but there could be a medical condition causing him to act strangely. I'll check him out, if you want. What's his name?"

"Thanks, I'd appreciate it," the officer says. "The DL (driver's license) says that his name is John Bradford."

Ray walks over to the car carefully, checking for any damage to the vehicle. There does not appear to be any. The driver is standing on the passenger side of the car, leaning against the door. Observing the position of the man's hands and his general appearance, Ray decides that he does not appear to be threatening.

"Hello, Mr. Bradford," he says, slowly reaching for the driver's radial pulse. "I understand that you might not be feeling well. Can I help you?"

A long pause follows. Finally, Mr. Bradford mumbles, "I'm fine. I need to get home."

As he feels the patient's radial pulse, Ray spies a large metal bracelet on the man's wrist. Part of the bracelet is shaped like a tag. Ray lifts the man's arm. He sees the word "diabetic" embossed on the tag.

Questions: How might this finding figure into the patient's condition? What questions should Ray ask the patient now? What are some of the management tasks Ray should perform as he works up the patient's condition?

EMS personnel frequently are called upon to care for patients with an **altered mental status (AMS)** or a change in the **level of consciousness (LOC)**. The causes of these conditions range from intoxication with alcohol or other drugs to medical or traumatic conditions that must be quickly identified and treated. These causes may develop and cause an altered mental status very quickly, or they may develop slowly. Most often, an altered LOC is caused by a reduction in the blood flow to the patient's brain. This reduction in blood flow causes hypoxia (lack of oxygen) of the brain. It can occur as a result of a number of conditions, which are described in this chapter. This situation frequently is temporary, but it can be permanent, as in a patient who has suffered a stroke. The emergency medical services (EMS) provider must always identify any condition that may be contributing to a change in the patient's LOC. For patients who appear to be intoxicated with alcohol or drugs, it is critical that the EMT evaluate the patient extensively to determine whether other medical or traumatic conditions also may be contributing to the changes in the patient's mental status.

Possible causes of altered mental status in patients include hypoxia, respiratory problems, head trauma, poisoning (alcohol or drugs/chemicals, whether accidental or intentional), diabetes, syncope, seizures, stroke, and central nervous system (CNS) or general body infection, especially if the patient has a fever.

The general initial care of these patients is the same regardless of the cause of the AMS:

1. Proper patient positioning
2. Airway maintenance
3. Oxygenation and ventilation
4. Body temperature maintenance
5. Expeditious transport to the hospital
6. ALS care if available
7. Consultation with medical control, if appropriate
8. Glucose administration, if the cause of the AMS is known and if allowed in the protocol, especially in patients who have diabetes

This chapter specifically discusses issues related to the more common causes of altered mental status: diabetes, syncope, seizures, and stroke. Other possible causes mentioned earlier are covered elsewhere in this text.

ALTERED LEVEL OF CONSCIOUSNESS

Patients with a normal LOC are awake, alert, and able to talk with you and converse appropriately. Patients who do not show these capabilities require rapid evaluation and care. Evaluation of mental status includes assessing patients for factors such as who they are (person), where they are (place), the correct day and time (time), and what is going on around them/what has recently happened to them (events). Patients who cannot respond appropriately to questions about these factors have an altered mental status or altered level of consciousness. The condition may range from slightly confused to completely unresponsive. In some patients, the person's mental status may be abnormal because of a previous illness or injury (e.g., Alzheimer's disease, stroke, or brain injury). In these situations, it is important for the EMT to determine whether the current mental status is different from the patient's baseline status.

You should be able to assess the patient's mental status generally based on the way the patient responds to your initial assessment and questioning. The patient may be slightly confused in orientation, may have difficulty remembering or explaining things, may provide only inappropriate responses to various levels of stimulation (normal talking, loud voice, painful stimulus), or may not respond at all. It is important to combine the information from this assessment with other information obtained from your patient assessment, including vital signs. Abnormal vital signs (high or low blood pressure, abnormal pulse or respirations) may be either a cause or a result of the AMS.

Two assessment tools frequently are used to describe a patient's LOC. The more general one is the **AVPU** assessment tool (Box 20-1). The AVPU method can be used very quickly during the assessment. The assessment tool that is used more commonly in medicine is the **Glasgow Coma Scale** (Tables 20-1 and 20-2). This scale measures three components of the patient's neurologic status: eye opening, speech function, and motor function. It provides for a more detailed assessment of the patient's neurologic status and frequently is used for describing that status in the hospital. Repeated examination of the GCS also al-

---

BOX 20-1

AVPU Assessment Tool

A—Alert (spontaneously awake)
V—Responds to verbal stimulus (reacts to loud voice)
P—Responds to painful stimulus (reacts to skin pinch)
U—Unresponsive (does not respond to painful stimulus)

TABLE 20-1

Glasgow Coma Scale for Adults

Criteria	Patient Response	Score
Eye opening	Spontaneously	4
	To speech	3
	To pain	2
	None	1
Verbal response	Oriented	5
	Confused	4
	Inappropriate words	3
	Incomprehensible words	2
	None	1
Motor response	Obeys commands	6
	Localizes pain	5
	Withdraws to pain	4
	Flexion to pain	3
	Extension to pain	2
	None	1

---

lows health care providers to follow a patient's progress over time.

In addition to the evaluation of the patient's mental status, other components of the physical examination can provide clues as to the cause of the alteration. The eyes should be examined, not only for their response to stimuli, as in the GCS, but also for their size and equality. For example, pinpoint pupils may indicate a patient who has overdosed on narcotics. Unequal pupils may suggest increased intracranial pressure. The motor examination may reveal a patient with weakness or paralysis of one side, suggesting a stroke or transient ischemic attack.

TABLE 20-2
Modified Glasgow Coma Scale for Children and Infants

Criteria	Child	Infant	Score
Eye opening	Spontaneous	Spontaneous	5
	To verbal stimuli	To verbal stimuli	4
	To pain only	To pain only	3
	No response	No response	2
Verbal response	Oriented, appropriate	Coos and babbles	5
	Confused	Irritable, cries	4
	Inappropriate words	Cries to pain	3
	Incomprehensible sounds	Moans to pain	2
	No response	No response	1
Motor response*	Obeys commands	Moves spontaneously and purposefully	6
	Localizes painful stimuli	Withdraws to touch	5
	Withdraws in response to pain	Withdraws in response to pain	4
	Flexion in response to pain	Abnormal flexion posture to pain	3
	Extension in response to pain	Abnormal extension posture to pain	2
	No response	No response	1

From Aehlert B: *Pediatric advanced life support study guide*, ed 2, St Louis, 2005, Mosby.
*If the patient is intubated, unconscious, or preverbal, the most important part of this scale is motor response. Motor response should be evaluated carefully.

GENERAL CARE OF PATIENTS WITH ALTERED MENTAL STATUS

The approach to general care applies to all patients with AMS or altered LOC, regardless of the specific cause. Usually, you should place the patient in the supine position. Do not allow the person to stand. Some patients experiencing respiratory distress may not want to lie flat. In these situations (and if no trauma is involved), it may be better to have the patient sit up and assume a position of comfort. If the possibility of trauma is a concern, maintain spinal stabilization. If the patient is unresponsive and trauma is not a concern, place the patient in the recovery position.

Immediately address the patient's airway, breathing, and circulation (ABCs). Maintain the airway, oxygenation, and ventilation. All patients with AMS should be placed on oxygen after the EMT has made sure the airway is clear and patent. Assess the circulation. If appropriate, perform cardiopulmonary resuscitation (CPR). A full history and physical assessment, including vital signs, are appropriate. Always try to maintain the patient's body temperature. If advanced life support (ALS) is available and protocols

ASK YOURSELF

Have you ever wondered how many of your friends or family members are diabetic? Maybe they have a seizure disorder or have had a stroke at some time. Would you be able to manage this type of incident? Would you be able to tell the difference between these conditions?

allow for activation or intercept, initiate the ALS response. Immobilize the trauma patient. Initiate transport to a hospital as quickly as possible.

SPECIFIC CAUSES OF ALTERED MENTAL STATUS

As noted earlier, a number of causes of AMS may require specific assessment or treatment considerations. This chapter discusses specific issues (cause, assessment [signs and symptoms], and treatment) for diabetes, syncope, seizures, and stroke. Other causes (e.g., infection, trauma, and alcohol and drug intoxication) are covered in other chapters.

Diabetes

Glucose is the body's primary source of energy. It is a simple sugar that is obtained from digestion of foods and must be incorporated into the body's cells to supply energy. **Insulin** (a hormone produced by the pancreas) is needed to transport glucose into the cells. Many cells in the body are able to store glucose (in the form of glycogen) and are able to survive for short periods with a decreased blood flow and decreased glucose supply. However, the brain has no mechanism for storing glucose. Therefore, when glucose is not supplied by a constant blood flow, energy is quickly lost and the patient loses consciousness. Without glucose, brain cells start to die within a few minutes.

If the body does not have enough insulin, glucose cannot get into cells, including brain cells. This results in high blood glucose **(hyperglycemia)** and AMS. If too much insulin is present and not enough glucose, low blood glucose **(hypoglycemia)** results, causing decreased LOC. Both of these conditions can occur in people with diabetes. Generally, hyperglycemia with AMS occurs more gradually; hypoglycemia with AMS or unresponsiveness occurs more rapidly.

Diabetes is a disease in which the pancreas does not produce enough insulin. The two types of diabetes are type I diabetes (insulin-dependent/juvenile onset diabetes) and type II diabetes (non-insulin-dependent/adult onset diabetes).

In **type I diabetes,** the pancreas either does not produce enough insulin or does not produce any insulin at all. Type I diabetes usually develops during childhood and requires the patient to take insulin shots. (Insulin cannot be absorbed via the gastrointestinal tract, therefore it cannot be given as a pill.) In **type II diabetes,** not enough insulin is produced for the body's needs, or the insulin receptors in the body do not work well. Type II diabetes usually occurs in adulthood and frequently is associated with obesity. It may be controlled with a specific diet, increased exercise, or oral medications that stimulate the pancreas to make more insulin or that make the body's cells more receptive to the insulin produced by the pancreas.

As noted previously, two types of problems can occur in people with diabetes: either a blood glucose level that is too low (hypoglycemia) or a blood glucose level that is too high (hyperglycemia). Both of these conditions are more common in people with type I diabetes because these individuals are more likely to have greater fluctuations in blood glucose.

SPECIAL Considerations

Take a Look
If you suspect that a patient with a decreased level of consciousness may be an insulin-dependent diabetic, check the refrigerator. Insulin must be refrigerated, so look for a vial of insulin or for syringes that are filled and ready for administration.

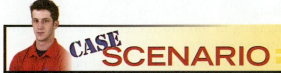

CASE SCENARIO
continued

The patient grimaces at Ray's treatment. "Yuck!" he exclaims. "This stuff tastes something awful!"

"I know it does," Ray replies with a laugh. "It's oral glucose paste, and it does taste bad. But really try to squirt as much of it as you can into your mouth, okay?"

Mr. Bradford puts the tip of the tube back into his mouth and squeezes the tube again. A little bit of the reddish paste comes out on his lip.

Questions: *What does Ray need to be most concerned about in this situation? After Mr. Bradford finishes taking the medication, what should Ray reassess?*

When assessing a patient you think may have diabetes, it is critical that you obtain certain information. This can be done by asking the following questions:

- "Do you have diabetes?" (Confirm that the patient has diabetes.)
- "Do you take medications for it? If so, what?" (Insulin or pills [hypoglycemic medication])
- "Have you taken your medications today? When? Was it the correct dose?"
- "When did you last eat?"
- "Have you had any unusual activities? Any recent illnesses?"

It is important that you try to find the patient's medications. Record the names and strengths of the medications on your patient care report and take the medications with the patient to the hospital.

Hypoglycemia

Hypoglycemia is the more common reaction with diabetes and occurs with both type I and type II diabetes. Hypoglycemia generally is more worrisome in people with type II diabetes, because the oral medications have a longer duration of action. This makes it more difficult to correct the low blood glucose level and to maintain the proper glucose level.

Hypoglycemia usually develops fairly quickly and can occur for a number of reasons, such as the following:

- Taking the regular dose of medication and not eating
- Engaging in too much exercise (using up glucose too quickly)
- Taking too much insulin or oral medication
- Suffering from an illness (not absorbing food/glucose, producing stress on the body, and using up glucose more quickly)

Hyperglycemia

As mentioned previously, hyperglycemia (high blood glucose level) results either because not enough insulin is present in the body or because the body's receptor cells do not respond to the insulin. Consequently, insulin does not transport glucose into cells, and the glucose builds up in the bloodstream (hyperglycemia) and spills over into the urine (glycosuria). Because of the increased glucose in the urine, more urine is produced, and the patient urinates more frequently (polyuria). This leads to dehydration and causes the patient to be thirsty and to drink more fluids (polydipsia). Because the body cannot use glucose for energy, it starts to break down fat for energy. This causes ketones and acids to form in the body and leads to a condition called **diabetic ketoacidosis (DKA).** This is a dangerous condition if allowed to continue, one that leads to coma. It usually develops over several hours to days and requires more complicated treatment than is available in the field.

Signs and Symptoms

Generally, patients with a diabetic emergency (either hyperglycemia or hypoglycemia) have the following signs and symptoms:

- AMS
- Rapid pulse
- Rapid, deep respirations (more common with hyperglycemia)
- Weakness
- Sweating and warm, dry skin (hyperglycemia) or cool, moist skin (hypoglycemia)

- Nausea/vomiting (hyperglycemia)
- Headache
- Seizures (in severe cases of hypoglycemia)
- Coma

Patients with diabetes frequently use a portable **glucose monitor** to measure their glucose levels at certain times of the day and to watch trends. If allowed in the protocol and you have the appropriate equipment, measuring the patient's blood glucose level is an important part of the assessment. The glucose monitor can give you an indication of the patient's glucose level and help with the assessment of whether the patient is experiencing hyperglycemia or hypoglycemia. An important aspect of the use of glucose monitors is to make sure they are tested frequently and calibrated to ensure that the reading is accurate.

Treatment

As noted earlier, the treatment for **hyperglycemia** is complicated and beyond an EMT's ability to treat in the field. Instead the patient must be transported to the closest appropriate emergency department for evaluation and treatment. The goal of treatment for **hypoglycemia** is to increase the patient's blood glucose level. Depending on the patient's mental status, you may be able to give liquids with sugar added or even some food or glucose bars. Have the patient consume these items if the person is able to do so. If the protocol allows, you may also use **glucose gel,** which is concentrated glucose in a paste form. The gel is placed in the mouth and quickly absorbed through the oral mucous membranes into the bloodstream. Oral glucose gel (Fig. 20-1) may be given to patients who are confused but awake, but you must be able to

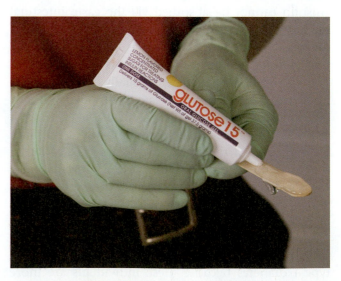

Fig. 20-1 Oral glucose gel.

SKILL 20-1
◎ *Administration of Oral Glucose*

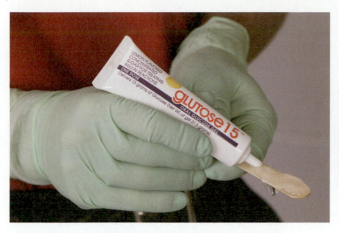

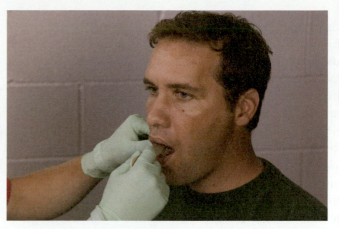

1. Consult medical control for authorization to administer oral glucose.
2. Check to make sure the patient is responsive and able to swallow.

3. Place the glucose on a tongue depressor and administer the full tube between the patient's cheek and gum, allowing the mucous membranes to absorb the glucose.
4. Reassess the patient and document the time of administration and any changes in the patient's condition.

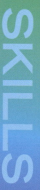

instill the gel carefully inside the cheek or under tongue. Position the patient on his or her side to allow secretions to drain and watch the airway closely. You may be able to squirt small amounts of the gel under the patient's tongue, or you can put small amounts of the gel on a tongue depressor and gently place it inside the cheek or under the tongue. Whether you are giving the patient food, liquid with glucose added, or glucose gel, the patient must be awake enough to swallow as well as protect the airway. Never put anything into the mouth of an unconscious patient, as he or she may aspirate it into his or her lungs.

Syncope

EMS providers frequently are called up to care for patients who faint. **Syncope** (a sudden, temporary loss of consciousness without residual neurologic deficits) is caused by a temporary decrease in blood flow (with decreased oxygen supply) to the brain. Remember, the brain has no mechanism for storing oxygen or glucose. Therefore it must have a constant supply of blood to get oxygen and glucose to maintain consciousness. Syncope may occur for many reasons, such as blood pooling in lower parts of the body (abdomen or lower extremities), with less flow going to the brain (situations in which a person gets up too quickly from a lying or sitting position); events that cause dilation of the body's blood vessels and shunts blood away from the brain (emotional experiences); overexertion; or heart abnormalities (low cardiac output, dysrhythmias). The elderly often have a decreased ability to compensate for changes in body position and are more prone to abnormal changes of the vascular system and to dysrhythmias.

Signs and Symptoms

Because syncope is a temporary condition, EMTs may arrive to find the patient normal or slightly confused but improving. Syncope often is preceded by sensations of lightheadedness; dizziness; tunnel vision; nausea; pale, cool, moist skin; an abnormal heart rate (either fast [dysrhythmia] or slow [vasovagal episode—emotional response]); abnormal respirations; or numbness or tingling of the extremities.

Treatment

Syncope usually resolves on its own, especially after the patient becomes supine and blood can more easily get to the brain. If the patient continues to experience AMS, you should consider other possible causes and investigate those.

If the person fell, evaluate for injuries, especially of the spine. With all syncope patients, loosen restrictive clothing; administer oxygen; elevate the legs, if appropriate; and assess and record vital signs frequently. As the patient's condition improves (and if possible injury is not a concern), you may allow the patient carefully to sit up, if appropriate. Continue to monitor vital signs closely, keeping in mind that an elevated pulse rate (especially in a syncopal patient) may be a more sensitive indicator of hypovolemia than blood pressure. Always try to figure out the reason for the syncope. In unusual cases call for ALS assist (especially if the patient is elderly or you are concerned about dysrhythmia) and transport the patient to the hospital for evaluation. Patients who faint or "pass out" and quickly return to normal and feel fine often want to refuse further care and transport. If this occurs, you should contact medical control before allowing the patient to refuse transport. Any case of a patient who has experienced an AMS and wants to refuse care or transport should be discussed with your medical oversight physician at the time.

Seizures

A **seizure** (also known as a **convulsion**) occurs when the electrical activity of the brain is altered for some reason, causing random electrical discharges that lead to the seizure. Seizures can be demonstrated in many different ways (e.g., partial or whole body muscle jerking, staring off into space), depending on how the brain is affected and how the impulses affect the body. The seizure causes a change in the patient's LOC, behavior, and/or muscle activity. Seizures have many possible causes, such as fever (especially in young children), infection (CNS or other), hypoglycemia, hypoxia, and injury. In some patients, the cause of a seizure cannot be determined with certainty. When the seizures are recurrent or chronic, the condition is referred to as **epilepsy.** Patients with seizure disorders most often are treated with anticonvulsant medications, which they usually have to take daily.

Seizures are classified according to how the seizure manifests in the patient.

- **Partial seizure:** Only part of the body is affected (e.g., arms or facial movement).
  - *Simple partial seizure:* A particular part of the body is affected (e.g., the arm may have tingling, spasms, or rigidity).
  - *Complex partial seizure:* The patient exhibits abnormal behavior (e.g., confusion, pacing, staring, or seeming intoxication).
- **Generalized seizure:** Also called a **tonic-clonic seizure** or a **grand mal seizure.** This type of seizure may be preceded by an *aura* (an unusual feeling or sensation that indicates to the patient the seizure is going to occur).
  - *Tonic phase:* The patient experiences rigidity of the muscles that lasts seconds to minutes.
  - *Clonic phase:* The patient experiences severe muscle contractions/spasms that usually last several minutes.
- Absence seizure: Also called a **petit mal seizure.** Usually, the patient blankly stares off into space, and no obvious muscle contractions occur. These seizures normally last seconds to minutes.

Signs and Symptoms

The signs of a seizure can range from mild to severe. As noted previously, the patient may experience an aura (a sensation of light, sound, smell, or colors) that indicates to the patient a seizure will occur. With simple seizures (e.g., petit mal seizures), the patient appears to stare off into space as though daydreaming. With more severe seizures, loss of consciousness occurs, along with localized or general muscle activity (contraction and relaxation) or tonic-clonic activity, with diffuse movement of the patient's arms and legs. The patient may have bladder and bowel incontinence. Seizures generally last a few seconds to a few minutes. If the seizure occurs, stops, and then recurs without the patient regaining consciousness, the patient is experiencing **status epilepticus,** a serious and potentially life-threatening condition that may result in permanent neurologic damage. These patients should be transported quickly, and ALS services should be requested, if available.

After the seizure, the patient may often appear to be resting or sleeping, in a postictal state. The person may appear unresponsive. This may last a few minutes to 30 minutes. Upon awakening, the patient may be confused or combative and often complains of being tired or of having a headache or sore muscles. The patient may have been incontinent. Patients often feel self-conscious or embarrassed after having had a seizure. Seizures can be frightening to the patient and to bystanders. However, they usually are self-limited and do not pose a problem for the patient.

Treatment

The following general treatment for patients experiencing a seizure should be provided, regardless of the type of seizure.

- Protect the patient from getting hurt. Place the patient on the floor, if the person is not already there. Move objects and furniture away from the patient.
- Place the patient in the recovery position if possible.
- During the seizure, do not place anything in the patient's mouth. The jaw usually is clenched tightly. Allow secretions to drain.
- Loosen any restrictive clothing.
- Support the patient and bystanders. Console, calm, and reassure them.
- Provide supplemental oxygen if possible. The patient may not appear to be breathing during the seizure, but there will be some air movement.

- Request ALS resources if available, especially if the seizure is prolonged or if it appears the patient is in status epilepticus.
- Transport the patient to the hospital for evaluation. Many patients have recurrent seizures because of poor medication compliance. They also should be evaluated for injuries that may have occurred during the seizure.

Many patients who have seizures (especially those whose seizures occur frequently despite proper medication use) may want to refuse further care or transport after they awaken. If this occurs, it is important that the EMT contact online medical control before allowing the patient to leave.

Stroke

Stroke, also called cerebrovascular accident (CVA), is the third leading cause of death in the United States. It frequently leads to residual mental and physical disability in patients. A stroke is caused by a permanent interruption of blood flow to the brain, either from a clot blocking blood flow (ischemia) or bleeding (hemorrhage) from a ruptured or leaking blood vessel. A clot can be a result of either a thrombus (a clot that forms in the blood vessel in the area of the damage) or an embolus (a clot that forms elsewhere in the body and travels through the bloodstream until it lodges in and blocks the blood vessel). The result of either a clot or hemorrhage is the loss of blood supply to a particular area of the brain. This leads to the symptoms and signs the patient experiences, depending on the area of the brain affected.

In some situations the decreased blood flow to an area of the brain may be temporary yet still cause symptoms similar to those of a stroke. This is called a transient ischemic attack (TIA). TIAs usually last minutes to hours and resolve without permanent problems. A TIA is a warning sign of a possible stroke, and all patients who experience a TIA must be evaluated at the hospital. These patients should not be allowed to refuse care and transport.

In the past it generally was believed that once a stroke had started, little could be done to prevent permanent residual neurologic problems. However, progress has been made in recent years in the treatment of patients experiencing strokes, at least those with ischemic strokes. If these patients are transported to the hospital and evaluated quickly, clot-dissolving medications (thrombolytics) can be administered in some cases to try to dissolve the clot and restore blood flow to the affected area of the brain. This is why a stroke is sometimes referred to as a *brain attack*. It is very important that patients experiencing a stroke get to the hospital as quickly as possible for evaluation and treatment. However, not all patients who have a stroke are treated with thrombolytics.

Signs and Symptoms

As noted earlier, it is important for EMTs to recognize the signs and symptoms of a stroke as soon as possible in order to obtain rapid hospital care for the patient. Any of the following should cause you to consider the possibility of a stroke in your patient: sudden behavior changes, AMS, difficulty speaking (inability to say what is meant, slurred speech), difficulty walking or maintaining balance, weakness of the arms or legs, unusual feelings (numbness or tingling), facial droop, visual changes, pupil differences, and difficulty swallowing. Any of these signs and symptoms should prompt early transport and further evaluation.

Treatment

Early recognition of signs or symptoms, leading to consideration of the possibility of a stroke, is paramount. Generally, the care you provide is supportive. Assess the ABCs, provide oxygen, assess the patient's neurologic status, talk with the patient about what is going on (the patient may have difficulty talking or responding but may easily hear and understand what you are telling him or her), and request ALS services if available. Place the patient in a position of comfort.

With the development in recent years of specialized evaluation and treatment of patients having a stroke, the EMS system may have identified specific hospitals to which the patient should be transported or stroke centers with specific resources for rapid assessment, diagnosis, and treatment of appropriate patients. Follow your local protocols and work within the EMS system to address the needs of these patients.

■ SUMMARY

Many conditions can result in an AMS. By using a structured approach to the assessment and treatment of these individuals, you can support your patients and provide them with appropriate stabilizing care and transport to the hospital.

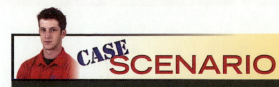

CASE SCENARIO

conclusion

"Yeah, the last thing I remember was drinking that can of cola because I knew my sugar level was very low," says Mr. Bradford as Ray rechecks his blood pressure. It has been 20 minutes since Mr. Bradford finished eating the oral glucose paste. His LOC has steadily improved. He is now oriented to person and recognizes where he is, although he can't remember how he got there. He also lost track of time for a couple of hours.

Letting the air out of the blood pressure (BP) cuff, Ray looks over at Mr. Bradford's car. In the rear seat, he spies an aluminum can. "Is that it?" he asks.

Mr. Bradford reaches in to get the can. "Yes, I think so," he says. They both look at the can. It is a diet cola. They both immediately understand what happened. "Well, that would explain it now, wouldn't it?" Ray comments. ■

TEAMWORK

As discussed in this chapter, EMTs can find themselves in various situations in which the patient may have a condition that results in altered mental status. Whether you are working with law enforcement at the local jail, as a firefighter at an accident scene, or in a fifth grade classroom, every-

one depends on you to assess the patient accurately, determine the problem, and make sure the proper care is initiated. Cooperation with other responders ensures that the patient care team works toward a positive patient outcome.

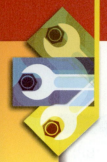

Critical Points

- The EMT must be able to differentiate between the possible causes of altered mental status.
- The EMT's assessment skills are crucial for determining the cause of a patient's problems in a wide variety of situations.
- EMTs must remember to request an ALS intercept early. Do not wait until your patient's condition has deteriorated to request assistance.

Learning Checklist

❑ EMS providers often are called upon to care for a patient with AMS or changes in LOC. Causes ranges from alcohol or drug use to medical or traumatic conditions that must be promptly identified and treated. The most common cause of AMS is reduced blood flow to the patient's brain.

❑ Conditions that may result in AMS include hypoxia, respiratory problems, head trauma, poisoning (alcohol or drugs/chemical), diabetes, syncope, seizures, stroke, and CNS or general body infection.

❑ Patients with a normal LOC are awake, alert, and able to talk and converse appropriately. Patients should be oriented to person, place, time, and events. AMS can range from slight confusion to complete unresponsiveness.

❑ Information from the assessment of the patient's mental status should be combined with other patient assessment findings, including vital signs.

❑ The AVPU assessment tool is useful for assessing mental status. The acronym stands for *a*lert, *v*erbal (response), *p*ainful (response), and *u*nresponsive.

❑ The Glasgow Coma Scale is used to measure three components of the patient's neurologic status: eye opening, speech function, and motor function. A score is derived by adding the components of the scale. The highest score is 15; patients with scores of 13 or lower are considered to be in critical condition.

❑ Patients with AMS usually are placed in the supine position. However, patients with respiratory distress may be better transported in a seated position. Those with potential trauma should have spinal stabilization. Patients who are unresponsive (and trauma is not a concern) should be placed in the recovery position.

❑ Diabetes results from a deficiency or complete lack of insulin secretion by the pancreas or from resistance to insulin. There are two types of diabetes. Type I usually develops during childhood and requires insulin shots. Type II usually develops in adults and often is associated with obesity. Type II diabetes may be controlled with diet, exercise, or oral medications.

❑ Glucose, a simple sugar, is the primary form of energy used by the body.

❑ Hyperglycemia is caused by blood glucose levels that are too high. Hypoglycemia results from blood glucose levels that are too low. Both conditions can occur in individuals with diabetes.

❑ It is important to ask patients with diabetes about the time of their last medication, last meal, and any unusual activities or recent illness. Record the names and strengths of the patient's medications in the patient care report. Take the medications to the hospital when the patient is transported.

❑ Patients with diabetes use portable glucose monitors to measure their blood glucose levels at certain times of the day. EMTs may use monitors to check the patient's blood glucose levels as part of their patient assessment. Follow local protocols regarding the use of glucose monitors.

❑ The treatment for hypoglycemia is to increase the patient's blood glucose level. The patient may be able to drink liquids with sugar added or eat some food or glucose bars. If allowed by protocol, the EMT may use glucose gel, which is placed in the patient's mouth and rapidly absorbed by the bloodstream.

❑ Syncope, or fainting, results from a temporary decrease in blood flow to the brain. Elderly patients may have a decreased capa-

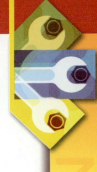

bility to compensate for sudden changes in body position, which can lead to syncope.

❑ Treatment for syncope includes evaluating the patient for possible injuries, particularly if the patient has fallen. For all syncope patients, the EMT should loosen restrictive clothing, administer oxygen, elevate the legs if appropriate, and assess and record vital signs frequently. The reason for the syncope should be determined. If a patient refuses further care and transport, the EMT should contact medical control and document the refusal of care.

❑ Seizures (convulsions) occur as a result of altered electrical activity in the brain. Seizures can change a patient's LOC, behavior, or muscle activity, or a combination of these factors. Signs of a seizure can range from mild to severe. Patients with seizure disorders usually are treated with anticonvulsant medications, which generally are taken daily. Epilepsy is a condition in which seizures are recurrent or chronic.

❑ In more severe seizures, loss of consciousness and localized or general muscle activity occurs. The patient may be incontinent. Seizures usually last a few seconds to minutes.

❑ Status epilepticus (a condition in which seizures occur, stop, and then recur without the patient regaining consciousness) is a life-threatening event that can cause permanent neurologic damage. Patients in status epilepticus should be transported quickly, and ALS services should be requested if available.

❑ A stroke, or CVA, is caused by a permanent interruption of blood flow to the brain. Strokes are the third leading cause of death in the United States. They can cause residual mental and physical disability.

❑ Signs of stroke include sudden behavior changes, AMS, speech difficulties, difficulty walking or maintaining balance, weakness of the arms or legs, unusual feelings or sensations (numbness or tingling), facial droop, visual changes, pupil differences, and difficulty swallowing.

❑ Early recognition and treatment of stroke are vital. Stroke care usually is supportive: assess the ABCs; provide oxygen; assess the patient's neurologic status; advise the patient what is happening; and request ALS assistance if available. The patient should be transported to a stroke center if one is available.

Key Terms

Altered mental status (AMS) Any mental state that differs from a conscious person's normal state of awareness or competence.

AVPU A mnemonic assessment tool used to determine a person's mental status. The acronym stands for *a*lert (the person is alert, awake, and oriented); *v*erbal (the person responds to voice); *p*ainful (the person responds only to a painful stimulus); and *u*nresponsive (the person is not awake and is completely unresponsive to any type of stimulation).

Cerebrovascular accident (CVA) An abnormal condition of the brain caused by occlusion of a blood vessel by an embolus, thrombus, or hemorrhage or vasospasm; also known as a *stroke.*

Convulsion Hyperexcitation of neurons in the brain, leading to sudden, violent, involuntary contractions of the muscles; also known as a *seizure.*

Diabetic ketoacidosis (DKA) Diabetic coma; an acute, life-threatening complication of uncontrolled diabetes.

Epilepsy A group of neurologic disorders characterized by recurrent episodes of convulsive seizures, sensory disturbances, abnormal behavior, loss of consciousness, or all of these.

Generalized seizure A tonic-clonic or grand mal seizure.

Glasgow Coma Scale A quick, practical, standardized system for assessing the degree of impairment of consciousness in critically ill patients. It also is used to predict the duration and ultimate outcome of a coma. This scale is used primarily in patients with head injuries.

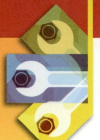

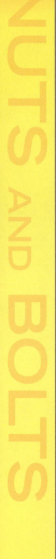

Glucose A simple sugar present in certain foods, especially fruits. It is a major source of energy that can be measured in the blood.

Glucose gel Concentrated glucose in a paste form.

Glucose monitor A battery-powered instrument used to calculate blood glucose levels from as little as one drop of blood.

Grand mal seizure A condition characterized by generalized involuntary muscle contractions and cessation of respiration, followed by tonic and clonic muscle spasms. Breathing returns with noisy respirations. The condition also is known as a *tonic-clonic seizure.*

Hyperglycemia A greater than normal amount of glucose in the blood.

Hypoglycemia A state of low blood sugar levels.

Insulin A naturally occurring hormone, secreted by the pancreas, that regulates the metabolism of glucose.

Level of consciousness (LOC) A degree of cognitive function involving arousal mechanisms in the brain. Levels of consciousness range from unconsciousness to full attention.

Partial seizure A seizure in which only part of the body is affected.

Petit mal seizure A seizure in which the patient usually has a blank stare with no obvious muscle contractions; it usually lasts for seconds to minutes. This type of seizure is also known as an *absence seizure.*

Status epilepticus A condition in which seizures occur, stop, and then recur without the patient regaining consciousness.

Seizure Hyperexcitation of neurons in the brain, leading to sudden, violent, involuntary contractions of the muscles; also known as a *convulsion.*

Stroke An abnormal condition of the brain caused by occlusion of a blood vessel by an embolus, thrombus, or hemorrhage or vasospasm; also known as a *cerebrovascular accident.*

Syncope Fainting; a brief lapse in consciousness. Syncope may be preceded by a sensation of lightheadedness.

Tonic-clonic seizure A seizure characterized by generalized involuntary muscle contractions and cessation of respiration, followed by tonic and clonic muscle spasms. Breathing returns with noisy respirations. The condition is also known as a *grand mal seizure.*

Transient ischemic attack (TIA) An episode of cerebrovascular insufficiency, usually associated with partial obstruction of a cerebral artery by plaque or an embolus.

Type I diabetes A type of diabetes in which the body is unable to metabolize carbohydrates because of insulin deficiency. The condition usually develops during childhood and requires the patient to take insulin shots.

Type II diabetes A type of diabetes in which the person is not insulin dependent or prone to ketosis, although insulin may be used to correct symptoms and persistent hyperglycemia. The onset usually occurs during adulthood. The condition often is associated with obesity.

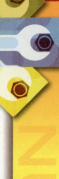

National Standard Curriculum Objectives

Cognitive Objectives

After completing this lesson, the EMT student will be able to do the following:

- Identify the patient taking diabetic medications who has an altered mental status and the implications of a diabetes history.
- State the steps in the emergency medical care of a patient taking diabetic medications who has an altered mental status and a history of diabetes.
- Establish the relationship between airway management and the patient with altered mental status.
- State the generic and trade names, medication forms, dose, administration, action, and contraindications for oral glucose.
- Evaluate the need for medical direction in the emergency medical care of the diabetic patient.

Affective Objective

After completing this lesson, the EMT student will be able to do the following:

- Explain the rationale for administering oral glucose.

Psychomotor Objectives

After completing this lesson, the EMT student will be able to do the following:

- Demonstrate the steps in the emergency medical care of a patient taking diabetic medications who has an altered mental status and a history of diabetes.
- Demonstrate the steps in the administration of oral glucose.
- Demonstrate the assessment and documentation of the patient's response to oral glucose.
- Demonstrate how to complete a prehospital care report for patients with diabetic emergencies.

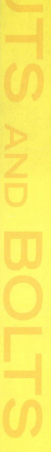

CHAPTER OUTLINE

OUTLINE

LESSON GOAL

As an emergency medical technician (EMT), you must be able to identify, assess, and treat patients who are having allergic reactions and their complications appropriately. This chapter presents information on allergic reactions, including their causes, signs, symptoms, and treatment. The information on assessment emphasizes early identification and airway management. The chapter also includes a description of the use of epinephrine in the form of an intramuscular injection, which can be used for anaphylaxis, a severe allergic reaction. ■

GOAL

Allergies

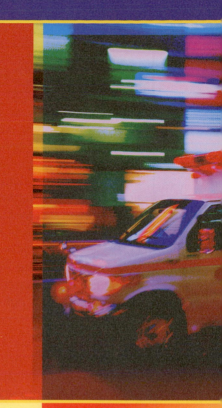

CHAPTER OBJECTIVES

After completing this chapter, the EMT student will be able to do the following:

1 Recognize when a patient is having an allergic reaction.

2 Discuss the role of histamine released during an allergic reaction.

3 Describe the mechanisms of an allergic response.

4 Describe the proper assessment of a patient having an allergic reaction.

5 Describe the emergency medical care of the patient having an allergic reaction.

6 Establish the relationship between the patient having an allergic reaction and airway management.

7 State the generic and trade names, medication forms, dose, administration, action, and contraindications for the EpiPen autoinjector.

8 Differentiate between the general category of patients having an allergic reaction and the specific subcategory of patients having an allergic reaction who require immediate medical care, including immediate use of an epinephrine autoinjector.

9 List the signs and symptoms of anaphylactic shock.

10 Describe the pathophysiology of anaphylactic shock.

11 Describe the emergency medical care of the patient in anaphylactic shock.

12 Demonstrate the emergency medical care of the patient having an allergic reaction.

13 Demonstrate the use of the epinephrine autoinjector.

14 Demonstrate the emergency medical care of the patient in anaphylactic shock.

21

OBJECTIVES

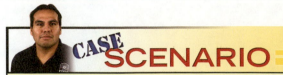

CASE SCENARIO

It's a gorgeous day, so Rafael decides to go surfing early in the morning, shortly after he goes off shift. The water is nearly perfect—not too cold, with large enough swells to give a few good rides back to the beach. All the regulars are there, too. Alan, for example, is a cabinetmaker Rafael has known for years. Rafael watches Alan catch the next one in, and then Rafael finds his own wave to ride. At the surf line, Rafael picks up his board to head back out. Looking up, he sees Alan sitting in the sand just beyond the water's edge. Sensing something wrong, Rafael jogs out of the water over to Alan.

"Are you okay, buddy?" Rafael asks. Up close, it's very apparent to him that Alan, in fact, is not okay. He is pale and is having breathing difficulty.

"I...got...stung by...a jellyfish...I think," pants Alan, who has difficulty speaking.

"Okay, Alan," Rafael says. "Just try to relax while I find my cell phone and call 911." Rafael can see Alan's face starting to swell.

Question: *What are Rafael's immediate priorities in managing Alan's condition?*

Allergies are a common problem that affect millions of Americans.[1] Acute allergic reactions are a serious manifestation of allergy that can affect many organ systems. The causes of allergies include a variety of environmental stimuli. A person may have an allergic reaction as a result of ingestion, inhalation, cutaneous contact (absorption through the skin), or injection. In addition, the reaction may range from a mild rash to severe shock and even death. Each reaction and the accompanying symptoms vary from individual to individual. However, the body's underlying response to these stimuli is similar in all cases.

■ THE IMMUNE SYSTEM

An **antigen** is any substance that causes the immune system to recognize it as foreign. Antigens induce a state of sensitivity and immune system responsiveness. An **allergen** is any substance that acts as an antigen. When the body senses an allergen/antigen, the immune system is triggered. The **immune system** normally protects the body from foreign invaders, including bacteria and viruses, as well as toxins. Its overreaction to a substance (an allergen) is called a **hypersensitivity,** or allergic, reaction. Almost anything can trigger an allergic reaction.

Common Causes of Allergic Reactions

The most common causes of allergic reactions can be broadly categorized as drugs and biologic agents, insect bites and stings, and foods and food additives. Specific causes are listed in Box 21-1.

Antigens, Antibodies, and the Allergic Reaction

The body's immune system produces **antibodies.** Antibodies detect, locate, and destroy the foreign invader (antigen). This production of antibodies occurs when the body is exposed to an antigen. With exposure, a series of reactions begins that results in the formation of an antibody specific to the particular antigen. The initial exposure of the immune system to the antigen is called *sensitization*. Antibodies are the soldiers that provide protection upon re-exposure to the antigen.

The immune system produces a wide variety of chemical mediators that are responsible for the symptoms a person has during an allergic reaction. These mediators affect local tissues and organs. The most important mediator of allergic reactions is **histamine.** Histamines cause the blood vessels to leak fluid and to dilate, leading to **edema** (swelling). Histamines also cause the smooth muscle of the bronchial tree and gastrointestinal tract to contract, leading to shortness of breath and problems such as nausea, abdominal cramping, vomiting, and diarrhea. In addition, they cause an increase in secretions and tearing and rhinorrhea (runny nose).[2]

Histamine

The membrane of the capillary holds blood within the confines of the blood vessel, just as a garden hose holds water. Histamine causes the small pores of this membrane to open, and fluid leaks out of the capillary into the surrounding tissues. This is similar to a

BOX 21-1

Common Causes of Allergic Reactions

Drugs and Biologic Agents
Antibiotics
Aspirin
Chemotherapeutics/anticancer agents
Insulin
Latex gloves
Local anesthetics
Muscle relaxants
Nonsteroidal antiinflammatory agents (e.g., ibuprofen)
Opiates
Vaccines

Insect Bites and Stings
Bees
Fire ants
Spiders
Wasps, hornets

Foods
Cod, halibut, shellfish
Egg whites
Peanuts, soybeans
Strawberries

Food Additives
Cottonseed oil
Mango
Milk
Sesame and sunflower seeds
Wheat, buckwheat

SPECIAL Considerations

Allergic to nuts and byproducts

You arrive at the scene of a call to find a patient who tells you that he is having an allergic reaction to peanuts. He has just eaten a cookie made with peanut oil. He says that he feels fine but that normally he has a reaction that affects his breathing.

What is a critical action for this patient?

It is critical that the patient's airway be monitored during an allergic reaction. Histamine causes swelling and constriction (narrowing) of the bronchial tree. Edema (swelling) of the mucous membranes causes constriction of the respiratory tract. This can occur at any time during an allergic reaction, or it may not occur at all. It is very important to reassess the airway frequently during an allergic reaction.

---

hole being punctured in the garden hose and water leaking out. This process causes a decrease in the circulating blood volume, which leads to hypotension. The other physiologic effects seen as a result of histamine release include cutaneous (skin) flushing, urticaria (hives), and edema (swelling) of mucous membranes. These symptoms most commonly occur on the skin but also can occur on mucous membranes. Most important, these effects can occur in the mouth and respiratory tract. The soft tissue swelling and bronchial constriction that histamine causes in the respiratory tract is responsible for respiratory distress. This distress can manifest as an increase in the breathing rate, wheezing, cyanosis, or complete respiratory failure.

Signs and Symptoms

Individuals who suffer from an allergic reaction may have symptoms that manifest differently from patient to patient. Some individuals may not even realize they have an allergy. Therefore it is important that EMTs recognize the signs and symptoms of allergic reactions (Box 21-2).

Important Points

Urticaria is a cutaneous manifestation of histamine release in an allergic reaction. Urticaria is associated with red, raised, circular lesions on the skin, known as *hives* (Fig. 21-1). Severe itching generally is associated with the lesions. When swelling occurs in the deeper capillaries and subcutaneous tissue, the condition is called **angioedema** (Fig. 21-2). It may involve the face and mucous membranes of the mouth, which may put these patients at increased risk for rapid deterioration. Angioedema, which often appears similar to an acute allergic reaction, is not a true allergic reaction. It may occur in patients who have been taking certain medications (e.g., lisinopril for high blood pressure) for a long time. The exact reason these patients develop angioedema is not known.

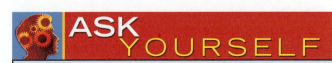

ASK YOURSELF

Think of a friend or family member who is allergic to certain foods, medications, or stings. All of a sudden, something happens; they have difficulty breathing and break out in a rash. Now what?

BOX 21-2

Signs and Symptoms of Allergic Reactions and Anaphylaxis

Upper Airway (Nose and Pharynx)
- Hoarseness
- Stridor
- Laryngeal or epiglottic edema
- Rhinorrhea

Lower Airway (Bronchi and Lungs)
- Bronchospasm
- Increased mucus production
- Accessory muscle use
- Wheezing
- Decreased breath sounds

Cardiovascular System
- Tachycardia
- Hypotension
- Dysrhythmia
- Chest tightness

Gastrointestinal System
- Nausea
- Vomiting
- Abdominal cramps
- Diarrhea

Neurologic System
- Anxiety
- Dizziness
- Syncope
- Weakness
- Headache
- Seizure
- Coma

Cutaneous System
- Angioedema
- Pruritus
- Erythema
- Edema
- Tearing of the eyes

From Sanders MJ: *Mosby's paramedic textbook*, ed 2, St Louis, 2001, Mosby.

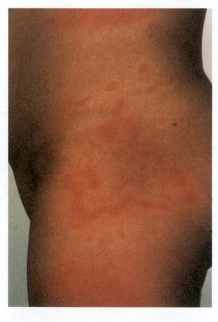

Fig. 21-1　Urticaria caused by an allergic reaction.

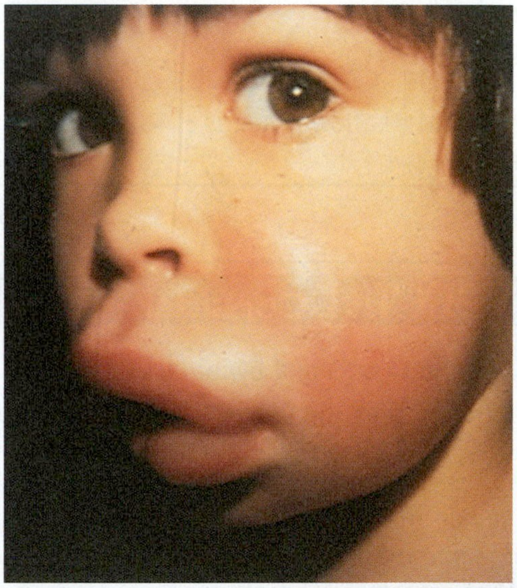

Fig. 21-2　Angioedema caused by an allergic reaction.

Anaphylaxis

Anaphylaxis is the most extreme form of an allergic reaction. It accounts for hundreds of deaths each year and has an overall annual mortality rate of 3%. Therefore rapid recognition and aggressive therapy are essential.[2] Anaphylaxis occurs when the immune system reacts rapidly. A rapid, powerful release of chemical mediators causes this life-threatening response after repeated exposure to an allergen. This reaction can lead to anaphylactic shock, which involves hypoperfusion of critical organ systems.

■ ASSESSMENT

Assessment of the allergic reaction begins with the initial assessment. If the patient is stable, the next step is to obtain the patient history and perform a physical examination. Allergic reactions and anaphylaxis are similar in origin, but differ in terms of the severity. What appears to be an allergic reaction may progress rapidly to anaphylaxis if not treated appropriately. The patient should be assessed for airway, breathing, and circulation abnormalities. As described previously, the findings of the initial assessment may be abnormal because of the immune system response and the release of histamine.

Initial Assessment

An initial assessment should include evaluation of the patient's airway. This, in turn, should include an inspection for edema in the oropharynx and face. Breathing should be evaluated for increased work, distress, or impending failure. Circulation should be evaluated by capillary refill, a pulse check, skin temperature, and skin color. If you note edema in the face or oropharynx, respiratory distress or wheezing, obvious redness or hives on the skin, and alteration in the peripheral pulse, your patient is having a moderate to severe allergic reaction.

History

If the patient's condition is considered stable after the initial assessment, a thorough history should be obtained. This step should not be taken lightly. It is important to get as much history as possible. If the patient cannot provide the history because of respiratory difficulty, family members or bystanders can be asked to provide pertinent information.

The chief complaint should be determined. (The SAMPLE mnemonic [i.e., *s*igns, *a*llergies, *m*edications, *p*ast medical history, *l*ast oral intake, and *e*vents preceding the current incident] can be used for this.) Signs and symptoms can be very helpful. Known allergies and possible exposure to one of these allergens is crucial. Medications also can cause allergic reactions. Some medications, such as epinephrine, can be used to treat allergic reactions. It is important to know whether the patient has been prescribed this medication and whether the person has it with him or her or has used it. These details are important for documentation and treatment. Past medical history is also helpful. The patient should be asked about the last reaction, how it was

---

BOX 21-3
Pertinent History Questions

- What causes the reaction?
- How long have you been experiencing symptoms?
- Are you having trouble breathing?
- Do you feel like your chest is tight?
- Do you feel like your throat is closing off?
- Do you feel like your tongue is swelling?
- What normally happens when you have this reaction?
- Do you carry an epinephrine autoinjector (EpiPen)?

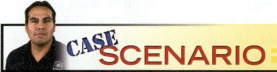

CASE SCENARIO
continued

Rafael helps Alan out of his wet suit. He notices the red rash and welts throughout Alan's upper body. He quickly locates the jellyfish stinger, still stuck in the posterior aspect of Alan's upper thigh. Looking back to Alan's face, Rafael can see that his friend is struggling to breathe. "Alan, do you carry any medication with you?" he asks urgently.

Question: To what medication is Rafael referring? How would this help Alan's condition?

---

treated, and its severity. While this information can provide a guide as to the current allergic reaction, remember that the patient becomes more sensitized with each exposure and the current episode may well be more severe than the prior one. It also is important to get additional medical history, such as illnesses (Box 21-3). Other useful information includes the last meal eaten and events leading up to the onset of the reaction.

Secondary Survey and Physical Examination

The patient's vital signs are critical and should be assessed as soon as possible. If the patient is having trouble communicating, you should search for medical alert tags. Inspect the patient's face for edema, rash, erythema (redness of the skin), tearing, and rhinorrhea. Evaluate the skin for erythema, swelling, and urticaria.[3]) The lungs should be assessed for respiratory rate, work of breathing, retractions, intercostal muscle use, and abnormal respiratory sounds, such as wheezes heard on auscultation. It is important to repeat vital signs frequently, because the initial vital signs may change rapidly as the reaction progresses. NOTE: It is crucial to remember that any allergic reaction, no matter how benign appearing, may progress to hypotension and cardiac arrest.

■ TREATMENT

The initial treatment of any allergic reaction begins with management of the airway. This may include monitoring an open airway or, in an unresponsive patient, placing an airway adjunct. The airway adjunct may be an oral pharyngeal airway or a Combitube, depending on local protocols. The importance of this step cannot be overstated. Airway edema can develop at any time. In unresponsive patients, the tongue may be larger than normal because of edema caused by histamine release. An airway adjunct helps provide the best possible airway in this life-threatening situation.

Oxygen should be administered based on the assessment of the patient. If respiratory and circulatory failure occur secondary to anaphylactic shock, follow the treatment guidelines for shock outlined in Chapter 25. The patient should be given maximum oxygenation with assisted ventilations as necessary. A blanket should be used to cover the patient to protect against heat loss. Elevating the legs of a supine patient improves the circulating blood volume and assists with vital organ perfusion.

In anaphylactic shock, the patient begins to show signs of deterioration. The person may be severely tachycardic and hypotensive and eventually may succumb to complete cardiopulmonary arrest. It is imperative that vital signs be monitored continually for changes. Moreover, the patient must be treated aggressively. Rapid transport for definitive medical care should be arranged.

Pharmacology

In addition to ventilatory support (e.g., metered-dose inhalers), many people with severe allergic reactions carry an autoinjectable syringe filled with epinephrine. **Epinephrine** is a drug that stimulates the body to increase the blood pressure, dilate the airways, and increase cardiac function. Because it has a rapid onset of action, it is the best pharmacologic agent for treating severe allergic reaction and anaphylaxis. Your

---

BOX 21-4
Epinephrine Administration

Indication for use: Severe allergic reaction after exposure to medication, food, insect bite or sting, other allergen
Dosage: *Adult dose:* 0.3 cc 1:1000 (adult EpiPen) intramuscularly
Pediatric dose: 0.15 cc 1:1000 (pediatric EpiPen [EpiPen Jr]) intramuscularly
Contraindications: Patient with prior history of myocardial infarction (heart attack)

Important Points

Like most drugs, the medication used to counter an allergic reaction has two names. Its generic name is *epinephrine*. Its trade name is *Adrenalin*. The **generic name** is the name given to a drug when it is originally manufactured. This name remains the same, regardless of who manufactures the drug. The **trade name,** on the other hand, is assigned by each manufacturer of the drug. Therefore a drug has only one generic name, but it may have many trade names.

SPECIAL Populations
Geriatric Perspectives

Elderly patients who have an anaphylactic reaction often are given the pediatric dose of epinephrine to prevent injury to the cardiovascular system. Be sure to provide medical control with a complete cardiovascular history if you are requesting orders to treat an elderly patient with epinephrine.

---

practice parameters may require you to be knowledgeable about various models of autoinjectable syringes and their use (Box 21-4).

Epinephrine Autoinjectable Syringe
Commercially available autoinjectable syringes often come in both adult and pediatric dosages. These syringes are available by prescription only. As with any other drug, they should be stored out of sunlight and at room temperature. The syringes have an expiration date, which should be checked prior to use. Each syringe has a set of instructions that come with it. It is important to remember that although these devices

SKILL 21-1

◉ *Using the Epinephrine Autoinjector*

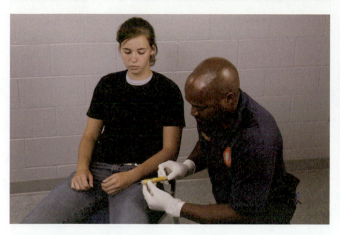

1. Remove the syringe/autoinjector from the package. Check the expiration date.

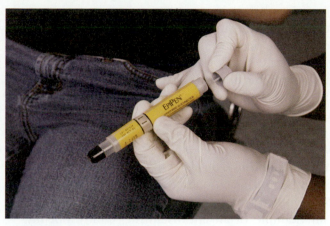

2. Expose the patient's thigh whenever possible and clean it with an alcohol prep, if available. Remove the safety mechanism on the syringe.

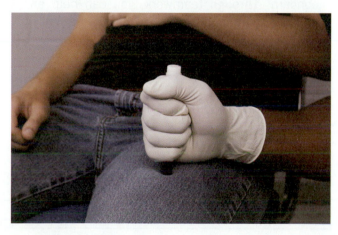

3. Place the syringe with the needle side against the thigh at a 90-degree angle. Activate the syringe, either by depressing a button or through actual skin pressure. The syringe should be kept against the thigh for several seconds to allow complete delivery of the medication. When the injection is finished, remove the syringe and massage the area for a few seconds. Place the used syringe in an appropriately labeled sharps container.

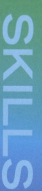

SKILLS

are manufactured with safety in mind, a needle is involved. The risk of puncture and body fluid exposure for the EMT is very real. Therefore personal protective equipment is absolutely necessary.

Intramuscular Injection

The epinephrine in an autoinjectable syringe is meant to be administered as an **intramuscular injection**. The preferred location is the thigh muscle, through bare skin. If administration through bare skin would be difficult or would cause a significant delay, the needle may be inserted through clothing.

Antihistamine

An **antihistamine** is an agent that blocks the action of histamine. Antihistamines are given for allergic reactions. Diphenhydramine (Benadryl is the trade name) is an example of an antihistamine. Oral diphenhydramine is available over the counter and does not require a prescription.

Transport

All patients with an allergic reaction require transport to the closest appropriate emergency department for treatment and continued monitoring. Even if you are permitted to treat the patient with epinephrine and the patient appears to be improving, the patient still requires transport for observation to assure that the patient does not relapse once the epinephrine wears off.

SPECIAL Considerations

Knowing your scope of practice
It is important to check your local protocols and practice parameters for specific guidelines on the use of epinephrine in the form of a prefilled syringe to treat an allergic reaction. Specifications may vary by location or by medical control authority.

SPECIAL Considerations

Be familiar
Several manufacturers make prefilled epinephrine syringes. These syringes do not all work in a similar manner. Make sure you read the instructions carefully when using these devices.

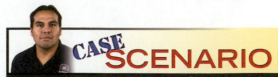

CASE SCENARIO
conclusion

The beach rescue unit comes rolling up the beach and stops a few feet from the scene. Rafael rechecks Alan's pulse. It's still high, about 130 beats per minute. Alan's respiratory rate is 26, and he seems able to take deeper breaths. Rafael identifies himself as an off-duty EMT-firefighter. He reports his findings to the medic and stays to help the team further stabilize Alan's condition. ◼

TEAMWORK

As an EMT, you may be asked to assist another EMT or other licensed health care provider. It is important to remember that safety is the primary concern. Through teamwork, you can help ensure the safety of all providers and the patient in the following ways:
- Assist with monitoring the patient's airway and vital signs. This is a critical step in caring for a patient with an allergic reaction.
- Assist with reading and relaying instructions for the autoinjectable syringe. This may be very helpful, particularly if the provider administering the injection is not familiar with the prescribed syringe's features.
- Keep the scene safe by properly disposing of all sharps in their appropriately marked containers.

Reference

1. WebMD Health: Allergies health center. Available at: http://my.webmd.com/medical_information/condition_centers/allergies/default.htm. Accessed October 10, 2004.
2. Sanders MJ: *Mosby's paramedic textbook*, ed 2, St Louis, 2001, Mosby.
3. Fitzpatrick RB, Johnson RA, Wolff K et al: *Color atlas and synopsis of clinical dermatology: common and serious diseases*, New York, 2001, McGraw-Hill.

Resource

Young SH, Dobozsin BS, Miner M: *Allergies: the complete guide to diagnosis, treatment, and daily management*, 1999, Plume.

NUTS AND BOLTS

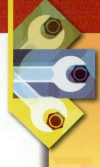

Critical Points

As an EMT, you will see a range of allergic reactions in a variety of patients. Many reactions are not life-threatening. However, it is critical that EMTs be able to differentiate between minor and more severe reactions. The importance of being able to manage an airway, use a prefilled medication syringe, and treat for shock cannot be overemphasized.

Learning Checklist

❏ An allergic reaction (hypersensitivity reaction) is the body's response to an allergen (antigen).
❏ The allergic reaction may range from a mild rash to severe shock and even death.
❏ An antigen is a foreign substance that causes the immune system to react.
❏ Common causes of allergic reactions include drugs, insect bites and stings, and food additives.
❏ The body's immune system produces antibodies in response to the foreign antigen.
❏ Histamine is released during an allergic reaction and causes vascular permeability.
❏ Histamine is responsible for urticaria and angioedema.
❏ Signs and symptoms of allergic reaction involve the airway (upper and lower), and cardiovascular, gastrointestinal, and neurologic systems.
❏ Anaphylaxis is the most extreme form of an allergic reaction.
❏ Anaphylaxis occurs when the immune system responds rapidly to the antigen. This response can result in hypoperfusion and shock.
❏ Treatment begins with the assessment of the patient and the primary survey.
❏ The assessment should focus on the airway, because edema can cause the tongue and mucous membranes to swell.
❏ A thorough history should be obtained if the patient is stable.
❏ A secondary survey should include an investigation for any type of urticaria, rash, or sting mark.

❏ Treatment should include airway assessment and breathing.
❏ If the patient appears to be deteriorating the treatment for shock should be initiated.
❏ Use of an epinephrine autoinjector should be considered for severe allergic reactions and anaphylaxis.
❏ The patient should be reassessed frequently after treatment because the person may improve and then deteriorate again.

Key Terms

Allergen An antigenic substance.
Anaphylaxis A severe, life-threatening hypersensitivity reaction to a previously encountered antigen that results in vasodilation and subsequent hypotension.
Angioedema Localized, edematous reaction of the deep dermis or submucosal tissues.
Antibodies Proteins that react with antigens.
Antigen Any substance that induces a state of hypersensitivity when it comes into contact with appropriate cells.
Antihistamine Drugs that block the action of histamine, thus preventing or alleviating the major symptoms of an allergic response.
Edema An abnormal accumulation of fluid in tissues; swelling.
Epinephrine A catecholamine hormone secreted by the adrenal medulla. It is also a neurotransmitter. *Epinephrine* is also the generic name of a synthetic pharmacologic agent used to treat severe allergic reactions. This agent counteracts the actions that cause respiratory distress and hypoperfusion.
Generic name The name assigned to a drug during development of the pharmacologic agent.
Histamine A chemical released by the immune system during an allergic reaction that causes many of the signs and symptoms of the reaction.
Hypersensitivity An inappropriate immune response to a generally harmless antigen.
Immune system The system responsible for protecting the body from disease.
Intramuscular injection An injection of medication or toxin that enters the muscle.

419

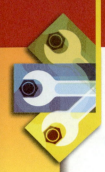

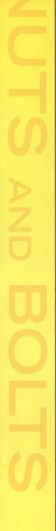

Trade name The name given to a drug by the manufacturer.

Urticaria Red, raised, circular lesions on the skin; also called *hives*.

National Standard Curriculum Objectives

Cognitive Objectives

After completing this lesson, the EMT student will be able to do the following:

- Recognize the patient having an allergic reaction.
- Describe the emergency medical care of a patient having an allergic reaction.
- Explain the relationship between a patient with an allergic reaction and airway management.

- Describe the mechanisms of allergic response and the implications for airway management.
- State the generic and trade names, medication forms, dose, administration, action, and contraindications for the epinephrine autoinjector.
- Evaluate the need for medical direction in the emergency medical care of a patient having an allergic reaction.
- Differentiate between the general category of patients having an allergic reaction and the specific subcategory of patients having an allergic reaction who require immediate medical care, including immediate use of an epinephrine autoinjector.

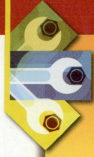

Affective Objective

After completing this lesson, the EMT student will be able to do the following:

- Explain the rationale for administering epinephrine using an autoinjector.

Psychomotor Objectives

After completing this lesson, the EMT student will be able to do the following:

- Demonstrate the emergency medical care of a patient having an allergic reaction.

- Demonstrate the use of an epinephrine autoinjector.
- Demonstrate the assessment and documentation of the patient's response to an epinephrine injection.
- Demonstrate proper disposal of equipment.
- Demonstrate the completion of a prehospital care report for patients with allergic emergencies.

CHAPTER OUTLINE

OUTLINE

LESSON GOAL

GOAL

This chapter provides the emergency medical technician (EMT) with some fundamental information on poisonings. Although EMTs may have to deal with a vast array of poisons in their work, an understanding of the commonly encountered clinical effects enables them to care for most poisoning patients successfully. ■

Poisoning and Overdose

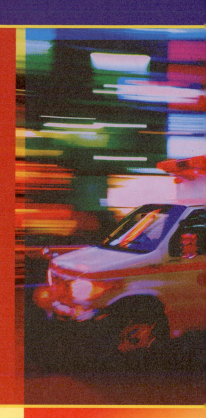

CHAPTER OBJECTIVES

After completing this chapter, the EMT student will be able to do the following:

1 Describe the effects of several common poisonings.

2 Recognize several clinical effects caused by poisonings.

3 Give the steps in the emergency care of a patient who may have overdosed.

4 Give the steps in the emergency care of a patient with suspected poisoning.

5 Describe a situation in which a patient suffering from poisoning or overdose requires airway management.

6 State the generic and trade names, indications, contraindications, forms, dosages, administration, actions, side effects, and reassessment strategies for activated charcoal.

7 Identify the need to seek medical direction in caring for the overdose patient.

8 Explain when and why the EMT might administer activated charcoal.

9 Explain the importance of contacting medical control early in the course of patient management.

10 Demonstrate the emergency medical care of a suspected overdose patient.

11 Demonstrate the emergency medical care of a suspected poisoning patient.

12 Demonstrate the proper administration of activated charcoal.

13 Demonstrate the proper disposal of equipment used to administer activated charcoal.

14 Demonstrate the assessment and documentation of a patient's response to treatment.

15 Demonstrate the proper way to give a report on a patient suffering from poisoning or overdose.

OBJECTIVES

CASE SCENARIO

Ray can see the lights of the patrol car parked near the gate to the high school football stadium. Beyond the gate he sees a police officer waving at him with her flashlight, signaling her location. Ray and his partner walk up to the scene, the gurney and medical bags in tow.

"What's happening, Gloria?" Ray asks.

The officer points at a young man sitting slumped over on one of the benches.

"This is John Wall. Seventeen years old," she says. "He was passed out when I came out here. I was able to wake him, but he's confused and slurring his speech, so I wanted him checked out for any medical problems."

Ray looks around. "How did you know he was out here?" he asks.

"Someone called it in," the officer replies.

"Guess they left before I got here. Not unusual."

Ray turns to the patient. "John? Hey buddy, wake up," he says.

John does not respond. Ray applies a trapezius pinch to John's left shoulder, and the young man groans lightly and tries to turn away from Ray. Ray can smell beer on John's breath. Feeling for the radial wrist, Ray determines that John's pulse rate is fast, about 110 beats per minute.

Ray pulls his penlight out of his shirt pocket. Flashing the light into John's eyes, Ray notices that the pupils are constricted and slow to react.

Questions: *Is this pupil reaction a normal, expected reaction? What other observations should Ray make?*

Poisonings and overdoses are relatively common problems for emergency medical services (EMS) providers. The incidents range from minor exposures that produce no symptoms to major exposures that can kill patients and also put providers at risk. The ultimate outcome of an exposure is determined by three main factors: (1) the poison, (2) the patient, and (3) the treatment. Each of these factors has a particular effect on the prehospital management of poisoning patients.

■ ROUTES OF EXPOSURE

The four main pathways by which poisoning occurs are ingestion, inhalation, absorption, and injection. Some toxins can enter the body by more than one route. The patient should always be asked specifically for the route of poisoning.

Ingestion occurs when a poison is swallowed and enters the gastrointestinal (GI) tract. Many toxins can enter the body by this route. They include medications, plants, household products, and illicit drugs. After ingestion, the poison is absorbed through the lining of the GI tract and brought into the bloodstream. Once in the bloodstream, the poison exerts

its toxic (poisonous) effects. Often, depending on the time of ingestion, the patient may be asymptomatic when EMTs arrive. The only evidence of poisoning may be the history or residual items found at the scene (e.g., pill bottles, empty household containers, plant residue). Ingestion of poisons may also cause burns around or in the mouth or in the esophagus, as well as nausea, vomiting, diarrhea, or abdominal pain. Children 1 to 3 years of age account for 80% of all accidental ingestions.[1] Children in this age group are inquisitive and often put things in their mouth as a means of investigation.

Poisons also can enter the body through **inhalation**. This occurs when a person is in an environment in which a poisonous gas or vapor can be inhaled.

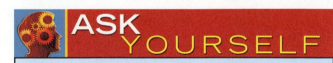

ASK YOURSELF

You and your partner are dispatched to a reported overdose. What can you do to prepare yourself for this call? Was it intentional or accidental? Where do you begin? What questions will you ask the patient or bystanders?

These patients generally have some symptoms of pulmonary toxicity, because many of the inhaled toxins are irritating to the respiratory tract. This class of poisons can include ammonia, chlorine, smoke from a fire, or carbon monoxide. Carbon monoxide is odorless and tasteless. In fact, people often are not aware that they are being poisoned. Some inhalation poisons can have a delayed onset. This is important to consider if your patient has pulmonary complaints and a history that may be consistent with a toxicologic cause. Because some of the pulmonary toxins are odorless and tasteless, make sure the scene has been evaluated for safety before you enter.

Inhaled toxins cause symptoms through several mechanisms of toxicity. Some inhaled toxins displace oxygen. This prevents the transfer and delivery of oxygenated blood. Symptoms in such cases include shortness of breath, chest pain, dizziness, altered mental status, or any manifestation of hypoxia. Inhaled toxins also can cause a systemic response. For example, hydrogen sulfide, a gas commonly found in sewers, smells of rotten eggs. It is a particularly toxic gas that can cause respiratory and central nervous system (CNS) depression, leading to rapid death. After the scene has been deemed safe, always remove a patient to fresh air as quickly as possible. Some toxins irritate the respiratory tract. These cause coughing, sputum production, shortness of breath, or even burns.

Dermal (skin) absorption is very common, especially with occupational exposures. The skin, which is the largest organ system, is a very effective barrier in most cases. It stops many toxins from entering the body. However, some poisons can be absorbed through the skin. These poisons can cause both direct skin injury and systemic toxicity. Chemicals that are absorbed through the skin include aniline, hydrogen cyanide, organic mercury, nitrobenzene, organophosphate insecticides, and phenol. Dermal toxins can cause a local reaction, such as a rash or burn, and systemic reactions. Hydrogen fluoride is a weak acid that dissociates after absorption through the skin. Small exposures cause pain in the affected area. Large surface area exposures can cause hypocalcemia, possibly resulting in cardiac dysrhythmias. It is important to irrigate the affected area to try to stop the exposure. In most cases a generous amount of water is adequate. However, some compounds can cause an exothermic (heat-creating) reaction (e.g., dry lime), and these require large amounts of water for irrigation. Therefore it is best to call your local poison control center or some other resource if you are unsure of a potential reaction.

> ## SPECIAL Considerations
>
> ### Multiple Medications
> Accidental overdose can affect anyone who takes more than one medication. However, it is much more common in the elderly. Elderly people often see several doctors for overlapping complaints that require *polypharmacy* (taking multiple medications for different conditions). Often they fail to keep all their doctors informed about medications prescribed by other doctors. Accidental overdose becomes an even greater risk for patients with confusion or short-term memory loss. These individuals often don't remember taking their medication and may repeat a dose without realizing it. Differentiating accidental overdose from other possible causes of a patient's condition may be difficult, but the EMT should be thorough in checking patients' medications.

Injection is the least common form of toxic exposure. It occurs with a needle stick or skin puncture, which allows a toxic substance to enter the body. This route is less clinically relevant. It generally is seen in either health care workers or intravenous (IV) drug users. Injected poisons have the most rapid absorption, because the drug goes directly into the bloodstream. Decontamination with charcoal is ineffective, because the toxin bypasses the GI tract altogether.

Poisonings by injection can also occur from the bites of arthropods, reptiles, and hazardous marine life. These injections may produce a wide variety of physiologic reactions. Venom is the toxic substance that many animals inject for protection. *Envenomation* is a common term that means to be injected with venom.

EMS calls regarding poisoning patients usually take one of two forms: poisoning with a known history of exposure or ingestion or suspected poisoning with no history of exposure or ingestion (discussed later in the chapter). The obvious cases involve a history of exposure or ingestion. In these cases, knowledge of the poison allows you to provide appropriate care and anticipate possible effects. The following sections cover commonly encountered poisons and their clinical effects. It is important to remember that even patients with clinically insignificant ingestions should be transported if you suspect the person intended to harm himself or herself.

■ COMMON POISONINGS

Ethanol (drinking alcohol) is the most commonly abused drug. It is easily available, socially acceptable, and often taken in overdose for fun. It is a direct CNS depressant and a respiratory depressant. As people chronically drink more, they develop a tolerance and can function, although often impaired, at very high alcohol levels. In contrast, some patients, particularly young adults who do not drink regularly, are at risk for alcohol toxicity when they binge drink. Patients can show a wide range of clinical effects. These range from euphoria, slurred speech, difficulty with coordination, impaired judgment, and decreased reaction time with mild intoxication to altered mental status, coma, respiratory depression, and death with major toxicity. Intoxicated patients are at risk for vomiting, aspiration of stomach contents into the lungs, and airway compromise. They also are at risk for falls and other trauma. Often the effects of the alcohol may mask significant injuries. If you suspect that your patient is intoxicated, transport the person to a medical facility for evaluation to rule out any concurrent injury or illness. It is important to remember that these patients can have traumatic injuries. Therefore a low threshold for instituting spinal immobilization is warranted.

Acetaminophen (Tylenol) is a commonly available, over-the-counter **analgesic** and **antipyretic** (fever-reducing medication). It often comes in combination with other drugs, such as multisystem cold and allergy medications. It is very safe in recommended doses. However, it can cause fatal liver damage in overdose. Patients who have ingested large amounts of acetaminophen often are asymptomatic for the first 24 to 36 hours. They then may develop nausea, vomiting, abdominal pain, and jaundice. In the hospital, these patients are given a specific antidote to acetaminophen. However, the effectiveness of the antidote decreases over time. Therefore patients should be treated as soon as possible. Evaluation in a health care facility is important for all patients who may have overdosed on acetaminophen, either to harm themselves or because of therapeutic error.

Carbon monoxide poisoning is one of the most common causes of unintentional poisoning and death. The gas is odorless, colorless, and tasteless. It is a byproduct of the combustion of fossil fuels. Carbon monoxide (CO) often is released by faulty equipment or fires. Only a few minutes of exposure to high levels of the gas can cause significant toxicity or death. Carbon monoxide prevents the blood from delivering

oxygen to the cells. This may result in symptoms such as headache, irritability, confusion, cardiac disturbances, difficulty with coordination and, eventually, seizures, coma, and death. CO detectors are becoming increasingly common in homes. These devices probably prevent many accidental exposures.

People also may use carbon monoxide in attempts to harm themselves (e.g., running a car engine in a closed garage to commit suicide).

The initial treatment for CO toxicity is to remove the person from the contaminated environment and administer high-flow oxygen. This enhances elimination of the CO. Depending on the patient's clinical presentation and status and on determination of the person's carboxyhemoglobin level in the hospital, the patient may be treated with hyperbaric oxygen. This further increases the elimination of CO. Hyperbaric oxygen is provided in a special chamber that increases the atmospheric pressure, thus providing much higher concentrations of oxygen to the patient.

It is important to consider CO toxicity as a possibility if your patient has an altered mental status or nonspecific symptoms, such as a headache. This is particularly important in the autumn and early winter, when many people first turn on their furnaces and heating systems, which may prove to be faulty and leak CO into the home.

Acetylsalicylic acid (aspirin) is another commonly used over-the-counter medication. It is used as an antipyretic and analgesic and for cardiac and neurologic disease prevention. Many people are on a regimen of an aspirin a day. However, patients often forget to list aspirin as one of the medications they are taking. Aspirin is very safe in appropriate doses. However, people often overdose on aspirin by mistake because they consider it so safe. Aspirin also is commonly used in suicidal gestures because it is easy to get. People who overdose on aspirin may be asymptomatic or may have abdominal pain, nausea, tinnitus (ringing in the ears), hyperventilation, or hyperpnea (rapid breathing). In severe or delayed presentations, the patient may have an altered mental status or pulmonary edema. Patients hyperventilate because the aspirin directly affects the respiratory center in the CNS, causing them to breathe quickly. Over time, the patient may develop a metabolic acidosis. This further increases the respiratory rate. EMTs must be very careful not to assume that this hyperventilation is caused by anxiety. In fact, having the patient slow the respirations or breathe into a paper bag may make the condition worse. The body is using the rapid breathing as a defense mechanism. Aspirin-toxic patients should have airway support and should be transported to the hospital for evaluation and further treatment. It is important to bring in the bottles from which these patients took the medications, because aspirin often is mistaken for acetaminophen or ibuprofen, and the treatment is vastly different for those drugs.

Household Products

Common household products frequently are the focus of a poisoning call. Children often find these products and ingest them in varying amounts. Literally hundreds of products found around the home may be ingested, but most are not toxic with small exposures.

Laundry Bleaches

Household bleach products generally are a 5% sodium hypochlorite solution. Most accidental ingestions of household bleach cause no symptoms. However, ingestion of a large amount can cause corrosive injury of the GI tract. In the past it was recommended that a patient be made to vomit to help remove the toxic bleach. However, having the patient vomit is no longer advised for ingestion of these products, because that can worsen injury of the gastric system. The absence of burns around the mouth does not exclude a more significant injury. Therefore all patients suspected of a sizable ingestion should be brought to the hospital for evaluation. If hypochlorite is mixed with ammonia, chloramine or chlorine gas can form, which can be very irritating to the respiratory tract and mucous membranes. In general, patients improve when they are removed from the source of the exposure and placed in fresh air. With extended exposure, the patient may require evaluation and treatment for chemical injury of the lungs.

Dish and Laundry Detergents

Dish and laundry washing products generally are a combination of a cationic **detergent** and an anionic detergent. They can cause nausea, vomiting, diarrhea, and irritation of the mucous membranes. GI burns and corrosive injury may occur with significant ingestion or if the product is very alkaline. Electronic dishwasher detergent is considerably more alkaline than other detergents and can cause significant injury. Patients who have ingested these products should be evaluated in a health care facility.

Mothballs

Mothballs can be made of either naphthalene or paradichlorobenzene. Naphthalene is an older product and can cause significant toxicity if eaten. Children often think mothballs look like candy and eat them. Naphthalene toxicity manifests as agitation, lethargy, seizures, and coma. These patients need support for the airway, breathing, and circulation (ABCs) and transport to the hospital. Ingestion of paradichlorobenzene mothballs is rarely a problem. However, it may cause nausea and vomiting. It is almost impossible to distinguish between naphthalene and paradichlorobenzene by looking at the mothballs. Therefore any patient who may have mothball toxicity should be transported to the hospital for further evaluation and treatment.

Chemicals

Many substances at work sites and in the home can cause chemical burns. The two most common classifications are **acid** and **alkali.** Acids have a low pH and alkalis have a high pH. Common acids include automotive tire or metal cleaners and rust removers or cleaning solvents, such as muriatic acid or hydrochloric acid. Alkalis generally include products such as drain cleaners and some electric dishwashing detergents. Acids cause damage by breaking down proteins on contact. A *coagulum* (a clot or lump of material in the middle of liquid) forms, and the damage stops at that point. Alkali burns are marked by liquefaction necrosis. This means that the alkaline agent "melts" the tissue, causing injury. There is nothing to stop the damage, which progresses into deeper and deeper tissues, even after the substance appears to be gone. This is why alkali burns generally are worse than acid burns.

Both of these types of exposure can cause obvious burns; however, the lack of visible burns does not rule out a significant injury. Some acids (e.g., hydrofluoric acid) can cause significant effects without outward signs of injury. Patients should be aggressively decontaminated. However, maintaining the safety of the responding EMS providers is also important. Decontamination often is done at the scene to prevent contamination of personnel and equipment en route and at the health care facility. If the eyes are the area of exposure, you should irrigate them with water for at least 20 minutes and possibly longer, depending on the agent (check with medical control or the poison center). This can be done en route and continued upon arrival at the emergency department (ED). Cover obvious burns on the body with a sterile, dry dressing. For burns of the airway or face, institute oxygen or other airway interventions as needed.

Antifreeze and Radiator Fluid

Antifreeze and radiator fluid often are found not only in bottles, but also in a puddle in the driveway or on the garage floor. This makes it easy for a small child to ingest the product or to be exposed to it while playing. It is important to bring the product to the hospital or to record the ingredients. The main ingredient often is ethylene glycol or methanol. In children, these alcohols are extremely toxic in small amounts. Children may appear asymptomatic for many hours after ingestion. However, these products cause a profound metabolic acidosis, as well as renal failure that may require dialysis. Patients can have abdominal pain, nausea, vomiting, or altered mental status. Patients who seek treatment late may have a worse clinical course than those treated early. These patients are treated with either ethanol or fomepizole, which prevent the toxins from being broken down into their toxic metabolites.

Drug Abuse

Drugs of abuse are an increasing problem in many communities. *Substance abuse* is the use of any substance or substances to induce an altered mental state or feeling of euphoria. The substance is not used for its intended purpose. The means of substance abuse include prescription medications, illegal drugs, cigarettes, alcohol, and naturally occurring herbs and plants. Substance abuse can start out as a recreational activity, such as drinking an alcoholic beverage at a restaurant. It can escalate into *psychologic dependence*, a condition in which the person relies on the substance for its pleasurable effects, and (or) *physical dependence*, a physiologic state in which the body becomes so used to the substance that its absence results in withdrawal symptoms. The patient may experience seizures, hallucinations, changes in mental status, and malnutrition.

EMS providers are often called to transport patients suspected of some type of illicit ingestion. Some drugs of abuse can cause patients to become violent and difficult to restrain. Therefore it is imperative that responding providers have adequate backup, including police officers, as necessary to secure the scene and the patient.

Many signs and symptoms of abuse are specific to the particular substance ingested (discussed later in the chapter). However, certain signs and symptoms should raise suspicion of substance abuse. Patients

who are intoxicated often lose control of their coordination. The patient may have an unsteady gait and may be unable to follow commands. Some substances affect vital signs and may alter the respiratory rate, pulse, or blood pressure. Patients may experience hallucinations or, as mentioned earlier, may become combative or unresponsive or develop seizures.

Marijuana is the most commonly encountered illegal drug of abuse. These patients usually are sleepy and have mild tachycardia and red eyes. Marijuana intoxication generally is not dangerous. However, patients have slow reaction times and impaired judgment. Consequently, accidents and injuries are common.

Cocaine, amphetamine, and **methamphetamine** are the most common **stimulant** drugs of abuse. Patients may snort, smoke, or inject these drugs. Patients may also ingest methamphetamine or amphetamine. The symptoms of stimulant intoxication include euphoria, anxiety, paranoia, agitation, and delirium. Physical findings include tachycardia, hypertension, dilated pupils, diaphoresis, and restlessness. Because most patients take these drugs only to get high, more serious effects are uncommon. However, overdose of these medications may produce life-threatening effects, such as seizures, cardiac dysrhythmias, and severe hyperthermia. The initial treatment is to prevent these patients from injuring themselves or health care providers. When the patient is safely controlled, high-dose **benzodiazepines** (administered by advanced life support [ALS] providers or in the hospital) are used to control agitation and seizures. Cocaine intoxication usually resolves over 2 to 3 hours. Symptoms of methamphetamine or amphetamine intoxication, however, may last for many hours. Methylenedioxymethamphetamine (MDMA), which has the street name **Ecstasy,** is an amphetamine derivative. It produces mild stimulant effects and hallucinations at "recreational" doses. Overdose of MDMA appears similar to amphetamine intoxication. **Phencyclidine (PCP)** is another drug that can have stimulant effects. However, PCP also causes a *dissociative state*. In such a state the patient has decreased pain sensation and awareness. These patients classically are extremely agitated. They often are very difficult to restrain. In fact, some patients on PCP have been able to fight despite extremity fractures. Other clinical findings of PCP intoxication may include roving eye movements, small pupils, and increased salivation. Treatment is similar to that for other stimulant drugs, but very high doses of benzodiazepines may be required.

Opiates are another group of drugs that patients commonly abuse. The most frequently encountered drug in this group is heroin. Heroin usually is injected, but it also may be snorted or smoked. Many of the other drugs of abuse in this group are prescription painkillers. Commonly encountered medications include morphine, codeine, hydrocodone, oxycodone (OxyContin), hydromorphone (Dilaudid), fentanyl, meperidine (Demerol), and many others. Opiates are combined with acetaminophen or aspirin in products such as Tylenol 3, Vicodin, Percocet, and Tylox. The symptoms of opiate intoxication include somnolence (sleepiness), respiratory depression, small pupils, and vomiting. Severe intoxication may result in coma and respiratory arrest. The initial treatment involves managing the airway, administering oxygen, and assisting ventilation. The effects of opiates can be rapidly reversed with administration of naloxone (Narcan) by ALS providers or in the hospital. In fact, administration of naloxone to opiate-dependent patients may put them into opiate withdrawal. Opiate withdrawal causes body aches, diarrhea, and muscle cramps. Opiate withdrawal is not life-threatening, but patients are often miserable for several days.

Other drugs of abuse are less common. **Hallucinogens** include lysergic acid **(LSD)** and **psilocybin** mushrooms. MDMA (and similar amphetamine derivatives) also has some hallucinogenic properties. These drugs alter sensory input and produce visual hallucinations, such as increased color intensity, color changes, or halos around lights. A sensation of depersonalization may occur, in which the patient feels separate from his or her environment or body. The patient usually is aware that the effects are caused by the drug, and the person generally responds appropriately to questions. Occasionally patients may have a "bad trip" and become frightened. This is best treated by providing reassurance and removing the patient from excess stimulation.

Huffing (glue sniffing) results in hydrocarbon intoxication. In the brain hydrocarbons act in a way similar to inhaled anesthetic medications. They produce somnolence, dizziness, and euphoria. The effects usually are short-lived (often resolving by the time the patient reaches a hospital). The main danger is that these patients will asphyxiate themselves while trying to get high. In many cases, the abuser puts the hydrocarbon into a plastic bag which they place over their nose and mouth in order to inhale the fumes. Unfortunately, they also rapidly deplete the available oxygen at the same time. These drugs also can cause arrhythmias by making the heart more sensitive to adrenalin. The term *sudden sniffing death* has been used to describe arrhythmias that occur when a hydrocarbon abuser is startled and the

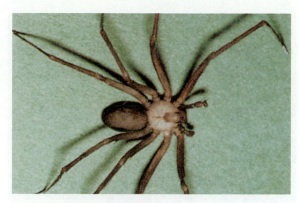

Fig. 22-1 Brown recluse spider.

sudden adrenalin surge causes ventricular tachycardia or fibrillation.

Common Bites and Stings

Brown Recluse Spider

The brown recluse is known for the fiddle on its back (Fig. 22-1). It is most often found in the Mississippi/Ohio/Missouri river basin in hot, dry, abandoned areas, including closets. The brown recluse is beige to dark brown and approximately $1/2$ to 1 inch long. These spiders are most active from April to October. They generally attack only if threatened.

Signs and Symptoms

The initial injection by the spider often is painless and may be minor. However, the venom can cause localized inflammation, edema, and erythema in 1 to 2 hours (Fig. 22-2). After 1 to 2 days, a blister may form. This blister may be surrounded by an area of necrosis or erythema, giving it a bull's-eye appearance. Over the next 1 to 3 days, the area of necrosis may expand and the center may become sunken and black. This bite can result in serious systemic infections, including muscle involvement. It is slow to heal and should be managed medically by a physician. Some bites take months to heal, and some even require skin grafting. If the venom becomes systemic, the patient has nausea, vomiting, chills, fever, generalized rash, and hypotension. Brown recluse bites occasionally are fatal.

Treatment

Treatment generally is supportive. The wound may be cleaned with soap and water, and cold compresses may be applied for pain relief. The patient should be transported. If the patient is evaluated days after the bite and has systemic complications, oxygen should be administered and the patient transported immediately.

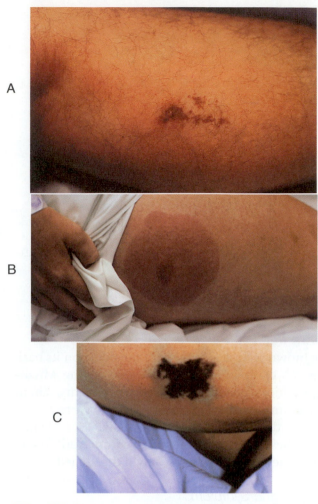

Fig. 22-2 Brown recluse spider bite. **A,** Brown recluse spider bite after 6 hours, showing hemorrhagic vesicle and gravitational spread of venom. **B,** Bite after 24 hours, showing central ischemia and rapidly advancing cellulitis. **C,** Bite after 48 hours, showing incipient central necrosis.

Black Widow Spider

The typical adult female black widow spider is black and has a red hourglass on the underside of the abdomen. These spiders usually are about 1 inch long (Fig. 22-3). Interestingly, the male is brown and is not venomous to human beings. The black widow usually is found under stones or logs and only rarely in dwellings. The initial bite has been described as resembling a pinch or a pin prick. Two small fang marks about 1 mm apart may be seen. The presence of multiple bites helps rule out spiders as the source. Spiders generally bite only once.

Signs and Symptoms

Within 1 hour after the patient is bitten, the neurotoxin in the venom causes muscle spasms and

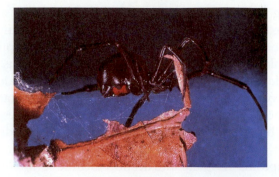

Fig. 22-3 Black widow spider.

cramps. This can progress to muscle rigidity and intense pain, particularly in the abdomen. A burning sensation may develop in the feet, the hands, or the entire body. The patient may have dizziness, nausea, vomiting, swelling and, in severe cases, respiratory depression.

Treatment

Treatment generally is supportive. The initial assessment is critical. Make sure the airway is patent and the patient is breathing adequately. If the primary survey reveals any abnormalities, breathing and circulation should be assisted per protocol. The affected area should be cleaned with soap and water. Antivenin is available but should be administered only in a hospital ED. Antivenin is a substance that either slows or stops the action of the venom (Box 22-1). Most patients recover completely in 36 to 72 hours. It is important to know that severe toxicity can cause vomiting, hypertension, and severe headache. The EMT should be aware of the symptoms and prepared to treat them.

Scorpions

The bark scorpion, also called the sculptured scorpion, is the only species of scorpion dangerous to human beings that is found in the United States and Mexico (Fig. 22-4). It favors wooded areas along the edges of the desert. This scorpion has

---

BOX 22-1

Antivenin and Antidote

Antivenin is a product that neutralizes or lessens the effect of an injected toxic venom. It is often made from horse serum. **Antidotes** are drugs or other substances that oppose the action of another drug or toxin.

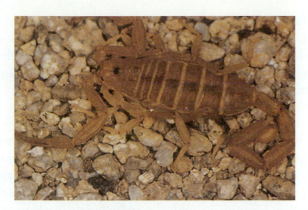

Fig. 22-4 Bark scorpion.

been known to invade homes. It is about 1 to 1½ inches long. It is yellow to brown and may have stripes near the tail. Bark scorpions are most active from April to August.

Signs and Symptoms

The scorpion's venom is released from a stinger. It affects the nervous system, causing hyperactivity. Other signs and symptoms may include local swelling, ecchymosis (bruising), and erythema (redness). Pain, tingling, and burning are common at the site. The patient may have muscle twitching, which can progress to convulsions. Signs and symptoms indicating stimulation of the parasympathetic nervous system also may occur (Box 22-2). Most of the toxic effects manifest within 5 hours.

Treatment

Patients should be transported for evaluation by the ED staff. The most important complication is interference with the airway and breathing. The toxin in scorpion venom can cause significant mucus and saliva production in the mouth. Bronchospasm also may occur, and the patient's breathing may be rapid. Continuous monitoring is vital, and each of the ABCs should be addressed and treated. Application of cool compresses to the site of the envenomation may provide some comfort.

BOX 22-2

Symptoms Caused by Stimulation of the Parasympathetic Nervous System

Stimulation of the parasympathetic nervous system produces *s*alivation, *l*acrimation, *u*rination, *d*efecation, *g*astrointestinal distress, and *e*mesis (vomiting). These symptoms can be remembered by the mnemonic SLUDGE.

Pit Vipers

The pit viper family includes rattlesnakes, cottonmouths, water moccasins, and copperheads (Fig. 22-5). This family received its name because these snakes have a heat-sensing pit near the eye. The fangs of these snakes are long and hollow. Venom is delivered through a canal in each fang. The purpose of the venom is to immobilize and kill prey.

Signs and Symptoms

Localized effects may be seen at the site of the bite, including edema and erythema. Milder effects include ecchymosis, diaphoresis, nausea, and vomiting. Severe systemic effects include alterations in blood coagulation, acute renal failure, convulsions, and hypotension accompanied by shock.

Treatment

Scene safety is critical, and this includes making sure the snake is no longer present. The primary survey is crucial and should be performed immediately. The ABCs should be monitored closely. The bitten extremity should be immobilized in a manner similar to that for a fracture. This may delay systemic absorption of the toxin in the venom. Also, movement of the patient should be minimized, and approved patient handling methods should be used to transfer the person. Keeping the patient calm may help reduce systemic spread of the toxin. According to current guidelines, incision of the bite wound should not be performed. There is conflicting evidence regarding use of the Sawyer extraction device at the wound site. EMTs should review their local protocols and contact medical control. Antivenin may be administered in the hospital.

Coral Snakes

The coral snake has a distinctive appearance. It has round eyes and multiple bands of color (Fig. 22-6). The coral snake, which is poisonous, can be identi-

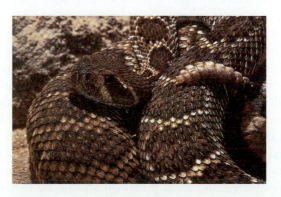

Fig. 22-5 Pit viper.

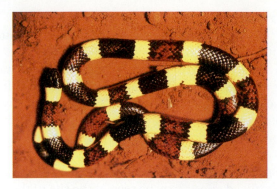

Fig. 22-6 Coral snake.

fied by red and yellow stripes that border one another. If a black stripe separates the red and yellow stripes, the snake is not a coral snake and usually is not poisonous. A common saying can help you remember this difference: "Red on yellow, kill a fellow; red on black, venom lack."[2]

Signs and Symptoms

Unlike the pit viper, which strikes and releases, the coral snake tends to hang on when it bites. Coral snake venom is primarily neurotoxic. The bite itself may cause little or no pain and minimal edema. Signs and symptoms of a bite include slurred speech and dilated pupils. If the venom spreads systemically, the patient's condition may progress to flaccid paralysis and death. Death usually is caused by respiratory failure that occurs secondary to muscle paralysis.

Treatment

It is imperative to continuously monitor for signs and symptoms of impending respiratory failure. You should conduct a primary survey and continuously monitor vital signs. Immobilize the extremity. Also, try to keep the patient calm and still. This can prevent further spread of the venom. Some evidence suggests that for bites from this family of snakes (Elapidae), the extremity should be immobilized with an elastic bandage or air splint. This immobilization and compression method, also known as the Commonwealth Serum Laboratory technique, slows the uptake of this type of venom in human beings.[2] This also may be referred to as a *venous tourniquet*. The elastic bandage or air splint is placed with the goal of slowing venous blood flow back to the heart. However, it should be just tight enough to slow venous blood flow but not interfere with arterial flow. The best way to assess this is to check for a distal pulse. Medical control should be contacted and local protocols should be reviewed before any technique is initiated.

Marine Animals

Marine species are many and varied. However, in U.S. coastal waters, most human poisonings are caused by coelenterates (jellyfish), echinoderms (sea urchins and starfish), and stingrays.

Coelenterates (Jellyfish)

Coelenterates have nematocysts, which often are long cells that contain venom. The jellyfish is a common coelenterate found in the warm coastal waters of the United States (Fig. 22-7). The actual nematocysts are found on tentacles, which can reach up to 100 feet in length. Any swimmer who comes in contact with these nematocysts can be injected with their poison. A sufficient amount of venom can cause systemic effects. Nematocysts can remain embedded in the skin. Interestingly, even if a jellyfish loses its tentacle, the venom in the nematocysts can remain potent for months.

Signs and Symptoms

Symptoms often include a reaction on the skin similar to an allergic reaction. The patient initially may feel a stinging sensation, and raised, red lesions may appear. This may be followed by numbness, tingling, and itching. If enough of the body surface area is affected, the patient may have nausea, vomiting, abdominal pain, bronchospasm, hypotension and, finally, respiratory arrest.

Treatment

The patient should be stabilized. The initial assessment should be conducted, and the patient's

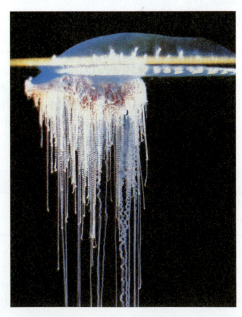

Fig. 22-7 Man-of-war jellyfish.

symptoms should be managed as appropriate. Monitor the vital signs continuously for changes. Also, remove any visible nematocysts. Wear gloves and use forceps to do this to avoid contaminating yourself. Rinse the wounds with seawater or vinegar if available. Do not use fresh water, because it causes the nematocysts to discharge more toxin into the patient's body. Isopropyl alcohol also may be used to inactivate the nematocysts. After inactivating the nematocysts, apply shaving cream and then remove it using the edge of a credit card or a shaving razor. This removes very small nematocysts. The patient should be transported for further evaluation. This is particularly important if the person demonstrates any significant systemic signs caused by this toxic venom.

Echinoderms (Sea Urchins, Starfish)

Sea urchins (Fig. 22-8) and starfish have tiny spines that inject venom. This can be a particular problem because these spines are fragile and can break off in the skin.

Signs and Symptoms

Immediate pain, bleeding, and mild swelling occur when the spines are injected into or become lodged in the skin. If the number of spines is significant, a systemic reaction may result. Systemic effects include nausea, vomiting, respiratory paralysis, and complete muscle paralysis.

Treatment

The initial assessment is very important and focuses on repeating vital signs. The respiratory component is critical. Most marine animals toxins lose their toxicity with an abrupt change in environment, including changes in temperature and humidity. Management of these types of injected toxins includes immersion of the affected extremity in warm water. The water should be as warm as the person can tolerate. It is important to note that these patients may have numbness and tingling in the affected extremity, and they may find it difficult to determine whether the water is too hot. Use caution for this reason. Transport the patient, keeping the affected extremity in the warm water if possible.

Stingrays

Stingrays are commonly seen on diving and snorkeling adventures. They generally are harmless unless a swimmer or diver accidentally steps on the venomous tail (Fig. 22-9). Stingrays often are difficult to see, because they may be buried in the sand. Sting wounds are common on the foot and lower leg. The stings are purely defensive, as these animals do not attack human beings as prey. As with the echinoderms, the spine may break off in the patient's skin.

Signs and Symptoms

Immediate pain, edema, and bleeding are common. Necrosis (tissue death) can occur. If the envenomation is severe enough and becomes systemic, the patient may have weakness, nausea, vomiting, diarrhea, vertigo, seizures, cardiac abnormalities, paralysis, and hypotension accompanied by shock. Death also is possible.

Treatment

Conduct a complete primary survey. Monitor vital signs continuously. The wound may be irrigated with large amounts of fresh water or normal saline. If a spine is visible, remove it with forceps to avoid contaminating yourself. Contact medical control if necessary and transport the patient for evaluation. Keep the affected body part immersed in warm water during transport.

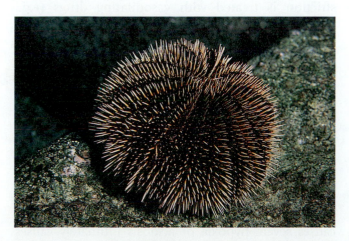

Fig. 22-8 Sea urchin.

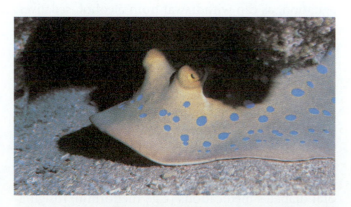

Fig. 22-9 Stingray.

■ COMMON CLINICAL EFFECTS CAUSED BY POISONS

As mentioned previously, the second type of EMS poisoning call involves patients who have symptoms that may appear to be caused by poisoning, but no history of exposure is available or provided. With these calls, the EMT must consider poisoning as a possible cause of these symptoms.

Poisoning Symptoms with No Known History of Exposure

Coma

Coma can occur because of direct effects on the brain. It also can be the result of effects on another system, which in turn affects the brain (e.g., a drug causes hypotension, therefore the brain is not perfused). Common drugs that cause coma by direct effects on the brain include alcohols, opiates, sedatives, muscle relaxants, antiseizure medications, antipsychotic medications, and antidepressant medications.

Seizures

Seizures most often are the result of poisoning from stimulant drugs, such as cocaine or amphetamine. Seizures caused by these drugs usually last only a short time and are self-limited. Other drugs that can cause seizures include the antidepressants, isoniazid, and theophylline. In addition, seizures can occur when a patient is in withdrawal from alcohol or sedative drugs.

Agitation

Agitation is commonly caused by sympathomimetic drugs, such as cocaine, amphetamine, and PCP. Anticholinergic poisons (e.g., jimson weed, antihistamines, and some muscle relaxants) may also cause agitation, as can withdrawal from alcohol, sedatives, or narcotics.

Hypoglycemia

The most common cause of hypoglycemia is insulin overdose. Other medications that may cause hypoglycemia include the sulfonylurea oral hypoglycemic medications, beta blockers, ethanol (especially in children), and salicylate. Hypoglycemic events are all treated initially with oral or IV administration of dextrose. It is worth noting that the non-sulfonylurea oral diabetes medications (e.g., metformin, rosiglitazone) do not cause hypoglycemia in overdose.

Hypotension

The three main mechanisms of hypotension from poisoning are cardiac dysrhythmias, dilation of the blood vessels (vasodilation), and decreased cardiac contraction. When a patient with a dysrhythmia is hypotensive, evaluation and treatment should be directed at the dysrhythmia (see Bradycardia and Tachycardia in the following text). Vasodilation is commonly caused by nitrates (nitroglycerin, amyl nitrate "poppers"), antihypertensive medications (alpha-adrenergic blockers, calcium channel blockers), and tricyclic antidepressants. Hypotension caused by vasodilation initially is treated with IV fluids. Patients who do not improve with IV fluids may require vasoconstrictive medications (e.g., dopamine), which are given by ALS providers or in the hospital. Poisons that decrease cardiac contraction include antihypertensives (beta blockers, calcium channel blockers), tricyclic antidepressants, and cyanide. This type of poisoning is difficult to treat, because patients often do not respond to dopamine or epinephrine. The most effective treatment is to give an antidote to the poison if one is available.

Hypertension

The most common cause of hypertension in a poisoning patient is agitation. This is the major cause of hypertension in cocaine, amphetamine, and PCP intoxication. Withdrawal from alcohol or sedative medications may also cause agitation and hypertension. Patients with hypertension associated with agitation should be treated with sedatives (benzodiazepines). Another major cause of hypertension is vasoconstriction. This is the mechanism of hypertension with pseudoephedrine and ergot migraine medications. Occasionally patients take enough cocaine or amphetamine to experience direct vasoconstrictive effects. Hypertension caused by vasoconstriction is treated with vasodilating drugs (e.g., nitroprusside).

Bradycardia

Bradycardia commonly is caused by antihypertensive drugs (beta blockers, calcium channel blockers, clonidine), digoxin, and **cholinergic substances** (e.g., organophosphate pesticides). In addition, many sedating drugs (ethanol, benzodiazepines, opiates) may cause mild bradycardia. Bradycardia that causes symptoms such as hypotension requires ALS treatment, initially with atropine. Most cases require cardiac pacing or antidote therapy. Any poisoning that causes severe hypoxia or acidosis ultimately causes bradycardia.

Tachycardia

Tachycardia is commonly seen with sympathomimetic medications (cocaine, amphetamine), antidepressants, and **anticholinergic medications** (e.g., jimson weed, antihistamines, and some muscle relaxants). Sinus tachycardia does not require specific treatment. Therapy usually is directed at other manifestations (e.g., agitation). Ventricular or supraventricular tachycardia may be treated with cardioversion by ALS providers or in the hospital. However, because the underlying poisoning is still present, this treatment often is only temporarily effective.

In addition to the previously mentioned general symptoms, poisoning patients may show a set of several symptoms that suggest a specific poison. This collection of findings is called a **toxidrome.** Some of the more common poisoning toxidromes are listed in Table 22-1.

When found on the physical exam, a toxidrome may be used to identify poisoning as the cause of a patient's symptoms. However, not all poisonings produce a recognizable toxidrome. For example, a patient poisoned by a mixture of cocaine and heroin may have features of both sympathomimetic and opiate toxidromes. It is important for EMTs to take care not to exclude a toxic ingestion even if the physical exam findings do not exactly match the expected findings based on the substance the patient was reported to have ingested.

■ EVALUATION OF POISONING

History and Physical Exam

As in all medical emergencies, a good history and physical exam can yield very helpful information. Some patients freely talk about a possible toxic ingestion. However, these incidents often are concealed for fear of embarrassment, legal ramifications, or social stigma. It is important to be sensitive to the current situation and to the patient's needs as the person is evaluated. As noted previously, the patient should always be transported to the hospital if evidence indicates that the person intended to harm himself or herself or if abuse of some sort is a concern. This rule applies even if the exposure appears inconsequential. If intent to harm oneself is suspected, the patient should not be allowed to refuse medical transport. These patients do not have the capacity to refuse. All pill bottles and containers should be transported with the patient.

TABLE 22-1

Common poisoning toxidromes

Toxidrome	Findings	Poisons
Sympathomimetic	Agitation Tachycardia Hypertension Dilated pupils Diaphoresis	Stimulant drugs, including cocaine, amphetamine, MDMA, and ephedrine
Opiate	Coma Respiratory depression Small pupils Decreased bowel sounds	Morphine, codeine, heroin, oxycodone, hydrocodone, methadone
Cholinergic	Drooling, tearing, nasal drainage Vomiting Diarrhea Weakness Seizures Small pupils Bradycardia	Organophosphate and carbamate pesticides, some mushrooms, medications for myasthenia gravis (e.g., edrophonium)
Anticholinergic	Dry mucous membranes Dilated pupils Tachycardia Delirium	Antihistamine, some muscle relaxants, jimson weed

The focused history and physical exam are virtually the same for toxic exposures as for other medical emergencies. However, some specific questions should be asked to try to identify the substance and to ensure the appropriate treatment (Box 22-3). The additional history questions in Box 22-4 also are important. They may reveal a potential toxin or assist the evaluation and treatment of an unknown toxic exposure.

The physical exam should help identify components that may be elements of the various toxidromes listed previously. A full physical evaluation is always important. However, the EMT should pay close attention to mental status, respiratory effort, pupillary size, skin findings, bowel sounds, and the neurologic exam. It is important to re-evaluate these patients continuously. Exam findings can change rapidly, and the original findings may be very important to the diagnosis and treatment. Vital signs should always be recorded and re-evaluated during evaluation and transport.

■ TREATMENT OF POISONED PATIENTS

The treatment of poisoned patients first requires recognition that a toxic exposure has occurred. In many cases, the toxic exposure comes to light while the patient is being evaluated for another reason. For example, a patient may be evaluated for dental pain and admit to taking four acetaminophen tablets every hour for the past 2 days. Table 22-2 lists some common toxins and their antidotes.

The first step is to ensure that the patient can be treated without danger to the providers. This is rarely an issue with any exposure except industrial or intentional exposures to hazardous chemicals. For example, patients with a dermal exposure to an organophosphate require decontamination before medical treatment. If a patient's skin or clothes have a significant amount of poison, decontamination should be done before resuscitation. Keep in mind that contamination of EMS providers or the ED prevents effective treatment of victims. In addition, a contaminated ED may become a secondary hazardous materials site (see Chapter 36). The patient's clothes and other personal items (e.g., watches, wallets) should be removed. Certain toxins (e.g., organophosphates and carbamates) can be absorbed by leather and can recontaminate the patient if the contaminated articles are left in place. In most jurisdictions, decontamina-

BOX 22-3

Important Questions to Ask Poisoning Patients

If EMTs suspect a toxic exposure, they should be sure to ask questions specific to the exposure, such as the following:
- What is your chief complaint (if any)?
- What is the substance?
- How long ago was the exposure?
- How much did you ingest (with ingestion exposure)?
- How long were you in the environment (with inhalation exposure)?
- How long was it in contact with the skin (with dermal exposure)?
- What have you done so far to treat the exposure?
- Have you called the poison center? If so, what were their recommendations?

BOX 22-4

Additional History That May Be Relevant in Poisoning Patients

- Past medical history
- Past surgical history
- Current medications (including over-the-counter medicines, vitamins, herbs, **homeopathic remedies,** and so on)
- Allergies and reactions
- Occupation (if applicable to exposure)
- Hobbies (if applicable to exposure)

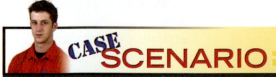

CASE SCENARIO *continued*

With the police officer's help, Ray and his partner pick up John and lay him on the stretcher. The officer asks, "Do you want him on his back or his front, Ray?"

Ray responds, "Actually, I want him to be lying on his left side."

Question: *Why would Ray want the patient to be lying on his left side rather than in one of the other two positions?*

TABLE 22-2

Common toxins and their antidotes

Toxin	Antidote
Acetaminophen	N-acetylcysteine
Crotalid snakes	Antivenin (Crotalidae) polyvalent
Black widow spider	Antivenin (*Latrodectus mactans*)
Organophosphate insecticide	Atropine sulfate and pralidoxime (PAM)
Cyanide	Cyanide antidote kit (amyl nitrite, sodium nitrite, sodium thiosulfate)
Iron	Deferoxamine
Digoxin or natural cardiac glycoside product (e.g., lily of the valley, foxglove)	Digoxin immune Fab
Arsenic, inorganic mercury, or lead	Dimercaprol
Lead	Ethylenediamine tetra-acetic acid (EDTA)
Ethylene glycol or methanol	Ethanol or fomepizole
Benzodiazepines	Flumazenil
Methemoglobinemia	Methylene blue
Opioids	Naloxone

tion is performed by qualified fire department hazardous materials teams (see Chapter 36).

After scene and provider safety has been ensured, resuscitation begins with evaluation of the airway. Burns, edema, or foreign bodies can compromise an airway. While establishing an airway, consider the use of spinal immobilization if trauma is a possibility. If any corrosive injury or burns to the airway are present, it is important to obtain ALS services and provide rapid transport to the hospital. Patients with such injuries can deteriorate quickly. They require advanced airway intervention. Patients who are not breathing, who are taking fewer than 12 breaths per minute, or who do not have an adequate respiratory effort should be assisted with a bag-valve-mask.

All patients with a symptomatic inhalation exposure should receive supplemental oxygen. Otherwise, a clinical judgment can be made on whether supplemental oxygen is necessary. In general, unless signs of hypoxia are present, oxygen given by nasal cannula is sufficient. If hypoxia is a possibility, administer high-flow oxygen with a nonrebreather mask.

Monitor vital signs frequently during evaluation and treatment. Also, keep hypotensive patients lying flat to minimize symptoms. These patients can become dizzy or syncopal when upright. Patients with significant tachycardia or bradycardia also can become hypotensive if the heart rate is too fast or too slow to allow efficient pumping of the heart. In addi-

tion, try to keep the patient's body temperature normal, because the body is metabolically more stable at normal core temperature.

Patients with an altered mental status or coma should be monitored closely for airway and breathing difficulties. Intervention should be based on the clinical presentation. Different toxins can result in a varying ability to protect the airway. An example of this can be seen in patients who have ingested **gamma hydroxybutyrate (GHB)**, which causes an altered mental status and has been used as a "date rape" drug. These patients appear comatose, but often they can protect the airway with minimal stimulation. Monitor the vital signs closely for improvement or deterioration, because the clinical situation can change rapidly.

Place and maintain patients with seizures in a position that keeps the airway clear and patent. Administer oxygen and check the vital signs frequently. If the patient is still seizing when you arrive, place the person in a position of safety that prevents self-injury. Never try to force anything into the patient's mouth. Also, do not try to stop the seizure with physical force.

It is important to involve ALS services if a patient suspected of poisoning or overdose has unstable vital signs, potential airway compromise, or altered mental status, including seizure activity. These patients may require intubation, IV access and fluids, and vasopressors, depending on the exposure and the patient's condition. Transport the patient to the closest appropriate facility. If a particular poison requires an antidote, contact the receiving hospital to give the staff time to prepare the required antidote (antidotes may be stocked in the pharmacy rather than the ED). The prehospital report should be concise but should provide enough information to allow the hospital to prepare for the patient's arrival (Box 22-5).

Activated charcoal (AC) is used to bind ingested poisons. It works by adsorbing (soaking up) the ingested poison before it can be absorbed from the GI tract. AC often is given in the emergency department if the patient is seen within the first hour after the ingestion. Some EMS systems use AC in the prehospital care setting. However, this should be done only with an order from medical control either online (real

---

SPECIAL Considerations

Pediatric Perspectives

Activated charcoal is available as a sorbitol or an aqueous mix. The aqueous mix should always be used for children. Sorbitol, which is intended to move the charcoal through the digestive tract faster, can cause serious diarrhea and dehydration in children.

---

time) or off-line (standing orders with guidelines). AC is given by mouth, usually as slurry (activated charcoal premixed in water) (Fig. 22-10). It is commercially available in plastic bottles containing 50 g of activated charcoal. AC also comes in a powdered form that must be mixed. This form should not be used in the field, because it is difficult to measure and mix. The usual adult and pediatric dosage is 1 g of AC per kilogram (2.2 pounds) of body weight. The usual adult dose is 25 to 50 g, and the usual pediatric dose is 12.5 to 25 g.[1] The premixed bottle must be shaken, because the AC may settle out. The medication looks like mud, consequently you often will have to cajole and encourage the patient to drink the preparation. Sometimes you can aid the process by putting the solution in a covered cup with a straw. That way, the charcoal cannot be seen. ***Never* give a patient with altered mental status charcoal (or *anything*) by mouth.** This may cause vomiting, which can lead to aspiration. Also, do not give charcoal or *anything* by mouth to any patient who is unable to swallow properly. AC also is contraindicated if the ingested substance might be an acid or an alkali. These agents are not adsorbed, and they can cause further injury or damage. It is important to document that the patient

---

BOX 22-5
Syrup of Ipecac

Ipecac syrup is made from a plant extract. When swallowed, it irritates the stomach and causes vomiting. For decades, syrup of ipecac was a standard remedy used not only by EMS personnel and hospital emergency departments but also by parents at home after ingestion of a poison. However, the use of ipecac has been called into question. In 2003, the American Academy of Pediatrics issued a position statement recommending that parents no longer use or store ipecac in the home.[2] The American Academy of Medical Toxicology also has recommended against its use in emergency departments.[3] These decisions were based on growing evidence that ipecac may not be helpful and that it may affect other treatments for the poisoning. In addition, airway compromise is always a possibility, and aspiration may occur in vomiting patients with an altered level of consciousness. Over the years, many EMS systems have stopped using ipecac. It should be reserved for special situations under direct, online medical control. As with charcoal, nothing should ever be given by mouth if the patient has an altered mental status, if the ingested substance may be caustic, or if the patient cannot swallow properly.

The adult dose of ipecac is 30 ml by mouth, followed by 8 to 10 ounces of water. In children younger than 1 year of age, the dose is 5 to 10 ml by mouth, followed by water 10-20 ml/kg. In children older than 1 year, it is 15 ml, followed by water 10-20 ml/kg up to 250 ml.

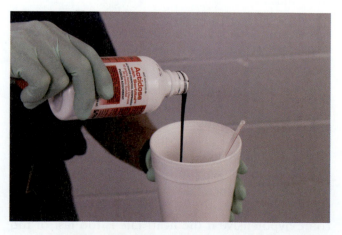

Fig. 22-10 Activated charcoal.

SKILL 22-1
◉ *Administering Activated Charcoal*

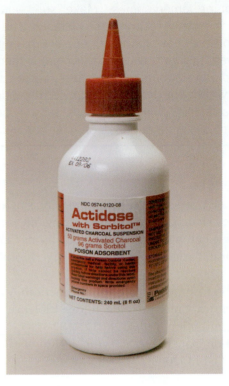

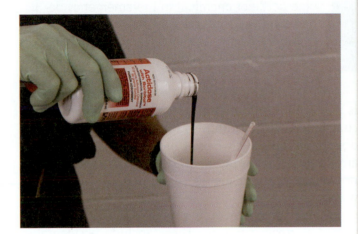

1. Obtain an order from medical control to administer activated charcoal. Based on local protocols, the directing physician will help you determine the appropriate dose. As a general rule, you may give 25 to 50 g to adults and 12.5 to 25 g to children, depending on the patient's weight.

2. Make sure that the medication has been properly suspended, then pour it into a container.

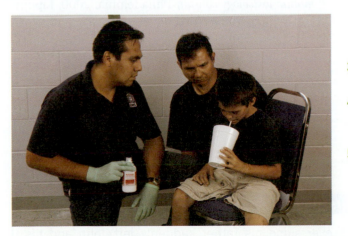

3. Explain the drug's action and the potential side effects to the patient.

4. Encourage the patient to drink the full dose. If the charcoal settles, shake or stir it back into suspension.

5. Reassess the patient, recording the time and any changes in the patient's condition.

SKILLS

SPECIAL Considerations

Shake That Bottle

Activated charcoal in containers sinks to the bottom, leaving a layer of liquid on top. Shake the container vigorously for 1 minute to ensure thorough mixing.

SPECIAL Considerations

Bring It Along

With a suspected ingestion, take the medicine bottle or chemical to the emergency department with the patient if it is safe to do so. This often is very helpful for identifying and quantifying the ingestion.

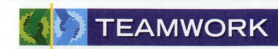

TEAMWORK

As previously discussed, EMTs must be prepared to deal with a multitude of possible causes of poisoning emergencies. Make sure you work with the other responders. Listen to the information they have gathered, or have them get the answers to your questions from family members, friends, bystanders, or witnesses. Make sure you stay within the limits of your certification; ask for assistance from ALS crews early. A positive patient outcome depends on your actions.

is alert and not vomiting before you administer the charcoal. After AC administration, it is important to document the dose, whether the patient vomits, and any respiratory symptoms. The charcoal container is not hazardous and may be discarded with medical waste.

EMS personnel encounter many different types of potential toxic exposure. These include accidental home ingestion, occupational exposure, use of illicit drugs, and attempts at self-injury. Some toxins have specific antidotes. However, in general, good symptomatic and supportive care form the mainstay of treatment. It is important to remember to treat the patient, not the poison. Moreover, recognition of a potential toxic exposure frequently can make diagnosis and treatment much faster and more effective. The best way to treat a poisoning is to prevent it in the first place. Often this can be accomplished through education and vigilance.

References

1. Chyka PA, Seger D: Position statement: single-dose activated charcoal, American Academy of Clinical Toxicology; European Association of Poisons Centres and Clinical Toxicologists, *J Toxicol Clin Toxicol* 35:721-741, 1997.
2. Poison treatment in the home, American Academy of Pediatrics, Committee on Injury, Violence, and Poison Prevention, *Pediatrics* 112:1182-1185, 2003.
3. Position paper: Ipecac syrup, *J Toxicol Clin Toxicol* 42:133-143, 2004.

Resources

Dart RC, Caravati EM, McGuigan M et al, editors: *Medical toxicology*, ed 3, Philadelphia, 2004, Lippincott Williams & Wilkins.
Dart RC, Hurlbut KM, Kuffner EK, Yip L, editors: *The five minute toxicology consult*, Philadelphia, 2000, Lippincott Williams & Wilkins.

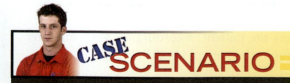

CASE SCENARIO

conclusion

At the hospital, Ray relays his findings to the receiving nurse. He then helps the ED staff transfer John from the ambulance stretcher to the hospital bed. Later during his shift, Ray finds out that John has gotten into trouble with narcotics and alcohol ever since his father suddenly left John and his mother a couple of months ago. This was the worst episode thus far, and a licensed social worker has been called in to evaluate John's situation. ■

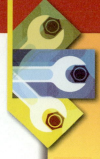

Critical Points

The effects of poisoning are determined by the poison, the dose, and the patient. An exposure that may have life-threatening effects in one patient may have minimal effects in another. Likewise, a poison that may have such effects at high doses may be less damaging at lower doses. Poisoning is a dynamic process. Patients must be monitored constantly for changes.

Learning Checklist

❑ Poisoning and overdose cases range from minor exposures that produce no symptoms to major exposures that can kill patients and put providers at risk. Three factors determine the outcome of an exposure: (1) the poison, (2) the patient, and (3) the treatment.

❑ The four main pathways of poisoning are ingestion, inhalation, absorption, and injection.

❑ Common poisonings include abuse of ethanol (drinking alcohol), acetaminophen and aspirin; carbon monoxide poisoning; and ingestion or exposure to household products.

❑ Substance abuse is the use of any substance or substances to produce an altered mental state or a feeling of euphoria. Sources of substance abuse include prescription medications, illegal drugs, cigarettes, alcohol, and naturally occurring plants and herbs.

❑ Cocaine, amphetamine, and methamphetamine are the most common stimulant drugs of abuse.

❑ The most commonly encountered opiate is heroin. Other medications in this group are morphine, codeine, hydrocodone, oxycodone, hydromorphone, fentanyl, and meperidine.

❑ Marijuana is the most common illegal drug of abuse.

❑ Less common drugs of abuse include hallucinogens (LSD and psilocybin mushrooms), MDMA, and hydrocarbons (glue sniffing/huffing).

❑ Common insect and animal bites and stings include those of the brown recluse spider,

black widow spider, scorpions, pit vipers, coral snakes, and marine animals (jellyfish, sea urchins, starfish, and stingrays).

❑ Poisonings can cause a wide range of symptoms, including coma, seizures, agitation, hypoglycemia, hypotension, hypertension, bradycardia, and tachycardia.

❑ Toxidromes are collections of findings associated with poisoning.

❑ Evaluation of poisoning includes a patient history and physical examination, with a focus on identifying potential toxins or exposures.

❑ The first step in the treatment of a poisoned patient is to make sure the patient can be treated with no danger to the provider. Once safety has been ensured, resuscitation begins with evaluation of the ABCs.

❑ All patients with symptomatic inhalation exposures should receive supplemental oxygen.

❑ Vital signs should be monitored frequently during evaluation and treatment. Patients with an altered mental status or coma should be monitored closely for airway and breathing difficulties.

❑ ALS providers should be involved if the patient has unstable vital signs, potential airway compromise, or altered mental status, including seizures.

❑ Poisoned patients should be transported to the closest appropriate facility.

❑ Activated charcoal binds ingested poisons by adsorbing them before they are absorbed from the GI tract.

❑ *Antidotes* are substances that counter the effects of a toxin or poison.

Key Terms

Acetaminophen A nonprescription drug with analgesic and antipyretic effects similar to aspirin. The trade name for acetaminophen is Tylenol.

Acetylsalicylic acid Chemical name for aspirin.

Acid Chemical that has pH less than 7, the opposite of an alkali.

Activated charcoal (AC) Substance used to adsorb toxins from the gastrointestinal tract.

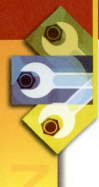

Alkali A chemical that has a high pH (greater than 7); the opposite of an acid.

Amphetamine A drug used as a central nervous system stimulant.

Analgesic A medication given to relieve pain.

Anticholinergic medications Drugs that block the action of acetylcholine (neurotransmitter) at receptor sites. Symptoms produced by these drugs can include dry mouth, hot skin, delirium, flushed skin, and big pupils.

Antidote A remedy that counteracts a poison.

Antipyretic A medication given to treat a fever.

Antivenin A product that neutralizes or lessens the effect of the injected toxic venom.

Benzodiazepines A group of medications used to treat seizures and calm patients. Examples include diazepam, midazolam, and lorazepam.

Carbon monoxide poisoning Poisoning caused by inhalation of carbon monoxide.

Cocaine A crystalline alkaloid used medically as a local anesthetic and illegally for its euphoric effects.

Cholinergic substances Substances that have physiologic effects similar to those of acetylcholine. These substances cause symptoms such as diarrhea, lacrimation, bronchorrhea, drooling, vomiting, seizures, weakness, and a slow heart rate.

Dermal (skin) absorption Uptake of a substance into or across the skin.

Detergent A chemical that binds a molecule and allows it to be dissolved in water. Detergents are categorized as cationic or anionic, depending on the type of molecules they bind.

Ecstasy A drug similar to amphetamine that causes mild hallucinations as well as stimulant effects. The chemical name is methylenedioxymethamphetamine (MDMA).

Ethanol Drinking alcohol; the most common drug of abuse.

Gamma hydroxybutyrate (GHB) An illicit "rave drug" originally used as an anesthetic and muscle-building aid. It now is abused for its euphoric effects. It also is one of the "date rape" drugs, used for its ability to rapidly incapacitate a person with small doses.

Hallucinogens Drugs that cause hallucinations (e.g., MDMA, lysergic acid diethylamide [LSD], and psilocybin mushrooms).

Homeopathic remedies Small doses of medicines or herbs or both that are believed to stimulate the immune system.

Huffing (glue sniffing) Deliberate inhalation of hydrocarbons to produce intoxication.

Ingestion Taking food, medicines, or drink into the body by mouth.

Inhalation Drawing air or other substances into the body by way of the nose and trachea.

Injection Forcing a liquid into a body part, such as into the subcutaneous tissues, the vascular tree, or an organ.

Ipecac syrup A substance used to induce vomiting with overdose and certain poisonings.

LSD The street name for lysergic acid or "acid"; a potent hallucinogen.

Marijuana A crude preparation of the leaves and flowering tops of *Cannabis* plants. It usually is made into cigarettes and inhaled as smoke for its euphoric effects.

Methamphetamine A derivative of amphetamine used both medically and illicitly as a central nervous system stimulant.

Opiates Drugs or substances that contain opium or an opium derivative (e.g., heroin, morphine, codeine, and fentanyl).

Phencyclidine (PCP) A stimulant drug that also induces a state in which the pain sensation is diminished.

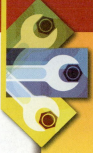

NUTS AND BOLTS

Psilocybin The chemical found in some mushrooms that causes hallucinations.

Stimulant A drug or medication that causes an increase in the activity of the sympathetic nervous system (fight or flight). Common stimulants include cocaine, amphetamine, and PCP.

Toxidrome A constellation of signs and symptoms characteristic of intoxication with a specific poison.

National Standard Curriculum Objectives

Cognitive Objectives

After completing this lesson, the EMT student will be able to do the following:

- List various ways poisons enter the body.
- List signs and symptoms associated with poisoning.
- Discuss the emergency medical care of the patient with a possible overdose.
- Describe the steps in the emergency medical care of a patient with suspected poisoning.
- Describe a situation in which a patient suffering from poisoning or overdose would require airway management.
- State the generic and trade names, indications, contraindications, medication form, dose, administration, actions, side effects, and reassessment strategies for activated charcoal.

- Recognize the need to contact medical control while caring for a patient with poisoning or overdose.

Affective Objectives

After completing this lesson, the EMT student will be able to do the following:

- Explain the rationale for administering activated charcoal.
- Explain the rationale for contacting medical control early in the prehospital management of a poisoning or overdose patient.

Psychomotor Objectives

After completing this lesson, the EMT student will be able to do the following:

- Demonstrate the steps in the emergency medical care of the patient with a possible overdose.
- Demonstrate the steps in the emergency medical care of the patient with suspected poisoning.
- Perform the steps required to administer activated charcoal to a patient.
- Demonstrate the assessment and documentation of the patient's response to treatment.
- Demonstrate proper disposal of the equipment used to administer activated charcoal.
- Demonstrate the completion of a prehospital care report for patients with a poisoning or overdose emergency.

443

CHAPTER

23

OUTLINE

GOAL

LESSON GOAL

As an emergency medical technician (EMT), you often will have to deal with environmental emergencies. This chapter will teach you to recognize the signs and symptoms of heat and cold exposure and the emergency medical care of these conditions. It also provides information on aquatic emergencies and bites and stings. ■

Environmental Emergencies

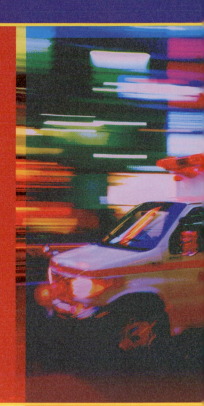

CHAPTER OBJECTIVES

After completing this chapter, the EMT student will be able to do the following:

1 Describe the different ways the body can lose heat.

2 List the signs and symptoms of exposure to cold.

3 Explain the type of medical care a patient exposed to cold should receive.

4 List the signs and symptoms of exposure to heat.

5 Explain the type of medical care a patient exposed to heat should receive.

6 Identify the signs and symptoms of near-drowning.

7 Describe the things that can go wrong with a near-drowning patient.

8 Discuss the emergency medical care of bites and stings.

9 Demonstrate the type of assessment and emergency care the cold exposure patient should receive.

10 Demonstrate the type of assessment and emergency care the heat exposure patient should receive.

11 Demonstrate the type of assessment and emergency care the near-drowning patient should receive.

12 Demonstrate the proper way to give a report on a patient suffering from an environmental emergency.

23

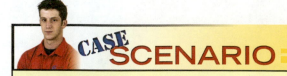

CASE SCENARIO

Ray's ambulance arrives at the scene just as fire-fighters pull a boy out of a freezing pond. Lucas and Jacob, both 9 years old, had been out on the ice since early morning, playing hockey with their recent holiday gifts, skates and sticks. The pond had finally frozen over the night before, or so the boys had thought. By noon the ice had begun to thaw, but the boys hadn't noticed as they skated from one side of the pond to the other. Abruptly the ice had cracked, and Lucas had plunged into the freezing water. Jacob ran back to the house to get help. Within minutes, firefighters from Liberty Fire Company and county police officers had converged on the scene.

Questions: In addition to a jump bag and airway kit, what other items should Ray bring down to the scene? Before leaving the ambulance, what can he do to prepare it for this patient?

Extremes of environment are a danger to both the patient and the rescuer. The extremes of temperature and pressure to which the patient is exposed often are the same conditions the EMT must endure to treat the patient. Therefore EMTs must be able to protect themselves and the patient while treating the patient's problems. It is important to note that these extremes do not occur just in the wide-open wilderness. They also can be factors in suburban and urban emergency medical services (EMS) situations. For example, a collision on icy suburban roads with entrapment, in which the extrication takes time, or a sporting event in humid, hot city weather each can involve patients with environmental injuries. The elderly and the very young are particularly vulnerable to these types of injuries. An older patient who lives in an apartment without air conditioning in the summer or one who cannot afford enough heat in the winter is at high risk.

The human body can function only within a narrow range of temperature and atmospheric pressure conditions. If the patient's temperature rises or falls only a few degrees, the chemical processes and metabolism of the body no longer work efficiently. At environmental extremes, they may not work at all. For example, sudden changes in pressure can cause severe problems. **Barotrauma** is an illness or injury caused by a sudden change in pressure, such as during a quick ascent to the surface while scuba diving; this may overexpand a lung and cause a pneumothorax. A weekend ski trip in the mountains can cause altitude sickness, which can be life-threatening or can mask or worsen underlying illness. These are examples of barotrauma in the everyday world of patient care.

■ THERMOREGULATION AND HEAT TRANSFER

To treat or prevent conditions caused by excessive heat or cold exposure, the EMT must understand how heat is gained or lost by the body. Heat is gained by the body in two ways: by internal means and by external means. The internal means is a byproduct of metabolism. Heat is a side product that occurs when sugar combines with oxygen to produce energy for cells in the body. This mechanism is responsible for the normal baseline body temperature. Heat is produced by muscular activity, such as shivering or exercise, or by other activities, such as strenuous work. The muscular activity related to shivering is the body's response to cold and is a method of raising the body's temperature.

The external means by which the body gains heat comes into play when the environment is warmer than the body's core temperature of 98° F (37° C). In this case, the five mechanisms that normally remove heat from the body (which are discussed in the following section) work in reverse, adding heat to the body. Under normal conditions, the body balances the gain and loss of energy by reducing heat gain or loss to the environment. This occurs mostly through changes in blood flow through the skin. To conserve heat in the body, blood vessels in the skin constrict, preserving heat internally. If heat needs to be dissipated, the blood vessels in the skin dilate, allowing warm blood to move closer to the body surface and thus lose heat to the external environment.

Mechanisms of Heat Transfer

Heat always flows from warmer to cooler. If the environment is cooler than the body, heat is lost from the body. If the environment is warmer than the body, heat is transferred into the body. There are five mechanisms by which the body loses or gains heat, depending on the conditions. They are conduction, convection, evaporation, respiration, and radiation (Fig. 23-1).

Conduction is the transfer of heat energy from a warmer object to a cooler one as a result of direct contact. This direct transfer of energy may be from the patient or EMT to the cold air or water or the ground on which the patient is lying. If the object with which the patient is in contact is warmer than the patient, heat flows into the body rather than out of it. This can either warm a patient or cause a heat injury. Water is 25 times more conductive than dry air. This means that a patient loses heat 25 times faster in the water or when wet than in the air or when dry. In fact, moderately cool but wet weather is far more dangerous than severely cold conditions because most people do not realize how fast they are losing heat. Any water in contact with the patient (or rescuer) absorbs tremendous amounts of heat energy.

Convection is the heating of a colder fluid or gas by air movement over the heat source. Baseboard heating elements heat a room this way. Wind chill also works this way. The wet suit worn by scuba divers prevents heat loss from the movement of the water over the diver's body. In a naked human body, given an ambient environmental temperature of about 81° F (27° C) and almost no wind (conditions known as a *natural environment*), 40% of heat loss occurs by convection. The windproof outer layer of a jacket prevents heat loss from convection. The concept of wind chill is derived from the idea that increased wind speed increases convection (Fig. 23-2).

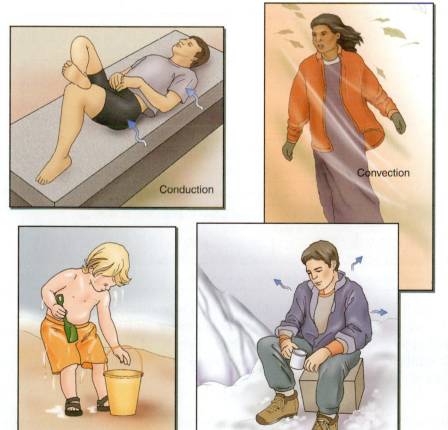
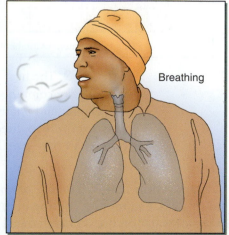

Fig. 23-1 Five mechanisms of heat loss in a patient.

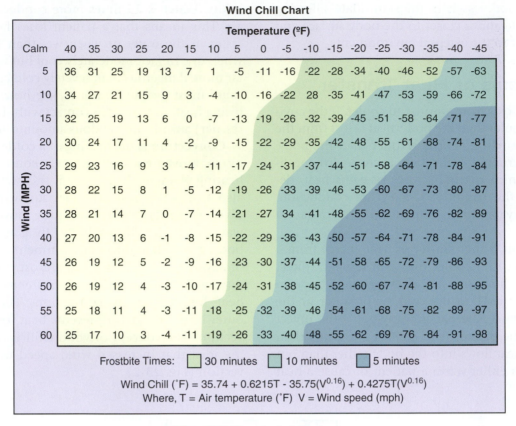

Wind Chill Chart

Temperature (°F)

Calm	40	35	30	25	20	15	10	5	0	-5	-10	-15	-20	-25	-30	-35	-40	-45
5	36	31	25	19	13	7	1	-5	-11	-16	-22	-28	-34	-40	-46	-52	-57	-63
10	34	27	21	15	9	3	-4	-10	-16	-22	28	-35	-41	-47	-53	-59	-66	-72
15	32	25	19	13	6	0	-7	-13	-19	-26	-32	-39	-45	-51	-58	-64	-71	-77
20	30	24	17	11	4	-2	-9	-15	-22	-29	-35	-42	-48	-55	-61	-68	-74	-81
25	29	23	16	9	3	-4	-11	-17	-24	-31	-37	-44	-51	-58	-64	-71	-78	-84
30	28	22	15	8	1	-5	-12	-19	-26	-33	-39	-46	-53	-60	-67	-73	-80	-87
35	28	21	14	7	0	-7	-14	-21	-27	34	-41	-48	-55	-62	-69	-76	-82	-89
40	27	20	13	6	-1	-8	-15	-22	-29	-36	-43	-50	-57	-64	-71	-78	-84	-91
45	26	19	12	5	-2	-9	-16	-23	-30	-37	-44	-51	-58	-65	-72	-79	-86	-93
50	26	19	12	4	-3	-10	-17	-24	-31	-38	-45	-52	-60	-67	-74	-81	-88	-95
55	25	18	11	4	-3	-11	-18	-25	-32	-39	-46	-54	-61	-68	-75	-82	-89	-97
60	25	17	10	3	-4	-11	-19	-26	-33	-40	-48	-55	-62	-69	-76	-84	-91	-98

Wind (MPH)

Frostbite Times: ☐ 30 minutes ☐ 10 minutes ☐ 5 minutes

Wind Chill (°F) = $35.74 + 0.6215T - 35.75(V^{0.16}) + 0.4275T(V^{0.16})$
Where, T = Air temperature (°F) V = Wind speed (mph)

Fig. 23-2 Wind chill chart.

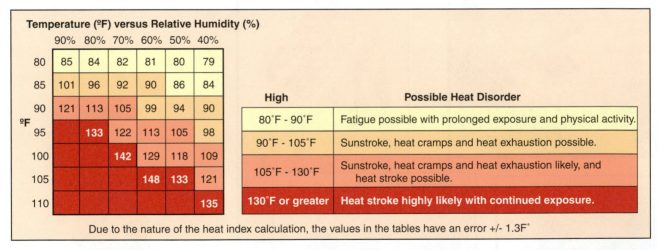

Temperature (°F) versus Relative Humidity (%)

°F	90%	80%	70%	60%	50%	40%
80	85	84	82	81	80	79
85	101	96	92	90	86	84
90	121	113	105	99	94	90
95		133	122	113	105	98
100			142	129	118	109
105				148	133	121
110						135

High	Possible Heat Disorder
80°F - 90°F	Fatigue possible with prolonged exposure and physical activity.
90°F - 105°F	Sunstroke, heat cramps and heat exhaustion possible.
105°F - 130°F	Sunstroke, heat cramps and heat exhaustion likely, and heat stroke possible.
130°F or greater	Heat stroke highly likely with continued exposure.

Due to the nature of the heat index calculation, the values in the tables have an error +/- 1.3F°

Fig. 23-3 The heat index (HI) is the temperature the body feels when heat and humidity are combined. This chart shows the HI that corresponds to the actual air temperature and relative humidity. The chart is based on shady, light wind conditions. Exposure to direct sunlight can increase the HI as much as 15° F. (The values in the chart have a margin of error of ±1.3° F.)

Evaporation is the changing of water from a liquid to a gas. Evaporative cooling occurs when perspiration or water on the skin is changed into a vapor by the heat of the body. In the neutral environment, mentioned previously, about 15% of heat loss occurs through evaporation. To prevent this, clothing next to the skin must be dry.

Respiration causes the loss of heat from inhaled air that has been warmed to body temperature and then exhaled. Water is also lost from the body this way. In a temperature-neutral environment, this accounts for half of the 15% heat loss of evaporative cooling.

Radiation is the direct transfer of energy from one object to another without the use of a medium such as water or air. All objects above absolute zero temperature ($-273°$ C) give off energy (heat) by radiation. In the neutral conditions noted previously, this loss may be as much as 45% of total heat lost from the body. Reflective blankets ("space blankets") are supposed to reduce heat loss from radiative cooling, but are also metallic and therefore will cause conduction of body heat at the same time.

The combination of heat and humidity is called the **heat index** (Fig. 23-3). The heat index is a better indicator of the potential for heat illness than the absolute temperature alone. As the humidity increases, the ability of many of the heat transfer mechanisms' to disperse heat is diminished.

■ HYPOTHERMIA

A patient is said to be hypothermic when the core temperature begins to fall because heat loss to the environment exceeds heat production through metabolism. **Hypothermia** can be caused by environmental exposure, such as falling into cold water or lying on the cold ground. It also can have a metabolic cause, such as cancer or infection. As a person gets colder, the body tries to protect itself by constricting superficial blood vessels and shunting warm blood away from the skin and periphery back into the central part of the body. The reduced blood flow in this "shell" means that the temperature falls faster in the periphery than in the core of the body. The speed of cooling determines the degree of difference in temperature and blood chemistry between the core and the shell. Acute hypothermia, sometimes called *immersion hypothermia*, occurs if a lightly clothed person falls into cold water and the body temperature drops quickly. The type of hypothermia associated with being lost in the woods is called *subacute hypothermia*. It occurs over several hours to days and often is accompanied by dehydration; this condition has been referred to as *exposure*. Chronic hypothermia takes weeks to months to occur and is a problem mostly of the elderly living in conditions of inadequate heat for their age. The elderly generally have less body fat and therefore less insulation.

Aging also reduces the body's thermoregulatory capability. This form of hypothermia should be suspected whenever EMTs respond to a call involving altered mental status in an elderly person in the winter, especially if the room in which the patient is found is a comfortable temperature. This temperature nonetheless may be too cold for the person.

Risk Factors

Certain risk factors can increase a patient's susceptibility to hypothermia or may increase the severity of mild or moderate hypothermia. The consumption of alcohol (ethanol) causes vasodilation increasing heat loss, thereby defeating the body's own mechanism for reducing heat loss through the skin. Patients with underlying diseases such as cancer, hypothyroidism, or sepsis are also at risk for hypothermia because of reduced metabolism, even in relatively warm weather.

Younger children also are at particular risk for hypothermia. However, the onset may occur much faster than in elderly patients. Young children have less muscle mass and body fat. Therefore they have less insulation and a limited ability to shiver. Infants cannot shiver at all and certainly cannot cover their own heads when cold.

Removing the patient from the offending environment and completing the initial assessment and initial treatment are the first priority.

Hypothermia is described as mild, moderate, or severe, depending on the signs and symptoms. In most EMS situations, taking a temperature is difficult, and getting an accurate core temperature is even more difficult. Therefore the severity and treatment of the hypothermia must be determined primarily by the clinical signs and symptoms. It is also worth noting that most traditional glass and mercury-filled medical thermometers do not read a low enough temperature for hypothermic patients. Moreover, many of the newer electronic thermometers need to be stored in a warm place before use.

Mild hypothermia occurs when the body temperature drops below $95°$ F ($35°$ C) to as low as $89.6°$ F ($32°$ C). Signs include shivering, cold skin from vaso-

> **SPECIAL** Populations
>
> **Geriatric Perspectives**
>
> The elderly are at increased risk for developing hypothermia. Deterioration of the nervous system diminishes older adults' ability to recognize that they are getting cold. Also, aging reduces mobility and metabolism. Cardiovascular disease and medications can further inhibit some compensatory mechanisms.

constriction, poor judgment, difficulty speaking (dysarthria), and difficulty walking (ataxia); these patients also may withdraw into themselves and become apathetic. The patient exhibits "the umbles"—the person fumbles, bumbles, mumbles, stumbles, and grumbles. This lack of judgment means that patients do not realize they are becoming hypothermic and therefore take no self-protective action. A hypothermic person's joint fluid thickens, making the joints stiff. Difficulty walking because of this can make cold hikers, for example, more prone to falls and fractures. Fine motor tasks become so difficult that the patient cannot zip up a jacket or dial a phone, as in the case of an elderly individual who has fallen and is lying on the cold kitchen or bathroom floor.

The first line of treatment for a patient with mild hypothermia is to remove the patient from the hazardous environment or to stop the heat loss. This can be done by drying the patient, insulating the person from wind and wet, and getting the patient off the ground. Remember that the patient may be losing more heat through the ground on which the person is lying than through the air. Because the patient in this stage is still conscious, warm, sweet, sugary liquids should be given. Caffeine and alcohol should be avoided. The use of nicotine promotes frostbite and should be avoided in all cold environments. Do not give liquids if the patient has an injury that may require surgery or if the person is unable to swallow on his or her own. Heat packs wrapped so as to prevent skin burns and heaters in the ambulance can be safely used at this stage of hypothermia.

Moderate hypothermia occurs when the core temperature drops below 89.6° F (32° C) to as low as 78.8° F (26° C). At these temperatures, the patient has stopped shivering and is stuporous. The pulses are slow (bradycardia) and become irregular (atrial fibrillation). Respirations also are slow. The level of consciousness decreases progressively. The pupils become slow to react. Occasionally patients may undress during this phase, although no one can explain this paradoxic behavior. During this phase of cooling, the heart becomes very unstable, and any bumping or rough handling may put the patient into ventricular fibrillation.

The first line of treatment for a patient with moderate hypothermia is to ensure the airway, breathing, and circulation (ABCs) and remove the patient from the hazardous environment or stop further heat loss. Warmed inspired air from a pocket mask or warmed humidified oxygen is always good. It may prevent or reduce the chance of ventricular fibrillation from rough handling and movement. It is important to make sure that a patient is truly in cardiac arrest before starting cardiopulmonary resuscitation (CPR). The patient's pulse should be carefully checked for at least 1 minute to ensure pulselessness before compressing the chest. Any cardiac activity, even just one or two beats a minute, is better than artificial circulation. Performing CPR on a bradycardic hypothermic patient may put the patient into ventricular fibrillation. Recently, most EMS systems changed their standard protocols for using automated external defibrillators (AEDs) to treat hypothermic patients with ventricular fibrillation. Instead of providing multiple sets of stacked shocks, the American Heart Association recommends that a maximum of three shocks (one set of stacked shocks) be delivered and that further shocks be withheld until the patient has been rewarmed.

Severe hypothermia occurs when the core temperature drops below 78.8° F (26° C). The patient has no reflexes and no response to pain. No pupil responses occur, and a bradycardic rhythm progresses to flatline. The patient has stiff joints and cold skin. Respirations and pulses are so slow and weak they cannot be detected. The patient appears dead, but he or she may not be. Consequently, a hypothermic patient is not considered dead until the person is *warm and dead*. In this stage of hypothermia, it is imperative to move the patient gently to avoid triggering ventricular fibrillation. Field treatment (warm packs to arm pits and groin area and conservation of body heat) is the same as for moderate hypothermia (Fig. 23-4).

In all cases of hypothermia, it is important that rewarming be done carefully and in an environment that protects the patient from the cold and refreezing.

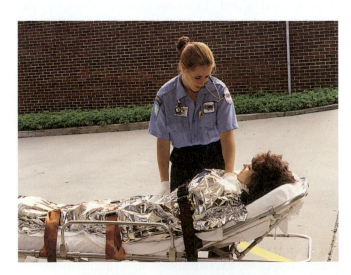

Fig. 23-4 Hypothermia wrap.

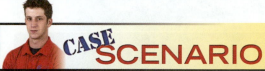

CASE SCENARIO

continued

Ray throws wool blankets and warm packs onto the gurney in addition to the medical bags. He also turns the patient compartment heater on high before closing the doors. As he approaches the scene, he can see the firefighters wrapping the boy in blankets that his mother brought down from the house. Lucas's lips are blue, and he appears to be unresponsive. Kneeling beside Lucas, Ray opens the boy's airway with a modified jaw thrust maneuver. He cannot hear or feel any breathing, nor can he feel a carotid or brachial pulse.

Questions: *What should the rescue crew do now? What are some special circumstances Ray should consider in managing this case?*

■ LOCAL COLD INJURY

Trench Foot, Cold Urticaria, and Frostbite

Hypothermia is a systemic problem that affects the whole body and all its systems. Cold injury can also affect specific parts of the body. This generally is referred to as a local injury. Areas farthest from the core of the body or with poor circulation and insulation are most vulnerable. Hypothermic patients are also at great risk because of the shunting of blood away from the periphery. People who use nicotine are at greater risk for local cold injury because nicotine also causes vasoconstriction. As a result, small parts of the body,

such as the fingers, toes, ears, and tip of the nose, are common sites of cold injury. This is why mittens actually provide more warmth than gloves.

Cold but nonfreezing injury of the lower extremities is called **trench foot,** also known as *immersion foot.* It takes its name from World War I soldiers who stood for long periods in cold, wet trenches. EMTs now see it in anyone who stands for a long time in cold, wet conditions. The affected part tingles or is numb and the skin may be wrinkled, as if the patient had been in the bath too long. It is cold to the touch and may be blanched white, without capillary refill. A less severe form of trench foot is called **chilblains.** Chilblains are more common in women. The affected part is red and blue and may itch or burn. These patients can be warmed in lukewarm, soapy water. They should be advised to keep the affected part clean.

Cold urticaria appears to be a local allergic reaction to the cold. It manifests as localized redness, wheals, itching, and edema in cold-exposed skin. Systemic symptoms may include fatigue, headache, dyspnea, tachycardia and, in rare cases, full-blown anaphylactic shock.

Frostbite results when the water in and around the skin cells starts to freeze. Frostbite is characterized by the depth of damage or in degrees, much like burns (Fig. 23-5). Superficial frostbite is also called frostnip, which ultimately does not result in tissue loss. In both cases, the affected area is initially painful. The injury is first red and then progresses to pale. The condition may be aggravated if it occurs in combination with windburn. When frostbite progresses from painful to numb, it is classified as first-degree frostbite. Often the stages, or degrees, are confused with one another.

Second-degree, or partial thickness, frostbite can be diagnosed only during thawing, as blisters develop. Third-degree, or full thickness, frostbite is characterized by skin that develops a purple/black

ASK YOURSELF

Imagine that you and your EMT partner are on duty during a winter storm. You have responded to multiple vehicle accidents throughout the night. Your partner tells you that her toes are numb, and you notice that she is shivering. Do you ignore her? Should you go out of service? Is your partner experiencing an environmental emergency?

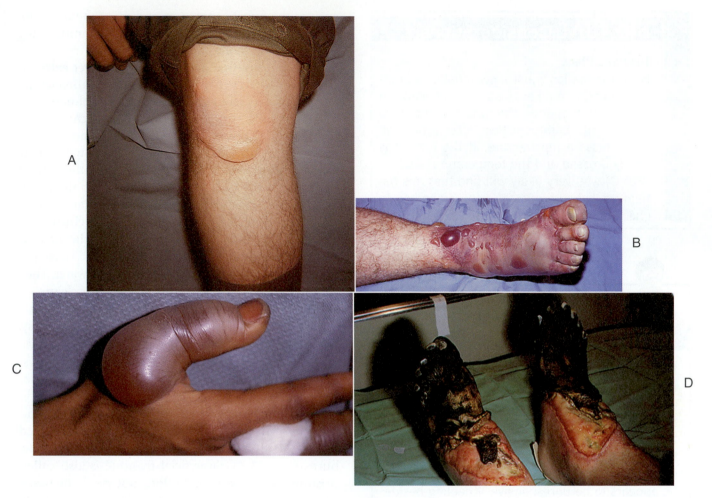

Fig. 23-5 Frostbite. **A,** First-degree frostbite of the knee, 12 hours after thawing. The person was kneeling to change a tire. **B,** Edema and blister formation 24 hours after frostbite injury in an area covered by a tightly fitting boot. **C,** Deep second- and third-degree frostbite with hemorrhagic blebs, 1 day after thawing. **D,** Gangrenous necrosis 6 weeks after frostbite injury shown in **B.**

color, indicating tissue necrosis or death. Second-degree frostbite creates a hard skin layer with a little give underneath. In third-degree frostbite, the skin and underlying tissues are more solid to the touch through and through. Fourth-degree frostbite involves the underlying muscle and bone. This depth of frostbite may result in mummification. In children, frostbite to this depth can affect the growth plate, interfering with bone development. Some classification systems refer to first- and second-degree frostbite as superficial frostbite and to third- and fourth-degree frostbite as deep frostbite.

Treatment begins with removal from the cold. Anything wet or restricting, including jewelry, should be carefully removed from the patient. Loose, sterile dressings and extremity splinting should be used for transporting the patient. Never rub a frostbitten area

or use anything cold on it, even if the patient complains of a burning sensation. This is like putting a burn back into the fire. Blisters usually do not develop until thawing has begun, but once they develop, they should be protected from breaking. Sterile dressings should be used to reduce the chance of infection.

In all frostbite treatment, it is most important to prevent the part from thawing and then refreezing. Freeze-thaw-refreeze causes mummification and greater tissue loss. Therefore most EMS systems with short transport times do not attempt any form of field thawing of the frozen part. If refreezing can be absolutely prevented and transport is prolonged or delayed, rewarming should be done in a warm water bath at a temperature of 104° to 108° F (40° to 42.2° C). Never use dry heat, such as from a fire or heater. A thermometer must be used to monitor the water temperature. Areas of skin damaged by frostbite are particularly susceptible to burns at temperatures lower than usual. If the water is too cold, thawing will be too slow and unnecessarily painful. A container large enough that the affected part does not touch the side walls should be used, and fresh, warm water should be added to the side as the water cools. All thawing causes considerable pain. Therefore, if pain management is not available, it may be preferable to delay thawing until pain control is available. Aspirin is useful for preventing clotting. As always, check your local protocols or call medical control for advice.

■ HEAT EMERGENCIES

In a hot or humid environment, the body may not be able to off-load enough heat to maintain the core temperature below a dangerous level. When the body temperature rises because of the environmental temperature and humidity, heat illness and a life-threatening emergency may result. Heat illness is more common in unacclimated individuals. People are more prone to heat illness when heat waves occur early in the season or when a person is suddenly exposed to environmental heat and humidity. As with cold, the very young and the elderly are at greatest risk, as are people taking certain medications. Most cases involve several days of heat exposure, although a relatively short exposure to high temperatures, often associated with overexertion, also can cause heat illness.

Heat illness is a spectrum of disease that can range from relatively mild (heat cramps) to severe and life-threatening (heatstroke).

Heatstroke

The severest but rarest form of heat illness is **heatstroke.** This often is a life- or brain-threatening illness. The two types of heatstroke are **classic heatstroke,** which affects mostly the very young or the elderly, and **exertional heatstroke,** which is caused by excessive exercise. The two forms of heatstroke are equally deadly if left untreated, and both are preventable.

Classic Heatstroke

Classic heatstroke has a slower onset, which may occur over several days during a heat wave. The onset can occur much more quickly in infants (who are at higher risk because of their immature thermoregulatory system), in children left in hot cars, or in adults who have been riding for extended periods in poorly ventilated vehicles in the summer heat. Sim-

ilar conditions may occur in closed spaces, such as machinery rooms or attics. Groups at risk include individuals without air conditioning, those with a chronic illness, the malnourished, and those with substance addictions. The number of classic heatstroke cases increases significantly in early season heat waves, when people are less acclimated. Signs and symptoms include disorientation, incoherence, confusion, and skin that is usually red, hot, and dry. Other signs may include rapid respirations and a rapid heart rate. Treatment must include removing the patient from the hot environment and cooling the body core as quickly as possible, but not to the point of inducing shivering (which will only serve to produce more heat). One of the most effective cooling techniques is performed as follows: (1) remove the patient's clothing; (2) cover the person with a sheet; (3) soak the sheet with cool water; (4) position a fan so that it blows air over the patient, enhancing evaporative heat loss. You should consider contacting advanced life support (ALS) services, if available, for fluid hydration and possible seizure control.

Exertional Heatstroke

Exertional heatstroke occurs during muscular activity, often in otherwise fit or well-conditioned individuals. The victims frequently are very motivated to continue the activity despite the hot, humid environment—and this group can include rescuers and EMTs. As with classic heatstroke, it often is important to know the temperature of the day before the signs and symptoms develop. If the day is hot and humid, an increased risk of heatstroke exists even if the patient is well hydrated. The signs and symptoms are similar to those of classic heatstroke: the patient becomes disoriented, incoherent, confused, and red and warm to the touch. These patients may have seizures. Moreover, patients with exertional heatstroke usually are still sweating and wet.

Rapid treatment of this true medical emergency is vital. Early transport should be considered after removing the patient from the offending environment and completing the initial assessment and initial treatment After ensuring any life-threatening conditions have been identified and treated, the next important treatment of both types of heatstroke is to rapidly cool the patient's core temperature back to normal. Many opinions exist on the best way to do this, but the fastest is immersion in cold or iced water. No proof exists that this is detrimental in any way. However, immersion may be impractical in the field and certainly is in the back of an ambulance. In the

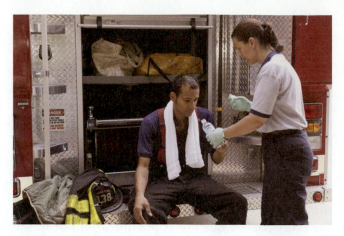

Fig. 23-6 Cooling a patient suffering from heat illness.

latter setting, turning up the air conditioning, removing excess clothing, wetting down the patient, and increasing evaporation by moving air over the person are the best measures (Fig. 23-6). Cold packs on the neck, in the armpit, and in the groin also may help.

Heat Exhaustion

Different types of **heat exhaustion** have been described. All forms of heat exhaustion involve excessive loss of water or salts. During continuous exercise, water loss from sweat may amount to as much as 1 to 4 liters per hour. Patients usually are pale, cool, and clammy, and they may have "goose bumps." They may complain of dizziness, headache, nausea, fainting, or simply fatigue. If the patient has altered mental status, consider heatstroke or another medical emergency as the cause. Treatment for all heat emergencies begins with getting the patient out of the heat. If the protocol allows, small sips of water may help patients who are not nauseated. Intravenous rehydration by an ALS unit or at the hospital is the definitive treatment. Patients should not be allowed to return to hot environments or to exercise for several days.

Heat Cramps

Heat cramps may be part of one type of heat exhaustion. Heat cramps often occur after several hours of sustained activity in hot environments with excessive sweating. Painful cramps occur in the large muscle groups of the abdomen and legs, usually after the patient has stopped exercising. They may even occur in a cooler, air-conditioned environment. Treatment involves removing the patient from the offending en-

vironment, rehydration of the patient, generally by allowing the patient to drink fluids. Gentle massage with the palm of an open hand may help temporarily. Salt tablets should always be avoided because they are gastric irritants.

■ ALTITUDE ILLNESS

People live under a blanket of air. This blanket has weight. At sea level, the weight of this blanket is 14.7 pounds per square inch, or 760 mm Hg (torr). As a person travels from sea level up into the mountains, the weight of the air declines. Although the percentage of oxygen in the air remains the same, the pressure of oxygen drops lower and lower as the altitude increases. As a result, less oxygen moves into the bloodstream from the lungs. Rapid ascent to altitude can cause illness even in well-conditioned and healthy people. This occurs more often than it might seem. Millions of visitors drive or fly to the mountains for recreation year round. Often these are short jaunts or weekend trips. Fatigue, exertion, diet, and dehydration, along with the speed of ascent, all play a role in determining whether altitude illness strikes.

The mildest form of altitude illness is **acute mountain sickness (AMS).** Signs and symptoms include lightheadedness, loss of appetite, shortness of breath, headache, nausea, and vomiting. This illness may begin within hours of reaching elevations as low as 8,000 feet. Most AMS is self-limited, but the effects may last for weeks. If symptoms do not resolve shortly with rest, fluids, and staying at the current altitude, treatment involves oxygen administration and descent to a lower altitude.

High altitude pulmonary edema (HAPE) and **high altitude cerebral edema (HACE)** are more severe forms of altitude sickness. These disorders usually require ascent to elevations above 12,000 feet. HAPE resembles congestive heart failure. It begins with a dry cough, shortness of breath, and wet lung sounds. It may progress to life-threatening pulmonary edema with frothy sputum and hypoxia. Treatment includes administration of oxygen, obtaining ALS help, and getting the patient to a lower altitude. HACE is marked by swelling of parts of the brain. It may resemble a stroke or seizure. Early signs include unsteady gait (ataxia), dizziness, Cheyne-Stokes respiration while sleeping, nausea, vomiting, and lack of energy. Again, the most important treatment is to take the patient to a lower altitude. En route to the lower altitude, oxygen and supportive care for the ABCs are the only real treatments EMTs can offer.

WATER-RELATED ENVIRONMENTS

Dysbarism (Decompression Sickness)

Altitude-related illnesses arise with decreases in atmospheric pressure. However, increases in pressure also can cause problems. This most often occurs when a person goes scuba diving. The United States has more than 4 million certified recreational scuba divers. As a diver descends deeper in the water, the weight of the water compresses any gases the diver breathes in. As a result, gases that normally do not cross from the lungs into the blood readily go into solution. When the diver ascends to the surface, the gas expands. Gas which was in solution in the blood and tissues expands to form bubbles. Bubbles in the joints exert a painful pressure, which forces the individual to bend the joints. This is called **decompression sickness,** commonly referred to as *the bends.* Decompression sickness can develop days after a dive and may not show up until a patient has returned from vacation. Bubbles can also form in the blood and can block blood vessels to the heart or brain, causing a heart attack or stroke. If the diver is holding his or her breath, a pneumothorax may result from the expanding air in the lungs.

Administration of high-flow oxygen with a nonrebreather mask is very important for patients with decompression sickness. Try to gather the history of the dive, such as the number of dives, the length and depth of each dive, when the signs and symptoms first started, and whether the patient has flown in an airplane since the dive. Make sure the hospital staff knows that this may be a scuba diving illness. Definitive care of this type of emergency often involves treating the patient in a hyperbaric chamber. Local protocols may dictate direct transport of these patients to a hospital with such a chamber.

Drowning

A far more common water-related emergency is drowning. **Drowning** is defined as suffocation that occurs from submersion in a liquid. The term *near-drowning* is commonly used, but it is no longer the recommended term; *submersion incident* is preferred. It is estimated that 80,000 submersion incidents occur each year in the United States, with about 9,000 deaths.

It is particularly important to ensure rescuer safety in water incidents. EMS personnel may also become victims if they are not well trained in water rescue and protected by personal flotation devices (PFDs) when appropriate. If rescue is to be attempted, every effort must be made by the rescuer to stay out of the water or away from a struggling, awake victim. More tragic than an unnecessary drowning is the double drowning of a victim and a potential rescuer. The following rule is important: *Reach, throw, row, and only then go.* This means that rescue should first be attempted by extending your reach to a victim using a pole, a branch, or an article of clothing. Most drownings occur within reach of safety. If the victim cannot be reached safely, throw an item that will float and can support the individual. The item should be soft, if possible, and should have a rope attached for retrieval. If the individual is too far from the shore for these measures, a boat-based rescue is preferable to a swimming rescue. All these rescue techniques require practice to be done safely. They should be drilled frequently if water rescue or water hazards are part of the EMT's responsibilities (Fig. 23-7).

Drowning does not occur only around large bodies of water. Washing machines, bathtubs, and even 5-gallon buckets are particularly dangerous to one of the age groups at highest risk for drowning: children under 5 years of age. Teenagers and people who have been drinking alcohol are also well represented among victims of submersion incidents. Several preventative measures can be taken that may lower the incidence of drowning, which is the third most common cause of accidental death in the United States. These measures include erecting fences around swimming pools, having rescue equipment readily accessible, and using water motion alarms.

Survival after submersion is primarily related to the duration of the submersion. The longer the patient goes without oxygen, the smaller the chance of survival. Therefore the sooner artificial ventilation can be started, the better. This may mean starting ventilations while the patient is still in the water. It is recommended that chest compressions be started only after the patient is on a firm surface. Another factor that affects survival is the cleanness of the water. The more polluted the liquid, the worse the outcome is likely to be. A much discussed factor is the temperature of the water. Water temperature may be a protective factor for young patients if the water temperature is below 70° F (21° C).

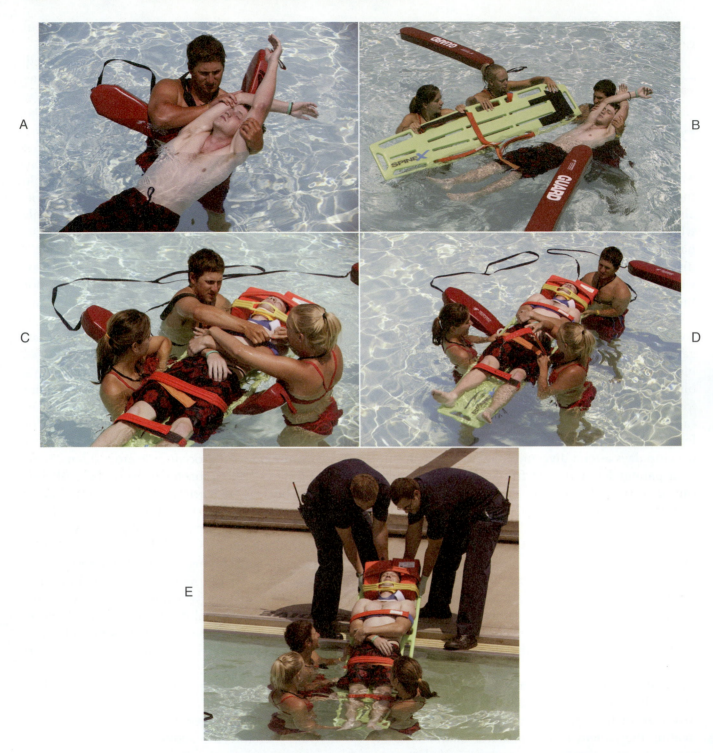

Fig. 23-7 Water rescue requires special training. **A,** Lifeguards find an unrespon-sive young man floating face down in a community pool. One rescuer reaches the victim, secures the man's head and neck between his arms, and rolls the patient's face out of the water. **B,** Two other lifeguards bring a backboard, a cervical collar (C-collar), and head blocks to the first rescuer and the patient. **C,** The backboard is floated under the patient, and the man is secured to it. **D,** After the man has been secured to the backboard, the lifeguards float the patient to the side of the pool, where EMTs are waiting. **E,** EMTs help remove the patient from the pool.

Another concern in submersion incidents is the risk of trauma. If a diving board is present or if the patient may have dived or fallen into the water from a height, spinal precautions should be taken when turning the patient over in the water and when removing the patient from the water on a backboard. This technique requires practice in both shallow and deep water before it is attempted on actual patients. Submersion patients or patients found in the water also may have other traumatic injuries, such as fractures or soft tissue injuries resulting from boat versus boat or boat versus swimmer collisions.

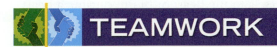

TEAMWORK

As previously discussed, EMTs work in all climates and conditions. It is extremely important that, as a member of the health care team, you keep alert to the well-being of police officers, firefighters, and others. In performing a rescue, these care providers themselves may experience an environmental emergency. As an EMT, you have an important obligation to take care of the team, including yourself.

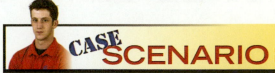

CASE SCENARIO
conclusion

Lucas is loaded into the ambulance, and Ray and a firefighter climb in with him. Although it is below freezing outside, Ray is sweating profusely, because the temperature in the back of the ambulance is quite warm by now. Ray continues to ventilate Lucas with the bag-mask device and high-flow, humidified oxygen. The firefighter continues to provide chest compressions, steadying himself with one hand braced against the ambulance wall as they rush to the hospital. Although Lucas is attached to the AED, Ray keeps the lid closed to prevent the unit from inadvertently defibrillating the patient.

Shortly after the ambulance arrives at the emergency department (ED), the attending physician takes Lucas's rectal temperature. She decides that the boy is warm enough to try one more defibrillation attempt. One shock converts the ventricular fibrillation. As blood flow returns to the heart muscle, it begins to contract more forcefully. The ED nurse soon is able to detect a brachial pulse. Although a challenging recovery lies ahead, Lucas has taken the first big step toward surviving what could have been a tragic event. ■

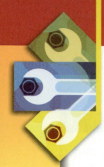

NUTS AND BOLTS

Critical Points

- EMTs must be able to recognize the signs and symptoms of possible heat and hypothermia emergencies.
- EMTs must be aware of risk factors (e.g., age, prior medical history, and medication use) and how they may affect a patient subjected to an environmental emergency.
- EMTs must be aware of the risks involved in many environmental emergency situations and must take steps to protect themselves and other members of the health care and rescue teams.

Learning Checklist

- ❏ Extremes of environment are a danger to both the patient and the rescuer. They can occur not only in the wilderness but also in suburban and urban EMS settings.
- ❏ The elderly and the very young are particularly vulnerable to environmental injuries.
- ❏ The five mechanisms by which the body removes or gains heat are conduction, convection, evaporation, respiration, and radiation.
- ❏ Hypothermia often is caused by environmental exposures such as falling into cold water or lying on the cold ground. It also can have a metabolic cause, such as cancer or infection.
- ❏ The three types of hypothermia—mild, moderate, and severe—are based on the patient's signs and symptoms. In all cases of hypothermia, it is important that rewarming be done carefully and in an environment that protects the patient from the cold and refreezing.
- ❏ Small parts of the body, such as the fingers, toes, ears, and tip of the nose, are common sites of cold injury.
- ❏ The most common forms of local cold injury are frostbite, chilblains, and cold urticaria.
- ❏ Heat illness can range from relatively mild (heat cramps) to severe and life-threatening (heatstroke).
- ❏ Classic heatstroke has a slower onset, which may occur over several days during a heat

wave. Exertional heatstroke occurs quickly during muscular activity, often in otherwise fit or well-conditioned individuals.
- ❏ Fatigue, exertion, diet, and dehydration, along with the speed of ascent, all contribute to altitude illness.
- ❏ The mildest form of altitude illness is acute mountain sickness (AMS). More severe forms are high altitude pulmonary edema (HAPE) and high altitude cerebral edema (HACE).
- ❏ Decompression sickness, a condition commonly seen in scuba divers that is caused by increased pressure, can develop days after a dive. Bubbles in the blood can block blood vessels to the heart or brain, causing a heart attack or stroke.
- ❏ It is estimated that 80,000 submersion incidents occur each year in the United States, with about 9,000 deaths. It is particularly important to ensure rescuer safety in water incidents.
- ❏ Survival of submersion is primarily related to the duration of the submersion. The longer the patient goes without oxygen, the smaller the chance of survival. Therefore the sooner artificial ventilation can be started, the better.

Key Terms

Acute mountain sickness (AMS) The mildest form of altitude illness.

Barotrauma Illness or injury caused by a sudden change in pressure.

Chilblains Redness or swelling of the skin caused by excessive exposure to cold.

Classic heatstroke A form of heatstroke that has a slower onset, possibly occurring over several days during a heat wave.

Cold urticaria Wheals caused by exposure to cold.

Conduction The transfer of heat energy from a warmer object to a cooler one as a result of direct contact.

Convection The transfer of heat through a gas or liquid by the circulation of heated particles.

Decompression sickness A painful, sometimes fatal condition caused by the formation of nitrogen bubbles in the tissue of divers, caisson workers, and aviators who move too rapidly from a higher to a lower atmospheric pressure.

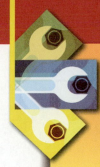

Drowning Asphyxiation caused by submersion in a liquid.

Evaporation Change in a substance from a liquid to a gas.

Exertional heatstroke A form of heatstroke that occurs during muscular activity, often in otherwise fit or well-conditioned individuals.

Frostbite The traumatic effect of extreme cold on skin and subcutaneous tissues. The first sign is distinct pallor of exposed skin surfaces, particularly the nose, ears, fingers, and toes.

Frostnip Superficial frostbite.

Heat cramps Any cramp or painful spasm of the voluntary muscles in the arms, legs, or abdomen that occurs after several hours of sustained activity in hot environments with excessive sweating.

Heat exhaustion A heat-related emergency that involves excessive loss of water or salts.

Heat index The combination of heat and humidity.

Heatstroke The severest but rarest form of heat illness. It results from failure of the temperature-regulating capacity of the body, which can be caused by prolonged exposure to the sun or to high temperatures.

High altitude cerebral edema (HACE) The severest form of acute high altitude illness. It is characterized by a progression of global cerebral signs in the presence of acute mountain sickness

High altitude pulmonary edema (HAPE) A form of pulmonary edema that occurs in people who move rapidly to higher altitudes. Fluid accumulates in the lungs as atmospheric pressure decreases.

Hypothermia An abnormal and dangerous condition in which the body temperature falls below 95° F (35° C), and the body's normal functions are impaired. This occurs because heat loss to the environment exceeds heat production by metabolism.

Radiation Movement to another area; often used to describe pain that moves from one location to another.

Respiration The physiologic process by which oxygen drawn into the lungs is delivered to tissues and cells throughout the body and exchanged for the waste products of cell metabolism.

Trench foot Moist gangrene of the foot that is caused by freezing of wet skin; also known as *immersion foot*.

National Standard Curriculum Objectives

Cognitive Objectives
After completing this lesson, the EMT student will be able to do the following:

- Describe the various ways the body loses heat.
- List the signs and symptoms of exposure to cold.
- Explain the steps in providing emergency medical care to a patient exposed to cold.
- List the signs and symptoms of exposure to heat.
- Explain the steps in providing emergency medical care to a patient exposed to heat.
- Recognize the signs and symptoms of water-related emergencies.
- Describe the complications of near-drowning.
- Discuss the emergency medical care of bites and stings.

Affective Objectives
No objectives identified.

Psychomotor Objectives
After completing this lesson, the EMT student will be able to do the following:

- Demonstrate the assessment and emergency medical care of a patient with exposure to cold.
- Demonstrate the assessment and emergency medical care of a patient with exposure to heat.
- Demonstrate the assessment and emergency medical care of a near-drowning patient.
- Demonstrate the completion of a prehospital care report for patients subjected to environmental emergencies.

NUTS AND BOLTS

CHAPTER OUTLINE

LESSON GOAL

"It has been estimated that as much as 20% of the U.S. population has some form of a mental health problem and that one person out of every seven will require treatment at some point in their life for an emotional disturbance."[1] As an emergency medical technician, you will encounter individuals who are experiencing behavioral emergencies. Approaching these situations requires a special set of skills. Understanding the causes of these behavioral emergencies will help you to recognize these patients and to manage their condition effectively. Strong communication skills are essential to providing support to the patient and preventing the situation from escalating. The emergency medical technician must be able to identify, assess, and treat patients with behavioral emergencies appropriately. This includes those patients with a psychiatric history and substance abuse. This chapter presents information on the causes, signs, symptoms, and the treatment for behavioral emergencies. ■

Behavioral Emergencies

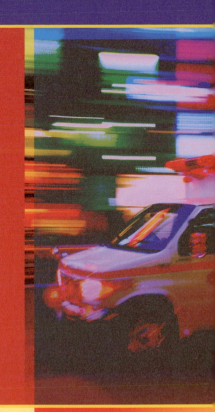

CHAPTER OBJECTIVES

24

After completing this chapter, the EMT student will be able to do the following:

1 Define these terms:

Suicide	Homicidal patient	Crisis
Depression	Mania	Delusions
Disorganization	Paranoia	Hallucinations
Disorientation	Phobia	Psychosis
Disruptive behavior	Regression	Hysteria
Domestic violence	Schizophrenia	Catatonia

2 Define behavioral emergencies.

3 Discuss the general factors that may cause a change in a patient's behavior.

4 State the various reasons for psychological crises.

5 Discuss the special considerations for assessing a patient with behavioral problems.

6 Explain the role drugs and alcohol play in behavioral emergencies.

7 Explain how substance abuse affects a patient's behavior.

8 List physical problems that can be caused by psychiatric problems.

9 Discuss the general elements of an individual's behavior that suggest he or she is at risk for violence.

10 Discuss methods to calm behavioral emergency patients.

11 List steps to initiate crisis management procedures.

Continued

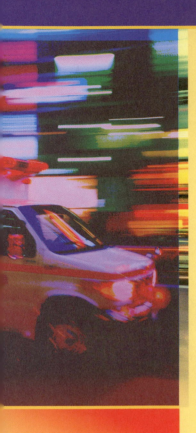

Chapter Objectives—cont'd

12 Discuss the characteristics of an individual's behavior that suggest the patient is at risk for suicide.

13 Discuss special medical/legal considerations for managing behavioral emergencies.

14 Describe the actions to take for the following situations:

Aggressive behavior   Assault

Domestic violence   Rape

Suicide attempt

15 Identify and describe the signs and symptoms for the following:

Anxiety   Depression   Domestic violence

Mania   Schizophrenia   Suicidal tendencies

16 Describe the emergency medical treatment for the patient experiencing the following:

Anxiety   Depression   Domestic violence

Mania   Schizophrenia   Suicide attempt

17 List the indications and procedures for restraining a violent patient.

18 Explain the rationale for learning how to modify your behavior toward the patient who is experiencing a behavioral emergency.

19 Demonstrate the assessment and emergency medical care of the patient who is experiencing a behavioral emergency.

20 Demonstrate various techniques safely to restrain a patient who is having a behavioral problem.

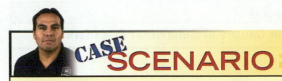

CASE SCENARIO

Rafael and his crew could hear the patient screaming from inside the apartment as they stepped off the engine. They also could hear the crashing of plates, glasses, and larger objects. The captain picked up the radio to request a speedy police response to their location while the rest of the engine crew gathered their gear and waited. Within a minute a patrol car pulled up behind the engine, followed by another patrol car.

"Well, this ought to be interesting," the captain said as they followed the police officers up to the door. An older man met them there. He appeared disheveled, with some cuts to his face and arms. Waving off any assistance, the man quickly relayed the story of his wife, who was apparently tearing up the house. "She doesn't know what's she's doing. This happens when she stops taking her medications. I've told her psychiatrist this, but he never follows up!"

They carefully enter the house. One of the police officers calls out, "Mrs. Gainer! Mrs. Gainer! This is the police and fire departments! We are coming in!" This elicited more screaming from the patient, who was somewhere toward the back of the home.

As Rafael moved toward the sounds with the rest of the rescuers, he saw broken glass, furniture, and pictures strewn around the floor.

In the back bedroom, an older woman was in the corner, her back toward the police officers. In one hand she held what appeared to be a broken broomstick. She appeared to be mumbling to herself, her eyes focused on the floor in front of her.

"Mrs. Gainer, can we help you?"

She screamed again and smashed the stick against the wall, as if trying to hit something. "Kill these spiders! Kill them! They're all over the place!" she cried out.

Question: *How should Rafael approach this situation? What communication skills should he use to gain the trust of the patient?*

BEHAVIORAL EMERGENCIES

Mental illness accounts for a significant number of adults who are disabled, either permanently or temporarily, in the United States. Mental illness is a lay term for a psychiatric disorder. This includes but is not limited to any changes in perception of the environment, thought disturbance, **paranoia, depression,** or a psychotic break. A simpler definition of mental illness might include abnormal thought. However, what "normal" thought entails is difficult to define exactly. Most persons would define "normal" as behavior that is accepted in their culture. "Abnormal behavior" would include any one of the following criteria:

1. An act that deviates from the norm of a specific culture.
2. An act that is disruptive to an individual's functioning or health.
3. An act that is harmful to oneself or others.

A behavioral emergency is defined as any behavior that results in one of these three "abnormal" criteria being met and requires immediate attention to ensure the safety of everyone involved. Behavioral emergencies may range from an individual having thoughts of **suicide** to a paranoid individual holding hostages. The behavioral emergencies may be caused by multiple factors (Box 24-1).

BOX 24-1
Vocabulary

Psychosis is a mental disorder involving disorganization of thought to the point that the person may be unable to care for himself or herself and poses a risk to himself or herself or others. This disorder commonly occurs in schizophrenia and severe mania.

General Factors Causing Altered Behavior

Genetic, chemical imbalances in the brain and social stressors are a few of the suspected causes for altered behavior. Exactly when or what will cause a behavioral emergency for a particular individual is currently unknown. An important note is that not everyone experiencing a behavioral emergency will present in exactly the same manner.

Specific Reasons and Causes for Altered Behavior

Psychological Causes

Psychological causes, also termed *functional causes,* may trigger a change in the behavior of a normally functioning individual. Certain mental illnesses present at various ages throughout the development of an individual. For example, **schizophrenia,** a disease discussed later in this chapter, has a tendency to show symptoms in men in their 20s and women in their 30s. Genetics also is believed to play a role, and depression actually may be an inheritable disease. In other instances, a social situation or life-altering situation may cause depression to manifest in a person with no previous symptoms.

Medical Causes

Medical causes of altered behavior are termed *organic.* These causes tend to be sudden changes resulting from a medical event. Box 24-2 highlights the most common medical causes of behavioral disorders. Changes in thought and emotion are not uncommon in these cases.

Intracranial Causes

Any intracranial process that causes bleeding, increased pressure, or loss of function of a portion of the brain may cause a change in an individual's behavior. Examples of such processes include tumors (cancer), traumatic or nontraumatic intracranial bleeds, dementia (loss of functioning brain tissue), and loss of blood flow (stroke). A specific example is an individual suffering from a brain tumor. As the tumor increases in size, considerable pressure is put on areas of the brain, which causes the behavioral abnormality.

Infectious Causes

Infectious illness also may cause a change in behavior because of swelling (edema). An example of such an infectious illness is meningitis, inflammation of

---

BOX 24-2

Medical Causes of Behavioral Disorders

Metabolic
Electrolyte disturbance (sodium, glucose, potassium, magnesium)
Hypoxia
Renal failure (kidney failure)
Liver failure

Infectious Disease
Encephalitis
Meningitis
Brain abscess
Sepsis (severe systemic illness)

Drug Reactions
Alcohol abuse
Narcotics
Hallucinogens (LSD [lysergic acid diethylamide])

Cardiovascular Emergencies
Hypotension
Abnormal heart rhythm

Intracranial Process
Brain tumor
Dementia (or Alzheimer's disease)
Stroke
Postseizure
Traumatic bleed

---

the lining of the brain and spinal cord. Another infectious illness that may cause abnormal behavior is encephalopathy (inflammation of the brain).

Metabolic Causes

Metabolic causes for altered behavior include diabetic emergencies, a change in electrolytes (blood salts), hypoxia, and failure of major organs. Many persons may suffer from a disease process for years before suffering any metabolic emergency. As with other causes of behavioral emergencies, the reaction of each individual will be unique. Therefore, one must obtain a history of prior illnesses, for this may provide a clue to the cause.

Psychosocial/Situational Causes

Mental illness may result from a wide variety of psychosocial causes. Traumatic events are a common cause for a change in behavior. A specific example is a posttraumatic stress reaction of a soldier who was involved in violent combat. Another example is an individual who was the victim of child abuse and is unable to cope as an adult.

Alcohol and Drug Use and Abuse

Alcohol and drugs play an important role in medical, toxicologic, and behavioral emergencies. Alcohol and drugs interfere with the ability of the brain to process and evaluate environmental stimuli. These substances also alter behavior. Patients may use such substances as a means to self-medicate or sometimes as a means to commit suicide.

Certain substances can induce **hallucinations** and **delusions.** These substances also may cause erratic and violent behavior. All patients with suspected drug or alcohol ingestion should be suspected to have behavioral abnormalities. For more information, see Chapter 22.

Assessing a Patient with a Behavioral Emergency

The fact that scene safety is the most important step in assessing a patient who is experiencing a behavioral emergency cannot be overemphasized. Many dangers arise when one is dealing with patients in these situations. These patients are often not aware that they are experiencing changes in their perception of events. It should be a common dispatch center practice for all known behavioral emergencies that the police be sent to and present at the scene. If this is impractical, one should take every precaution to ensure the safety of the crew and bystanders.

When responding to a call involving a behavioral emergency, the emergency medical technician (EMT) may have time to plan and prepare. One must remember that any emergency medical services (EMS) call may involve a behavioral emergency. Many individuals will call for help but may be too embarrassed to state the actual reason they are calling. For example, a patient may state that he or she is bleeding but fail to mention he or she slit his or her wrists intentionally with a razor blade.

After reviewing dispatch information and assessing overall scene safety, carefully observe the patient from the door of the room or residence. Pay special attention to the patient's condition, posture, speech, and possession or presence of weapons. Remember, any object may become a weapon if a patient feels threatened.

The EMT should approach the patient carefully. A suicidal patient actually may want to receive medical treatment, whereas another individual who is para-

noid may feel threatened when approached. Therefore, movements should be slow and calculated. Moreover, maintain an easy exit at all times.

Talking to the patient is important. This provides valuable information about the condition and mental state of the patient. Begin by introducing yourself and others who are part of the response team. Attempt to build confidence with the patient by creating a good rapport.

Also important is to remember that physical ailments can result from psychiatric problems. Patients with psychiatric problems may not seek medical attention and therefore also may have medical conditions that have not been treated. Examples of such conditions include untreated diabetes mellitus, poor hygiene leading to abscess and gangrene, poor nutrition, and organ failure. Therefore, when one is responding to behavioral emergencies, it is critical to treat the emergency and any medical conditions.

Initial Assessment

The primary survey is as important for the patient experiencing a behavioral emergency as for any other non-psychiatric patient. This step should not be overlooked. Remember, a number of causes of behavioral emergencies are due to medical emergencies. If you note any abnormalities, address them.

Focused History

Conduct the secondary survey with special attention to history. Ask about the standard information such as name, age, medical history, and medications. Additionally, it is important to ask specific questions in terms of psychiatric history. An example is to ask the patient, "Do you have a history of depression?" If the answer is yes, it would be appropriate to ask about medications and compliance with taking those medications. To ask what situation caused the patient's current state also would be appropriate.

Calming and Crisis Management Techniques for Behavioral Emergencies

Some patients are difficult to assist when they are experiencing a behavioral emergency. However, it is important to keep in mind that many situations can be defused with a few simple techniques:

1. Anticipating any changes in scene safety is the first step to eliminating tension in any environment. Enlist law enforcement as needed (Fig. 24-1).
2. Designate one contact person for the patient/EMS provider interaction.

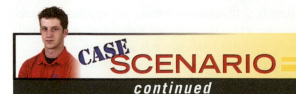

CASE SCENARIO
continued

Mrs. Gainer sat on the edge of the bed. Rafael used a low-key, nonconfrontational approach, taking care that his mannerisms and voice were nonthreatening. As he spoke with the patient, she became less animated but remained openly hostile. However, with encouragement and reassurance, she did what Rafael asked in putting down the potential weapon. Rafael continued to speak with her calmly, making sure not to appear aggressive.

One of the police officers quietly asked Rafael, "Do you want us to take her now?"

Question: *Should Ray allow the police to take the patient to the hospital? What are some techniques or procedures Rafael should perform now?*

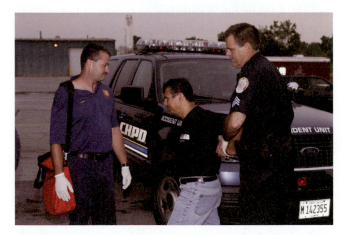

Fig. 24-1 Emergency medical technicians should foster good working relationships with law enforcement personnel because they can assist with violent and uncooperative patients.

3. Speak in a slow, relaxed tone. Do not insult, antagonize, or mimic any patient who is experiencing a behavioral emergency. This can escalate the situation.
4. If the patient is experiencing hallucinations or delusions, explain what truly is occurring. Do not play into the patient's delusions or hallucinations in an attempt to earn trust or to coerce. This is dangerous.

5. Finally, use restraints only as a last resort. Attempt to negotiate and explain all procedures clearly. Enlist medical control and follow protocols.

■ SPECIFIC BEHAVIORAL EMERGENCIES

Anxiety

Anxiety is a condition that everyone experiences at some time in his or her life. Anxiety is characterized by feelings of fear that often are accompanied by physiologic symptoms. Anxiety is a normal response in certain situations. The diagnosis of anxiety is given to those individuals who experience severe and persistent feelings of fear. Other subcategories of anxiety include phobias and panic attacks. A **phobia** is an irrational fear that often provokes anxiety; therefore, it is included in this discussion of anxiety. A panic attack is the sudden onset of anxiety when a person is placed in a stressful situation.

Signs and Symptoms

Physical symptoms of anxiety include difficulty in breathing, chest discomfort, sweating, shaking, and syncope (Box 24-3). Treatment begins by dealing with the patient respectfully. The patient's symptoms are a real physiologic response. Although it may appear that he or she is overreacting or that his or her fears are unfounded, it is important to remember that the patient feels all of these physical symptoms (Boxes 24-4 and 24-5).

Assessment and Treatment

Approach the patient cautiously. One EMT should talk with the patient and try to establish good communication. The patient may be taking medication for this condition. Antidepressants and anxiolytics commonly are prescribed as preventative medications. Benzodi-

BOX 24-3
Physical Symptoms and Medical Conditions Associated with Anxiety
Hyperventilation Dyspnea Choking, difficulty swallowing Numbness and tingling in hands, feet, and around the mouth Racing or pounding heart Dizziness Fainting Sweating

azepines often are used in acute situations. When taking a medical history, be sure to document the medications taken and the amount. If the anxiety is severe, a patient possibly may overmedicate himself or herself in an attempt to treat his or her symptoms.

If a patient is experiencing a phobia, attempt to remove the patient from the environment or remove what is causing the anxiety (i.e., a spider). Certain patients fear crowds; therefore, be aware that an entire crew may cause the situation to worsen. Limiting contact to one EMS provider may help alleviate anxiety in these patients.

Depression

Depression is a common impairment. This condition often affects a person's normal daily functioning. Depression can interfere with a patient's ability to interact with friends and family and to perform work functions. The symptoms are defined by the *Diagnostic and Statistical Manual of Mental Disorders*, fourth edition (DSM-IV),[2] which is written by psychiatrists who specialize in the treatment and diagnosis of mental illness. Box 24-6 contains a summary of

symptoms that typically are noted in depression. Depression is characterized by at least five symptoms for a minimum of 2 weeks.[3] These symptoms should not be attributed to substance abuse, a general medical condition, or a life event such as bereavement.

Signs and Symptoms

Symptoms of depression include feelings of despair, failure, worthlessness, and isolation; weight loss/gain; and sleep disturbances or disorders (Box 24-7). Some symptoms may be minor. These include changes in normal activities or loss of interest in activities. With this depression comes an increased risk of suicide.

SPECIAL Populations

Elderly patients are particularly at risk for what some practitioners refer to as the "3 Ds"—depression, dementia, and delirium. The emergency medical technician should always try to determine whether the presentation is of new onset, because a number of medical emergencies can have a similar presentation.

Assessment and Treatment

One must assume that a patient may be suicidal when he or she states that he or she is depressed. The EMT should approach these patients carefully. One EMT should talk with the patient and attempt to establish a good rapport. Asking direct questions such as "Do you want to hurt yourself?" and "Do you have a plan?" is important (Box 24-8). Asking these questions does not increase the risk of suicide but does allow the EMT to assess the potential severity of the patient's depression. These patients need to be transported to the hospital for further medical evaluation (Box 24-9).

Mania

Mania often is found in patients with bipolar disorder. This disorder is characterized by periods of depression alternating with improved mood and increased activity. These patients often seem to be euphoric and have inflated views of their importance.

Signs and Symptoms

Characteristics of mania include excessive mood elevation, talkativeness, increased activity, risk taking, and expressions of grandeur. These patients often en-

gage in risky behavior because they feel they are invincible and incapable of getting hurt.

Assessment and Treatment

Patients experiencing mania should be approached carefully, and the EMT should be firm. These patients often will make statements indicating that they do not need help; however, this is not true. In fact, they are at risk of harming themselves. One EMT should communicate with the patient. In addition, environmental stimulation should be minimal. Minimal stimulation includes, for example, quiet transport with no lights and sirens. Loud sounds, bright lights, or voices can irritate these individuals further. These patients pose a significant risk to themselves, and transport is necessary.

Schizophrenia

Schizophrenia is actually a group of disorders that often demonstrate psychotic behavior characterized by disturbances in thought processes, including disorganized or bizarre thoughts. The disease can be genetic. Patients who suffer from schizophrenia account for a large percentage of the homeless population. These patients often make poor decisions. In fact, others may take advantage of them. Medications are available and have been used with success. Generally, exacerbations occur when the patient does not take medications or when patients attempt to self-medicate with alcohol or street drugs. This is called **regression** (Boxes 24-10 and 24-11).

Signs and Symptoms

A primary symptom of schizophrenia is disturbances in the normal thought process. Patients may have hallucinations, delusions, and paranoia. These patients often have bizarre thoughts that they firmly believe to be fact. They also may have thoughts that are not based in reality. Such disorganized thought is common in these patients. They often do not process information in a logical progression, and this causes their patterns of thought to be random.

When a psychotic event or **psychosis** occurs, the individual often will not be able to take care of himself or herself. Moreover, some specific conditions may develop. One of these is **catatonia**, a state in which a patient has changes in physical and emotional symptoms. With this condition, the patient may have a rigid posture or appear to be in a coma-like state. Patients also may have intense emotions, including **hysteria.**

BOX 24-10
Vocabulary

Catatonia: A disturbance that is characterized by physical and emotional symptoms. These symptoms may include rigidity, negativity, stupor, and noncommunicative states. Catatonia can occur in patients with schizophrenia. Catatonic patients may be sitting and staring into space and not communicating. Medications used to treat schizophrenia when reaching toxic levels may cause similar symptoms. Therefore transport of symptomatic patients is imperative.

Delusion: A false belief. An example of a delusion is a patient who believes that he is God or that a spaceship is landing and coming to get him.

Hallucinations: The perception of an event that is auditory or visual but not actually occurring in reality. Examples of hallucinations include the feeling of bugs crawling on the skin, one hearing voices telling him or her to hurt someone, or hearing God speak to them.

Hysteria: A disorder in which a loss of physical functioning occurs. It is often the sign of a psychological conflict or need. An example of hysteria is when an event overwhelms an individual. This includes, for example, rape, homicide, abuse, battering, and mass tragedy.

Mania: An emotional disorder characterized by euphoria, irritability, and grandiose thoughts.

Paranoia: A disorder in which a person is plagued with bizarre thoughts of persecution. An example of paranoia is a patient who thinks you are with the CIA and are coming to take him to prison for espionage.

Psychosis: A mental disorder in which there is disorganization of thought to the point that the person may be unable to take care of himself or herself. This may occur in schizophrenia or other disorders. These patients are often unaware of their psychosis.

Regression: A relapse or return of symptoms. This commonly is seen when patients discontinue therapeutic medications for schizophrenia.

BOX 24-11
Facts about Schizophrenia[1]

- More than 2 million adult Americans are affected by schizophrenia.
- In men, schizophrenia usually appears in the late teens or early 20s.
- In women, schizophrenia usually appears in the 20s to early 30s.
- Schizophrenia affects men and women with equal frequency.
- Most persons with schizophrenia suffer chronically throughout their lives.
- One of every 10 persons with schizophrenia eventually commits suicide.
- Schizophrenia costs the nation more than $32 billion annually.

and state your title. You may need to repeat this information. One must speak to the patient and not just to his or her family members as if the patient were not even there. Speaking only to family members could diminish the patient's sense of control. Finally, do not feed into the patient's delusions or hallucinations. These patients actually believe that what they are seeing and hearing is fact. One must try to discuss only real sights and sounds. Transport is imperative for further medical management because these patients may pose a harm to themselves and others.

Domestic Violence

Domestic violence consists of physical, emotional, or sexual abuse. This form of violence may be directed toward any person who is in a family relationship with the abuser. Common types of abuse include spousal, child, and elder abuse (Fig. 24-2). Abuse is a common problem. Abuse often results in the manipulation of the abused individual. The abuser often has issues with control, power, and feelings of superiority. Many abused individuals see their situation as hopeless and that they have no way out. As an EMS provider, you must understand domestic violence, abuse, and battering syndromes. Often the EMS provider helps the abused individual to seek help to terminate this cycle.

Signs and Symptoms

Victims of abuse often display multiple injuries in various stages of healing. They may not report their injuries immediately. This delay is often an attempt to protect the abuser and to see whether their injuries will heal spontaneously. In addition, the abused may

Assessment and Treatment

One must approach any patient in a behavioral emergency carefully. If the patient feels like he or she is being pursued or threatened, the patient may attempt to harm the EMT. Many patients experiencing behavioral emergencies are prone to paranoia, which aggravates or creates a perceived threat. Clear communication with these patients is important. Introduce yourself

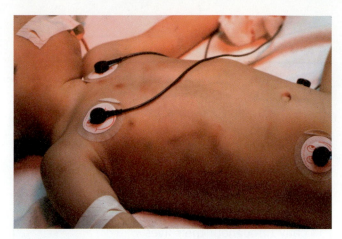

Fig. 24-2 Signs of child abuse.

be a substance abuser as a method of dulling the pain or hiding from his or her situation. Suicidal gestures are often a cry for help from the abused. Moreover, frequent calls and cancellations for EMS assistance are common for domestic violence situations.

A trait often found in the abuser is impulse control. Abusers often cannot control their rage or anger. They commonly appear concerned and apologetic after they have hurt someone for whom they care. This sets up the cycle for verbal exchange, abuse, and apologies.

Assessment and Treatment for General Domestic Violence

One must be sympathetic and kind to patients who have sustained any form of abuse. Reprimanding these patients for returning to their abuser is not helpful. In fact, it actually may further harm the patient's self-esteem. The patient should receive a standard assessment, beginning with the initial assessment. Treat physical injuries. Arrange transport so that further medical care can be rendered. It is critical not to confront the abuser or to assume that a partner or parent is the guilty party. Confrontation only will escalate an already tense situation. Moreover, scene safety must be a priority with these calls because they tend to be violent situations. Follow local protocols for regulations and rules regarding police involvement.

Assessment and Treatment for Rape Victims

Rape is defined as unwanted sexual contact. Rape victims can be of any age and either gender. Patients may be afraid to discuss their situation with multiple care providers present. The EMT must be sensitive to this and ensure that a single caregiver communicates with the patient in as private a setting as possible and appropriate in the situation. The patient may have a preference as to the gender of the EMT who is going to communicate and examine him or her. Cooperation regarding this is helpful

in establishing trust and helping to calm the patient in an already overwhelming situation.

Examine the patient with careful attention to evidence preservation. Notify the police of this violent crime, and they will handle the evidence. In the event that the arrival of law enforcement is delayed, place any clothing that may have been removed from the patient or other evidence in a paper bag (Fig. 24-3). If a biohazard bag is to be used because paper is unavailable or there are hazard concerns, leave the top open. Humidity and moisture trapped in a plastic bag may destroy DNA evidence.

The focus of the patient care should be attention to medical problems and traumatic injury. The EMT should avoid specific questions regarding the details of the sexual assault. Most hospitals have trained doctors, nurses, police officers, or counselors who can obtain that information. The priority for the EMT must be patient safety and treatment of all medical and emotional conditions.

Assessment and Treatment for Assault Victims

Assault is a threat of any kind. This includes verbal, physical, or emotional threats. Battery is the unwanted touching of another person. All patients who have been assaulted should be encouraged to file a police report. The EMS provider or hospital is responsible to notify the police in any case in which assault is suspected. Treatment of assault victims should be similar to that of sexual assault victims. All medical and traumatic injuries should be treated. The provider should attempt to preserve evidence as well.

Suicidal Patients

Most EMS providers have responded to an emergency involving a suicidal patient. A suicide attempt is a sign that an individual is in **crisis.** The attempt may

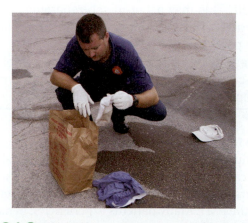

Fig. 24-3 Evidence, such as any clothing removed from the patient, may be placed in paper bags if police arrival is delayed.

be a cry for help or a real attempt to end one's life. These individuals commonly suffer from other emotional issues (Box 24-12). If the patient has developed a plan or has made a previous attempt, it is important to take the person seriously and not to minimize his or her actions.

Women attempt suicide more often than men. However, men are more successful. This is often because men use more violent and rapid means. Those who are successful at completing suicide often have made an unsuccessful attempt in the past.

Signs and Symptoms

Suicidal patients often suffer from depression, anxiety, or a particular stress. They may complain of feelings of hopelessness or feeling like they have no way out of a particular situation. These patients may try violent methods of ending their life, such as cutting their wrists, using a firearm, wrecking or crashing a motor vehicle, or hanging themselves. Other methods include toxic ingestion, overdose, and substance abuse.

Assessment and Treatment

Approach suicidal patients with caution. They may have a weapon or be in a toxic environment (i.e., carbon monoxide). Complete a full initial and secondary assessment. Treat all injuries and medical conditions. Once all medical conditions are treated and the patient is stabilized, complete a specific history similar to the one listed under depression. Transport all suicidal patients for definitive medical care. Documentation should be a priority.

Violent and Aggressive Patients

Violent and aggressive behavior is increasing in society every day. The reasons for the increase are numerous. However, identification is the most important step in preventing injury resulting from the violence

and aggression. There are many predictors of violent behavior. One of the most significant predictors is any individual who has a history of violence or has been violent in the past. Because substance abuse alters the perception of environmental stimuli and behavior, it is important to anticipate violence in drug and alcohol abuse. Another indicator of impending violence is the posture and tone of voice of the patient. Often rage is present and can be observed from a distance. Finally, the actual bodily or physical movement of a patient is important to observe. Patients who are moving or who appear to be anxious are prone to violent outbursts.

Homicidal patients are those who wish to harm others. They are at the extreme of violent behavior. An important note is that these patients often are not operating under the same social guidelines and restraints as most patients who will be encountered. Moreover, they may not value life. Call for law enforcement for all situations involving a **homicidal patient.**

Indications for the Use of Restraint

Individuals who pose a threat to themselves or others should be restrained. No situation exists for which the EMT should place the crew in danger from a potentially violent patient. Involvement of law enforcement early is important for any call or situation that has the potential for violence. The keys to success are early preparation and anticipation. Generally, restraint of a patient who is an immediate or potential threat to himself or herself or others is acceptable.

Patients also may be deemed incompetent to refuse treatment. This is common in those patients who attempt suicide, who suffer from schizophrenia or mania, and who have consumed drugs or alcohol. You must realize that you are an advocate for these patients. If a patient is refusing transport and is incompetent, follow local protocols or contact medical control for permission to restrain the patient.

Legal Considerations

Any physical assault is a crime. Most states have mandatory reporting requirements. These mandatory requirements include the reporting of abuse, domestic violence, sexual assault, physical assault, battery of any type, and any violent crimes. If there is any question about the nature of the situation, consult medical protocols, medical control, or law enforcement. The reporting of any situation by EMS does not require that the victim press charges. Reporting is simply a method of notifying the authorities of the situation.

Documentation is also critical. An important concept medically and legally is as follows: "If it isn't writ-

---

BOX 24-12

Predictors of Suicide

History of depression
History of previous attempt
Substance abuse
Financial distress/loss of a job
Loss of a loved one
History of abuse
Divorce/widow
Older age
Male gender
Specific plan

SPECIAL Considerations

Procedures for Restraint Application

If permission is given to restrain a patient, restraint must be done with as little force as possible. Injury to a patient is generally unacceptable unless there is immediate danger to the emergency medical technician and crew. Preparation, planning, and familiarity with restraint devices is critical to the success of restraint application.

Restraint Procedures

1. Enlist the assistance of law enforcement if possible. For any homicidal patient, law enforcement should be present.
2. Anticipate that the patient can use any object as a potential weapon to defend himself or herself. If at all possible, get the patient to a safe location with no objects and with ample space. Always assume the patient is carrying a weapon, such as a pocketknife, gun, or lighter.
3. Always keep yourself between the patient and the door.
4. Always have a backup plan.
5. Be sure that adequate help and support are available. If the patient is physically strong, it may be important to wait for backup assistance.

Many commercial restraint devices are available. The emergency medical technician should become familiar and comfortable with the use of the particular kind that is carried in his or her area. If no restraint devices are available, other materials may be used. For instance, small towels, triangular bandages, webbed straps, roller bandages, and blanket rolls may be used.

When applying the restraints, move swiftly and carefully. The team should have a plan for how to approach the patient. Simultaneous restraint of all of the patient's limbs is important. This will prevent the combative patient from having the upper hand.

Once the patient is restrained, ensure that he or she is fastened securely to a fixed object, such as the stretcher or backboard. The patient's respiratory and circulatory status should be checked frequently and never compromised. Patients should never be restrained in a prone position.

When restraints are used, the process of documentation is important. On the run report, include a detailed description of the events. In addition, carefully document any attempts at negotiation and the enlistment of cooperation.

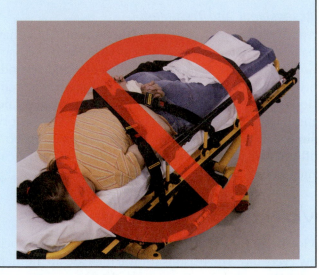

ten down, it didn't happen." This is important regarding evidence and scene preservation. Documenting findings on the run report is an effective method for ensuring that all information is going to be kept for legal proceedings. This includes documentation of the scene, witnessed altercations, wounds, traumatic injuries, and facts surrounding the incident. Place any subjective comments in quotation marks, and identify by name the person making those comments in the run report. To ensure accurate reporting, complete all run reports as soon as possible following the incident.

Patient confidentiality is critical in the establishment of trust with a patient. Confidentiality is also the law. However, there are mandatory reporting requirements that supersede the usual need to maintain confidentiality. For example, it is imperative that police be notified if any threat is made to another individual in your presence.

Because of the wide variation in state, national, and local protocols, you must become familiar with the requirements in your area.

■ VIEWS ON BEHAVIORAL EMERGENCIES

Often EMS personnel find behavioral emergencies to be a burden. The actions of the patients experiencing behavioral emergencies are difficult to comprehend and are stress provoking for others. These patients can be extremely demanding and difficult to deal with. These situations actually can cause workplace stress and burnout. The division of medicine that deals with emotional and behavioral disturbances is psychiatry. Therefore, it is appropriate to consider these patients medical patients. They have a definable illness according to the medical community. These patients often are unaware of their actions. In fact, they may require therapy or medication in order to function within societal norms. Prioritization of scene safety and that of the entire crew is important. Also crucial is to treat every individual with respect and dignity in the hope of making a difference.

SPECIAL Populations

Elderly Concern

Confused and disoriented elderly patients sometimes are found wandering or driving around without purpose and without identification. Always check for items such as a bracelet, clothing label, lapel pin, or "dog tag" to determine whether the person is enrolled in one of the increasingly popular identification programs, such as the Alzheimer's Association Safe Return program. Such tags and bracelets provide a toll-free phone number to contact the patient's relatives or caregivers.

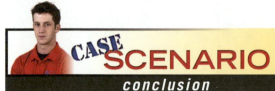

CASE SCENARIO

conclusion

The patient was sobbing, holding her hands to her face as Rafael helped load her into the back of the waiting ambulance. When she became calmer, Rafael could complete his history taking and physical exam. Her vital signs, though elevated, were within normal limits. She was confused as to time and date, although she knew she was inside her house and could recognize her husband. She did not understand when Rafael tried to explain that she had not taken her medication; however, she did not react in an aggressive way either. When the medics arrived, Rafael gave a report of what had happened. The ambulance crew continued to provide supportive care and was careful to restrain the patient's arms and legs gently once she was on the ambulance stretcher. This was to protect her and the attending medic while en route to the facility. ■

TEAMWORK

In your role as an emergency medical technician, you will encounter many types of behavioral emergencies. This may include patients who suffer from psychiatric conditions and those patients who are abused. Scene safety must remain a top priority.

These types of emergencies often involve many different facets of the emergency response system. For everyone to work well as a team and use the skills in which he or she has been trained is important. A number of ways exist by which teamwork will promote the safety of all providers and the patient. Some of these follow:

- Scene safety is critical. Patients often are unaware of their actions. Moreover, they may be under the influence of a substance. Keeping the line of communication open between the patient and the emergency medical technician is important.
- Assist with monitoring the patient's airway and vital signs. This is a critical step in caring for a patient with a behavioral emergency. The patient may have a toxic ingestion that is contributing to his or her symptoms.
- Assist with taking a thorough history.
- Contact the police if there is any indication of overdose or a scene that is unsafe.
- When restraining a patient, make sure there is adequate support for the safety of emergency medical services providers.

References

1. Sanders MJ: *Mosby's paramedic textbook*, rev ed 2, St Louis, 2001, Mosby
2. American Psychiatric Association: *Diagnostic and statistical manual of mental disorders*, ed 4, Washington, DC, 1994, The Association.
3. Rosen P, Barker FJ, Braen R: *Rosen's emergency medicine concepts and clinical practice*, ed 5, St Louis, 2002, Mosby.

Resources

American Psychiatric Association: *American Psychiatric Association practice guideline for the treatment of psychiatric disorders: compendium 2004*, Washington, DC, 2004, The Association.

Berry DB: *The domestic violence sourcebook*, ed 3, New York, 2000, McGraw-Hill.

Jamison KR: *Night falls fast: understanding suicide*, New York, 1999, Vintage.

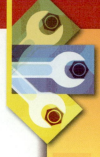

Critical Points

As an emergency medical technician, you will see various forms of behavioral emergencies. Some of these emergencies may involve life-threatening injuries and conditions of the patient. To stay focused and ensure the safety of the scene for yourself and that of your crew is critical. Remember, patients with behavioral emergencies are patients with a medical condition. They may not be aware of their actions and can be dangerous. Use restraints only when absolutely necessary. When using restraint devices, make sure that you are prepared and have adequate help. Contact the police as necessary for assistance. When treating any patient, focus on all parts of the assessment, beginning with the primary survey.

Learning Checklist

❑ Mental illness accounts for a significant number of disabled adults in the United States.
❑ A behavioral emergency consists of any patient exhibiting a behavior that is abnormal or that endangers himself or herself or others.
❑ Multiple factors may cause a behavioral emergency. These include biologic, medical, intracranial, infectious, metabolic, and psychosocial factors, as well as substance use and abuse.
❑ When assessing a patient with a behavioral emergency, one must keep scene safety as the top priority. Contact law enforcement before any call that appears to be dangerous.
❑ All patients experiencing a behavioral emergency should receive a full assessment. This includes a primary and secondary survey. A complete history is also helpful.
❑ When approaching a patient with a behavioral emergency, always assume that he or she has a weapon.
❑ One emergency medical technician should approach and talk with the patient. Use of a quiet voice may be calming to the patient.
❑ Anxiety develops when a fear causes a physical reaction.

❑ Symptoms of anxiety include changes in breathing, chest pain, racing heartbeat, and sweating.
❑ A phobia can provoke symptoms similar to those exhibited in anxiety.
❑ Depression can cause physical symptoms, such as weight loss and sleep abnormalities.
❑ Depression is defined by the loss of interest in activities and feelings of despair and hopelessness.
❑ Mania is defined by feelings of euphoria and grandeur.
❑ Schizophrenia can occur with signs of disorganized thought, random thoughts, delusions, hallucinations, catatonia, hysteria, or violence.
❑ Schizophrenic patients often are homeless if their disease is untreated. They also may be incapable of taking care of themselves.
❑ Regression occurs when a relapse is in a process. This often occurs when a schizophrenic patient does not take his or her medication.
❑ Paranoia occurs when a person feels threatened.
❑ Domestic violence is a national problem. Situations involving domestic violence can escalate. One should take extreme caution.
❑ Any form of abuse should be reported to the police.
❑ Any violent act should be reported to the police.
❑ Restraints should be used as a last resort.
❑ Documentation is essential for all behavioral emergencies.
❑ Remember, individuals suffering from behavioral emergencies have a medical condition.

Key Terms

Catatonia A disturbance characterized by physical and emotional symptoms. These symptoms may include rigidity, negativity, stupor, and noncommunicative states.
Crisis An overwhelming event.
Delusions False beliefs.
Depression A mental state characterized by feelings of loneliness, sadness, low self-esteem, and self-reproach.

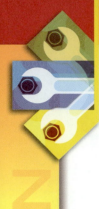

Disorganization Interruptions in normal thought process or randomization of thought process.

Disorientation Loss of familiarity with one's surroundings.

Disruptive behavior Any behavior that is deemed inappropriate for the environment or that others find disturbing.

Domestic violence Intentionally inflicted injury caused by family members or those of close relation.

Hallucinations Perception of an event, often auditory or visual, that actually is not occurring in reality.

Homicidal patient A person who has the intention of harming another person.

Hysteria A disorder in which a loss of physical functioning occurs. It is often the sign of a psychological conflict or need.

Mania An emotional disorder characterized by euphoria, irritability, and grandiose thoughts.

Paranoia A disorder in which a person is plagued with bizarre thoughts of persecution.

Phobia An irrational fear.

Psychosis A mental disorder in which there is often disorganization of thought to the point that the person may be unable to care for himself or herself.

Regression A relapse or return of symptoms.

Schizophrenia A psychotic disorder characterized by distortions of reality. Disturbances in language and communication may occur. The patient also may have bizarre thoughts, including those of persecution, paranoia, and hallucinations.

Suicide An attempt by a person to end his or her life.

National Standard Curriculum Objectives

Cognitive Objectives

After completing this lesson, the EMT student will be able to do the following:

- Define these terms:

Suicide	Homicidal patient	Crisis
Depression	Mania	Delusions
Disorganization	Paranoia	Hallucinations
Disorientation	Phobia	Psychosis
Disruptive behavior	Regression	Hysteria
Domestic violence	Schizophrenia	Catatonia

- Define behavioral emergencies.
- Discuss the general factors that may cause a change in a patient's behavior.
- State the various reasons for psychological crises.
- Discuss the special considerations for assessing a patient with behavioral problems.
- Explain the role drugs and alcohol play in behavioral emergencies.
- Explain how substance abuse affects a patient's behavior.
- List physical problems that can be caused by psychiatric problems.
- Discuss the general factors of an individual's behavior that suggest he or she is at risk for violence.
- Discuss methods to calm behavioral emergency patients.
- List steps to initiate crisis management procedures.

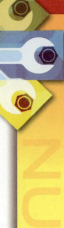

- Discuss the characteristics of an individual's behavior that suggest the patient is at risk for suicide.
- Discuss special medical/legal considerations for managing behavioral emergencies.
- Describe the actions taken by the emergency medical technician for the following situations:

  Aggressive behavior   Assault
  Domestic violence   Rape
  Suicide attempt

- Identify and describe the signs and symptoms for the following:

  | Anxiety | Depression | Domestic violence |
  | Mania | Schizophrenia | Suicidal tendencies |

- Describe the emergency medical treatment for the patient experiencing the following:

  | Anxiety | Depression | Domestic violence |
  | Mania | Schizophrenia | Suicide attempt |

- List the indications and procedures for restraining a violent patient.

Affective Objective

After completing this lesson, the EMT student will be able to do the following:

- Explain the rationale for learning how to modify your behavior toward the patient who is experiencing a behavioral emergency.

Psychomotor Objectives

After completing this lesson, the EMT student will be able to do the following:

- Demonstrate the assessment and emergency medical care of the patient who is experiencing a behavioral emergency.
- Demonstrate various techniques to restrain a patient safely who is having a behavioral problem.

References

1. Sanders MJ: *Paramedic Textbook*, ed 2, St. Louis, 2001, Mosby
2. Rosen P, Barker FJ, Braen R: *Rosen's Emergency Medicine Concepts and Clinical Practice*, ed 5, St. Louis, 2002, Mosby.
3. Modified from *The Diagnostic and Statistical Manual of Mental Disorders*, ed 4-TR, Washington, DC, 2000, American Psychiatric Association

Resources

Jamison KR: *Night Falls Fast: Understanding Suicide*, 1999, Vintage, First Vintage Books Edition, Random House

American Psychiatric Association Practice Guideline for the Treatment of Psychiatric Disorders: Compendium 2004

Berry DB: *The Domestic Violence Sourcebook*, ed 3, New York, 2000, McGraw-Hill.

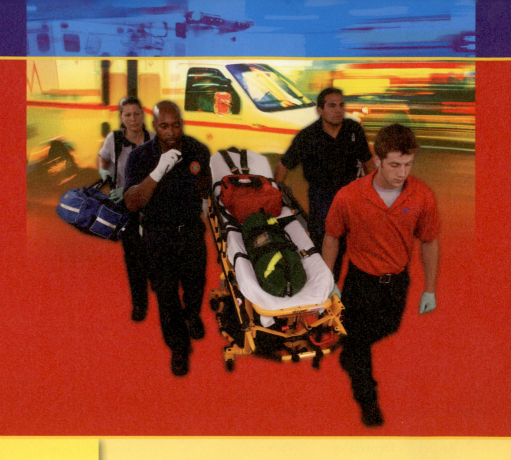

CHAPTER

25

OUTLINE

LESSON GOAL

This chapter reviews the cardiovascular system and describes the care of the patient with internal and external bleeding, signs and symptoms of shock (hypoperfusion), and the emergency medical care of shock. ∎

GOAL

Bleeding and Shock

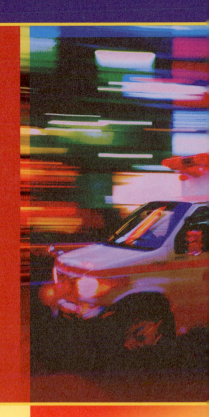

CHAPTER OBJECTIVES

After completing this chapter, the EMT student will be able to do the following:

1 List the different parts of the circulatory system and how they work.
2 Describe the differences between arterial, venous, and capillary bleeding.
3 Discuss the different ways to treat external bleeding.
4 Discuss the importance of wearing protective equipment when caring for the patient who is bleeding actively.
5 Establish the importance of airway management in the trauma patient.
6 Relate how the patient was injured to internal bleeding.
7 List the signs of internal bleeding.
8 List the steps of emergency care the patient with internal bleeding should receive.
9 List signs and symptoms of shock (hypoperfusion).
10 State the steps of emergency care the patient in shock should receive.
11 Explain the importance of rapid transport of patients with signs of shock.
12 Demonstrate the proper way to control external bleeding using direct pressure.
13 Demonstrate the proper way to control external bleeding using diffuse pressure.
14 Demonstrate the proper way to use pressure points and tourniquets to control external bleeding.
15 Show the type of emergency care the patient with internal bleeding should receive.
16 Show the type of emergency care the patient suffering from shock should receive.
17 Demonstrate the proper way to give a report on a patient with bleeding and shock.

25

OBJECTIVES

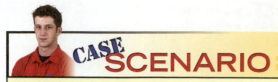

CASE SCENARIO

"Rich, what hurts you the most?" Ray asked hurriedly. Ray and his partner were working on Rich Tomasado, who had fallen off his painter's ladder about 30 minutes earlier. From the initial assessment, Ray knew that Rich was having a serious problem. His skin was cool, clammy, and pale. His heart rate was high, and his pulse weak at the wrist. He also was breathing at an accelerated rate. Judging from eyewitness reports, Rich fell about 25 feet, landing on his side partially on the sidewalk and partially on the adjacent grass. It did not appear that Rich lost consciousness. In fact, he tried to pick himself up off the ground almost immediately but had some pain to his back and left side. At first Rich did not want to go to the emergency department, but the pain grew steadily worse. In addition, he felt nauseated and progressively weaker. Using a cell phone, worried co-workers called 911. Shortly thereafter, Ray arrived with his partner and began the assessment.

"My side doesn't feel too good." Rich grimaced as Ray gently palpated through the area. Already exposed, Rich's left lateral quadrant had begun to bruise.

Question: *What could explain Rich's skin signs and other assessment findings? In addition to the abdominal injury, what other problems might Rich have that Ray will have to manage?*

In this chapter you will become familiar with the basics of the **circulatory system** and **cellular metabolism.** In addition, you will become familiar with the resulting consequences when the circulatory system is unable to function adequately, resulting in **shock.** Shock is the condition in which the cardiorespiratory system is unable to meet the oxygen and nutrient demands of the body. This leaves the cells of the body unable to produce sufficient energy to survive. This affects every organ system, tissue, and cell in the body. Some organs are more susceptible than others to the deprivation of oxygen and nutrients. Moreover, some patients may respond very differently to the same circulatory insult or injury. The patient's degree of signs or symptoms depends a great deal on his or her baseline status and the presence or absence of preexisting illness. Your goal is to become familiar with some of the causes of shock, recognize the state of shock, understand its consequences, and treat the patient based on the presumed cause. Even without aggressive intravenous fluid therapy and pharmacotherapy, numerous early interventions can improve a patient's outcome from a shock state.

■ CELLULAR METABOLISM

Every cell in the body requires nutrients and oxygen to function efficiently. The circulatory system is responsible for delivering oxygen and nutrients to the tissues. The process by which cells use the nutrients and oxygen to produce energy is called cellular metabolism or cellular respiration. When oxygen is available in sufficient amounts to the cells, **aerobic metabolism** is used to produce energy. This process of energy production using oxygen is more efficient and produces up to 18 times more energy than trying to produce energy without oxygen. Cellular metabolism is possible without oxygen for short periods of time. This is termed **anaerobic metabolism.** It results in far less energy production and in the formation of toxic metabolites. Anaerobic metabolism can continue only for a limited time before cell death ensues.

When cells are deprived of oxygen for a sufficient period of time, it is termed **hypoxia,** or lack of oxygen. Tissue hypoxia results when the tissues are no longer receiving an adequate oxygen supply from the circulatory system. This can result from decreased oxygen content in the bloodstream or reduced supply of oxygenated blood to the tissues. Under these conditions the cells can no longer produce sufficient en-

ASK YOURSELF

Have you ever wondered what we mean when we say someone is in shock? Were they electrocuted? Scared? Bleeding? Can the emergency medical technician do anything to stop shock?

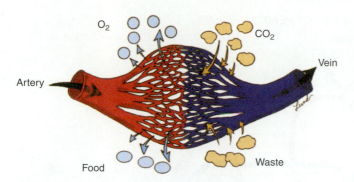

Fig. 25-1 Perfusion is the process by which the blood delivers oxygen and nutrients to and removes waste carbon dioxide from the organs.

ergy to continue functioning. Tissue hypoxia can be reversed if it is treated early. However, if it has been persistent, irreversible cell death ensues. **Perfusion** is a term used to describe the process of oxygenated blood reaching the tissues, whether in adequate or inadequate amounts (Fig. 25-1). Normal perfusion is a state in which the tissues are receiving an adequate supply of oxygenated blood. Decreased tissue perfusion refers to a poor or absent blood supply reaching the tissues.

■ CIRCULATORY SYSTEM

To understand the shock state and its treatment, you will need to become familiar with the fluid compartments of the body, including the circulatory system. The circulatory system includes the intravascular space, or space within the blood vessels. The two other fluid spaces (the **intracellular space** and the extracellular or interstitial space) are covered later in this chapter. Understanding the function of the circulatory system under normal conditions will help you understand the causes and consequences of decreased perfusion of the organs and tissues.

Intravascular Space

For cells to receive oxygenated, nutrient-rich blood, several things must take place. Oxygen is carried on the hemoglobin molecule contained within the red blood cell. These red blood cells, with their oxygenated hemoglobin, need to be circulated to all the tissues of the body. The complex circulatory system is in place to accomplish this. White blood cells that fight infection and platelets that aid in clotting also are transported in the bloodstream.

The cardiorespiratory, or circulatory, system is essentially a closed-pump system. The heart, the central pump in the machinery, needs to pump blood adequately to the lungs for the blood to become oxygenated. The lungs need to be receiving and transferring sufficient oxygen to the hemoglobin in the red blood cells of the bloodstream. The heart then needs to pump oxygenated blood returning from the lungs to the organs and tissues of the body. The **vasculature,** or blood vessels, needs to be intact and able to respond to changes in pressure. The blood vessels are the pipes for this pumping system. The tissues then will receive oxygen delivered by the circulatory system, leaving the deoxygenated blood to return to the heart and lungs to begin the cycle again. The system needs to remain a closed system without "leaks." In addition, the system needs to respond to changes that affect volume, pump strength, oxygenation, and changes in demand.

Now, follow the path of blood as it travels through the circulatory system (Fig. 25-2). Although the heart is one organ, it is essentially two pumps attached side by side. The heart consists of four chambers, the right atrium attached to the right ventricle and the left atrium attached to the left ventricle. A healthy heart is muscular and is able to contract forcefully and rhythmically. The heart should be the approximate size of the patient's own fist, regardless of his or her age. The atria are essentially volume, or collection, chambers. The ventricles are pumping chambers. To illustrate, begin at the right atrium of the heart. Deoxygenated blood returns from the body via the venae cavae; these large veins empty into the right atrium. The right atrium is essentially a volume chamber, as mentioned previously. The blood crosses the tricuspid valve that separates the right atria from the right ventricle and enters the right ventricle.

The heart valves separate each heart chamber. They also separate each ventricle from adjacent blood vessels. They include the tricuspid, pulmonic, mitral, and aortic valves. The valves are necessary to ensure forward, or one-way, flow of blood as it is pumped through the heart.

From the right ventricle, the blood then is pumped through the pulmonic valve and into the pulmonary artery on its way to the lungs. The right side of the heart and the pulmonary arteries and veins compose the pulmonary circulation. The pulmonary circulation is responsible for loading the hemoglobin molecule with oxygen and unloading carbon dioxide, a significant by-product of aerobic metabolism. The pulmonary circulation is a low-pressure system. Because the pressure is low, the

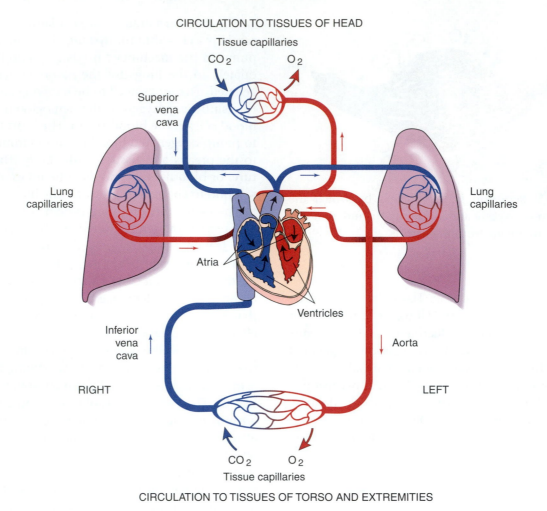

CIRCULATION TO TISSUES OF HEAD

Fig. 25-2 Blood flow through the circulatory system.

right side of the heart, notably the right ventricle, is not as thick or muscular as the left ventricle. The pulmonary arteries branch and divide into progressively smaller and smaller vessels, eventually forming capillary beds that surround each of the alveoli of the lungs. Capillaries are the smallest blood vessels carrying blood in the body. To visualize the progressively smaller vessels of the circulatory system, picture the branching of a large tree trunk into limbs and into smaller and smaller branches. The smallest stems would represent the alveolar capillaries. At the level of the alveolar capillaries, the red blood cells receive oxygen from the inhaled air with oxygen content that has filled the alveoli. The oxygen is attached to the hemoglobin molecule carried in the red blood cell. The oxygenated blood then returns to the heart through progressively larger and larger vessels, eventually reaching the largest pulmonary veins and emptying into the left atria. Imagine the transition from the smallest branches of the tree returning to the trunk of the tree.

The pulmonary, or lung, circulation is normally the only location in which deoxygenated blood is present in an artery, and oxygenated blood is present in a vein. Arteries often are thought of as carrying only oxygenated blood. However, the term *artery* more accurately is defined as a vessel that carries blood away from the heart. Arteries are thick-walled, muscular vessels that branch to become smaller arterioles and eventually microscopic capillaries. Similarly, veins often are thought of as carrying only deoxygenated blood. However, the pulmonary veins carry oxygenated blood from the lungs back to the heart. Veins, in fact, carry blood to the heart. The venous system begins as small venules that collect blood from the capillaries. The blood in the venules flows into larger and larger veins, which ultimately flow into the vena cava and then to the right atrium.

The oxygenated blood that is leaving the pulmonary circulation has hemoglobin molecules that have been saturated with oxygen. This causes a color change of the hemoglobin, giving it a bright red color. Later, when the hemoglobin in the red blood cells has transferred its oxygen content to the cells, it will appear dark red.

Now, return to the course of blood throughout the circulatory system. The newly oxygenated blood now has returned to the left atrium from the lungs and will move quickly from the left atrium to the left ventricle, crossing the mitral valve between the chambers. The left ventricle is the workhorse chamber of the heart. The left ventricle is responsible for pumping this oxygenated blood to the entire body and all of the tissues and organs. The left ventricle is pumping against higher resistance; therefore the left ventricle is necessarily much thicker and more muscular than the right ventricle. Blood leaves the left ventricle by passing through the aortic valve and into the aorta. The aorta is the largest artery in the body and has a thick and elastic wall. This part of the circulatory system begins the arterial systemic circulation. A higher pressure is necessary for blood to reach the most remote tissues. To help accomplish this, the arterial system has elasticity and muscle layers built into the vessel walls. This results in recoil and propagation of pressure waves generated by each contraction of the left ventricle. If the vessels were rigid or flaccid, they would be poorly equipped to maintain a pressure gradient. The vessel walls of the venous system lack this elasticity. Thus the venous system is a low-pressure and slow-flow system. Finally, after the smallest branches of the arterial systemic circulation, the capillaries, have brought blood to the tissues, the blood returns to the right atrium of the heart through the venules and progressively larger and larger veins. While the blood is coursing through the systemic circulation, it picks up glucose and other nutrients from the gastrointestinal tract and liver. In addition, it eliminates waste products and by-products of cellular metabolism primarily through the kidneys.

You might be wondering how the oxygen and nutrients are able to traverse the blood vessel walls. The large arteries have thick, muscular, elastic walls. The walls become thinner and have fewer cell layers as the vessels divide into smaller and smaller arteries. Ultimately, when at the level of the capillaries, the walls are only one cell thick, and nutrients and oxygen can traverse the capillary wall with ease. In addition, hemoglobin that is returning from the body and has given up its oxygen now has an increased affinity for oxygen, which improves the ability of the oxygen to cross the alveolar cell wall and capillary cell wall to attach to the hemoglobin.

Intracellular Space

The second fluid space to be covered is the intracellular space. This is the space within each of the cells. The cells also contain the machinery for cellular metabolism: proteins, lipids, and electrolytes. Their exact content is beyond the scope of this text. However, one must understand the relationship between the fluid spaces. The third fluid space is the **interstitium,** or **interstitial fluid.** This space is composed of everything that is not within the cell or within a blood vessel. In other words, the fluid is located between and surrounding all of the cells, but not within the bloodstream. The interstitial fluid and the intravascular fluid (within the blood vessels) collectively are referred to as the extracellular fluid (outside of the cells). Water can move freely between all of these spaces, but other substances cannot. For instance, electrolytes need to be actively pumped into or out of the cells; however, many proteins and sugars selectively are prevented from entering or leaving the cells unless a carrier is present. A good example is glucose. Glucose is unable to enter most cells across the cell wall unless insulin is present to act as the carrier. These processes maintain the integrity of the cell and maintain the appropriate concentrations of fluid, electrolytes, and proteins necessary for cell function. In the shock state, however, the cell wall, pumps, and carriers begin to deteriorate and fail. This allows fluid shifts and leakage of intracellular substances out into the interstitial space. It also allows extracellular fluids and substances to leak into the cell in abnormal concentrations. This leads to rapid cell death.

■ CIRCULATORY COMPROMISE

After reviewing this brief description of the closed-pump circulatory system, you can imagine several scenarios that would impair the ability of the system to function adequately. Any process that "opens" the system eventually will cause loss of pressure and decreased circulation of oxygenated blood. This most often results from a traumatic injury to the vessels, allowing them to lose blood volume. This is referred to as volume loss, or **hypovolemia.** Any process that affects the ability of the lungs to deliver oxygen to the alveoli and thus to the alveolar capillaries results in inadequate oxygen delivery to the tissues. (Specifics regarding this process are covered in Chapter 17.) If there is inadequate hemoglobin in the blood cells of the bloodstream, oxygen-carrying capacity is insuffi-

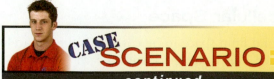

CASE SCENARIO
continued

The rescue crew worked quickly to immobilize Rich onto a long backboard, using a properly fitted cervical collar, 9-foot-long board straps, and a head immobilization device. Rich was breathing high-flow oxygen via a non-rebreather mask. Despite the care being provided, Rich began to feel cold, shivering even though it was not cold out.

Question: *What could be causing Rich to feel this way? What could Ray do to help manage this condition?*

cient and tissues receive poorly oxygenated blood. Similarly, if the hemoglobin molecule is abnormal and therefore cannot take on oxygen present in the alveoli, the blood remains deoxygenated. When the oxygen content of the blood is low, it is referred to as **hypoxemia.** When oxygen content of the tissues is low, it is referred to as tissue hypoxia.

If the heart weakens or fails, there is no pump for the system. The heart can be damaged by disease, infection, or trauma. If blood cannot travel through intact blood vessels, it cannot reach the tissues to deliver oxygen as needed.

This section covers some of the specific compromises of the circulatory system and how they can result in shock.

Volume Loss

Volume loss resulting in insufficient circulatory volume is termed *hypovolemia.* Volume loss can occur by several mechanisms. The major categories include increased fluid loss, decreased fluid intake, or decreased blood production. Increased fluid losses are most common. Fluid losses result from problems such as prolonged vomiting, diarrhea, and profuse sweating such as may occur with heat exposure. **Hemorrhage** is the loss of blood volume and may be easily visible or occult (hidden). Traumatic wounds often cause visible hemorrhage from severed blood vessels. Occult blood loss is also common. In the setting of trauma, occult blood loss occurs in the chest, abdomen or in association with pelvic or femur fractures. The patient can reach the shock state rapidly

from uncontrolled hemorrhage into the chest or abdomen from organ or vessel injuries. A large amount of blood volume also can be lost into the soft tissues as a result of a long bone fracture.

Bleeding can occur in the brain, but if the skull remains intact, the volume loss is limited. If a patient with a head injury is in shock but the skull is intact, never assume that the head injury is responsible. The closed space of the intact skull does not have sufficient capacity to account for hypovolemic shock.

As mentioned before in this chapter, the same circumstances do not affect every patient in the same way. The same amount of volume loss may affect two persons differently because of their condition before the volume loss. If a person is already dehydrated, is **anemic,** or has coexisting medical problems (such as diabetes, heart disease, or respiratory disease), he or she will have a decreased ability to compensate for additional stressors affecting his or her circulatory status. For instance, a previously healthy patient can tolerate a significant amount of volume loss without detrimental effects. The patient's body compensates for the volume loss by increasing the heart rate and respiratory rate and vasoconstricting appropriate vessels in order to maintain an adequate blood pressure. However, a patient who is already anemic (decreased or abnormal hemoglobin) will have a decreased oxygen-carrying capacity as a baseline (Fig. 25-3). The patient's heart rate and respiratory rate already may be increased. If this patient suffers even a modest amount of volume loss in the form of a hemorrhage, he or she may exhibit significant signs and symptoms because of the lack of reserve capacity. Another example is the patient who already has preexisting heart disease and therefore may be unable to increase his or her heart rate in response to hypovolemia and now lacks an important compensatory mechanism.

Gynecologic causes of hemorrhage and volume loss include ruptured or leaking ectopic pregnancy (pregnancy that is growing in one of the tubes leading to the uterus rather than in the uterus as normal), and postpartum (after-delivery) uterine or vaginal hemorrhage from retained placenta. When treating shock in a female of childbearing age, consider ruptured ectopic pregnancy, even if the patient does not report being pregnant. Rupture of an ectopic pregnancy most often occurs between 4 to 6 weeks of gestation, often before the patient knows that she is pregnant.

Gastrointestinal causes of volume loss occur as well. Peptic ulcer disease, tumors, and abnormal blood vessels can result in slow bleeding or acute hemorrhage from the lesion. This can appear as bloody emesis or bloody stool. Some patients, how-

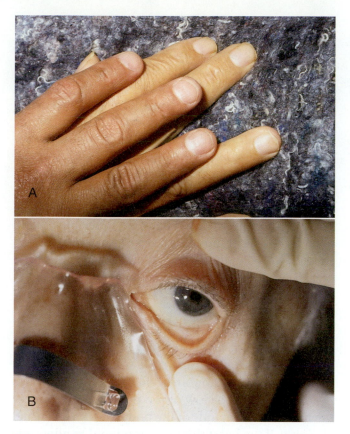

Fig. 25-3 Anemia. Check the nail beds and conjunctivae for pallor. Pale coloring of the nail beds and conjunctivae can indicate a deficiency of red blood cells and their pigment, hemoglobin. **A,** The patient *(bottom hand)* has half the normal amount of red blood cells. Note the contrast of the patient's nail beds with the examiner's hand *(top hand)*. Regardless of skin pigment, the nail beds provide a quick check during the respiratory and circulatory assessment. **B,** Note the pallor of conjunctiva in the patient with severe anemia (low blood hemoglobin).

ever, will have shock from gastrointestinal blood loss without outward signs of hemorrhage. A large amount of blood can be in the stomach and intestines without emesis or visible blood in the stool. Fluid loss without bleeding, in the form of emesis or diarrhea, also can be responsible for hypovolemia. The fluids that are lost in the form of emesis or diarrhea are replenished at the expense of the intravascular, or circulating, blood volume. This leads to hypovolemia without decreased blood cell mass or hemoglobin.

Additional causes of hypovolemia without blood loss include increased respiratory and skin losses resulting from fever. Heat exposure also causes increased loss through sweating. Uncontrolled diabetes can cause significant volume depletion because of in-creased urinary losses in an attempt to compensate for elevated blood sugar. Countless other causes of hypovolemia exist, but the end result is similar. If there is insufficient circulating blood, or intravascular volume, the tissues will not be perfused with oxygenated blood, and serious consequences will ensue.

Another concept is *relative volume loss.* Imagine the vascular system as a closed system of pipes (the container) with a fixed amount of liquid (volume) in the pipes. If you increase the size of the pipes (increase the capacity of the container), without increasing the volume of fluid occupying the container, you will have a relative volume loss. Examples of this scenario include **sepsis, anaphylaxis,** and the effects of some medications.

Sepsis is infection that overwhelms the body. It results in dilation of the blood vessels, sometimes by toxin formation. This dilation results in increased intravascular capacity. If this increased capacity is not met with increased blood/serum volume, relative hypovolemia exists.

Anaphylaxis is a severe, life-threatening allergic reaction. The blood vessels dilate in response to an allergen. Some medications also can result in vasodilation by intention or by side effect. If the vasodilation surpasses the intended effect of the medication, relative hypovolemia again occurs.

■ COMPENSATORY MECHANISMS

As mentioned previously, the healthy body will attempt to compensate for volume loss. The perfusion of the tissues depends on adequate **cardiac output.** Cardiac output is the amount of blood pumped by the heart in 1 minute. A normal value is approximately 5 L/min for a 70-kg adult. Cardiac output depends on the amount of blood pumped with each contraction (stroke volume) of the left ventricle, and the number of times the ventricle beats in 1 minute (heart rate). To maintain cardiac output in the setting of blood loss, the heart rate or stroke volume will have to increase. The blood vessels also will constrict in order to reduce the volume of the "container." Blood vessels that supply nonessential tissues are constricted preferentially before others. This reduces blood supply to the skin, muscles, and gastrointestinal tract before other critical organs.

The compensatory mechanisms have a limit. Each individual has a maximum heart rate and maximum stroke volume. Also, the faster the heart rate, the less time there is for ventricular filling. As a result, the stroke volume is reduced to less than normal with very rapid heart rates. This causes further compromise of the circulation.

Patients in compensated shock have a normal or near normal blood pressure because of the increased heart rate and vascular constriction. These mechanisms, however, are at the expense of tissue perfusion. Uncompensated shock refers to the patient who can no longer maintain his or her blood pressure because of lack of, or exhaustion of, the compensatory mechanisms.

Another mechanism to compensate for hypovolemia involves fluid shifts between the intracellular, interstitial, and intravascular fluid compartments. If the volume loss has occurred over several hours or days, fluid shifts can compensate partially. Initially, interstitial fluid shifts to the intravascular space. This begins within an hour of **hypoperfusion.** If the hypovolemia persists, intracellular fluid shifts to the interstitial space and in turn shifts to the intravascular space. For this reason, a rapid fluid loss of 1000 mL usually results in shock because there is insufficient time for fluid shifting. The same fluid loss occurring over several hours or days may be compensated fully and reversed if the fluid is regained within several hours. As you would imagine, the fluid shift places additional metabolic stress on the cell and affects cellular metabolism.

All of the compensatory mechanisms in shock are intended to be short term. If prolonged, the compensatory response becomes part of the cellular insult. One also must remember that some patients cannot compensate for shock as well as others; for example, the elderly.

■ PUMP FAILURE

The heart must be able to adequately pump blood to the lungs and to the body organs and tissues to maintain perfusion. If the heart, as a pump, fails, perfusion will stop. If the pump is weakened but has not failed, compensation may be possible. If oxygen consumption is conserved, as with rest, symptoms may be minimal. However, with exertion, oxygen consumption and oxygen demand will increase. If the heart is unable to meet this demand, the patient will become symptomatic.

Many causes of pump failure have a gradual onset and therefore have a more gradual onset of symptoms. If the pump failure is sudden, symptom onset may be dramatic because of the limited ability of the body to compensate. If shock is a result of pump failure, it is referred to as **cardiogenic shock.**

One of the more dramatic causes of pump failure is heart attack, or myocardial infarction. When blood flow to an area of heart muscle is blocked, that area of heart muscle will die unless the blood flow is restored quickly. If a large enough area of muscle is involved, the wall motion of the ventricular contraction will be compromised and pump failure will occur. In this circumstance, other compensatory mechanisms have little opportunity to work, and shock may be quickly evident.

Pump failure also can result from dysrhythmias. Dysrhythmias are abnormal heart rhythms. If the heart rhythm is too slow or too disorganized to meet the metabolic demands of the body, shock will ensue. Similarly, if the heart rhythm is too rapid to allow adequate ventricular filling time, shock may ensue.

Finally, two additional situations often are referred to as shock states, although they do not truly represent shock on a cellular level. The first is psychogenic, more commonly referred to as a simple faint. The patient may experience a drop in blood pressure and heart rate from an emotional upset. This is believed to result from increased output from the vagus nerve. This incident is also called **vasovagal syncope.** It does not represent shock because cellular metabolism is not affected.

The second is **neurogenic shock.** In the case of severe spinal cord injury, the nervous system is unable to communicate with the vascular system. Because the nervous system mediates the vasoconstriction that maintains blood pressure, the vessels dilate, increasing the volume of the container and decreasing the blood pressure. In this case, the heart rate does not increase in response to the low blood pressure because of the disconnect with the nervous system. Tissue perfusion, however, remains normal unless traumatic blood loss has accompanied the spinal cord injury.

■ ASSESSMENT OF SIGNS AND SYMPTOMS

Symptoms are the complaints reported by the patient. Signs are the objective findings on physical assessment. A patient experiencing shock may complain of few or numerous symptoms. The patient also may be unable to report any symptoms. In this situation, physical findings are the only clues to the patient's status.

Conscious patients who are in shock most often report feelings of diffuse weakness, fatigue, dizziness, shortness of breath, palpitations, visual disturbance, and sweating (Fig. 25-4). Patients often complain of nausea. They may complain of a feeling of impending doom. If the patient has preexisting heart or lung disease, he or she may report chest pain and more severe shortness of breath. The symptoms are due to decreased perfusion of body organs and tissues. Decreased perfusion of the brain is responsible for mental status changes, confusion, and even agitation. This is followed by unresponsiveness. While still responsive, the patient may report these as symptoms, or you may identify them during your assessment as signs of hypoperfusion.

Physical exam findings are numerous. Remember to evaluate the airway, breathing, and circulation first. Perhaps the first signs identified will be the general appearance of the patient as you approach him or her.

SPECIAL Considerations

When a pediatric patient is suffering hypoperfusion, compensatory mechanisms in the patient will run at maximum until exhausted. When they fail, the failure is rapid. Always remain on your guard.

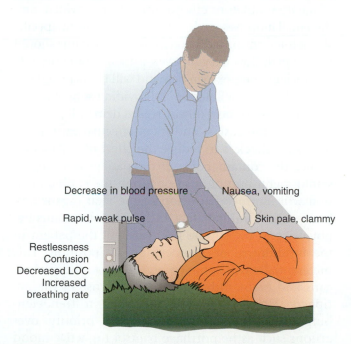

Decrease in blood pressure

Nausea, vomiting

Rapid, weak pulse

Skin pale, clammy

Restlessness
Confusion
Decreased LOC
Increased
breathing rate

Fig. 25-4 Signs and symptoms of shock. *LOC*, Level of consciousness.

A patient in shock will appear pale, even without hemorrhage. Paleness results from the decreased perfusion of the skin and periphery in an attempt to maintain perfusion to the vital organs. The patient also may have cool, moist skin. **Capillary refill** also will be slowed. This refers to the amount of time it takes for blood to refill capillaries that have been emptied, normally less than 2 seconds. Capillary refill time is a reliable measure only in patients younger than 6 years of age. It should not be used for adult patients or older children. To assess capillary refill time, compress the skin of the thumb, ear lobe, or great toe briefly until it turns white. Release the compression and monitor the time for the compressed area to return to a pink color. The longer it takes, the slower the tissues are being perfused, and the more likely that tissue hypoxia is present. The skin may take on a bluish hue as tissue hypoxia ensues. The patient may appear apprehensive, restless, agitated, or confused. This is a result of decreased perfusion of the brain.

The patient typically will have rapid breathing, which may or may not be labored. The normal adult ventilatory rate of 12 to 20 breaths per minute usually is increased to greater than 20. The patient is attempting to increase the oxygenation of the blood, necessary to meet the increased oxygen demand by the heart and tissues. The increased ventilatory rate is also necessary to blow off the increased amounts of carbon dioxide through the lungs that were produced by cells that are using anaerobic (without oxygen) metabolism.

Assessment of the patient's vital signs offers additional information. The pulse rate most often is increased. If the patient appears to be in shock but the heart rate remains within the normal range, medications may be responsible for the inability to mount a tachycardic response. Patients in spinal shock also usually have a normal heart rate, as previously described.

Pump impairment caused by bradycardia also may be responsible. The amount of oxygen available to the central circulation may affect the ability of the heart to beat faster.

The pulse may be weak and difficult to palpate because of a reduced pressure wave with decreased blood pressure. The pulse may not be palpable in the extremities because these vessels have vasoconstricted to shunt blood preferentially to the vital organs in the central core. You should assess more central pulse points, such as the carotid or femoral pulse, in these patients (Fig. 25-5). If the central pulses are palpable and the peripheral pulses (radial and foot) are not, this is an indication of significant shunting to compensate for the shock state. These patients must be treated aggressively.

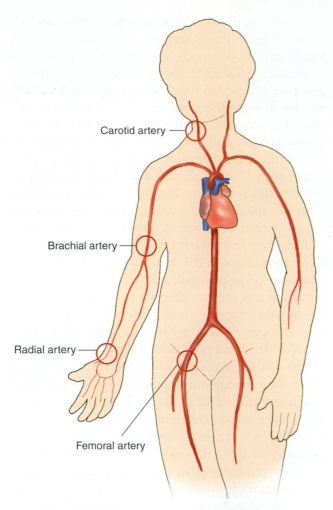

Carotid artery

Brachial artery

Radial artery

Femoral artery

Fig. 25-5 Easiest places to locate a pulse.

One of the last steps of your assessment of the patient in possible shock is blood pressure. The patient's blood pressure will be lower than his or her baseline. If the patient has low blood pressure (hypotension) but has no signs of hypoperfusion (decreased perfusion of the brain and other organs), he or she is not in shock. The blood pressure may be one of the last vital signs to change in patients with shock.

Whenever possible, make a comparison to the patient's baseline blood pressure. Asking the patient whether he or she knows his or her previous blood pressure, for comparison, is helpful. For instance, a young, healthy female may have a systolic blood pressure of 80 mm Hg in the supine position. This value alone does not indicate shock. If there are no signs of hypoperfusion, the patient is not in shock. It is common for young, healthy persons to have a systolic blood pressure less than 100 mm Hg in the supine position. Similarly, an elderly patient with a systolic blood pressure of 110 mm Hg, but with signs of hypoperfusion, is in fact in shock. This patient may have a baseline systolic blood pressure of 180 mm Hg, the

pressure necessary to perfuse the vital organs and brain. Reduction of the blood pressure to 110 mm Hg has dramatically decreased the patient's ability to perfuse organs and tissues, and the patient may no longer be meeting the minimum blood pressure necessary.

■ TREATMENT

Recognition of shock in its earliest stages allows one an opportunity to treat the patient aggressively and possibly avoid the most serious complications. These include brain and organ injury and ultimately death. One must recognize the patient at risk of developing shock and must intervene before shock develops.

Unfortunately, many patients already are in shock before the arrival of emergency medical care. If the patient is already in shock, your treatment will need to stop the process that caused it and attempt to reduce the impact of decreased perfusion on the organs and tissues. Having already reviewed some of the more common causes of shock, interventions used to treat shock now are covered.

Prior to treating any patient consider the need for body substance isolation based on the presenting situation. At a minimum disposable gloves should be utilized for the protection of the providers as well as for the patient. If there is a chance for body fluids exposure, eye protection and gowns should be utilized.

During the initial assessment pay attention to airway and breathing, followed by assessment of the circulation. After a patent airway has been confirmed, an adequate ventilatory rate confirmed or provided, and the circulation assessed, you can move on to specific shock interventions. All potential shock victims should receive high-flow oxygen. Even if their ventilatory rate is sufficient, their oxygen demand will be increased significantly at the cellular level. Providing supplemental oxygen helps to meet this increased demand.

One of the easiest and most effective early treatments for shock is to reduce the effect of gravity and reduce the container size. If the patient is sitting or semiupright, putting him or her in the supine position will improve perfusion of the vital organs and brain almost immediately. If the patient remains hypotensive in the supine position, put the patient in the head-down, or Trendelenburg's, position. This preferentially will enhance circulation to the vital organs and brain, although at the expense of the periphery. However, placing a patient in Trendelenburg's position should never take priority over actions such as hemorrhage control for active blood loss or the initiation of transport to an appropriate receiving hospital.

Control any visible source of hemorrhage. Visible sites of hemorrhage are usually from trauma, including lacerations. Most often this control can be accomplished by applying direct pressure to the bleeding vessels or tissue (Fig. 25-6). Maintain the pressure until further control of the bleeding can be completed.

If the hemorrhage is visible, coming from an extremity, but cannot be controlled with direct pressure, a **tourniquet** may be successful (Skills 25-1 and 25-2). Apply the tourniquet proximal to the wound to control arterial bleeding. Arterial bleeding will be pulsatile and rhythmic with the contraction phase of the left ventricle (Table 25-1). Although venous (low-pressure) bleeding can be profuse, arterial bleeding involves higher pressure and is usually much more dramatic and leads to greater blood loss. The use of a tourniquet carries significant risk of tissue hypoxia. The arterial blood supply will be reduced or eliminated to the tissues beyond the tourniquet. The tourniquet should be applied only tight enough to control the hemorrhage and should be removed by qualified personnel as soon as it is safe to do so. If you apply a tourniquet, record the date and time and communicate these clearly to the next caregivers receiving the patient.

If a long bone fracture, such as a femur fracture, is responsible for significant blood loss, applying a trac-tion splint may reduce movement of the fracture site and decrease further bleeding. Pelvic fractures can be responsible for extensive occult hemorrhage because of large pelvic vessels being torn by the bone edges. Stabilizing the pelvic fracture may reduce the ongoing bleeding. Stabilization can be accomplished with the bed sheet technique or with application of the **pneumatic antishock garment.**

If there is no visible blood loss but the patient has suffered from a traumatic mechanism, suspect occult or internal bleeding. A massive amount of hemorrhage can be concealed in the chest, abdominal, and pelvic cavities. If the site or suspected site of bleeding is not visible, control is more difficult or impossible. In these situations, the pneumatic antishock garment may be appropriate (Skill 25-3).

TABLE 25-1

External Bleeding

Source	Color	Flow
Arteries	Bright red	Pulsatile, rapid
Veins	Dark red	Steady, continuous
Capillaries	Dark red	Oozing, continuous

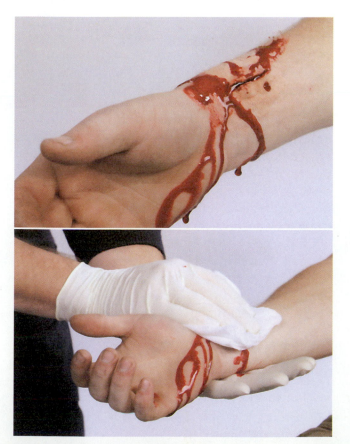

Fig. 25-6 Apply direct pressure to control hemorrhage.

SKILL 25-1

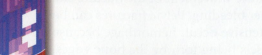

Application of a Tourniquet Using a Blood Pressure Cuff

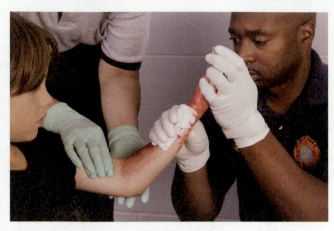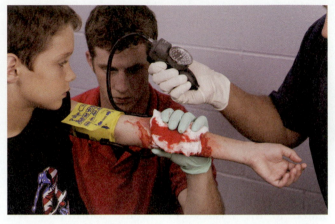

1. Apply a pressure dressing to the wound while elevating the extremity.

2. Wrap a blood pressure cuff above the wound and inflate the cuff until bleeding is controlled without obliterating the distal pulse.

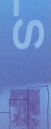

SKILLS

SKILL 25-2

Application of a Tourniquet Using a Triangular Bandage

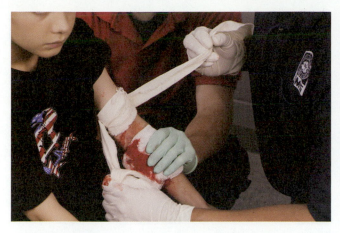

1. Apply a pressure dressing to the wound and wrap a triangular bandage around the extremity above the wound.

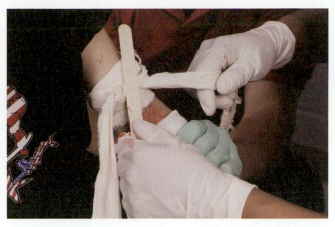

2. Tie a single knot in the bandage and place a stick or tongue blade over the knot.

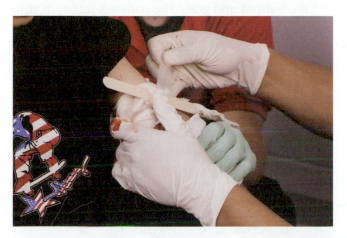

3. Tie a second knot over the stick or tongue blade and turn it until bleeding is controlled without obliterating the distal pulse. Secure the blade with tape or by wrapping and tying the remaining length of bandage.

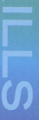

SKILLS

SKILL 25-3
Application of a Pneumatic Antishock Garment

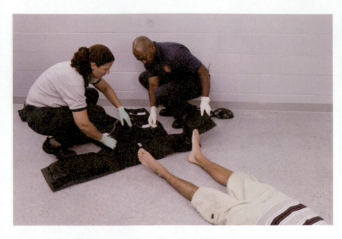

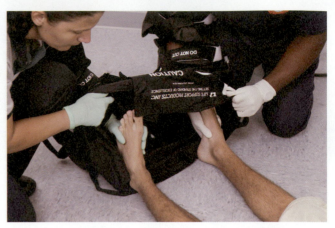

1. First, obtain authorization from medical direction to use a pneumatic antishock garment. Keep in mind that the application of a pneumatic antishock garment will prevent further inspection of the abdomen, pelvis, and lower extremities.
2. Remove the patient's clothing from the waist down. Unfold the pneumatic antishock garment and place it at the feet of the patient. Separate the Velcro strips to make the pants as big as they can be.

3. The two emergency medical technicians should be placed at the patient's feet. Use the arm located nearest the feet to slide the pants up from the bottom and grasp the patient's feet with your hand. Then lift the legs and pull the garment up onto the patient's legs.

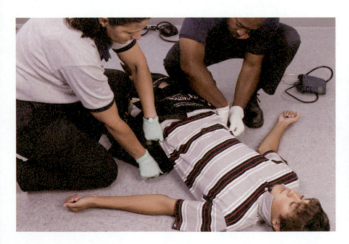

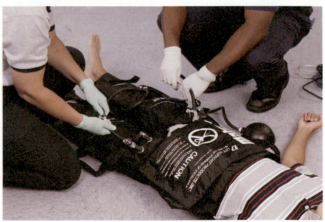

4. Pull the pants up to the patient's diaphragm by lifting up the buttocks and pulling upward.

5. Secure the Velcro closures on the garment. Connect the tubing to the valves on the garment.

SKILLS

SKILL 25-3

◉ *Application of a Pneumatic Antishock Garment—cont'd*

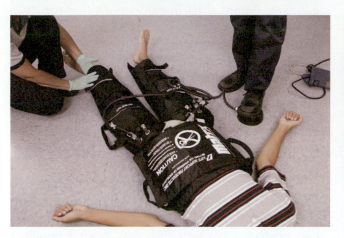

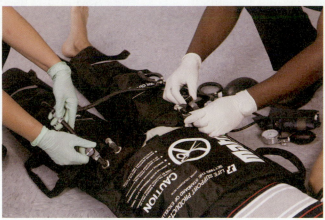

6. Open the valves for inflation. Inflate the garment.* Ensure that the garment is inflated properly by listening for pops in the Velcro as the bladders reach full inflation.

7. Close the valves.

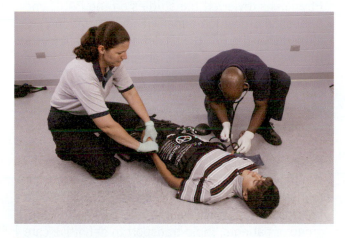

8. Reassess the patient.

---

*Please note that some protocols recommend inflating the legs and then the abdomen, or some may indicate inflating the whole suit at one time.

SPECIAL Considerations

Pneumatic Antishock Garment

The pneumatic antishock garment (PASG) is a device intended to increase the blood pressure in certain patients in shock. The PASG also is used to stabilize unstable pelvic fractures because these patients can suffer serious hemorrhage from lacerated pelvic blood vessels. The PASG originally was known as the military antishock trouser (MAST). The military antishock trouser were developed for jet fighter pilots in order to maintain blood flow to their brains (G-suits). The concept then was applied for use in trauma patients. The PASG has fallen out of favor over the past several years for various reasons. Once a frequently used piece of equipment on the ambulance, the PASG now seldom is used other than in rural areas with prolonged transport times. Pros and cons are attributed to its use. Several studies have attempted to find the appropriate group of patients who would benefit from the PASG, but opinion still varies.

The PASG serves to increase the resistance applied to the peripheral vascular system of the lower extremities by inflating air-filled compartments surrounding the legs and pelvic region. This causes direct compression of the vascular bed, primarily the venous system. This results in increased venous return, increased cardiac output, and increased afterload. This effect is temporary and decreases with time. At higher pressures, arterial compression and occlusion may occur. When arterial occlusion occurs, cellular ischemia and cell death will occur. The potential for pressure injury must be considered.

The studies that have been performed have been on animals and human beings. Study size has been relatively small, and it has been difficult to obtain statistically significant and reproducible results. Limitations include difficulty randomizing the patients, inability to design a double-blind study, disparity in patient groups and initial status, measurement difficulties, and multiple different outcome measures. Animal studies have shown benefit in hemorrhagic shock, with the exception of hemorrhage above the diaphragm or thoracic hemorrhage. Reproducible data indicate improved outcomes in patients with ruptured abdominal aortic aneurysm treated with the PASG. This is the subgroup of patients that showed most consistent benefit when using the garment. Potential harm can occur when the device is used on patients with diaphragmatic injuries or penetrating thoracic injury. Patients with abdominal evisceration also failed to show benefit. Patients in cardiogenic shock or with pulmonary edema have worsened with application of the PASG because of increased afterload and increased myocardial oxygen demand. Pregnant patients also are put at increased risk with application of the garment.

Controversy also exists regarding the use of the PASG in head-injured patients. It has been shown that the garment increases the intracranial pressure; however, this has been compensated by the improved cerebral perfusion pressure following increased venous return and increased cardiac output.

In summary, the National Association of EMS Physicians reviewed the studies on the PASG and published a position paper.[1] The association concluded that the PASG was definitely beneficial for ruptured abdominal aortic aneurysm and if there would be a delay in surgery and possibly beneficial in patients with hypotension caused by pelvic fracture. The PASG also was considered acceptable in patients with anaphylactic shock refractory to standard therapy, as well as in patients with lower extremity hemorrhage uncontrollable by standard means and in patients with severe traumatic hypotension with a pulse but without blood pressure. Even when using the PASG on this subgroup of patients, rapid transport to definitive care is paramount to a successful outcome.

Patients with femur fractures are best treated with traction splints, and patients with pelvic fractures can be immobilized with spine boards or other stabilizing devices.

The position paper was intended to be used as a resource, not to dictate standard of care. Local emergency medical services medical direction should determine which patient groups should be considered for PASG application and also should indicate which patient groups could benefit from online medical control regarding the decision.

Attempt to conserve body heat by covering the patient. Do not cover the patient in such a manner that compromises your ability to reassess him or her continually.

■ CONSEQUENCES OF SHOCK

If the cells of the body do not receive sufficient oxygen and nutrients, their ability to produce energy quickly deteriorates. Although the cells can produce energy briefly in the absence of oxygen, this creates toxic by-products, which further damage the cell. Under these conditions, the cells begin to die. When a sufficient number of cells of the particular organ have died, the organ then fails or dies. When a sufficient number of critical organs in the body have died, the patient dies.

Remember that shock is not defined by the visible signs and symptoms that it causes but rather the underlying condition in which cellular metabolism is not producing sufficient energy to support life. It is important to note that the patient may not die until critical organs have died. For instance, kidney failure caused by shock may not result in death of the patient for several days, even if untreated. However, if the heart or brain is significantly injured from shock, death will be more immediate.

If the patient in prolonged shock is treated aggressively, and perfusion improves, a second phase of shock may be seen. Because of the anaerobic metabolism (without oxygen) that was occurring at a cellular level, toxic and acidic by-products have accumulated. When circulation is restored, these substances are washed into the central circulation and result in acidosis. This is termed **reperfusion acidosis.**

The enzymes necessary for cellular metabolism function in a narrow pH range. As the acidic by-products cause the pH to fall to a more acidic level, enzyme function and therefore cellular function are affected. During the low-flow shock state, red blood cells also may have stagnated in small arterioles and capillaries. As blood flow to these areas is restored, these roulettes of red blood cells become numerous small emboli in the circulation. They can stick together, forming larger emboli and eventually causing blockages in blood vessels supplying other organs and tissues. This blockage reduces or halts oxygen delivery to the affected organ and ultimately may cause organ failure or organ death.

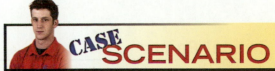

CASE SCENARIO
conclusion

Ray reassessed Rich's vital signs as they quickly moved to the hospital. Although the patient was still tachycardic, his blood pressure was not as low as before, and he was breathing a bit easier. Rich was covered with a heavy blanket, and the foot of the board was slightly raised to promote blood return to the central circulation. Later on, Ray found out that during the fall, Rich had injured his kidney, which was bleeding into the retroperitoneal space. Trauma surgeons were able to stop the bleeding and save the kidney and Rich from premature death. ■

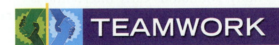

TEAMWORK

Many times bleeding and shock emergencies take place at unstable scenes. Be sure to conduct a proper scene size-up to ensure everyone's safety. Once the scene is determined to be safe, enter, begin assessing, and implement treatment for your patient. Work with other responders because sometimes these calls require that multiple tasks be done simultaneously. Using all available resources effectively and efficiently will ensure a positive patient outcome.

Reference

1. O'Connor RE, Domeier R: Use of the pneumatic antishock garment: position paper of the National Association of EMS Physicians, *Prehosp Emerg Care* 1(1):32-35, 1997.

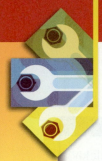

NUTS AND BOLTS

Critical Points

- Emergency medical technicians must have an understanding of the different types of shock, their causes, and treatments.
- Emergency medical technicians must know how to interpret correctly the signs and symptoms discovered.
- Emergency medical technicians must realize when to request advance life support assistance.

Learning Checklist

❑ Shock is the condition in which the cardiorespiratory system is unable to meet the oxygen and nutrient demands of the body. Numerous early interventions can improve a patient's outcome from a shock state.

❑ The circulatory system delivers oxygen and nutrients to the tissues so that cells can produce energy in a process called cellular metabolism (cellular respiration).

❑ Oxygen is carried on the hemoglobin molecule in the red blood cell. These red blood cells, with their oxygenated hemoglobin, need to be circulated to all the tissues of the body by the circulatory system.

❑ The cardiorespiratory, or circulatory, system is a closed-pump system that needs to remain a closed system and respond to changes that affect volume, pump strength, oxygenation, and changes in demand.

❑ The heart consists of four chambers, the right atrium attached to the right ventricle and the left atrium attached to the left ventricle. The atria are volume chambers, whereas the ventricles are pumping chambers.

❑ The three types of fluid spaces are intravascular space, intracellular space, and extracellular (interstitial) space.

❑ The major categories of volume loss include increased fluid loss, decreased fluid intake, and decreased blood production.

❑ A patient with preexisting medical problems will have a decreased ability to compensate for additional stressors affecting his or her circulatory status.

❑ The patient's body compensates for the volume loss by increasing the heart rate and respiratory rate and vasoconstricting appropriate vessels in order to maintain an adequate blood pressure.

❑ The perfusion of the tissues depends on adequate cardiac output.

❑ The compensatory mechanisms are limited because each patient has a maximum heart rate and stroke volume. Also, the faster the heart rate, the less time there is for ventricular filling, which further compromises the circulation.

❑ The two types of shock are compensated and uncompensated shock.

❑ The compensatory mechanisms in shock are intended to be short term. If prolonged, the compensatory response can do further damage.

❑ The heart should be able to pump blood to the lungs adequately and to the body organs and tissues to maintain perfusion. If the heart fails, perfusion will stop.

❑ A patient in shock most often reports feelings of diffuse weakness, fatigue, dizziness, shortness of breath, palpitations, visual disturbance, and sweating, and complains of nausea and a feeling of impending doom. This is due to decreased perfusion of body organs and tissues. Decreased perfusion of the brain is responsible for mental status changes, confusion, and agitation, followed by unresponsiveness.

❑ A patient in shock will have a blood pressure lower than his or her baseline.

❑ To treat a patient in shock, the focus is to stop the process that caused it and attempt to reduce the impact of decreased perfusion on the organs and tissues.

❑ Shock is not defined by its signs and symptoms but rather by the condition in which cellular metabolism is not producing sufficient energy to support life. The patient will not die until critical organs have died.

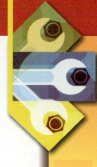

Key Terms

Aerobic metabolism Metabolism that occurs in the presence of oxygen.

Anaerobic metabolism Metabolism that occurs in the absence of oxygen.

Anaphylaxis A severe, life-threatening hypersensitivity (allergic) reaction to a previously encountered antigen that results in vasodilation and subsequent hypotension.

Anemic A decrease in hemoglobin in the blood to levels below the normal range of 12 to 16 g/dL for women and 13.5 to 18 g/dL for men.

Capillary refill The time it takes for the capillary bed to refill after it is compressed and the pressure is released.

Cardiac output The amount of blood expelled by the ventricles of the heart with each beat (the stroke volume) multiplied by the heart rate.

Cardiogenic shock Shock caused by dysfunction of the heart.

Cellular metabolism The process by which cells use the nutrients and oxygen to produce energy. Also called *cellular respiration.*

Circulatory system The network of channels through which blood circulates.

Hemorrhage The loss of a large amount of blood volume in a short period, either externally or internally.

Hypoperfusion Decreased or inadequate perfusion that results in insufficient delivery of oxygen and nutrients necessary for normal tissue and cellular function; also known as *shock.*

Hypovolemia An abnormally low circulating blood volume.

Hypoxemia A deficiency in the concentration of oxygen in arterial blood.

Hypoxia Inadequate cellular oxygenation.

Interstitial fluid The fluid in the space between cells.

Interstitium The space between cells

Intracellular space The fluid space within a cell.

Intravascular fluid space The fluid space within a blood vessel.

Neurogenic shock A form of shock that results from peripheral vascular dilation.

Perfusion The passage of a fluid through a specific organ or an area of the body.

Pneumatic antishock garment A garment designed to produce pressure on the lower part of the body, thereby preventing the pooling of blood in the legs and abdomen.

Reperfusion acidosis A form of acidosis that results when circulation is restored and the acidic substances are washed into the central circulation.

Sepsis A systemic response to a blood infection that results in hemodynamic instability, usually manifested by tachycardia and hypotension.

Shock The inadequate delivery of oxygen and nutrients to cells, resulting in organ system malfunction. Eventually shock is detectible with abnormal vital signs. It can lead to death.

Tourniquet Constricting band placed above an injured extremity to stop the flow of blood. Tourniquets should be used only as a last resort.

Vasculature Blood vessels.

Vasovagal syncope A sudden loss of consciousness generated by a transient vascular and neurogenic reaction; it may be triggered by pain, fright, or trauma.

National Standard Curriculum Objectives

Cognitive Objectives

After completing this lesson, the EMT student will be able to do the following:

- List the structure and function of the circulatory system.
- Differentiate between arterial, venous, and capillary bleeding.
- State methods of emergency medical care of external bleeding.
- Establish the relationship between body substance isolation and bleeding.
- Establish the relationship between airway management and the trauma patient.
- Establish the relationship between mechanism of injury and internal bleeding.
- List the signs of internal bleeding.

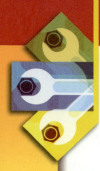

- List the steps in the emergency medical care of the patient with signs and symptoms of internal bleeding.
- List signs and symptoms of shock (hypoperfusion).
- State the steps in the emergency medical care of the patient with signs and symptoms of shock (hypoperfusion).

Affective Objective

After completing this lesson, the EMT student will be able to do the following:

- Explain the sense of urgency to transport patients who are bleeding and show signs of shock (hypoperfusion).

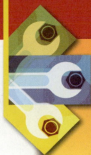

Psychomotor Objectives

After completing this lesson, the EMT student will be able to do the following:

- Demonstrate direct pressure as a method of emergency medical care of external bleeding.
- Demonstrate the use of diffuse pressure as a method of emergency medical care of external bleeding.
- Demonstrate the use of pressure points and tourniquets as a method of emergency medical care of external bleeding.

- Demonstrate the care of the patient exhibiting signs and symptoms of internal bleeding.
- Demonstrate the care of the patient exhibiting signs and symptoms of shock (hypoperfusion).
- Demonstrate completing a prehospital care report for the patient with bleeding and/or shock (hypoperfusion).

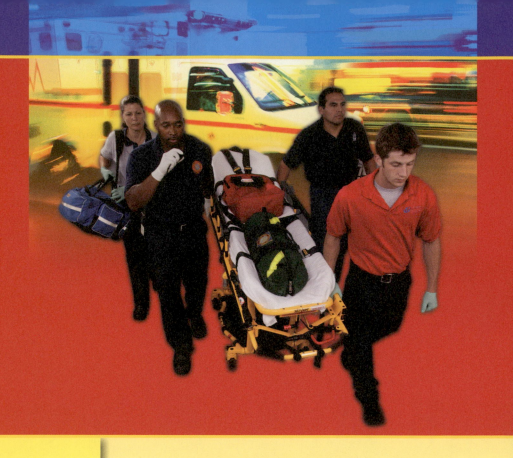

CHAPTER

26

OUTLINE

LESSON GOAL

All soft tissue injuries insult the circulatory system of the body in one way or another. As you know, circulation is one of the big three: the ABCs. Therefore, a thorough knowledge of soft tissue injuries is necessary to function effectively as an emergency medical technician. This chapter takes you through the various types of soft tissue injuries and their treatments. ∎

GOAL

Soft Tissue Trauma

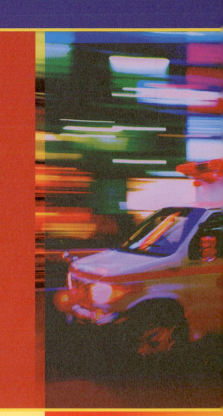

CHAPTER OBJECTIVES

After completing this chapter, the EMT student will be able to do the following:

1 State the function of the skin.

2 List and describe the three layers of the skin.

3 Explain why body substance isolation is a critical safety element when treating a patient with soft tissue injuries.

4 Explain the rule of nines and how it relates to soft tissue injuries.

5 Differentiate between the three types of bleeding: arterial, venous, and capillary.

6 Differentiate between a closed and an open soft tissue injury.

7 Identify and treat the different types of closed soft tissue injuries.

8 Identify and treat the different types of open soft tissue injuries.

9 Explain the difference between a dressing and a bandage and what the functions and purposes are for each.

10 Demonstrate the various methods for controlling bleeding.

11 Differentiate between penetrating trauma to the chest and penetrating trauma to the abdomen, and explain what the emergency medical technician may expect to see from each.

12 Define and be able to treat partial-thickness burns.

13 Define and be able to treat full-thickness burns.

14 Explain how electrical and chemical burns are different from thermal burns.

15 Explain how to treat an electrical burn and the complications associated with that type of burn.

16 Explain how to treat a chemical burn and the complications associated with that type of burn.

26

OBJECTIVES

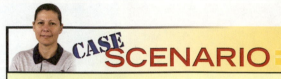

CASE SCENARIO

Elizabeth could hear the squeal of tires coming to an all-too-quick stop in front of the station. Sure enough, a couple of seconds later there was a frantic knocking on the front door glass. As Elizabeth headed to the front door, she could see a car parked on the apron, with the driver's door open. There appeared to be a passenger in the back seat of the car, leaning his head against the back of the seat.

The driver almost literally pulled Elizabeth through the front doorway. "My friend just got bat-tery acid all over him. He's burned bad!" Elizabeth called to her crew members to open the garage door and get the first aid bag. She then followed the driver over to the car.

Question: *What are some of the safety concerns that Elizabeth will face? Based on the mechanism of injury, what are potential injuries with which the rescue crew will have to deal?*

Not surprisingly, soft tissue injuries are one of the most common traumatic injuries the emergency medical technician (EMT) encounters. The skin is the largest of the human organs. Moreover, it makes up a large percentage of the overall body mass. Therefore, not surprisingly, the skin is the first to feel the effects of trauma. Traumatic insults can be minor or emergent. This depends on how much tissue has been injured, how much blood has been lost as a result of active bleeding, and most importantly, how much damage the organs and structures beneath the soft tissue have sustained.

During the assessment of the trauma patient, the EMT must answer several key questions:

- Is this an isolated injury, or could other organs or structures beneath this area be affected?
- How much blood has been lost?
- What types of injuries are present?
- Is the patient in shock as a result of these injuries?
- If the soft tissue injury is to the face or neck, is it compromising the patient's ABCs (airway, breathing, circulation), or *could* it compromise them as a result of swelling?

The answers to these questions will help determine the course of action the EMT will take to care for this patient. Consequently, the EMT must possess the knowledge and skills to be able to answer the questions and intervene appropriately to the best of his or her level of training. The following statement is a good rule of thumb to follow to keep yourself motivated during your training: "You can't find out what's wrong unless you know what's *right.*"

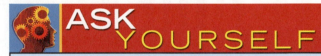

ASK YOURSELF

You and your partner arrive on the scene of a motor vehicle collision. You note that a car has hit a utility pole and has sustained extensive front-end damage. The driver is still inside the vehicle, head back against the neck rest, not moving. From a distance, you can see the patient bleeding from several head wounds. You also note a motorcycle lying on its side in the middle of the street. The rider of the motorcycle, a young male, approaches you. You note that his T-shirt is torn and he is limping. He tells you he was the one who called 911 from his cell phone. He states that he was riding behind the car when he saw it start to swerve out of control and head toward the utility pole. The motorcyclist tells you that in an effort to avoid hitting the car, he laid his bike down. He states that he was wearing a helmet and denies any loss of consciousness. Police and fire department personnel have arrived on the scene. What is your first priority? How would you delegate to the personnel at your disposal? What other resources would you need? What other information do you need? Should these patients be triaged? If so, how? If not, why not? What are both patients' possible injuries?

■ THE SKIN

Importance of Body Substance Isolation

As you know, the primary concern on any emergency medical services call is always scene safety. Therefore your first priority will be your own protection, not the patient's. The functions of the skin are covered in greater detail in the next section, but one of the most important functions of the skin is to act as a barrier or shield to protect the body. So the EMT must take steps to protect his or her own skin from blood-borne pathogens that could be carried by the patient. **Body substance isolation** is the main method of protecting oneself from potential exposure. You should be wearing gloves and eye protection while assessing and treating *all* patients (Fig. 26-1). In situations in which there is a great deal of blood loss or active bleeding and the EMT's mouth, eyes, open wounds, or clothing could become contaminated, the use of an approved face mask or shield and gown is highly recommended, in addition to gloves and eye protection (Fig. 26-2).

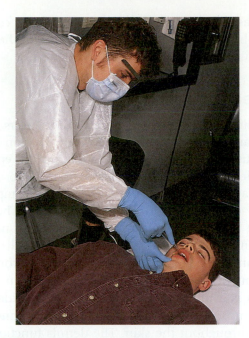

Fig. 26-2 If excessive bleeding or the risk of exposure to other body fluids is great, the emergency medical technician should wear all the body substance isolation gear shown.

Major Functions of the Skin

The functions of the skin can be summarized in three words: protect, prevent, and maintain:

Protect: The skin protects the body from invading microorganisms that could lead to infection. While the skin is intact, bacteria are held outside the body where they can do little harm. However, in the case of an open soft tissue injury, where the integrity of the skin has been breached, bacteria have an open pathway into not only the tissue directly under the open wound but also the entire body once the bacteria invade the bloodstream. Another way the skin protects the body is through the nerve endings found in the skin. When these nerve endings sense a change in the environment, they send a signal to the brain to react. For example, when a person gets too near a heat source, a flame for instance, the nerves sense the sudden rise in temperature and signal the brain to draw away from the heat source.

Prevent: The skin prevents the loss of body fluid. It serves as a protective barrier to prevent drying out of the underlying tissues.

Maintain: The skin maintains the body temperature through the same method it uses to prevent body fluid loss. By constricting or dilating pores and vessels based on messages sent from the nerve endings in the skin to the brain and from the brain to the nerve endings, the body regulates its temperature. When the body is too hot or stressed, the vessels and pores dilate and give off fluid in the form of perspiration (diaphoresis). When the body is too cold or already has lost some of its circulating volume, the vessels and

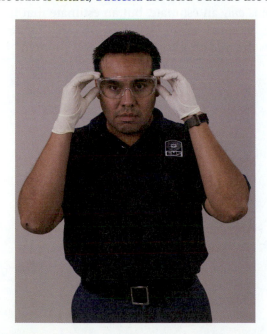

Fig. 26-1 Wear basic body substance isolation equipment while assessing every patient.

pores constrict, sending fluid back to the core of the body where it is needed to maintain the vital organs within (shunting).

Layers of the Skin

The skin is composed of three distinct layers, each performing a role in the functions of the skin listed previously (Fig. 26-3). These layers are the **epidermis, dermis,** and **subcutaneous tissue.** The outermost layer of the skin, the epidermis, is composed mostly of dead cells called epithelial cells. The epidermis has no vessels through it, so it does not receive any blood. However, these epithelial cells form the frontline defense, protecting the body from the invasion of infection-causing microorganisms. The dermis is a much thicker layer than the epidermis. The dermis is composed of cells that form connective tissue throughout the skin. The dermis functions as

the "control center" of the skin. Within the dermis are blood vessels, lymphatic vessels, nerve endings, and the dermal appendages: sebaceous glands, hair follicles, and sweat glands. Sweat glands also may be found in the deepest layer of the skin, the third layer, subcutaneous tissue. Subcutaneous tissue, also called the hypodermis, is composed of elastic connective tissue and fatty tissue. The fatty tissue provides a layer of insulation to protect body temperature and a ready source of energy for the body to burn.

Rule of Nines

Certain soft tissue injuries can cover large sections of skin: burns, abrasions, and contusions. (These are covered in greater detail later in this chapter.) The EMT must be able to judge the amount of damage done to the soft tissue when these potentially large injuries occur. This judgment is important for future treatment options. The EMT can use a tool to estimate the amount of damage incurred. Every patient is "built" differently; thus the tool is helpful but not an absolute. The tool is the **rule of nines.** The rule of nines is based on the **body surface area** of adults and children. The tool is an estimation of the percentage of damaged tissue based on the entire surface area of skin on the body equaling 100%. For example, the amount of intravenous fluid a burn patient is to receive in the hospital is based on the amount of burned skin. While usually utilized to estimate the extent of a burn, it can also be used for other soft tissue injuries as well. Granted, this figure is *only* an estimate, but an estimate that has become accepted as the standard of care. Figure 26-4 shows the rule of nines for adults and children.

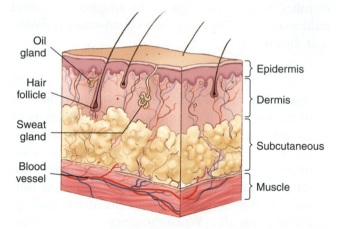

Fig. 26-3 Layers of the skin.

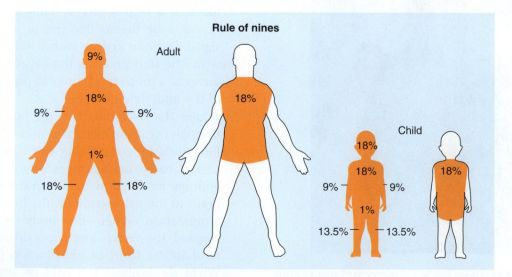

Fig. 26-4 The rule of nines is an effective tool for determining the approximate size of soft tissue damage.

■ BLEEDING

External Bleeding

All injuries to soft tissue result in external or internal bleeding (hemorrhage). This section focuses on the three types of external bleeding and how to identify the characteristics of each type. Although the treatment for each is the same, the EMT must be able to identify the nature of the bleed in order to understand the need for rapid intervention in some cases. Also, the EMT must be able to identify the nature of the bleed to relay that information to the receiving hospital.

Of the three types, **arterial bleeding** is the most significant and dangerous soft tissue bleed. With this type of bleeding, an artery has been cut, and oxygenated blood is not able to reach the body distal to where the cut has occurred. Not only could the patient lose a lot of blood with this injury, but also this injury is extremely time sensitive. That distal area can survive only a limited amount of time without oxygenated blood. Arterial bleeding is identifiable by bright red blood that spurts or pumps as it bleeds. If left untreated, death could occur within minutes depending on the size of the artery.

Venous bleeding can also be significant with regards to the amount of blood that can be lost. That amount depends on the size of the vein that was cut. The larger the vein, the greater the blood loss *and* the less time one has before the significant loss of circulating volume puts the patient into a state of shock and potentially leads to death, as is the case with the arterial bleed. You can identify venous bleeding by free-flowing, dark red blood from the wound site.

Capillaries are the smallest of the vessels. They ooze when they are cut. **Capillary bleeding** is not life threatening. However, the EMT must bear in mind where the capillary bleeding originates. An arm or leg will not have a dense grouping of capillaries (less vascular) and hence will not bleed as much as an area such as the face or the hand, which has considerably more vessels in the same amount of space (highly vascular). Consequently, a facial cut may cause the patient a great deal of stress who sees all that blood. Moreover, the cut also may cause the EMT to focus on that area and miss a more critical injury somewhere else. A solid knowledge base of soft tissue injuries and a good assessment will prevent this **tunnel vision.**

Internal Bleeding

External bleeding is easily identifiable and relatively easy to treat, unlike internal bleeding. For the most part, internal bleeding is hidden from view. It can

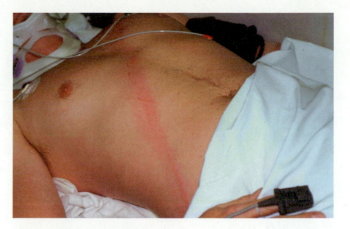

Fig. 26-5 Bruising to the torso should alert the EMT to the possibility of more extensive damage beneath the soft tissue bruise.

be minor, as in the case of a bruise. It can be critical, as in the case of a bleeding internal organ. It can be both. The seat belt bruise across a patient's abdomen could be an indicator that something more serious is going on beneath that bruise (Fig. 26-5). The EMT cannot just "look inside the patient" and see what is going on inside. Therefore several key elements will go a long way in helping the patient survive. First, the EMT must maintain a high index of suspicion based on the mechanism of injury and must possess a good knowledge base of applying the principles of force transference to the human body. The EMT also must perform a complete and thorough assessment and recognize the presence of life-threatening situations. Moreover, the EMT must intervene rapidly, provide rapid transport to a trauma center, and recognize that this patient may need a surgeon.

■ CLOSED SOFT TISSUE INJURIES

Contusions

Simply put, a **contusion** is a bruise. A contusion is a closed soft tissue injury (skin remains intact despite the trauma). It results when vessels within the skin are ruptured from a direct blunt force. As the vessels bleed, blood spreads out through the tissues under the site of the impact. As that blood coagulates, it leaves the distinctive mark of a contusion. The greater the force, the deeper the damage and the more likely that larger vessels also could be ruptured (Fig. 26-6). This is why contusions can be light in color, a light

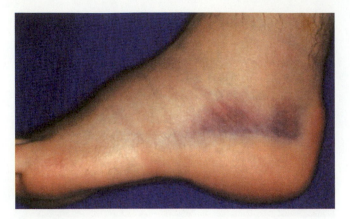

Fig. 26-6 Depending on the location and the vessels involved, contusions could result in extensive circulating blood loss.

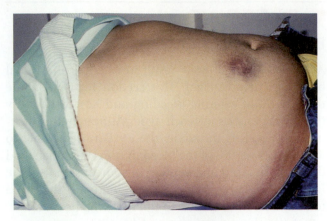

Fig. 26-7 A hematoma could hold a considerable amount of blood trapped, depending on its location.

blue, or deep in color, a dark purple. Likewise, if the blunt trauma covers a large area of the body, more vessels will be broken. As a result, larger contusions would be present. Contusions are characterized by pain and swelling to the injury site. After some time, the discoloration sets in. The ICE principle (ice, compression, and elevation) is the best method for treating contusions. Apply a cold pack directly to the area injured. Hold the cold pack in place with a loose **dressing,** and try to keep the affected area above the level of the heart to minimize the blood flow to that area.

Hematomas

A **hematoma** is another closed soft tissue injury. It also results from direct blunt force trauma that causes blood vessels to rupture. However, with the hematoma, the bleeding vessels form a pool of blood under the surface of the skin, instead of spreading out like a contusion. This pooling of blood causes considerable localized swelling and pain to the injury site (Fig. 26-7). The treatment for a hematoma is identical to the treatment of a contusion. Apply a cold pack, apply gentle pressure, and keep the area above the level of the heart if possible.

Crush Injuries

A **crush injury** results when a body part is caught between two compressing surfaces. The two surfaces have a density that is greater than that of the body part. Crush injuries may not look serious at

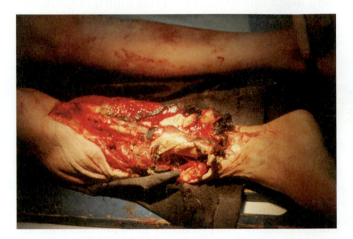

Fig. 26-8 Severe crush injuries to extremities could result in the surgical amputation of parts if the damage is extensive.

first. However, they can prove to be life threatening. The amount of internal bleeding from soft tissue damage could cause the patient to go into shock. Underlying organs (if any), muscle and bones could be damaged. Crush injuries also can cause significant injuries to areas distal to the actual injury site. The increase in pressure from the compressing surfaces forces blood to the distal areas, engorging those vessels to the point of possible rupture (Fig. 26-8). Crush injuries occur with extensive swelling, pain, and deformity. If the injury is to an extremity, cold packs and elevation may help the swelling and pain (Skill 26-1). If possible, allow the patient to assume a position of comfort for the transport to the hospital.

SKILL 26-1
Application of Ice for Swelling

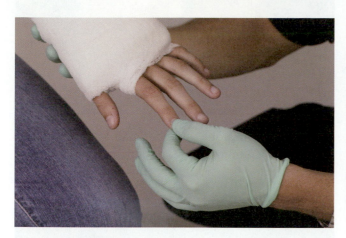

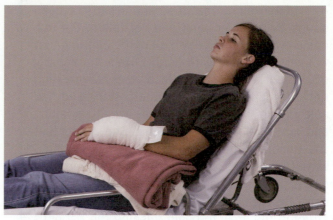

1. Extremities will swell after a soft tissue injury. Applying ice will help reduce the swelling.
2. Apply a pressure dressing tightly enough to hold an ice pack in place but not so much that it cuts off circulation.
3. Check for the presence of circulation by checking the capillary refill time after the application of the pressure dressing.

4. Elevate the extremity with a pillow or blanket during transport.

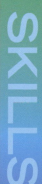

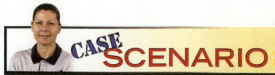

After determining that the patient had not been struck by an object and had not fallen, the rescue crew worked to cut off all of the clothing that was contaminated with acid. Elizabeth carefully inspected the patient's face, oropharynx, and neck to make sure none of the battery acid had splashed in those areas and was causing swelling and potential airway problems. She noted that the patient's chest and abdomen were covered with burns that looked red and blistered. His hands also had been splashed as he had tried to cover his face during the explosion. Elizabeth instructed the crew to begin flushing the patient's hands, arms, and torso with water.

Question: How much of the patient's body is involved in the burn? Why are the injuries to the hands especially critical? What are the management procedures necessary in this case?

■ OPEN SOFT TISSUE INJURIES

Abrasions

An **abrasion** is a shear injury where the skin is dragged across a rough surface with enough force to scrape the epidermis and often the dermis. Abrasions have minimal or no bleeding, yet they are always characterized by pain because nerve endings are closer to the surface than blood vessels. Abrasions that are small, less than a few square inches, usually are not serious (Fig. 26-9). However, when abrasions are large, as in the case of someone falling off a bicycle onto a parking lot, the area of abrasion could be substantial. Although the wound is not life threatening by itself, the resulting infection could present a problem in the future. It would be prudent for the EMT to estimate the size of the abrasion using the rule of nines and report those findings to the receiving hospital.

Lacerations

Tears in the skin as a result of forceful contact with a sharp object are **lacerations.** The sharper the object or the greater the force applied, the deeper the lacer-

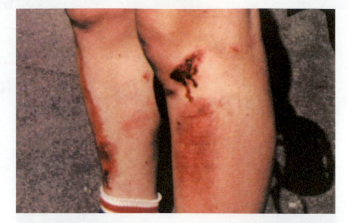

Fig. 26-9 Abrasions could be small, such as this one, or large depending on the amount of shearing force involved.

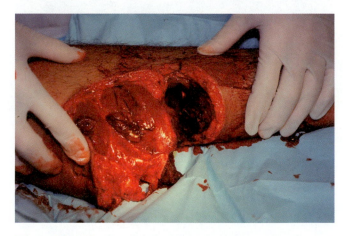

Fig. 26-10 Lacerations are the most common soft tissue injuries the emergency medical technician encounters.

ation. In either case the laceration will have more bleeding than the abrasion. The laceration bleeds more because it goes through all levels of the skin (full thickness), whether the wound presents as a straight cut (**linear laceration**) or a jagged cut (**stellate laceration**). Deep lacerations can have extensive bleeding. If a major vessel is involved, the patient could lose enough blood to go into shock. The EMT must be able to recognize this, control the bleeding, and prevent further contamination of the wound (Fig. 26-10).

Punctures and Impaled Objects

Penetrating injury results whenever any object is forced into the soft tissues of the body causing injury to the tissues underneath. Examples of this type of injury include stab wounds, gunshot wounds, shrapnel injury from an explosion, and falling onto a pointed object. The significance of all of these types of injuries relates to the potential injury to the organ that lies underneath the open wound and along the pathway of the penetrating object.

A **puncture wound** is the result of a sharp, pointed object penetrating the skin. For example, a stab wound caused by a knife is a good example for explaining the potential damage that can be done. If the knife were to be removed after the stabbing, an initial assessment would reveal an external wound that is relatively small. However, the damage beneath the wound could be significant, depending on several factors:

- How long was the knife blade?
- What direction did the knife take? Downward? Upward? Straight in?
- Was the knife twisted after it was impaled into the patient?

These are important questions to ask and answer when treating a puncture wound of this nature. If the knife were 1-inch wide at its widest part and 6 inches long, the external wound would be relatively small. However, that knife could have penetrated the full 6 inches into the body, far deep enough to hit a vital organ. Moreover, if the knife were twisted, instead of a straight jab, the damage could extend into a much greater area, the **cone of damage** (Fig. 26-11).

If the knife (or other penetrating object) remains in the patient's body, that injury is called an **impaled object.** Impaled objects can take on many forms: knives, scissors, pieces of wood or debris, or metal.

Any object that can penetrate the skin can be an impaled object. The primary rule the EMT must follow is that he or she must *never remove an impaled object unless it interferes with the patient's airway or chest compressions during cardiopulmonary resuscitation* (Fig. 26-12). Removing the object could cause further injury to the patient. The EMT should stabilize the object in place as best as possible using bulky bandaging before moving or transporting the patient (Fig. 26-13).

Avulsions

When a large amount of force is transferred to a compact area of the skin, the skin often will tear or be pulled loose, creating flaps of skin, or the force will

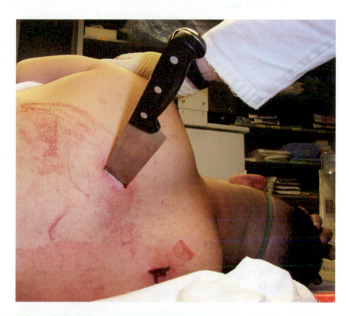

Fig. 26-12 Never remove an impaled object unless it interferes with the patient's airway or prevents chest compressions during cardiopulmonary resuscitation.

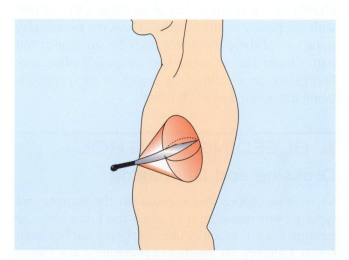

Fig. 26-11 Cone of damage. The length and movement of the knife blade determine the amount of damage inside the body.

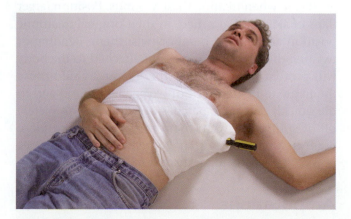

Fig. 26-13 Use bulky dressings to stabilize an impaled object during treatment and transport.

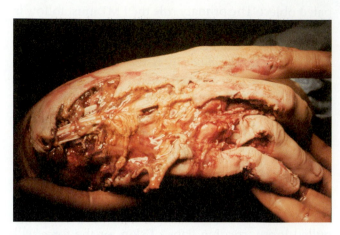

Fig. 26-14 Avulsion of large skin flap from the posterior surface of hand

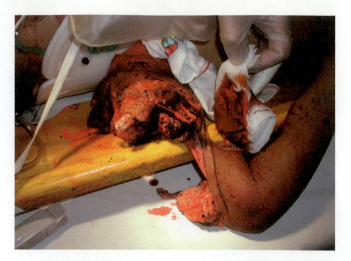

Fig. 26-16 Partially amputated arm.

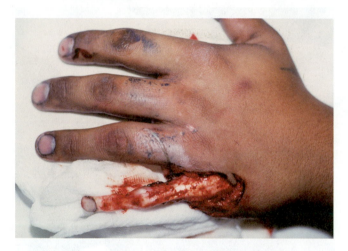

Fig. 26-15 Large areas of skin can be torn completely off, exposing the tissue beneath.

tear off the skin completely (Fig. 26-14). This **avulsion** can be serious, depending on the size and location of the injury. Bleeding also can be extensive, depending on the depth of the avulsion. You must take great care when treating these wounds. Position larger flaps of skin, still attached, in their original anatomic position and do not bend or twist them. Bending or twisting the part of the skin still attached to the body will prevent blood flow to the flap and could cause the tissue to be deprived of oxygenated blood and to die quickly. For large patches of skin torn completely off, if still intact, wrap them in dry gauze and place them in a plastic bag (Fig. 26-15). Set the bag on ice or a cold pack during transport to the hospital.

Amputations

An **amputation** occurs when a part of an extremity, the entire extremity, or other body part is completely severed from the body. When *some* connective tissue remains attached to the body, this is known as a partial amputation (Fig. 26-16). Bleeding from the amputation site may be severe or limited, depending on whether the vessels within the site can constrict enough to suppress the flow of blood through the tear. This constriction is a natural phenomenon within the body. Amputations usually look horrific and are often the patient's focus of attention. The EMT must not be distracted by this injury but must focus first on airway and then breathing. Once airway and breathing have been established, *then and only then* should the EMT focus on the amputation and controlling the bleeding. Once the bleeding is controlled, the EMT must find the severed appendage quickly if there is to be a chance of reattaching the appendage. Wrap the severed appendage in sterile gauze and place it in a plastic bag. Keep the bag cool. Never immerse an amputated body part in water, and never place it directly on ice. If found, transport the amputated part with the patient to the hospital. However, never delay transport of the patient to search for an amputated part. Others left on scene such as police officers or firefighters can continue the search as the patient is being transported to the hospital.

■ BLEEDING CONTROL
Dressing and Bandaging

So far, this chapter has focused on the sources and types of soft tissue injuries. Now the focus shifts to treating the soft tissue injuries beyond what has been covered already. As was noted previously, the risk of contamination and potential infection are two areas of which the EMT needs to be cognizant when dealing with open soft tissue injuries. Dressings are sterile material placed directly over an open wound to re-

SPECIAL Considerations

WARNING: Do not waste time looking for an amputated body part if the patient is in critical condition. The primary considerations are rapid intervention and rapid transport. Have other responding units look for the amputated part and bring it to the hospital if they know how to handle such a situation. The emergency medical technician may have to take a minute or two to explain the procedure and give the other unit(s) the necessary equipment, but he or she should let them find the part.

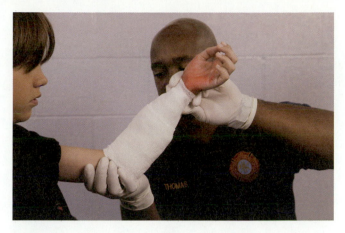

Fig. 26-17 Bandages are used to hold dressings in place and to apply pressure.

duce the chances of further contamination. This material can be gauze pads, petroleum jelly pads, trauma dressings, or a variety of other products available. Whatever dressing is chosen, it must be large enough to cover the open wound and surrounding skin completely. To apply a dressing that is considerably larger than the wound is better than to use one that just barely covers it.

Bandages serve two purposes. First, they hold dressings in place when used on open soft tissue injuries. Second, they are used to apply pressure to a closed soft tissue injury to aid in the reduction of swelling. Self-adhering bandages have tape on them to hold them in place (Fig. 26-17). They come in a variety of sizes and shapes and are used for different purposes, but generally they are used on smaller wounds. For larger wounds or closed soft tissue injuries, bandages made of gauze, elastic material, cloth (as in the case of a triangular bandage), or adhesive tape are needed. They help to hold dressings effectively in place on open wounds and apply pressure to closed injuries.

Bleeding Control Techniques

The EMT has five techniques within his or her arsenal of skills to control active bleeding, depending on the severity of that bleeding. These techniques include elevation, **direct pressure, pressure dressing, proximal pulse point,** and **tourniquet.** If a wound is located on an extremity, simply elevating the injury above the level of the heart may be beneficial. Gravity will pull the blood down and slow its progress, allowing the EMT some time to get a direct dressing prepared.

As its name implies, direct pressure involves placing a dressing over an open wound and applying firm pressure (Fig. 26-18). If the wound bleeds through

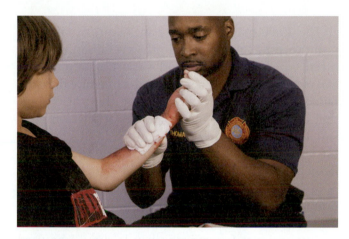

Fig. 26-18 Elevate an injured extremity and apply pressure directly on the wound with a sterile dressing. If the wound bleeds through, add more dressing and continue applying pressure.

the original dressing, the EMT should apply more dressing material while maintaining pressure on the wound. Direct pressure is the *best* way to control any external active bleeding regardless of where the bleed originates.

If direct pressure fails to control the bleeding or there are multiple bleeding sites, the EMT can use a pressure dressing. To create a pressure dressing, place a dressing over the wound and wrap a bandage around the dressing. The bandage should be wrapped tightly enough to stop the bleeding but not so much that it cuts off blood flow past the injury site. A pressure dressing that is wrapped too tightly may become a tourniquet and cause severe damage to healthy tissue distal to the injury. The EMT should always assess for the presence of a distal pulse after applying a pressure dressing or splint.

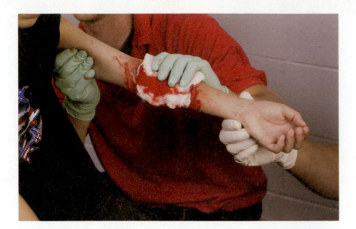

Fig. 26-19 Apply continuous pressure to the closest proximal pulse for 5 minutes to slow bleeding to a manageable level.

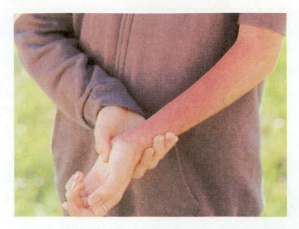

Fig. 26-20 First-degree burns are characterized by red, painful skin.

The EMT may consider using a proximal pulse point to slow the bleeding in the event of an arterial bleed, where bright red blood is spurting or pumping *and* elevation, direct pressure, and a pressure dressing failed to stop the bleeding. Locate the pulse point that is just above the injury site and apply firm pressure to it to reduce the blood flow. Hold this pressure for 5 minutes (Fig. 26-19). (Blood flow to the distal tissue should not be interrupted for more than 5 minutes.) Slowly release pressure on the pulse point while observing the wound. If the wound continues to bleed, reapply pressure.

A tourniquet (constricting band) should be used *only* as a last resort to stop massive bleeding from a severed extremity. The function of the tourniquet is to cut off virtually all the blood supply to the bleeding site in the extremity in order to keep a patient from bleeding to death. When a tourniquet has been used, the chances of reattaching a severed extremity are minimal. Therefore a tourniquet should be used only when the choice to save the patient's life must take precedence over saving the patient's extremity. If the decision is made to use a tourniquet, place it above and as close to the injury site as possible and document the time of application. Skill 26-2 demonstrates different methods for controlling external bleeding.

■ BURNS

Assessment and Classification

The EMT is faced with several challenges when treating any burn victim. These challenges include determining the size, type, and depth of the burn and the source of the burn and identifying and treating

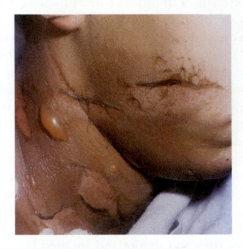

Fig. 26-21 Be careful not to break the blisters intentionally on second-degree burns.

any injuries or conditions that result from the burn. Burn types are expressed in degrees, and their severity is determined by their depth into the skin and underlying tissue. **Superficial burns** have the least penetration into the skin. Most **first-degree burns** fall into this category. First-degree burns have pain and reddened skin (Fig. 26-20). A mild to moderate case of sunburn is a good example of a superficial first-degree burn.

A **partial-thickness burn** goes slightly deeper into the skin. More severe first-degree burns and some **second-degree burns** are partial-thickness burns. Second-degree burns have blisters—opened, closed, or both—and pain to the burn area (Fig. 26-21).

Full-thickness burns go all the way through the skin into the tissue beneath. Deep second-degree and **third-degree burns** are full-thickness burns. Third-degree burns have charring of the skin (black, white,

SKILL 26-2
● *Bleeding Control*

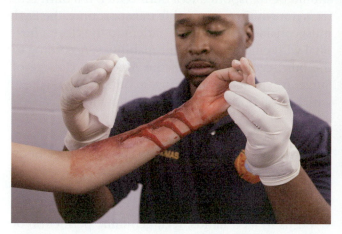

1. *Elevation.* Elevate the extremity above the level of the heart.

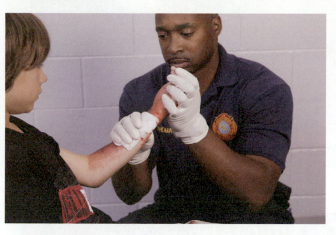

2. *Direct pressure.* Apply a gauze pad to the wound and apply direct pressure with your gloved hand to decrease blood flowing from the wound.

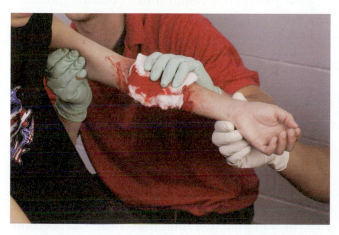

3. *Pulse point pressure.* Locate the strongest pulse point immediately proximal to the injury and apply deep pressure to obstruct blood flow to the wound.

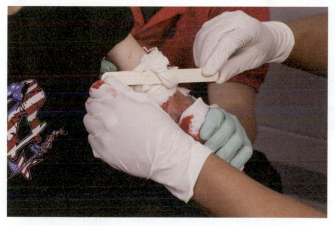

4. *Tourniquet.* Place the tourniquet as close as possible to the point of injury and tighten the stick (or pen) only until the bleeding stops. Secure the stick and write the date and time of application on the tourniquet. Only hospital personnel should remove the tourniquet. To ensure that the tourniquet is not overlooked, write the letters "TK" on the patient's forehead or on a piece of tape placed on the forehead.

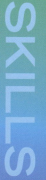

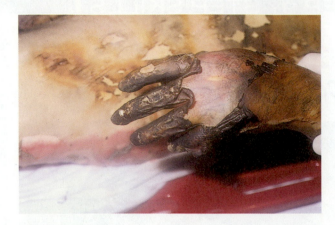

Fig. 26-22 Third-degree burns are not painful. However, burns of lesser degree often surround the third-degree burn and cause pain.

SPECIAL Populations

PEDIATRIC Considerations

Because young children have thin skin layers, they get serious burns much more rapidly than an adult would from the same mechanism. For example, 1 second of 160° F water contact, a liquid temperature one would get from a freshly poured cup of coffee or tea, will cause a full-thickness burn on the pediatric patient.

---

or gray) and little or no pain because the nerves in the skin have been destroyed (Fig. 26-22).

One should note that often more than one type of burn may be present with partial- or full-thickness burns. The central part of the burn may be a full-thickness burn and partial-thickness burns may surround it. So although the patient may not experience any pain directly to the third-degree burn, the surrounding second-degree burn would cause a considerable amount of pain.

In addition to the type and depth of a burn, the size or how much body surface area has been involved also plays an equal role in determining its severity. As was stated previously, burn sizes are estimated by using the rule of nines. Often the rule of nines is only an estimation of the initial burns. In a majority of cases, the original rule of nines assessment has been determined to have underestimated the total body surface area damaged once the burn reached its maximum exposure level.

Identifying the type, depth, and size of a burn is only one part of the assessment of the burn patient. The EMT also must determine whether the patient is in critical condition as a result of those burns. Patients meeting the criteria for critical status ideally should be transported to a burn center. If a burn center is not within a reasonable transport time, the EMT must consider bringing the patient to the closest hospital with emergency room capabilities. According to the burn center criteria of the American College of Surgeons, patients requiring a burn center (those with critical burns) include the following[1]:

- Inhalation injury
- Partial-thickness burns of greater than 10% body surface area
- Full-thickness (third-degree) burns in any age group
- Burns to face, hands, feet, genitalia, perineum, or major joints
- Electrical burns (including lightning)
- Chemical burns
- Burn injury in a compromised patient (preexisting illness)
- Burn patients with concomitant trauma where burn is the greatest threat to life
- Burned children in the presence of inadequate resources
- Burn injury in patients requiring special social, emotional, or long-term rehabilitation

Burn Treatments

The primary rule of treating a burn patient is to *stop the burning.* Removing the heat source is only the first step in stopping the burning. Heat can become trapped in layers of clothing. Therefore, at the very least, all burn victims should have the area around the burn free from clothing. If part of the clothing has become melted to the skin, do not pull at it. Leave the melted part attached to the skin and cut the material around it. Remove all jewelry because swelling may develop if the burn is on or near an extremity.

If evidence of burning about the face (e.g., singed hairs or soot in the mouth or nose) or burns on the face exist, the EMT must be prepared to treat the airway aggressively. Inhalation of superheated gases could irritate or damage the upper or lower airway, causing edema and obstructing the airway rather quickly. Time is critical when dealing with a burn victim's airway. Supplement breathing with high-flow oxygen or assisted ventilations with a bag-valve-mask and supplemental oxygen if inadequate breathing is observed. Evaluate circulatory status and provide support as needed. Burns can have devastating effects on the circulatory system if they are left untreated and the burns are significant. Damaged skin from a large burn or several smaller burns may result in a patient being unable to maintain body temperature or fluid balance. Keep the patient warm as you treat the burns.

Superficial burns need little or no treatment in the prehospital setting. The EMT should never apply an ointment or salve to a burn area. However, to help relieve pain, use moist dressings on superficial and partial-thickness burns that cover no more than 10% of the body surface area. Use of moist dressings on patients with more than 10% burns could result in the patient losing body heat more quickly. The moisture from the dressings acts as a wicking effect and draws the body heat from the patient. Cover partial-thickness burns of more than 10% body surface area or any full-thickness burn in dry, sterile dressings. Exercise great care to maintain the integrity of unbroken blisters on second-degree burns. Blisters should never be broken intentionally in the prehospital setting. Burn blisters can be opened in the hospital using sterile technique. To maintain a sterile environment in the prehospital setting is almost impossible; however, exercise as great care as possible to keep the burn areas clean. Before transport, it is a good idea to wrap the patient in a burn sheet before wrapping the patient in a blanket for warmth.

SPECIAL BURN SITUATIONS

The EMT must be aware of two situations that require special consideration when dealing with burn victims: chemical burns and electrical burns.

Chemical Burns

A chemical burn results when the body is exposed to a caustic substance (Fig. 26-23). As you know, the EMT's primary responsibility is scene safety. Therefore the EMT must be aware of the chemical to which the patient has been exposed and the way in which that chemical could affect the EMT's ability to treat the patient. The EMT may not be equipped to care for a patient who has been exposed to certain chemicals until the patient has been decontaminated properly by a hazardous materials response team. The EMT can obtain information about a particular chemical by requesting to see the **material safety data sheet.** Every business or industry is required to have a ma-

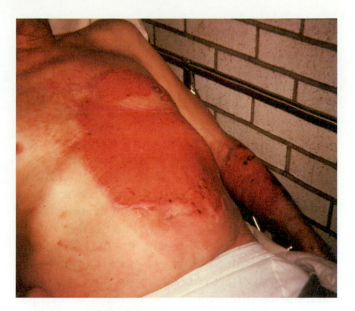

Fig. 26-23 Chemical burn.

terial safety data sheet on hand for each chemical it stores. If one is not available, the EMT could contact a local poison center or call **CHEMTREC** at 1-800-424-9300. Chapter 35 goes into greater detail in dealing with these situations. This section covers smaller, more manageable exposures.

The first objective before treatment is to remove all the contaminant from the patient. Anyone who will be coming in contact with the patient must be protected. These persons must don approved personal protective equipment. Remove the patient's clothing and shoes and place them in a biohazard container. If the exposure is a dry chemical, brush as much of the chemical off the patient as possible, and then flush the area with copious amounts of water. Irrigation should begin as quickly as possible. Most minor exposures to powders and liquids can be treated effectively in this manner, provided there is enough water to maintain irrigation from initial treatment through delivery at the hospital. The EMTs also must remember to protect themselves from possible runoff of the diluted chemical during irrigation. Never use neutralizing agents in the prehospital setting. Some agents may cause a chemical reaction with the initial chemical and cause additional exothermic (heat) injuries. Notify the receiving hospital as soon as possible of the exposure. This will help the hospital prepare a safe environment to accept and treat the patient without contaminating the entire emergency room. The quick notification also allows the hospital to make preparations for antidotes or special treatments, depending on the chemical involved. Therefore it is imperative that the EMT notify the hospital of the correct name of the chemical and even spell out the name if necessary.

Electrical Burns

Electricity always will take the path of least resistance. The damage caused, when electricity comes into contact with the human body, depends on the amount of energy delivered and the length of time it was delivered. The EMT first must determine whether the patient is still in contact with the source of the electricity. If the patient is still in contact with the source, the EMT must not approach the patient, keeping a safe distance away, until the power is shut off. The EMT can begin assessing and treating the patient once the patient is safely accessible. While physically assessing the patient, the EMT should attempt to determine the type of electrical injury that has occurred: **direct contact burns, arc injuries,** or **flash burns.** Direct contact burns result when a patient has had an electric current pass through his or her body. Direct contact burns often have a charred entrance wound, extensive internal damage along the pathway of the electricity, and an exit wound where the electricity grounded itself. This exit wound may appear as a section of the body that seems to have exploded, if the current was strong enough. In contrast, the external wounds could be small, but the internal damage caused could be extensive. The EMT must assume that extensive damage to body parts has occurred along the pathway. When electricity arcs between two contact points and those contact points are near exposed skin, the skin could be exposed to extreme temperatures (4500° F to more than 5000° F). Arc injuries, caused by this extreme heat, could affect the whole body or an isolated area. In either situation, extensive soft tissue damage will be evident. Open electrical sources could cause flash burns to unprotected skin or the eyes if the source is within proximity.

When treating an electrocuted patient, the EMT must remember not to become part of the problem. Stay clear until it is safe to enter and approach the patient. Because much of the damage of an electrical burn is internal and hidden from view, the EMT must be prepared for the worst. Electricity often disrupts the natural electrical activity of the heart. Thus the EMT should be prepared to begin cardiopulmonary resuscitation and defibrillate as early as possible if the patient is pulseless and not breathing. The EMT also should look for associated injuries such as injuries to bones, organs, and nerves. When reporting to the hospital, report discovered injuries and, if possible, the amount of current to which the patient was subjected and the duration.

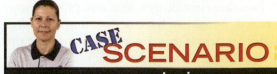

CASE SCENARIO
conclusion

After wrapping the patient's hands with dry, sterile gauze, the rescue crew carefully covered his chest and abdomen area with additional dressings. Then they covered the patient with several light sheets to prevent heat loss. Oxygen was given as a precaution. A member of the crew reassessed the patient's blood pressure on the patient's least affected arm as the ambulance began to travel toward the trauma center. ■

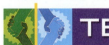

TEAMWORK

Although soft tissue injuries are common in the prehospital setting, they sometimes are so extensive that the patient is at risk of going into shock from blood loss or even at risk for death. The emergency medical technician (EMT) must be able to recognize when such life-threatening situations exist. Transport to an appropriate receiving facility, such as a trauma center, should be initiated as soon as possible. The EMT also must know to call for advanced life support intervention if providing fluid intravenously or if other interventions are needed for the patient and are outside the scope of his or her practice. The EMT must possess the skills necessary to attempt to stabilize the patient until such advance life support help arrives. If advanced life support intervention is not available, the EMT is responsible to provide all necessary care and to deliver the patient safely to the appropriate facility. By performing a thorough assessment, recognizing the presence of potential life threats, and providing meaningful intervention, the EMT will have the information at hand to relay to the trauma center of their upcoming arrival. Then the trauma center can be prepared with the specific information provided by the EMT in the field.

Reference

1. Committee on Trauma, American College of Surgeons: *Resources for optimal care of the injured patient: 1999,* Chicago, 1998, The College.

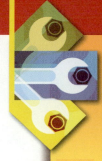

Critical Points

Protect yourself. Identify whether a scene is safe for entry. The emergency medical technician is primarily responsible for himself or herself and his or her partner. *If you don't know, don't go.* Open soft tissue injuries bleed, sometimes profusely. Always wear some form of body substance isolation when in contact with a patient who is bleeding actively.

Assess the patient completely. The primary objective in dealing with soft tissue injuries is to identify the possibility of underlying life-threatening conditions. The wise emergency medical technician lets soft tissue injuries guide him or her in identifying those life threats. Am I dealing with an isolated soft tissue injury, or could more significant multisystem injuries be present? The answer to this question is critical in the overall success of the call. Once the possibilities of life threats have been eliminated, the emergency medical technician then can use his or her skills in treating those injuries as described in this chapter. Any penetrating injury to the torso should be considered a life threat in the prehospital environment. Treat such an injury appropriately by providing rapid intervention on the scene and then rapid transport to the closest trauma center.

Learning Checklist

❑ Be able to determine what level of body substance isolation is needed and to don the appropriate wear.

❑ Describe the functions of the skin.

❑ Identify the layers of the skin and the components in each layer.

❑ Be able to calculate body surface area involvement by using the rule of nines.

❑ Differentiate between arterial, venous, and capillary bleeding.

❑ Identify and treat the following closed soft tissue injuries: contusions, hematomas, and crush injuries.

❑ Identify and treat the following open soft tissue injuries: abrasions, lacerations, punctures, impaled objects, avulsions, and amputations.

❑ Define *dressing* and its role in bleeding control.

❑ Define *bandage* and its role in bleeding control.

❑ Be able to demonstrate the following bleeding control techniques: elevation, direct pressure, pressure dressing, proximal pulse point, and tourniquet.

❑ List injuries associated with penetrating trauma to the upper torso and the treatment for each injury.

❑ List injuries associated with penetrating trauma to the lower torso and the treatment for each injury.

❑ Be able to classify and identify burns by thickness and degree.

❑ Be able to treat a burn victim.

❑ Describe how electrical burns are unique and how to treat them.

❑ Describe how chemical burns are unique and how to treat them.

Key Terms

Abrasion Open soft tissue injury characterized by scraping.

Amputation Complete avulsion where a body part has been removed from the body.

Arc injuries Burns caused by exposed skin being too close to two contact points of electricity.

Arterial bleeding Bleeding characterized by pumping or spurting of bright red blood.

Avulsion Open soft tissue injury characterized by skin being torn and leaving a flap or being completely removed.

Bandages Devices used to hold a dressing in place or provide pressure to an injury.

Body substance isolation Protective equipment worn to prevent exposure to blood-borne pathogens or body fluids.

Body surface area Amount of body skin damaged by burns, abrasions, or other injury. Body surface area is expressed in terms of percentage.

Capillary bleeding Bleeding characterized by the oozing of blood.

CHEMTREC The Chemical Transportation Emergency Center, continuously accessible via phone (1-800-424-9300). CHEMTREC

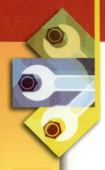

provides immediate online advice to emergency and rescue personnel on site at hazardous materials incidents.

Cone of damage Amount of internal damage caused by the movement of an impaled object, such as a knife.

Contusion Closed soft tissue injury characterized by discoloration beneath the surface of the skin; a bruise.

Crush injury Closed soft tissue injury where a body part is compressed between two sources with densities that are greater than that of the skin.

Dermis Middle layer of the skin serving as the "control center" of the skin.

Direct contact burns Injuries sustained from coming in contact with electricity.

Direct pressure Bleeding control technique that involves applying pressure; the best way to control active bleeding.

Dressing Sterile material placed over an open wound.

Epidermis Outermost layer of the skin, made up mostly of dead skin cells.

First-degree burns Minor burns characterized by reddened skin.

Flash burns Burns from an open electrical source to exposed tissue.

Full-thickness burns Burns that penetrate all three layers of the skin and into the tissue below.

Hematoma Closed soft tissue injury characterized by blood pooling at the injury site, producing swelling.

Impaled object Pointed object that has penetrated the skin.

Lacerations Open soft tissue injuries characterized by a jagged cutting of the skin.

Linear laceration A laceration in a straight line.

Material safety data sheet Information on the characteristics, uses, and medical consequences of chemical exposure.

Partial-thickness burn Burn that penetrates the epidermis and part of the dermis.

Pressure dressing Dressing applied to help reduce swelling or control excessive bleeding.

Proximal pulse point Bleeding control technique that involves applying manual pressure to the most proximal pulse of an injury site.

Puncture wound Open soft tissue injury resulting from a pointed object penetrating the skin.

Rule of nines Method of determining the amount of damage done to body surface area as a result of burns, abrasions, or other injury.

Second-degree burns Partial- to full-thickness burns characterized by pain and the formation of blisters.

Stellate laceration Laceration that is jagged.

Subcutaneous tissue Innermost layer of the skin.

Superficial burns First-degree burns that affect only the outermost layers of skin.

Third-degree burns Full-thickness burns characterized by charred, white, or gray skin, with no pain involved.

Tourniquet Constricting band placed above an injured extremity to stop the flow of blood. Tourniquets should be used only as a last resort.

Tunnel vision Focusing on horrific-looking injuries instead of identifying possible life-threatening injuries.

Venous bleeding Active bleeding characterized by large amounts of dark red blood steadily flowing from a wound site.

National Standard Curriculum Objectives

Cognitive Objectives

After completing this lesson, the EMT student will be able to do the following:

- State the major functions of the skin.
- List the layers of the skin.
- Establish the relationship between body substance isolation and soft tissue injuries.
- List the types of closed soft tissue injuries.
- Describe the emergency medical care of the patient with a closed soft tissue injury.
- State the types of open soft tissue injuries.
- Describe the emergency medical care of the patient with an open soft tissue injury.
- Discuss the emergency medical care considerations for a patient with a penetrating chest injury.
- State the emergency medical care considerations for a patient with an open wound to the abdomen.

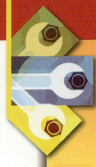

- Differentiate the care of an open wound to the chest from an open wound to the abdomen.
- List the classifications of burns.
- Define *superficial burn*.
- List the characteristics of a superficial burn.
- Define *partial-thickness burn*.
- List the characteristics of a partial-thickness burn.
- Define *full-thickness burn*.
- List the characteristics of a full-thickness burn.
- Describe the emergency medical care of the patient with a superficial burn.
- Describe the emergency medical care of the patient with a partial-thickness burn.
- Describe the emergency medical care of the patient with a full-thickness burn.
- List the functions of dressing and bandaging.
- Describe the purpose of a bandage.
- Describe the steps in applying a pressure dressing.
- Establish the relationship between airway management and the patient with chest injury, burns, and blunt and penetrating injuries.
- Describe the effects of improperly applied dressings, splints, and tourniquets.
- Describe the emergency medical care of a patient with an impaled object.
- Describe the emergency medical care of a patient with an amputation.
- Describe the emergency care for a chemical burn.
- Describe the emergency care for an electrical burn.

Affective Objectives

No affective objectives identified.

Psychomotor Objectives

After completing this lesson, the EMT student will be able to do the following:

- Demonstrate the steps in the emergency medical care of closed soft tissue injuries.
- Demonstrate the steps in the emergency medical care of open soft tissue injuries.
- Demonstrate the steps in the emergency medical care of a patient with an open chest wound.
- Demonstrate the steps in the emergency medical care of a patient with open abdominal wounds.
- Demonstrate the steps in the emergency medical care of a patient with an impaled object.
- Demonstrate the steps in the emergency medical care of a patient with an amputation.
- Demonstrate the steps in the emergency medical care of an amputated part.
- Demonstrate the steps in the emergency medical care of a patient with superficial burns.
- Demonstrate the steps in the emergency medical care of a patient with partial-thickness burns.
- Demonstrate the steps in the emergency medical care of a patient with full-thickness burns.
- Demonstrate the steps in the emergency medical care of a patient with a chemical burn.
- Demonstrate completing a prehospital care report for patients with soft tissue injuries.

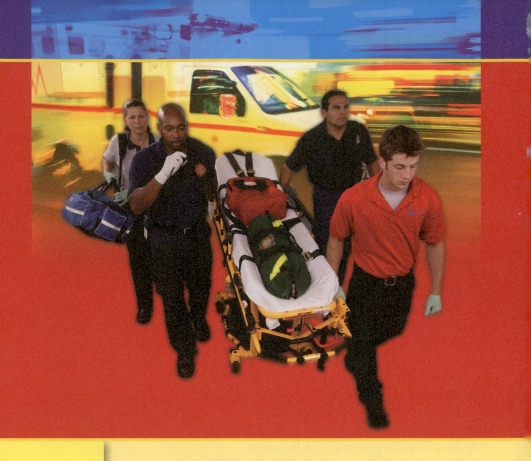

CHAPTER

27

OUTLINE

GOAL

LESSON GOAL

Many patients who sustain serious or life-threatening injury to the chest and abdomen receive their initial trauma care by emergency medical technicians. It is critical for the emergency medical technician to be able to recognize the mechanisms and patterns of injury and assess and stabilize these injuries.

These injuries can result in major hemorrhage and a shock state for the patient. Definitive treatment of these injuries and shock requires rapid transport to a trauma center for surgical intervention. This chapter identifies common injuries to the chest and abdomen. In addition, the chapter examines the initial lifesaving care these patients often require. Assessment clues often can help to identify those patients who need advanced intervention immediately. ■

Chest and Abdominal Trauma

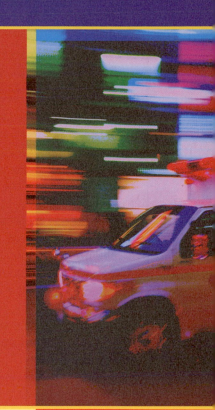

CHAPTER OBJECTIVES

After completing this chapter, the EMT student will be able to do the following:

1 Identify patients at risk for significant chest or abdominal injuries based on the mechanism of injury.

2 Recognize the importance of obtaining appropriate basic vital signs and a general physical assessment.

3 Recognize signs and symptoms of the shock state in victims of chest and abdominal trauma.

4 Demonstrate the physical exam of the chest and abdomen.

5 Recognize patients who need high-priority transport and tiered response with advanced prehospital care.

6 Describe how to bandage and protect open chest and abdominal injuries.

7 Describe how to make trauma patients more comfortable using nonpharmacologic means.

8 Describe how to recognize and preserve forensic evidence that is involved in penetrating trauma care.

OBJECTIVES

Jack could see the flashing blue and red lights of multiple police cars bouncing off the walls of the neighboring buildings as Elizabeth and her crew pulled up to the bar. As the crew assembled their equipment, one of the police officers indicated that there were several victims inside the establishment that needed medical attention. However, one seemed "critical," as the officer pointed him out.

Taking direction from Elizabeth, Jack knelt down near the young man, who was sitting propped up against a wall. Even though it was dark inside the bar, Jack could make out dark stains of blood on the man's shirt and pants. Reaching for the patient's radial pulse, Jack asked him, "What's your name?"

"Manuel," he replied, with difficulty. Jack noted that he was tachypneic, with a rapid radial pulse. "What happened?"

"I've been stabbed. It hurts!" Just then the officer shined his light on the patient. Jack could clearly see that the patient was pale.

Questions: *Based on the initial assessment, how serious is Manuel's condition? What steps should the ambulance crew perform next? What precautions should the crew consider during their care of the patient?*

After airway emergencies, injuries to the chest and abdomen are leading causes of death and serious outcomes for trauma victims. Appropriate, rapid, and accurate prehospital recognition and treatment of chest and abdominal trauma injuries can minimize the development of postinjury **shock** and the worsening of internal injury. The most common cause of serious chest and abdominal injuries is motor vehicle trauma. However, falls and **penetrating trauma** are also significant causes. Even more rare but perhaps more complex are **blast injuries.** These can produce not only blunt force injuries of virtually every organ system as the victim is thrown against fixed objects but also penetrating injury from flying debris. This chapter examines the assessment, treatment, and transportation of these patients.

■ INJURY AND SHOCK

Chest and abdominal injuries can involve damage to any of the soft tissues, solid organs (liver, spleen, and kidneys), and hollow organs (stomach and intestines) (Fig. 27-1). The heart and the lungs also can suffer direct injury from blunt and penetrating trauma. Blood loss from direct injury or laceration to organs or blood vessels or "**third-spacing**" of fluid as commonly occurs after crush injury or burns can cause shock as the available volume in the circulatory system drops. Third-spacing occurs when fluid leaves

ASK YOURSELF

- Is the scene safe?
- Where do I begin?
- Do I need backup?

the blood vessels (first space) and even leaves the cells (second space) to be trapped uselessly in the tissues between cells and organs (third space). Thus not all fluid loss is visible as external hemorrhage. In addition, volume loss can result from internal bleeding into the chest or abdominal cavity. As fluid is lost from the circulation, the patient's level of alertness, sense of well-being, and even mental clarity can decline. Ultimately, the patient will lose consciousness as blood flow to the brain decreases. Your ability to evaluate the patient and the extent of his or her injuries is complicated by this declining mental status. Your assessment begins with a scene size-up (see Chapter 8).

■ MECHANISM OF INJURY

Sudden deceleration and impact on the chest or abdomen with the internal structures of the motor vehicle result in predictable patterns of internal injury

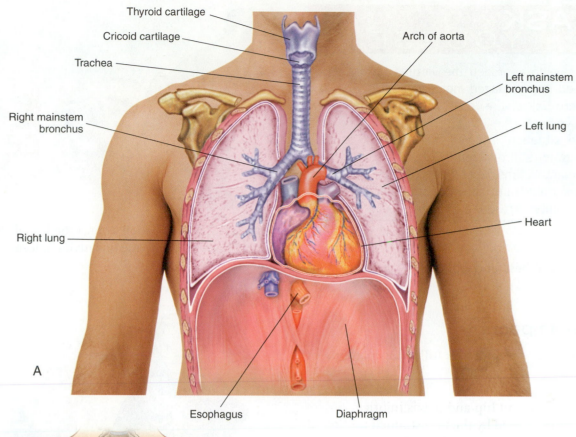

Thyroid cartilage

Cricoid cartilage

Trachea

Right mainstem bronchus

Right lung

Arch of aorta

Left mainstem bronchus

Left lung

Heart

A

Esophagus

Diaphragm

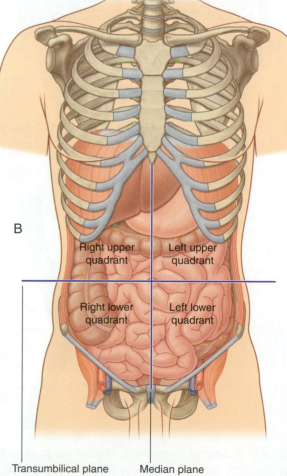

B

Right upper quadrant

Left upper quadrant

Right lower quadrant

Left lower quadrant

Transumbilical plane

Median plane

Fig. 27-1 **A,** Chest cavity and related anatomic structures. **B,** Four-quadrant topographic map.

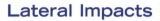

ASK YOURSELF

- Is it safe to approach the victims, or are they trapped in a damaged motor vehicle?
- Is there risk of fire, electric shock, or air bag deployment?
- If the situation involved an assailant, is the perpetrator still on scene?
- How many victims or potential patients do I have?
- Are they alert and able to communicate, or is their ability to respond impaired?

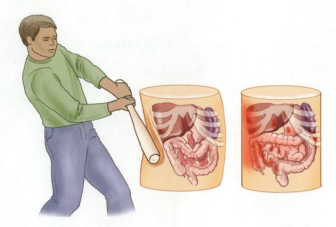

Fig. 27-2 Compression against the lateral chest and abdominal wall injures the underlying spleen, liver, and kidney.

to the trunk (chest and abdomen) of the patient (Figs. 27-2 to 27-4).

Lateral Impacts

Lateral impacts produce the following patterns of injury:

- Shoulder, rib, and hip and pelvis injuries
- Neck injury caused by the unrestrained motion of the victim's head, even without direct impact

Recently developed side restraint air bags lessen these injuries.

Frontal Impacts

Frontal impacts produce the following patterns of injury:

- Anterior chest injuries (Fig. 27-5)
- Lower extremity injuries caused by impact with the dashboard
- Abdominal injuries from impact with the lower rim of the steering wheel or misapplied seat belts (Fig. 27-6)
- Neck injuries caused by the unrestrained motion of the head, particularly if there is no head rest or the head rest is positioned improperly.

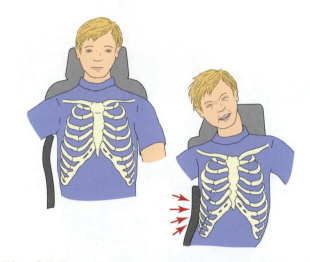

Fig. 27-3 Lateral impact to the chest will produce rib fractures and possible injury to underlying organs.

Rollover Impacts

Rollover impacts produce the following effects:

- Depending on the restraint use of the victim, injuries may occur to any area.
- Ejection from the vehicle is common if the patient is unrestrained.

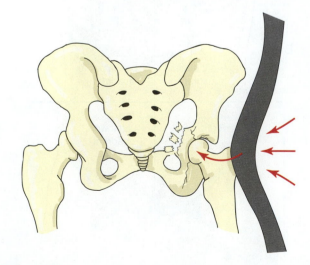

Fig. 27-4 Lateral impact on the femur pushes the head through the acetabulum or fractures the pelvis.

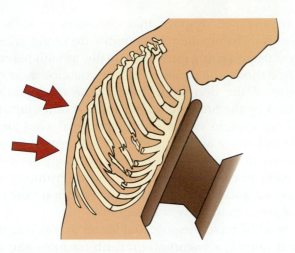

Fig. 27-5 Ribs forced into the thoracic cavity by external compression usually fracture in multiple places, producing the clinical condition known as flail chest.

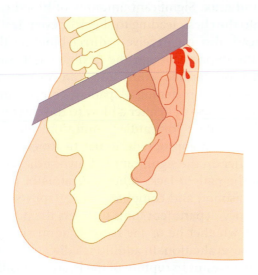

Fig. 27-6 Abdominal injury can result from a seat belt that is positioned incorrectly. If the belt is positioned above the brim of the pelvis, the abdominal organs can be trapped between the moving posterior wall and the belt. Injuries to the pancreas and other retroperitoneal organs and blowout ruptures of the small intestine and colon result.

■ CHEST INJURY

Blunt Injury

As impact to the chest occurs, the soft tissues of the chest wall have limited capacity to absorb energy before transmitting it to the internal structures. Ribs and **intercostal muscles** are pliable but eventually yield to the force applied to them, leading to rib fractures. The underlying lungs, **great vessels,** and heart can sustain contusions and can rupture. Blood seeping from damaged capillaries in the lungs can fill the **alveolar air spaces,** creating **pulmonary contusion** and decreased ventilation of the involved **alveoli** and resultant dyspnea and **hypoxia** for the patient.

Rib fractures worsen the patient's situation by adding significant pain to the breathing process. The resulting splinting, or attempt to limit motion of the injured area of the chest wall, can worsen the hypoventilation and oxygenation problem. Splinting can lead to **atelectasis,** or collapse of the hypoventilated areas of the lung. This is visible on x-ray films within 1 or 2 days of the chest injury. Supplemental oxygen is *always* appropriate for chest trauma victims, even those with a history of chronic obstructive pulmonary disease. In addition, ribs may fracture in more than one place. When multiple ribs are broken in multiple places, the structural ability of the chest to breathe normally is compromised, leading to further difficulties with dyspnea and hypoxia. This condition is referred to as flail chest. When a patient with an uninjured chest breathes in, the chest expands and the ribs move outward, allowing the lungs to expand. However, when a patient has a flail chest, the segment of the chest that is fractured is no longer attached to the rest of the rib cage. When a patient breathes in, the intact portion of the chest moves normally, but the ribs that are broken move inward instead because of the negative pressure inside the chest. This results in compromise of the patient's ability to breathe.

Rib fractures also can create a serious problem by collapsing the adjacent lung, creating a **pneumothorax** (Fig. 27-7). Air leaks from the damaged lung into

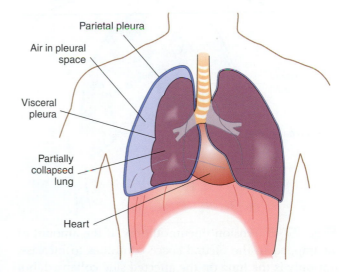

Fig. 27-7 Pneumothorax. Air in the pleural space forces the lung to collapse, decreasing the ability to ventilate and therefore decreasing the oxygenation of the blood leaving the lung.

the normally nonexistent pleural space between the lung and the chest wall. This can collapse the lung further and compromise air exchange.

A pneumothorax frequently can occur without rib fracture. The impact to the chest when the patient's body strikes the inside of the vehicle can cause an instantaneous rise in the intrathoracic pressure, popping the lung like an inflated brown paper bag.

A pneumothorax also can progress to a **tension pneumothorax** (Fig. 27-8). Normally, the air leaking into the pleural space eventually will stop as the pressure in that space equals the pressure in the rest of the chest cavity. However, sometimes the air leaks out from the airways, but a naturally occurring flap valve prevents it from escaping out of the source of the leak. This allows the pleural space to keep getting inflated at higher and higher pressures, creating tension. Eventually the increasing pressure not only fully collapses the affected lung, but also actually begins to displace the heart and great vessels into the opposite side of the chest. When this occurs, the large veins returning blood to the heart become kinked, blood return to the heart decreases, and the patient develops signs of shock. This situation can be rapidly fatal if the increasing pressure is not relieved by a medical procedure, **needle decompression.** This condition presents to the emergency medical technician (EMT) as a patient with spontaneous or

trauma-related dyspnea that continues to worsen. This is accompanied by rapidly declining blood pressure and rising pulse. Eventually, as with hemorrhagic shock, the patient will lose consciousness because of the decreasing blood flow to the brain caused by the pressure on the aorta. If other injuries do not explain considerably abnormal vital signs and tachypnea and the patient has decreased breath sounds in one side of the chest, strongly consider tension pneumothorax as the cause. Promptly involve advanced care providers to perform needle decompression to prevent loss of life.

In addition to the potential for air to leak into the chest causing a pneumothorax, rib fractures also directly may tear blood vessels that are located immediately adjacent to the ribs (intercostal arteries or veins) or blood vessels of the lungs, producing hemorrhage into the chest cavity. This condition is known as a **hemothorax.** Significant amounts of blood can be lost into the chest, leading to shock or even death.

The heart also can receive a direct blow by the force of the impact through the flexible chest wall. Myocardial or **cardiac contusion** can vary from harmless to life threatening. A patient complaining of angina-like chest pain after a blow to the chest is a potential candidate for cardiac contusion. Supplemental oxygen is appropriate initial treatment. Authorities differ on the significance of myocardial contusions if the patient lacks other indicators of chest injury. Ultrasound and computed tomography scans are emergency department tools to assess the patient and decide whether he or she requires admission or other cardiac evaluation. In addition, a direct blow to the chest may result in rupture of the heart. Typically, rupture of the heart leads to rapid development of pericardial tamponade and death.

An uncommon but serious injury caused by deceleration is traumatic aortic tear produced by the motion of the flexible portion of the aorta next to the fixed ligamentous area of the aorta (Fig. 27-9). This rupture kills 90% of its victims at the scene of the accident because of massive hemorrhage into the chest cavity. Patients who survive to the hospital are at increased risk of sudden death from the aortic tear if the injury is not discovered and promptly repaired surgically. Tremendous chest pain and different blood pressure readings in each arm are potential initial assessment findings. Routine chest computed tomography of significant trauma victims in the emergency department virtually has eliminated this preventable cause of death from chest trauma, at least for those victims who survive to reach a hospital with surgical capabilities.

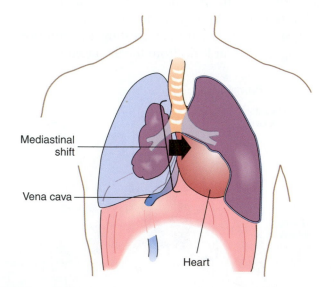

Fig. 27-8 Tension pneumothorax. If the amount of air trapped in the pleural space continues to increase, not only is the lung on the affected side collapsed, but the mediastinum also is shifted into the opposite side. The lung on the opposite side then collapses and intrathoracic pressure increases, which decreases capillary blood flow and kinks the vena cava.

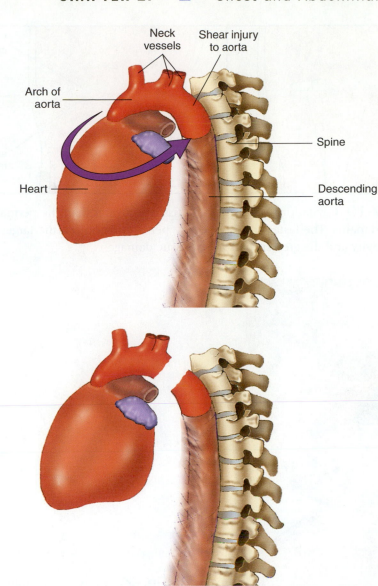

Fig. 27-9 Aortic injury. The descending aorta is affixed tightly to the thoracic vertebrae. The arch of the aorta and the heart are not attached to the vertebrae. Disruption from shear force usually occurs at the junction of the arch and the descending aorta.

Penetrating Injury

Penetrating injuries to the chest are due largely to **gunshot wounds** and to accidental or intentional knife wounds. Even more rarely, an object will penetrate the chest cavity and remain impaled. Depending on the weapon used and the path of the projectile(s), the injury can be to the soft tissue of the chest wall only, can produce pneumothoraces or hemothoraces of varying severity, or can result in injury to the great vessels and heart that is rapidly fatal. High-velocity projectiles can create tissue damage at distances many times their diameter because of the shock wave

that is created by their supersonic travel. **Cavitation,** the shock wave–created space in tissues struck by the bullet, can tear and disrupt tissue and adjacent blood vessels and nerves (Figs. 27-10 and 27-11). Bones in the direct path or close by can be shattered, even creating secondary projectiles of bone.

In the case of a knife injury, the potential for organ injury is described as the **cone of injury** (Fig. 27-12). This cone of injury represents the sites in the body that were potentially reachable by the tip of the knife and could have been penetrated (Fig. 27-13). Thus tissues and body cavities apparently remote from the point of entry still can be damaged severely.

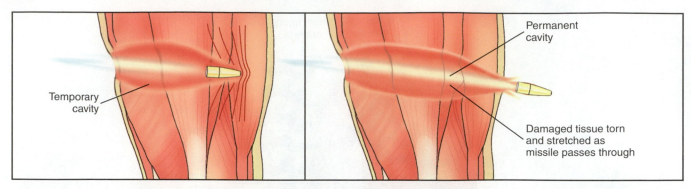

Fig. 27-10 Cavitation. Damage to the tissue is greater than the permanent cavity that remains. The faster and heavier the penetrating object, the larger the temporary cavity and the greater the zone of tissue damage.

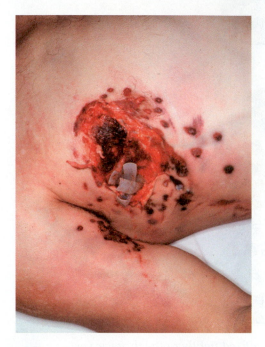

Fig. 27-11 Shotgun blast to chest.

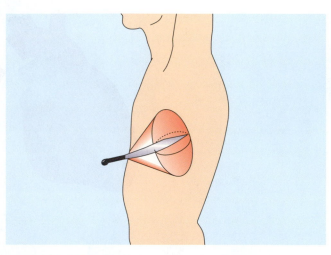

Fig. 27-12 Cone of injury from knife wound. The damage produced by a knife depends on the movement of the blade inside the victim.

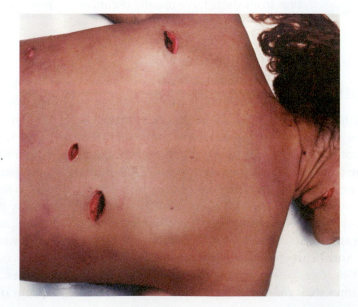

Fig. 27-13 Multiple stab wounds.

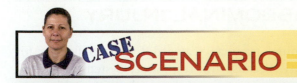

CASE SCENARIO

continued

Elizabeth opened the oxygen bag and fished out a non-rebreather oxygen mask. Jack took her shears out of his pocket and quickly cut off Manuel's shirt, being careful to not cut through the areas where the knife was used to stab him. Performing a rapid trauma assessment, Jack observed that there appeared to be an open wound on the left lower lateral side of the chest, a second wound to the left lower quadrant of the abdomen, and slashes across both hands and arms. Blood was coming out of the abdominal injury, and Jack could see frothy blood oozing out of the chest wound. The arm wounds were bleeding as well, but not quickly. The patient's breath sounds were diminished on the left side, and no jugular venous distention was noted.

Questions: Which of the injuries is most life threatening to Manuel? Why? How should Jack treat each of these injuries? When should transport be initiated?

SPECIAL Populations

Pediatric Considerations

A child's ribs are more pliable than those of an adult. Children are less likely to have rib fractures, but because the ribs provide much less protection for the vital organs in the chest, children are more likely to have internal organ damage in blunt trauma to the chest.

Assessment and Treatment

Assessment of chest injury begins as you approach the patient. Ask yourself whether the patient is breathing spontaneously. Does the patient have the ability to speak and answer questions? If so, your tasks are greatly simplified. If not, initiate support of airway and breathing immediately. Next, expose the patient's chest and assess for injuries. First, observe the exposed chest wall. This observation can reveal significant findings. If a large bruise or a penetrating wound is visible, this will substantially increase the probability of serious internal chest injury. Palpate the chest wall gently to determine whether there are any points of tenderness or pain. Auscultate the patient's breath sounds and note whether they are equal or unequal. Rales, coarse breath sounds, or stridor (whistling noises) suggest fluid in the lungs or obstruction to the airways.

Immediate assessment and transport of victims of penetrating trauma to the chest is vital. Attempting to determine exit and entrance wounds is often impossible in the field. However, disrobing and logrolling of the patient to search for additional injuries is es-

sential. A patient with one anterior stab wound noted prehospital could have 15 or more posteriorly when disrobed at the emergency department.

If an open wound is found on the chest or back, the EMT must pay extra close attention to it. Penetrating trauma to the upper torso could interrupt the airtight seal around the lungs provided by the chest wall. When this happens, the patient will have an open chest wound, or sucking chest wound. The wound has a sucking sound each time the patient breathes. Bubbles of blood may also form on the surface of the wound. The patient, if conscious, will complain of extreme difficulty in breathing. As the patient inhales, air is drawn into the chest cavity (the cavity, not the lungs) through the penetrating hole. As the amount of air in the cavity increases, so does the pressure inside the chest if the air cannot escape. This pressure then pushes against the involved lung, which pushes against the heart and good lung. This development is called a tension pneumothorax. Tension pneumothorax will lead quickly to the patient's death if it is not assessed and treated appropriately. The EMT must act quickly by applying an occlusive dressing over the penetrating wound. The foil packet that holds a petroleum gauze pad or a double layer of aluminum foil serves as an excellent occlusive dressing. The purpose of an occlusive dressing is to stop air from being drawn into the chest cavity when the patient inhales, yet allow for some air to escape during exhalation. Place the dressing over the wound and tape it on *three* sides. As the patient inhales, the dressing is pulled tighter over the wound, blocking the further entry of air. As the patient exhales, the dressing allows for air to move out of the chest cavity. This process reduces some of the pressure that would build up in the chest cavity, but not all of it. Occasionally, the patient's respiratory status may worsen because of the increased pressure. When this occurs, the EMT temporarily removes the dressing until the problem is resolved but then quickly reapplies the dressing. The EMT repeats this process as often as necessary.

Penetrating trauma to the chest also can cause a pericardial tamponade. This is a life-threatening injury that may develop quickly. A tough layer of membrane, the pericardium, covers the heart. This layer can be penetrated, but blood may not be able to exit through the entry hole. The space between the heart and the pericardium is usually a small space filled with a tiny amount of fluid to help lubricate the heart as it beats within the pericardium. If a knife penetrates the pericardium and a wall of the heart, blood will leak into the pericardium as the heart beats. As blood accumulates, there is less room for the heart to expand and fill with blood and then contract and pump blood to the body. This results in a decrease in the overall output of blood, depriving the body of oxygen. Several signs and symptoms for which the EMT should look when assessing a patient who may have a pericardial tamponade are the following:

- *Tachycardia:* In an effort to maintain an adequate blood flow, the heart will beat faster to increase its output.
- *Narrowing pulse pressure:* Pulse pressure, the difference between the systolic and diastolic pressures, decreases.
- *Paradoxical pulse:* If the systolic blood pressure drops more than 10 to 15 mm Hg with each inspiration, the EMT can feel the radial pulse diminish or even disappear.
- *Jugular vein distention:* The heart is not effectively pumping, so blood may back up in the vascular system.
- *Muffled heart tones:* As the pericardium fills with blood, the heart sounds as if it is being heard through fluid.

The EMT should look for these signs if a pericardial tamponade is suspected based on the mechanism of injury. In addition, the EMT must transport the patient rapidly to a trauma center and notify the center of the patient's status.

Give supplemental oxygen to all patients with blunt or penetrating chest injury. Treat any penetrating injuries of the chest by covering the opening with an airproof dressing or packaging materials secured on three sides. Allow air to escape via the open side, which should pull itself shut when the patient inhales, preventing more air from entering the chest cavity. In any penetrating chest wound, initiate a tiered response with advanced emergency medical services providers.

■ ABDOMINAL INJURY

Abdominal trauma creates different challenges for the EMT. Because the respiratory system is not involved, injuries to the abdominal cavity and its contents are rarely fatal in the abbreviated time frame sometimes seen with chest injuries. However, severe and life-threatening hemorrhage and shock can occur. Thorough and repeated assessment of the patient who has sustained abdominal injuries is essential.

The buffer zone between the chest and the abdomen created by the diaphragm and the overlap of the ribs with the upper abdomen frequently results in trauma involving both body cavities. Injury to the chest also can result in liver, spleen, and kidney lacerations. Forces applied to the abdomen can cause diaphragmatic rupture that allows abdominal organs to enter the chest and can affect ventilation adversely.

The patient who has sustained blunt trauma to the abdomen often has other injuries that may be more obvious and painful. These more obvious injuries may include, for example, long bone fractures. As a result, such a situation requires a systematic approach to avoid overlooking the abdominal injuries.

Patients with abdominal trauma frequently will have significant pain but cannot always localize the source. The nerves to the internal organs do not have the ability to localize pain. Only when the lining of the abdominal cavity is irritated by blood, pus, or contaminants does the pain become localized.

Solid organ injury most commonly involves the spleen, liver, and kidneys and less commonly the pancreas. These organs are firm and do not tolerate a direct blow without risk of tearing. When tearing occurs, bleeding into the abdominal cavity can occur and can be life threatening. The hollow intestinal organs and stomach can tolerate some compression, but when squeezed against a solid object, such as the small intestine pressed against the spine by a misapplied seat belt, they can be ruptured. This rupture results in bleeding and allows intestinal contents to spill into the normally sterile abdominal cavity. This can have disastrous results if it is not corrected surgically.

SPECIAL Populations

Pediatric Considerations

The child's abdominal musculature is much less developed than in adults and cannot provide the same protection for that area of the body. Children are more likely to suffer internal organ damage in blunt trauma to the abdomen.

Assessment and Treatment

Assessment of the patient with abdominal injury requires removing the patient's clothing and warming the diagnostic tools. Placing an ice-cold hand or stethoscope on someone's abdomen guarantees a firm abdominal wall. After performing the primary assessment and ensuring adequate airway and breathing, inspect the abdominal wall for obvious injury or penetration. Look for distention, which is the abnormal increase in size of the abdomen from extra gas or fluids being present. In cases involving penetrating trauma, look to see whether any of the abdominal contents have come out through the penetrating wound.

Many textbooks traditionally teach that part of the examination involves assessing for bowel sounds. Unfortunately, it usually takes time for absent bowel sounds to occur. In addition, the prehospital setting is not conducive to listening for bowel sounds because of other distracting noises. Therefore listening for bowel sounds is not really applicable in the field. Feel each of the four quadrants of the abdomen gently, checking for firmness or spontaneous pain with palpation. Rough or rapid handling may give falsely abnormal results. Your goal is to determine which, if any, areas are tender. Upper abdominal tenderness suggests spleen or liver injury. Lower abdominal tenderness can be from many causes but suggests bowel injury or abdominal wall injury. Omit the palpation of the abdomen if a penetrating injury is present. You will always find tenderness, and the palpation could result in **evisceration** of abdominal contents through the wound (Fig. 27-14). Cover any exposed organs found with moistened sterile dressings to avoid having them adhere to the exposed tissues (Fig. 27-15).

Provide patients with signs of abdominal injury with supplemental oxygen and provide rapid transport to an appropriate receiving hospital, preferably a trauma center. Identification of the specific organ injuries and the extent of those injuries or provision of

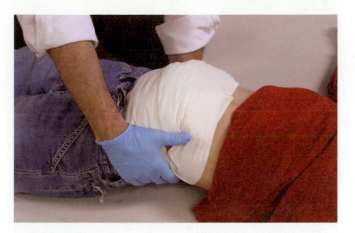

Fig. 27-15 An evisceration is covered with a thick, moist dressing and then is covered with a dry, sterile dressing.

definitive care are not possible in the field. Delay in transport only allows for continued hemorrhage into the abdominal cavity and may result in a patient who is at serious risk of death from blood loss.

Logroll the patient to determine whether there are contusions, deformities, or penetrating injuries to the back that are not seen anteriorly. Note all your findings in your report.

■ CRIME SCENE ASSESSMENT

Assaults and penetrating injuries can create an extra burden for the EMT if the scene and the victim are part of the investigation of a criminal act. In addition to your normal assessment, careful handling of clothing and other items at the scene so as not to damage or contaminate potential evidence can be crucial to the successful prosecution of the crime. Whenever possible, do not cut clothing through the point of entry caused by a weapon. This will serve only to damage potential evidence. In addition, do not place clothing or other items removed from the victim in sealed plastic bags. Instead, use paper bags because any moisture wicking off the clothing will not diffuse the gunpowder or other chemicals imbedded in the fabric.

Avoid entering any areas of the scene that are not absolutely essential to the care of your patient. Footprints, fingerprints, and other evidence may be disturbed easily. Lastly, if your patient is already clearly deceased as a result of his or her injuries, contact your medical control and avoid disturbing the body and scene. Do not even begin resuscitation efforts. When in doubt, perform potentially lifesaving services while seeking medical control advice. Once death is verified

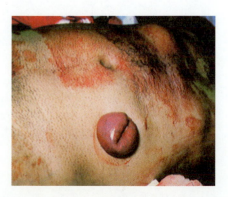

Fig. 27-14 Evisceration.

and further efforts are considered futile, law enforcement agency staff who are present at the scene can assist you in contacting the medical examiner or coroner to assume control and responsibility for the victim's body and can maintain control of the crime scene.

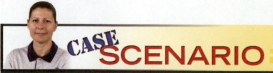

CASE SCENARIO

conclusion

The patient compartment doors slammed shut, and the rig almost immediately began to move to the hospital. Manuel was seat belted to the gurney, lying in the semi-Fowler position, with a non-rebreather mask providing oxygen. Jack finished dressing the wounds on Manuel's arms; he already had placed an occlusive dressing over the chest wound and another crew member was applying manual pressure to a bulky dressing covering the abdominal wound. As Elizabeth was obtaining the blood pressure and other vital signs, she noted that Manuel still was having difficulty breathing and was becoming increasingly tired. Elizabeth knew that time was of the essence and hoped they would get to the trauma center soon. ■

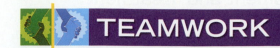

TEAMWORK

The emergency medical technician often functions as the first of many trained responders in initiating the chain of survival for the patient with chest and abdominal trauma. Prompt transport and involvement of advanced care response when appropriate, as well as rapid transfer to trauma services, can be lifesaving. The involvement of paramedics, helicopter emergency medical services, and trauma centers reflects the team effort needed to ensure the best outcome for the victim of these serious injuries.

Resources

Chapleau W: *Emergency first response: making the difference,* St Louis, 2004, Mosby.

Cox JF: Complexities of blunt chest trauma, *JEMS* 29(11):44-55, 2004.

National Association of Emergency Medical Technicians: *PHTLS: basic and advanced prehospital trauma life support,* ed 5, St Louis, 2003, Mosby.

O'Keefe MF, Limmer D, Grant HD, et al: *Emergency care,* ed 8, Saddle River, NJ, 1998, Prentice-Hall.

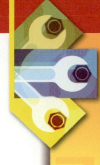

Critical Points

Chest and abdominal trauma can be rapidly fatal to trauma victims.

Many presentations of chest and abdominal trauma are not immediately obvious. They require systematic assessment to detect. Distracting painful injuries can divert attention from the more serious internal injuries.

For seriously injured trauma patients, rapid assessment and appropriate tiered response with advance care services are vital.

For patients who have expired already from their traumatic injuries, contact the medical examiner authorities and do not disrupt the death scene.

Learning Checklist

❏ The chest and abdomen frequently are involved in traumatic injury.

❏ The mechanisms of injury can be motor vehicle collisions or penetrating wounds by knives, gunshots, or blast debris.

❏ Injuries to the organs of the chest and abdomen frequently can lead to the shock state and become life threatening for the patient.

❏ The chest includes the skin, ribs, muscles of the chest wall, the heart and great vessels, the lungs, the trachea, and the bronchi and air passages.

❏ The abdomen contains solid organs—such as the liver, kidneys, and spleen—and hollow organs, including the stomach, small and large intestine, and the rectum. The kidneys and ureters also are considered abdominal organs.

❏ Shock is the inadequate delivery of oxygen and nutrients to the cells of the body.

❏ Decreased circulating blood volume caused by injury is a major cause of shock.

❏ Fluid can be lost from the circulation without hemorrhage; this is called third-spacing.

❏ Blood loss and shock can lead to decreased levels of consciousness in the victim.

❏ The thin rib cage cannot tolerate large impacts without bony and soft tissue injuries.

❏ Painful rib fractures can compromise a patient's respiratory effort.

❏ Pneumothorax can result from rib fractures or pressure increase in the chest with impacts.

❏ Simple pneumothorax can progress to tension pneumothorax, which causes severe buildup of air within the chest cavity that can prevent the function of the heart and the remaining lung.

❏ The heart can be bruised because of a blow to the chest.

❏ The aorta can be torn by rapid deceleration. This is frequently a fatal injury.

❏ Penetrating injuries to the chest and abdomen are primarily due to gunshot wounds. The injured tissues may be remote from the site of entry of the bullet. Knife wounds also can cause remote injury.

❏ Open wounds of the chest should be covered by occlusive dressing (closed on three sides) with a small flap to allow air to exit but not enter the chest.

SPECIAL Considerations

When your patient requires an occlusive dressing, you often can accomplish that task without hunting for plastic wrap or vasoline gauze. Simply use the inside (sterile side) of the plastic wrapper in which many of the dressings and roller bandages come. For wounds that require bleeding control and an occlusive dressing, simply remove the paper side of the wrapper and place the dressing and wrapper over the wound.

❏ Eviscerations should be covered with warm saline-moistened dressings. Do not attempt to replace the eviscerated organs back into the abdominal cavity.

❏ Abdominal pressure in traumatic injury may rupture the diaphragm, pushing abdominal contents into the chest. As a clue to this condition, bowel sounds may replace breath sounds. The patient may be in respiratory distress.

❏ Solid organs of the abdomen can split and bleed extensively with blunt injury to the abdomen.

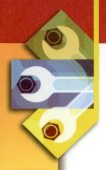

❏ Hollow organs can be ruptured by pressure between the anterior abdominal wall and the spine.

❏ Abdominal injuries do not result in localized pain, but diffuse pain. Gentle palpation to localize the area of maximum pain is best.

❏ Victims of penetrating trauma nearly always are involved in a crime scene. Whenever possible, the treatment of the victim must be sensitive to avoiding disturbing any evidence.

Key Terms

Alveoli Small air sacs within the lungs formed by elastic, highly vascularized membrane. Oxygen delivered to the alveoli during inspiration diffuses across the membrane and into the bloodstream. In the bloodstream, oxygen is taken up by red blood cells, bound to hemoglobin, and transported to tissues throughout the body. At the same time, carbon dioxide dissolved in the blood diffuses in the opposite direction, crossing the membrane and accumulating within the alveoli to be exhaled.

Alveolar air spaces The gas-filled spaces of the alveoli.

Atelectasis Collapse of underventilated areas of lung because of inadequate chest motion and lung expansion.

Blast injuries Created by explosions of all types, these injuries can create penetration by any involved materials. The patient even may become a projectile and be injured by impact with fixed objects. Additionally, any nearby materials may be accelerated by the blast and strike nearby victims.

Cardiac contusion Injury to the heart muscle from a direct blow; bruising.

Cavitation The shock wave–created space in tissues struck by a bullet. This space can be many times the diameter of the bullet that causes it.

Cone of damage Any internal tissues within reach of a knife inserted at the point of entry. This can be far more distant and extensive than evident at first.

Evisceration Protrusion of abdominal contents through a wound in the abdominal wall.

Great vessels Aorta and inferior and superior venae cavae and their largest branches.

Gunshot wounds Wounds resulting in penetrating trauma and organ injury from a gunshot.

Hemothorax Injury to blood vessels of the lungs or rib cage and subsequent bleeding into the chest cavity.

Hypoxia Inadequate cellular oxygenation.

Intercostal muscles The muscles that lie between the ribs and assist respiration by raising and lowering the adjacent ribs with each breath.

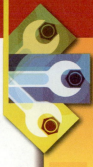

Needle decompression Insertion of a large intravenous-style needle between the ribs to relieve a tension pneumothorax.

Penetrating trauma Stabbing, gunshot wounds, or other injuries created by the entry of a sharp object into the body.

Pneumothorax Development of air in the normally empty space between the lung and the chest wall.

Pulmonary contusion Lung injury that results in fluid or blood seeping into the alveolar air spaces, preventing that area from exchanging oxygen and carbon dioxide with the blood.

Shock The inadequate delivery of oxygen and nutrients to cells, resulting in organ system malfunction. Eventually shock is detectible with abnormal vital signs. It can lead to death.

Tension pneumothorax Pressure increase inside the chest from a natural one-way valve that allows air into the chest cavity but with no escape. Eventually this pressure increase can result in compression of the heart and the unaffected lung to the point of circulatory failure and death.

Third-spacing Loss of fluid from the blood vessels (first space) and even the cells (second space) to be trapped uselessly in the tissues between cells and organs. In this location, the fluid is of no physiologic value to the patient.

National Standard Curriculum Objectives

Cognitive Objectives

After completing this lesson, the EMT student will be able to do the following:

- Discuss the emergency medical care considerations for a patient with a penetrating chest injury.
- State the emergency medical care considerations for a patient with an open wound to the abdomen.
- Differentiate the care of an open wound to the chest from an open wound to the abdomen.
- Establish the relationship between airway management and the patient with chest injury.

Affective Objectives

No affective objectives identified.

Psychomotor Objectives

After completing this lesson, the EMT student will be able to do the following:

- Demonstrate the steps in the emergency medical care of a patient with an open chest wound.
- Demonstrate the steps in the emergency medical care of a patient with open abdominal wounds.

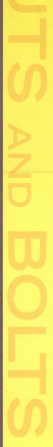

NUTS AND BOLTS

CHAPTER

28

OUTLINE

GOAL

LESSON GOAL

This chapter teaches the emergency medical technician (EMT) student how to recognize and treat musculoskeletal trauma. You must be able to perform the skills presented and be ready to act on the knowledge you will gain. Mastering the basic principles discussed in this chapter will help you significantly as your education and career in emergency medical services (EMS) advance. ■

Musculoskeletal Trauma

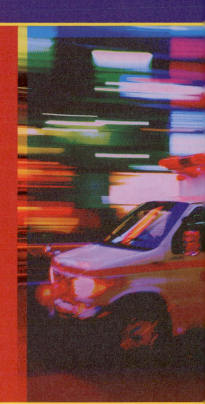

CHAPTER OBJECTIVES

After completing this chapter, the EMT student will be able to do the following:

1   Describe the function of the muscular system.
2   Describe the composition of the muscular system.
3   Describe and compare and contrast the different injuries to the muscular system.
4   Describe the function of the skeletal system.
5   Describe the composition of the skeletal system: the bones of the head, spinal column, thorax, upper extremities, and lower extremities.
6   Describe the structures within a joint.
7   Compare and contrast the different types of joints.
8   Distinguish between open and closed skeletal injuries.
9   Define splinting.
10   List the reasons for splinting.
11   List the rules for splinting.
12   Explain and demonstrate the procedures for splinting.
13   Explain the complications of splinting.
14   Explain the situations in which splinting on the scene is not acceptable and why.

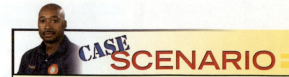

Fact: In the year 2000, musculoskeletal conditions and injuries accounted for 146 million visits to physicians' offices, 14 million visits to hospital outpatient departments, and 30 million visits to emergency departments.[1]

Fact: In the year 2000, more than 7 million people were hospitalized for musculoskeletal conditions.[2]

Fact: In the year 2000, more visits were made to physicians' offices for musculoskeletal conditions than for any other reason.[3]

Considering these facts, it's not surprising that musculoskeletal injuries are one of the most common types of injuries encountered by the EMT. Isolated musculoskeletal injuries generally are not life-threatening. However, when musculoskeletal trauma is present, the EMT must evaluate those musculoskeletal injuries as possible indicators of other life-threatening injuries. Remember, trauma is the result of force applied to the body and the transference of energy from that force to the body. Ask yourself, "If the energy transferred here was enough to insult the integrity of the bone, wouldn't it stand to reason that the same energy could severely damage the structures underneath?" The answer is a resounding *yes!* Therefore, it is essential that you become not only comfortable with but also proficient in your knowledge of the musculoskeletal system in order to perform a good, accurate assessment of the trauma patient (Box 28-1). Moreover, you must develop the special skills needed to treat musculoskeletal injuries.

■ THE MUSCULAR SYSTEM

Muscular Function

The exact number of muscles is unknown, because anatomists' opinions vary. However, almost everyone agrees on the roles the muscular system plays. The muscular system serves a variety of purposes in the human body, all of them vital to existence:

BOX 28-1

DCAPBTLS Assessment Tool

The DCAPBTLS mnemonic, discussed in earlier chapters as an assessment tool, also can help the EMT student learn about soft tissue and musculoskeletal injuries. Remember, the acronym stands for

D = Deformities
C = Contusions
A = Abrasions
P = Punctures or penetrations
B = Burns
T = Tenderness
L = Lacerations
S = Swelling

- Muscles give the body its shape.
- Muscles protect the internal organs by providing a layer between them and the inner aspect of the skin.
- Muscles provide motion.
- Muscles move blood through the body, delivering needed oxygen.
- Muscles move food through the digestive tract.

Muscle Composition

Because of the variety of roles they play, muscles are classified by anatomic location (Fig. 28-1) and by function. The three types of muscle are **skeletal muscle, cardiac muscle,** and **smooth (visceral) muscle.** When classified by function only, muscles are either **voluntary muscles** (consciously controlled) or **involuntary muscles** (unconsciously controlled). Muscles also are classified by their appearance under a microscope. **Striated muscles** appear to have lines running through them, whereas **nonstriated muscles** do not have this appearance. Combining all these classifications, the ultimate differentiation among muscles can be summarized as follows: (1) striated voluntary muscles are skeletal muscles (the group predominantly discussed in this chapter); (2) striated involuntary muscle is cardiac muscle; and (3) nonstriated involuntary muscle is smooth muscle, such as that found in the gastrointestinal tract.

Muscles cause motion and mobility. Moreover, they allow the body to perform a variety of actions. Consequently, muscle groups need to work together

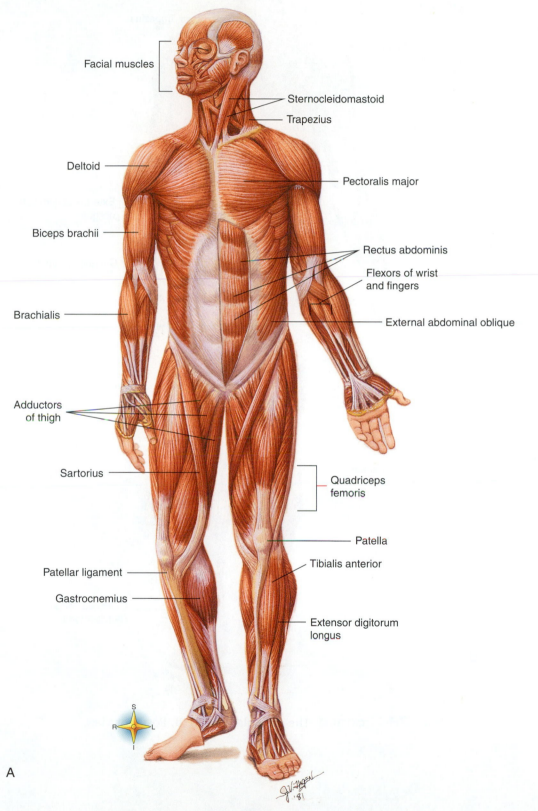

Fig. 28-1 The muscular system. **A,** Anterior view.   *Continued*

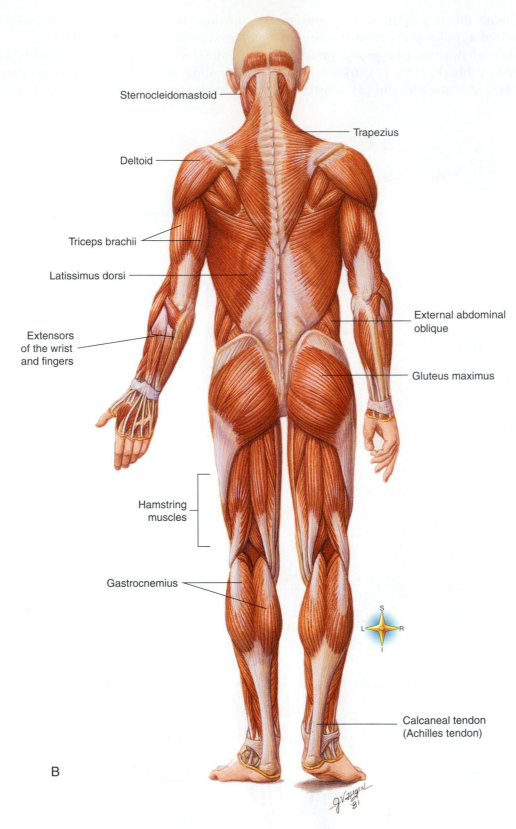

Fig. 28-1, cont'd The muscular system. **B**, Posterior view.

to accomplish these actions. For example, as you read the words on this page, your eyes focus on the words as the muscles that move your eyes shift them from left to right. Your lip muscles may form the words your eyes read. Your neck muscles move your head as you read. Your arm and hand muscles are ready to turn the page when you reach the bottom right-hand corner. This cooperative effort on the part of the muscles is the result of the communication between them via **nerves,** which receive signals from the brain, and **tendons,** which connect muscles to bones and to other muscles. Tendons are tough, durable, cordlike structures known for their strength and durability. The last component of the musculature is the thin layer of membrane over each muscle, the **fascia.** The fascia gives the muscle its shape.

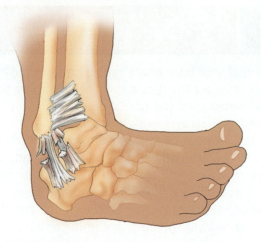

Fig. 28-2 A sprain is an injury in which ligaments are stretched or partially torn.

Injuries of the Muscular System

Trauma to the musculature can result in a variety of injury types and patterns. Fascia, tendons, and muscles can be torn by shearing forces. Tendons and muscles can be stretched beyond their normal **range of motion.** When a muscle is stretched beyond its normal range of motion, the injury is known as a **strain.** When a tendon or ligament is stretched beyond its normal range of motion, the injury is known as a **sprain** (Figs. 28-2 and 28-3). Any part of the musculature can be lacerated, punctured, contused, avulsed, crushed, or amputated. Injured musculature bleeds, and bleeding causes swelling. Depending on the size of the muscle involved, swelling can be very significant. In fact, swelling can be so significant that pulses distal to the injury site can be affected or even nonexistent. Injuries to the musculature cause pain. Pain can be minimal or unbearable, depending on the extent of damage. Nearby nerves can be damaged and the normal electrical activity disrupted, causing loss of sensation or movement in that part of the body. In addition, nearby blood vessels can be damaged, resulting in hematomas or significant blood loss.

During the assessment of an isolated, painful, swollen extremity, the EMT should assess for the **six Ps of musculoskeletal assessment:**

- *Pain* or tenderness in the extremity, as well as the level of pain (1 to 10).
- *Pallor,* or skin color—Is the extremity pale? Does it have poor capillary refill?
- *Pulses*—Are pulses present or absent?
- *Paresthesia*—Does the patient have a "pins and needles" sensation?

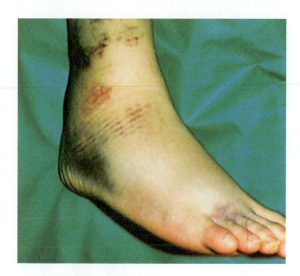

Fig. 28-3 An example of a bad sprain.

- *Paralysis*—Can the patient move the extremity? (Wiggling fingers or toes is appropriate.)
- *Pressure* or *puffiness*—Is swelling present at the injury site?

In addition to assessing the injury, you should determine how it occurred and what type of force was involved. **Direct force** results in damage to the body at the point of contact. A knee hitting the dashboard during a motor vehicle collision is an example of a direct force injury (Fig. 28-4). **Indirect force** is energy that is transferred from the point of contact and travels along the extremity, causing damage farther away. In the example of the knee hitting the dashboard, the patient will have a knee injury, but the person also may have a hip injury because of the transference of energy (Fig. 28-5).

ASK YOURSELF

You and your partner are returning from the hospital after a call. It is a cold, windy, rainy Sunday morning. As you pass a church, you notice a crowd gathered, waving you down. As you approach, several people move away, and you notice an elderly lady supine on the ground. She appears awake and alert and answers your questions appropriately. She says she was going into church, slipped on the bottom step, and fell. She denies any difficulty breathing and has a radial pulse of 90 and irregular. She complains of severe pain in her left hip.

1. Based on your initial assessment, is this patient critical or noncritical?
2. What would you do next?
3. What would you do after that?
4. What other treatments should be done?
5. Are there any confounding factors? If so, what are they?

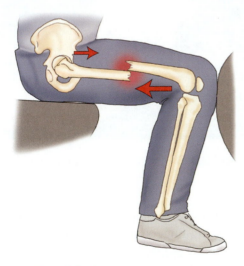

Fig. 28-4 A direct force injury.

Twisting force occurs when the extremity acts as a pivot point that is planted. As the body twists, the energy of the twisting body causes the pivot point to give way to injury. For example, a football player plants his foot to make a quick move laterally and twists his ankle. This is twisting force.

Armed with this information, the EMT can relay the complete assessment findings about the patient's status to the receiving hospital after the patient has been completely evaluated and treated.

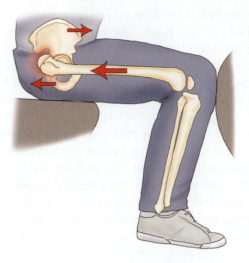

Fig. 28-5 An indirect force injury.

The treatment of a patient with an isolated, painful, swollen extremity is similar to that for a patient with a soft tissue injury; however, it requires an additional step. The musculature of the extremities covers the underlying bones. The EMT must maintain a high index of suspicion that the bony structures under the muscles also may have been injured. In many cases, x-ray films are the only means of determining the integrity of a bone. Therefore you must treat every musculoskeletal injury as if the bone were not intact. The painful, swollen extremity should be elevated, and cold packs should be applied. In addition, you should generally splint the extremity in the position in which you find it (the fundamentals of splinting are covered later in the chapter).

■ THE SKELETAL SYSTEM

Function of the Skeletal System

The bones of the human body support and protect it. Anyone who has visited a large city has been able to look up and marvel at a skyscraper. The construction of a skyscraper is not unlike that of the human body. The outer surface of the building, which may be glass, metal, concrete, or some other material, is very much like the human skin. However, the strength of the building and its ability to rise many stories lie in the infrastructure of steel. The infrastructure of the human body is the skeletal system (Fig. 28-6). Bones are made up of minerals, mostly calcium, and living cells that give them strength and durability. Within the bones are channels, or cavities, filled with **marrow.** Yellow marrow consists mostly of fat cells. Red mar-

Axial skeleton   **Appendicular skeleton**   **Axial skeleton**

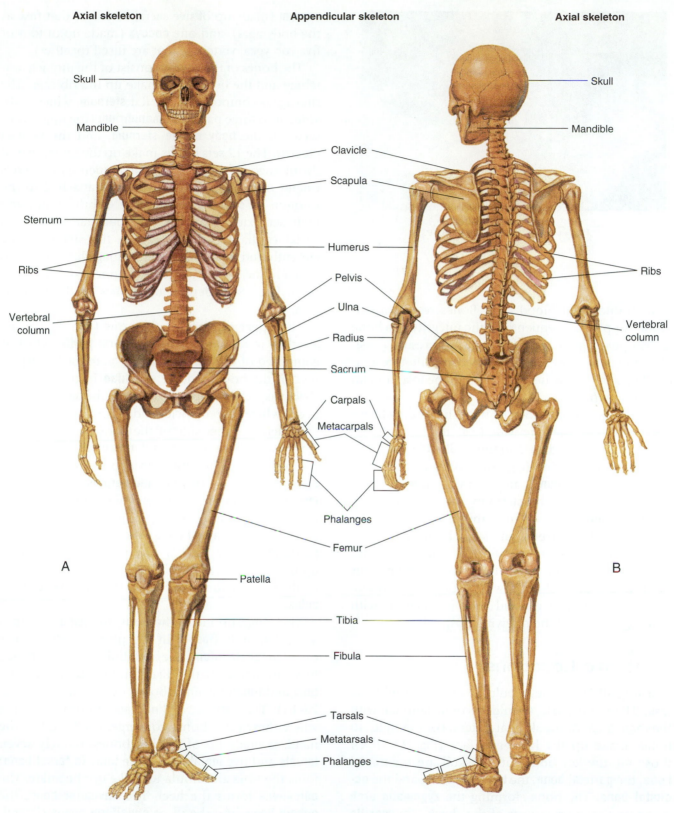

Skull

Mandible

Clavicle

Scapula

Sternum

Humerus

Ribs

Pelvis

Ulna

Vertebral
column

Radius

Sacrum

Carpals

Metacarpals

Phalanges

Femur

A

B

Patella

Tibia

Fibula

Tarsals

Metatarsals

Phalanges

Skull

Mandible

Ribs

Vertebral
column

Fig. 28-6 Anterior (**A**) and posterior (**B**) views of the skeleton.

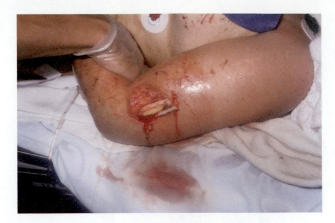

Fig. 28-7 An open fracture.

row produces red blood cells. Bones receive a rich blood supply. Consequently, if the integrity of a bone is disrupted, significant bleeding could result, possibly enough to cause shock and become life-threatening. Fig. 28-7 shows how blood could be lost from an open bone injury.

Bones also are classified by their shape. **Long bones** are longer than they are wide (e.g., the femur, tibia, fibula, humerus, radius, and ulna). **Short bones** are as long as they are wide (e.g., the bones of the wrists and ankles). **Flat bones** are bones such as the ribs, some skull bones, the sternum, and the scapulae. **Irregular bones** don't fit into any of the other categories (e.g., the vertebrae and facial bones).

You should become comfortable with the names and locations of the major bones in the body. This information can help you with your patient assessments. Moreover, it can aid your interactions with other agencies and the receiving hospital.

Anatomic Locations

Learning all 206 bones would be quite a formidable task. Therefore EMTs should become familiar with the main areas of the skeletal system. For example, 40 bones make up the head and face (Fig. 28-8). Of those 40, the key bones of the skull are the **frontal bone,** the **parietal bone,** the **temporal bone,** and the **occipital bone.** The bones forming the **zygomatic arch** make up the outer aspects of the cheek. The **maxilla** and **mandible** are the upper and lower jawbones, respectively.

The **spinal column,** also called the *vertebral column* (Fig. 28-9), is composed of seven **cervical vertebrae,** 12 **thoracic vertebrae,** five **lumbar vertebrae,** one

sacrum (made up of five sacral vertebrae that fuse as the body ages), and one **coccyx** (made up of four or five coccygeal vertebrae that are fused together).

The bones of the thorax consist of the thoracic vertebrae and the bones that make up the rib cage. The rib cage is composed of the flat **sternum,** which is divided into three parts: the **manubrium** (the uppermost section), the **body of the sternum,** and the **xyphoid process.** The 12 sets of **ribs** make up the remainder of the rib cage. Of those 12, the top (superior) seven sets extend from the spine, and each is attached to the sternum by **costal cartilage.** The eighth, ninth, and tenth sets extend from the spine but share a common costal cartilage that attaches to the sternum. The eleventh and twelfth sets are **floating ribs;** these ribs attach at the spine but are not connected to the sternum. Fig. 28-10 depicts the bones of the thoracic area.

The upper extremities, the arms (Fig. 28-11), are attached to the body by the **pectoral girdle,** which is composed of the **clavicles** in the anterior (front) aspect of the body and the **scapulae** in the posterior (back) aspect. The upper arm bone, the **humerus,** connects where the clavicle and scapula join at the shoulder on either side of the body. The forearm is composed of the **radius** and the **ulna.** The wrist is composed of eight **carpals** in two rows of four. The hand is made up of five **metacarpals,** and 14 **phalanges** make up the five fingers of each hand (two in the thumb and three in each finger).

The legs are attached to the lower torso by the **pelvic girdle** (Fig. 28-12). The pelvic girdle is made up of two **coxae,** or hip bones. Each coxa is formed by three fused bones: the **ilium,** the **ischium,** and the **pubis.**

The longest bone in the body, the **femur,** fits into a cup-like hole **(fossa)** in the pelvis. Each fossa is called an **acetabulum.** The acetabulum allows the leg to swing freely. At the distal end of the femur, the **tibia** and **fibula** form the bones of the lower leg (Fig. 28-13). The **patella,** or kneecap, protects the area where these three bones converge. The foot, like the hand, is made up of smaller bones, namely seven **tarsals** and five **metatarsals.** The **talus (a tarsal bone)** joins the tibia and fibula to make up the ankle. The **calcaneus** forms the heel. The **navicular bone,** the **cuboid bone,** and the three **cuneiform bones** (lateral, medial, and intermediate), plus the five metatarsals, form the remainder of the foot. The toes are made up of 14 phalanges, which are arranged as in the hand: the great toe has two, each of the other toes has three.

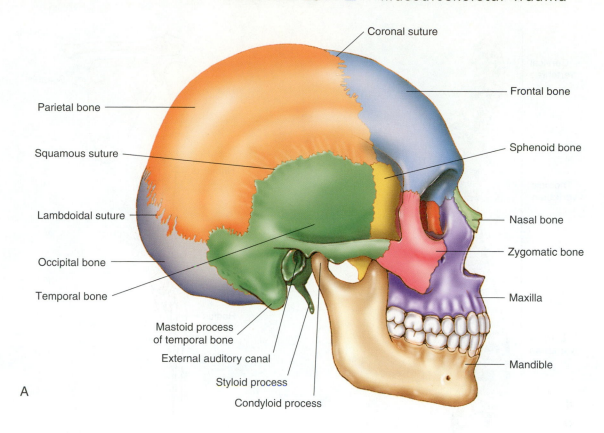

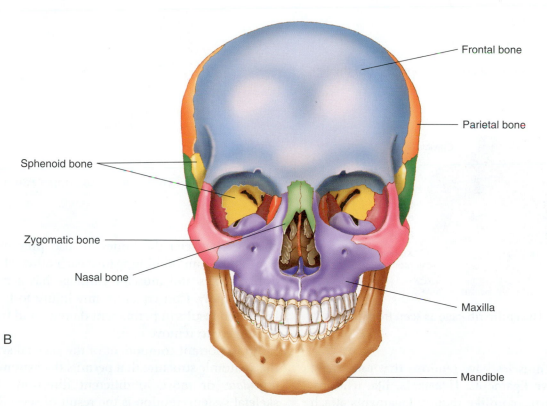

Fig. 28-8 The skull viewed from the right side (A) and from the front (B).

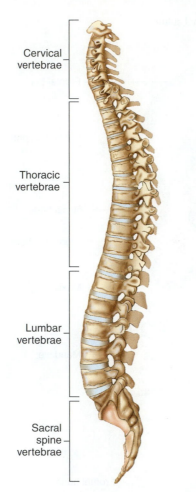

Fig. 28-9 The vertebral column viewed from the left side.

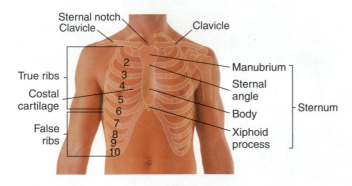

Fig. 28-10 The entire rib cage as seen from the front.

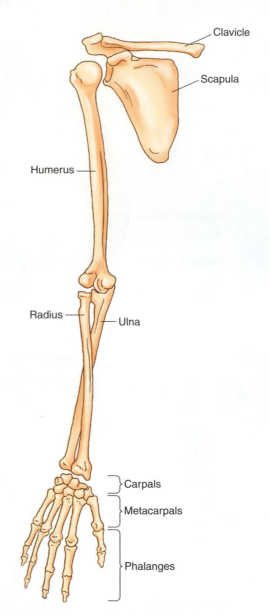

Fig. 28-11 The bones of the upper extremity.

Just as the muscles have tendons that join them, the bones have ligaments. **Ligaments,** like tendons, are tough, elastic, cordlike tissues. Ligaments attach bones to each another and give greater support to the body. They also keep the bones aligned in their proper anatomic positions. When the body is in motion, **cartilage,** a soft, spongy tissue, acts as a shock absorber between the bones. It also prevents hard bone ends from rubbing against each other. However, unlike bones and muscles, cartilage has a minimal blood supply. Consequently, any injury to the cartilage often results in permanent damage and the need for surgery to remove it.

An important component of the skeletal system is the anatomic structure that permits the extremities to *articulate*, or move in different directions. In the skeletal system, motion is the result of several bones and muscles working together. Except for the **hyoid bone,** which is a free-floating bone between the mandible and the larynx, every bone is connected to at least one other bone. The convergence of two or

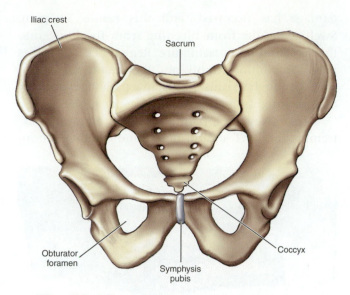

Fig. 28-12 Anterior view of the pelvic girdle.

more bones is called a **joint.** Joints are classified by the type of tissue that connects them and the amount of motion they allow. The three classes of joints are fibrous joints, cartilaginous joints, and synovial joints. **Fibrous joints** have little or no movement (e.g., the bones of the skull). **Cartilaginous joints** allow some motion but not a great range of motion. For example, the cartilaginous tissue that attaches the ribs to the sternum allows for expansion and contraction of the chest wall during inspiration, but no more than that. **Synovial joints,** which are the focus of this discussion, allow a much greater range of motion than the other two types. They are the most frequently affected of the three types, as a result of trauma arising from their extensive range of motion. The bone ends of synovial joints are covered by a thin layer of cartilage and enclosed in a **joint capsule.** The joint capsule is composed of an outer fibrous capsule and an inner synovial membrane. The synovial membrane lines the inside of the capsule and produces **synovial fluid,** which lubricates the joint, allowing smooth motion.

Synovial joints are divided into six categories:

- **Plane (gliding) joints.** This type of joint is found in the area between flat-surfaced bones; an example is the vertebrae.
- **Saddle joints.** In a saddle joint, two bone surfaces converge at a 90-degree angle, allowing motion on two planes; an example is the thumb joint.

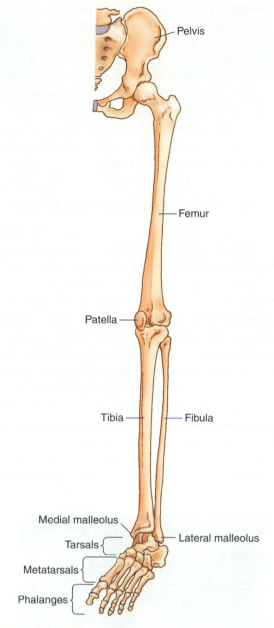

Fig. 28-13 The bones of the lower extremity.

- **Hinge joints.** As the name implies, a hinge joint flexes or extends; examples are the knee and elbow.
- **Pivot joints.** This type of joint is composed of a round bone that rotates within a ring of bone and ligament; an example is the forearm near the elbow where the radius and ulna meet.
- **Ball-and-socket joints.** In this joint, the ball end of one bone fits into a socket in the adjoining bone, allowing a wide range of motion in almost any direction; examples are the hip and shoulder joints.

- **Ellipsoid joints.** An ellipsoid joint is a pseudo-ball-and-socket joint in which the converging bone ends are elliptic rather than round. This shape limits the joint's range of motion, which is similar to that of a hinge joint. However, ellipsoid joints can move on two planes. An example is the joint where the occipital bone of the skull converges with the first vertebra (referred to as the atlas); this joint permits the neck to flex, extend, or turn.

Injuries of the Skeletal System

As is the general rule in all forms of trauma, injuries of the skeletal system are classified as closed or open. A **closed skeletal injury** (Fig. 28-14) is one in which the integrity of the skin has not been compromised, regardless of the damage beneath it. In contrast, an **open skeletal injury** (Fig. 28-15) involves a break in the skin, which creates a soft tissue injury in addition to the skeletal injury. Whether open or closed, skeletal injuries may involve bones, joints, or possibly both. If enough force is applied to any bone or joint in the skeletal system, the integrity and continuity of that bone or joint becomes suspect. This type of injury produces pain, swelling, and possibly deformity. The pain results from nerve endings that run along the bone (or bones). These nerve endings sense that

damage has occurred, and this results in pain. Swelling results from bleeding from the bone into the surrounding musculature. Remember that bones have a rich blood supply, and they can bleed significantly, enough to cause shock in a patient. Deformity of a fractured bone may be obvious or subtle.

When assessing a painful, swollen, deformed extremity, the EMT should determine whether the in-

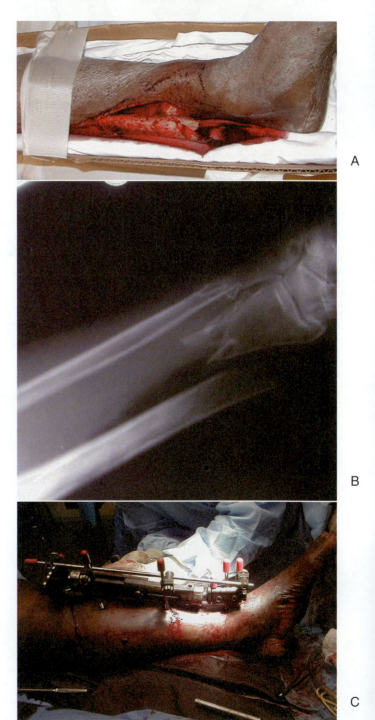

A

B

C

Fig. 28-15 **A,** An open fracture. **B,** X-ray film of an open fracture. **C,** Repair of an open fracture with an external fixator.

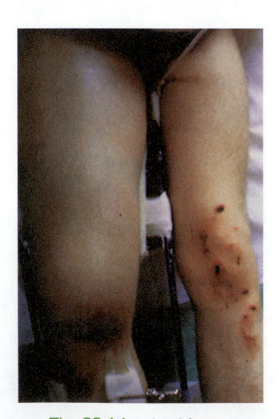

Fig. 28-14 A closed fracture.

jury is open or closed. A soft tissue wound near the injury site could indicate that a bone has breached the outer surface of the skin. In some cases, the bone may still protrude, or it may have slid back under the skin as the patient moved. In addition to pain, swelling, deformity, or the lack of an open wound, you may note crepitus. **Crepitus** is the sound produced when two ends of a broken bone rub together; it is an unmistakable sound, and once heard, it is difficult to forget. You must exercise great caution to prevent continued movement of the broken ends of a bone by properly splinting the extremity (discussed in the next section). Proper splinting will help minimize ongoing blood loss from the fracture as well as the potential for injury to adjacent structures. Once the patient has been appropriately treated and transported to the hospital, a physician can confirm the loss of integrity and continuity of the painful, swollen, deformed extremity with an x-ray film. At that time, the injury is recognized as a **fracture** if a bone is broken or as a **dislocation** if a joint was injured. Dislocation occurs when one or more bones that compose a joint become separated from the point of articulation with the other bone or bones (Fig. 28-16). Most dislocations cause significant pain, moderate to severe swelling and, usually, gross deformity (Fig. 28-17).

Assessing a painful, swollen, deformed extremity can be a challenging task. Patients with these injuries often are in considerable pain and reluctant to allow

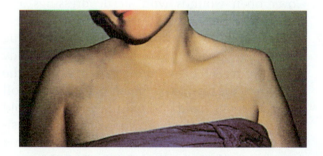

Fig. 28-16 Anterior dislocation of the shoulder.

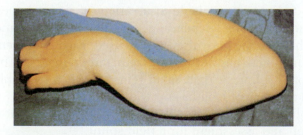

Fig. 28-17 A greenstick fracture with marked deformity.

the EMT to touch the injury site. However, you must assess the extremity to the best of your ability. As stated previously, the six *P*s of musculoskeletal assessment serve as an important tool in these situations. Moreover, you must know how those assessment points relate to the injury and the damage caused. Although rating pain is subjective and based on the patient's tolerance and stress level, you may be able to determine the degree of force to which the patient was subjected. Pallor, or skin color, is very important to assess. Blanched, gray, or pale skin distal to the injury site may indicate a lack of blood flow to the area. Fractures and dislocations can damage or occlude blood vessels, creating limb-threatening conditions as a result of oxygen deprivation in the distal tissue. By checking for the presence and strength of distal pulses or evaluating the capillary refill time, you can determine whether the extremity is receiving the circulation it needs. If the pulse is absent, you must recognize the severity of the situation and act accordingly. Nerves, like blood vessels, can be impinged upon or destroyed in traumatic injuries. If impingement or destruction of a nerve has occurred, the patient may not have sensation beyond the injury site. The person may claim that the extremity feels like "pins and needles." This sensation may be temporary or permanent, depending on the severity of the injury.

Next, you must assess for mobility or paralysis. *Do not have the patient move the extremity!* Rather, ask the patient to wiggle the toes (if the injury is to a lower extremity) or the fingers (if an upper extremity was injured). If the patient can wiggle the digits on the injured extremity, nerve function is intact. Finally, check for swelling. Consider how much swelling exists and how quickly the swelling has occurred.

You can easily accomplish the six *P*s evaluation during your assessment by doing the following:

- Ask the patient, "On a scale of 1 to 10, with 1 being very little pain and 10 being the worst pain you have ever experienced, how would you rate this pain?" (Pain assessment)

- Feel for a distal pulse. While doing this, assess skin temperature, moisture, and sensation. Ask, "Can you feel me touch you here?" Touch other areas of the extremity while asking the same question. (Pallor, pulse, paresthesia, and puffiness assessment)
- Ask the patient, "Could you please wiggle your fingers (toes) for me?" (Paralysis assessment)

Extreme pain, lack of a distal pulse, or lack of sensation or motion (or both) should alert you that a serious situation has developed or is about to develop. In cases of isolated musculoskeletal trauma, it's time to splint.

■ SPLINTING

It is prudent to err on the side of treatment. In other words, it is better to overtreat an injury than to undertreat it. With *every* patient, always assess airway, breathing, and circulation (ABCs) before treating the specific injury. EMTs who take the time to properly splint the injuries of a patient who is not breathing only succeed in transporting and delivering a well-splinted corpse. Once the ABCs have been assessed, you may focus on splinting the isolated musculoskeletal trauma. The objectives of splinting are as follows:

- To stabilize the injury to prevent movement
- To prevent further injury to the site by stabilizing bone ends
- To provide some pain relief through stabilization
- To restore or maintain circulation to the extremity
- To provide padding during transport

The rules for splinting extremity injuries are simple:

- If it's painful, splint it.
- If it's swollen, splint it.
- If it's deformed, splint it.

To splint a bone effectively:

- The joint above the injury and the joint below the injury must be immobilized with the bone in question.
- The bone (or bones) above the injury and the bone (or bones) below the injury must be immobilized with the joint in question.
- The *most* important rule: The splint must completely immobilize the injury and the surrounding area.

Before applying a splint to an isolated extremity injury, you should do the following as part of the assessment and treatment:

1. Support the area of the injury.
2. Remove or cut away clothing and jewelry.
3. Assess for pulse, motion, and sensation distal to the injury and record those findings on the patient care form.
4. If a pulse *is* present, take a ballpoint pen and mark the site where the pulse was detected. This will help you in your reassessment of the patient later.
5. If a pulse is *not* present, if the skin distal to the injury is cyanotic, or if gross deformity is present, gently apply inline traction to the limb and attempt to restore the extremity to its normal anatomic position. If the injury is an open injury with a bone end protruding, do not push the bone end back in. However, applying traction sometimes allows the bone end to slip back below the surface of the skin, and this is acceptable.
6. Cover open wounds with sterile dressings and control bleeding.
7. Pad each splint before applying it. If you are using a long spine board, pad voids between the body and the arms and between the patient's legs. If the injury is to the forearm or hand, place a gauze roll in the patient's hand and tell the patient to hold onto it by curling the fingers around it. This **position of function** allows the hand to relax rather than tensing during splinting (Fig. 28-18).
8. When possible, splint before moving the patient.

Splints are available in a variety of sizes, shapes, and materials, depending on their purpose and where on the body they will be used. Each type mentioned here has both advantages and drawbacks. The board splint, or **rigid splint** (Fig. 28-19), is available in a variety of lengths and widths and works well for splinting long bones. Skill 28-1 shows the application and assessment for a rigid splint.

A **ladder splint** is made of sturdy yet lightweight metal that can easily bend around joints and still be long enough to splint long bones (Fig. 28-20).

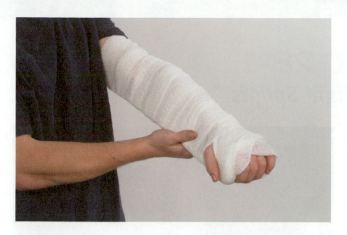

Fig. 28-18 Immobilization of the forearm.

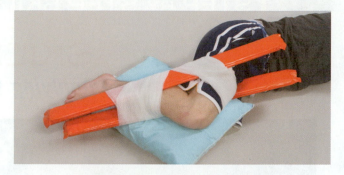

Fig. 28-19 Rigid splint.

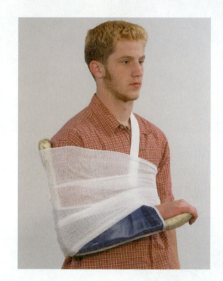

Fig. 28-20 Formable ladder splint.

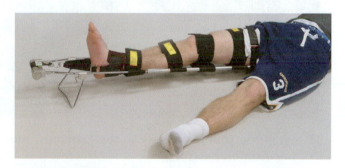

Fig. 28-21 Traction splint.

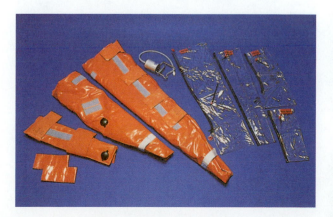

Fig. 28-22 Air splints.

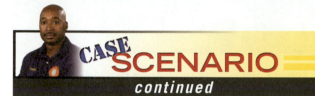

CASE SCENARIO
continued

After palpating around the patient's neck and head, Jack determined that there were no injuries; the helmet had done its job in protecting the girl from the impact of the fall. Jack then turned to the patient's left wrist that looked painful. Comforting the girl, Jackie gently palpated around the deformity site. It was shaped like a spoon, just as she had learned it in the class, a classic sign of a Colles fracture.

Question: What important finding should Jack assess that is related to the injury? Why is it important?

A **traction splint** (e.g., the Hare, Thomas, or Sager) is specially designed for use on midshaft fractures of the femur (Fig. 28-21). These splints apply constant traction to the upper leg to stabilize and align the femur. Skill 28-2 shows the application and assessment for a traction splint.

These splints are effective at maintaining immobilization of an extremity. Their main drawback is that they must be removed before the extremity can be x-rayed, because the composition of the splints obscures the bone in the x-ray film.

X-rays can be taken through soft splints such as an **air splint** (Fig. 28-22), pillow splint, or a **vacuum splint.** These splints provide good immobilization to an extremity, provided the injury is below the elbow or the knee. Skill 28-3 shows the application and assessment for a vacuum splint.

SKILL 28-1
◉ *Applying Rigid Splints*

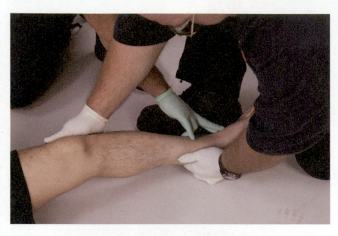

1. Check the distal pulses and stabilize the extremity above and below the fracture site before manipulating the extremity.

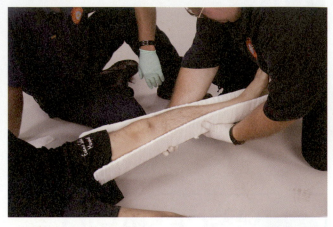

2. Apply rigid splints on at least two sides of the extremity.

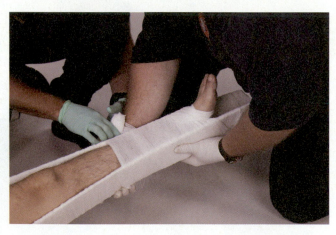

3. Wrap the splints securely to the extremity, moving distal to proximal.

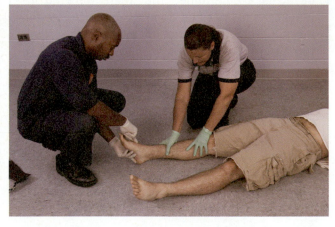

4. Recheck the distal pulses after applying the splints.

SKILL 28-2
◎ *Applying a Traction Splint*

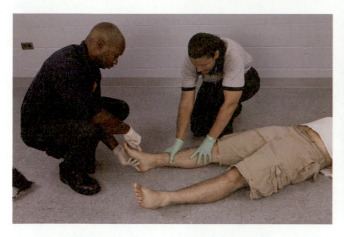

1. Check the distal pulses while supporting the injured extremity.

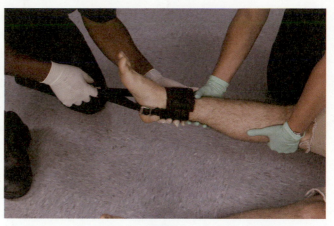

2. Attach the ankle strap and apply manual traction. Check the distal pulse after applying the traction.

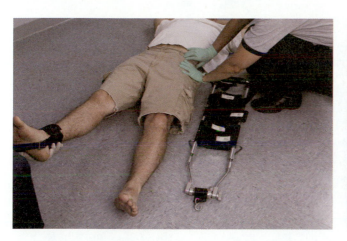

3. Adjust the traction splint to the proper length using the uninjured extremity as a guide.

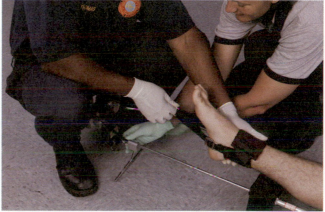

4. Slide the splint under the injured extremity and fasten the strap at the top of the splint. Recheck the distal pulse.

Continued

SKILLS

SKILL 28-2
⊚ *Applying a Traction Splint—cont'd*

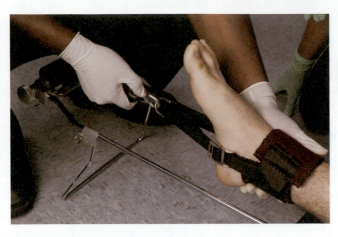

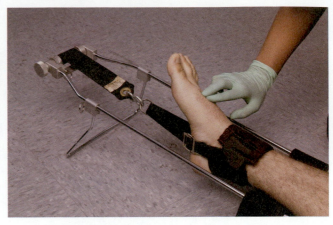

5. Attach the traction device to the ankle strap and ratchet up the traction until the device takes the traction away from the EMT applying manual traction.

6. Recheck the distal pulse after traction is turned over to the device.

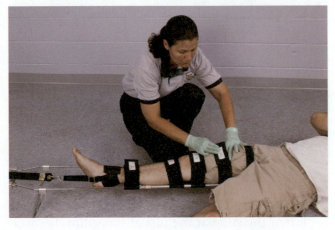

7. Attach the leg straps to secure the leg in the splint.

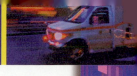

SKILL 28-3
◉ *Applying a Vacuum Splint*

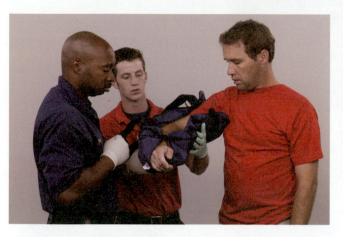

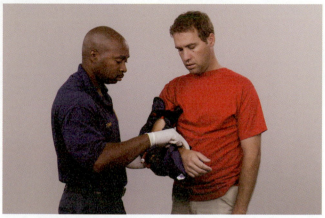

1. Lay the splint on a flat area. Smooth it out until the plastic beads are evenly distributed. Remove some air from the splint so that the sides do not collapse when the splint is shaped.

2. Place the splint underneath the extremity and then bend it into a U-shape around the extremity. Fasten the Velcro fasteners. Then, form each major curve around any bend in the extremity so that the extremity is held completely in place.

4. Check the distal circulation on the extremity.

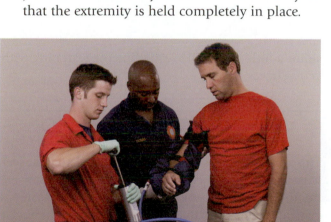

3. Use the pump to remove the remaining air to leave the splint rigid.

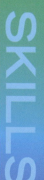

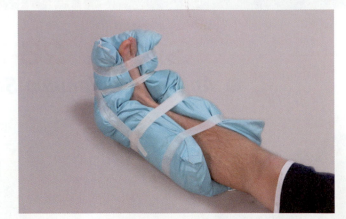

Fig. 28-23 Pillow splint.

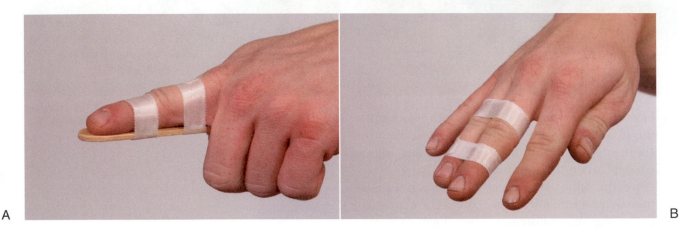

A   B

Fig. 28-24 **A,** Immobilization of a single finger. **B,** Splinting of an injury to two fingers.

A soft, **formable splint,** such as a pillow, blanket, stiff foam splint, or some cardboard splints, can be molded and secured to an extremity (Fig. 28-23). Pillows and blankets are readily available on all ambulances, and all these splints can be left in place when the extremity is x-rayed. However, like air and vacuum splints, these splints should be used only below the elbow or knee.

In certain situations, an **anatomic splint** is a wise choice. These splints prevent movement by securing the injured extremity to the patient's body. For example, the EMT can *buddy-tape* injured fingers to provide immobilization (Fig. 28-24). Skill 28-4 shows how to secure an injured arm with a **sling and swathe** using either triangular bandages or rolled gauze.

Regardless of the type of splint used, once it has been applied, you must reassess the distal pulse, motor function, and sensation frequently. Even a properly applied splint initially can become constricting, impeding circulation or compressing the nerves, because of swelling or movement (of the patient and during transport). A watchful EMT looks for these situations and responds accordingly by loosening the splint a little or slightly realigning the extremity with gentle traction.

■ OTHER CONSIDERATIONS

This discussion has focused on the isolated musculoskeletal injury, the painful, swollen, deformed extremity. What happens when multisystem trauma is evident? **Multisystem trauma** involves more than one of the body's systems, creating the possibility of life threats. These life-threatening injuries must be detected in the initial assessment. If a life threat is detected, you must shift the focus from the obvious fracture and external injuries to what is actually going to kill the patient. What kills trauma victims? *Any compromise to airway, breathing, and circulation kills trauma victims.* Fractures then become a low priority, and the call becomes a load-and-go situation. So how *do* you deal with those fractures in light of the life threats? The answer is anatomic splinting. By completely immobilizing a patient on a long spine board, securing the extremities to the body and board, keeping the patient

SKILL 28-4
Applying a Sling and Swathe

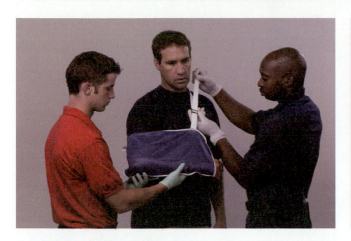

1. Check the distal pulse and sensation. Then, apply the sling.

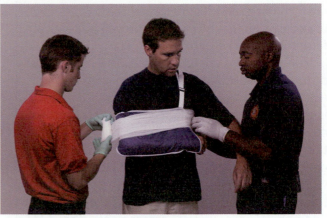

2. Wrap the upper arm to the chest without restricting breathing.

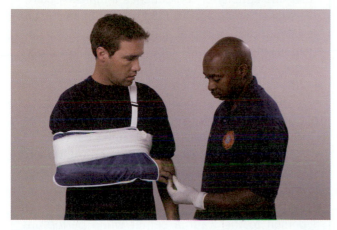

3. Recheck the distal pulse and sensation after securing the sling.

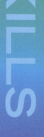

BOX 28-2

No Job Is Complete Until the Paperwork Is Done!

A critical component of the EMT's responsibilities is documentation. Documentation must be accurate, concise, and legible (if written). EMTs need to become familiar with the approved patient care forms used in their area.

For musculoskeletal trauma, the EMT must document the initial assessment. For example, Is it an isolated injury or multisystem trauma? If it is determined to be a multisystem, "load and go" case, what initial findings led to that determination? What was done on the scene? What was done en route? Are the times correct?

Documentation of isolated musculoskeletal trauma, on the other hand, is more detailed. In addition to the initial assessment, the EMT should record the distal pulse, motor functions and sensation, the type of splint used, and how often the patient was reassessed.

Remember, be as thorough with documentation as you are with assessment and treatment.

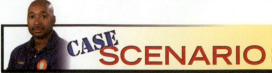

CASE SCENARIO
conclusion

The ambulance had arrived to take over care of Jennifer. With care and attention, the crew placed the wrist into a padded board splint and applied ice at the deformity site. They reassessed her motor-pulse-sensory status in the fingers before and after they were done with the splinting, to make sure that they were not compromised. ■

TEAMWORK

Once scene safety has been established, the first arriving unit on the scene of any trauma must determine the severity of the patient's injuries. A basic life support ambulance should be able to handle an isolated musculoskeletal injury. However, if the patient is critical, the EMT faces a formidable barrage of questions, which must be answered quickly:

- Why is this patient critical?
- Is the problem something I can fix (e.g., basic airway maneuvers, assisted ventilations)?
- How far is it to the closest trauma center?
- Should I call for advanced life support (ALS) help?
- How long will it take ALS services to get here?
- Is ALS intercept possible?
- Is it better for the patient if we transport the person to the trauma center while performing basic life support or should we wait a few minutes for an ALS unit to respond?

No one answer is correct 100% of the time. No answer is written in stone. However, this *is* written in stone: the first arriving unit at any trauma incident *must* be able to assess the patient properly. Assessment skills must be sharp. The responder on the scene must be decisive, always acting in the patient's best interest. EMTs must be familiar with local protocol. They also must be able to communicate effectively with the hospital to "paint the picture" of what is going on with the patient. Other agencies, such as hospitals, ALS ambulances, and air medical services, are willing and always ready to be called upon for help. However, it is the EMT, the first one on the scene, who must be the most prepared of all and must know when to call!

warm, rapidly transporting the patient to a trauma center, and completing other treatment en route, you give your patient the most important thing needed at that instant—time. The sooner the patient gets into surgery, the greater the person's chance of survival.

References

1. National Center for Health Statistics, National Ambulatory Medical Care Survey, 2000.
2. National Center for Health Statistics, National Hospital Discharge Survey, 1996, 2000.
3. National Center for Health Statistics, Advance Data: National Ambulatory Medical Care Survey, 2000 Summary.

Resources

Sanders MJ: *Paramedic textbook*, ed 2, St Louis, 2001, Mosby.

McSwain N, Paturas J: *The basic EMT*, ed 2, St Louis, 2003, Mosby.

Prehospital trauma life support (PHTLS), ed 5, St Louis, 2005, Mosby.

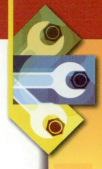

Critical Points

Assessment is the key to determining the severity of a musculoskeletal injury.

- EMTs must have a basic knowledge of the musculoskeletal system to perform a good assessment.
- EMTs must have the skills to assess and treat musculoskeletal injuries.
- EMTs must be able to communicate their findings and treatments, both orally and through documentation, to other agencies involved.
- EMTs must be able to demonstrate the use of various splinting options and must know the indications and contraindications for each, as well as the complications of splinting.

Learning Checklist

❑ Musculoskeletal injuries are one of the most common injuries EMTs encounter.

❑ The three types of muscles are skeletal muscle, cardiac muscle, and smooth (visceral) muscle. Muscles also are classified as either voluntary or involuntary.

❑ The six *P*s of musculoskeletal assessment are pain, pallor, pulses, paresthesia, paralysis, and pressure or puffiness.

❑ Bones are classified by their shape into one of four categories: long bones, short bones, flat bones, and irregular bones.

❑ The key bones of the skull are the frontal bone, parietal bone, temporal bone, and occipital bone.

❑ The spine is made up of seven cervical vertebrae, 12 thoracic vertebrae, five lumbar vertebrae, one sacrum, and one coccyx.

❑ The sternum is divided into three parts: the manubrium, the body of the sternum, and the xiphoid process.

❑ Ligaments attach bones to one another and give greater support to the body. They also keep the bones aligned in their proper anatomic positions.

❑ Synovial joints are divided into six categories: plane (gliding) joints, saddle joints, hinge joints, pivot joints, ball-and-socket joints, and ellipsoid joints.

❑ Injuries of the skeletal system are classified as closed or open and are recognized as a fracture or a dislocation.

❑ A variety of splints may be used for musculoskeletal trauma, including board (rigid) splints, ladder splints, traction splints, air and vacuum splints, and formable splints.

❑ After a splint is applied, the distal pulse, motor functions, and sensation must be reassessed frequently.

Key Terms

Acetabulum A large, cup-shaped articular cavity that contains the head of the femur.

Air splint A splint that has a cavity that is filled with air, thus providing support for an injured extremity.

Anatomic splint A splint in which the body is used as a self-splint.

Ball-and-socket joints Joints in which the head of one bone (the ball) fits into a cup (socket) in the articulating bone (the socket), allowing a wide range of motion in almost any direction. The hip and shoulder joints are examples of this type of joint.

Body of the sternum The central part of the sternum between the manubrium and the xiphoid process.

Calcaneus One of seven tarsals in the foot; the heel bone.

Cardiac muscle One of three muscle types; the specialized striated muscle of which the heart is composed.

Carpals Eight bones that make up the structure of the wrist.

Cartilage A spongy material on the ends of bones that provides cushioning and prevents bone ends from rubbing together.

Cartilaginous joints One of three major classes of joints; cartilaginous joints have limited motion.

Cervical vertebrae The first seven vertebrae of the spinal column.

Clavicles The bones that extend from the sternum and join with the scapulae to form the pectoral girdle; the collar bones.

Closed skeletal injury An injury that does not breach the outer surface of the skin.

Coccyx The most distal part of the spinal column; it is composed of four or five coccygeal vertebrae that are fused.

Costal cartilage Cartilaginous tissue that connects the eighth, ninth, and tenth ribs to the sternum.

Coxae The hip bones; the hip bone is composed of the ilium, the ischium, and the pubis.

Crepitus A crunching or grating sound heard when broken bone ends rub together.

Cuboid bone The most lateral of the seven tarsals of the foot.

Cuneiform bones Three tarsals (medial, lateral, and intermediate) that make up part of the foot.

Direct force Force applied directly to the body as a result of contact.

Dislocation A medical diagnosis indicating disruption of the integrity of a joint in which one or more bones separate from each other.

Ellipsoid joints Modified ball-and-socket joints in which the bones are elliptic rather than round. An ellipsoid joint is similar to a hinge joint; its range of motion is limited, but movement takes place on two planes. The joint where the occipital bone of the skull converges with the first vertebra is an example of this type of joint.

Fascia The fibrous tissue that covers a muscle.

Femur The longest bone in the body; the thigh bone.

Fibrous joints One of the three major classes of joints; fibrous joints have little or no motion.

Fibula A non-weight-bearing bone of the lower leg located next to the tibia.

Flat bones A bone classification; flat bones characteristically are more flat than round (e.g., the ribs).

Floating ribs The eleventh and twelfth ribs, which connect to the spinal column but do not attach anywhere else.

Formable splint A soft splint that can be shaped to fit the contours of the area being splinted.

Fossa A large depression formed by the juncture of two bones.

Fracture A medical diagnosis indicating interruption of the continuity or integrity of a bone.

Frontal bone One of the main bones of the skull; it forms the forehead.

Hinge joints Joints in which a concave bone and a convex bone merge; this type of joint flexes and extends on one plane. The knee and elbow are examples of this type of joint.

Humerus The bone of the upper arm.

Hyoid bone A free-floating bone in the neck (i.e., it is not attached to any other bone).

Ilium One of three bones that make up half of the pelvis. The superior end of the ilium is known as the *iliac crest*.

Indirect force Force that travels through the body and causes damage in an area or areas away from the contact site.

Involuntary muscles Muscles that move without conscious effort.

Irregular bones A bone classification; irregular bones are characterized by their nonspecific shape (e.g., the facial bones).

Ischium One of three bones that make up half of the pelvis.

Joint The convergence of two or more bones.

Joint capsule The layered tissue that surrounds and protects a joint. The joint capsule is composed of a tough, outer fibrous capsule and an inner membrane that produces synovial fluid.

Ladder splint A durable, lightweight splint made of metal that can be bent to conform to the shape of long bones.

Ligaments Tough, elastic, cordlike tissues that connect bone to bone.

Long bones A bone classification; long bones characteristically are longer than they are wide (e.g., the femur).

Lumbar vertebrae Five vertebrae of the spinal column (L20 to L24).

Mandible Lower jawbone.

Manubrium Uppermost section of the sternum.

Marrow A spongy material in the center of bones. Yellow marrow is mostly fat cells. Red marrow produces red blood cells.

Maxilla Upper jawbone.

Metacarpals Five bones that form the structure of the hand.

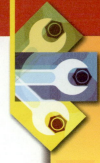

Metatarsals Five bones that form the structure of the foot.

Multisystem trauma Significant trauma involving more than one system of the body.

Navicular bone The most medial of the seven tarsal bones.

Nerves Fibers and connective tissue located outside the brain that send and receive signals from the brain.

Nonstriated muscles Muscles characterized by the absence of lines in the muscle tissue.

Occipital bone A major (and the most posterior) bone of the skull.

Open skeletal injury Trauma that breaches the integrity of the outer surface of the skin.

Painful, swollen extremity A descriptive EMS field observation.

Parietal bone A major bone of the skull; it constitutes the top of the skull.

Patella The kneecap.

Pectoral girdle The union of the clavicle and the scapula where the upper extremity attaches to the body.

Pelvic girdle The union of the ilium, the ischium, and the pubis where the lower extremity attaches to the body.

Phalanges The fourteen bones in each hand and foot that make up the structures of the fingers and toes, respectively. Each thumb and great toe consists of two phalanges, each other finger or toe has three.

Pivot joints Round bones that rotate within a ring of bone and ligament. The forearm near the elbow, where the radius and ulna meet, is an example of a pivot joint.

Plane (gliding) joints Joints formed by two flat-surfaced bones (the carpal bones of the wrist).

Position of function The natural position of the hand (i.e., with the fingers slightly curled).

Pubis One of three major bones that make up half of the pelvis.

Radius The larger of the two bones of the forearm.

Range of motion An extremity's ability to move based on the type of joint involved. Injuries limit range of motion.

Ribs Flat bones of the thoracic cavity that protect the lungs, heart, great vessels, and diaphragm.

Rigid splint A splint that cannot be bent or conformed to the body. Rigid splints are used to stabilize long bones; also called a *board splint.*

Sacrum A distal part of the spinal column; it consists of five sacral vertebrae that fuse as the body ages.

Saddle joints Joints in which two saddle-shaped bones converge at a 90-degree angle, allowing movement on two planes. The thumb joint is an example of this type of joint.

Scapulae Large, flat bones that form the structure of the back and the pectoral girdle.

Short bones A bone classification; short bones characteristically have an approximately equal length and width (e.g., the bones of the wrists and ankles).

Six *Ps* of musculoskeletal assessment Assessment factors for evaluating musculoskeletal trauma; they are pain, pallor, pulse, paresthesia, paralysis, and puffiness or pressure.

Skeletal muscle One of three muscle classifications; skeletal muscle is *striated*, which means the muscle tissue appears to have lines running through it.

Sling and swathe An immobilization technique for an upper extremity injury in which the forearm is placed in a sling and a bandage, and the swathe secures the humerus to the body.

Smooth (visceral) muscle A major class of muscle that includes involuntary muscles, such as those that move food through the digestive tract.

Spinal column A series of 26 bones that support most of the body's weight and protect the spinal cord. It is the main nerve pathway to and from the brain; also called the *vertebral column.*

Sprain An injury to a tendon or ligament.

Sternum The breast bone.

Strain An injury to a muscle.

Striated muscles Muscles in which the tissue appears to have lines.

Synovial fluid Fluid produced in the joint capsule to lubricate the bone ends of a joint.

Synovial joints One of the major classes of joints; synovial joints allow a wide range of motion.

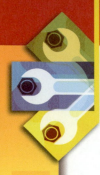

Talus One of seven tarsals; the ankle bone.

Tarsals Seven bones that make up the ankle and proximal aspect of the foot.

Temporal bone A major bone of the skull; it forms the side of the skull.

Tendons Durable, elastic tissues that join muscle to muscle and muscle to bone.

Thoracic vertebrae The 12 central vertebrae of the spinal column (T8 to T19).

Tibia The long bone of the lower leg; the shin bone.

Traction splint A special splint for midshaft fractures of the femur that applies gentle but constant pressure to keep the lower extremity aligned.

Twisting force Force applied where a body part acts as a pivot point and twists beyond the normal range of motion.

Ulna The smaller of the two bones in the forearm.

Vacuum splint An extremity or full body splint; air is drawn out of the splint so that it contracts and conforms to the body to maintain immobilization.

Voluntary muscles Muscles that move as a result of conscious effort or direction.

Xyphoid process Cartilaginous tissue located at the distal end of the sternum.

Zygomatic arch A bony structure that forms the lateral aspect of the eye socket.

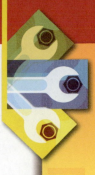

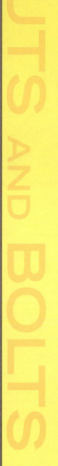

National Standard Curriculum Objectives

Cognitive Objectives

After completing this lesson, the EMT student will be able to do the following:

- Describe the function of the muscular system.
- Describe the function of the skeletal system.
- List the major bones or bone groupings of the spinal column, the thorax, the upper extremities, and the lower extremities.
- Differentiate between an open and a closed painful, swollen, deformed extremity.
- State the reasons for splinting.
- List the general rules of splinting.
- List the complications of splinting.
- Explain the emergency medical care of a patient with a painful, swollen, deformed extremity.

Affective Objectives

After completing this lesson, the EMT student will be able to do the following:

- Explain the rationale for splinting at the scene versus load and go.
- Explain the rationale for immobilizing a painful, swollen, deformed extremity.

Psychomotor Objectives

After completing this lesson, the EMT student will be able to do the following:

- Demonstrate the emergency medical care of a patient with a painful, swollen, deformed extremity.
- Demonstrate the completion of a prehospital care report for patients with musculoskeletal injuries.

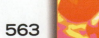

CHAPTER

29

OUTLINE

GOAL

LESSON GOAL

Head and spinal injuries affect millions of people each year. The long-term effects of these injuries depend to some degree on the ability of the emergency medical technician (EMT) to recognize and treat them appropriately. By learning good assessment skills and the appropriate treatment for patients with head and spinal injuries, EMTs can make a significant difference in these individuals' lives. This chapter teaches you what to look for when assessing a patient who has or may have a head or spinal injury. It also teaches you how to treat such injuries effectively. ■

Head and Spinal Trauma

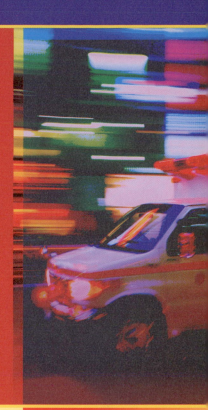

29

CHAPTER OBJECTIVES

After completing this chapter, the EMT student will be able to do the following:

1 State the components of the nervous system.
2 List the functions of the central nervous system.
3 Define the structure of the skeletal system as it relates to the nervous system.
4 Relate the mechanism of injury to potential injuries of the head and spine.
5 Describe the implications of not properly caring for potential spine injuries.
6 State the signs and symptoms of a potential spinal injury.
7 Describe the method of determining whether a responsive patient may have a spinal injury.
8 Relate the airway emergency medical care techniques to the patient with suspected spine and head injuries.
9 Describe how to stabilize the cervical spine.
10 Discuss the indications for immobilizing the spine using various devices (e.g., cervical immobilization device, spine board)
11 Identify different types of helmets and state the circumstances in which a helmet should be left on the patient and when a helmet should be removed.
12 Explain the preferred and alternate methods for removing a helmet.
13 Demonstrate how to open the airway in a patient with a suspected spinal cord injury.

Continued

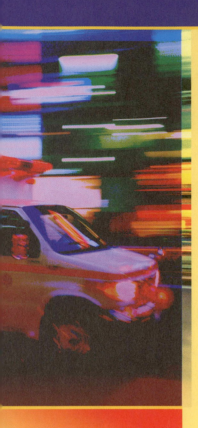

Chapter Objectives—cont'd

14 Demonstrate the evaluation of a responsive patient with a suspected spinal cord injury.

15 Demonstrate stabilization of the cervical spine.

16 Demonstrate, with help, the four-person log roll for a patient with a suspected spinal cord injury.

17 Demonstrate, with help, the two-person log roll for a patient with a suspected spinal cord injury.

18 Demonstrate how to secure a patient to a long spine board.

19 Demonstrate the short board immobilization technique.

20 Demonstrate the procedure for rapid extrication.

21 Demonstrate the preferred methods for stabilizing a helmet.

22 Demonstrate helmet removal techniques.

23 Demonstrate alternative methods for stabilizing a helmet.

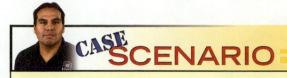

CASE SCENARIO

The motorcyclist is still lying on the ground when the engine crew pulls up at the scene. The site is on a long, windy stretch of mountain road, a favorite among Sunday morning motorcycle riders. The road has claimed its fair share of riders who went down after misjudging a turn. This appears to be another casualty. As Rafael begins his scene assessment, other riders state that they saw the motorcyclist ride a bit too close to the edge of the roadway and hit a sandy patch. The motorcycle went down almost immediately, they say, tossing the rider onto the road. The witnesses think the rider was going about 40 miles per hour when the motorcycle went down. The rider slid for about 75 feet and tumbled a few times before coming to a stop in the middle of the road, they report. Other riders immediately pulled off the road and blocked traffic in both directions. One of them called the state patrol on her cell phone.

Rafael had stepped off the engine with the first-in bag. Another member of the crew had grabbed the airway bag. The third crew member began to pull out the long backboard. The captain calls for an estimated time of arrival (ETA) on the rescue ambulance as Rafael kneels beside the rider and guides a coworker in maintaining manual stabilization of the patient's head and neck. The patient is unconscious. Rafael applies a sternal rub to the chest, but the patient does not respond. His respirations are irregular and marked by gasping sounds. Rafael feels for a radial pulse; it is strong and regular but surprisingly slow.

Question: *What steps should the engine crew take for the initial management of this patient?*

I njuries to the head and spine can be extremely devastating to your patient. The potential for a life-altering outcome, such as permanent disability or even death, should make EMTs aware of how important their role is in the management of these patients. Using thorough and proper assessment techniques and appropriate treatment, the EMT can have a positive effect on the outcome for a patient with a head or spinal injury. This is the EMT's second most important responsibility, surpassed only by the management of airway, breathing, and circulation (ABCs).

■ REVIEW OF THE NERVOUS SYSTEM

For all practical purposes, the nervous system controls all functions in the body. Through a complex network of nerve cells, the nervous system sends and receives information from the body and the environment. After the brain receives and processes information, nerve impulses are sent throughout the body to implement whatever changes the brain deems necessary. Because the nervous system is so important to the body's well-being, it is fairly well protected from injury by the skull and the spinal

column. However, injuries can occur if significant force is applied to the body.

The nervous system is divided functionally into two parts: the central nervous system (CNS) and the peripheral nervous system (PNS). The CNS consists of the brain and the spinal cord. The PNS consists of pairs of nerves that exit and enter the spinal column, as well as all motor and sensory nerves throughout the body.

The Central Nervous System

As mentioned, the CNS consists of the brain and the spinal cord. This is where higher level functions take place, such as memory, emotions, and communication. The brain also receives sensory data and coordinates motor control throughout the body.

The brain itself is divided into the cerebrum, the cerebellum, and the brainstem (Fig. 29-1). The **cerebrum** makes up the largest portion of the brain (approximately 75% to 80%). It controls many functions of the body, such as visual impulses for the eyes, speech, balance, hearing, and emotion. The **cerebellum** coordinates body movements. Without the control of the cerebellum, a person would not be able to accomplish fine motor skills such as writing,

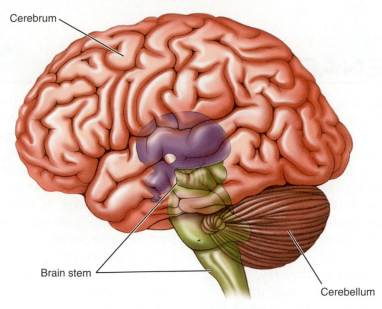

Cerebrum

Brain stem

Cerebellum

Fig. 29-1 The major areas of the brain are the cerebrum, the cerebellum, and the brainstem.

typing, or sewing. The **brainstem** lies at the base of the brain. This is where all the body's "vegetative" functions reside. Certain activities necessary for life, such as control of the heart rate and respirations, may be affected if the brainstem is injured.

The spinal cord extends from the brainstem down through the spinal column to the level of the second lumbar vertebra. Other nerves continue on to the sacral level.

Nervous system tissue cannot regenerate if it is injured; therefore it is fortunate that the CNS is reasonably well protected. The brain (Fig. 29-2) lies within the cranium and has various layers of protection. Starting from the outside, the skin of the scalp provides the first layer of protection. This skin is extremely vascular, which means that scalp lacerations can sometimes cause dramatic blood loss (Fig. 29-3). The next layer of protection is a fascia and muscle layer, followed by the skull (bone) itself. Directly beneath the skull lie the meninges. The meninges are three distinct layers of tissue that surround and protect the brain. The first layer is the **dura mater.** The dura mater is a tough, leatherlike covering that forms a sac around the brain. Next is the **arachnoid layer,** followed by the very thin **pia mater,** which rests on the surface of the brain. Between the arachnoid layer and the pia mater run various blood vessels that feed the brain. Cerebrospinal fluid (CSF) is also produced in this area and provides a cushion of protection for the brain and spinal cord.

The Peripheral Nervous System

The PNS is made up of spinal nerves and cranial nerves. It is divided functionally into the autonomic (involuntary) nervous system and the somatic (voluntary) nervous system.

Involuntary functions, such as respirations, the heart rate, blood vessel size, and bladder and bowel control, are all controlled by the **autonomic nervous system** (meaning "automatic"). These are all functions that do not require any active effort or decision making on the part of the individual. They are considered vegetative functions.

As the brain interprets sensory information from the environment, nerve impulses are sent throughout the body, directing it to take action, such as walking, for example. All body functions that can be voluntarily controlled come under the **somatic nervous system** (meaning "voluntary").

The PNS can be divided into sensory, motor, and connecting nerves. Twelve pairs of cranial nerves pass directly from the brain, through an opening in the skull, to the head and face. These nerves control functions such as facial expressions, sight, taste, and smell. The 31 pairs of spinal nerves conduct sensory and motor impulses from the spinal cord to all parts of the body. Sensory nerves include nerve endings that sense heat, cold, pressure, pain, and visual sensations. Sensory nerves carry those impulses back to the brain via the spinal cord. The brain then interprets the information and directs the body to act accordingly.

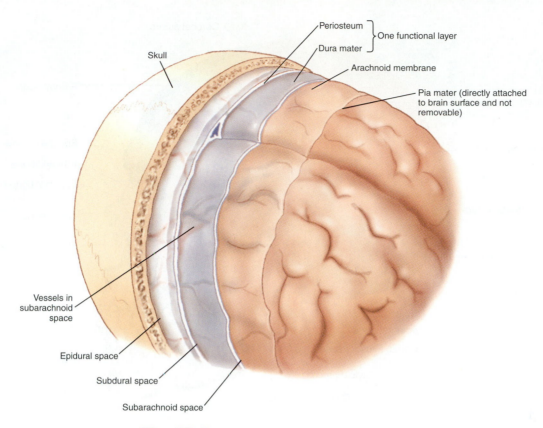

Skull
Periosteum
Dura mater } One functional layer
Arachnoid membrane
Pia mater (directly attached to brain surface and not removable)
Vessels in subarachnoid space
Epidural space
Subdural space
Subarachnoid space

Fig. 29-2 Meningeal coverings of the brain.

All muscles in the body have motor nerves that stimulate the muscle by means of electrical impulses, causing the muscle to contract. Connecting nerves are found in both the brain and spinal cord. They connect the sensory and motor nerves directly. In effect, this creates a shortcut of sorts for nerve impulses. Say, for example, that someone pokes your finger with a needle. You immediately withdraw your finger from the source of pain. The sensation of pain in your finger travels from your sensory nerve endings, through the connecting nerve system, and onto the motor nerve system in your finger. The motor nerves immediately stimulate the muscles in your finger and hand to contract and move away from the stimulation. This shortcut is referred to as a *reflex arc*. Reflex arcs help protect the body from injury.

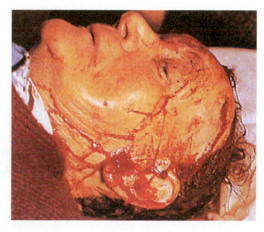

Fig. 29-3 Even a small scalp wound can bleed profusely.

■ REVIEW OF THE SKELETAL SYSTEM

The skeletal system provides the human body with form. It also protects the vital internal organs and allows a person to move. This chapter covers the skull and spinal column. The skull (cranium) consists of numerous thick, fused bones (Fig. 29-4). These

bones form a shell that houses and protects the brain. At the base of the skull is a large opening called the *foramen magnum*. This is where the brainstem and spinal cord connect. The spinal cord continues down through the spinal column to the second lumbar vertebra.

The spinal column serves a number of functions. First, it provides support for the body and allows the body to bend and twist. The spinal column also provides protection for the spinal cord.

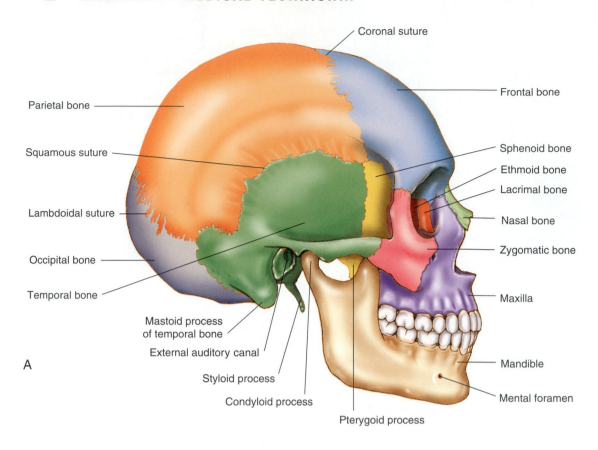

A

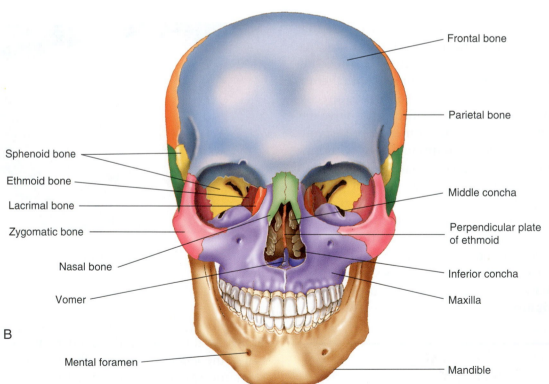

B

Fig. 29-4 The skull viewed from the right side (**A**) and from the front (**B**).

Thirty-three irregularly shaped bones, called *vertebrae*, make up the spinal column (Fig. 29-5). Most of the vertebrae are stacked one on top of another, with a cartilaginous intervertebral disk (Fig. 29-6) separating them (the bottom nine vertebrae are fused). As the spinal cord travels down through the spinal column, spinal nerves branch off and run to all parts of the body (Fig. 29-7). Injury to any part of the spinal column can damage the spinal cord or nerves.

The vertebrae are divided into five sections. The seven **cervical vertebrae** make up the neck region, with the skull resting on top. This area is quite flexible, allowing for a wide range of motion. Support of the cervical region is provided by a number of muscles and ligaments. The 12 **thoracic vertebrae**

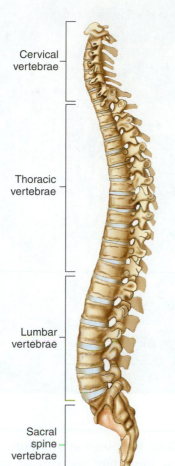

Cervical vertebrae

Thoracic vertebrae

Lumbar vertebrae

Sacral spine vertebrae

Fig. 29-5 The vertebral column viewed from the left side.

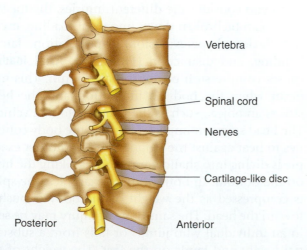

Vertebra

Spinal cord

Nerves

Cartilage-like disc

Posterior   Anterior

Fig. 29-6 The cartilage found between two vertebral bodies is called an *intervertebral disk*. These disks act as shock absorbers. If damaged, the cartilage may protrude into the spinal canal, compressing the cord or the nerves that pass through the intervertebral foramina.

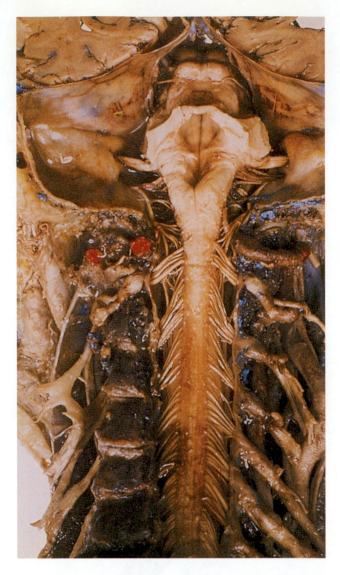

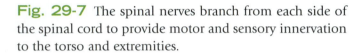

Fig. 29-7 The spinal nerves branch from each side of the spinal cord to provide motor and sensory innervation to the torso and extremities.

(sometimes referred to as the *dorsal spine*) make up the thoracic spinal region. Attached to each thoracic vertebra is a pair of ribs that reach around to the anterior side of the body. There they join the sternum to form the rib cage. The five **lumbar vertebrae** are next. Because they support the most weight, they are the largest of the vertebrae. The lumbar region is frequently injured by improper lifting techniques. The five **sacral vertebrae** are fused together to make up the posterior portion of the pelvic girdle. Last are the four **coccygeal vertebrae,** which form the tailbone (coccyx).

■ INJURIES OF THE SPINE

The spinal column can withstand a significant amount of force. However, many everyday activities create enough energy to cause injury. Crashing a vehicle, playing a contact sport, or simply jumping off a ladder all have the potential to injure the spine. As an EMT, it is important for you to recognize the mechanism of injury and to use that information to help determine your patient's possible injuries.

As you consider the different injuries, the mechanisms can be broken down into axial loading, excessive flexion, hyperextension, hyperrotation, lateral bending, and distraction (Fig. 29-8). **Axial loading** causes compression of the spinal column. This may occur when the body is in motion and the head strikes an object, such as the windshield of a vehicle. The head stops on impact; however, the body continues to bear against the stopped head. Another example is diving into shallow water and striking the head on the bottom. In both of these examples, the spine is compressed as the weight of the body is pushed toward the head. The same type of injury may be seen in an individual who jumps or falls from a substantial height and lands on the feet. The weight of the head and upper body drives down onto the lumbar

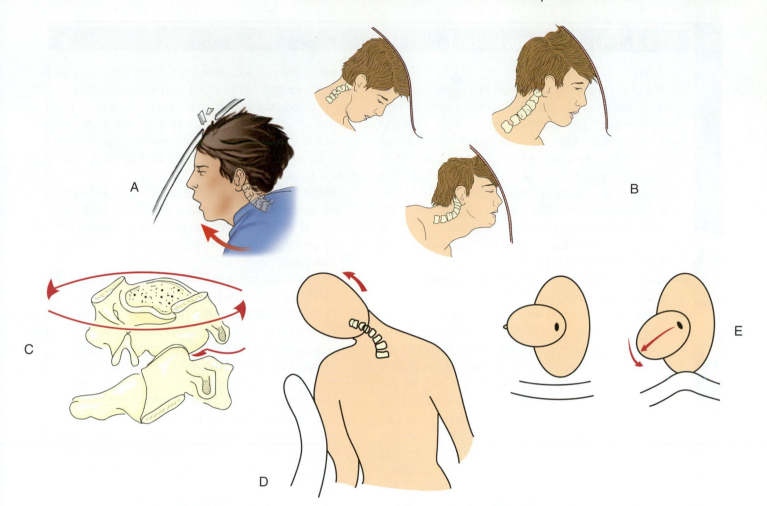

Fig. 29-8 A, The skull frequently stops its forward motion, but the torso does not. Just as the brain compresses within the skull, the torso continues in its forward motion until its energy is absorbed. The weakest point of the forward motion is the cervical spine. **B,** The spine can be compressed directly along its own axis or angled either into hyperextension or hyperflexion. **C through E,** The center of gravity of the skull is anterior and superior to its pivot point between the skull and cervical spine. During a lateral impact when the torso is rapidly accelerated out from under the head, the head turns toward the point of impact, both in the lateral and anterior-posterior angles. Such motion separates the vertebral bodies from the side of opposite impact and rotates them apart. Jumped facets, ligaments, tears, and lateral compression fractures result.

spine, causing compression. This compressive force may be significant enough to rupture intervertebral disks, fracture vertebrae, or both. These injuries may result in pressure on or damage to the spinal cord. Therefore your patient may experience pain and show signs of a neurologic deficit. The most common causes of compression injuries are vehicle crashes, shallow water diving accidents, motorcycle crashes, and falls.

The head, which weighs approximately 16 to 17 pounds, sits atop the spinal column. The neck is supported by the cervical spine and by numerous strong muscles and ligaments. When forces exceed what

these structures can support, the result is **excessive flexion** (forward movement of the head), **hyperextension** (rear movement of the head), or **hyperrotation** (sideways turning of the head). As you examine a motor vehicle crash, consider what your patient's head must have done on impact. With impact from the front, the head would fly forward, causing excessive flexion. Impact from the back causes the head to fly backward, causing hyperextension (commonly called *whiplash*). What about impact on the right front corner from the side? This could certainly cause a hyperrotation. The body would turn with the vehicle, whereas the head would not. Any situation in

SPECIAL Considerations

Helmets

EMTs often treat patients who are wearing a helmet of some kind. Many different types of helmets are worn for various events. These helmets can be categorized into two basic types: those that typically are open anteriorly (e.g., sports helmets) and those that are considered full face models (e.g., motorcycle and snowmobile helmets). Regardless of the type of helmet, the EMT must answer three important questions:

- Is the patient able to breathe adequately with the helmet in place?
- Can I access and control the patient's airway without removing the helmet?
- Does the helmet fit well enough to ensure that the patient's head will not move inside it?

Sometimes leaving the helmet on is in the patient's best interest. If the patient is wearing a helmet that has been appropriately sized for the person and if there is little or no movement of the head within it, you may consider leaving the helmet on. If you are able to access, assess, and control the patient's airway by removing the face mask or shield, you also may leave the helmet in place. Removing the helmet can cause movement of the spine, which in turn aggravates injuries or causes new ones. If you can adequately manage the patient's airway and immobilize the patient appropriately with the helmet in place, it should be left on.

Remember, however, that a patient's status can change at any time, possibly requiring removal of the helmet. When a patient's airway status deteriorates to the point that you cannot manage it adequately with the helmet in place, the helmet must be removed. It also must be removed if the patient is in or goes into cardiac arrest. Some general rules must be followed when removing a helmet:

1. Make sure that adequate padding is available to place under the patient's head after removal of the helmet, especially if the person is wearing bulky clothing or any type of shoulder pads.
2. The removal technique depends on the type of helmet (Skills 29-1 to 29-3).
3. One EMT stabilizes the helmet by placing the hands on each side to prevent motion.
4. A second EMT loosens and removes the chin strap. This EMT then places one hand on the mandible at the angle of the jaw and the other hand against the occipital region of the head.
5. The first EMT moves to the side edges of the helmet and gently spreads the helmet, carefully slipping it halfway off. The helmet may need to be rotated slightly forward to accomplish this.
6. The second EMT repositions so as to maintain control of the head once the helmet has been removed.
7. The helmet is completely removed.
8. Padding is placed underneath the patient's head as indicated.

---

which the forces applied exceed the limits of the supporting structures may cause bone damage of the vertebrae, tearing of the muscles and ligaments, or stretching of the cord.

Much less movement is required to cause a **lateral bending** injury than a flexion/extension injury. For example, say your patient's vehicle is struck broadside. The vehicle and your patient's body tend to move away from the impact. The head has a tendency to remain in place until it is "pulled" along by the cervical spine, muscles, and ligaments. In addition, because the head's center of gravity is more anterior, the head has a tendency to roll sideways and down. These motions cause lateral bending, which may result in vertebral fractures or dislocations.

Injuries that cause a "pulling apart" of the spinal column are called **distraction injuries.** These injuries occur when the head and body are moving in one direction and the head is abruptly stopped. Such an injury might occur in a child playing on the monkey bars who falls and catches the chin on a bar. Another example would be an intentional or unintentional hanging. These circumstances cause a separation of the vertebrae with stretching or tearing (or both) of the cord.

Maintaining a high index of suspicion and examining the mechanism of injury can help you determine the likelihood that your patient has a spinal injury. Assume that the patient has a spinal injury in any of the following situations:

- Any significant, violent force striking the head, neck, torso, or pelvis
- A vehicle or motorcycle crash
- A pedestrian-vehicle collision
- Any situation involving sudden acceleration, deceleration, or lateral bending forces

SKILL 29-1
◎ *Motorcycle Helmet Removal*

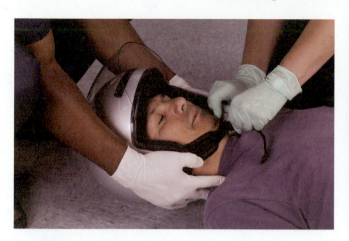

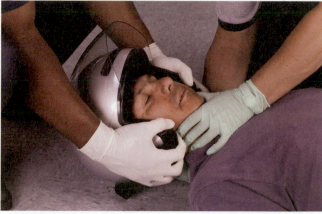

1. One EMT takes position above the patient's head and stabilizes the helmet, head, and neck in as close to a neutral inline position as the helmet allows. A second EMT kneels at the patient's side, opens or removes the face shield, if necessary, and undoes or cuts the chin strap.

2. The second EMT grasps the patient's mandible between the thumb and the first two fingers at the angle of the mandible. The EMT's other hand is placed under the patient's neck, on the occiput of the skull, to take control of manual stabilization. The EMT's forearms should be resting on the floor, the ground, or his or her thighs for additional support.

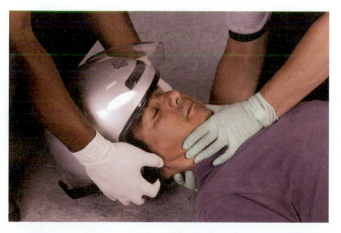

4. Continue manual stabilization after removal of the helmet. Place padding behind the patient's head to maintain a neutral inline position and apply a properly sized cervical collar.
   NOTE: Two key elements are involved in helmet removal:

   - While one EMT maintains manual stabilization of the patient's head and neck, the other EMT can move. At no time should both EMTs be moving their hands.
   - The EMT must rotate the helmet in different directions, first to clear the patient's nose and then to clear the back of the patient's head.

3. The first EMT pulls the sides of the helmet slightly apart, away from the patient's head, and rotates the helmet with up-and-down rocking motions while pulling it off the patient's head. The helmet is moved slowly and deliberately, and care is taken as the helmet clears the patient's nose.

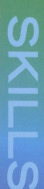

SKILLS

SKILL 29-2

⊙ *Bicycle Helmet Removal*

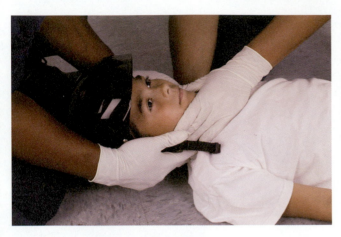

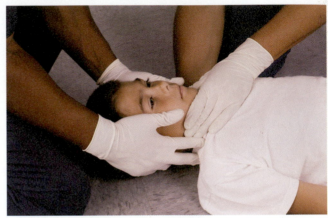

1. While one EMT stabilizes the head and cervical spine, a second EMT releases the chin strap.

3. After the helmet is removed, the second EMT continues to support the patient's head and neck. The first EMT applies a cervical collar and uses padding to stabilize the head and neck.

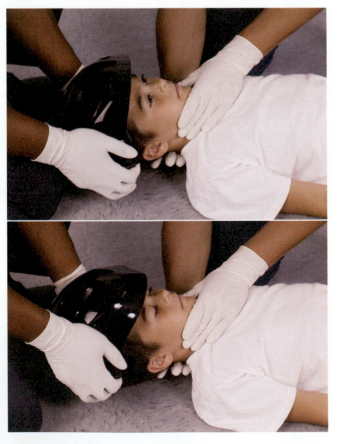

2. The second EMT supports the back of the head and the chin so that the first EMT can remove the helmet.

SKILLS

SKILL 29-3
◉ *Football Helmet Removal*

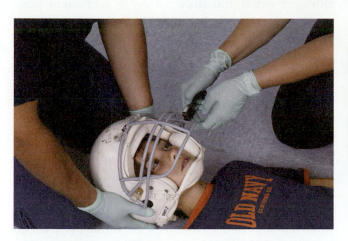

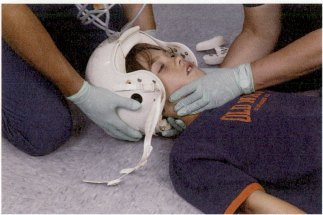

1. While one EMT stabilizes the head and neck, a second EMT releases the face piece by unscrewing the clasps or cutting them.

2. After the face piece has been cleared, the second EMT supports the head and neck so that the first EMT can remove the helmet.

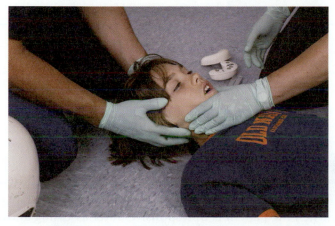

3. After the helmet is removed, the first EMT stabilizes the head and neck while the second EMT provides padding and applies a cervical collar.

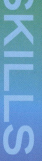

- A fall from a significant height (normally considered to be 15 feet or higher) in which the patient landed on the feet or the head
- A fall in which one part of the body is suddenly stopped
- An unrestrained victim in a rollover accident or a person ejected from a vehicle
- A victim of an explosion
- Any shallow water diving accident
- Blunt or penetrating trauma to the head, neck, or torso
- An unconscious trauma victim

In addition to the preceding situations, maintain a high index of suspicion if your patient has any of the following:

- A head injury with any change in the level of consciousness
- Significant helmet damage
- Fractures of the legs and hips caused by an impact
- Injuries directly to the spinal area

Assessing the Patient with a Possible Spinal Injury

Begin your assessment as you approach the patient. By observing the scene, you may obtain clues as to what happened and what specific mechanisms were involved. These are very important observations that will help as you continue with the patient assessment. Once you have established that the patient's ABCs have been addressed, you must determine whether your patient is conscious and responsive. You can do this by asking the person questions. First, determine whether the patient knows his or her name, the day, and the location. This provides a good baseline for the patient's mental status. Remind your patient to remain still as you ask the following questions:

- Does your neck or back hurt?
- Do you know what happened?
- Where does it hurt?
- Can you move your hands and feet?
- Do you feel me touching your fingers?
- Do you feel me touching your toes?

Next, proceed with the focused physical exam. Spinal cord injuries can produce numerous signs and symptoms. It is your responsibility to gather as much information as possible. Asking appropriate questions can help you determine your patient's needs. As you examine the patient's body, note any swelling, contusions, lacerations, punctures or penetrations, or deformities. Palpate areas of tenderness or deformity; however, keep any movement to a minimum. Testing a patient's grip helps determine whether the two sides are equal and strong. Have your patient push against your hand with each foot. Document your findings. Remember that the ability to walk or to move the extremities and/or a lack of pain do not rule out a spinal injury. Patients who require surgical repair for an unstable spine are often found walking around at the scene. If the mechanism of injury exists, immobilize the patient.

Tenderness in an affected area indicates an injury. Is there pain with movement? Even though this is an important finding, do not ask or allow your patient to move excessively. Is there pain without movement? Along the spine? In the legs? Is it constant or does it come and go? As you examine the patient, note any obvious deformities of the spine. Does the patient have soft tissue injuries in the head and neck area? Did trauma to the shoulders, back, abdomen, or lower extremities occur? Is weakness or tingling present in any of the extremities? Has the patient lost sensation or is paralysis present below the suspected injury level or in the extremities? Remember that patients who have lost sensation below a spinal injury will also not feel the pain from other injuries such as a fracture or intra-abdominal bleeding. Has the patient had an episode of incontinence? It is important that you gather information with these questions and document the answers on the prehospital care report.

With regard to assessment, an unresponsive patient presents more of a challenge. Determining the mechanism of injury becomes even more important when the patient is unresponsive. After assessing and managing the ABCs, proceed with the focused exam just as you would with a responsive patient. Make sure to ask family members or bystanders, if available, for additional information. Did they see what happened? What was the patient's mental status before the incident? Has the person's mental status changed since the incident? This type of questioning may yield additional clues about your patient. With an unresponsive trauma patient, **always** assume that the patient has a spinal injury and immobilize the person.

Spinal cord injuries may lead to some very serious complications. Paralysis below the level of injury may leave the patient unable to walk (paraplegic) or unable to use the upper extremities (quadriplegic). Depending on the level of the injury, a patient's breathing may also be affected. The diaphragm is innervated between the third and fifth cervical verte-

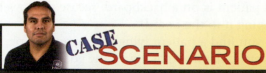

CASE SCENARIO
continued

As Rafael ventilates the patient with a bag-mask device, the crew carefully but quickly begins to secure the patient to the long backboard. After securing the torso and legs with the board straps, the crew members use the head immobilizing device to secure the head and neck. After the device is applied, Rafael finds it more difficult to manage the patient's airway with the jaw thrust maneuver.

Questions: *Which is more important, ventilating the patient or controlling the cervical spine? What can Rafael do to best manage this situation?*

SPECIAL Populations

Infants and Children

Immobilization of infants and children requires adjustments to the customary adult immobilization techniques. Infants' and children's body structures are not fully mature and therefore are proportionally different from those of an adult. This becomes evident when the EMT tries to lay a pediatric patient supine on a long backboard. In infants and children, the head is more posterior than in an adult (see Fig. 29-11). Laying these patients flat forces the head forward (flexion) and may close the airway. To prevent this, you should place padding beneath your patient's shoulders. This raises the torso, allowing the head to be in a neutral position.

Next, select and apply an appropriately sized cervical collar. Although these collars are available in a range of sizes, EMTs often find that they do not fit a pediatric patient appropriately. In such cases, use rolled towels to secure the patient's neck. Both the towel rolls and the patient's head must be secured to the backboard. Remember, an improperly fitting cervical collar does more harm than good.

brae. However, the intercostal muscles of the rib cage receive their nerve impulses lower in the spine. If an injury occurs between these two areas, the diaphragm operates normally, but the intercostal muscles do not expand the rib cage. You may see that, as the patient tries to breathe, the abdomen expands while the chest collapses. As the abdomen collapses, the chest expands. The patient therefore is unable to bring air into the lungs adequately. Consequently, the person has poor air exchange and becomes hypoxic.

■ IMMOBILIZATION

After the EMT establishes that a spinal injury is possible, the next step is to protect the spine. It is imperative that the patient be immobilized; this minimizes the chance of aggravating existing injuries or causing new ones. The rule of immobilization above and below the injury also holds true with the spine. Because you cannot be sure at which level the injury exists, you must immobilize the total spine. This can be accomplished only by securing your patient to a long backboard.

As with all patient care, EMTs first must make sure that the ABCs have been managed and that the appropriate body substance isolation (BSI) precautions are taken to protect themselves and the patient. One EMT then should apply manual inline stabilization (Fig. 29-9). This can be done in a number of ways. The goal is to have the patient's head and neck in a neutral inline position. If the patient's head is not in

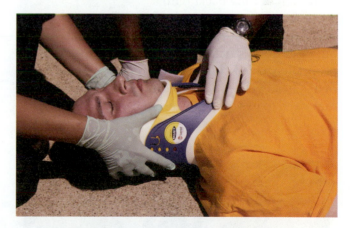

Fig. 29-9 Manual inline stabilization.

this position, gently turn the head until it is. If the patient complains of pain or if the head is not easily moved, stop and secure the head and neck in the position found. It is important to maintain the manual inline stabilization until the patient is securely fastened to a long backboard.

Motor function and sensation must be assessed in all extremities before and after immobilization. With the patient's eyes closed, lightly touch the hands, fingers, toes, and feet. Does the patient respond to light touch? Does the person require a stronger touch? If the patient does not respond to touch, you may need to prick the person gently with an object that does not penetrate the skin. If possible, have the patient squeeze your fingers with both hands, if it does cause the patient pain. Note the strength in the two extremities. Sensation and strength should be equal on the two sides of the patient's body. Also, with a conscious patient, ask whether the person has any weakness, tingling, numbness, paresthesia, or "shooting" pain.

Assess the cervical spine and neck. Obvious spinal deformities are rare; however, you should consider the patient to have a serious spinal injury if you feel unusual gaps, bone fragments, or bulges as you palpate the spinal column. If soft tissue injuries can be seen in the neck region, consider the potential for a spinal column or spinal cord injury (or both).

The cervical spine should be maintained in as close to a neutral position as possible. To assist with this, a cervical collar should be sized and applied to the patient. Cervical collars come in various types and sizes (Fig. 29-10). Remember, a cervical collar alone does not provide complete immobilization. It is merely an adjunct to help limit flexion, extension, and lateral movement of the neck. A cervical collar must be used in conjunction with another spinal immobilization device, such as a short backboard and, eventually, a long backboard.

An improperly sized cervical collar may do more harm than good. A properly sized collar fits snugly but does not restrict the patient's breathing. If an appropriately sized collar is not available or if the patient's head is not in the neutral inline position, you may need to use rolled towels to help secure the neck.

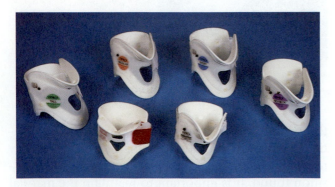

Fig. 29-10 Cervical collars in various sizes.

Once the patient is on a backboard, secure the towel roll by taping it to the board.

When you find a patient lying supine and suspect that the person has a spinal injury, the goal is to have the patient totally immobilized on a long backboard. Therefore, how do you transfer the patient to the backboard with the least amount of movement? Log rolling the patient as a single unit can minimize movement of the spine (Skills 29-4 and 29-5). The procedure is as follows:

- Make sure that the ABCs are assessed and any problems addressed, that BSI precautions are taken, that one EMT is stabilizing the spine manually, and that a properly fitted cervical collar has been or is being applied. Assess the patient's pulse, motor function, and sensation in all extremities. Place the patient's arms at the sides.
- Position the long backboard next to the patient. If the backboard is equipped with a head immobilizer, make sure all the straps and cushions have been removed or moved out of the way.
- One to three EMTs then position themselves at the patient's shoulders, waist, and knees on the side opposite the backboard.
- The first EMT (the one providing manual inline stabilization) gives the order to roll the patient toward the other EMTs. On the first EMT's count, the patient is rolled, as a unit, toward the other EMTs. Continue to roll the patient until the person is resting against the EMTs' legs. It is very important to keep the spine inline as the patient is rolled onto his or her side.
- After the patient has been rolled onto his or her side, the EMTs assess the posterior body. Quickly check for any spinal deformities, obvious injuries, or bleeding and treat accordingly.
- Next, position the backboard as close to the patient as possible. If room allows, the head of the board should extend approximately 16 inches beyond the patient's head.
- The first EMT gives the command to roll the patient back onto the board. Typically the patient is not centered on the backboard at this point. Do not push the patient laterally to center the person on the board. Instead, an EMT faces the patient's head and puts his or her hands in or near the patient's armpits. A second EMT puts his or her hands on the patient's hips. A third EMT controls the legs. As the first EMT gives the command to move, the other three slide the patient up and toward the cen-

SKILL 29-4
● Log Roll with Suspected Spinal Injury

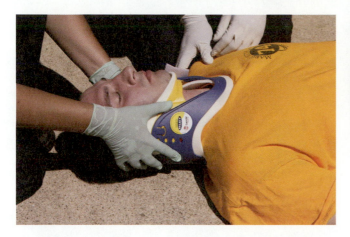

1. While one EMT stabilizes the head and neck, a second EMT applies a cervical collar.

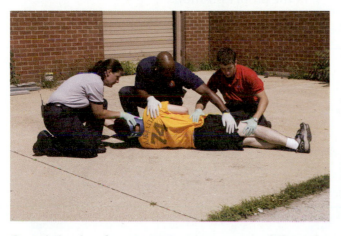

2. While the first EMT continues to stabilize the head and neck, the second and third EMTs position themselves on the patient's side, placing their hands in positions to evenly distribute the patient's weight.

3. With the first EMT stabilizing the head and neck and the second and third EMTs in position at the patient's side, the patient is rolled onto the side on a 3-count.

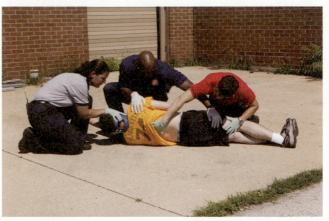

4. While the patient is in this position, an EMT should examine the person's back.

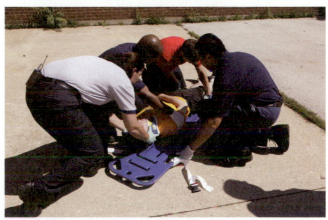

5. A fourth EMT moves a backboard into position, and the patient is lowered onto the board on a 3-count.

Continued

SKILLS

581

SKILL 29-4

◎ *Log Roll with Suspected Spinal Injury—cont'd*

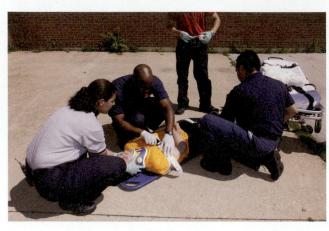

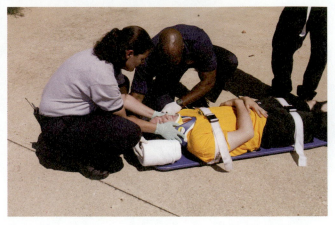

6. Once positioned on the backboard, the patient is strapped to the board in this order: chest, pelvis, legs, and head.

7. The head and neck are stabilized by placing head blocks or towel or blanket rolls to maintain them in the proper position.

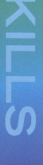

SKILLS

SKILL 29-5

Log Roll with Suspected Spinal Injury from a Prone Position

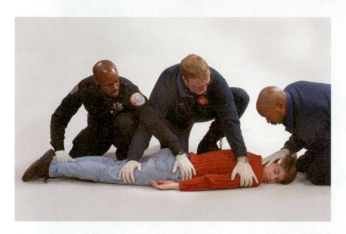

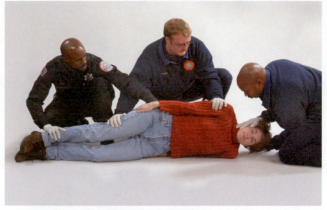

1. While one EMT maintains manual inline stabilization of the head and neck, two other EMTs line up on one side of the patient and position their hands at the shoulder, hip, and upper and lower leg.

2. On the first EMT's count, the patient is rolled toward the other two EMTs as a single unit.

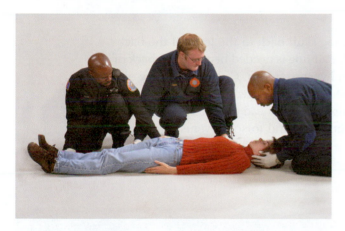

3. On the first EMT's count, the patient is rolled further onto the back as a single unit. Manual stabilization of the head and neck is continued throughout.

SKILLS

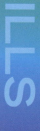

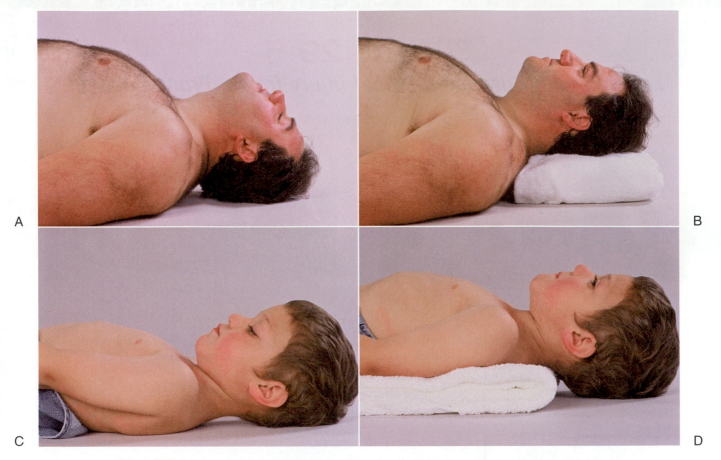

Fig. 29-11 **A,** In some patients, pulling the skull back to the level of the backboard can produce severe hyperextension. **B,** Padding is needed between the back of the head and the backboard to prevent such hyperextension. **C,** The larger size of a child's head relative to body size, combined with the reduced development of the posterior thoracic muscles, produces hyperflexion of the head when a child is placed on a backboard. **D,** Padding beneath the shoulders and torso prevents this hyperflexion.

ter of the board. This motion keeps the patient's spine inline while centering the person on the board. This may also be accomplished by using a patient slide or scoop stretcher, if available.

- Once the patient is positioned on the board, fill all voids with padding and place a pad under the head. Avoid excessive motion. With pediatric patients, pad beneath the shoulders. The head of a pediatric patient lies more posterior than the head of an adult. Therefore lying flat on a backboard forces the pediatric patient's head forward and may close the airway (Fig. 29-11, *C*).

- You are now ready to secure the patient to the long backboard (Fig. 29-12). The patient's torso should be secured first, followed by the legs, with the head last. Although there are many strapping techniques, it is important to remember that the

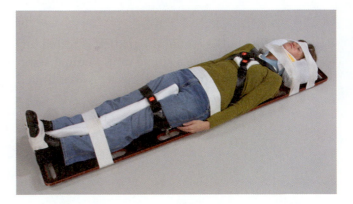

Fig. 29-12 A patient fully immobilized to a long backboard.

ultimate goal is to have the patient completely immobilized, which simply means that the person cannot move. At a minimum, secure the torso, the pelvis, the legs, and the head. Also remember that circumferential straps (around the patient) do not stop the patient from moving up or down on the backboard. Straps placed over the shoulders and around the bottom of the feet help eliminate this movement. As straps are applied across the knee area, you should slide a pad under the patient's knees. Most patients find it more comfortable with padding filling this void.

- Reassess pulse, motor function, and sensation in all extremities. Compare these new results with those obtained before immobilization and record what you find. Note any differences and forward that information to the receiving facility.

Often the patient is found in a sitting position, such as in a motor vehicle crash (MVC). The MVC certainly provides the EMT with enough evidence of the potential for a spinal injury. It is your responsibility to move the patient from a sitting position to supine on a long backboard without aggravating existing injuries or causing additional damage. To accomplish this, you must use a short spine immobilization device (Skill 29-6). The exception to this is a case in which the patient must be moved immediately, perhaps because the person's condition is deteriorating rapidly, the scene is dangerous, or immediate access to others in the vehicle is vital. Under any of these circumstances, a technique called *rapid extrication* is used.

Often EMTs find a patient standing when they arrive at the scene. If the mechanism of injury (e.g., an MVC) tells you that this patient has experienced enough force to cause a spinal injury, you must immobilize the person. This is done by immobilizing the patient to a long backboard in a standing position (Skill 29-7).

Some common mistakes made during immobilization include the following:

- The patient is not adequately secured to the immobilization device. If the device is allowed to move significantly in any fashion, the head may also move. This could aggravate existing spinal injuries and cause new ones.
- The head is not immobilized in a neutral position. Not providing padding behind the patient's head puts the person in a hyperextended position; placing too much padding behind the head puts the patient in a hyperflexed position.

SPECIAL Considerations

Use of Rapid Extrication

With a seated patient, the best method of immobilization is a short spine immobilization device. However, in some situations the time required to apply such a device may be harmful to the patient's condition. Examples of such situations include the following:

- The scene is unsafe for the patient and rescuers.
- The patient is in unstable condition and requires immediate interventions that cannot be provided in the person's current position.
- A seated patient obstructs access to a more seriously injured patient.

In any of these situations, the rapid extrication technique is used. *It is important to note that rapid extrication should not be used instead of a short spine immobilization device unless the situation (such as those described) dictates.* The choice is based on the time available and the patient's condition, not on the EMT's personal preference.

- Torso straps are not sufficiently snug before the head is secured. Adjusting the torso straps after securing the head may create movement of the device and may cause the head to move.

■ INJURIES OF THE BRAIN AND SKULL

The brain and skull can be injured in a number of ways. Some injuries are obvious (e.g., scalp lacerations), whereas others cannot be seen. With unseen injuries, determining what has happened (e.g., brain injury) may be difficult. EMTs must keep in mind that whenever a significant force has been applied to the head, both skull injury and brain injury are possible.

Head Injuries

All head injuries should be considered serious and evaluated appropriately. Even a seemingly insignificant injury may prove life-threatening. On the other hand, many head injuries are minor and have little or no long-term effect.

SKILL 29-6
◉ Short (Seated) Spine Board Immobilization

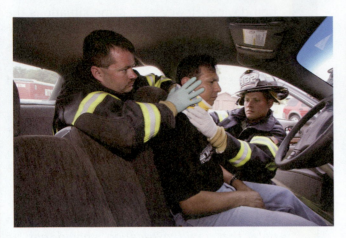

1. Make sure that body substance isolation (BSI) precautions are taken, that the spine is immobilized manually, and that a properly fitted cervical collar has been or is being applied. Assess the patient's pulse, motor function, and sensation in all extremities. Document these baseline findings.

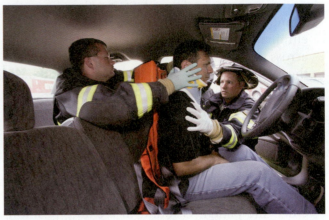

2. Slide the immobilization device behind the patient. Position the device so that the top is level with the top of the patient's head. If the device has body flaps, fold them toward the front of the patient and lift the device so that they fit securely in the armpits. Throughout this process, minimize patient movement as much as possible.

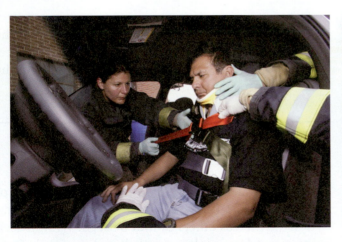

3. Secure the patient's torso to the device using its own straps. If the device has leg straps, they may be secured at this time. Verify that the device is securely fastened to the torso by checking the tightness of all straps. Adjust them as needed, again without excessive movement of the patient.

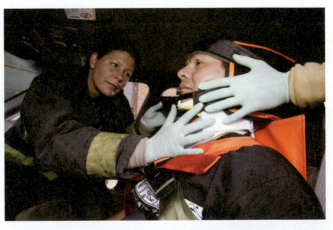

4. Pad behind the patient's head as needed to maintain a neutral inline position. This can be accomplished by using padding provided with your immobilization device or folded towels or other available padding. You are now ready to secure the patient's head to the device. Typically, head straps are provided with the immobilization device. If not, you may use elastic bandages, roller bandages, cravats, or other materials to secure the head to the device. *Note: The head is always secured last.*

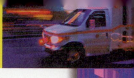

SKILL 29-6
◎ *Short (Seated) Spine Board Immobilization—cont'd*

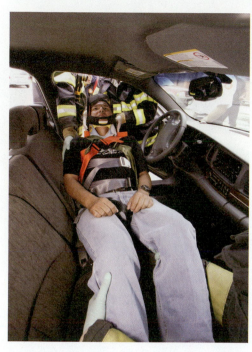

5. You are now ready to move the patient to a long backboard. If possible, place the end of the backboard under the patient's buttocks. Using the short immobilization device, rotate your patient and lay the person down on the backboard. If you are unable to slip the backboard under the patient's buttocks, you may need to lift the person to the backboard using the short immobilization device.

6. Reassess the patient's pulse, motor function, and sensation in all extremities. Compare these results with your previous ones and document what you find. Forward this information to the receiving facility.

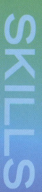

SKILLS

SKILL 29-7
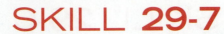
Standing Long Board Application

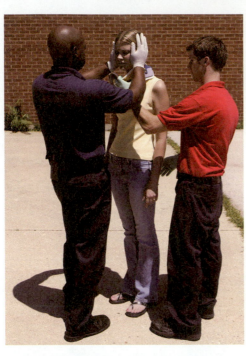

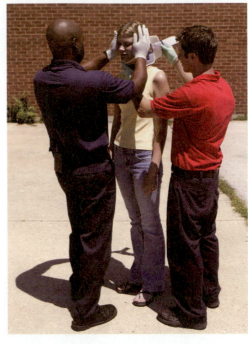

1. Make sure that body substance isolation (BSI) precautions are taken. Apply manual inline stabilization by approaching the patient from the front and placing your hands on each side of the patient's head.

2. Have a second EMT assess the patient's pulse, motor function, and sensation in all extremities. The second EMT also sizes the patient for a cervical collar, assesses the neck and spine area for injury, and applies the collar.

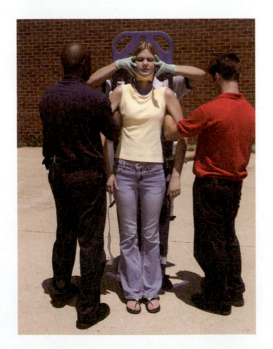

3. The second EMT positions a long backboard behind the patient, between the first EMT's arms, while the first EMT continues holding the patient's neck inline. Additional EMTs place their arms under the patient's armpits and grasp the backboard. The backboard then is placed against the patient's back.

SKILLS

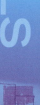

SKILL 29-7
◉ *Standing Long Board Application—cont'd*

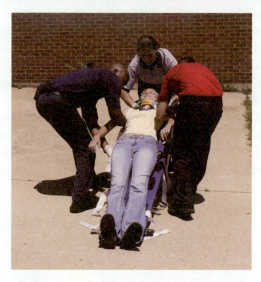

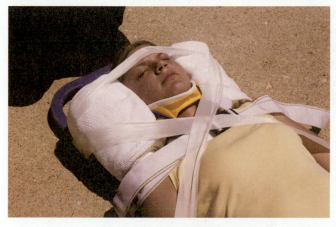

4. Inform the patient that you will be leaning him or her backward. Once all are ready, the EMT in back gives the order to lean the patient toward him or her and onto the ground.

5. Reassess the patient's pulse, motor function, and sensation. Secure the patient to the backboard as previously described.

Scalp Lacerations

EMTs will treat many scalp lacerations during their careers. Many of these injuries are just that, a scalp laceration without any additional damage to the skull or brain. Because the scalp is very vascular, even a small laceration can cause dramatic blood loss. This blood loss may be significant enough to cause hypovolemia in a patient (particularly in a child). To control the bleeding, fold any skin flaps back into place and apply direct pressure to the wound with a sterile dressing. Keep in mind that applying too much pressure could push bone shards into the brain if the skull has been fractured. If the dressing becomes soaked with blood, do not remove it. Simply apply additional dressings. Secure the dressings in place with a roller bandage.

Skull Fractures

Skull fractures are classified as open or closed. An open fracture indicates that enough force was applied to the skull to fracture the "bone" and create an opening. Causes can include penetrating injuries (e.g., bullets) or blunt force sufficient to fracture the skull (e.g., MVC, baseball bat to the head) (Fig. 29-13). X-ray films must be taken to determine the severity of these injuries. However, you should suspect an open fracture whenever you see a deformity of the skull.

Also suspect a skull fracture if your patient has **ecchymosis** (bruising) around the eyes and orbits **(raccoon's eyes)** (Fig. 29-14) or behind the ears over the mastoid process **(Battle's sign)** (Fig. 29-15). Leakage of blood or fluid (CSF) from the nose or ears is another indication that the skull may have been fractured.

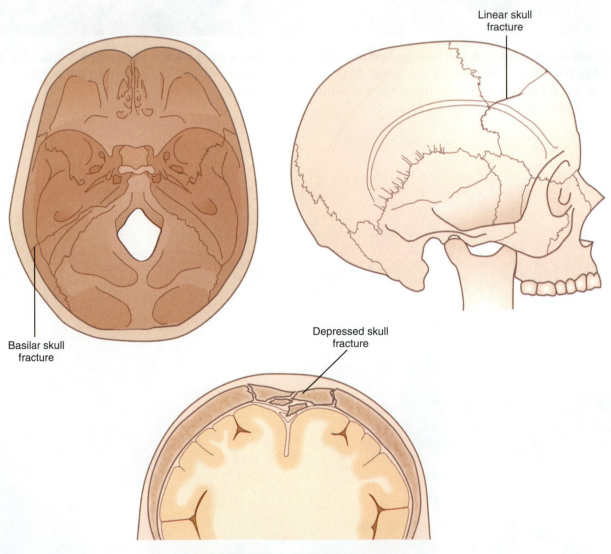

Fig. 29-13 Types of skull fractures.

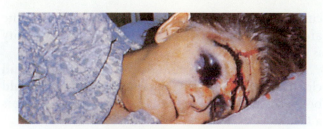

Fig. 29-14 Raccoon's eyes.

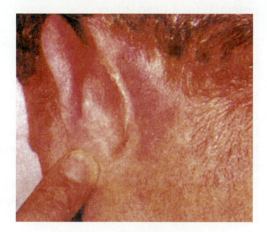

Fig. 29-15 Battle's sign.

Brain Injuries

Injuries to the brain are classified as direct or indirect. A direct injury to the brain occurs with an open head injury. The brain is lacerated, punctured, or bruised by bone fragments or by any other foreign object. An indirect injury can occur with an open or closed head injury. Forces applied to the head cause the brain to strike the skull. Contusions and concussions are common indirect injuries.

A **concussion** is difficult to define precisely. However, when a patient has a concussion, temporary loss or alteration of the brain's ability to function is clear. Although the brain does not suffer any gross physical damage, it is incapable of functioning normally for a time. After the injury or incident, the symptoms may be as minor as the patient temporarily "seeing stars." On the other hand, the symptoms may be as serious as the patient losing consciousness for a period of time. The patient also may have loss of memory (amnesia), either **retrograde amnesia** (loss of memory of events leading up to the incident) or **anterograde amnesia** (loss of memory of events that occurred immediately after the incident). These symptoms usually are short-lived. In fact, they may be gone by the time the EMT arrives. Nevertheless, it is important for the EMT to ask the patient about other symptoms, such as dizziness, nausea, or weakness.

A **contusion,** like any other soft tissue bruise, causes blood to accumulate in the traumatized area. A brain contusion is far more serious than a concussion because the brain suffers actual physical injury. This injury may cause increased **intracranial pressure** (ICP) as a result of bleeding into the tissue and may cause permanent damage to the brain tissue. These patients have many of the same signs and symptoms as other patients with a head injury.

Intracranial bleeding may occur as a result of direct or indirect trauma. As the name indicates, intracranial bleeding involves bleeding into the cranium, which causes a hematoma to develop. The hematoma can develop in different areas, such as between the skull and the dura (epidural hematoma), beneath the dura but outside the brain (subdural hematoma), or within the brain tissue itself (intracerebral hematoma) (Fig. 29-16). Regardless of the location, as a hematoma develops and expands, ICP increases, the brain is compressed, and tissue damage occurs.

An **epidural hematoma** typically results when the blood vessels that run between the skull and the brain are stretched or torn. An epidural hematoma normally is caused by a low-velocity impact to the head or a sudden deceleration in which the dura is pulled away from the skull. The skull, being a rigid structure, does not move. However, the brain inside the skull moves away from the force, stretching and tearing blood vessels (typically arteries), and a hematoma results. An epidural hematoma may de-

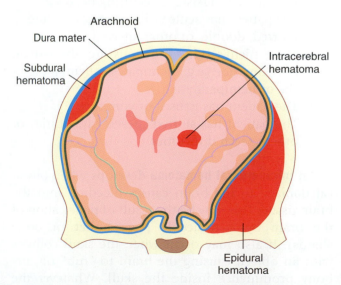

Fig. 29-16 Types of intracranial hemorrhage.

velop fairly rapidly. Signs and symptoms include the following:

- Loss of consciousness followed by a lucid period
- Secondary depression of consciousness
- Hemiparesis on the side opposite the impact
- Fixed and dilated pupil on the affected side

Recognizing that the patient may have a head injury and transporting the person rapidly to an appropriate facility increase the chance of a positive outcome.

A **subdural hematoma** occurs when, as a result of an injury, blood accumulates beneath the dura but outside the brain itself. Individuals who have a subdural hematoma have a higher mortality rate (50% to 60%) than those with an epidural hematoma. Because the injured vessels (usually veins) bleed slowly, a subdural hematoma may take much longer to develop. Therefore symptoms may not appear until several hours or days after the injury incident. As a result of this delay of symptoms, the patient may not to connect them to the incident. Therefore it is important for the EMT to question the patient (or family members and friends) about any injuries in the recent past. A subdural hematoma should be considered with any of the following signs and symptoms:

- The patient has a change in personality or level of consciousness (e.g., confusion, disorientation, unconsciousness).
- The patient has the worst headache of his or her life or a persistent, recurring headache.
- The patient has acute vision changes, including blurred, double, or other affected vision.
- The patient's body functions are affected on only one side (e.g., hemiparesis, hemianesthesia, or hemiparalysis).
- The patient has nausea or vomiting.
- The patient has slurred speech (dysarthria) or other speech difficulties.

An **intracerebral hematoma** develops when physical damage to the brain causes bleeding into the brain tissue. This may be the result of penetration of the brain by a projectile (e.g., bullet or bone shards). It also may occur when the skull collides with an object, causing the brain to "rub" on any bony prominence inside the skull. Whatever the cause, the brain tissue is damaged, and bleeding oc-

curs. Signs and symptoms vary, depending on the area of the brain affected, although seizure activity is common.

Many of the signs and symptoms of open and closed head injuries are the same. The patient should be evaluated for head injury if any of the following is a factor:

- A mechanism of injury (e.g., a broken windshield or helmet damage) that indicates the potential for a head injury
- Irregular breathing patterns
- Contusions, lacerations, or hematomas of the scalp
- Any deformity of the skull
- Soft or depressed areas on palpation
- Exposed brain tissue
- Bleeding from an open fracture
- Blood or fluid (CSF) leaking from the ears or nose
- Bruising (discoloration) around the eyes (raccoon's eyes) or behind the ears (Battle's sign)
- Nausea or vomiting
- Seizure activity
- Increased blood pressure with a decreasing pulse rate

In addition to these factors, the single most important observation in a patient with a head injury is any change in the person's level of consciousness (LOC). A change in the LOC corresponds with some type of injury or damage within the brain. Therefore, if the patient with a head injury is in unstable condition, it is extremely important for the EMT to establish a baseline LOC and re-evaluate it every 5 minutes using the AVPU (alert, verbal, painful, unresponsive) assessment tool or the Glasgow Coma Scale (see Chapter 10). The patient's LOC may fluctuate between improving and diminishing, or the patient may simply deteriorate over time with no improvement. This is a sign of a serious brain injury, and the patient needs aggressive treatment.

Another sign you may see is a change in pupil size. The nerves that control pupil size are very sensitive to ICP changes. Unequal pupil size normally indicates increased pressure on one side of the brain (Fig. 29-17). It is important to note the size of both pupils and to re-evaluate them in light of your assessment of the patient's LOC. Make sure to report any changes.

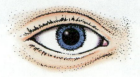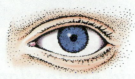

Fig. 29-17 Suspect injury to the brain whenever a patient's pupils are unequal in size.

Nontraumatic Conditions

A number of medical conditions, such as blood clots, hemorrhage from weakened blood vessels, high blood pressure, and others, may cause spontaneous bleeding into the brain. The end result of these non-traumatic conditions is significant bleeding and swelling within the brain. As the ICP within the skull increases, the patient begins to display an altered mental status. This change in LOC may be the first sign of a brain injury. Other signs and symptoms mimic those of traumatic injuries, but there is no evidence of trauma and no mechanism of injury.

Management of the Patient with a Head Injury

Identification of the potential for a head injury is very important to the patient's long-term prognosis. Once the potential for a head injury is suspected, the EMT must provide the appropriate care. This care includes the following:

- Take appropriate BSI precautions to protect yourself and your patient.
- Assess the ABCs and correct any life-threatening problems.
- Provide manual stabilization of the spine while completing your initial assessment. Complete the focused exam en route.
- With any head injury, suspect spinal injury and immobilize the spine.
- Closely monitor the patient's airway, breathing, pulse, and mental status for deterioration. For an unstable patient, reassess every 5 minutes. Support breathing and ventilation as needed or indicated.
- Be very observant for changes in the patient's condition.
- Document your findings and transport the patient immediately to an appropriate facility.

SPECIAL Considerations

Pediatric Patients in Car Seats

EMTs often are called to treat pediatric patients who are in car seats. If the car seat has not been damaged and you can manage your patient's injuries with the child sitting in the seat, immobilize the patient in the seat (Fig. 29-18). In effect, you are using the car seat as a splint. However, *the car seat should never be reused as a car seat.* Place the car seat and patient on a long backboard, secure them, and move them to your stretcher.

Sometimes the patient must be removed from the car seat. Numerous pediatric immobilization devices are available for use in these cases (Fig. 29-19). Unfortunately, not all ambulance services carry pediatric immobilization devices. If you do not have this equipment, slide the patient out of the car seat directly onto a short immobilization device or a long backboard (Fig. 29-20). When adequate padding is used to fill all voids, these devices work nicely to immobilize pediatric patients.

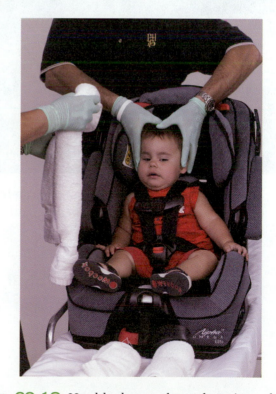

Fig. 29-18 Use blankets and towels to immobilize an infant in a car seat.

SKILL 29-8
◉ *Three-person Rapid Extrication*

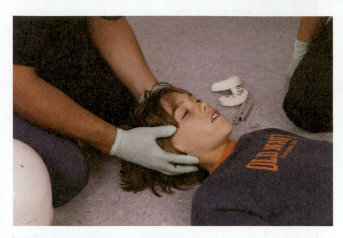

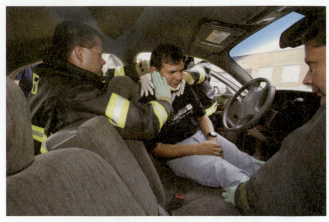

1. One provider holds manual inline stabilization of the head and neck while another applies a cervical collar.

2. While manual stabilization is maintained, the patient's upper torso, lower torso, and legs are rotated in a series of short, controlled movements until the patient is in such a position that manual stabilization can no longer be maintained.

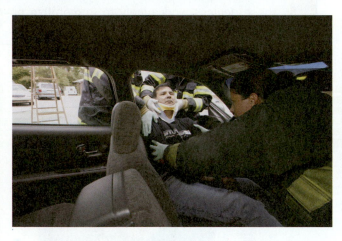

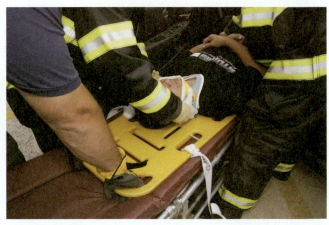

3. The patient is rotated until he or she can be lowered out of the vehicle door opening and onto a long backboard.

4. The patient is moved onto the long backboard and then secured to the long backboard.

SKILLS

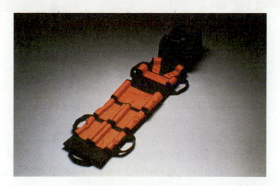

Fig. 29-19 Infant and pediatric immobilization board.

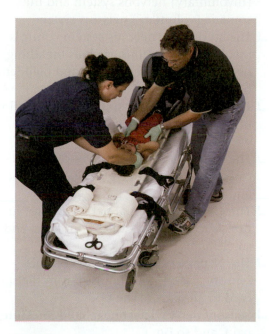

Fig. 29-20 A pediatric patient is slid out of a car seat onto a long backboard.

Rapid Extrication

Occasionally the EMT is faced with having to care for a critical patient in a confined space (e.g., inside a vehicle). When faced with an unstable patient where time is critical, a safe scene is becoming unsafe, or when a stable patient must be moved to attend to a more seriously injured patient, the EMT should rely on **rapid extrication**. *It is important to note that rapid extrication should not be substituted for the use of a short spine immobilization device unless situations, such as those described, dictate.* It is based on time and the patient, not the EMT's personal preference. Rapid extrication is the quick, but safe, manner to remove a pa-

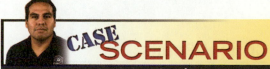

CASE SCENARIO
conclusion

With one of the firefighters manually stabilizing the patient's cervical spine, Rafael is easily able to ventilate the patient once again. It requires some coordination, but the crew is able to manage the patient well with this two-person technique until the medic ambulance arrives to take over care. ■

TEAMWORK

EMTs must deal with a variety of head and spinal trauma emergencies. Responding to accident scenes, trench rescues, and a variety of other scenes requires a good working relationship with other responders. The limitations of your equipment, certification, or licensure may require you to request assistance early in the emergency call.

tient from an area to provide meaningful intervention. Rapid extrication can be performed with two or more rescuers. Skill 29-8 explains three person rapid extrication in detail.

Resources

Chapleau W: *Emergency first responder: making the difference,* St Louis, 2004, Mosby.

McSwain NE et al: *The basic EMT: comprehensive prehospital patient care,* St Louis, 1997, Mosby.

National Association of Emergency Medical Technicians: *PHTLS: basic and advanced prehospital trauma life support,* ed 4, St Louis, 1999, Mosby.

Sanders MJ et al: *Paramedic textbook,* ed 2, St Louis, 2000, Mosby.

Seeley RR et al: *Anatomy and physiology,* ed 2, St Louis, 1992, Mosby.

US Department of Transportation, National Highway Traffic Safety Administration: *EMT-Basic: National Standard Curriculum* 1999.

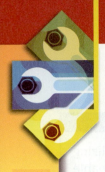
Critical Points

Injuries of the head and spine can be life altering for your patient. Your role in managing these injuries is crucial. Using thorough and proper assessment techniques and appropriate treatment, you can have a positive effect on the outcome for a patient with a head or spinal injury. Second only to management of the ABCs, this is your most important responsibility.

Learning Checklist

❏ The nervous system controls all functions in the body. It is divided into the central nervous system and the peripheral nervous system.

❏ The CNS consists of the brain and spinal cord.

❏ Functions such as memory, emotions, and communication take place in the CNS.

❏ The brain also receives sensory data and coordinates motor control throughout the body.

❏ The brain is divided into the cerebrum, the cerebellum, and the brainstem.

❏ The cerebrum makes up 75% to 80% of the brain and controls functions such as the visual impulses of the eyes, speech, balance, hearing, and emotion.

❏ The cerebellum coordinates body movements.

❏ The brainstem controls the body's vegetative functions, such as the heart rate.

❏ The spinal column extends from the brainstem to the level of the second lumbar vertebra.

❏ Nervous system tissue cannot regenerate if it is injured.

❏ The brain lies within the cranium; it is protected by the skin, fascial muscle, the skull bone itself, and the meninges.

❏ The skin of the scalp is extremely vascular, and scalp lacerations sometimes can cause dramatic blood loss.

❏ The meninges comprise three distinct layers of tissue: the dura mater, the arachnoid layer, and the pia mater.

❏ The dura mater is a tough, leatherlike covering that forms a sac around the brain.

❏ The arachnoid layer and the pia mater rest on the surface of the brain. Between these two layers run the various blood vessels that feed the brain. Cerebrospinal fluid is also produced in this area and provides a cushion of protection for the brain and spinal cord.

❏ The PNS is divided into the autonomic (involuntary) nervous system and the somatic (voluntary) nervous system.

❏ The autonomic nervous system controls involuntary functions, such as breathing, the heart rate, blood vessel size, and bladder and bowel control.

❏ The somatic nervous system controls all voluntary functions of the body, such as walking or typing.

❏ The cranial and spinal nerves of the PNS are categorized into three types: sensory, motor, and connecting.

❏ The 12 pairs of cranial nerves control functions such as facial expression, taste, and smell.

❏ The 31 pairs of spinal nerves conduct sensory and motor impulses from the spinal cord to all parts of the body.

❏ Sensory nerves detect heat, cold, pressure, pain, and so on.

❏ Motor nerves stimulate muscles, causing them to contract.

❏ Connecting nerves connect the sensory and motor nerves directly, enabling the protective reflex arc reaction.

❏ A reflex arc occurs when a stimulus (usually pain) is applied to the body, and the sensory nerves send an impulse through the connecting nerves directly to the motor nerves, causing a reflexive reaction. (For example, if someone poked your finger with a pin, you might reflexively pull your hand away.)

❏ Reflex arcs protect the body from injury.

❏ The skeletal system gives the body form, provides protection for the internal organs, and enables movement.

❏ The skull consists of numerous thick, fused bones that form a shell that houses and protects the brain.

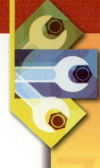

- The brain connects with the spinal cord through a large hole in the skull called the *foramen magnum.*
- The spinal column provides support for the body, enables it to bend and twist, and provides protection for the spinal cord.
- The spinal column consists of 33 vertebrae, which are divided into five sections: cervical vertebrae (seven), thoracic vertebrae (12), lumbar vertebrae (five), sacral vertebrae (five), and coccygeal vertebrae (four).
- Mechanisms of injury to the spine include axial loading (compression of the spinal column), excessive flexion (forward movement of the head), hyperextension (rear movement of the head), hyperrotation (sideways turning of the head), lateral bending (sideways bending of the spinal column), and distraction (expansion or stretching of the spinal column).
- It is important to assess the mechanism of injury. When the mechanism of injury is a concern, the patient should be suspected of having a spinal injury.
- Signs and symptoms of spinal injury include the mechanism of injury, altered mental status, swelling, contusions, lacerations, punctures, tenderness, deformity, weakness or tingling in the extremities, incontinence, paralysis, and difficulty breathing.
- If a spinal injury is suspected, the entire spine should be immobilized. Apply manual stabilization of the head and neck, use the jaw thrust method to open and maintain the airway, assist ventilations if necessary, and complete a detailed assessment as necessary.
- Head injuries may be open or closed. Open injuries may involve profuse external bleeding. Closed injuries may involve internal bleeding.
- Signs and symptoms of possible head injury include pain, swelling, deformity, or open wounds to the head; altered mental status; loss of consciousness after trauma; irregular breathing pattern; pupils that are unequal, slow, or nonreactive to light; loss of normal speech; weakness or paralysis of the extremities; bleeding or fluid loss from the ears;

exposed brain tissue; bruising around both eyes; and bruising behind one or both ears.
- If a patient is suspected of having a head injury, assume that the person also has a spinal injury. Do not probe open wounds or depressions in the skull, assist ventilations if necessary, provide supplemental oxygen if possible, control bleeding and dress wounds, and monitor the patient's mental status.

Key Terms

Anterograde amnesia Loss of memory of events that occurred immediately after the event that precipitated the amnesia.

Arachnoid This is a thin layer of tissue which is located under the dura mater of the brain.

Autonomic nervous system This part of the nervous system involves all automatic and involuntary functions, such as respirations, the heart rate, blood vessel size, and bladder and bowel control. These are all functions that do not require any active effort or decision making on the part of the individual. They are considered vegetative functions.

Axial loading Vertical compression of the spine.

Battle's sign Bruising or bluish discoloration of the bone behind the ear, indicating a basilar skull fracture.

Brainstem Located at the base of the brain. This is where all the body's "vegetative" functions reside such as control of the heart rate and respirations

Cerebellum Located under the cerebrum, it coordinates body movements

Cerebrum The largest portion of the brain (approximately 75% to 80%). It controls many functions of the body, such as thought, visual impulses for the eyes, speech, balance, hearing, and emotion.

Concussion Damage to the brain caused by violent jarring or shaking, such as a blow or an explosion.

Contusion A closed soft tissue injury characterized by discoloration beneath the surface of the skin; a bruise.

Distraction injuries Injuries that cause a "pulling apart" of the spinal column.

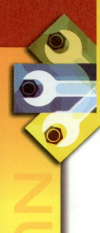

Dura mater The dura mater is a tough, leather-like covering just under the skull that forms a sac around the brain.

Ecchymosis Bluish discoloration of an area of skin or mucous membrane caused by the leakage of blood into the subcutaneous tissues as a result of trauma.

Epidural hematoma An accumulation of blood in the epidural space caused by damage to and leakage of blood from the middle meningeal artery; this causes compression of the dura mater and therefore of the brain.

Intracerebral hematoma A localized collection of extravasated blood within the cerebrum associated with a cerebral laceration caused by a contusion.

Pia mater This is a very thin, tissue paper-like layer which rests on the surface of the brain.

Raccoon's eyes Bilateral bruising around the eyes, often associated with a basilar skull fracture.

Retrograde amnesia The loss of memory of events that occurred before a particular time in a person's life, usually before the event that precipitated the amnesia.

Somatic nervous system The portion of the nervous systems that controls all body functions that are voluntary, such as movement.

Subdural hematoma An accumulation of blood in the subdural space, usually caused by an injury.

National Standard Curriculum Objectives

Cognitive Objectives

After completing this lesson, the EMT student will be able to do the following:

- State the components of the nervous system.
- List the functions of the central nervous system.
- Define the structure of the skeletal system as it relates to the nervous system.
- Relate the mechanism of injury to potential injuries of the head and spine.
- Describe the implications of not properly caring for potential spine injuries.

- State the signs and symptoms of a potential spinal injury.
- Describe the method of determining whether a responsive patient may have a spinal injury.
- Describe the airway emergency medical care techniques for a patient with a suspected spinal injury.
- Describe how to stabilize the cervical spine.
- Discuss indications for sizing and using a cervical spine immobilization device.
- Explain the relationship between airway management and the patient with head and spine injuries.
- Describe a method for sizing a cervical spine immobilization device.
- Describe how to log roll a patient with a suspected spinal injury.
- Describe how to secure a patient to a long backboard.
- List instances when a short spine board should be used.
- Describe how to immobilize a patient using a short spine board.
- Describe the indications for the use of rapid extrication.
- State the circumstances in which a helmet should be left on the patient.
- Discuss the circumstances in which a helmet should be removed.
- Identify different types of helmets.
- Describe the unique characteristics of sports helmets.
- Explain the preferred methods for removing a helmet.
- Discuss alternative methods for removing a helmet.
- Describe how the patient's head is stabilized for removal of a helmet.
- Compare the methods for stabilizing the head with and without a helmet.

Affective Objectives

After completing this lesson, the EMT student will be able to do the following:

- Explain the rationale for immobilization of the entire spine when a cervical spinal injury is suspected.

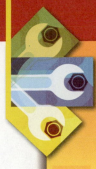

- Explain the rationale for using immobilization methods apart from the straps on the cots.
- Explain the rationale for using a short spine immobilization device when moving a patient from the sitting to the supine position.
- Explain the rationale for using rapid extrication approaches only when they will make the difference between life and death.
- Give the reasons for leaving a helmet in place for transport of a patient.
- Give the reasons for removing a helmet before transporting a patient.

Psychomotor Objectives

After completing this lesson, the EMT student will be able to do the following:

- Demonstrate how to open the airway in a patient with suspected spinal cord injury.

- Demonstrate the evaluation of a responsive patient with a suspected spinal cord injury.
- Demonstrate stabilization of the cervical spine.
- Demonstrate the four-person log roll for a patient with a suspected spinal cord injury.
- Demonstrate the two-person log roll for a patient with a suspected spinal cord injury.
- Demonstrate how to secure a patient to a long backboard.
- Demonstrate the short board immobilization technique.
- Demonstrate the preferred methods for stabilizing a helmet.
- Demonstrate helmet removal techniques.
- Demonstrate alternative methods for stabilizing a helmet.
- Demonstrate the completion of a prehospital care report for patients with head and spinal injuries.

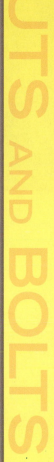

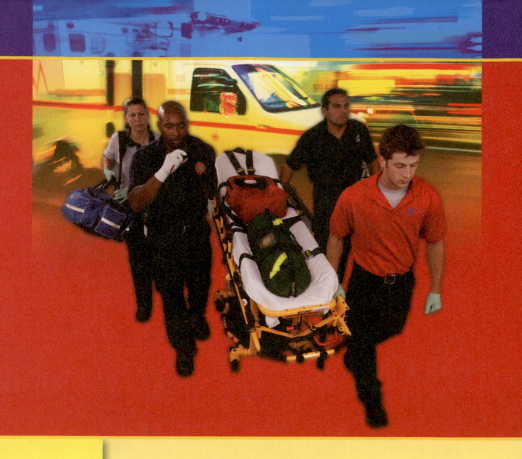

CHAPTER

30

LESSON GOAL

Childbirth is a natural part of the human life cycle. As an emergency medical technician (EMT), you're very likely to be called to assist in a delivery that happens rapidly or unexpectedly. This chapter helps prepare you to deal with normal childbirth and with some of the possible complications of pregnancy and delivery. It also discusses the management of traumatic injuries in a pregnant woman and the immediate postdelivery care of the mother and the newborn. ■

Obstetrics and Gynecology

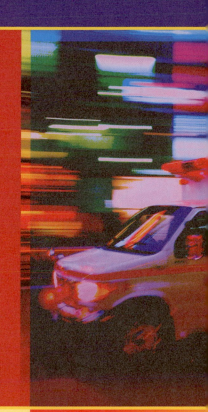

30

CHAPTER OBJECTIVES

After completing this chapter, the EMT student will be able to do the following:

1 Identify the anatomic structures of the female reproductive tract.
2 Define the terms *bloody show, crowning, labor,* and *miscarriage.*
3 Describe the contents and use of an obstetrics kit.
4 Identify complications of early pregnancy.
5 State the indications of imminent delivery.
6 List the steps of predelivery preparation of the mother.
7 Establish the relationship between body substance isolation (BSI) and childbirth.
8 List the steps for assisting a delivery, including care of the baby as the head appears, when and how to cut the umbilical cord, and delivery of the placenta.
9 List the steps in the emergency medical care of the mother after delivery.
10 Summarize the resuscitation of the newborn.
11 Describe the signs and symptoms of three complications of late pregnancy.
12 Describe the procedures for abnormal deliveries, specifically breech birth, shoulder dystocia, prolapsed cord, and limb presentation.
13 Describe the special considerations for meconium, multiple births, and premature deliveries.
14 Describe special considerations for a pregnant trauma patient.

OBJECTIVES

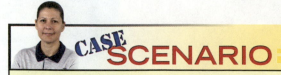

Elizabeth and the crew are met at the door of the house by a very anxious but angry woman, who exclaims, "Well, I told her that if she wasn't gonna be careful, she'd get knocked up. So does she listen? 'Course not. Serves her right." Elizabeth looks back at her crew and grits her teeth. This is going to be a tense situation.

Inside the home, Elizabeth sees a teenage female, whose name is Mary, in the hallway near the bathroom. Mary is crying and supporting herself by grasping both sides of the doorway. Elizabeth can see that the girl is obviously pregnant. She is dressed in only an oversized T-shirt. Beyond her, blood can be seen on the floor and in the toilet.

Questions: *What are some of Elizabeth's concerns at this point? For what should the ambulance crew be preparing?*

Women have given birth to babies for thousands of years without the assistance of medical providers. In fact, most childbirths on this planet take place with little or no medical assistance. Most of these deliveries proceed without complication. However, when complications do occur, they can be terrifying and disastrous for the mother and her infant. In this country, patients who deliver in the prehospital setting are more likely to face the following circumstances:

- They have had previous deliveries.
- They call for emergency medical services (EMS) because of an unexpected complication, such as premature labor or bleeding.
- They have psychosocial issues, such as lack of access to medical care, drug or alcohol abuse, or domestic violence.

Because of these issues, mothers and infants who experience delivery in the prehospital setting have much higher rates of complications and death than those that have a hospital delivery.[1]

As an EMT, you must be prepared to deal with a normal or a complicated delivery in the field. This chapter introduces you to the anatomy and physiology of pregnancy, the stages of labor and delivery, and the postdelivery care of the mother and the newborn. It also discusses some of the complications of pregnancy and delivery.

ANATOMY OF THE FEMALE GENITAL TRACT

The female reproductive structures include the uterus, vagina, fallopian tubes, ovaries, and perineum (Fig. 30-1). The **ovaries** are a pair of organs that release eggs and hormones. Normally one of the ovaries releases an egg each month. The egg travels down its adjacent **fallopian tube** into the uterus. The **uterus (womb)** is a pear-shaped organ where the **embryo,** or fertilized egg, implants and develops. The fertilized egg implants in the lining of the uterus, where it grows and matures. The neck of the uterus, or **cervix,** inserts into the **vagina,** which leads to the outside of the body. Together, the lower part of the uterus, the cervix, and the vagina often are referred to as the **birth canal.** The tissue between the vaginal opening and the anus is called the **perineum.**

■ ANATOMY AND PHYSIOLOGY OF PREGNANCY

Pregnancy is a normal event in the life cycle of human beings. However, unique changes in anatomy and physiology take place during pregnancy. You can better assess and treat a pregnant patient if you understand these normal changes.

The fertilized egg is called an *embryo* during the first 8 weeks of pregnancy. After that it is called the **fetus.** During its growth in the uterus, the fetus is encased in a protective bag, called the **amniotic sac (bag of waters).** The fetus receives nutrition and oxygen and eliminates waste through the **umbilical cord.** The umbilical cord has three vessels, two arteries and a vein. It connects the fetus to the **placenta (afterbirth)** (Fig. 30-2)**.** The function of the placenta, which attaches to the wall of the uterus, is to provide nutrients for and remove waste from the fetus.

The normal length of pregnancy is about 40 weeks. For ease of reference, the pregnancy typically is divided into three parts, or *trimesters*, each lasting about 3 months.

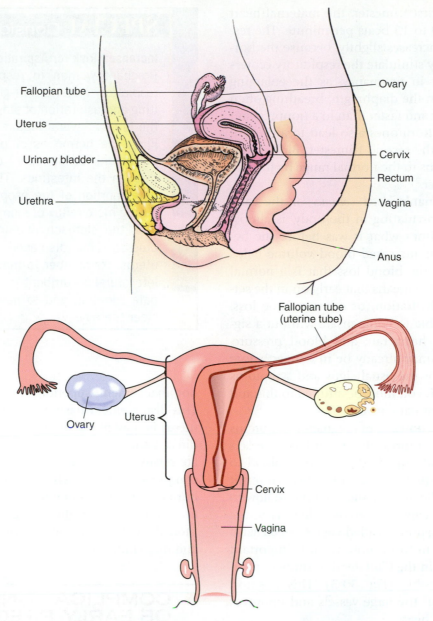

Fallopian tube

Uterus

Urinary bladder

Urethra

Ovary

Cervix

Rectum

Vagina

Anus

Fallopian tube
(uterine tube)

Ovary

Uterus

Cervix

Vagina

Fig. 30-1 Anatomy of the female genital tract.

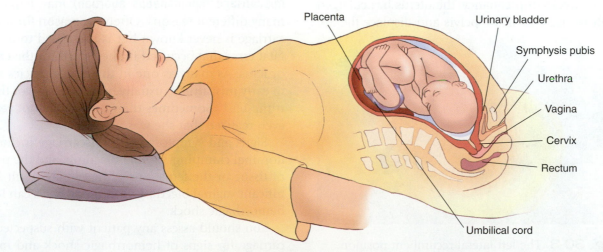

Placenta

Urinary bladder

Symphysis pubis

Urethra

Vagina

Cervix

Rectum

Umbilical cord

Fig. 30-2 Anatomy of the pregnant female.

As early as the first trimester, the maternal heart rate increases by 10 to 15 beats per minute. The respiratory rate also increases slightly, because the hormones of pregnancy stimulate the respiratory centers of the brain. Later in pregnancy, as the enlarging uterus pushes up on the diaphragm, breathing often is slightly shallower and faster than in a nonpregnant patient. Pregnancy hormones also lead to a drop in blood pressure by the second trimester. Blood pressure gradually returns to the normal range by the end of the third trimester.[2]

A pregnant woman's *blood volume*, or the total amount of blood circulating in the body, is almost one-and-one-half times what it was before she became pregnant. This increased blood volume helps her body adjust to the blood loss that is a normal part of delivery. It also means that early on in the setting of trauma, dehydration, or other volume loss, her body may be able to compensate without a significant change in heart rate and blood pressure. However, her fetus may already be in danger before the mother develops the usual signs and symptoms of shock. As an EMT, you must be attuned to this and monitor all pregnant patients closely.

During the third trimester of pregnancy, the uterus is large enough to compress the major blood vessels in the abdomen and impede the return of blood to the heart when the patient is supine. This can result in hypotension in the mother and poor blood flow to the uterus, which means poor oxygen delivery to the fetus. This phenomenon is called **supine hypotensive syndrome.**[3] To prevent this syndrome, it is important to keep the patient in the left lateral recumbent position whenever possible (Fig. 30-3). This position moves the uterus off the large vessels and improves blood return to the heart.

During the first trimester, the uterus is still small enough to be entirely protected by the pelvis. After about 13 weeks of pregnancy, the uterus has enlarged enough to rise out of the pelvis and displace the ab-

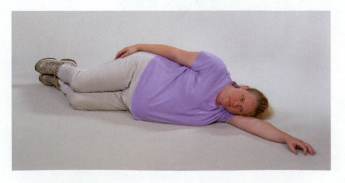

Fig. 30-3 The left lateral recumbent position.

dominal contents superiorly, laterally, and posteriorly. This displacement has several implications. First, the uterus is now much more susceptible to injury from direct trauma, whereas the other abdominal organs are relatively protected. Second, the enlarging uterus compresses the stomach and contributes to the heartburn that is common in pregnancy. Third, pressure on the diaphragm from the enlarging abdomen makes it more difficult for a pregnant woman to breathe deeply and may contribute to shortness of breath.

■ COMPLICATIONS OF EARLY PREGNANCY

Miscarriage

Miscarriage (spontaneous abortion) may happen for many different reasons. Often the reason for the miscarriage is never known but is presumed to be some fatal error that occurred in the growth of the embryo or fetus. As many as one in three pregnancies results in early miscarriage, usually before the end of the first trimester.[4,5] Sometimes the woman may not yet have even realized that she was pregnant.

Signs and symptoms of a miscarriage include abdominal cramping, vaginal bleeding, and the passage of tissue or the fetus. Miscarriages may result in significant vaginal bleeding and in rare cases can lead to hemorrhagic shock.

You should assess any patient with suspected miscarriage for signs of hemorrhagic shock and manage her accordingly. Assess airway, breathing, and circulation (ABCs). Provide oxygen and treat the patient for shock, if necessary. If the patient has passed tissue or the fetus, place this in a clean plastic bag or other container and transport it to the hospital with the mother.

A miscarriage can be an emotionally traumatic experience for parents, even if it is early in the pregnancy or if the pregnancy was unplanned. Offer compassion and psychologic support, if needed.

Ectopic Pregnancy

An **ectopic pregnancy** is one that occurs outside the uterus, usually in the fallopian tube. If the fertilized egg implants in the tube instead of the uterus, it stretches the tube as it grows, causing pain and sometimes vaginal bleeding. Eventually it may cause the tube to rupture, producing severe and even life-threatening intraabdominal bleeding. Symptoms of an ectopic pregnancy usually begin during the second or third month of pregnancy.

An ectopic pregnancy is a potentially life-threatening emergency. Usually the woman does not know her pregnancy is ectopic, and in fact she may not know she is pregnant. Therefore any sudden or severe lower abdominal pain or vaginal bleeding in a woman of childbearing age should be taken seriously. Transport the patient to a hospital for further evaluation.

■ COMPLICATIONS OF LATE PREGNANCY

Placental Abruption

Placental abruption (abruptio placentae) is defined as separation of part of the placenta from its normal attachment to the inner wall of the uterus. This leads to bleeding from the site of separation. It usually is accompanied by painful uterine contractions and sometimes vaginal bleeding.

Studies have shown abruption to be correlated with certain conditions, including abdominal trauma, high blood pressure, maternal cocaine and tobacco use, poor nutrition, advanced maternal age, and infection of the uterus or placenta. The most common causes of abdominal trauma in pregnancy are motor vehicle accidents and domestic violence.[4]

Abruption may not always be an obvious diagnosis. Although significant separation of the placenta may result in vaginal bleeding, the bleeding may be contained between the uterine wall and the placenta. Also, the signs and symptoms normally associated with blood loss may not be obvious, because the normal increase in blood volume during pregnancy initially protects the mother from developing overt shock.[4] In the case of abruption from abdominal trauma, the patient may show little or no external bruising or injury even with a significant abruption.

Abruption may be a life-threatening event for both the mother and baby. Some studies have shown mortality rates as high as 25% to 30% in fetuses and newborns with placental abruption.[4] If a woman has vaginal bleeding and abdominal pain in the third trimester of her pregnancy, you should always consider this diagnosis. Ask about risk factors for abruption and be aggressive about treating shock.

Placenta Previa

Placenta previa is abnormal placement of the placenta such that it partly or completely covers the cervix. When the cervix begins to dilate during labor, the placenta separates at the edge of the cervix and causes vaginal bleeding, sometimes massive and life threatening. This accounts for 20% of bleeding episodes in the second half of pregnancy.[5] The blood is often bright red, and the episode is painless. Consider the diagnosis of placenta previa in any woman with third trimester bleeding. Placenta previa can be difficult to distinguish from abruption.

As with any vaginal bleeding in pregnancy, monitor the mother closely for shock and transport to a facility with obstetric capabilities.

Pre-eclampsia

Pre-eclampsia, or pregnancy-induced hypertension, is a potentially life-threatening condition that occurs in about 5% to 7% of pregnancies.[6] Although the causes are not fully understood, pre-eclampsia appears to be related to abnormal blood vessel constriction, which leads to multiple complications after 20 weeks of pregnancy. Symptoms of this disorder can include headache; severe swelling of the hands, feet and face; abdominal pain; nausea and vomiting; visual disturbances; and, in severe cases, seizures.

Remember that blood pressure in pregnancy should be normal or slightly lower than normal. A blood pressure of 140/90 mm Hg, which might be considered normal in a nonpregnant woman, may indicate pre-eclampsia. A woman with signs and symptoms of pre-eclampsia should be positioned on her left side and transported to a hospital with obstetric capabilities.

Seizures in pregnancy should be assumed to be eclampsia until proven otherwise. Treatment in the field is the same as for any other seizure (see Chapter 20). Manage the patient's airway, provide oxygen, and transport her on her left side.

■ LABOR

Labor is defined as the onset of regular, coordinated **contractions** of the uterus, combined with opening **(dilation)** of the cervix, which ultimately lead to delivery of the infant and the placenta. The time course of labor varies greatly, ranging from a few hours to longer than a day. Labor tends to be longer with the first pregnancy and shorter with subsequent pregnancies.

Normally labor is divided into three stages: Fig. 30-4.

First Stage

The first stage begins with the onset of contractions and ends when the cervix is fully dilated. Contractions usually start out shorter in duration and farther apart. They become longer, more intense, and closer together as labor progresses. The contractions of true labor usually are painful. Measuring the **contraction time** (the length of each contraction) and the **contraction interval** (the time between contractions) can help you determine whether delivery is imminent. Contractions that last longer than 1 minute or that are closer than every 2 or 3 minutes may indicate that birth is very near.

SPECIAL Considerations

Treat it as the Real Thing
Braxton-Hicks contractions, also called *false labor*, are normal during the second half of pregnancy. They help prepare the uterus for the work of delivery. Typically these are mild, irregular contractions that are not associated with dilation of the cervix. However, in the field, Braxton-Hicks contractions cannot be distinguished from early labor. You should assume that any patient with contractions may be in labor and treat her accordingly.

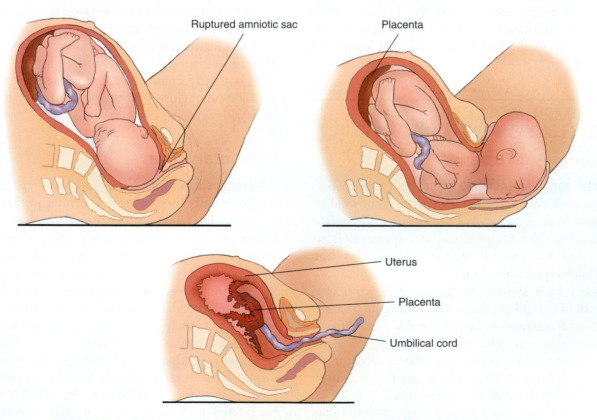

Fig. 30-4 As labor progresses, the amniotic sac ruptures and the baby begins to move along the canal to birth. As the head emerges, the baby will turn slightly, allowing the shoulder to emerge. Once the baby has been born, the placenta will separate from the uterine wall and be expelled.

Another clue to the first stage of labor may be the presence of **bloody show.** This is the passage of a small amount of mucus and blood from the vagina. It indicates that the protective mucous plug that normally seals the cervix has been released as a result of dilation of the cervix. Bloody show consists of only a small amount of blood. Any significant or persistent bleeding is abnormal and may indicate a serious complication (see Complications of Late Pregnancy earlier in this chapter).

Second Stage

The second stage of labor is defined as the interval from complete dilation of the cervix to delivery of the infant. During the second stage of labor, the EMT should use BSI, including gown and mask. During this stage, the infant moves out of the uterus and down into the birth canal. This causes a strong pressure sensation in the perineal area. The mother usually has an overwhelming urge to bear down or push. The contractions are very intense and very close together, sometimes with a contraction interval of less than 1 minute. As the baby moves down the birth canal, the presenting part becomes visible at the vaginal opening. The **presenting part,** or first part of the baby's body to come into view, is usually the head. When the head is visible at the vagi-nal opening, the infant is said to be **crowning.** The second stage ends after the baby is delivered.

Third Stage

The third stage of labor begins after the infant is delivered and ends with delivery of the placenta. This stage usually lasts only 10 to 15 minutes but can last as long as 30 to 45 minutes.

■ DELIVERY

Decision to Transport versus Delivery in the Field

Obviously, transporting the mother to the hospital before delivery is preferable if time allows. However, in some cases delivery may be likely to occur before you can safely transport the mother. When deciding whether to transport the patient immediately or deliver the infant in the prehospital setting, you should consider several factors. These include the estimated transport time to the closest hospital and whether the mother's condition is complicated by other immediate life threats, such as active vaginal bleeding, hypotension, seizures, or trauma. Box 30-1 presents some questions you can ask to help determine whether delivery is imminent.

BOX 30-1

Questions to Help Determine Whether Delivery Is Imminent

First, identify any urgent signs and symptoms:

- *Do you feel like you need to push or have a bowel movement?* (Women often feel the sensation of "needing to push" when the baby's head has moved into the birth canal. They may also describe this as an urge to have a bowel movement or as intense pressure in the vaginal area.)
- *Are you bleeding or having any vaginal discharge?* (Bloody show may indicate the start of labor. Significant bleeding in labor is *not* normal and should prompt immediate stabilization and transport.)
- *Has your water broken?* (The amniotic sac usually ruptures at some point during labor. If the sac has already ruptured, delivery may be imminent.)

Next, gather other important pieces of the patient's history:

- *Is this your first pregnancy?* (Labor and delivery usually occur more rapidly with each successive pregnancy. If the woman has had babies before, ask how long her previous labors lasted.)
- *How long have you been having contractions?* (Contractions become more forceful and last longer as labor progresses.)
- *How far apart are your contractions?* (As a woman gets closer to delivery, the contractions come closer together.)
- *What is your due date?* (Delivery more than 2 weeks before the due date is considered preterm or premature. This information is important for anticipating the needs of the infant after birth.)
- *Is there any chance you're having more than one baby?* (A woman who has had regular prenatal care probably will know this. If more than one infant is expected, you may need to call for additional resources.)

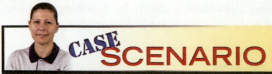

CASE SCENARIO *continued*

In Mary's bedroom, Elizabeth quickly lays absorbent sheets and towels on the bed and helps the patient lie down on her back. Mary keeps saying, "I have to go to the bathroom! It hurts so bad!" Lifting the T-shirt, Elizabeth checks the girl's vaginal area. Right at that moment, the top of a baby's head appears at the opening of the birth canal.

Questions: What should Elizabeth get out of the obstetrics kit now? What procedure should she perform next?

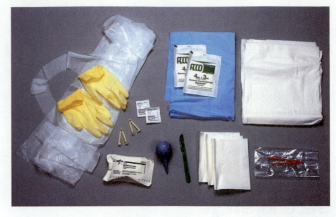

Fig. 30-5 Supplies in a typical delivery kit.

- 2 plastic umbilical cord clamps
- Gauze sponges
- 1 pair of scissors
- Container for the placenta

If delivery appears to be imminent, particularly if the mother says that she has an urge to bear down, you should strongly consider visually inspecting the mother's perineum. To do this, find or create a private area for the mother to remove her pants or undergarments. Have her lie on her back with her knees flexed and spread apart to allow inspection. If you see crowning or bulging, you should prepare for delivery.

Preparation for Delivery

Preparation for delivery involves preparing the mother, yourself, and your surroundings. Begin by finding a private, protected place for the delivery to occur, if possible. If you cannot move the mother to your ambulance and if no private area is available, consider creating some privacy by draping sheets and blankets to form visual barriers.

As always, use proper BSI techniques. These include wearing gloves, a mask, a gown, and eye protection. If you have a commercially prepared obstetrics kit, these items are probably included. If you do not have a kit, prepare the following supplies (Fig. 30-5):

- Gown, gloves, mask, and protective eyewear
- Clean towels and blankets
- 1 bulb syringe (bulb wrapped with gauze to prevent slipping)

Next, help the mother position herself for delivery (Fig. 30-6). Have her remove her underwear if she has not done so already.

To best assist the mother with the delivery, have her lie on her back with her knees flexed and her feet flat on the stretcher or some other surface. Place a clean sheet or towel under her buttocks to elevate her hips slightly. You can drape a sheet over her lower abdomen and upper legs for modesty's sake if time permits, but make sure it is not in your way for the actual delivery.

If the mother feels the urge to push, encourage her to keep her chin down and her knees flexed. She can push more effectively if her head and back are elevated to a partial sitting position. Encourage her to push for about 10 seconds, then rest and breathe for 10 seconds. Long, sustained pushing (for longer than 10 seconds) can rupture blood vessels and tear the perineum.

Delivery Procedure

Once the baby's head is crowning, use the following steps to help you deliver the infant (Skill 30-1):

1. Allow the head to emerge in a controlled, gradual manner. This allows the mother's perineum to stretch more and therefore tear less. To do this, put one hand on the baby's head and the other hand, covered by a towel or a

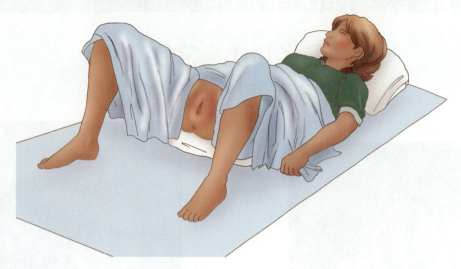

Fig. 30-6 The position for delivery.

piece of gauze, on the perineum. Exert very gentle pressure on the baby's head with your hands to avoid an explosive delivery. The head most often faces downward at this point.

2. Once the head has been delivered, suction the baby's mouth and nose with the bulb syringe. To do this, first squeeze all the air out of the syringe. Then, with the syringe still compressed, place the tip into the infant's mouth and release the compression to suction out any fluids. Move the syringe away from the baby's face and squeeze it several times to expel the contents. Repeat this procedure one or two times for the mouth and each nostril. If you do not have a bulb syringe, use a gauze pad to wipe any fluid off the mouth and nose area.

3. Check around the infant's neck to see whether it is encircled by a loop of umbilical cord. If the cord is there, gently hook your finger under the loop and pull it over the baby's head. You may have to repeat this procedure if more than one loop is present. If the loop of umbilical cord is too tight to be pulled over the baby's head, quickly clamp and cut the cord before delivering the rest of the baby.

4. During the previous steps the baby's head probably will have started to turn toward one side or the other. Gently direct the head downward to allow the anterior shoulder to slip out from under the pubic bone. Once the anterior shoulder has been delivered, the rest of the baby's body usually is born quickly (Box 30-2).

5. Keep the infant at about the level of the vagina while you use a gauze pad to wipe off any remaining secretions around the mouth and nose.

6. Dry the infant to reduce loss of body heat and to stimulate the baby to breathe. The easiest way to do this is simply to place the infant on the mother's abdomen and rub the baby dry with a towel. If necessary, you can also stimulate the baby by flicking the soles of the feet.

7. Cut the umbilical cord. Place the first of two cord clamps on the umbilical cord 3 or 4 inches from the baby's abdomen. Place the second clamp 4 or 5 inches from the first clamp, toward the mother. Cut *between* the two clamps.

8. Wrap the infant in clean towels or blankets. This step is important for preventing hypothermia (see Box 30-2).

9. Note the time of delivery.

10. If you expect multiple births, prepare for the next delivery.

11. Watch for the placenta to be delivered. This can take 30 to 45 minutes. *Do not pull on the umbilical cord to help deliver the placenta.* Also, transport the mother and infant as soon as possible; do not wait in the field for delivery of the placenta.

12. If the placenta is delivered, place it in a clean container and transport it to the hospital with the mother and infant.

SKILL 30-1
Assisting a Normal Delivery

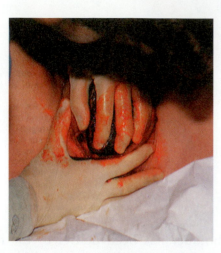

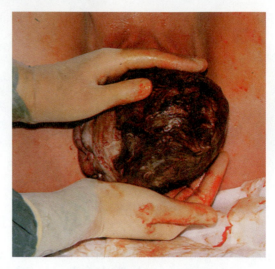

1. Apply gentle pressure to the infant's head during crowning to allow a gradual, controlled delivery.

4. Support the infant's head as it rotates.

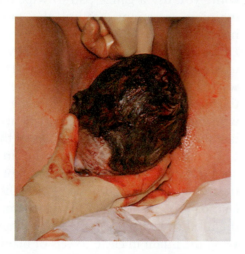

2. Suction the baby's mouth and nose with a bulb syringe.

3. Use your index finger to feel for and remove a loop of umbilical cord if it is around the infant's neck.

SKILL 30-1
Assisting a Normal Delivery—cont'd

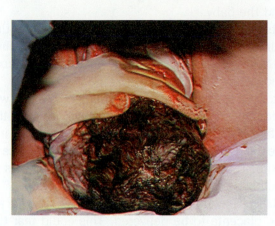

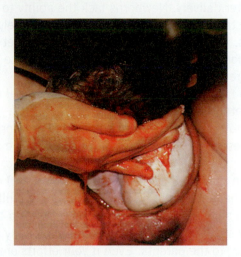

5. Gently guide the infant's head downward to deliver the anterior shoulder.

6. Guide the infant's head upward to deliver the posterior shoulder and the rest of the body.

BOX 30-2

Do's and Don'ts of Delivery

Do's

Do: Dry, cover, and warm the baby as soon as possible after delivery. Newborns lack the ability to regulate their body temperature as effectively as adults. In addition, the newborn emerges wet into a cooler environment than the womb. These factors predispose newborns to hypothermia.

Do: With multiple births, clamp each umbilical cord separately. Also, more than one placenta may need to be delivered after the babies are born. If so, preserve and transport all of them to the hospital.

Do: Begin cardiopulmonary resuscitation (CPR) on a baby that appears to be very premature or stillborn unless signs of death are obvious. Loss of a baby at any stage of pregnancy can be emotionally devastating to the parents. Even if your efforts are unsuccessful, they may be one of the kindest things you can do for the survivors.

Don'ts

Don't: Put the mother's legs together in an effort to delay the birth. This will not stop the delivery and is in fact extremely dangerous to both the mother and the baby.

Don't: Pull hard on the infant's head or extremities during the delivery process. You can break bones or cause permanent damage to the spinal cord and nerves.

Don't: Drop the baby! Remember, the baby will be wet and slippery. One effective maneuver is to let the infant be delivered into your hands and then immediately tuck the baby under your arm (like a football) as you wipe off the face and body. As in football, a fumble is considered poor form.

Don't: Pull on the umbilical cord while waiting for the placenta to be delivered. This could tear the cord. If the placenta has not been delivered by the time you arrive at the hospital, simply note this in your report to the hospital care providers.

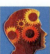 **ASK** YOURSELF

You are called to the ninth floor corner office of a 33-year-old advertising executive. She tells you that she is 39 weeks pregnant with her third child and has had worsening contractions all day, but she wanted to finish a project and thought she could wait till after work to call her obstetrician. She is starting to feel the urge to push, and her secretary called emergency medical services because the patient does not think she can walk downstairs to the parking lot.

1. What questions can you ask to determine whether she is close to delivering?
2. What physical assessment might be helpful?
3. If you determine that she is about to deliver, what are some specific issues to address, given the location of the patient?

■ COMPLICATIONS OF DELIVERY

Vaginal Bleeding

Bleeding during and after delivery is a normal part of childbirth. Remember that the mother's blood volume is increased during pregnancy, and this allows her body to compensate for the expected blood loss. Up to 500 ml of blood loss is considered normal, but more than 500 ml is considered excessive. Do not be alarmed by the normal bleeding that occurs, but watch for signs of excessive bleeding. If bleeding is brisk and does not slow within several minutes of delivery, take appropriate steps. Excessive vaginal bleeding is the most common complication of labor and delivery.[7]

To help slow vaginal bleeding and to reduce the risk of excessive bleeding, you can massage the abdomen over the uterus (see Postdelivery Care of the Mother later in this chapter). You can also encourage the mother to breast-feed, if she is able. Watch for signs and symptoms of shock. Provide oxygen, keep the mother warm, and transport as soon as possible.

Meconium

Meconium is a dark green substance that represents a newborn's first bowel movement. Normally a newborn does not produce stool until after delivery. However, occasionally an infant passes meconium while still in the uterus. This is important to recognize for two reasons. First, meconium passage in utero means that the baby may already be in some distress as a result of lack of oxygen, infection, or some other cause. Second, the infant may aspirate meconium into the lungs when taking the first breath. Meconium aspiration syndrome can result in pneumonia and lung damage.

If the infant has passed meconium in the uterus, you or the mother may note a greenish tint to the amniotic fluid. You may also see a thick, dark greenish substance coming from the vagina or covering the baby as the head emerges.

Routine intrapartum suctioning of infants born to mothers with meconium-stained amniotic fluid is not necessary if the infant is active and vigorous. Monitor the baby closely after delivery for breathing difficulties and provide oxygen. Be sure to inform hospital personnel of your suspicions on arrival at the hospital.

Preterm Delivery

Preterm (premature) delivery is defined as any delivery before the thirty-seventh week of pregnancy. Only about 10% of babies are born preterm, but 80% of newborn deaths are related to prematurity.[8] It is important to ask the mother how far along she is in her pregnancy and whether she has noticed fluid leakage that might indicate her amniotic sac has broken.

If you must deliver a preterm infant in the field, expect that the baby may need more aggressive resuscitation. You more likely will need to provide ventilatory assistance with a bag-mask device, and you must take particular care to keep the infant warm.

The age at which a fetus generally is considered old enough to survive is about 24 weeks. However, unless the baby is showing clear and obvious signs of death, you should begin resuscitative measures even if you think the infant is unlikely to survive. A mother may be unsure or incorrect as to how far along she is. Also, by making every attempt to save the baby, you may help the family to cope with the loss later.

Breech Delivery

A **breech presentation** means that either the baby's buttocks or the lower extremities are the first part of the body to enter the birth canal. This occurs in about 4% of deliveries[7] and is the most common abnormal presentation. Often the baby is delivered uneventfully, although the process may be slower because the head, which is the largest part, is the last to be delivered. As the infant's body is delivered, support the legs and pelvis with your gloved hands. Do not grasp the infant around the abdomen, because this can lead to damage of the internal organs. Instead, grasp the infant over the bony part of the pelvis to help guide the body out. Do not pull on the body. If the head is not delivered shortly, you can assist the delivery as follows:

1. Support the baby's body on your forearm.
2. Place the mother in a knee-chest position (Fig. 30-7). This position creates the widest possible diameter of the mother's pelvis and allows more room for the baby's head to pass.
3. Use your fingers to create an airway for the baby (Fig. 30-8). Do this by placing two fingers inside the vagina, one on either side of the baby's nose. Bend your fingers slightly to push the birth canal away from the baby's face and create a breathing space.

ASK YOURSELF

You are called to a downtown apartment for a report of a pregnant female with vaginal bleeding and abdominal pain. You arrive to find an 18-year-old woman and her boyfriend. She says that she is pregnant and has been bleeding for an hour. She is not sure how far along she is but thinks she is at least 7 months into the pregnancy. The apartment is a shambles, and drug paraphernalia is strewn on the kitchen table. She admits to smoking crack cocaine today with her boyfriend and says that the abdominal pain began shortly after she started smoking.

1. What questions can you ask to determine whether she is close to delivering?
2. What physical assessment might be helpful?
3. What unique challenges does this case pose?
4. What life-threatening conditions must you consider in your list of possible diagnoses?

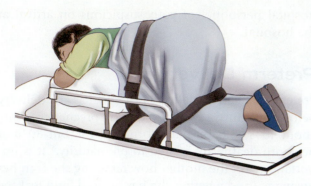

Fig. 30-7 The knee-chest position, which is used for shoulder dystocia, breech delivery, prolapsed umbilical cord, and limb presentation.

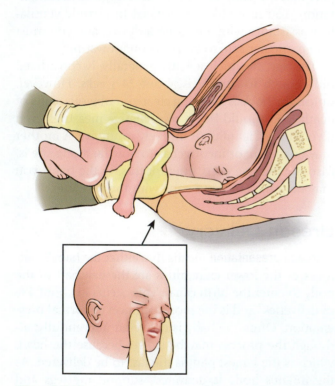

Fig. 30-8 Creating an airway for the infant during a breech birth.

4. With the next contraction, lift the baby's body upward slightly to create a better angle for delivery of the head.
5. Provide blow-by oxygen to the area near the baby's nose to increase the oxygen concentration. You may also provide oxygen to the mother if you have not already done so.

Shoulder Dystocia

Shoulder dystocia occurs when the head has been delivered but the shoulder is trapped under the mother's pelvic bone and the infant's body does not easily slide out. This is the second most common abnormal presentation and is more likely with a very large infant or a mother whose pelvis is very small.

If the baby's body does not slide out easily with very limited traction on the head, *do not* pull hard to deliver the shoulder. This not only worsens the shoulder impaction, it may also cause serious, permanent nerve damage in the baby. Instead, place the mother in the knee-chest position (see Fig. 30-6) as discussed previously for breech presentation. You can also press downward with your fingers on the baby's shoulder through the mother's abdominal wall just above the pubic bone. Together these maneuvers often dislodge the wedged shoulder and allow the baby to be delivered.

If these maneuvers are unsuccessful, it is important to stay calm and keep the mother calm. Transport her immediately and call ahead to let hospital personnel know of your arrival.

Prolapsed Umbilical Cord

With **umbilical cord prolapse,** the umbilical cord is in front of the presenting part and becomes compressed, cutting off the blood supply and oxygen to the baby (Fig. 30-9). This is more likely to happen when the presenting part is something other than the head (e.g., breech or shoulder presentations). This is a rare but potentially catastrophic event in which the baby will die quickly without intervention.

If the umbilical cord protrudes from the vagina before the baby has been delivered, immediately place the mother in the knee-chest position (see Fig.

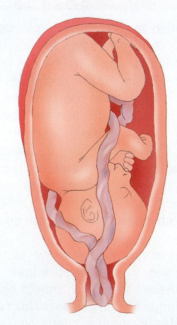

Fig. 30-9 A prolapsed umbilical cord.

30-7). If possible, place the bed in the Trendelenburg position. Both these maneuvers reduce pressure on the cord. Insert your gloved hand into the vagina and push upward on the presenting part to reduce pressure on the cord further. Keep upward pressure on the presenting part during transport. Cover the cord with wet dressings but do not manipulate it.

Umbilical cord prolapse often requires an emergency cesarean section to save the infant's life. The infant's survival is directly related to the time from prolapse to surgical intervention.[7] Your top priority is to transport the mother immediately. Notify hospital personnel of the prolapsed cord during transport so that they can prepare for immediate surgery.

Limb Presentation

An arm or a leg is rarely the presenting part. However, when this happens, specialized intervention usually is required for delivery, and the baby is unlikely to be born outside the hospital. If this occurs, do not pull on the extremity to try to help deliver the infant. Place the mother in the knee-chest position (see Fig. 30-6), give her oxygen, and prepare to transport. Stay calm and try to keep the mother calm.

Multiple Births

Most mothers expecting more than one baby know this before delivery and tell you during your evaluation. However, if the mother has not had prenatal care, she may not realize she is carrying multiple fetuses. If a woman still has a markedly enlarged abdomen after delivery and has had no prenatal care, consider the possibility of multiple births. You can try to auscultate for fetal heart sounds over the abdomen with a stethoscope.

The procedures for delivering multiple babies are the same as those for a single baby. It is important to keep in mind that infants of multiple births are more likely to be born prematurely and often are smaller than a single full-term infant. This means that they are at greater risk for breathing difficulties and hypothermia. Be ready to resuscitate them and continue close observation and assessment during transport.

Fetal Death

Loss of a child is probably one of the worst traumas human beings can experience. Although indications of something wrong may have been noted ahead of time, it may also be an unexpected tragedy, especially in trauma cases.

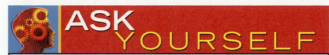

Unless signs of death are obvious, err on the side of performing cardiopulmonary resuscitation (CPR) and attempting resuscitation. Family members may find it easier to cope with the loss if they feel that everything possible was done. Be ready to offer emotional support to the parents and be prepared for a range of responses from the family.

■ POSTDELIVERY CARE OF THE MOTHER

It is normal for the mother to feel quite weak and tired after delivery. Occasionally women have involuntary trembling in the legs or the entire body after the infant is born. This resolves on its own in a few minutes. During this time it is important to continue regular monitoring of the blood pressure and heart rate. Keep the mother warm and watch for signs of shock.

As mentioned previously, the average amount of blood lost with a vaginal delivery is about 500 ml. Because of the increase in blood volume that occurs in pregnancy, most women can tolerate this blood loss without any symptoms. Monitor the amount of blood lost; if needed, provide clean pads or bedding. If blood loss continues or seems excessive, massage the uterus to promote uterine contraction and to reduce bleeding (Fig. 30-10). Place your fingers flat on the mother's abdomen, just above the pubic bone, and massage in a circular fashion. You probably will feel the enlarged uterus through the abdominal wall under your fingers. The mother will experience a cramping sensation; this is a sign of effective massage. If the mother and baby are able, you can also encourage the mother to breast-feed her newborn to

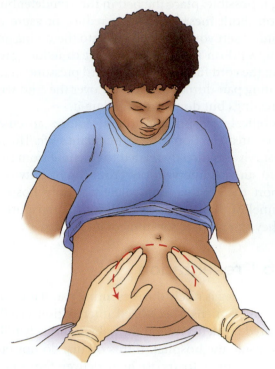

Fig. 30-10 Uterine massage can help control post-delivery bleeding.

promote uterine contraction and slow the bleeding. Breast-feeding stimulates the release of oxytocin, a hormone that causes the uterus to contract.

Remember that delivery of the placenta can take 30 to 45 minutes. Do not delay transport to await delivery of the placenta.

■ POSTDELIVERY CARE OF THE INFANT: ABCs

Newborn babies usually are bluish or purplish immediately after delivery. As they begin to breathe, they normally "pink up" within several minutes. If the mother is frightened by this, reassure her that the color change is normal.

The newborn should be assessed continually for the first few minutes after delivery. Most EMS systems use the appearance, pulse, grimace, activity, and respirations (APGAR) scoring system (Table 30-1) for initial assessments. APGAR scoring is done minimally at 1 minute and 5 minutes after delivery. The scores from the five assessment areas are totaled and reported to the receiving facility.

Your priorities in caring for a newborn are the same as for any other patient: the ABCs.

- *Airway.* You should have already cleared the baby's airway immediately after the head was delivered. Check again to make sure no more mucus or other material is blocking the airway. Repeat bulb suctioning, if necessary, and position

TABLE 30-1

APGAR Score

Assessment Factor	Score		
	0	1	2
Appearance (skin color)	Blue, pale	Body pink, extremities blue	Completely pink
Pulse rate	Absent	<100 beats per minute	>100 beats per minute
Grimace	No response	Grimace	Cough, sneeze, cry
Activity	Limp	Some flexion	Active motion
Respirations	Absent	Slow, irregular	Good, crying

the child on his or her side. During this time you should also dry the infant and cover the baby with a clean, dry blanket to prevent heat loss.

- *Breathing.* Usually clearing the airway and drying the baby will have stimulated the infant to begin breathing independently. If not, you can stimulate the baby further either by rubbing the back vigorously or by flicking the feet with your fingers. If the infant still is not breathing after these maneuvers, make sure that the airway is open with a chin lift or jaw thrust maneuver. Provide bag-mask breaths for about 30 seconds at a rate of 40 to 60 breaths per minute and re-evaluate.

Once the infant is breathing, check to make sure the respiratory rate is at least 30 breaths per minute (the normal rate for a newborn is about 40 breaths per minute). If the baby is not taking at least 30 breaths per minute or is having trouble breathing, assist with bag-mask ventilation.

- *Circulation.* Check for a pulse in either the umbilical cord or the brachial artery. If there is no pulse or if the pulse rate is lower than 60 beats per minute, begin chest compressions at a rate of 120 compressions per minute, with bag ventilations at a rate of at least 30 per minute at a 3:1 ratio (compressions to ventilations). These actions are summarized in Fig. 30-11.[9]

The frequency of need for resuscitative measures for newborns is represented by the inverted pyramid of neonatal resuscitation (Fig. 30-12).

INITIAL STEPS OF RESUSCITATION OF THE NEWLY BORN

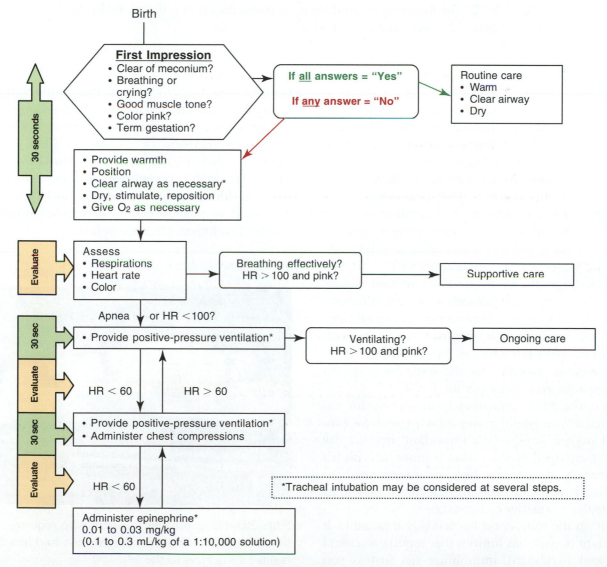

Fig. 30-11 Initial steps of resuscitation of the newly born.

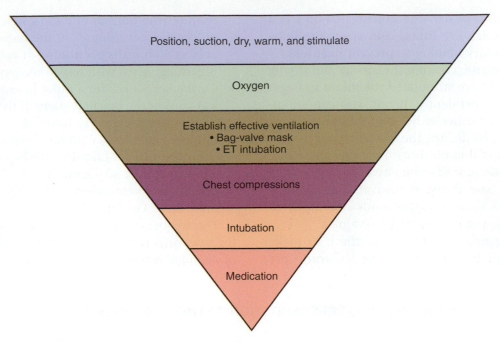

Fig. 30-12 The frequency of need for resuscitative measures is illustrated by the inverted pyramid of neonatal resuscitation.

■ TRAUMA IN PREGNANCY

Trauma is the leading cause of death among pregnant women in the United States.[10] Motor vehicle accidents account for most injuries and injury-related deaths in pregnant women (see Motor Vehicle Accidents later in this chapter). In motor vehicle accidents, the most common cause of death of the fetus is death of the mother. Domestic violence should also be considered as a possible cause of injury (see Domestic Violence later in this chapter).

Trauma in pregnancy means that you have two patients—the mother and her unborn infant. Although it is important to remember this axiom, it is also important to remember that, in general, the best treatment for the baby is to take care of the mother. Therefore treatment priorities are the same for pregnant and nonpregnant trauma victims.[11]

Assess the ABCs immediately in a pregnant patient, just as you would in any other patient. Supplemental oxygen is especially important, because the mother's enlarged uterus makes it more difficult for her to breathe deeply. She therefore is more prone to becoming hypoxic. In addition, the developing fetus is particularly sensitive to hypoxia.

Position the mother on her left side if possible. If a pregnant patient has injuries that require a cervical collar and backboard, immobilize her just as you would a nonpregnant patient. Remember that placing a pregnant woman flat on her back reduces blood flow to the uterus and blood return to the mother (supine hypotension of pregnancy). This problem can be avoided by tilting the backboard 15 degrees to the left. To do this, place linens or other items under the right side of the backboard (Fig. 30-12). You may also need to place a pillow or blanket under the mother's abdomen for her comfort.

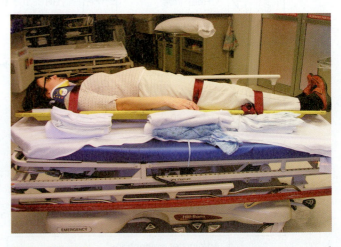

Fig. 30-13 A pregnant woman who requires spinal immobilization should be placed on a backboard that is tilted 15 degrees to the left.

Even relatively minor trauma to the abdomen can cause injury to the placenta and uterus. Placental abruption can be life-threatening for the mother and baby (see Complications of Late Pregnancy earlier in this chapter). Any pregnant patient with possible abdominal or chest trauma, no matter how trivial, should be transported to the hospital for further evaluation.

■ GYNECOLOGIC EMERGENCIES

Vaginal Bleeding

Although vaginal bleeding is a normal part of the monthly menstrual cycle, at times it may be very heavy or irregular. It may also be accompanied by severe cramping pain. Vaginal bleeding in a nonpregnant patient usually is not life-threatening. However, a woman may not yet realize she is pregnant if the bleeding occurs very early in the pregnancy. An ectopic pregnancy is a life-threatening cause of vaginal bleeding in early pregnancy (see Complications of Early Pregnancy earlier in this chapter). Therefore, assume that any woman with vaginal bleeding has a potentially life-threatening condition until proved otherwise.

Treat this patient as you would any other patient with the potential for hemorrhagic shock (see Chapter 25). Keep the patient warm, administer oxygen, watch vital signs carefully, and give the patient high priority for transport and treatment.

Sexual Assault

A sexual assault can be a terrifying and traumatic experience. A person who has been sexually assaulted may respond in a variety of ways. Some patients may be agitated or hysterical; others may react with fear and withdrawal. Obtaining a detailed history may not be possible or desirable with a patient who has been sexually assaulted. Be prepared to respond with compassion and patience.

A person who is sexually assaulted may have physical injuries other than those of the genital tract. Head injuries, abdominal trauma, strangulation injuries, chest trauma, and extremity lacerations or fractures are all reported in the context of sexual assault. Assess and manage this patient as you would any other trauma patient.

Remember that the scene of an alleged assault is a crime scene, and law enforcement officials may want to gather evidence. It is important to work with law enforcement to preserve the scene whenever possible. However, your primary responsibility is to attend to the physical and emotional needs of your patient.

Motor Vehicle Crashes

As mentioned before, motor vehicle crashes account for most of the injuries and injury-related deaths in pregnant women in the United States. As many as one third to one half of all pregnant women do not use seat belts or do not use them properly.[12] Yet the evidence is clear: maternal injuries from car accidents can be effectively reduced or prevented by three-point restraints.[13] There is no evidence that properly worn restraints increase the chance of fetal injury. A properly positioned lap belt fits snugly and comfortably under the abdomen and across the thighs. The shoulder belt is positioned between the breasts (Fig. 30-14).

Women who receive information from a health care professional on seat belt use during pregnancy are more likely to use seat belts and use them properly.[12] As a health care professional, you should emphasize the use of three-point restraints for all passengers, including pregnant women.

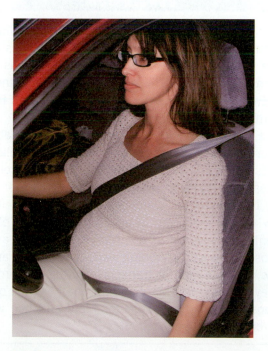

Fig. 30-14 Proper positioning of the seat belt during pregnancy. The lap belt goes over the pelvis and under the abdomen. The shoulder harness is positioned between the breasts.

Domestic Violence

Pregnant women appear to be at increased risk for domestic violence.[14] The abuser often is the father of the child.[15] The most common injury from domestic violence in a pregnant woman is blunt trauma to the abdomen.[16] Other common sites of injury are the face, head, and breasts. A pregnant woman who has been abused usually does not tell health care providers what really happened, at least not initially.[17] You should suspect domestic violence when the patient's injuries do not match the mechanism or the story is confusing or changes over time. As the first member of the health care team to contact the patient outside the hospital or at her home, you may be able to gather valuable information not available to hospital personnel. If you arrive at an uncontrolled scene where you suspect domestic violence has occurred, try to avoid confronting those involved. Your top priority is safety, yours and your patient's.

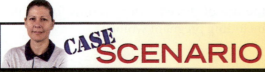

CASE SCENARIO
conclusion

The baby, a boy, is crying now, his lungs filling with air for the first time. Elizabeth watches as the baby's skin, initially blue, rapidly begins to turn pink, first in the nose and face and then outward from the center of the chest toward the extremities.

Elizabeth quickly finishes drying the baby. She then wraps him up in several cotton blankets and puts a cap on his head. She encourages Mary to take her new son to her breast to try to breast-feed, which would help with delivery of the placenta. Shortly afterward the placenta is delivered intact. Mary's vital signs and those of her son are doing well, so Elizabeth and the crew prepare for transport. During this time, they discuss with Mary and her mother what options might be available for Mary and her son through social services. ■

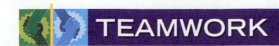

TEAMWORK

Although childbirth is a natural process, birth out of the hospital may signal problems for the mother, the baby, or both. Complications with the pregnancy can result in premature birth. Premature deliveries might result in newborns in need of tracheal suctioning and ventilatory support. It is possible that the mother may be in distress as well. Consider ALS assistance when available for out-of-the-hospital situations.

References

1. Brunette DD, Sterner SP: Prehospital and emergency department delivery: a review of eight years experience, *Ann Emerg Med* 18(10):1116-1118, 1989.
2. Morrison LJ: General approach to the pregnant patient. In Marx JM, editor: *Rosen's emergency medicine: concepts and clinical practice*, ed 5, St Louis, 2002, Mosby.
3. Cunningham FG: *Williams' obstetrics*, ed 19, Norwalk, CT, 1993, Appleton & Lange.
4. Simpson JL: Fetal wastage. In Gabbe SG, Niebyl JR, Simpson JL, editors: *Obstetrics: normal and problem pregnancies*, ed 4, New York, 2002, Churchill Livingstone.
5. Houry D, Abbott JT: Acute complications of pregnancy. In Marx JM, editor: *Rosen's emergency medicine: concepts and clinical practice*, ed 5, St Louis, 2002, Mosby.
6. Wagner LK: Diagnosis and management of preeclampsia, *Am Fam Physician* 70(12):2317-2324, 2004.
7. Mallon WK, Henderson S: Labor and delivery. In Marx JM, editor: *Rosen's emergency medicine: concepts and clinical practice*, ed 5, St Louis, 2002, Mosby.
8. Gianopoulos JG: Emergency complications of labor and delivery, *Emerg Med Clin North Am* 12(1):201-217, 1994.
9. Hazinski MF, Zaritsky AL, Nadkarni VM et al: *PALS provider manual*, Dallas, 2002, American Heart Association.
10. Fildes J, Reed L, Jones N et al: The leading cause of maternal death, *J Trauma* 32:643-645, 1992.

11. Van Hook JW: Trauma in pregnancy, *Clin Obstet Gynecol* 45(2):414-424, 2002.

12. Pearlman MD, Phillips ME: Safety belt use during pregnancy, *Obstet Gynecol* 88:1026-1029, 1996.

13. American College of Obstetricians and Gynecologists: Trauma during pregnancy, *ACOG Technical Bulletin* 161, 1991.

14. Shah KH, Simons RK, Holbrook T et al: Trauma in pregnancy: maternal and fetal outcomes, *J Trauma* 45:83-86, 1998.

15. Poole GV, Martin JN Jr, Perry KG Jr et al: Trauma in pregnancy: the role of interpersonal violence, *Am J Obstet Gynecol* 174(6):1873-1877, 1996.

16. Webster J, Sweett S, Stolz TA: Domestic violence in pregnancy: a prevalence study, *Med J Aust* 161(8):466-470, 1994.

17. Stewart DE, Cecitto A: Physical abuse in pregnancy, *Can Med Assoc J* 149:1257-1263, 1993.

Resources

Abbott J: Obstetric and gynecologic emergencies. In Pons PT, Markovchick VJ, editors: *Prehospital emergency care secrets*, Philadelphia, 1998, Hanley & Belfus.

Abbott J, Gifford MJ: *Prehospital emergency care: a guide for paramedics*, ed 3, New York, 1996, Parthenon.

Doan-Wiggins L: Emergency childbirth. In Roberts JR, Hedges JR, editors: *Clinical procedures in emergency medicine*, ed 4, Philadelphia, 2004, Elsevier.

Pons PT: Prehospital considerations in the pregnant patient, *Emerg Med Clin North Am* 12(1):1-7, 1994.

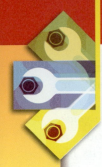

NUTS AND BOLTS

Critical Points

Remember that childbirth is a normal event in the human life cycle and usually progresses without difficulty, no matter where it happens. However, when complications occur, they often happen rapidly and can result in disastrous outcomes for the mother and baby. In this country, most deliveries occur in hospitals or birthing centers with medical professionals in attendance. If you are called to help with a delivery, reassure the mother, prepare for delivery, assist with the birth, and then monitor the mother and baby closely after delivery. The ABCs apply in these cases as they do with any other patient. Also remember that the most common cause of death in pregnant women is not pregnancy, but trauma. In cases involving trauma, the best treatment for the fetus is effective treatment of the mother.

Learning Checklist

❏ The female reproductive structures include the uterus, ovaries, fallopian tubes, and vagina.

❏ When an egg is fertilized, it travels down the fallopian tube and implants in the lining of the uterus. The egg develops into an embryo, which is attached via the umbilical cord to the placenta. The placenta is the organ that serves to exchange nutrition and toxins for the embryo. After 8 weeks of age, the embryo becomes a fetus.

❏ The enlarging uterus causes physiologic changes unique to pregnancy. The heart rate and respiratory rate increase slightly, and blood pressure decreases slightly. Blood volume increases significantly. The enlarging uterus can compress the major blood vessels in the abdomen and cause supine hypotension syndrome. To avoid this, transport a woman on her left side during the second half of pregnancy whenever possible.

❏ Vaginal bleeding and abdominal pain in pregnancy may be signs of a miscarriage or an ectopic pregnancy. Both conditions may cause life-threatening bleeding. Monitor these patients closely for shock and transport as soon as possible.

❏ Labor is divided into three stages. The first stage begins with the onset of contractions and ends when the cervix is fully dilated. The second stage is the time from complete dilation of the cervix until the delivery of the infant. The third stage begins after the infant is delivered and ends with delivery of the placenta.

❏ Some indicators that delivery may be imminent include the mother's sensation of needing to push, rupture of the amniotic sac, and contractions that last longer than 1 minute and are closer than 2 or 3 minutes apart. If you suspect delivery is imminent, you should examine the mother for crowning or perineal bulging.

❏ If you must deliver the infant in the prehospital setting, try to find a private and protected place. Remember to use proper BSI techniques, including wearing a gown, gloves, mask, and protective eyewear.

❏ Supplies for delivery include clean linens, a bulb syringe, umbilical cord clamps, gauze sponges, scissors, and a container for the placenta.

❏ Position the mother on her back with her knees bent and her feet flat. You can elevate her hips by placing a sheet or towel under her buttocks. Place pillows behind her to support her back so that she can push more effectively.

❏ Allow the head to emerge in a gradual, controlled manner. Check for an umbilical cord wrapped around the baby's neck and, if present, pull the cord over the baby's head. Immediately suction the infant's nose and mouth before the body emerges. If meconium is present, suction the mouth and nose thoroughly, provide oxygen, and watch for breathing difficulties.

❏ After the body is delivered, dry the baby, clamp the umbilical cord, and then cut the cord. Assess the baby's airway, breathing, and circulation. Stimulate the infant to breathe, if necessary, and provide oxygen as needed.

❏ If the placenta is delivered, place it in a clean container and transport it to the hospital with the mother and infant.

- Continue to reassess the ABCs in both mother and baby and provide support as needed.
- Placental abruption and placenta previa are complications of late pregnancy that may cause vaginal bleeding. Significant vaginal bleeding is *not* normal before delivery and should prompt careful monitoring for shock and rapid transport.
- Pre-eclampsia is a disorder of the second half of pregnancy that may include such signs as hypertension, severe swelling of the extremities, and vomiting, as well as symptoms such as abdominal pain and headaches. The most serious complication of pre-eclampsia is seizures. Any seizure in pregnancy should be assumed to be due to eclampsia and treated with careful airway management, supplemental oxygen, and prompt transport.
- Blood loss after delivery of up to 500 ml is normal and should be expected. If the mother continues to have brisk bleeding, massage the uterus through the abdominal wall to slow the bleeding.
- Preterm delivery is defined as any delivery before the thirty-seventh week of pregnancy. Preterm infants may need more aggressive resuscitation than term infants and are more prone to hypoxia, respiratory distress, and hypothermia. Keep the infant warm and provide ventilatory assistance as needed.
- Abnormal presentations include breech presentation, shoulder dystocia, limb presentation, and umbilical cord prolapse. In all of these situations, placing the mother in a knee-chest position provides the widest possible diameter of the pelvis and may expedite delivery. In the case of cord prolapse, it helps reduce pressure on the cord.
- Trauma is the leading cause of death among pregnant women in the United States. The best care for the fetus is good care for the mother. Treat her as aggressively as you would any other trauma victim. Always position a pregnant woman in the left lateral recumbent position when possible. If she requires a backboard, it can be tilted to the left to provide the same effect.

Key Terms

Amniotic sac (bag of waters) The fluid-filled protective sac that surrounds the fetus inside the uterus.

Birth canal The part of the female reproductive tract through which the fetus is delivered; it includes the lower part of the uterus, the cervix, and the vagina.

Bloody show Blood and mucus discharged from the vagina, often an early sign of labor.

Breech presentation Presentation of the buttocks or feet of the fetus as the first part of the infant's body to enter the birth canal.

Cervix The lowest part of the uterus; it connects to the vagina as part of the birth canal. The cervix must shorten and dilate during labor for the fetus to pass into the vagina.

Contractions Episodes of tightening of the muscular uterine wall that occur rhythmically during normal labor. This leads to expulsion of the fetus and placenta from the uterus.

Contraction interval The time from the beginning of one contraction to the beginning of the next contraction.

Contraction time The time from the beginning to the end of a single uterine contraction.

Crowning The appearance of the head of the infant at the vaginal opening during delivery.

Dilation Spontaneous opening of the cervix that occurs as part of labor.

Ectopic pregnancy A pregnancy that implants outside the uterus, usually in the fallopian tube.

Embryo The developing egg from about 2 weeks after fertilization until about 8 weeks of pregnancy.

Fallopian tube One of the paired structures that extend from each side of the uterus to each ovary. The tubes provide a way for the egg to reach the uterus.

Fetus The term used for an infant from about 8 weeks of pregnancy until birth.

Labor The process by which the fetus and placenta are expelled from the uterus. It usually is divided into three stages, starting from the first contraction and ending with delivery of the placenta.

Meconium A dark green substance that represents the infant's first bowel movement.

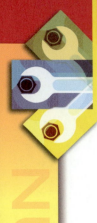

Miscarriage (spontaneous abortion) Loss of the products of conception before the fetus can survive on its own.

Ovaries The paired female reproductive organs found on each side of the lower abdomen.

Perineum The tissue between the mother's vaginal and rectal openings. This tissue may be torn during delivery.

Placenta (afterbirth) The organ inside the uterus that serves the function of exchanging nutrition and waste between the mother and the fetus.

Placental abruption (abruptio placentae) Separation of part of the placenta from the wall of the uterus.

Placenta previa Placement of the placenta such that it partly or completely covers the cervix.

Pre-eclampsia A complication of pregnancy that involves hypertension, swelling of the extremities and, in its severest form, seizures.

Presenting part The first part of the infant to appear at the vaginal opening; this is usually the head.

Preterm (premature) delivery Delivery before the thirty-seventh week of pregnancy.

Shoulder dystocia Impaction of the baby's anterior shoulder underneath the mother's pubic bone such that delivery is slowed or prevented.

Supine hypotensive syndrome A physiologic phenomenon in which the enlarged uterus compresses the inferior vena cava in the abdomen and impedes the return of blood to the heart. This can happen during the second half of pregnancy when a woman lies supine.

Umbilical cord The cord containing blood vessels that connects the fetus to the placenta.

Umbilical cord prolapse Appearance of the umbilical cord in front of the presenting part, usually with compression of the cord and interruption of the blood supply to the baby.

Uterus (womb) The muscular organ in which the fetus develops.

Vagina The lower part of the birth canal, extending from the uterus to the outside of the body.

National Standard Curriculum Objectives

Cognitive Objectives

After completing this lesson, the EMT student will be able to do the following:

- Identify the following structures: uterus, vagina, fetus, placenta, umbilical cord, amniotic sac, and perineum.
- Describe the contents and use of an obstetrics kit.
- Identify predelivery emergencies.
- State the indications of an imminent delivery.
- Describe the differences in emergency medical care between that provided to a patient with a predelivery emergency and that provided to a patient having a normal delivery.
- State the steps in the predelivery preparation of the mother.
- Describe the relationship between body substance isolation and childbirth.
- State the steps for assisting in delivery, including care of the baby as the head appears, delivery of the body, how and when to cut the umbilical cord, and delivery of the placenta.
- List the steps in the emergency medical care of the mother after delivery.
- Summarize neonatal resuscitation procedures.
- Describe the procedures for abnormal deliveries, specifically vaginal bleeding before birth, breech birth, prolapsed cord, and limb presentation.
- Describe the special considerations for multiple births, meconium, and the premature baby.
- Discuss the emergency medical care of a patient with a gynecologic emergency.

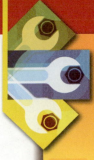

Affective Objective

After completing this lesson, the EMT student will be able to do the following:

- Explain the implications of treating two patients (mother and baby).

Psychomotor Objectives

After completing this lesson, the EMT student will be able to do the following:

- Demonstrate the steps in assisting a normal delivery.
- Demonstrate the necessary care of the fetus as the head appears.
- Demonstrate the postdelivery care of the infant

- Demonstrate how and when to cut the umbilical cord.
- Demonstrate the steps in the delivery of the placenta.
- Demonstrate the postdelivery care of the mother.
- Demonstrate the procedures for abnormal deliveries, specifically vaginal bleeding before birth, breech birth, prolapsed cord, and limb presentation.
- Demonstrate the steps in the emergency care of a mother who has excessive postdelivery bleeding.
- Demonstrate the completion of a prehospital care report for patients with obstetric or gynecologic emergencies.

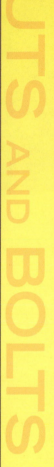

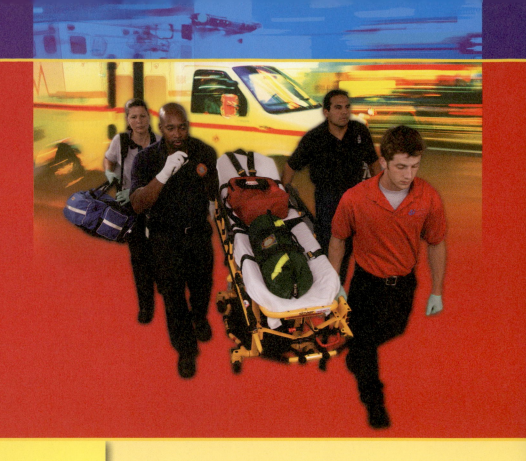

CHAPTER
31

LESSON GOAL

GOAL

The urgent treatment of infants and children presents unique challenges for the emergency medical technician (EMT). The saying "children are just small adults" couldn't be more incorrect, especially with regard to medical emergencies. Pediatric patients are different from adults, both anatomically and psychologically. Therefore they must be approached differently by emergency medical services (EMS) providers. These differences also make pediatric patients more prone to certain medical problems. The goal of this chapter is to familiarize EMTs with the special characteristics of infants and children so that they may become both comfortable and efficient in treating pediatric emergencies. ■

Pediatric Emergencies

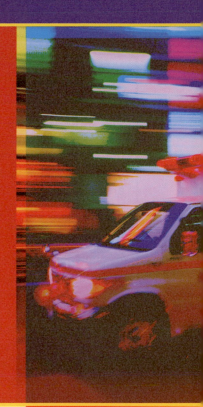

CHAPTER OBJECTIVES

After completing this chapter, the EMT student will be able to do the following:

1 Identify the physical and developmental differences between infants and children.

2 Recognize the unique anatomic characteristics of the pediatric airway and how pediatric airway management differs from adult airway management.

3 Identify and treat respiratory distress in pediatric patients.

4 Identify and treat respiratory failure in pediatric patients.

5 Identify and treat pediatric upper airway obstruction.

6 Identify and treat the pediatric patient in shock.

7 Identify and treat pediatric seizures.

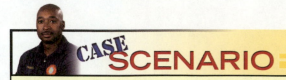

CASE SCENARIO

The winter evening is proving to be a cold one. It isn't anything unexpected; after all, it's 2 weeks before Christmas. Up to now, though, the days had been unseasonably warm. Strings of colored lights and other holiday scenes compete with the flashing lights of the ambulance as it rolls into the neighborhood. The call was for a "baby having trouble breathing," and Jack's mind is running through the materials his instructor had just covered only a week ago. Elizabeth calls into the back of the rig, "Hey, Jack, could you grab the pedi-kit when we get to the house?"

"I've got it," Jack responds as he looks at the red bag perched on the side shelf. He knows that the bag holds the pediatric bag-mask device, nasal cannula, and simple face masks, several small blood pressure (BP) cuffs, and a teddy bear with an unobtrusive oxygen outlet.

The unit makes one more left and comes to a gradual stop in front of the ranch-style home. Even though it is nearly midnight, most of the lights in the home are on, including the front porch light. Framed in the doorway is a woman who seems to be clutching a small bundle tightly against her chest. She begins walking quickly to the ambulance as Jack opens the side door to the passenger compartment. Getting out of the ambulance, Elizabeth quickly helps the woman into the vehicle, where she sits on the bench seat. Jack can see that the bundle is actually the patient, a baby who looks to be about 8 months old.

Working with pediatric patients can be especially challenging. Therefore EMTs should have a basic understanding of the developmental stages from infancy to adolescence. This knowledge can help ensure effective communication and appropriate treatment of pediatric patients. With this in mind, the chapter begins with a quick review of the basic developmental milestones of childhood and how these pertain to the EMS evaluation. A discussion of the basic principles for recognizing, approaching, and managing pediatric emergencies follows. Such emergencies include respiratory distress, upper airway obstruction, shock, and seizures. Emphasis is placed on how these emergencies may manifest differently with infants and children. Considerations in pediatric trauma also are covered, as are the difficulties EMTs encounter in caring for victims of child abuse.

■ DEVELOPMENTAL CONSIDERATIONS

The following sections provide a quick review of the basic developmental milestones of childhood and how these pertain to the EMS evaluation.

Infants

Infants (babies under 1 year of age) react to varying stimuli. Crying can be a response to many things, including cold, pain, hunger, discomfort, or a need for sleep. Infants easily lose heat. Therefore the EMT should make every effort to keep them warm and covered. In addition, EMTs should warm their hands and stethoscopes before examining the patient. When infants are difficult to console, a pacifier may help to soothe them. Because infants commonly have stranger and separation anxiety, they usually are best evaluated in the lap of the primary caregiver. If possible, they can be kept in the arms of the caregiver during transport (check your state and local laws for transport requirements).

Motor skills progress from head to toe and from trunk to extremities. Even in the first month of life, an infant can make eye contact. This is a reassuring sign of wellness. Young infants usually are found with the extremities in the flexed position. With time, the arms become less flexed, followed by the legs. A 3-month-old may have good head control, and a 6-month-old may be able to sit without support and pick up small objects.

Toddlers and Preschool-Age Children

The toddler years (1 to 3 years) are a time of rapid change. Toddlers become more autonomous and independent as their motor and verbal skills develop. Most toddlers can walk by the age of 18 months. This skill, along with toddlers' intense curiosity about their surroundings, can place the child in dangerous situations. The toddler may also have separation anxiety and may not cooperate with an examination out of fear of being touched or hurt. Distracting the toddler with a gamelike style of interaction can facilitate the examination (Box 31-1). Start your exam with the feet or trunk and work up to the head. This helps build confidence and trust. Optimally, a heart and lung exam should be attempted before the child becomes agitated. The caregiver can get involved with the exam by asking the child pertinent questions and/or by removing the child's clothing.

Preschool-age children (3 to 6 years) understand speech and follow commands at a higher level. Therefore these children often are more willing to cooperate with an exam. However, it is important to explain what you will be doing in simple terms and to respect the child's modesty. At this age, children are becoming aware of their sexual identity. One helpful technique is to ask the patient's permission to do the assessment examination.

School-Age Children and Adolescents

School-age children (6 to 12 years) have a better understanding of their bodies. They may have a fear of permanent injury, or they may be afraid of pain or blood. Any painful procedures should be explained before the procedure. This helps prevent unnecessary surprises.

Adolescents (12 to 18 years) should be spoken to as adults. They are relatively independent and have a good sense of the world around them. Moreover, they are likely to have their own opinions. Therefore, when reasonable, they should be allowed to make their own choices about certain aspects of care (i.e., which arm should have an intravenous line). However, unless a child or an adolescent is an **emanci-**

SPECIAL Populations

Know Your Rules

Each community sets its own rules for determining whether a young person should be declared an emancipated minor. The following factors are often considered:
- Marriage
- Judicial decree
- Military service
- Parental consent
- Financial independence
- Motherhood

The consent given by a minor is valid if the minor is considered capable of understanding the clinical consequences of the treatment options offered.

---

pated minor, he or she cannot consent or deny essential treatment without parental consent.

The Pediatric Airway

The anatomy of the pediatric airway differs from that of the adult airway in many ways. A child's airway is relatively shorter and smaller than that of the adult. Also, the pediatric airway is funnel shaped, whereas the adult airway is cylindric. In children, the tongue is larger relative to the **oropharynx.** The **larynx** is more cephalad (toward the head) and anterior (toward the front), and the **epiglottis** is long and floppy. The narrowest portion of the pediatric airway is the **cricoid ring;** in the adult airway, the narrowest portion is the glottic inlet (Fig. 31-1). The EMT must recognize and

---

BOX 31-1

Approaching the Pediatric Patient

1. Address the child by his or her first name. This reduces the anxiety of both the patient and the caregiver, because the child is being treated as an individual rather than a generic "patient."
2. Never tower over patients when interacting with them. Get down to the child's level to reduce intimidation.
3. With toddlers and children, examine the patient from toe to head. Examine the area of concern or injury (i.e., the painful area) last, because this gives you an opportunity to win the patient's trust.

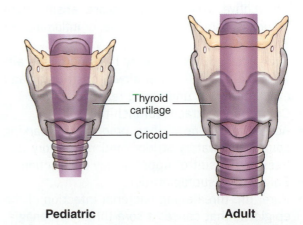

Pediatric   **Adult**

Thyroid cartilage

Cricoid

Fig. 31-1 The narrowest portion of the pediatric airway is the cricoid ring. In contrast, in the adult airway, the glottic inlet is the narrowest portion.

understand these differences to manage airway and breathing effectively in a pediatric patient.

■ RESPIRATORY DISTRESS

Respiratory distress is indicated by an increase in the work of breathing. Clinical signs may include tachypnea (increased rate of breathing), hyperpnea (increased depth of breathing), nasal flaring, accessory muscle use, or retractions (Box 31-2).

Upper Airway Considerations

With pediatric patients, EMTs should always have suction readily available for removal of large amounts of secretions. These secretions may be the sole cause of respiratory distress. This situation is particularly common in infants, who are preferentially nasal breathers. However, even in older children, small amounts of edema and secretions can increase airway resistance dramatically and therefore impede effective respirations. This is due to the child's narrow trachea, which is relatively more affected by changes in airway diameter than that of the adult. Age-appropriate suctioning devices should be readily available, and the EMT should be familiar with their use. In an infant, a bulb suction device may be most appropriate. In the child, on the other hand, rigid suction catheters may be applied to the oropharynx (Fig. 31-2). During quiet breathing, resistance is inversely proportional to the fourth power of the radius (Resistance $\propto$ 1/radius^4). During crying or turbulent airflow, resistance is inversely proportional to the fifth power of the radius (Resistance $\propto$ 1/radius^5) (Fig. 31-3).[1] Because of this phenomenon, you should make every possible effort to make the child physically and psychologically comfortable.

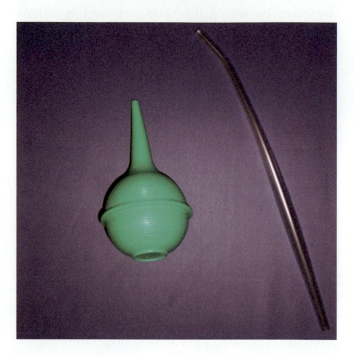

Fig. 31-2 Age-appropriate suctioning devices should be readily available and familiar to the EMT. In an infant, a bulb suction device may be more appropriate. In the child, more rigid suction catheters may be applied to the oropharynx.

BOX 31-2

Specific Pediatric Respiratory Emergencies

- Reactive airway disease (asthma)
- Obstructive lower airway disease arising from bronchospasm, mucosal edema, or inflammation
- Bronchiolitis
- Viral-induced inflammatory reaction of the airways that leads to lower airway obstruction and exacerbation of underlying reactive airways
- Croup (laryngotracheobronchitis)
- Acute viral illness that produces a barking cough, inspiratory stridor, and respiratory distress as a result of upper airway obstruction
- Epiglottitis (supraglottitis)
- Rare, life-threatening bacterial infection of the epiglottis that causes a sore throat, dysphagia, dysphonia, stridor, and rapid upper airway obstruction.

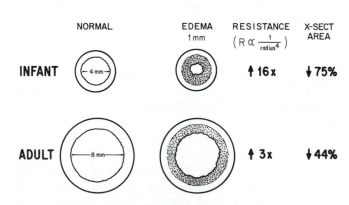

Fig. 31-3 During quiet breathing, resistance is inversely proportional to the fourth power of the radius (Resistance $\propto$ 1/radius^4). During crying or turbulent airflow, resistance is inversely proportional to the fifth power of the radius (Resistance $\propto$ 1/radius^5). Because of this phenomenon, every feasible effort should be made to make the child physically and psychologically comfortable.

If possible, allow the child to stay with the parent or guardian. Do not use unnecessary restraints or other external monitoring devices on a panicked child. Likewise, blow-by oxygen, rather than a face mask, may be more effective in delivering supplemental oxygen. If a paper cup is available, oxygen can be delivered by punching a hole in the bottom of the cup and inserting the oxygen tubing through this opening. Using the child's favorite toy or stuffed animal also may prove helpful. This provides the child with a familiar device by which to receive the oxygen. Having the caregiver hold the cup may also improve cooperation (Fig. 31-4). Ultimately, however, maximum oxygen delivery is the primary goal, because pediatric patients in respiratory distress may have compromised uptake and delivery of oxygen. The appropriate method of providing oxygen depends on the patient's age and clinical status.

Oxygen Delivery Systems

In general, oxygen delivery systems can be categorized as low-flow or high-flow systems. Nasal cannulas, blow-by oxygen, and simple masks are considered low-flow systems, because the oxygen flow is less than the patient's inspiratory drive. Low-flow systems generally provide an oxygen concentration of 23% to 80%.[2] The advantage of low-flow systems for an alert pediatric patient is that they are less threatening and anxiety provoking. In general, no more than 4 L/min of oxygen should be used with a nasal cannula. Higher flow rates can irritate the **nasopharynx** and reduce the efficiency of oxygen flow.

A simple mask can deliver 35% oxygen at 6 L/min and up to 60% oxygen at 10 L/min. A minimum of 6 L/min is needed to maintain an increased inspired oxygen concentration and prevent rebreathing of exhaled carbon dioxide. When a face mask is placed on the patient's face, it must be age appropriate so that it fits over the bridge of the nose and hugs the chin (Fig. 31-5).

> ### SPECIAL Considerations
>
> **Oxygen Delivery Systems and Patient's Age**
> Low-flow oxygen delivery systems may provide higher flow in an infant. For example, a nasal cannula may deliver more oxygen flow for an infant's inspiratory drive than it would in an adult.

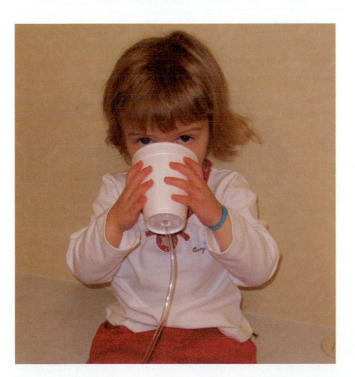

Fig. 31-4 Blow-by oxygen, rather than face masks, may be more effective in delivering supplemental oxygen. If a paper cup is available, oxygen can be delivered by punching a hole in the bottom of the cup and inserting the oxygen tubing through this opening. This provides the child with a familiar device by which to receive the oxygen.

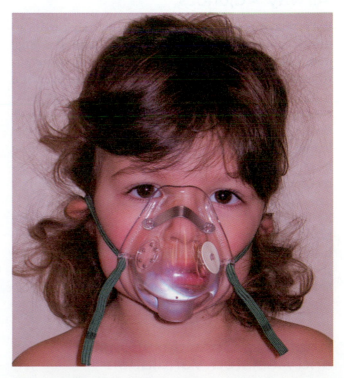

Fig. 31-5 When a face mask is placed on the patient's face, it must be age appropriate so that it fits over the bridge of the nose and hugs the chin.

High-flow systems include the partial **nonrebreather mask** and the complete nonrebreather mask. These devices consist of a mask with a reservoir bag. They involve less entrapment of room air. Moreover, they can reliably provide a 50% to 95% inspired oxygen concentration at a flow rate of at least 10 L/min.[2]

■ RESPIRATORY FAILURE

The EMT must be prepared at any time to take over management of the airway and breathing in case the patient decompensates (continues to gets worse) from respiratory distress. This need for intervention marks the progression of respiratory distress to **respiratory failure.**

Signs of respiratory failure include the following:

- Decreased or decreasing responsiveness
- Inability to recognize parents or caregivers
- Poor interaction with parents or caregivers
- Decreased muscle tone
- Use of accessory muscles for breathing
- Retraction of chest muscles
- Nasal flaring
- Cyanosis
- Head bobbing

Airway Adjuncts

EMTs may need to secure a temporary airway in an unconscious patient. In pediatric patients, the large pediatric tongue can itself occlude the airway. To correct this, use a two-handed jaw thrust maneuver or a tongue-jaw lift maneuver (Fig. 31-6). If this is unsuccessful, you can place a nasal or oral airway to relieve this anatomic obstruction. To determine the correct length of a nasal airway, measure from the tip of the nose to the earlobe of the ear. To determine the correct length of an oral airway, measure from the lips just cephalad to the angle of the mandible (Fig. 31-7). In placing the oral airway, you can use the tongue blade technique to push the tongue down, allowing insertion of the airway (Fig. 31-8). This technique should not be used in patients with an intact **gag reflex.** It would cause continuous discomfort and possibly emesis (vomiting) with aspiration.

Anatomic Considerations and Assisted Ventilation

Oral, Pharyngeal, and Tracheal Pediatric Axes
The EMT must assess anatomic, age-related differences to properly align the oral, pharyngeal, and tracheal axes of the pediatric patient. This is important

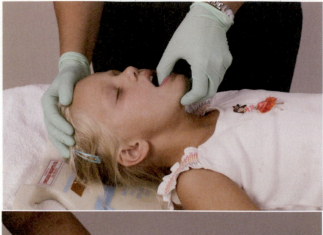

A

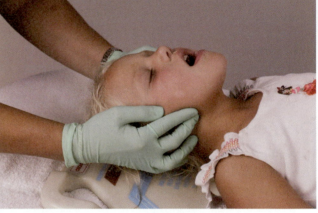

B

Fig. 31-6 In infants and children, the large pediatric tongue can occlude the airway. This can be corrected with a tongue-jaw lift maneuver (**A**) or a two-handed jaw thrust maneuver (**B**).

for helping to facilitate and maintain an open airway. For infants and sometimes toddlers, you can put a towel under the shoulders to accommodate the relatively larger **occiput.** For older children, putting the towel under the child's head probably will be more helpful. These maneuvers should put the patient in the sniffing position, with the external ear canal anterior to the shoulder (Fig. 31-9). An age-appropriate mask can then be selected, and active bag-valve-mask (BVM) assisted ventilation can be started. The mask should fit over the bridge of the nose and the cleft of the chin (Fig. 31-10).

Because upper airway structures in infants and children are immature and pliable, a small degree of hyperflexion or hyperextension can cause inadvertent airway obstruction. Keeping this in mind, make sure you bring the patient's jaw up to the mask, rather than the mask down to the patient. This prevents unnecessary neck flexion and helps prevent airway obstruction. This technique is particularly helpful for preventing neck movement when the cervical spine also must be immobilized.

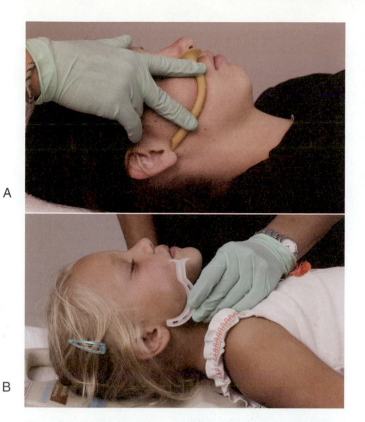

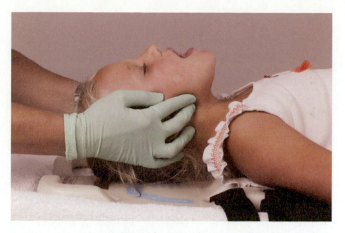

Fig. 31-9 To properly align the axis of the airway, put the pediatric patient in the sniffing position with the external ear canal anterior to the shoulder. With infants and sometimes toddlers, a towel may be placed under the shoulders to accommodate the relatively larger occiput.

Fig. 31-7 Anatomic upper airway obstruction can be relieved by **(A)** a nasal airway, measured from the tip of the nose to the earlobe for length, or **(B)** an oral airway, measured from the lips just cephalad to the angle of the mandible.

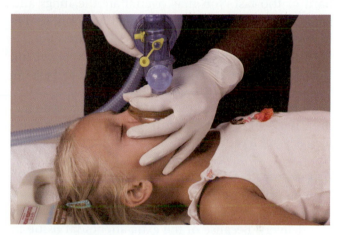

Fig. 31-10 An age-appropriate bag-mask should fit over the bridge of the nose and the cleft of the chin. To facilitate bagging, think of the E-C technique. In this technique, fingers three, four, and five form an **E** along the jawline and the thumb and index finger form a **C** that encircles the mask.

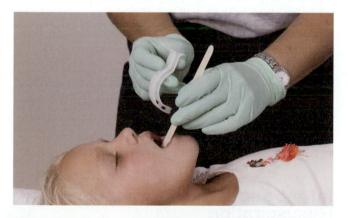

Fig. 31-8 For placement of the oral airway, the tongue blade technique can be used to push the tongue down, allowing insertion of the airway.

Bag-Mask Ventilation

Patients with respiratory failure need assisted ventilation for adequate gas exchange. A ventilation mask allows you to ventilate and oxygenate a patient. This is called *artificial ventilation*. Selecting the appropriate mask size and using good technique are important

for ensuring effective artificial ventilation. Without an airtight seal, both oxygenation and ventilation become less effective. As mentioned previously, the ventilation mask should fit along the bridge of the nose and the cleft of the chin. However, avoid unnecessary pressure on the patient's eye, because this can cause **bradycardia** (a slow heart rate).

Masks should be transparent. This allows you to make a number of observations: the color of the patient's lips; condensation on the mask, which indicates exhalation; and the need for suctioning in case of vomiting. Bags also are available in different sizes (infant, child, and adult).

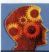

ASK YOURSELF

Question: Even though you have administered bag-mask ventilation using good technique, your patient still has poor oxygenation. What should you do next?

Answer: First, always administer 100% oxygen by using a reservoir bag. Also, always use a pulse oximeter to monitor the patient's oxygen status. If hypoxia persists despite good ventilation technique, check your tubing and make sure it is hooked up to an appropriate oxygen source.

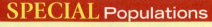

SPECIAL Populations

Tracheostomy Tubes

For an infant or a child with a tracheostomy tube, do not apply the oxygen source or bag-mask to the face. Instead, use the tracheostomy tube. Also, many of these patients will have airway obstruction or cyanosis. A thick mucous plug in the tracheostomy tube may be the culprit. Suction the obstructed tube immediately.

ASK YOURSELF

You are called to the home of a child who is known to have chronic asthma. You find that the child is having an acute asthma exacerbation. You have been called to this home three times over the past 2 months for similar episodes. The parent has not had an inhaler prescription filled for more than 3 months. Is this considered neglect?

Remember to squeeze the bag enough so each ventilation lasts 1 second and only enough to watch the chest rise adequately. If you squeeze the bag too hard or too fast, you may overinflate the lungs and possibly cause gastric inflation. This not only results in less effective ventilation, it may also cause the patient to vomit and aspirate gastric contents. During each bagging effort, watch the chest rise as you say "squeeze-release-release" to guide the rate of active ventilation. The ventilation rate for infants and children is 12-20 breaths per minute, and this rate is effectively achieved with this technique.

Bag-Mask "E-C" Technique

Patients in severe respiratory distress or respiratory failure need assisted ventilation in addition to oxygen delivery. Because of the extra adenoidal tissue in children, mask-to-face techniques should focus on putting pressure on the bony prominence of the jawline rather than on the **submandibular** or **submental** tissue. Pressure applied to the submandibular or submental areas can easily obstruct the child's larynx.

To aid bagging (if you are working by yourself), think of the E-C technique. Fingers three, four, and five form an E along the jawline, and the thumb and index finger form a C that encircles the mask (Skill 31-1). Two-person bag-mask ventilation is more effective and should be used if possible, especially if the patient has significant airway obstruction or poor lung compliance. If you encounter resistance to the ventilation efforts, try repositioning the patient's head, make sure the mask fits tightly, lift the jaw, and consider suctioning the airway.

Cricoid Pressure

To minimize aspiration, carefully apply cricoid pressure to a bagged pediatric patient. However, keep in mind that, because of the pliability of the pediatric upper airway, you can easily impede airflow with this maneuver. In adults, the rule of thumb for the amount of pressure to apply is that pressure which, when applied to the cartilage of the nose, starts to be painful. In a child, a relatively lesser degree of force should be applied and should be adjusted if it hinders effective bagging.

Always use 100% oxygen by using a reservoir bag. Also use a pulse oximeter to monitor the patient's oxygen status. If hypoxia persists despite good ventilatory technique, remember to check your tubing and make sure it is hooked up to an appropriate oxygen source.

Infant and Child Cardiopulmonary Resuscitation

In addition to oxygenation and ventilation, EMTs must be trained to perform CPR properly in case of loss of adequate circulation (Skills 31-2 to 31-4). After opening up the airway (using the techniques described previously), you must determine whether the patient is breathing. To do this, look, listen, and feel: *look* for rise of the chest and abdomen; *listen* at the child's nose and mouth for breath sounds; and *feel* for exhaled air. If respirations are agonal or nonexistent, deliver two rescue breaths using the bag-mask device. If the rescue breaths are successful, assess the circulation.

SKILL 31-1

Performing Bag-Mask Ventilation on Infants and Children

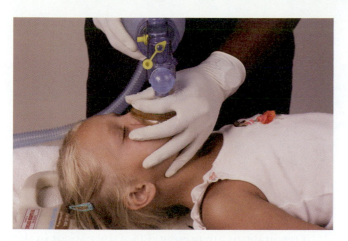

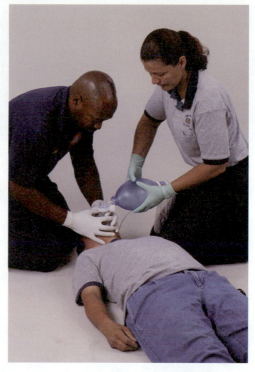

1. Kneel at the patient's head. If the patient does not have a neck injury, place a towel beneath the head (for a child) or the torso (for an infant).
2. If a neck injury is suspected, open the airway with the jaw thrust technique without head tilt.
3. Apply the mask to the patient's face. The mask should reach from the bridge of the nose to the cleft of the chin without overlapping the eyes.
4. Apply the E-C technique by placing the thumb and index finger on the mask to apply downward pressure. The remaining fingers are positioned along the angle of the mandible to lift the jaw up and forward.

5. Apply only the force and volume needed to cause the chest to rise visibly.
6. A two-person bag-mask technique may be more efficient.

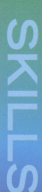

SKILLS

635

SKILL 31-2
Performing Cardiopulmonary Resuscitation (CPR) on Children

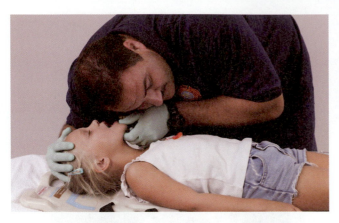

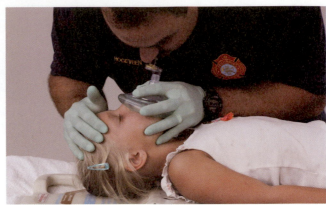

1. Shake the patient gently and shout; if there is no response, call for help. Open the airway using one of the following techniques: head-tilt chin-lift, jaw thrust, or tongue-jaw lift maneuver. Check for breathing: look, listen, and feel.

2. If respirations are present: Place the patient in the recovery position and continue to monitor.

3. If breathing is absent: Deliver two rescue breaths. If resistance is encountered, reposition the airway.

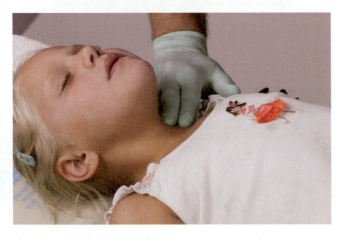

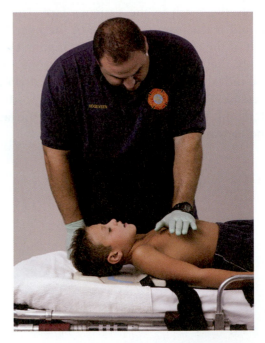

4. Check for a pulse for up to 10 seconds.

5. If a pulse is present (>60 beats per minute): Continue with rescue breathing at a rate of 12-20 breaths per minute.

6. If the pulse is absent or is slower than 60 beats per minute: Begin chest compression with hands placed at the lower half of the sternum. If a pediatric automatic external defibrillator (AED) is available and the child meets the machine's requirements, attach the patient to the machine and follow the AED protocol.

7. Chest compression depth should be one-third to one-half the depth of the patient's chest.

8. Use the appropriate compression-to-ventilation ratio: 3:1 for newborns; for all other children, the compression/ventilation ratio is dependent on the number of rescuers—30:2 for 1 rescuer, 15:2 for two rescuers.

9. Reassess the pulse after 5 cycles of compressions and ventilations (approximately 2 minutes).

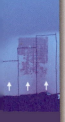

SKILLS

SKILL 31-3
Performing Chest Compressions on Infants

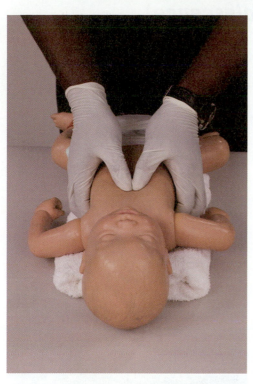

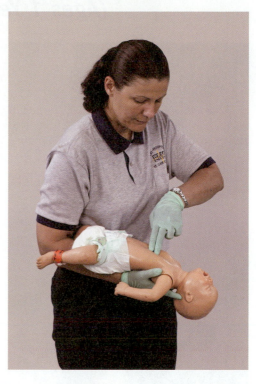

Two-Thumb Encircling Hands Technique (Used When There Are Two Rescuers)

1. Position yourself at the infant's feet or side.
2. Place your thumbs side by side over the lower half of the infant's sternum, approximately $\frac{1}{2}$ inch apart just below the level of the nipples. Support the infant's back with the fingers of both hands.
3. Use both thumbs to depress the sternum approximately one-third of the depth of a newborn's chest and one-third to one-half the depth of the infant's chest.
4. Deliver compressions at a rate of at least 100 per minute (about two compressions per second).
5. Use a compression-to-ventilation ratio of 3:1 in newborns and 15:2 in infants.

Two-Finger Compression Technique (Used if Single Rescuer)

1. Place two fingers of one hand over the lower sternum, approximately in the midline and approximately $\frac{1}{2}$ inch below the level of the nipples (be careful not to compress over the xiphoid process).
2. Deliver compressions at a rate of at least 100 per minute.
3. Use a compression-to-ventilation ratio of 3:1 in newborns and 30:2 in infants.

637

SKILL 31-4

Performing Chest Compressions on Children (Ages 1 Year to Adolescence)

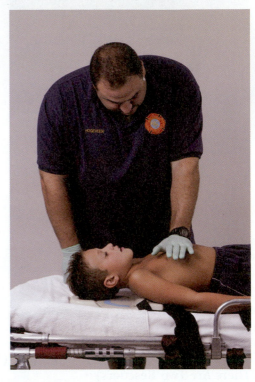

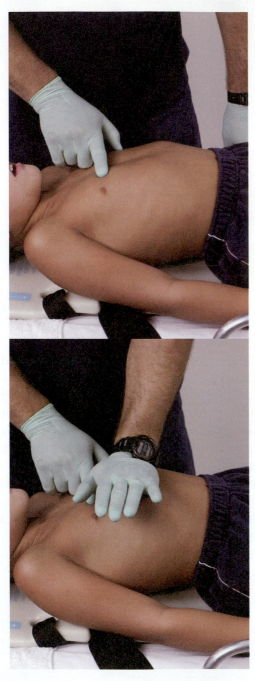

1. Place the heel of one hand over the lower sternum between the nipple line. Be careful not to compress over the xiphoid process. Lift your fingers off the chest.

2. Depress the sternum approximately one-third to one-half the depth of the victim's chest.

3. After delivering the compression, release the pressure to allow the chest to return to normal position before beginning the next compression. Do not lift your hand off the chest during compressions.

4. Deliver compressions at a rate of approximately 100 per minute.

5. Use a compression-to-ventilation ratio of 30:2 for one rescuer and 15:2 for two rescuers.

NOTE: For adolescents (12-14 years of age), use the same CPR technique as that used for adults with a compression-to-ventilation ratio of 30:2.

SKILLS

SPECIAL Considerations

Brachial versus Carotid
Checking the carotid pulse in infants is not recommended. Their short, chubby necks make the pulse difficult to locate. Moreover, it is easy to compress the airway and stimulate a vagal response while attempting to palpate a carotid pulse. It is best to check the brachial or femoral pulse in infants.

If the patient's chest does not rise with ventilation or if you feel resistance to bagging, an obstruction exists. Reposition the airway and make sure you have a good seal with the bag-mask device. If you still feel resistance, follow the protocol for an unconscious victim with foreign body airway obstruction.

Do not take longer than 10 seconds to check the pulse of an infant or a child. If the child has no pulse or if the pulse rate is below 60 beats per minute, start chest compressions. The patient should be on a hard, flat surface (e.g., a backboard) to facilitate compressions. The depth and rate of compressions are discussed further in Skills 31-2 to 31-4. In general, compressions are delivered at a rate of approximately 100 per minute. Guidelines for the compressions-to-ventilations ratio suggest a ratio of 30:2 for a single rescuer and 15:2 if there are two rescuers. Children older than 8 years of age are treated similar to adults, with a compressions-to-ventilations ratio of 15:2.

■ PEDIATRIC UPPER AIRWAY OBSTRUCTION

Respiratory emergencies in pediatric patients have numerous causes: upper airway foreign body obstruction, croup, epiglottitis, bronchiolitis, asthma, and pneumonia, to name a few. If a child is somnolent (semi-comatose) or unconscious, the airway may become obstructed from a combination of neck flexion, posterior tongue displacement, and collapse of the **hypopharynx.**[2]

Upper Airway Obstruction

Upper airway obstruction is relatively common. It requires prompt action by EMTs. Signs of upper airway obstruction include motioning by the victim toward the throat, known as the universal choking sign (Fig. 31-11); inability to speak or cry; **stridor;** weak cough; accessory muscle use; and ineffective retractions with

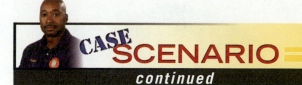

CASE SCENARIO
continued

Jerome is a 15-month-old male who, according to his mother Alice, had been experiencing a "cold" for the past 3 days. Alice had brought Jerome to the neighborhood clinic early that morning, but the wait was so long that Alice would have missed work. They left without being seen by the clinic pediatrician.

Alice returned home after work to find Jerome sleeping. Her mother-in-law said that he had been sleeping on and off through the day, and had relatively little to drink or eat. Alice was concerned but decided to let Jerome continue sleeping. About 20 minutes earlier, she could hear Jerome coughing and making an awful noise—it almost sounded like a harsh, barking sound when he breathed.

In the brightly lit patient compartment, Jack could see that Jerome was struggling to breathe. Pulling up the shirt, Elizabeth pointed out where the ribs appeared to stick out when Jerome took a breath – a sign of intercostal retractions. Still, he clung to his mother's arm tightly and had that tired, frightened look in his eyes. Each time Jack tried to place the bell of his stethoscope against his chest, he would pull away and cry weakly. As his respirations increased the "barking" sound reappeared.

Questions: *How should the EMTs proceed with their assessment? Should they try to separate the child from the mother? Why or why not? What treatments are indicated by this situation?*

subsequent **cyanosis.** With a partial upper airway obstruction, the patient remains conscious and has pink skin. To prevent progression to complete obstruction, allow the patient to maintain the position of greatest comfort without undue agitation. Once the diagnosis of a partial airway obstruction has been made, avoid any maneuver that may cause distress. This includes blood pressure measurements or other unnecessary examination efforts. Instead, focus your efforts on providing rapid transport to an emergency facility and administering supplemental oxygen (Skills 31-5 to 31-8).

Should the need arise, however, EMTs must be familiar with rescue techniques for upper airway obstructions.

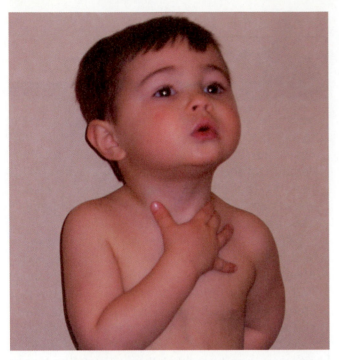

Fig. 31-11 Upper airway obstruction is relatively common. It requires prompt action on the part of the EMT. One sign of upper airway obstruction is motioning by the victim toward his or her throat, known as the universal choking sign.

Infant: Rescue Technique for Upper Airway Foreign Body Obstruction

For an infant (under 1 year of age), use back blows and chest thrusts to dislodge the obstruction. Hold the infant prone on your forearm. Because the head will be tilted slightly lower than the infant's torso, support the head at the chin without pressing on submental tissues. Using the heel of your free hand, forcefully deliver five blows to the middle of the back between the shoulder blades. Then, while constantly supporting the infant's head, transfer the infant to your other arm into the supine position. With the fingers of your free hand, deliver five chest thrusts on the lower third of the infant's sternum, using 1-second downward motions (Fig. 31-12). Repeat this sequence of maneuvers until the object is dislodged or the infant becomes unresponsive.

Text continued on p. 646

Important Points

Never attempt a blind sweep of the oropharynx. This may exacerbate the obstruction by causing the foreign body to migrate deeper into the airway.

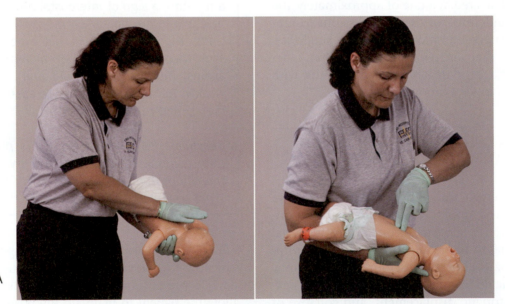

Fig. 31-12 A, With an infant (under 1 year of age), back blows and chest thrusts should be used to dislodge an upper airway obstruction. To do this, hold the infant prone on your forearm. Because the head is tilted slightly lower than the infant's torso, support the head at the chin without pressing on submental tissues. With the heel of your other hand, forcefully deliver five blows to the middle of the back between the shoulder blades. **B,** Next, while constantly supporting the infant's head, transfer the infant to the other arm into the supine position. With the fingers of your free hand, deliver five chest thrusts on the lower third of the infant's sternum, using 1-second downward motions. Repeat this sequence of maneuvers until the object is dislodged or the infant becomes unresponsive.

SKILL 31-5
Clearing a Foreign Body Airway Obstruction in the Responsive Infant

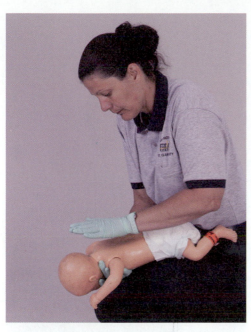

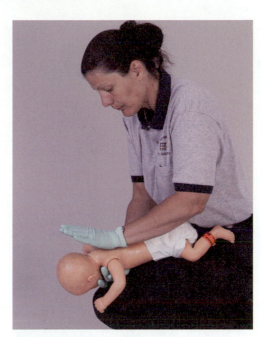

1. Sit or kneel. Hold the infant prone, with the body resting on your forearm and the head slightly lower than the chest. Support the infant's head with your hand under the jaw, taking care not to compress the soft tissues of the infant's mouth or throat. Rest your forearm on your thigh to support the infant's weight.

2. With the heel of your free hand, deliver five blows to the infant's back between the shoulder blades. Use enough force to attempt to expel the foreign body.

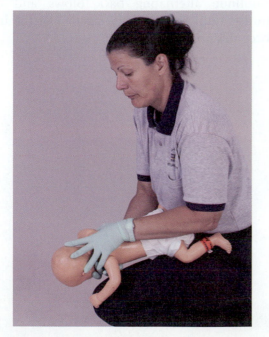

3. After delivering the five back blows, place your free hand over the infant's occiput (back of the head) and your forearm over the middle of the back. This should cradle the infant between both forearms, with one hand supporting the face and jaw and the other hand supporting the occiput.

Continued

SKILLS

SKILL 31-5

Clearing a Foreign Body Airway Obstruction in the Responsive Infant—cont'd

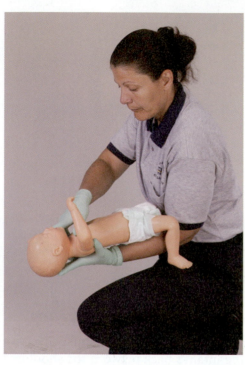

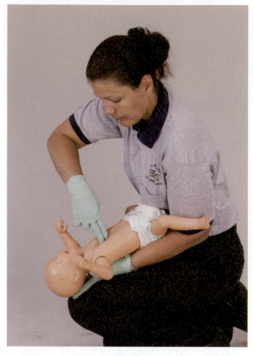

4. Turn the infant supine as a unit, supporting the head and neck at all times. Place the forearm supporting the infant's weight on your thigh. Keep the infant's head lower than the trunk.

5. Using the hand that was supporting the infant's face and jaw, deliver up to five chest thrusts in the same location as chest compressions (see Skill 31-2) at a rate of about 1 per second. Use enough force to attempt to expel the foreign body.

6. Continue alternating back blows and chest thrusts until the object is expelled or the infant becomes unresponsive.

SKILL 31-6
Clearing a Foreign Body Airway Obstruction in the Unresponsive Infant

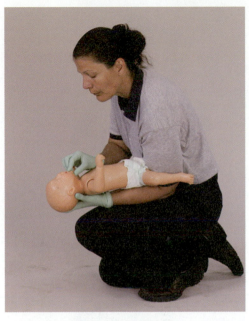

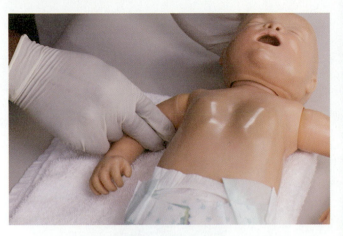

1. Open the infant's airway using the tongue-jaw lift maneuver. Look for an object in the mouth and throat. If you see the object, remove it. *Never* perform a blind finger sweep.

2. If no object is visible, open the airway with a head-tilt/chin-lift and attempt to provide two rescue breaths. If the breaths are ineffective, reposition the head and reattempt rescue breaths.

3. If the breaths still are not effective, give up to five back blows and chest thrusts (see Skill 31-5).

4. Repeat steps 1 through 3 until the foreign body is expelled and the airway is patent or until attempts have lasted at least 1 minute. If at 1 minute the patient is still unresponsive and the airway is still obstructed, transport the patient to the nearest medical facility while continuing steps 1 through 3.

5. If rescue breaths are effective, check for signs of circulation and continue cardiopulmonary resuscitation (CPR) as needed (see Skill 31-2).

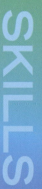

SKILL 31-7
Clearing a Foreign Body Airway Obstruction in the Responsive Child

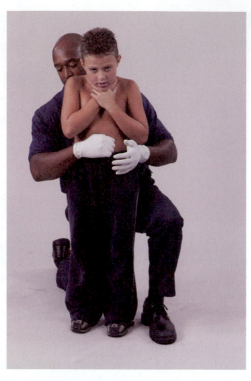

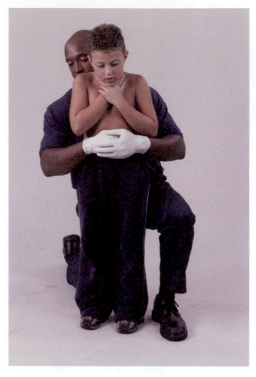

1. Stand or kneel directly behind the child. Put your arms under the axillae (armpits), encircling the chest.
2. Place the flat, thumb side of one fist against the victim's abdomen in the midline, slightly above the navel and well below the tip of the xiphoid process.

3. Grasp the fist with the other hand and deliver a series of up to five quick, inward and upward thrusts (Heimlich maneuver).
4. Deliver each thrust as a separate, distinct movement with enough force to attempt to expel the obstruction. Continue the series of five thrusts until the object is expelled or the child becomes unresponsive.

SKILLS

SKILL 31-8
Clearing a Foreign Body Airway Obstruction in the Unresponsive Child

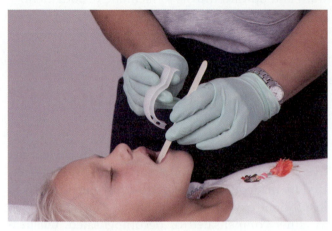

1. Lay the child on a flat surface and position yourself near the child's head.
2. Open the airway using the tongue-jaw lift maneuver and look for the foreign body. If the object is visible, remove it. *Never* do a blind finger sweep.
3. If no object is visible, open the airway with a head-tilt/chin-lift and attempt to provide two rescue breaths. If the breaths are not effective, begin CPR, checking the mouth for dislodged foreign objects before delivering breaths.
4. Continue CPR until the object is expelled and the airway is patent or until attempts have lasted approximately 1 minute. (If at 1 minute the patient is still unresponsive and the airway is still obstructed, transport the patient to the nearest medical facility while continuing steps 1 through 5.)
5. If rescue breaths are effective, check for signs of circulation and continue cardiopulmonary resuscitation (CPR) as needed (see Skill 31-2).

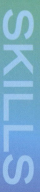

SKILLS

If the infant becomes unresponsive, carefully inspect the mouth for an obvious foreign body. To do this, you can use a tongue-jaw lift maneuver (see Fig. 31-6, *A*).

For an unresponsive infant with an upper airway obstruction, position the airway and provide two rescue breaths. If these are ineffective, try to reposition the head, possibly with a jaw thrust maneuver, and attempt rescue breaths again. If this is still ineffective, begin CPR until the object is expelled. These maneuvers can be done en route to the nearest emergency department (ED). A more definitive airway may need to be established by ED personnel. If the foreign body is dislodged and rescue breaths are effective, check for signs of circulation and provide additional steps of CPR as needed.[1] Continue to monitor the airway and respirations; be sure to keep oxygen, suction, and bag-mask equipment readily available.

Child: Rescue Technique for Upper Airway Foreign Body Obstruction

A similar sequence of maneuvers is used for the child (over 1 year of age) with a foreign body airway obstruction. However, instead of back blows and chest thrusts, abdominal thrusts (the Heimlich maneuver) should be used.

With a responsive victim, you can apply abdominal thrusts by standing behind the victim and encircling the victim's chest via the axillae (armpit). Make a fist with one hand and place the flat, thumb side below the victim's xiphoid process and just above the navel. Grasp your closed fist with the other hand and deliver five quick, inward and upward thrusts. If the child be-

---

SPECIAL Populations

Avoid Abdominal Thrusts

Abdominal thrusts are not recommended for infants. In infants the liver lies below the rib cage, making it susceptible to injury.

SPECIAL Populations

Avoid Abdominal Thrusts – Part 2

Do not perform abdominal thrusts on pregnant adolescent females. Instead, use chest compressions to dislodge a foreign body. If the patient is conscious, you can apply these from behind the individual, as with the Heimlich maneuver, but with your hands positioned over the sternum.

---

comes unresponsive, use a tongue-jaw lift maneuver to inspect for a foreign body; if one is obvious, remove it. As with infants, *never* attempt a blind finger sweep.

With an unresponsive child, begin CPR. To do this, straddle the victim's hips. Place the heel of one hand above the navel in the midline of the child's abdomen. Then use both hands to deliver quick, inward and upward thrusts to facilitate dislodgment.

■ **SHOCK (HYPOPERFUSION) AND RESUSCITATION OF THE INFANT AND CHILD**

Shock is defined as a mismatch between oxygen delivery and tissue metabolic demands. It is characterized by inadequate tissue perfusion, which results in insufficient oxygen delivery. Shock can be classified as either compensated or decompensated. **Compensated shock** is defined by the presence of a normal systolic blood pressure with signs and symptoms of inadequate tissue perfusion. **Decompensated shock** occurs when hypotension becomes evident.[3]

Causes of Shock

Shock can occur for a variety of reasons. It usually is categorized according to its cause. The three main categories of shock are hypovolemic shock, cardiogenic shock, and distributive shock. **Hypovolemic shock** refers to inadequate intravascular volume. This is the leading cause of shock in children worldwide. Diarrhea, vomiting, blood loss, and trauma all can lead to hypovolemic shock. **Cardiogenic shock** is less common in children. However, it can occur in patients with cardiac dysfunction. **Distributive shock** is characterized by inappropriate distribution of blood volume. It may be caused by **sepsis, anaphylaxis,** or spinal cord injury.[3]

SPECIAL Populations

Central Venous Lines

Some children have central venous catheters or long-term peripheral catheters for daily administration of medicines. These children are at increased risk for sepsis, because the catheter creates a portal of entry for bacteria into the blood. Other complications of central lines include bleeding at the site, clotting off, and a cracked or leaking line.

TABLE 31-1

Normal Vital Signs for Infants and Children

Age	Heart Rate (Beats per minute)	Blood Pressure (Systolic)	Respiratory Rate (Breaths per minute)
Newborn to 3 months	105-180	60-95	40-60
3 months to 1 year	110-185	65-110	20-40
2 to 4 years	75-150	70-110	20-30
5 to 14 years	60-135	80-130	12-25

Compensated versus Decompensated Shock

In compensated shock, blood is diverted from the skin, intestines, and kidneys to maintain perfusion of the heart and brain. An increased heart rate can be an early sign of shock. This occurs as the body attempts to increase cardiac output. An increased respiratory rate or tachypnea may be evident as well. The increased respiratory rate can arise from a primary respiratory disorder or as a compensatory mechanism for the metabolic acidosis observed in shock. The respiratory rate increases as the body attempts to maintain a normal acid-base status. Blood pressure is maintained in compensated shock because the peripheral blood vessels are constricted (Table 31-1). Any sign of hypotension should raise concern about cardiovascular decompensation.

Assessment of End Organ Perfusion

The infant or child in shock often shows signs of inadequate perfusion of end organs. As blood gets diverted to vital organs, such as the heart and the brain, other organs in the body are relatively hypoperfused. EMTs should be attuned to the early signs of shock, as evidenced in the distal pulses, skin, brain, kidneys, and mucous membranes.

Pulses

A patient in shock may have diminished or "thready" distal pulses as a result of decreased intravascular volume or impaired cardiac function associated with increased peripheral vasoconstriction. In contrast, a patient in early septic shock may have bounding pulses as a result of the heart's high-output state and vasodilation.

Skin

In early shock the skin may become cool and clammy. This may begin at the periphery and extend proximally as more blood is diverted to the vital or-

> **SPECIAL Considerations**
>
> **Pulse Checks**
> An infant's pulse is best evaluated at the brachial or femoral artery. The pulse of an older child can be assessed at the radial or carotid artery.

gans. Capillary refill is delayed (longer than 2 seconds), and the skin may become mottled, pale, or cyanotic. To measure capillary refill accurately, place the extremity you are testing at the level of the heart. Remember, capillary refill alone is not a reliable measure and should be assessed in the context of the patient's presentation.[3] Cyanosis that occurs secondary to cardiogenic shock often manifests as a **central cyanosis** (cyanosis involving the face or trunk or both).

Brain (Mental Status)

Early signs of shock may include irritability, agitation, confusion, or lethargy. With more severe shock, the patient may be unconscious and have poor muscle tone. With an infant, loss of eye contact or response to voice may be an early sign of shock. Lack of response to painful stimuli is particularly worrisome. The Glasgow Coma Scale (Tables 31-2 and 31-3) or the **AVPU** (alert, verbal, painful, unresponsive) assessment method (Box 31-3) may be helpful for establishing and following the patient's mental status.

Kidneys

The best measure of hypoperfusion of the kidneys is urine output. While an exact measurement of urine output is not possible in the field, the number of wet diapers the infant or child produces can be used to help determine perfusion status. However, this may be inaccurate in the early stages of shock.

TABLE 31-2
Glasgow Coma Scale for Pediatric Patients

Assessment Factor	Points
Eye Opening	
Spontaneous	4
To speech	3
To pain	2
None	1
Best Verbal Response	
Oriented, converses	5
Disoriented, confused	4
Inappropriate words	3
Incomprehensible sounds	2
No response	1
Best Motor Response	
Obeys verbal commands	6
Localizes to painful stimuli	5
Withdraws to pain	4
Abnormal flexion (decorticate rigidity)	3
Abnormal extension (decerebrate rigidity)	2
None	1

TABLE 31-3
Modified Glasgow Coma Scale for Infants

Assessment Factor	Points
Eye Opening	
Spontaneous	4
To speech	3
To pain	2
None	1
Best Verbal Response	
Coos, babbles	5
Irritable, cries	4
Cries to pain	3
Moans to pain	2
None	1
Best Motor Response	
Normal spontaneous movements	6
Withdraws to touch	5
Withdraws to pain	4
Abnormal flexion (decorticate rigidity)	3
Abnormal extension (decerebrate rigidity)	2
None	1

BOX 31-3
AVPU Assessment Method

A—alert (the patient is alert, awake, and oriented)

V—verbal (the patient responds to voice)

P—painful stimuli (the patient responds only to a painful stimulus)

U—unresponsive (the patient is not awake and is completely unresponsive to any type of stimulation)

SPECIAL Considerations

How Many Diapers?
Urine output can vary in toddlers and children. However, infants generally should produce 4 to 10 wet diapers a day. Fewer than this should raise concern about dehydration.

Mucous Membranes

With hypovolemic shock, the patient may have very dry **mucous membranes** and may not produce tears while crying.

Management of the Pediatric Patient in Shock

As an EMT, your role in caring for a patient in shock is to manage airway, breathing, and circulation (ABCs). Make sure the airway is patent and adminis-

ter 100% oxygen. Artificial ventilation may be needed if the patient's breathing is compromised. Manage any obvious bleeding with direct pressure. To stabilize a patient in early shock, elevate the legs and keep the patient warm. Finally, rapid transport is needed to ensure the patient's best outcome.

Pediatric Cardiac Arrest

Cardiopulmonary arrest in infants and children most often occurs as a result of a primary respiratory disorder. If a child can be resuscitated in the early stages of **pulmonary arrest**, before **cardiac arrest** develops, the prognosis is much better. Once the patient is in cardiac arrest, the chances of surviving the primary pulmonary disorder are about 20% at best. In the case of *primary cardiac arrest* (cardiac arrest that is *not* precipitated by a respiratory event), the outlook is even grimmer: in these cases, the percentage of patients who survive and are discharged is 2%. The rate for survival to discharge with a good neurologic outcome is even lower.

Fortunately, primary cardiac arrest is rare in infancy and childhood. The fact that survival is so low points to this being the direct result of a terminal condition, illness, or injury. Furthermore, the causes of cardiac arrest in pediatric patients differ greatly from those in adults. Primary cardiac arrest in adults commonly occurs secondary to **cardiac ischemia, arrhythmia,** or **structural cardiac abnormalities.** The most common causes of childhood cardiac arrest are **sudden infant death syndrome (SIDS),** trauma, submersion incident (near-drowning), and sepsis. Thus 75% of presenting pediatric arrest rhythms are the terminal rhythms of **bradyasystole.**

Unless signs of death are obvious (e.g., rigor mortis or lividity), always attempt resuscitative efforts for a pediatric patient in cardiopulmonary arrest. Once the child is in a terminal rhythm, the chances for survival are slim. However, EMTs must consider the family's emotional response and their need to see some attempt at rescue. Do not make any comments that might point an accusatory finger at the caregivers. This situation can be quite traumatic for them and requires a thoughtful, empathetic approach.

■ PEDIATRIC SEIZURES

Seizures are the most common neurologic disorder of childhood. Approximately 4% to 6% of children will have had a seizure by the age of 16 years. EMTs must be able to recognize and describe the characteristics of a seizure.

Most seizures in infancy and childhood are the **tonic-clonic seizure** type. This means that the patient may have a period of body stiffness (tonic) followed by a period of rhythmic shaking (clonic). Some seizures involve both sides of the body (generalized), whereas others involve only one side (partial or focal). A seizure may be a one-time event, or it may be part of a recurring seizure disorder **(epilepsy).** A patient may have an altered level of consciousness during a seizure and then may remain confused, irritable, or sluggish for minutes to hours after the seizure. This aftermath is called the **postictal period,** and it is usually proportional to the length of the seizure.[4] Not all patients who have a seizure have a postictal period. However, it is important that EMTs provide any information about this period to the receiving medical personnel. The seizure disorder **status epilepticus** is a life-threatening event. This disorder is characterized either by a prolonged seizure (one that lasts longer than 30 minutes) or by multiple seizures that occur without recovery to baseline consciousness between episodes.

A number of factors can cause seizures in pediatric patients. Many children have known seizure disorders. Always ask the caregivers if the patient's presentation is typical or if it is different from the usual seizure pattern, which would suggest a new problem. Also, always obtain a list of the patient's medications, because these children may have a subtherapeutic level of antiseizure medication. This can occur if the patient has not been taking the needed medication or if the child has not been absorbing the medicine because of vomiting or diarrhea.

In the trauma setting, assume bleeding within or a **contusion** of the brain. Check the patient for signs of external trauma, which may have occurred before or

SPECIAL Considerations

Fever Considerations

Fever in an infant or a child is a common reason for an ambulance call. A fever can arise from a number of causes, most of which are not life-threatening. However, certain findings should raise concern that the fever may be a sign of a potentially serious illness. A rash is a common finding with fever in viral illnesses. However, it may also be seen in children with serious bacterial infections. Also, any febrile infant or child with a central venous line, ventricular-peritoneal (VP) shunt, or gastric feeding tube is at risk of having a more serious infection.

SPECIAL Considerations

Ingestions

With suspected ingestion, take the medicine bottles or chemical to the emergency department (ED) with the patient. This is very helpful to the ED staff for quantifying and identifying the ingestion.

TABLE 31-4

Nonepileptic Events That May Mimic Seizures

Breath-holding spells	Acute dystonia
Syncope	Gastroesophageal reflux
Migraine	Night terrors
Jitteriness	Sleep paralysis
Benign myoclonus	Narcolepsy
Shuddering attacks	Pseudoseizures
Tics	

during the seizure. It is not uncommon for an infant or a toddler to have a brief period of seizure activity after a minor head injury (post-traumatic seizure). These patients need further evaluation in an ED.

If fever is present along with the seizure, consider brain infections, such as meningitis or encephalitis. Infants may also have a **febrile seizure,** in which the fever itself is the reason for the seizure. The exact mechanism of the seizure is unknown, but the fever is thought to lower the threshold for a seizure in children 6 months to 6 years of age. A **simple febrile seizure** is tonic-clonic in nature and lasts less than 15 minutes. This type of seizure usually causes no permanent injury. A **complex febrile seizure** is focal in nature or lasts longer than 15 minutes. This type of seizure is cause for greater concern.

Metabolic disturbances can lead to seizures. A common metabolic cause is **hypoglycemia.** EMTs must investigate the possibility that the infant or child ingested a toxic substance. Ask the caregivers about any medicines in the household. Alcohol and illicit drugs can lead to seizures and should also be considered in the pediatric age group.

Supplemental oxygen should be administered to a patient who is having a seizure or who is in the post-ictal period. This improves hypoxia (decreased levels of oxygen in the blood) in a patient in respiratory distress, which may have led to seizure activity.

Some seizures have no recognizable cause. These are called *idiopathic* (unknown cause) seizures.

It is worth noting that certain nonepileptic events may appear to be seizures to caregivers and medical personnel (Table 31-4). For example, **breath-holding spells** occur in children 6 months to 4 years of age, typically in response to an event that causes fear, anger, or agitation. The patient may cry vigorously and then hold his or her breath, turning pale or cyanotic. The patient may become stiff briefly and subsequently limp, which may lead to jerking movements. Breath-holding spells, however, are not followed by a postictal period. This helps to distinguish them from seizures. **Syncope,** or fainting, may also be confused with a seizure.

Treatment of Seizures

The first priority with a seizure patient is to assess the ABCs. Airway patency is the first step. A patient having a seizure may have an airway obstruction from secretions, emesis, or tongue position. Such an obstruction puts the patient at risk for aspiration and hypoventilation. Simply positioning the airway, using the jaw thrust maneuver, may help clear this obstruction. Remember to perform this maneuver with cervical spine precautions if trauma is a factor.

Suction is vital for clearing the airway of secretions or emesis (or both) and preventing aspiration. An airway adjunct (oral or nasopharyngeal) also may help keep the airway patent. However, do not place an oral airway, or anything else, in the mouth of an actively seizing patient. If no cervical spine trauma is suspected, the patient can be placed on his or her side to help drain secretions.

After the airway has been secured, administer 100% oxygen, because apnea and subsequent hypoxia are common with seizures. Moreover, hypoxia may be the very reason for the seizure in a patient in respiratory distress. BVM with cricoid pressure can facilitate ventilation in a patient with respiratory depression or apnea. A transient seizure is unlikely to cause the patient any permanent damage. However, rapid transport to an ED is essential, because the underlying condition that caused the seizure may lead to further seizures and clinical deterioration.

■ PEDIATRIC TRAUMA

In the United States, trauma accounts for more than 20,000 pediatric deaths each year. Most fatalities are caused by head injuries, followed by thoracic and abdominal injuries. Most traumatic injuries occur secondary to motor vehicle–related incidents, but falls, bicycle accidents, and child abuse are common causes.[5]

The head often takes the brunt of traumatic forces because it accounts for much of the pediatric patient's weight. Furthermore, the child's large head and weak cervical muscles result in higher cervical neck fractures than are found in adults. Other anatomic features make infants and children more susceptible to injury than adults. These include the pediatric patient's relatively smaller pelvis and rib cage and underdeveloped abdominal muscles. These features, as well as the child's proportionately larger solid organs, lead to a greater vulnerability to intraabdominal injury. Finally, the greater ratio of surface area to mass in infants and children results in increased oxygen demand and more rapid heat loss, creating a unique potential for hypothermia.[5]

For children who have suffered trauma, the EMT's main task is to stabilize the patient and rapidly transport the child to an emergency facility. Because the head and neck are particularly susceptible to injury in pediatric patients, you must be alert for signs and symptoms of intracranial injury. These include vomiting, confusion, agitation, and lethargy, as well as bradycardia and high blood pressure. If the patient needs airway protection because of an altered level of consciousness, perform a jaw thrust maneuver with cervical spine precautions and use airway adjuncts as needed to maintain patency. Age-appropriate cervical collars should be readily available. If an appropriate-

///CAUTION!

Never use sandbags to stabilize a patient's head and neck.

sized cervical collar is not available, use rolled towels and tape or small head blocks to maintain neutral head and neck alignment.

For an injured infant or child, a brief assessment includes checking for airway patency and ensuring adequate ventilation (using the AVPU assessment to determine the level of consciousness), ensuring cervical spine immobilization, and looking for any site of active bleeding that may require a compressive dressing during transport. These critical parts of the evaluation should be repeated intermittently during immediate, rapid transport of these victims.

■ CHILD ABUSE

The term *child abuse* is used to describe a range of behaviors that are destructive to the normal growth, development, and well-being of a child. Abuse may be divided into four categories: (1) physical abuse, (2) sexual abuse, (3) neglect, and (4) emotional abuse. Numerous factors can lead to child abuse, but the two primary causes are family stress and a lack of knowledge of child rearing.

EMTs are most likely to suspect physical abuse and neglect. Therefore they should become familiar with these conditions so that they are able to recognize a problem. EMTs often see an infant or a child in the home environment. For this reason, they have a unique advantage in assessing the situation and evaluating the possibility of abuse (Box 31-4).[6]

Physical Abuse

Physical abuse is the result of improper or excessive actions that injure or cause harm. The manifestations of abuse can affect any body system.

Skin

The skin is the most commonly injured organ with child abuse. Bruises and abrasions on the forehead, elbows, knees, and shins are common in active children and are not worrisome. However, bruises and abrasions that are more centrally located, such as on the buttocks, abdomen, back, or chest, are more suspicious for abuse. Bruises in various stages of healing

BOX 31-4
Risk Factors for the Development of Abuse

Familial Stress Factors
- Economic difficulty/low income
- Poor housing
- Joblessness/unemployment
- Illness of a family member
- Crowded living conditions

Psychological Factors (Parents)
- Impulse disorder
- Depression or other mental illness
- Alcohol/drug abuse
- Mental retardation

Child Factor
- Provocative behavior

Parenting Factors
- Lack of preparation for parenting role
- Poor parental role models
- Unrealistic expectations for the child
- Use of corporal punishment
- Unsupportive spouse
- Inconsistent parenting practices

Social Factors
- Social isolation
- Distant or absent extended family
- High societal expectations for all parents
- Acceptance of violence

Modified from Ludwig S: Child abuse. In Fleisher GR, Ludwig S, Henretig FM, et al: *Textbook of pediatric emergency medicine,* ed 4, Philadelphia, 2000, Lippincott Williams & Wilkins.

also raise concern, as do those with certain shapes or patterns, such as a belt buckle, an electrical cord, or the imprint of a hand. Burns and bite marks also are common nonaccidental lesions. Burns in particular account for approximately 5% of physical abuse cases.[7] These can be in the shape of a cigarette butt, or they may have an immersion pattern (typically, covering the buttocks and feet). Immersion injuries occur when an infant or a child is held down in hot water.

Bones

Broken bones are a common phenomenon in young children who are active and curious. Unfortunately, they are also common in child abuse. Certain fractures are associated with abuse, especially

SPECIAL Considerations

Is this Abuse?
A number of "red flags" should alert the EMT to suspect child abuse. These warning signs are as follows:
- The injury is not consistent with the mechanism described.
- EMTs make repeated calls to the same address.
- The parent or parents are inappropriately unconcerned about the child's injury.
- Conflicting stories are told about the circumstances of the injury.
- The child is afraid to discuss the injury.

when the history does not adequately explain the physical findings. Fractures associated with a twisting, pulling, or yanking force produce typical x-ray findings. For the EMT's purposes, the location of a fracture should trigger a suspicion of child abuse. A clavicle fracture or an elbow fracture is common in an active, ambulatory child. In contrast, a fracture of the femur, especially in a very young child (under 2 years of age), without a significant mechanism, is highly suspicious for abuse. Other injured areas that should raise concern are the ribs, sternum, vertebrae, skull, and pelvis.

Mouth

Injuries to the mouth may be a red flag for child abuse. A torn **frenulum** in infants, which can occur as a result of "bottle jamming," or dental trauma in older children may be caused by physical assault.

Brain

Brain injuries produce some of the most devastating effects of child abuse. Shaken baby syndrome occurs when an infant or a child is shaken violently, leading to diffuse brain damage. This ultimately may be lethal or at the very least may result in permanent developmental delay, blindness, deafness, or seizures.

Neglect

Neglect means giving insufficient attention or respect to someone who has a claim to that attention. It is the most prevalent form of child abuse.

SPECIAL Considerations

Health Care Provider Debriefing

The plight of a sick or injured child affects not only the family, but also the EMS providers and emergency department staff who care for the child. Sometimes the emotional response of these health care providers can be underestimated and unfortunately overlooked. This may result in suppressed and therefore unresolved anxiety about caring for children. For this reason, it is crucial that all members of the heath care team have a debriefing of the events in a particularly difficult case. At the debriefing, health care providers are allowed to voice their concerns and emotions. Making this a routine practice helps alleviate stress and gives the health care team a means of preventing unnecessary fear and burnout. However, with a particularly devastating pediatric case, health care providers, like the patient and family, may require extended time and possibly professional counseling to adjust.[8]

However, it often goes unnoticed for some time. A diagnosis of child neglect is difficult to make because it is more subjective and often lacks physical evidence.

EMTs must be able to recognize the manifestations of neglect. Failure to thrive or a lack of food and feeding skills is a common finding. A child who has very thin extremities and a protuberant abdomen likely is showing signs of malnourishment. *Medical neglect*, or the failure to provide needed health care, is a form of neglect.

Abandonment

Abandonment, or a total lack of supervision, is a safety hazard for children and infants. Abandonment is difficult to define. No societal standards have been established either for the appropriate age at which children can be left alone or for the length of time they can be left alone. Leaving a 2-year-old for 20 minutes may be considered abandonment, whereas leaving a 10-year-old for 8 hours may not be. Again, EMTs are in a unique position to evaluate for abandonment, because they often visit the home environment and can assess for parental supervision and overall safety. EMTs should be familiar with any laws in their state that may define at what age and in what conditions adolescents may be left without adult supervision.

Medical-Legal Responsibilities

When child abuse is suspected in good faith, physicians are required by law to report it. Likewise, EMTs also have the responsibility to report suspected child abuse to the receiving facility. Local regulations in each jurisdiction may more clearly define these specific responsibilities. EMTs should objectively relay any pertinent information to the receiving personnel, including concerns about abuse or neglect.

EMTs should not make accusations at the scene. This probably would alienate the family, fuel conflict, and delay transport of the patient. Careful documentation of the history and physical findings is very helpful, particularly regarding the caregiver's explanation of the mechanism of injury. ED personnel can use this documentation to support their own findings, because the caregiver's story may change when the suspicion of child abuse is raised.

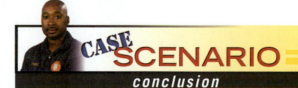

CASE SCENARIO
conclusion

As Alice comforted her son, Jack carefully held an oxygen teddy near Jerome, gently rocking it back and forth. Quickly, he quieted and gently reached for the bear. With Elizabeth's coaching, soon he was cradling the bear, and supplementing himself with oxygen in the process. The rest of the call went smoothly; later Jack and Elizabeth discussed how sometimes the best medicine is a caring touch. ■

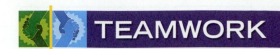

TEAMWORK

EMTs can take a crucial step toward improving the care of infants and children in their community by becoming involved in injury prevention programs. Teaching families how to create a safer environment for their children will reduce the number of childhood deaths caused by illness and injury. Vital subjects that EMTs can cover include the following:

- Helmet safety
- Proper use of infant and child car seats and restraints
- Smoke and carbon monoxide detectors
- Childproof containers for hazardous household materials
- Storage of firearms in locked containers
- Water safety (for pools, beaches, and bathtubs)
- Planning of escape routes in case of fire
- CPR

The EMT is in a unique position to see different patients in different environments. EMTs must work as a team to put together educational strategies and to lobby for changes in the law to make the world a safer place for children.

References

1. Hazinski MF et al: *PALS provider manual: basic life support for the PALS healthcare provider*, Dallas, 2002, American Heart Association.
2. Hazinski MF et al: *PALS provider manual: airway, ventilation, and management of respiratory distress and failure*, Dallas, 2002, American Heart Association.
3. Hazinski MF et al: *PALS provider manual: recognition of respiratory failure and shock*, Dallas, 2002, American Heart Association.
4. Chiang VW: Seizures. In Fleisher GR, Ludwig S et al, editors: *Textbook of pediatric emergency medicine*, ed 4, Philadelphia, 2000, Lippincott Williams & Wilkins.
5. Sanchez J, Paidas C: Childhood trauma: now and in the new millennium, *Surg Clin North Am* 79:1503-1535, 1999.
6. Ludwig S: Child abuse. In Fleisher GR, Ludwig S et al, editors: *Textbook of pediatric emergency medicine*, ed 4, Philadelphia, 2000, Lippincott Williams & Wilkins.
7. Gorelick MH: Neurologic emergencies. In Fleisher GR, Ludwig S et al, editors: *Textbook of pediatric emergency medicine*, ed 4, Philadelphia, 2000, Lippincott Williams & Wilkins.
8. Scott K: The psychological aspects of pediatric trauma: perspectives on patient, family and provider, *Surg Clin North Am* 82:419-434, 2002.

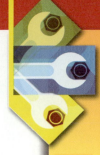

Critical Points

To provide optimal field care, the EMT must know the anatomic, physiologic, and emotional milestones of the pediatric patient. Pediatric patients present many challenges for the EMT, because children may be particularly vulnerable to hemodynamic changes that occur after specific illnesses and injury patterns. The EMT is in a unique position to assess the patient's social situation and initiate care of the patient with a positive, family-centered approach.

Learning Checklist

❑ Motor skills in infancy and early childhood progress from head to toe. EMTs will find it helpful to familiarize themselves with some normal developmental milestones.

❑ Crying may be a response to multiple external stimuli, such as cold, pain, hunger, or a need for sleep.

❑ In infants, the brachial artery should be used to assess the pulse; in children, the radial or carotid artery may be used.

❑ EMTs should assume that a lethargic baby who does not respond well to external stimulation is very ill. These patients need rapid transport to the hospital.

❑ Infants, especially, should be kept warm. They have an increased surface-to-mass ratio and therefore are susceptible to heat loss.

❑ Both infants and toddlers may have separation and stranger anxiety. They should be approached in a nonthreatening manner with the help of the caregiver.

❑ To build trust, the EMT should begin the assessment of the pediatric patient away from the area of pain or discomfort.

❑ Toddlers are often modest about undressing in front of strangers. At this age, they are becoming aware of their sexual identity.

❑ School-age children may be afraid of permanent disfiguration or injury.

❑ The child's airway is relatively shorter and smaller than the adult's airway. Also, the child's tongue is relatively larger.

❑ Respiratory distress in the pediatric patient may manifest as tachypnea, hyperpnea, nasal flaring, accessory muscle use, and retractions.

❑ An essential skill for managing the pediatric upper airway is age-appropriate airway suctioning.

❑ Airflow is highly dependent on the radius of the airway and the patient's work of breathing.

❑ Oxygen delivery systems include low-flow systems (blow-by oxygen, nasal cannula, and simple face masks) and high-flow systems (partial and complete nonrebreather masks).

❑ In respiratory failure, the EMT must take over management of the airway and breathing to provide adequate oxygenation and ventilation of the patient.

❑ Nasal and oral airway devices help maintain airway patency in a patient with an altered level of consciousness.

❑ The sniffing position is the best orientation for lining up the oral, pharyngeal, and tracheal axes.

❑ An infant may need to have a towel placed under the shoulders, whereas a child more likely will need one under the head to achieve an open airway.

❑ To avoid overinflation, EMTs can pace themselves by saying the words "squeeze-release-release" when bagging a pediatric patient.

❑ During active bagging, the E-C technique should be used to apply the face mask on the pediatric patient.

❑ Cricoid pressure should be applied during active ventilation to prevent insufflation of the pediatric stomach.

❑ Some common respiratory emergencies in pediatric patients are upper airway obstruction, croup, bronchiolitis, epiglottitis, asthma, and pneumonia.

❑ Shock is a mismatch between oxygen delivery and tissue metabolic demands.

❑ The pediatric patient may deteriorate rapidly from compensated to decompensated shock.

❑ The main categories of shock are cardiogenic shock, distributive shock, and hypovolemic shock.

NUTS AND BOLTS

- End organ perfusion may be assessed using pulses, capillary refill time, and level of consciousness (i.e., the Glasgow Coma Scale or AVPU assessment tool).
- Pediatric cardiac arrest usually occurs secondary to a primary respiratory event.
- Contrary to popular perception, primary cardiac arrest in a pediatric patient has a very poor prognosis.
- SIDS in infants under 1 year of age and trauma in all other age groups top the list of causes of pediatric cardiac arrest.
- Seizures are common in childhood.
- A seizure may be followed by a confused or postictal state.
- The mainstays of treatment of the seizure patient are airway protection and oxygenation.
- The EMT must maintain a high level of suspicion for head trauma with a pediatric patient who is having a seizure.
- Child abuse may take many forms, including physical and sexual abuse, neglect, and abandonment.
- The EMT is in a unique position to assess the social setting and level of suspicion for abuse.
- Skin, oral, genital, or head injuries may be clues to cases of child abuse.
- Inconsistencies between the physical findings and the explanations given for the patient's history should alert the EMT to the possibility of abuse.

Key Terms

Abandonment Loosely defined as a total lack of supervision leading to a safety hazard for the child or infant.

Anaphylaxis A severe, life-threatening hypersensitivity reaction to a previously encountered antigen. It results in vasodilation and subsequent hypotension.

Arrhythmia Any cardiac rhythm other than normal sinus rhythm, including bradycardias and tachycardias, of either atrial or ventricular origin.

AVPU A mnemonic assessment tool used to determine a person's mental status. The acronym stands for *a*lert (the person is alert, awake, and oriented); *v*erbal (the person responds to voice); *p*ainful stimuli (the person responds only to a painful stimulus); *u*nresponsive (the person is not awake and is completely unresponsive to any type of stimulation).

Bradyasystole A rhythm that is either slowed (brady) or completely absent (asystole).

Bradycardia A slow heart rate.

Breath-holding spells Episodes in which children hold their breath for approximately 30 to 60 seconds, resulting in cyanosis and sometimes syncope. This is rare before 6 months of age.

Cardiac arrest The halting of all functioning heart activity.

Cardiac ischemia A condition of inadequate oxygenation of the heart muscle, which results in heart dysfunction. It may be caused by decreased oxygen delivery or excessive cardiac demands.

Cardiogenic shock Shock caused by dysfunction of the heart.

Cardiopulmonary arrest Cessation of blood flow and respiratory function, either from a primary heart or lung event.

Central cyanosis Cyanosis that manifests as a bluish discoloration of the central areas of the body, indicating a more profound degree of hypoxia, or low-oxygen state.

Compensated shock Shock characterized by a normal systolic blood pressure with signs and symptoms of inadequate tissue perfusion.

Complex febrile seizure A febrile seizure that is focal and/or lasts longer than 15 minutes.

Contusion A closed soft tissue injury characterized by discoloration beneath the surface of the skin; a bruise.

Cricoid ring A cartilaginous ring at the junction of the larynx and the trachea.

Cyanosis Blue discoloration of the skin, signifying poor oxygen delivery to the tissues. The oxygen-carrying molecules in red blood cells (hemoglobin) take on a bluish color when not bound to oxygen. Therefore, when a high proportion of hemoglobin in the blood delivered to the tissues is not bound to oxygen, the tissues appear blue.

Decompensated shock The end stage of shock when hypotension is present.

Distributive shock Shock caused by a pathologic dilation of the blood vessels.

Emancipated minor A child who is released from the control of parents or guardians.

Epiglottis A curved flap of tissue that covers the opening of the trachea during swallowing to prevent food or liquid from entering the lower respiratory tract.

Epilepsy A group of neurologic disorders characterized by recurrent episodes of convulsive seizures, sensory disturbances, abnormal behavior, loss of consciousness, or all of these.

Febrile seizure A seizure caused by a rapid rise in body temperature.

Frenulum A small, midline flap of mucosal tissue on the inside of the lip or the bottom of the tongue.

Gag reflex The occurrence of gagging or vomiting as a result of stimulation of the posterior oropharynx.

Hypoglycemia A state of low blood sugar.

Hypopharynx The inferior portion of the larynx; it contains the superior openings of the larynx and the esophagus.

Hypovolemic shock Shock caused by a lack of adequate circulating volume. This can occur secondary to gastrointestinal losses, such as with vomiting and diarrhea, blood loss, or inadequate fluid intake.

Larynx The cartilaginous structure in the anterior neck that connects the posterior pharynx with the trachea in the upper airway; also known as the *voice box*.

Mucous membranes Layers of membranes found in the respiratory and digestive tracts.

Nasopharynx The air passageway immediately posterior to the nose that forms the upper portion of the pharynx.

Neglect Insufficient attention to or respect for someone who has a claim to that attention.

Nonrebreather mask A combination of a face mask, a bag reservoir, and a one-way flow valve that allows oxygen to flow from the reservoir into the mask without letting exhaled air into the reservoir. This ensures that a high concentration of oxygen is contained within the reservoir at all times and that a high concentration of oxygen is delivered with each inhalation.

Occiput The back of the skull.

Oropharynx The air cavity/passageway at the back of the mouth.

Postictal period The period immediately after a generalized seizure; it manifests as confusion, agitation, or somnolence.

Pulmonary arrest Cessation of respiratory function.

Respiratory distress An increase in the work of breathing. It may involve tachypnea (increased rate of breathing), hyperpnea (increased depth of breathing), nasal flaring, accessory muscle use, or retractions.

Respiratory failure A deterioration from respiratory distress; it requires the EMT to intervene and take over the work of breathing for the patient.

Sepsis A systemic response to a blood infection that results in hemodynamic instability, usually manifested by tachycardia and hypotension.

Shock A condition characterized by inadequate delivery of oxygen and nutrients to cells, resulting in organ system malfunction. Eventually shock is detectable through abnormal vital signs. It can lead to death. Five types of shock are cardiogenic shock, compensated shock, decompensated shock, distributive shock, and hypovolemic shock.

Simple febrile seizure A single tonic-clonic febrile seizure that lasts less than 15 minutes.

Status epilepticus A condition marked by seizures that persist or intermittently continue, without a return to a normal level of consciousness, for longer than 30 minutes.

Stridor A high-pitched, harsh, respiratory sound that indicates upper airway obstruction.

Structural cardiac abnormalities A condition marked by a grossly abnormal heart structure, including valve, muscle, and vessel positioning irregularities.

Submandibular Indicates the area under the mandible, or lower jaw.

Submental Indicates the area under the chin.

Sudden infant death syndrome (SIDS) The sudden, unexpected death of a previously healthy infant.

Syncope Fainting; a brief lapse in consciousness. Syncope may be preceded by a sensation of lightheadedness.

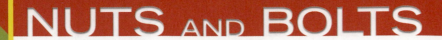
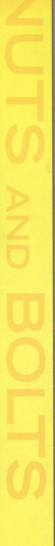

Tonic-clonic seizure A grand mal seizure. It is characterized by generalized involuntary muscle contractions and cessation of respiration, followed by tonic and clonic muscle spasms; breathing returns with noisy respirations.

National Standard Curriculum Objectives

Cognitive Objectives

After completing this lesson, the EMT student will be able to do the following:

- Describe the differences in anatomy, physiology, and development for infants, children, and adults.
- Explain how the differences in pediatric physiology become evident in the clinical presentation of the ill or injured infant or child.

- Define and identify respiratory distress and respiratory failure.
- Explain how to identify common causes of respiratory distress in the pediatric patient.
- Explain how to identify and treat a foreign body upper airway obstruction in an infant or a child.
- Describe the signs and symptoms of shock in the pediatric patient and explain how to perform a directed exam for end organ perfusion.
- List the common causes of cardiac arrest in pediatric patients.
- Describe the common causes and field management of pediatric seizures.
- Identify the unique injury patterns of the pediatric trauma patient.
- Describe the field management of the pediatric trauma patient.
- Describe the different categories of child abuse.

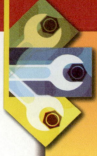

- List specific findings that lead to a suspicion of child abuse.
- Explain the need for EMT debriefing after a difficult case involving a pediatric patient.

Affective Objectives

After completing this lesson, the EMT student will be able to do the following:

- Understand the need for a thoughtful, sympathetic approach to dealing with the pediatric patient and caregivers.
- Understand and demonstrate responsiveness to the specific fears of the pediatric patient.
- Communicate openly, honestly, and empathetically with pediatric patients and caregivers.
- Understand the EMT's own emotional response to caring for ill or injured infants and children.

Psychomotor Objectives

After completing this lesson, the EMT student will be able to do the following:

- Demonstrate the assessment of an infant and a child.
- Demonstrate maneuvers for removing upper airway foreign body obstructions in an infant and in a child.
- Demonstrate oxygen delivery for an infant and for a child.
- Demonstrate bag-mask ventilations for an infant and for a child.
- Demonstrate chest compressions for an infant and for a child.
- Demonstrate the sequence of CPR for an infant and for a child.

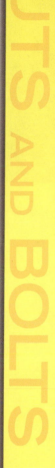

CHAPTER OUTLINE

Physiologic Changes with Age

Assessment

Reporting of Symptoms

Medical Emergencies

Trauma Emergencies

Abuse

LESSON GOAL

Interacting with, assessing, and treating geriatric patients are essential functions of an effective emergency medical technician (EMT). This chapter looks at the important differences between elderly patients and younger patients. It also explains the physiologic changes that occur with aging. Communications differences, the effects of medications, and common fears of older patients are discussed, as are common medical emergencies and traumatic injuries and their management ■

Geriatric Emergencies

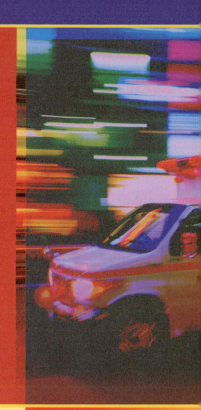

CHAPTER OBJECTIVES

After completing this chapter, the EMT student will be able to do the following:

1 Explain the normal physiologic changes that occur with aging.

2 Discuss common fears geriatric patients may have about obtaining health care.

3 Discuss the communications skills that should be used with an elderly patient.

4 Describe changes the EMT may need to make when assessing an elderly patient.

5 Discuss common medical emergencies that occur in the elderly.

6 Discuss common traumatic injuries that occur in the elderly.

7 Explain how medications can affect the patient's presentation.

8 Discuss changes the EMT may need to make in managing an elderly patient.

9 Describe signs of abuse of an elderly patient.

CASE SCENARIO

"Mrs. Applegard? Mrs. Applegard? Are you in there?" Elizabeth knocks on the door loudly one more time. The ambulance crew is at the senior citizen high-rise complex for a report of a "person down" inside one of the apartments. Not hearing anything, the crew chief motions the building superintendent to unlock the door. It opens onto a narrow, tidy hallway lit by several small ceiling lights. At the far end of the hallway, Elizabeth can see a bathroom, in which the light also is on. Faintly, she hears a woman calling for help.

After checking the scene for any unusual odors or other safety problems, the crew make their way to the bathroom. Mrs. Applegard, a 77-year-old woman with Parkinson's disease, is lying on the bathroom floor, still in her nightgown. The original report states that she had not been heard from for nearly 18 hours. She typically calls her daughter each morning and evening, but she had failed to call this morning. Kneeling beside the patient, Elizabeth sees that Mrs. Applegard has a bruise on the left side of her head and that her left leg is abnormally rotated inward. The patient also is incontinent of urine, and her nightgown is wet.

Questions: *What potential injuries should be suspected in this situation? What initial interventions are indicated? How might the patient best be removed from the apartment?*

As an EMT, you will interact with geriatric patients on a daily basis. Not only do the elderly (age 65 years or greater) use health care more than any other age group, they also are the fastest growing segment of society. Currently, older adults make up approximately 12% of the population. With the aging of the baby boomers, the elderly soon will account for approximately 33% of the population. This "graying of society" will pose several unique challenges for the health care system and for emergency medical services (EMS).

As an EMT, you must understand the factors that are unique to this age group so that important yet subtle information and findings are not overlooked (Fig. 32-1). You need a basic knowledge of the physiologic changes that occur in people as they age and of the ways these changes affect communication, your assessment, and the patient's presentation. An understanding of the ways medications can affect these factors also is important.

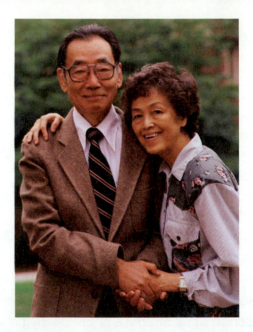

Fig. 32-1 The elderly are the largest population group served by emergency medical services. EMTs must understand the physiologic differences between the geriatric patient and the average adult.

PHYSIOLOGIC CHANGES WITH AGE

Do you know the saying, "After 30, you're over the hill"? Have you ever wondered where that saying originated? It actually arose from a medical fact. After the age of 30, the functions of a person's organs start to decline, and they continue to do so each succeeding year of life. By age 60, as much as 30% of organ function has been lost. As individual cells in an organ die, new cells replace them. However, eventually the rate of loss exceeds the rate of replacement, and the result is dysfunction or death of the organ. Based solely on the loss and replacement rates of

Physiologic Dead Space

Physiologic dead space is the term used for the amount of inhaled air that is unavailable for gas exchange and thus metabolic use. Physiologic dead space is made up of two components. One component is the **anatomic dead space;** in adults, this is the approximately 150 ml of air in the trachea and mainstem bronchi. The other component is the amount of space taken up by nonfunctional alveoli; these alveoli have been damaged by exposure to noxious gases or by the normal aging process, or they are ventilated but poorly perfused. Although anatomic dead space remains fairly constant among adults, the total physiologic dead space differs from person to person. To determine the potential effect of physiologic dead space, you should take into account your patient's age, the environment in which the person may have worked, and whether the patient has any history of smoking.

Minute Volume

To calculate the minute volume (MVa), subtract the amount of physiologic dead space (VD) from the tidal volume (TV) and multiply the result by the respiratory rate (RR), as stated in the following equation:

$$MVa = (TV - VD) \times RR$$

cells, the estimated human life span would be 115 to 120 years. However, the effects of disease cause most people to die of organ dysfunction much earlier than that. As an EMT, you must be able to differentiate the normal physiologic changes of aging from changes caused by a disease process that requires treatment.

The Respiratory System

With aging, the chest wall loses its elasticity and ability to expand fully. The alveoli also decrease in number, surface area, and effectiveness. These conditions lead to a reduction in tidal volume and vital capacity and an increase in physiologic dead space and residual volume.

As discussed in Chapter 7, **minute volume** (the amount of air reaching the alveoli each minute) is the critical component in determining the effectiveness of respiratory effort and respiratory status. Because the minute volume is equal to the tidal volume (minus physiologic dead space) multiplied by the respiratory rate, older patients must compensate for the decreased tidal volume.

Because of the inverse relationship of this formula, a decreased tidal volume results in an increased respiratory rate to maintain adequate minute volume. Therefore geriatric patients normally may

have a respiratory rate higher than 20 breaths per minute because their tidal volume is smaller. EMTs must keep in mind that an increased resting respiratory rate may be normal and may not necessarily be a sign of distress or disease. However, they also must remember that elderly patients are less able to compensate for respiratory distress by increasing the respiratory rate, because they are already doing so to maintain a normal minute volume.

The increase in residual volume (the amount of air left in the lungs after maximum exhalation) can lead to retention of carbon dioxide. This retention in turn can lead to confusion, altered mental status, and respiratory acidosis. Spinal curvature that leads to a dorsal hump **(kyphosis)** also reduces lung capacity and compliance.

The Cardiovascular System

Cardiac disease remains the leading cause of death among the elderly. As people age, the elasticity of the cardiovascular tissue decreases, and the heart is less able to circulate the blood efficiently to meet metabolic demands. Heart rate and **stroke volume** decline, resulting in a decrease in **cardiac output,** specifically during times of stress or exercise. (Remember: Cardiac output = Stroke volume × Heart rate.) The size of the heart may decrease as cells are lost faster than they can be replaced. However, in individuals with systemic hypertension, the myocardium in the left ventricle may be enlarged (left ventricular hypertrophy). In individuals with pulmonary hypertension, the myocardium of the right ventricle (right ventricular hypertrophy) may be enlarged.

The cells responsible for creating electrical impulses also decrease in number with age. As a result, abnormal pacemaker sites control the heart's electrical conduction system and cause abnormal heart rhythms (dysrhythmias). Approximately 80% of elderly patients have a pulse that is sometimes irregular. This is the result of a heart rhythm called **atrial fib-**

rillation, in which various cells of the atria fire randomly, generating the heart's electrical stimulus. This condition can have serious consequences. It causes loss of atrial filling (another name for atrial filling is *atrial kick*, which accounts for 25% to 30% of stroke volume). It also promotes the formation of clots (mural thrombi) on the atrial walls. If one of these clots breaks off and enters the circulation, the patient is at high risk for a pulmonary embolism or stroke.

In addition to the heart becoming stiff and inelastic, the peripheral blood vessels lose their elasticity. This results in a decreased ability to compensate for sudden changes in blood pressure or blood loss. Older patients may become lightheaded or dizzy when they move from the supine position to the sitting or standing position. The sudden change in position causes a drop in blood pressure for which the older body cannot compensate as quickly as can a younger body (Box 32-1).

Narrowing of the blood vessels caused by the buildup of fatty deposits (**atherosclerosis**) also occurs with aging. This can leave the circulatory system unable to provide blood to organs during times of increased metabolic demand. In addition, atherosclerosis increases the risk of heart attack, particularly in patients with other risk factors for heart disease, such as smoking. Older patients also are at increased risk of diseases such as aortic aneurysm or dissection (separation of the layers of the artery).

The Skin

As a person gets older, the amounts of elastin and collagen in the skin decrease, reducing the skin's elasticity (Fig. 32-2). The underlying subcutaneous tissue thins, and muscle atrophy occurs. This causes the loose skin and wrinkling commonly seen in the hands and over the joints of elderly patients. EMTs must keep in mind that this normal loose, wrinkled

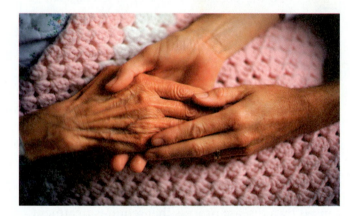

Fig. 32-2 Wrinkled, loose skin on the back of the hand is the result of a decrease in elastin and collagen; it should not be mistaken for poor skin turgor.

skin can give a false positive result if skin turgor is assessed inappropriately (Box 32-2).

Various glands that produce sweat and oils also become inactive with age. This leads to further drying of the skin. In addition, it reduces the body's ability to regulate the internal temperature. Pigments that provide color diminish, and the skin assumes a translucent appearance. As a result of all these changes, the skin becomes dry, thin, flaky, and brittle. Therefore it lacerates and tears much more easily than the skin of younger adults. Also, bleeding is not easily stopped and can result in external bleeding or large hematomas under the skin. Take care not to cause a **skin tear** when you move and handle an elderly patient. If a tear occurs, completely document the events surrounding the incident, your assessment of the tear, and your treatment.

BOX 32-2
Skin Turgor

Skin turgor can be a valuable means of assessing a patient's hydration status. You most likely were taught to perform this test on the back of the hand. However, consider the effects of normal aging on this procedure. As the skin loses its elasticity and underlying structures, tenting on the back of the hand can occur in a normally hydrated elderly individual. Assessing skin turgor in this location can give you a false positive result. In elderly patients, skin turgor is best assessed over the sternum or on the abdomen, where the skin retains its elasticity and underlying structure longer than it does on the back of the hand.

ASK YOURSELF

Picture your grandparents or an elderly person you know. Ever wonder, "Why do they move a little slower than me? Are they really that different from me? Do I need to speak louder to get my point across?"

The Nervous System

Normal changes with aging should not include changes in general intelligence and mentation until age 70 or later. Any significant changes at an earlier age should raise suspicion of an underlying disease, such as presenile dementia. As a person ages, the number of neurons declines, resulting in **atrophy** (shrinkage) of the brain. Also, neural impulses are transmitted more slowly, resulting in slowed responses and decreased sensation.

Sensory Changes

Hearing loss at the higher frequencies generally begins in the fifth decade of life. A further decrease in sound conduction to the inner ear can also occur as a result of loss of hair cells in the organ of Corti. Vision changes are more pronounced than hearing changes. The lens of the eye becomes thicker and more rigid with age, which can lead to loss of visual clarity and to cataract formation, which further impairs vision. The muscles of the iris become weaker, resulting in smaller pupils and difficulty seeing in dim environments. The peripheral visual fields narrow, causing "tunnel vision" and leaving the person unable to see people or objects to the sides.

Sensory losses can lead to unique challenges for EMTs during the patient interview. When speaking with an elderly patient, be sure to position yourself directly in front of the person and speak in a low tone of voice. If the patient has eyeglasses or a hearing aid, be sure to take them to the hospital with you (Fig. 32-3 and Box 32-3). (See Chapter 14 for more detailed information about communications issues in treating elderly patients.)

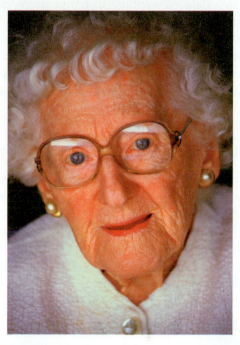

Fig. 32-3 Take a moment to retrieve any sensory aids; they are important to the patient.

BOX 32-3
Sensory Aids

Sensory aids, such as eyeglasses and hearing aids, and other items, such as dentures, are very important to the elderly patient. Not only do they represent a significant financial expense if they must be replaced, they also are critical for performing daily functions. Don't be surprised if patients remain fixated on the location of these items until they are given to them or until they are sure the items are in a safe place. If you do not leave the items in the patient's direct possession at the hospital, be sure to tell the person with whom you left them. These items, along with prescription medications and driver's licenses, are the belongings patients most often call to report as missing after an ambulance transport.

Thermoregulation

The hypothalamus is responsible for **thermoregulation** in the body. When the body temperature gets too low, shivering and vasoconstriction are stimulated in an attempt both to generate heat and to conserve heat in the core of the body. Conversely, when the temperature gets too high, the body uses the mechanisms of vasodilation and sweating to rid itself of excess heat. Several factors make the elderly more susceptible to heat- and cold-related emergencies. For example, the number and effectiveness of thermoreceptors in the body decline, resulting in a delayed response to temperature variances in the environment. Because of the decrease in muscle mass that occurs with aging, shivering is not as effective at generating heat as it is at a younger age. The loss of blood vessel elasticity diminishes vasoconstriction and vasodilation and does not allow for the conservation or dissipation of heat as in younger individuals.

The Immune System

The body's ability to fight infection declines with age as a result of diminished functioning of the immune system. The thymus gland (where T cells are produced) is very large at birth and during infancy but shrinks as a person ages. Septic shock arising from infection, often of the urinary tract, is a common cause of death in elderly individuals.

The Musculoskeletal System

In older people, new bone production is exceeded by bone resorption. This leads to a loss of bone mass and more fragile bones. Vertebral disks flatten, causing a decrease in height. Kyphosis also contributes to this loss of height (Fig. 32-4). The decrease in bone

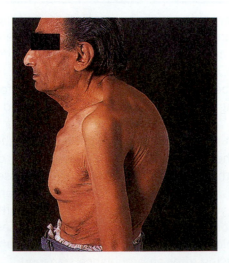

Fig. 32-4 Patient with kyphosis.

mass is accompanied by a decrease in underlying tissues around the joints, which causes the bony prominences to become more visible. In addition to the muscle atrophy mentioned earlier, the tendons lose their elasticity. Muscle fatigue can set in quickly in older patients, and the weight-bearing bones are more prone to fracture because of the loss of bone mass and muscular support.

■ ASSESSMENT

Assessment of a geriatric patient follows the same pattern and format as those used for any patient. However, certain differences must be taken into account with an elderly patient.

Scene Size-Up

The scene size-up for patients in this age group differs little from that for any EMT call. Assess the scene for your own safety and that of any other emergency responders. In addition, assess the scene for indicators of the underlying complaint. Check for clues to the patient's general condition. Is there a car in the driveway that looks as if it is driven daily? Is a wheelchair ramp attached to the house? What is the overall condition and maintenance of the exterior of the house? If the call is to a residence, you have a unique opportunity to observe the patient's living conditions and overall status. Is there food in the house? Is the house neat and clean? Are there overflowing ashtrays next to an oxygen tank? Is alcohol abuse a factor? Are there dirty dishes piled up and half-eaten food around the house? Are there trip hazards? What is the temperature? Are there pill bottles present, and if so, what are the medications? The answers to these questions can give you valuable insight into both the patient's general health and possible causes of the person's current distress.

Initial Assessment

The steps in the initial assessment are the same for all patients. The goal is to detect immediate life threats and determine the type of call to which you have responded.

General Impression

What is your general impression of the patient? Does the person acknowledge you as you enter the room, indicating a conscious and alert state? How is the patient dressed? Is the person well groomed or unkempt and unable to perform self-care? Is the person in obvious respiratory distress, as indicated by the use of accessory muscles and positioning? Is the patient leaning forward and clutching his or her chest (Levine's sign), which may lead you to suspect chest pain as the reason for the call? Are any signs of hemorrhage or other injury obvious? Information gathered from the general impression, combined with that from the scene assessment, can give you valuable clues to the patient's condition and general health status.

Mental Status Assessment

Determine the patient's level of consciousness. Is the patient conscious and alert? Does the person respond only to verbal or painful stimuli?

What is the patient's baseline score on the Glasgow Coma Scale? Determine whether the patient is conscious, alert, and responding to questions appropriately. In a younger adult, this often is done by determining the patient's orientation to person, place, time, and situation. In an elderly patient, however, you may have to alter your approach.

Determine the elderly patient's normal mental status by asking family members or caregivers and alter your line of questioning appropriately (Fig. 32-5). Patients rarely do not know their own name. However, if this is the case or if the patient's inability to remember his or her name is new, strongly consider a disease process such as stroke as the cause.

Answers to questions about place may vary based on the patient's normal mental status. Elderly patients may not know their exact address. However, they often can tell you whether they are at home, at

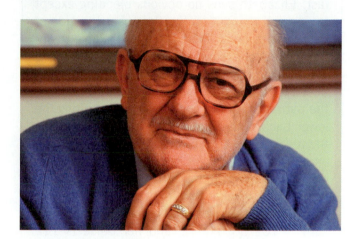

SPECIAL Considerations

Cultural Perspectives

Take care to avoid "invisible patient syndrome." As with any other patient, you need to talk to and with older patients, rather than talking about them. Talking to someone else in the room as though the patient were incapable of understanding or were not there shows disrespect.

Fig. 32-5 Determine the patient's normal mental status by asking family members or caregivers. Then alter your line of questioning appropriately when talking to the patient.

---

the hospital, or in an ambulance, or they can answer other questions appropriately. You must determine whether an answer is appropriate based on family members' or caregivers' response about the patient's normal mental status. If patients are unable to tell you their location, try to determine whether they recognize their surroundings and the people around them. Correct answers to these questions also indicate that the patient is oriented to place.

Elderly individuals often follow the same routine regardless of the day or date. Therefore these patients frequently do not answer correctly when you ask questions about the day or the date. First, determine whether the patient is normally aware of the day and date. If so, an inability to remember the day and date during your contact with the patient indicates an altered mental status that is new. If the patient does not normally know the exact day and date, alter your line of questioning appropriately. Most patients can recall the approximate time of day. Therefore asking whether it is early morning, morning, afternoon,

---

Important Points

During your training, you may have been taught to use a sternal rub to determine a patient's level of responsiveness. However, place yourself in the position of the bystanders for this procedure. You have been called to treat their elderly friend or family member and, as they see it, the first thing you do is beat on the patient's chest. Not only does this look barbaric, it also may create scene safety problems by upsetting the bystanders. In addition, this procedure has caused injuries in elderly patients. Rather than a sternal rub, use a subtler, less harmful application of a painful stimulus, such as a web space pinch or pressure on the nail beds.

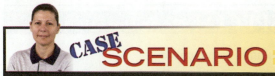

CASE SCENARIO

continued

While one crew member carefully stabilizes the patient's cervical spine, Elizabeth begins her assessment. Mrs. Applegard's airway appears patent, and her respiratory rate is 22 breaths per minute. Her wrist feels very cool when Elizabeth checks for the radial pulse, which is faint and fast. Elizabeth sees no obvious bleeding except for a small amount on the floor near the side of the patient's head. Mrs. Applegard is able to answer questions slowly, but her answers seem confused.

A rapid trauma assessment reveals pain in the patient's left hip and shoulder and along the lower back. There appears to be a deformity in the area of the left hip. Breath sounds are clear, and the patient denies any chest or abdominal pain. She cannot move her left leg, and the left hand seems weaker than the right hand. For the first set of vital signs, the patient's blood pressure is 102/68 mm Hg and her pulse is 112 beats per minute and regular.

Questions: *Is Mrs. Applegard's condition stable or unstable? What injuries and illnesses are more likely, given the physical findings? How might the environment affect the patient's condition?*

---

evening, or night can provide more accurate information about the patient's awareness of time.

Finally, determine the patient's awareness of the situation. This, too, varies based on the patient's normal mental status and ability. Simply asking, "What happened today?" often is enough to determine situation awareness. If the patient normally is unable to answer this type of question, you may have to ask the person what is going on around him or her or other such questions. Family members, caregivers, and others familiar with the patient are valuable assets in this situation. Be sure to enlist their help when you are determining whether an answer is correct or appropriate for the patient or a change in mental status and ability.

When documenting the findings of the mental status exam, EMTs generally use statements such as, "The patient is conscious and alert ×4, responding to all questions appropriately," or, "The patient is alert

to person and place only." These statements are based on the assumption that a patient normally is alert to person, place, time, and situation. However, EMTs often treat elderly patients whose normal mental status enables them to answer only certain questions correctly. In this situation, the EMT's documentation should reflect that a finding that would be considered abnormal in a younger patient is actually a normal finding for this patient. For example, you might note, "The patient is alert to person and place only; however, according to family members on scene, this is normal for the patient, and they deny any acute change in mental status."

Airway

The airway itself does not undergo many specific changes after 8 years of age. However, the EMT must consider a number of issues when ensuring the patency of the airway in a geriatric patient. For example, the cough and the gag reflexes diminish with age. This can result in an inability to clear secretions, leading to airway obstruction and a greater need for suctioning. The muscles of the upper airway weaken (as do all muscles), which can allow the tongue to occlude the airway more easily than in a younger adult. Dentures quickly can create complete airway obstruction if they become dislodged. Therefore EMTs should always ask about or assess for the presence of dentures in a geriatric patient. Dentures that are securely in place should be left in the mouth. Loose-fitting or partially dislodged dentures should be removed and brought in with the patient. With age, sensory stimuli to the hard palate diminish. This decrease in sensory input is even greater if a patient's dentures have a plate that completely covers the hard

---

Important Points

The origin of the term *café coronary* is unknown. The term is commonly used to describe choking incidents that occur when a person is eating. However, the term is a misnomer, because the condition is not related to the heart or to coronary circulation and function. The circumstances actually describe a foreign body airway obstruction, which occurs when a person tries to swallow a piece of food that is too large and a choking emergency results. This condition is more common in elderly patients. It often is associated with the presence of dentures, the consumption of alcohol, or both.

palate. The lack of palatal sensation often leads to a condition known as a *café coronary*. With this condition, the person cannot adequately sense the size of a piece of food in the mouth and swallows a piece that is too big; the result is an airway obstruction, which sometimes is fatal.

Breathing

As with younger patients, the goal of this part of the assessment is to determine the adequacy of the respirations and respiratory effort. Assess the rate, depth, and rhythm of the respirations. Remember that the respirations of elderly patients often are shallower than those of younger patients and have minimal chest rise because of decreased chest wall compliance. Therefore, in an older individual, a "normal" respiratory rate of 12 to 20 breaths per minute can result in inadequate oxygenation, and an increased rate may be perfectly normal. Chest wall expansion also may be more difficult to see because of the decreased movement and multiple layers of clothing.

Expose the chest as needed to confirm the adequacy of respirations and respiratory effort. If you still have trouble determining the respiratory rate and chest expansion, put your stethoscope on the chest as an aid. Look for use of accessory muscles or any abnormal movement of the chest wall. Accessory muscle use may not always be evident because of the stiffening of the chest wall muscles. After you expose the chest, check its shape, which can provide valuable clues to the patient's medical history.

Other valuable assessments of the patient's respiratory adequacy include the ability to complete sentences and the use of pursed-lip breathing or other methods to increase positive end expiratory pressure (PEEP).

Circulation

Determine the rate, rhythm, and quality of the pulse. Is it regular and strong or irregular and weak? Remember that elderly individuals have a high incidence of atrial fibrillation; don't be surprised if the pulse is irregular. As a result of the changes in the cardiovascular system, the heart rate may be slower and the pulse weaker in an elderly patient. Evaluate the radial and carotid pulses simultaneously to gain a true sense of the quality of the pulse. Compare bilateral pulses; this can help you distinguish bilateral weak pulses caused by decreased cardiac output from a unilateral weak pulse caused by occlusion of peripheral vessels.

Assess for any significant external hemorrhage. The bodies of elderly patients are less able to compensate for blood loss because of the circulatory changes that occur with age. Therefore they may become symptomatic earlier than younger patients. Significant hemorrhage can occur with minor scalp lacerations or with bleeding under the skin, which can cause large hematomas.

A quantitative determination of blood pressure is done later, during the physical exam. However, you can make a qualitative determination of blood pressure while assessing the circulation. Remember that in evaluating the blood pressure, you are assessing the circulatory system. As a result of the loss of blood vessel elasticity, the baseline blood pressure in an elderly patient may be higher than what you learned is normal for adults. Always try to find out what blood pressure is normal for the individual patient. In a patient with a high baseline blood pressure, a measurement of 120/80 mm Hg may indicate hypotension and that the patient is in a hypoperfused state. Depending on the medications the patient takes, his or her body may not be able to increase blood pressure to compensate for fluid loss. Critically evaluate any blood pressure findings and incorporate them into treatment decisions.

History, Physical Examination, and Ongoing Assessment

After the initial assessment, the focused history, physical exam, and ongoing assessment are completed in a manner similar to that for a younger adult. However, EMTs must always keep in mind the normal physiologic changes of aging, as discussed previously, and the effects they may have on the physical exam.

■ REPORTING OF SYMPTOMS

For a variety of reasons, elderly adults may underreport or falsely report symptoms. They often believe that aches, pains, and other sensations are simply "part of getting older." Consequently, they may not report symptoms because they do not feel they are significant or worth reporting. Moreover, elderly patients may have an increased tolerance to pain as a result of chronic conditions that create constant pain of some degree. Medications can alter the perception of pain and other symptoms, leading to underreporting of occurrences. In addition, sensation declines in elderly people because of the decrease in synapses of the nervous system and the decreased speed of impulse transmission. Consequently, an elderly individual may not be aware of symptoms until they have progressed considerably or started to affect other body systems. This may lead to vague rather than specific complaints. Damage to peripheral nerves (peripheral neuropathy) from aging, trauma, or disease further leads to undersensation of symptoms. The classic example of this is the elderly diabetic patient who, when having a heart attack, does not feel chest pain, because of decreased sensation, and complains only of general weakness.

Patients may also have fears about the health care system. They may view the hospital as a place where people go to die. They may fear losing their independence or have other quality of life concerns. These issues can lead to underreporting or falsification of symptoms. The patient may deny having an injury or illness in an attempt to avoid health care and what the person perceives goes along with it.

■ MEDICAL EMERGENCIES

As an EMT, you will encounter elderly patients with a variety of medical emergencies. Some of the more common conditions are altered mental status, chest pain, respiratory emergencies, abdominal pain, and patients with vague, nonspecific complaints.

Altered Mental Status

It is normal for an individual's problem-solving skills to deteriorate during the aging process. However, as mentioned previously, general intelligence typically does not decline before age 70 unless disease is a factor. If memory *is* affected, recent memory is affected before the memory of distant events.

As with all alterations in mental status, the cause in an elderly patient is a space-occupying structural lesion or a toxic metabolic state. EMTs should determine whether the altered mental status was sudden or gradual in onset. If possible, be sure to enlist the help of family members and caregivers to determine the patient's baseline, or normal, mental status. Acute changes in mental status can be caused by hypoglycemia or hypoxia, which are both quickly and easily corrected in the prehospital setting. Chronic carbon dioxide retention, such as occurs in patients with chronic obstructive pulmonary disease (COPD), can lead to hypercapnia (increased levels of carbon dioxide in the circulating blood), which can also lead to changes in mentation. Medications

may be a cause of altered mental status. The patient's presentation may be due to a side effect of a medication, too high or too low a level of medication in the bloodstream, or an interaction with another medication (Fig. 32-6). Always determine whether the patient is compliant with his or her medications. Also, find out if any recent change was made in doses or medications, including prescription, over-the-counter, and herbal forms. Treatable causes of altered mental status should be sought and reversed as soon as possible.

Normal aging involves some memory difficulties and lapses. **Dementia,** however, is a progressive condition marked by significant loss of memory that may be difficult to distinguish from amnesic disorders. Dementia often may cause personality changes, and it is accompanied by impairment of at least one other cognitive function, such as abstract thinking, judgment, or language. A key to recognizing dementia is that broad, severe, and excessive intellectual changes are symptomatic of the condition, and true dementia creates social impairments. Dementia has many causes (Box 32-4), but the most common form is

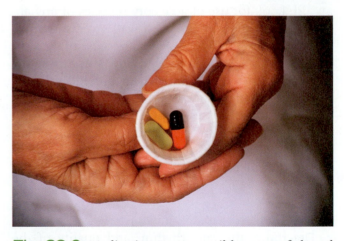

Fig. 32-6 Medications are a possible cause of altered mental status.

BOX 32-4
Causes of Dementia
Neurologic
Metabolic
Nutritional
Sensory
Vascular

BOX 32-5
Causes of Delirium

Fever
Stress
Nutritional factors
Head injury
Neurologic factors
Intoxication
Infection
Drugs

Alzheimer's disease. This disease generally occurs after age 65, and its prevalence increases dramatically late in the seventh decade and early in the eighth decade of life. It is important to note that Alzheimer's disease is a presumptive diagnosis; it can be truly diagnosed only after death, when an autopsy reveals an increased number of neurofibrillary tangles and senile plaques.

Delirium may be thought of more as a "clouding of consciousness." Unlike dementia, delirium is rapid in onset and may result in illusions, hallucinations, and misinterpretations. Patients with this disorder have great difficulty concentrating and maintaining a straightforward stream of thought, and they may be disoriented to place, time, and situation. Delirium, also, has many causes (Box 32-5), but it often is reversible with the correct diagnosis and treatment.

Chest Pain

Cardiovascular disease is a leading cause of death in the United States. It also is a common emergency in elderly patients. Chest pain in the elderly can be caused by numerous factors, including myocardial infarction, angina, pneumonia, and pulmonary embolus. When evaluating a patient with chest pain, try to determine whether the patient has had similar pain in the past and how this current pain compares. A patient who suffers from angina probably has recurring episodes and will be aware of the presentation. Pay close attention to the person's description of the pain, comparisons to previous events, and to the effect of nitroglycerin taken or given. The pain of a myocardial infarction may be very similar to that caused by angina, which can be misleading to both the patient and the EMT. Strong indicators of a myocardial infarction (as opposed to angina) include ineffective treatment with nitroglycerin (which nor-

mally works for the patient) or pain that is different or more severe than the patient's usual angina attack.

Respiratory Emergencies

Respiratory disorders also are common in elderly individuals. The approach to an elderly patient who complains of shortness of breath is similar to that for a younger patient. Older patients may have several underlying chronic respiratory problems, which may lead to calls for emergency medical care. Moreover, older people are susceptible to many acute causes of respiratory distress. The challenge for the EMT is to determine the cause of the respiratory distress and the best course of treatment. If the problem is chronic in nature, determine what changed that prompted the call to EMS. A classic sign of progressing left-sided heart failure (congestive heart failure) is progressing exertional dyspnea. This occurs as the lungs fill with fluid and less alveolar surface is available for oxygen exchange, leading to shortness of breath with minimal physical exertion. During the history and physical exam, also evaluate for several acute causes of shortness of breath. Remember, because older individuals have decreased pain sensation, shortness of breath may be the patient's only complaint during a myocardial infarction.

Abdominal Pain

Abdominal pain in an elderly person often represents a much more severe emergency than in a younger patient. Also, it more commonly results in hospitalization, surgery, and death. This is true because reduced pain perception often delays recognition of the abdominal emergency and also because of the nature of the conditions that cause abdominal pain. Abdominal pain may be caused by an abdominal aortic aneurysm, bowel ischemia, intestinal obstructions, and gastrointestinal bleeding. The exact cause of abdominal pain in any patient can be difficult to determine in the prehospital setting; however, you should have a high index of suspicion for a life-threatening condition with an elderly patient with abdominal pain. Also, make sure you transport the patient to a facility with immediate surgical capability.

Patients with Vague, Nondescriptive Complaints

Elderly patients often may have vague complaints that do not lead the EMT to a determination of the underlying problem. These complaints may include generalized weakness, dizziness, or malaise. Because of chronic illnesses or decreased pain perception, vague complaints may be the only presenting symptom of a serious medical emergency. Sudden arrhythmias can cause a sudden decrease in cardiac output, leading to weakness or a condition called **cardiac syncope,** in which the patient faints for a short period. Hypoxia, dehydration, and electrolyte imbalances also can lead to these symptoms. A thorough history and physical exam, including determining intake and output and whether the patient has sensations of palpitations in the chest, can provide valuable clues to the cause of the presenting symptoms. The most important point, however, is that EMTs should never dismiss vague complaints in an elderly person as minor or insignificant.

■ TRAUMA EMERGENCIES

Trauma is the leading cause of death in patients ages 1 to 44 years. Not until the fifth decade of life do medical conditions begin to cause more deaths than trauma. However, trauma remains one of the leading causes of death in older people. Several conditions predispose elderly individuals to traumatic injuries, including slower reflexes and reaction times, diminished eyesight and hearing, and a reduced ability to maintain balance. Pre-existing diseases also increase mortality in trauma, and the elderly have a greater proportion of pre-existing diseases.

EMTs must keep in mind that the normal aging process, as well as any medications the patient is taking, affect the person's response and presentation and the body's ability to compensate for traumatic emergencies. For example, in the elderly, because of the decreased heart rate and decreased elasticity of blood vessels caused by aging, the body cannot compensate as well or as quickly for blood loss and shock. If the patient is taking medications for blood pressure control (e.g., a beta blocker or an angiotensin-converting enzyme [ACE] inhibitor), the body is even less able to compensate for these conditions. Not only will this patient progress to decompensated shock much more quickly than a younger patient, he or she also may not show the classic signs of shock, such as an increased heart rate or skin color changes that occur secondary to vasoconstriction.

When you treat an elderly patient involved in a traumatic incident, make sure you do not cause any additional injury or harm. Spinal immobilization is a common difficulty in the management of elderly trauma patients. The curvatures of the spine caused by aging can make it difficult to place the patient flat on a long spine board. This condition can also exacerbate pre-existing medical conditions, such as congestive heart failure. Older patients may require more padding when they are immobilized. Other modifications that may need to be made include elevating the head of the board, placing towel rolls under the patient's head and neck, or modifying the cervical collar. When you immobilize an elderly patient, make sure you achieve the goal of maintaining normal neutral alignment for that patient.

Falls

Falls are a common cause of traumatic death in people over age 75 and a common emergency among all elderly individuals. The exact number of falls that occur among the elderly each year is unknown, because many are not reported to health care providers. When treating an elderly patient who has fallen, you must determine not only what traumatic injuries were caused by the fall, but also *why* the patient fell. Falls may occur because of changes in posture, balance, and vision, but medical emergencies also can cause them. Ask these patients whether they simply tripped over something or slipped on a slippery surface, or whether they had any medical symptoms (e.g., chest pain, dizziness, weakness, or respiratory distress) before, during, or after the fall. Just as important, determine whether the patient lost consciousness at any time by asking if he or she remembers all events before, during, and after the fall. You may quickly find that a medical condition caused the fall. In such cases the medical condition must be treated in conjunction with any traumatic injuries.

Head Injuries

Common intracranial hemorrhages in elderly individuals occur in a different location from those in younger adults. As people age, the dura mater comes to adhere tightly to the inside of the skull. Consequently, elderly people have a lower incidence of epidural hematomas than younger people. However, as the brain atrophies, the bridging veins in the subdural space are stretched, and trauma to the head may cause them to tear and bleed. Therefore older individuals are more likely to have a **subdural hematoma.** Because these intracranial hemorrhages generally result from venous bleeding, they can manifest slowly, with minimal signs and symptoms. Elderly patients also are susceptible to chronic subdural hematomas, which can manifest with initial signs and symptoms *months* after a seemingly insignificant incident, such as a minor fall or motor vehicle accident.

■ ABUSE

Unfortunately, abuse of the elderly is on the rise as indicated by the increase in reported cases. The reason for this is unknown. The exact incidence of elder abuse also is unknown, largely because it often goes unreported and essentially has been hidden from society. In addition, until recently the definition of abuse in the elderly age group has not been consistent. Moreover, different geographic locations have different reporting requirements, and elderly patients often do not report abuse for fear of revenge or embarrassment.

Abuse can be divided into three major categories: physical abuse, emotional abuse, and financial abuse (Fig. 32-7). Physical abuse involves inflicting physical injury, physical neglect, malnutrition, or poor sanitation and hygiene. Emotional abuse involves causing mental distress through fear, intimidation, verbal threats, and isolation. Financial abuse includes theft, embezzlement, or any other misuse of an elderly person's property or assets.

The signs of elder abuse can be difficult to spot and are often missed. This is one reason elder abuse has gone unrecognized and has largely been ignored by society. EMTs should carefully evaluate each scene for signs of abuse that may have led to the injuries being treated. Abuse can occur in the home and in medical facilities and adult care centers. Do not let a "professional" setting deter you if you suspect abuse. You must also be aware of warning signs of abuse. These may include the patient's living conditions. Is the residence clean, heated appropriately, and free of hazards? Is adequate food present? Is the patient's personal hygiene adequate? Look for patterns of injury or injuries caused by objects. Is there a history of frequent injuries, calls for emergency assistance, or visits to the emergency department? Injuries that do not match the history, or vague or differing histories from the patient and caregivers are indicators of abuse. Other indicators include a patient who appears fearful of caregivers, or caregivers who will not allow the patient to be alone with medical professionals.

A number of characteristics are common to patients who are abused and those who abuse them. Abused patients often are over 65 years of age and, in particular, women over 75 years of age. They usually have several medical problems, including dementia. They often are incontinent, and behaviors include sleep pattern disturbances, sleepwalking, and shouting in the middle of the night. Frequently the abused patient lives with the abuser. Abusers commonly were themselves abused as children, have addiction and dependency problems, are dependent on the victim for financial support or have financial and employment difficulties, and are over age 50. In addition, the abuser often is either the patient's spouse or a middle-aged daughter-in-law who is also caring for children and working outside the home.

When you suspect abuse, report it according to the laws of the state in which you work. In most states, reporting your suspicion to the emergency department physician fulfills this requirement. However, in other states, EMTs may need to call social services directly. Make sure you know the specific reporting requirements of the state in which you work. When documenting cases of suspected abuse, report your findings and observations objectively. For example, do not include subjective assumptions as to the cause of the patterned circular burns on the patient's back; instead, state that they are present and describe them carefully. Statements made by the patient should be written verbatim and placed in quotation marks.

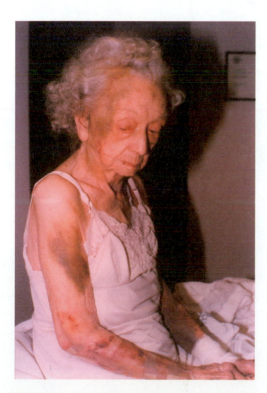

Fig. 32-7 Abuse can be divided into three major categories: physical abuse, emotional abuse, and financial abuse.

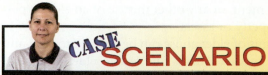

CASE SCENARIO
conclusion

Although Mrs. Applegard's condition is serious, Elizabeth and her crew devote extra time and attention to preparing her for transport. They remove her nightgown and cover her with a blanket to preserve body heat. They also apply a cervical collar and administer low-flow oxygen. A scoop stretcher padded with several blankets is used to lift the patient gently from the bathroom floor. After getting through the tight hallway, Elizabeth has the patient transferred to a backboard that had been placed on the gurney. The transfer takes a few minutes to complete; the crew wants to make sure the spinal precautions are handled correctly. They also want to avoid causing Mrs. Applegard any additional pain.

Later on, the crew finds out that Mrs. Applegard had suffered a stroke and had fallen during the night. Her left hip was dislocated in the fall. She ended up spending many months under the care of physical therapists to regain limited use of the left side of her body.

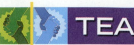

TEAMWORK

When encountering dependent elderly patients, EMTs may be required to interact with multiple individuals and/or agencies along with the patient. Family members, additional caregivers, and support agencies can be a source of information and assistance with certain elderly patients.

Resources

American Geriatrics Society: *Geriatric education for emergency medical services,* Sudbury, Mass., 2003, Jones & Bartlett.

Comer R: *Abnormal psychology,* ed 3, New York, 1998, WH Freeman & Co.

National Association of Emergency Medical Technicians: *Prehospital trauma life support,* ed 5, St Louis, 2003, Mosby.

Seidel HM et al: *Mosby's guide to physical examination,* ed 4, St Louis, 1999, Mosby.

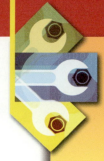

Critical Points

- The ability to examine and treat elderly patients is critical to your ability to be an effective EMT.
- You must understand and be able to differentiate between the normal changes that occur with aging and those that are the result of disease processes. Without this ability, you can easily miss subtle signs and symptoms that are essential to proper treatment. Also, you may not recognize findings associated with significant injury or illness.

Learning Checklist

- ❑ A number of key changes occur as people age:
- ❑ Tidal volume and vital capacity decrease, and physiologic dead space and residual volume increase.
- ❑ Cardiovascular elasticity diminishes, and heart rate and stroke volume decrease. The number of cells responsible for creating electrical impulses also declines.
- ❑ The skin loses its elasticity and becomes dry, thin, flaky, and brittle. The underlying subcutaneous tissue becomes thinner.
- ❑ General intelligence and mentation should not change until age 70 or later. However, slower transmission of neural impulses results in slower responses and decreased sensation. Hearing, vision, and thermoregulation deficiencies also develop.
- ❑ New bone production is exceeded by bone resorption, muscles atrophy, and tendons lose their elasticity.
- ❑ Assessment of the geriatric patient follows the same pattern and format as for any patient. However, certain differences must be taken into account:
- ❑ The EMT should always assess the scene for clues to the underlying complaint.
- ❑ When assessing mental status, EMTs should determine the patient's normal mental status by asking family members or caregivers; they should then alter their line of questioning appropriately.

- ❑ Cough and gag reflexes diminish with age, and dentures can quickly become a complete airway obstruction if they become dislodged.
- ❑ The respirations of elderly patients often are shallower than those of younger patients.
- ❑ Atrial fibrillation is not uncommon, and pulses should be assessed simultaneously.
- ❑ Medications can alter the perception of pain and other symptoms.
- ❑ Patients may view the hospital as a place people go to die; they may fear losing their independence, or have other quality of life concerns.
- ❑ Common medical emergencies include altered mental status, chest pain, respiratory emergencies, abdominal pain, and patients with vague, nondescriptive complaints.
- ❑ Falls, head injuries, and abuse are common traumatic injuries.
- ❑ Signs of elder abuse can include poor living conditions, inadequate food, patterns of injury, and a suspicious history. Abuse victims may fear their caregivers.

Key Terms

Anatomic dead space The amount of inhaled air in the trachea and mainstem bronchi, which therefore is not available for exchange (approximately 150 ml in adults).

Atherosclerosis Narrowing of the blood vessels that occurs secondary to the buildup of fatty deposits.

Atrial fibrillation A chaotic heart rhythm that results in an unusually irregular pulse; this condition is seen in many elderly patients.

Atrophy The wasting away, deterioration, or shrinking of a body organ, tissue, or part.

Cardiac output The amount of blood expelled by the ventricles of the heart with each beat (the stroke volume) multiplied by the heart rate.

Cardiac syncope A fainting episode caused by reduced cardiac output and the resulting hypotension, which occur secondary to tachycardia or bradycardia; the most dangerous cause of syncope in the elderly.

Delirium An acute, temporary state of confusion that may result in illusions, hallucinations,

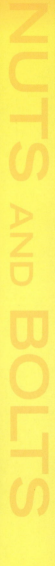

and misinterpretations. Delirium has many causes and often is reversible.

Dementia A progressive alteration of mental status associated with deterioration of at least one other cognitive function. It may be associated with emotional disturbances and emotional changes. Dementia has many causes and often is not reversible.

Hypertrophy An increase in the size of the cells of a tissue in response to an increased workload.

Kyphosis An abnormal outward curvature of the spine that creates a dorsal hump.

Minute volume The amount of air available for alveolar exchange each minute. The minute volume (MVa) is determined by subtracting the physiologic dead space (VD) from the tidal volume (TV) and multiplying the result by the respiratory rate (RR): $MVa = (TV - VD) \times RR$.

Orthostatic hypotension A fall in blood pressure of 20 mm Hg or more or an increase in heart rate of 20 beats per minute or more that results from a change in position; it often occurs secondary to hypovolemia.

Physiologic dead space A combination of the anatomic dead space and the amount of air in the alveoli that is not available for exchange. This amount of air varies from person to person based on the number of nonfunctional alveoli.

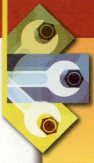

Skin tear A traumatic injury to an elderly person's skin that can be caused by minor circumstances. It occurs because of the loss of elasticity and the thinning of the skin that take place with aging.

Stroke volume The amount of blood ejected by the heart with each contraction.

Subdural hematoma An intracranial hemorrhage that occurs in the subdural space.

Thermoregulation The body's ability to regulate temperature despite changes in the environment. The hypothalamus is responsible for this process.

National Standard Curriculum Objectives

Cognitive Objectives
No objectives identified.

Affective Objectives
No objectives identified.

Psychomotor Objectives
No objectives identified.

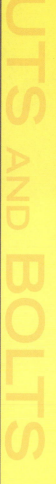

CHAPTER OUTLINE

Phases of an Emergency Medical Services (EMS) Response

Air Medical Considerations

LESSON GOAL

Nonmedical operational skills are as critical as competent patient care skills. As an emergency medical technician (EMT), you need to know the fundamentals and have a working knowledge of the skills required for all phases of an EMS response. In addition, you must understand your role and responsibility in each phase. ■

Ambulance Operations

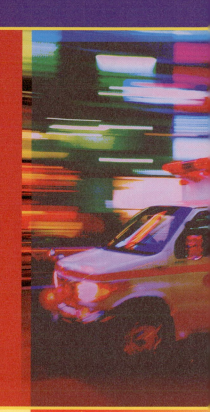

CHAPTER OBJECTIVES

After completing this chapter, the EMT student will be able to do the following:

1 Discuss the medical and nonmedical equipment needed to respond to a call.

2 List the phases of a prehospital call.

3 Describe the general provisions of state laws relating to the operation of the ambulance and privileges that concern speed, warning lights, sirens, right of way, parking, and turning.

4 List factors that contribute to unsafe driving conditions.

3 Describe the considerations that should be given to requesting an escort, following an escort vehicle, and navigating intersections.

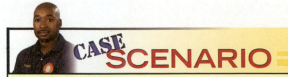

CASE SCENARIO

Traffic is at a standstill in front of the station as the garage door rises. Jim starts the diesel motor of the type III ambulance as Elizabeth gets into the front seat. Jim quickly checks the rear view mirror to make sure Jane and Jack are seated in the back of the unit. Dropping the transmission into drive, he eases the ambulance onto the apron and edges toward the driveway.

From the back, Jack can see that Jim has not yet turned on the emergency lights. Also, Jack doesn't hear the siren. In fact, Jim stops the unit at the edge of the driveway. "What's up?" Jack wonders to himself. "There's a lot of vehicles stopped in the roadway, but they should yield to the ambulance."

Questions: *Why would Jim wait to begin his code 3 response? Shouldn't Jim just move into the street quickly? Why would he slow down before reaching the street?*

■ PHASES OF AN EMS RESPONSE

A typical EMS response has nine stages, or phases:

1. Preparation for the call
2. Dispatch
3. En route to the scene
4. Arrival at the scene
5. Transferral of the patient to the ambulance
6. En route to the receiving facility
7. Arrival at the receiving facility
8. En route to the station
9. The postrun phase

Preparation for the Call

The preparation phase is the period before an EMS call when you should be getting ready to respond to an emergency. During this phase, you should be checking supplies and equipment in jumpkits, gear bags, and emergency vehicles (Box 33-1). Check that mechanical equipment, such as the automated external defibrillator (AED), is working properly and that your vehicle is fueled and operating without any problems.

In addition, make sure you are physically and mentally prepared to respond to any emergency call. It is important to have your supplies and your vehicle well prepared. However, you have an equally important responsibility to yourself, your family and, most important, your patient to be mentally and physically fit. Exercise and a balanced diet are key elements of both mental and physical fitness (see Chapter 2). Preparation also means practicing the skills you have learned and reviewing the knowledge you have gained to ensure that you are prepared to respond.

Whether you are using an EMS response vehicle or your private vehicle, it must be prepared to respond to any emergency call. It must always be stocked with both medical and nonmedical supplies and any medical equipment you are authorized to use. Your EMS system, along with state and local regulations, dictate the specific equipment required or allowed in EMS vehicles (Fig. 33-1). Most EMS systems and other agencies that require EMS training equip the typical emergency vehicle (e.g., ambulance, fire apparatus, police squad car) with an array of basic medical supplies (see Box 33-1).

Nonmedical equipment, such as gloves, gowns, masks, and protective eyewear, also is required for safe, efficient EMS operations. In fact, many states, as well

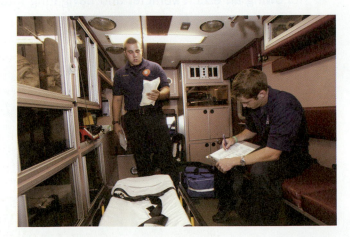

Fig. 33-1 Your EMS system, along with state and local regulations, dictates the specific equipment required or allowed in the EMS vehicle.

BOX 33-1
Emergency Vehicle Equipment

- Basic supplies
- Airways and masks (barrier devices)
- Artificial ventilation devices
- Suction equipment
- Basic wound care supplies

BOX 33-2
Personal Protective Equipment

- Protective eyewear (This equipment should have an elastic strap and vents to prevent fogging. The shield on a helmet is not considered protective eyewear.)
- Impact-resistant protective helmet with ear protection and chin strap
- Lightweight, puncture-resistant turnout coat and pants
- Leather gloves
- Boots with steel insoles and steel toes

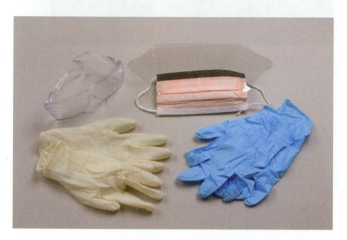

Fig. 33-2 Personal protective equipment (PPE).

as local government agencies, require specific personal protective equipment (PPE) (Fig. 33-2 and Box 33-2) and safety equipment. Appropriate gear for responding to a rescue/extrication situation is also needed.

Other helpful nonmedical supplies and equipment that should be available include local street maps, preplanned routes, patient care reports, the Department of Transportation's *Emergency Response Guidebook*, a protocol book, and traffic warning devices.

You should be aware of your role in the local EMS system. As an EMT working with EMS or the fire service, you may be the third pair of hands on the responding vehicle. If you are not associated with EMS/fire service, you may respond as a volunteer in your community, or you may just be first on the scene of a multiple-vehicle accident or medical emergency. Whatever role you play, you must be prepared to respond to an emergency at any time.

Continuing education is a very important element of EMS at all levels. It can take many forms, such as attending additional classes, attending locally sponsored conferences or symposiums (e.g., those provided by hospitals, EMS services, or EMT associations), or enrolling in an EMT continuing education course. Sharing patient care experiences with fellow first responders and advanced level providers is a great way to increase your overall patient care knowledge (re-

member not to use any patient names or any identifiers that may violate the regulations of the Health Insurance Portability and Accountability Act [HIPAA]). In the rapidly changing, ever-evolving field of prehospital emergency care, it is imperative that EMS teams at all levels be adaptable and open to new ideas and procedures emerging from ongoing scientific research.

Dispatch

Dispatch is a critical phase of any emergency response. Currently, no consistent mechanism exists for dispatching across the 50 states. However, most dispatch centers have a central access number, usually 911 or enhanced 911. In areas where this access number is not available (mostly rural areas), a specific, well-publicized number usually is available for reaching the EMS system (as well as police and fire assistance). The dispatch/communication center is staffed 24 hours a day with personnel who may be able to provide emergency medical instructions (prearrival instructions) to the caller before EMS or first responders arrive (Fig. 33-3). This system allows family, friends, or bystanders to begin basic emergency care while help is en route. Many dispatch systems have preplanned response policies that allow dispatchers to use computer-assisted dispatch (CAD) programs or cardex systems to determine individual unit or agency dispatch and give them a mode of response based on patient information.

If you are working as an EMT in an EMS agency or system, you are notified by the dispatcher that you have a call. You need very specific information to respond to the call. The information depends on your particular communication/dispatch center and the description of the incident provided by the caller. At a minimum, you should be informed of the patient's

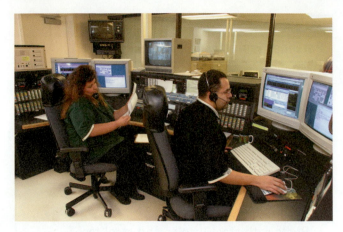

Fig. 33-3 911 Dispatch center.

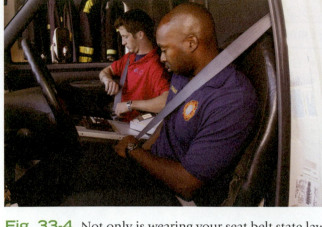

Fig. 33-4 Not only is wearing your seat belt state law in most states, it also may save your life.

location and the mechanism of injury or nature of the illness. In many systems the dispatcher provides the caller's name, location, and callback number. In systems with enhanced 911, addresses and phone numbers are displayed automatically on the dispatcher's computer screen. Additional information may be provided at the time of dispatch or may become available en route. This information may include the number of patients, severity of injuries, patient breathing or nonbreathing, patient conscious or unconscious, or other special problems, hazards or complications at the scene. Keep in mind that dispatch information may signal to you that more resources are needed, such as law enforcement or firefighters.

En Route to the Scene

To provide emergency care, you must arrive at the scene safely. Simple things can minimize your risk of injury, such as not running to the vehicle and not running while at the scene. The dispatch center should be notified when you respond and again upon your arrival at the scene. It is important to write down the information provided by dispatch in as detailed a manner as possible.

Wearing seat belts is critical for everyone in your EMS response or privately owned vehicle (Fig. 33-4). Not only is wearing your seat belt state law in most states, it also may save your life!

Whether you are driving an emergency vehicle or your own vehicle, you are responsible for knowing and following all state and local laws and regulations governing the use of emergency warning devices. If you are not the driver, obtain additional information from the dispatcher to help prepare for the scene size-up. Another task involves assigning specific duties and

considering special equipment needs. Any planning you do en route may save time at the scene. Also, you can use this time to select the initial equipment to take out at the scene, and prepare it if necessary.

Upon arrival, even before getting out of the vehicle, your first task is the scene size-up. Position your vehicle primarily for safety and then for departure from the scene. Safety considerations include parking uphill or upwind from any hazardous substance and at least 100 feet (30 m) from any wreckage or unknown spills. Local policy dictates whether to park the vehicle in front of or beyond the wreckage or spill.

Always position the vehicle to allow for safe loading of the patient and easy departure from the scene. Use the parking brake and turn on your warning lights to alert other vehicles of your presence. If it is dark, turn off the headlights to avoid blinding other drivers approaching the scene, unless the headlights are being used to illuminate the scene.

Arrival at the Scene

When you arrive at the scene, be sure to notify dispatch. Remember, *safety first!* This means sizing up the scene *before* entering it. Protect yourself from harm. If the scene appears to indicate a potential for violence or is unsafe for any reason, wait for law enforcement or appropriate fire apparatus for assistance before approaching. Is there a possible need for body substance precautions? Is a potential assailant still on the scene? A hazardous spill or vapor? Downed power lines? Fire? Is it safe to approach the victim? Is it necessary to move the victim or victims to remove them from some hazard?

Your next step should be noting the mechanism of injury or the nature of the illness. Additional re-

SPECIAL Considerations

Keep an Eye Out
Watch where you walk when carrying or moving patients through accident scenes. Walking through antifreeze spills in rubber-soled boots or shoes can be like walking on ice.

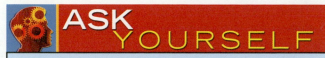

ASK YOURSELF

You and your partner are starting the shift. Off-going crews report that some new equipment, a stair chair, has been placed in service. You decide to eat breakfast at a local restaurant instead of checking the new equipment. While you're eating, the tones go off, and you're dispatched to a medical emergency. You find that you need the new stair chair, but you don't know how to use it. Now what? How can this situation be avoided?

sources and **triage** may be necessary if there are more patients than you and a partner can handle. (The principles of triage are covered in more detail in Chapter 35). If you have only one patient, begin your initial assessment with a general impression. If trauma is evident, provide inline spinal immobilization.

Remember: *All* your actions at the scene must be rapid, organized, and efficient.

Transferral of the Patient to the Ambulance

Using the principles you learned in Chapter 6, direct passersby or assist other EMS personnel in transferring the patient to a transport vehicle. Before handoff to an advanced life support (ALS) unit (if conditions warrant) and after performing all critical interventions, make sure that all dressings and bandages or splints are secure. Make sure your patient is covered for protection against the elements and secured to the appropriate lifting and moving device.

En Route to the Receiving Facility

En route to the receiving facility, a decision is made about the response mode (emergency or nonemergency) to be used while transporting the patient to the hospital. Recheck the patient's status to make sure that all life-threatening problems have been identified and treated. If time permits, you can perform a complete physical examination to identify other injuries or concerns. Appropriate treatments and interventions not accomplished at the scene may be performed during transport. You also should be thinking about the report you will give on arrival at the receiving facility.

Arrival at the Receiving Facility

Once you arrive at the destination, provide the hospital staff with a verbal report. Then prepare and leave a written report of the history and the assessment and treatment you performed during your time with the patient. In some EMS systems, this also is the time to prepare your ambulance for the next call and get it ready for the next patient encounter. In other systems, this preparation is postponed until the crew returns to the station.

En Route to the Station

The trip back to the station is a good time to review the particulars of the call with your partner to see whether you could have improved upon anything. It also gives you an opportunity to think about what items need to be restocked in the vehicle to get it ready for the next call.

The Postrun Phase

Depending on whether you used your own vehicle or an agency unit, you should use this phase of the emergency response to check fuel levels, restock supplies and equipment and, just as important, clean and disinfect equipment and the inside of the response vehicle. This is also the time to complete and file all paperwork from the call, as required by your service or agency. When all this is accomplished, the dispatch center should be notified of your availability.

■ AIR MEDICAL CONSIDERATIONS

Air medical transportation should be considered when the victim's condition warrants it and significant time can be saved or when a patient must be transported to a specialty care facility (e.g., trauma center, burn center, neonatal center, or other tertiary care facility).

Helicopter transport has become increasingly common for specific medical and trauma emergencies in most of the United States. The decision to request air medical transport must be made in consultation with the medical director of a hospital or an EMS system. Guidelines or protocols probably are in place for requesting a helicopter, or the arriving EMS personnel make the decision. It is important to remember that this aircraft has limitations. For instance, it cannot fly in certain weather conditions, and it requires maintenance, both scheduled and unscheduled, that may prevent its use when you need it.

You must help prepare the patient for air medical transport. Litter restraints must be secure, intravenous (IV) sites must be covered and stabilized, and the patient must be covered appropriately for the climate.

Landing zones are a key component of air medical transport. If trained personnel are available, one person should be identified as the communications officer, who sets up the landing zone. This individual should have a reasonably good sense of direction, be familiar with the area surrounding the landing zone, and not be directly involved with patient care. If the communications officer is in radio or cell phone contact with the air medical dispatch center, he or she should give the following essential information: (1) the unit or individual making the call and any call sign; (2) the radio frequency, if appropriate; (3) the number of patients; (4) whether more than one aircraft is needed; (5) the location of the incident; and (6) prominent landmarks in the area.

A landing zone should be set up. If possible, it should be 100 × 100 feet (30 × 30 m); at the very least, it should be 60 × 60 feet (18 × 18 m), depending on the type of aircraft (Fig. 33-5). It should be free of debris, obstructions, overhead wires, trees, fences, and any loose objects. Ideally, the ground should not slope. The communications officer should mark each corner of the landing zone with an independent light source, such as a flare, lightstick, adequately secured cone, or emergency or personally

owned vehicle. Vehicle headlights should point toward the center of the landing zone. If it is dark, make sure that headlights are turned off as the helicopter makes its final descent into the landing zone so as not to blind or distract the pilot.

If the designated communications officer is in radio or cell phone contact with the pilot or air medical dispatch center, this person should contact the pilot when he or she sees or hears the helicopter. At this point it is very important to provide good descriptive landmark information, such as water (lakes, rivers, and ponds), radio towers, schoolyards, tennis courts, high-power lines, or major roadway intersections. The clock face method is the preferred way to direct the pilot to the landing zone. The pilot is always facing the twelve o'clock position. Therefore, if you are facing the helicopter and it is heading toward you, you would use the three and nine o'clock positions for right-left directions. As the pilot makes the final approach, provide details on the surface of the landing zone, including the type of surface and, for example, whether it is a field, road, or construction site. Boundary information (e.g., trees, buildings, wires, fences, or towers) is also important. Most important is the proximity of power lines. If possible, illuminate potential hazards.

Safety is extremely important for those working around a helicopter. It is everyone's responsibility. If flight crews in your area offer continuing education courses, take advantage of this opportunity and attend one. When you are working around aircraft of any kind, common sense is crucial. Wear goggles or safety glasses to protect against flying debris or particles. Also, keep a safe distance from turning blades. This safe distance is 30 feet (9 m) from the landing zone for emergency vehicles, and 100 feet (30 m) for crowds. Do not run or smoke in or around the landing zone.

The pilot or flight crew will signal when you can approach the aircraft. *Do not approach unless directed to do so.* When directed, always make sure you are within view of the pilot by approaching from the front. The tail section is especially dangerous for

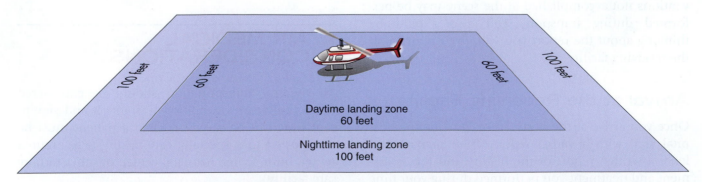

Fig. 33-5 Minimum landing zone dimensions.

ground personnel. The tail rotor blade usually is low to the ground and difficult to see when it is rotating. Whether the engine is running or not, *all* personnel should avoid the tail section. Remember: all movements around the helicopter must be between the nine o'clock and three o'clock positions, within the pilot's visual range. Never attempt to take shortcuts under the body, the rear section, or the tailboom. If you are assisting the flight crew, *do not* attempt to operate any of the aircraft doors. These are the responsibility of the flight crew.

It also is extremely important to stay low when approaching the helicopter. Wind gusts can unexpectedly change the height of the blades. Never wear or carry equipment on your head, even if you have ducked very low. This is very dangerous. Items such as hats or loose equipment can be blown about by the wind from the rotor blades. If the helicopter parks on a slope, always approach from the downhill side, because the main rotor blade will be lower to the ground on the uphill side. The flight crew is always in charge of activity around the helicopter; follow their directions for approaching and leaving the aircraft (Fig. 33-6).

If you are asked to help the EMS or flight crew load the patient, make sure all straps are secure and that no loose material is evident. Always follow the directions of the air crew when working around the helicopter (Figs. 33-7 and 33-8).

> ///**CAUTION!**
>
> Do not wear or carry equipment on your head around a helicopter, even if you have ducked very low. This is very dangerous. Items such as hats or loose equipment can be blown about by the wind from the rotor blades.

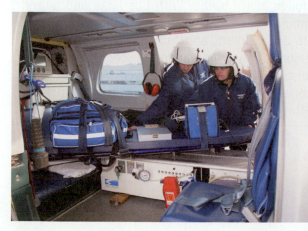

Fig. 33-6 Flight crew removing a stretcher from a helicopter.

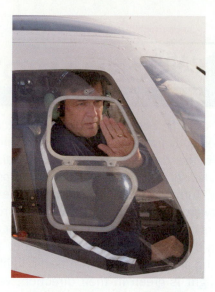

Fig. 33-7 Do *not* approach the aircraft until the pilot indicates that it is safe to do so.

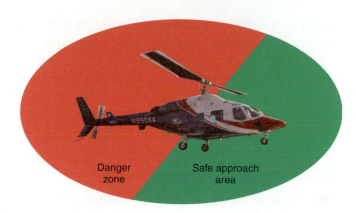

Danger zone   Safe approach area

Fig. 33-8 Always approach a helicopter from the front where the pilot can see you.

One additional safety note: If the pilot chooses a different departure route because of winds and/or obstacles, the aircraft may need to be turned while still close to the ground. It is critical that *all* personnel and equipment be clear of the landing zone.

You can get additional information on EMS helicopters from organizations or agencies such as the Association of Air Medical Services, the National Association of EMS Pilots, and your local EMS air medical provider.

■ SUMMARY

Response Phases

The nine phases of a typical EMS response are (1) preparation for the call; (2) dispatch; (3) en route to the scene; (4) arrival at the scene; (5) transferral of the patient to the ambulance; (6) en route to the re-

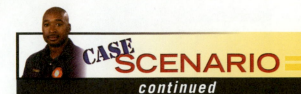

CASE SCENARIO
continued

Once the traffic begins to move, Jim switches on the emergency lights and waits for someone to let him into the traffic lane. Almost immediately a driver does so, and Jim eases the vehicle onto the roadway. Turning on the siren, he steers the ambulance toward the left innermost lane of the roadway as drivers begin to move to the right to clear a path.

From the back, Jack can see that they are approaching an intersection with traffic lights. The traffic light is green in their direction, yet Jack can feel the ambulance losing speed. He asks Jim why they are slowing down.

ceiving facility; (7) arrival at the receiving facility; (8) en route to the station; and (9) the postrun phase.

The EMT's roles and responsibilities are determined by each phase of the call and whether the EMT is responding alone or as part of an EMS squad or agency. Both personal and patient safety are critical components of each phase.

Air Medical Transport

Across most of the United States, a critically ill or injured patient is transported by air medical services when ground transport is prolonged or access is difficult. The two key determinants of possible use of air medical transport are the mechanism of injury and the transport time and distance. Generally, EMS systems have protocols or guidelines for making this decision. The landing zone and communications setup should be arranged by a person who is not involved in patient care. It is critical that the landing zone be clear of debris and wires and that the helicopter pilot be provided as much information as possible.

As in all aspects of on-scene prehospital care, safety must be the foremost consideration. Safety is the responsibility of everyone in and around the landing zone. The main rotor can dip as low as 4 feet (about 1 m) from the ground, and the tail rotor speed makes it virtually invisible. Always approach the aircraft between the nine and three o'clock positions and only when directed to do so by a member of the flight crew. Never walk near the tail rotor or under the tail boom. Always follow the flight crew's instructions regarding safe practices.

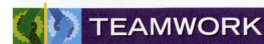

TEAMWORK

As discussed in this chapter, EMTs work in a wide range of settings with a variety of health care providers. Whether you are working with the flight crew from the local trauma center or with firefighters, you must not only understand the limitations of their equipment, but also their role in the "big picture." Also, EMTs must be confident in their skills, which means they must know how all assigned equipment works. Always check your equipment and report any defects—your patient is counting on you.

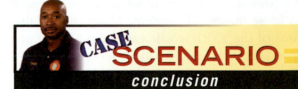

CASE SCENARIO
conclusion

"We can't help anyone if we don't get to the scene in one piece," Jim called back to Jack's question. "While it's true an emergency vehicle has right-of-way while responding, drivers often panic and do very unpredictable things with their cars, like stop right in front of you, pull to the left rather than the right, sometimes even follow you through heavy traffic. With this large and heavy ambulance we have a responsibility not to get into an accident, and hurt or even kill another person." They pulled up to the scene. "Besides," Jim concluded, "the time saved by racing to a scene is outweighed by the danger and risk of getting involved in an awful wreck." ■

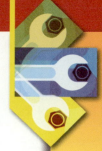

Critical Points

- Preparation and safety are the keys to a good response to any call.
- Regularly check supplies and equipment in jumpkits, gear bags, and emergency vehicles.
- Verify that mechanical equipment, such as the automatic external defibrillator (AED), is working properly and that your vehicle is fueled and operating without any problems.
- Make sure you are physically and mentally prepared to respond to any emergency call.
- Size up the scene before entering it. If there is any question of safety, call for support; do not enter the scene.

Learning Checklist

- A typical EMS call has nine phases: (1) preparation for the call, (2) dispatch, (3) en route to the scene, (4) arrival at the scene, (5) transferral of the patient to the ambulance, (6) en route to the receiving facility, (7) arrival at the receiving facility, (8) en route to the station, and (9) the postrun phase.
- The individual EMS system and state and local regulations dictate the specific equipment required or allowed in EMS vehicles. The typical emergency vehicle includes an array of basic medical supplies, nonmedical equipment (gloves, masks, gowns, and protective eyewear), and appropriate gear for rescue or extrication, in addition to maps, patient care reports, protocol books, emergency response guides, and traffic warning devices.
- Minimum information provided by dispatch should include the patient's location and the mechanism of injury or the nature of the illness. The EMT should notify the dispatch center as the unit responds and upon arrival. Dispatch information should be written down in as detailed a manner as possible.
- EMTs are responsible for knowing and following all state and local regulations regarding the use of emergency warning devices.
- On arrival at the scene, the first step is to perform a scene size-up and determine scene safety. If the scene appears to hold the potential for violence or is unsafe for any reason, wait for law enforcement, fire apparatus, or other assistance before approaching.
- Triage may be necessary if there are more patients than you and a partner can handle.
- Begin the initial assessment with a general impression. If trauma is evident, provide inline spinal immobilization.
- The postrun phase involves checking fuel levels, restocking supplies and equipment, cleaning and disinfecting equipment and the interior of the response vehicle, and completing and filing all paperwork from the call.
- The decision to request air medical transport must be made in consultation with the medical director of a hospital or EMS system. Follow local protocols.
- Landing zones should be marked at each corner with an independent light source, such as flares, lightsticks, secured cones, or emergency or personal vehicles. Provide good descriptive landmarks (e.g., water, radio towers, schoolyards, high-power lines, major intersections). Use the clock face method to direct the pilot to the landing zone. For night operations, make sure all headlights are turned off as the helicopter makes its final descent.
- Do not approach the helicopter unless directed to do so. All movement around the helicopter must be between the nine and three o'clock positions, within the pilot's visual range. Never approach from the rear of the helicopter. The flight crew is always in charge of activity around the helicopter; follow their directions.

Key Terms

911 This is a common and uniform number used in much of the United States to access emergency medical services.

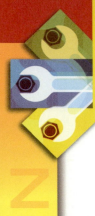

E-911 or Enhanced 911 This is an upgraded version of the 911 system which automatically displays the caller's telephone number and location for the telephone being used to call for assistance.

Prearrival instructions This is the process by which an EMS dispatcher will provide a caller needing medical assistance specific instructions on steps the caller can take to initiate providing care to an ill or injured party.

Triage This is the process of sorting patients for treatment and transport based upon the severity and survivability of the illness or injury.

National Standard Curriculum Objectives

Cognitive Objectives

After completing this lesson, the EMT student will be able to do the following:

- Discuss the medical and nonmedical equipment needed to respond to a call.
- List the phases of an ambulance call.

- Describe the general provisions of state laws relating to the operation of the ambulance and privileges in any or all of the following categories:
  - Speed
  - Warning lights
  - Sirens
  - Right of way
  - Parking
  - Turning
- List factors that contribute to unsafe driving conditions.
- Describe the considerations that should be given to the following:
  - Request for escorts
  - Following an escort vehicle
  - Intersections

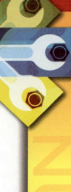

- Discuss the importance of due regard for the safety of all others while operating an emergency vehicle.
- State the information that is essential in order to respond to a call.
- Discuss various situations that may affect the response to a call.
- Differentiate the various methods of moving a patient to the unit based on injury or illness.
- Apply the components of the essential patient information in a written report.
- Summarize the importance of preparing the unit for the next response.
- Identify the essentials for completing a call.
- Differentiate the terms *cleaning, disinfection, high-level disinfection,* and *sterilization.*
- Explain how to clean or disinfect items after patient care.

Affective Objectives
After completing this lesson, the EMT student will be able to do the following:

- Explain the rationale for appropriate reporting of patient information.
- Explain the rationale for having the unit prepared to respond.

Psychomotor Objectives
No objectives identified.

CHAPTER

34

LESSON GOAL

The goal of this chapter is to familiarize the emergency medical technician (EMT) student with the basics of emergency rescue operations. When such operations are mounted by fire, rescue, and emergency medical services (EMS) agencies, the EMT is allowed access to the patient to provide prehospital emergency care. This chapter covers the basic rescue principles and practices used nationwide. It is recommended that EMT students obtain additional training in technical rescue. ■

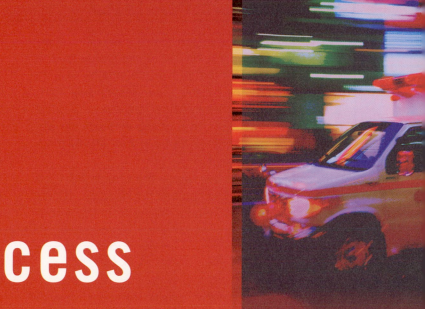

Gaining Access

CHAPTER OBJECTIVES

After completing this chapter, the EMT student will be able to do the following:

1 Discuss the role of the EMT in rescue operations.
2 List the seven rescue specialties and discuss the differences in the required safety equipment.
3 Identify the basic components of a rescue operation.
4 Discuss the steps that should be taken to protect the patient during a rescue operation.
5 Describe the different ways of gaining access to the patient.
6 Discuss the differences between a simple and a complex rescue.

OBJECTIVES

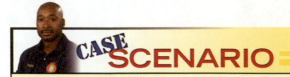

CASE SCENARIO

At the scene, Jack can see that the wrecked, mid-size car had been hit on the driver's side by the smaller vehicle. The patient in the smaller vehicle is being cared for by the other responding unit. Broken glass and pieces of car are strewn around the intersection. The driver of the mid-size car appears to be awake; Jack can see him slowly moving around in his seat.

Elizabeth makes her way to the vehicle from the front so that the driver can see her head-on. "Don't move, sir!" she commands. "We're from the ambu-lance service, and we want to check you over, okay?" The driver stops moving and sits still as Jane opens the rear passenger side door and climbs into the back seat. While Jane manually stabilizes the driver's head and neck, Elizabeth tries to open the driver's door. It is stuck.

Questions: *What are some of the extrication options the ambulance crew could explore in this situation? Should they be concerned about any other hazards?*

■ TECHNICAL RESCUE

Technical rescue generally consists of seven areas of specialty, as identified by National Fire Protection Association 1670: Standard on Operations and Training for Technical Rescue Incidents. The seven areas of specialty are

- Structural collapse rescue
- Rope rescue
- Confined space rescue
- Trench rescue and excavation
- Vehicle and machinery rescue
- Water rescue
- Wilderness search and rescue

The federal Occupational Safety and Health Administration (OSHA) has adopted operational features for these specialty areas. These operational features probably are enforced in your local area by OSHA or by your state Department of Labor. The basic component of Standard 1670 requires that all emergency medical personnel responding to a technical rescue incident be trained at minimum to the **Awareness level.** This specialized training usually can be obtained through local fire and rescue service organizations. The information in this chapter is provided as a reference to Awareness level training only. EMTs who want to become more versed in the field of technical rescue should seek follow-up training for the **Operations level** and the **Technician level** of technical rescue.

Technical rescue incidents have many unique hazards that can directly affect the victim and the emergency responder. Emergency responders tend to be action oriented, and may want to help the victim immediately. This is normally an asset; however, it also can turn the emergency responders into the biggest hazard on the rescue scene. When emotions take over, dangerous attempts at technical rescue often are made without the proper training, equipment, or resources for a successful outcome. In these haphazard attempts, the emergency responder frequently becomes another victim. It is important that all emergency responders develop a strong, competent, level-headed attitude. This helps them to gain control of the incident scene and prevent injury to one of their own.

As an EMT, you will work with other responding agencies. Therefore you should be familiar with and follow the personnel accountability system used by the agency charged with scene management. It is imperative that those responding to incident scenes be familiar with incident management and local emergency evacuation procedures and guidelines. The type of personal protective equipment (PPE) worn depends on the type of incident and the hazards that may exist.

As an emergency responder to a technical rescue, you must perform a hazard and risk assessment. You also must continuously size up the incident, because both the technical rescue situation and the environment can change rapidly. The initial hazard analysis sets the groundwork for the entire incident. However, expect the follow-up analysis to be dynamic. The incident may affect only local areas, or it may encompass a multicounty region. In the latter situation, resources could become compromised. In some areas the magnitude of the incident may not have been realized or anticipated through adequate planning.

A primary component of the size-up is locating and determining the number of victims involved in the incident. This can be aided by considering the time of day with regard to the location of the incident. Emergency responders must ask themselves questions that analyze risk versus benefit factors. For instance, what is the acceptable level of risk for this rescue? How will prolonged rescue efforts, coupled with extreme environmental conditions, influence victim survival? Are we using our resources to maximize the survivability of the majority of victims? These moral and ethical questions cause much concern among emergency responders. Moreover, there will come a time when no matter what efforts are put forth, the end result will not change.

Emergency responders can improve a victim's chances of survival by identifying and planning potential technical rescue scenarios in their response area. For instance, consider more than one way into an area that may be stricken, resulting in road closures caused by the event or by environmental conditions. Acquiring a knowledge of building layouts and hazard locations in your community before an event also improves the emergency response. Emergency responders should consider the resources available before an event and should know how to obtain additional resources when needed. The use of preplanned principles can also expedite patient contact. Can you see or hear the victim? Does the victim know you are there? Some invaluable resources for a technical rescue include two-way radios, hard line communications systems, specialized cameras, and listening devices. However, when establishing contact with victims, keep in mind that personal safety is paramount.

The Federal Emergency Management Agency's (FEMA) **National Incident Management System (NIMS)** has become widely accepted in North America as the basis for a standardized incident command system (ICS). As an EMT, you most likely will be concerned with elements associated with the following:

- Command
- Safety
- Rescue
- Medical care
- Control zones

You must become familiar with and practice the NIMS/ICS policies and procedures established in your area of operation. The web sites of the United States Fire Administration (USFA) and the FEMA provide useful links to educational resources that can help you build your understanding of NIMS concepts. Also, many local fire, rescue, and police agencies may provide NIMS/ICS training for emergency and government personnel in their region. A standardized ICS greatly improves emergency personnel safety, streamlines technical rescue operations, and increases the victim's chances of survival.

■ STRUCTURAL COLLAPSE RESCUE

Certain conditions and events affect structures worldwide. These include earthquakes, wind storms, floods, heavy snow or rain, substandard construction, explosions, fire, transportation accidents, and age-related decay. EMTs responding to a structural collapse incident must be aware that such emergencies present special hazards and challenges to rescuers attempting to reach victims. Gathering information and analyzing it are two crucial steps in the successful **extrication** of trapped victims. Rescue personnel should consider the following factors when determining a collapse rescue action plan:

- **Occupancy:** The activity performed in the structure and the number of potential occupants.
- **Structural type:** The type of structural materials involved and the type of collapse.
- **Collapse mechanism:** A determination of the reason for the structural failure and establishment of zones within the collapse that may prove to be more likely to support victim survival.
- **Time of day:** The time when the collapse occurred and the expected occupant load at that time.
- **Prior intelligence:** Information from occupants, the public, and local authorities that can predict the location of trapped victims.
- **Search and rescue resources:** The structural design or material may require resources beyond those already available.
- **Structural condition postcollapse:** The stabilization efforts needed to prevent further deterioration of the structure.

When a structural collapse occurs, rescue operations typically follow a four-phase pattern, depending on the seriousness of the collapse.

Phase 1

The first phase of the rescue operation is the initial spontaneous response. This phase consists of rescue activity by unskilled good Samaritans and civilians. These efforts usually are augmented and become managed by local fire and rescue personnel, who often act beyond their normal skill level. Typically, 75% of the lightly trapped victims are rescued during this phase. The survival rate for these victims is usually high, because the entrapment was minimal and they have prompt access to medical care.

Phase 2

The second phase is the planned community response. With strong leadership, this phase may be activated shortly after the initial rescue phase. Depending on the magnitude and cause of the incident, trained community response teams may be instructed to search for and rescue victims trapped by light debris or other objects that can be removed relatively easily. This phase also involves mitigation of active hazards (e.g., fires) and elimination of potential hazards (e.g., shutting down utilities). Throughout this phase, a well-defined ICS must be in use. ICS leaders gather information, analyze it, and direct community resources as needed. Their analysis determines the deployment of resources to subsequent phases of response. Operations during this phase can continue for days.

During phase 2, special identifiers may be used for streets and structures. As search, rescue, and damage assessment teams proceed into the stricken area, a uniform marking system that shows the hazards and history of the damaged structure may be used. These highly visible marks generally are spray painted (in international orange) adjacent to accessible entry points. The structure hazards mark is a 2-foot square box, which indicates that the structure is safe for search and rescue. Additional marks may include the following:

- One diagonal (/) inside the square box indicates that significant damage exists but the structure is relatively safe; shoring, bracing, and monitoring of hazards may be required before search and rescue.
- Two diagonals (X) inside the square box indicate that the structure is unsafe and may suddenly collapse. Rescue teams should not enter until measures have been taken to reduce the risk of injury to search and rescue personnel.
- An arrow near the square box directs search and rescue personnel to the safest entry point.
- An "HM" next to the square box alerts search and rescue personnel to the possible presence of hazardous material. Operations are deferred until the hazardous condition is better defined or eliminated.

Along with structure hazard marks, search assessment marks are painted at the entry point. A 2-foot diagonal, with the date and time above it, indicates entry. When the search and rescue team exits the structure, an alternating diagonal is painted, forming a large X. Information relating to the search team identifier is noted in the left margin of the X. Special information is noted in the right margin of the X, such as the presence of animals or unusual hazards. The lower margin of the X contains information about occupants, such as "NO VICTIMS," "3 DEAD," or "LOCATED." This information is valuable for directing resources to follow up search and recovery activities.

Phase 3

The third phase of the rescue operation involves the use of void space rescue forces. (Phase 2 search elements will have helped prioritize the use of these teams based on risk-benefit analysis.) Void space rescue teams have special training in structural stabilization and may use aspects of the collapsed structure to gain access to victims. They analyze the type of structural collapse and how it may relate to victims' chances of survival. Different types of structural collapse can be identified by their physical characteristics. Moreover, analysis of the collapse features allows prediction of some aspects of the void space rescue operation. Generally, there are five types of collapse: lean-to; vee; A, or inverted vee; pancake; and cantilever.

- **Lean-to collapse:** A vertical structural component rests against another vertical structural component, creating a triangular void between the vertical components.
- **Vee collapse:** A horizontal structural component collapses close to the center of the span, creating two triangular voids on either side of the collapse.
- **A (inverted vee) collapse:** A horizontal component collapses at one or both ends of its span, creating one triangular void that is supported close to the center by a vertical component.
- **Pancake collapse:** Horizontal structural components detach from vertical support systems, resulting in uniform downward collapse. Inverted vee voids may be created in this type of collapse by rigid furnishings in the occupancy or strong protruding vertical components in the collapse zone.
- **Cantilever collapse:** Limited detachment of a horizontal structure from the vertical support system, resulting in collapse usually to one side of the structure; this forms a triangular void toward the standing vertical component.

Many void space rescue teams have been established by intergovernmental mutual aid agreements. This means that teams may be dispatched to a stricken area within a few hours of an incident. All emergency personnel should be familiar with disaster plans designed for their region. They should pay special attention to identifying resources and the capabilities of those resources. Continued use of a strong ICS structure is imperative during phase 3.

Phase 4

The fourth phase of response calls for use of technical experts and **urban search and rescue teams (USARs).** These experts and teams may be dispatched from several regions across North America. In fact, they also may be drawn from overseas resources. At this level of response, state and federal agencies work with local authorities to obtain equipment and resources for prolonged operations that may take weeks. State and federal disaster plans usually have been instituted at this level.

EMTs can expect a wide variety of trauma injuries in victims of structural collapse, as well as exacerbations of pre-existing medical conditions.

■ ROPE RESCUE

Rope rescue generally can be divided into two categories: high angle (vertical) evacuation and low angle (slope) evacuation. In high angle rope operations, the entire weight of the rescuer and the victim is supported by rope systems. In low angle rope operations, the rescuers' weight is directed to the ground as they manipulate the victim in a litter or basket. In these operations rope is used to provide additional stability to rescuers (Fig. 34-1). Rope also may be attached

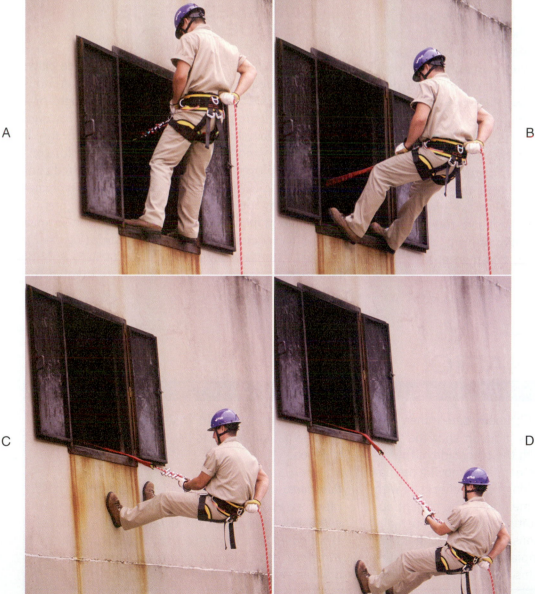

A
B
C
D

Fig. 34-1 Rope rescue.

to rescue baskets to facilitate smooth, safe movement of the victim and rescuers up or down from low angle inclines. The use of rope is not limited to low or high angle rescues. It also may be used in confined space, trench, water, and wilderness search and rescue operations.

Many hazards are possible with rope rescue operations. The most common hazard is falling. Any responder involved in such operations must be se-cured. Other hazards that may be encountered during a rope rescue include the following:

- Tripping
- Uneven or wet ground
- Entanglement or pinching by rope or equipment
- Falling objects
- Active utilities
- Atmospheric conditions
- Weather
- Untrained responders
- Hostile bystanders and victims
- Location-specific hazards

EMTs should work within the ICS structure and be prepared to provide care for the victim.

SPECIAL Considerations

Harness Suspension

Suspension trauma is a medical issue just gaining recognition. It is a concern for both victims and rescuers who are suspended by harnesses during high angle rescues. It can happen as quickly as 15 minutes after the victim has been suspended by a harness. Suspension trauma occurs when the legs are immobile while a person is in an upright position. Gravity pulls blood into the lower legs, which have a very large storage capacity. Eventually enough blood accumulates to reduce return blood flow to the right chamber of the heart. Because the heart can pump only the blood available, cardiac output begins to fall. The heart speeds up to maintain sufficient blood flow to the brain; however, if the blood supply to the heart remains restricted enough, circulation will cease to keep the victim awake, and then alive.

■ CONFINED SPACE RESCUE

OSHA has defined two types of **confined space entry:** non-permit-required and permit required. A non-permit-required confined space is large enough for a worker to enter to perform his or her duties. However, the worker may have limited or restricted means of entry or exit, and the space is not designed for continuous employee occupancy. A permit-required confined space may have hazardous atmospheres, material that may engulf the entrant, or a configuration that could trap the entrant. These spaces also may have other serious safety or health hazards (Fig. 34-2).

OSHA statistics have shown that 60% to 80% of fatalities in confined space accidents involve the

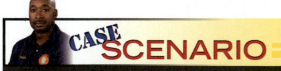

CASE SCENARIO

continued

Moving around the car, Elizabeth determines that the force of the crash has jammed shut the front passenger's side door. With the other side of the vehicle smashed in by the other car, removing the patient is going to be a challenge. Jack checks in with Jane and the other crew members. The patient appears to be in stable condition. He has an open airway, adequate respirations, and a strong radial pulse. However, he complains of neck and back pain, as well as pain in his left shoulder and arm.

Jack completes a rapid trauma exam and reports that the patient needs to be immobilized before extrication.

Questions: *Based on the patient's presentation, is rapid extrication necessary? What would be the safest way to extricate the driver from the vehicle? What equipment might be used to assist in the extrication? What safety precautions should the EMS crew consider during extrication?*

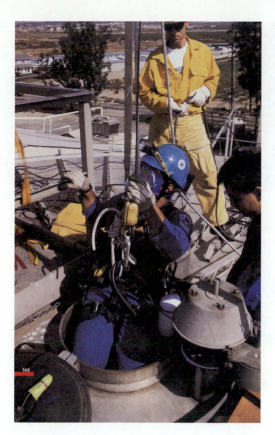

Fig. 34-2 Rescuer entering a confined space.

would-be rescuers. These individuals usually are bystanders or rescue personnel who are not trained in confined space rescue operations and who think they can quickly drag the victim out of danger. As many as 90% of these fatalities are the result of exposure to inhaled hazards. Other hazards encountered in confined space rescues include the following:

- Falls
- Slippery floors
- Tripping hazards
- Mechanical hazards
- Electrical hazards
- Pneumatic hazards (i.e., high-pressure gases)
- Drowning/engulfing
- Excessive temperatures (heat or cold)
- Predetermined hazards
- Hazards introduced by the rescuer

EMTs should never attempt to enter a confined space unless they have the proper training, resources, and authority to do so. EMTs can expect victims removed from a confined space to have suffered various traumatic injuries, along with respiratory injuries as a result of hazardous inhalation exposure.

■ TRENCH RESCUE AND EXCAVATION

A **trench** is an excavation that is less than 15 feet wide and is deeper than it is wide. OSHA publishes regulations governing the construction and human occupation of trenches if they are over 5 feet deep. Trenches less than 5 feet deep also may be regulated if special hazards are a factor. Trench incidents and confined space incidents have many similarities. Escape routes must be determined, air quality must be monitored, and other, similar protective measures must be taken. The most alarming similarity is that 65% of untrained would-be rescuers are killed in secondary trench collapses. Virtually all the hazards associated with trench rescue (Fig. 34-3) are hidden from the untrained rescuer. Some of these hazards are manmade, but most of them are present naturally in all trenches and cannot be eliminated. However, they can be anticipated.

The most lethal hazard in a trench rescue is **secondary collapse.** After the **initial collapse** traps a victim, the remaining sections of the trench may have less stability and can fall, causing successive collapses. There is little warning from falling soil. Trench walls can collapse in as little as one tenth of a second and can weigh as much as 145 pounds per cubic foot. A small cave-in usually involves 1.5 cubic yards of dirt weighing as much as 2 tons. The average man covered with 2 feet of soil could be under some 3000 pounds with as much as 1000 pounds crushing his chest area. Many secondary collapses occur while rescuers are trying to dig out the initial victim. It is imperative that untrained and unequipped rescuers never enter a collapsed trench.

The four basic types of trench collapses that may be encountered are as follows:

- *Slough in:* The lower portion of a side wall gives way into the trench, leaving an upper portion dangling.
- *Side wall in:* A complete side wall gives way into the trench.
- *Shear in:* A side wall falls downward, with the lower portion filling the trench first.
- *Soil in:* The soil removed from the trench is placed too close to the side wall boundary, overloading portions of the side wall, and slips back into the trench.

Trench rescues usually are 4- to 10-hour operations. The victim may be "frozen" in the position he or she was in when the collapse occurred. Often limbs

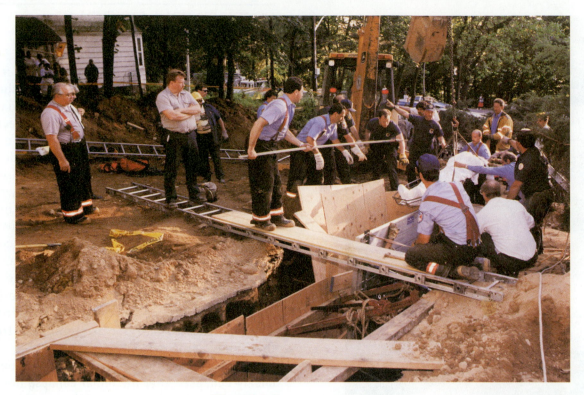

Fig. 34-3 Trench rescue.

are bent in odd positions, and in many cases the victim has fractures. Victims cannot merely be pulled out from under the dirt. They must be carefully uncovered with hand tools before being removed from the trench (Fig. 34-4); they cannot be yanked out. Moreover, the use of backhoes only results in additional injury or death. Many factors can complicate trench rescues, such as wet soils, loosely packed soils, buried utilities, and previously disturbed soils.

At a trench collapse scene, the most important initial measures involve keeping all vehicular traffic at a distance, limiting access by unnecessary personnel, preventing foot traffic adjacent to trench walls, and eliminating vibration by shutting down all mechanical equipment.

Establishment of a strong ICS structure and control zones ensures rescuer safety and expedites rescue operations. Workmen at the excavation site should be interviewed, because they may be able to offer vital information as to where the victim was last seen before the trench collapse.

Rescue personnel should never enter an unprotected trench. Only rescuers or engineers with proper technical training in this specialty rescue field should construct a protected trench. Three basic methods can be used to create a protected trench (Fig. 34-5):

- **Shoring** is a method of creating a support system inside the trench that places pressure

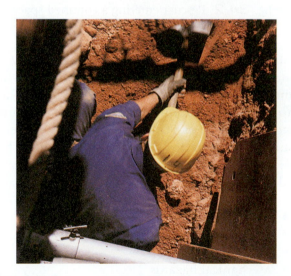

Fig. 34-4 In a trench collapse, rescuers often must dig the victim out by hand and with small hand tools.

against trench walls, preventing soil from moving. NOTE: Shoring does not stop currently moving soil.

- **Shielding** is a method of placing extremely strong metal boxes inside a trench. These boxes are engineered to withstand moving soil and protect workers inside the shield, or trench box.

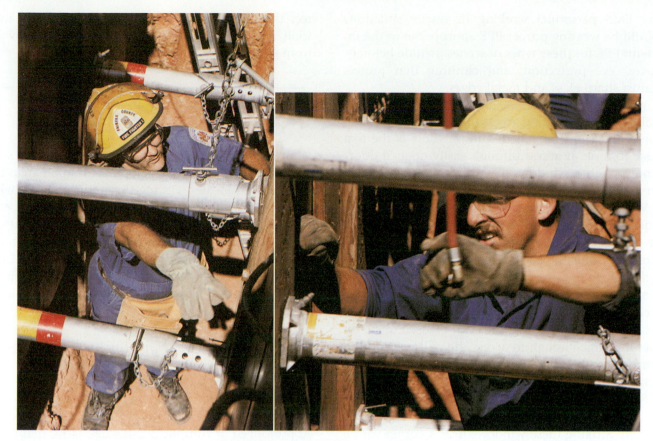

Fig. 34-5 In trench collapse operations, pneumatic rams are used with paneling to stabilize the walls of the trench. (From Smith B: *Rescuers in action*, St Louis, 1996, Mosby.)

- **Sloping** is a technique of cutting back the side walls of the trench to the angle of repose (i.e., the angle at which soil no longer slides).

EMTs should prepare for the following injuries in victims removed from trench and excavation collapses:

- Open and closed fractures
- Crush syndrome
- Traumatic asphyxia

- Hypothermia
- Head injuries
- Lung injuries
- Spinal injuries
- Hypoxia

SPECIAL Considerations

Bystanders at a Scene
Bystanders try to help at the scene of a trench or hole collapse. One of the most important things the EMT can do is clear the bystanders away from the hole. The added weight and movement can cause secondary collapses, possibly trapping more people in the hole. The more unstable the soil, the farther away the bystanders should be moved.

GAINING ACCESS

Although EMTs are always anxious to get to their patients as quickly as possible, it is important that the scene is made safe before entering. Fire and rescue personnel should isolate fire, electrical, and fluid hazards that are typical in vehicular events. As soon as possible, the first goal in rescue situations is gaining access to the patient for medical personnel. In most cases, gaining access for medical personnel will also establish a route to remove the patient; in some cases, extrication may require time and sophisticated skills and equipment. Gaining access allows aid to be given to the patient while the extrication is accomplished.

Ideally, specially trained rescue technicians will gain access to the patient for the medical responders.

Any EMS personnel working in rescue situations should be wearing proper PPE appropriate to the incident. PPE for these types of scenes include helmets, gloves, eye protection, and clothing that protect against sharp glass and metal edges.

When gaining access, simple things should be evaluated first. Gaining access to the patient through doors that can be opened without tools is the first place to look. If access through easily opened doors is not possible, windows may be a route for medical personnel to get to the patient.

When gaining access through windows, techniques are specific to the type of glass. Windshields are constructed out of safety glass, which has a laminate that holds the glass together when broken. It is preferable to remove the entire windshield, creating a clean route for personnel to get to the patient and, if need be, removing the patient from the vehicle. If necessary, axes or cutting tools can be used to cut an opening large enough to access the patient. Caution will need to be taken to protect rescuers or patients moving through the opening.

Side and rear windows are constructed of tempered glass, which shatters into small pieces when broken. Striking these windows near a corner with a tool or using a spring-loaded nail punch will easily shatter the glass, and precautions will need to be taken to protect the patient and rescuers from the glass fragments.

If the rescue operation is more complex, rescue technicians may also use tools to pry open doors or create openings by removing the roof of the vehicle. Rescue technicians will use a variety of cutting tools and rams to remove or push parts of the vehicle away from the patient and create the space EMTs will need to work.

Once access is gained to the patient, EMTs will assess the patient based on an understanding of the mechanism of injury. Immediate life threats may be addressed to some degree in the vehicle, but patients will need to be removed to be cared for. In the case of critical patients, it is particularly important to remove the patient from the vehicle as quickly as possible to continue care and get the patient to the trauma center. Assessment and treatment of trauma patients is covered more fully in Chapter 29.

EXTRICATION

Extrication (also called *disentanglement*) is the process of removing the vehicle from the patient rather than the other way around. Precautions are taken to protect the injured person while hydraulic and hand tools are used to cut, pry, and push the vehicle away from the patient.

■ VEHICLE AND MACHINERY RESCUE

Vehicle rescue and machinery rescue can occur in settings ranging from densely populated urban areas to remote rural locales. During their careers, EMTs will be called to multivehicle accidents with victim entrapment and emergencies involving entrapment of limbs in industrial machinery or farm equipment. In these situations, most extrications are performed by fire or rescue agencies. When emergency personnel arrive on the scene, effective incident management must prevail. This is the cornerstone of rescuer safety and efficient victim access.

The EMT's initial scene size-up should evaluate the environmental factors, the victim's injuries, and the conditions at the scene. Environmental extremes can adversely affect those involved in rescue operations. They also may create added problems for the victim. At prolonged or complicated rescues, tarps, blankets, fans, portable heaters, and hot and cold packs may be used to reduce the effects of environmental extremes. Heated or cooled rest areas and fluids must be provided to rescuers to protect them against environmental injury.

In vehicle and machinery rescues, the victim's injuries usually are the result of blunt force trauma. Injuries can be caused by a windshield, air bag, steering wheel, dashboard, side posts, rearview mirror, door, or roof in vehicle incidents and by an auger, a punch press, or a conveyer belt in machinery incidents. It is important that the EMT recognize the mechanism of injury, because it indicates the magnitude of force applied in the injury (Fig. 34-6). The victim may have external injuries, as indicated by bruises, lacerations, fractures, and amputations, and/or internal injuries,

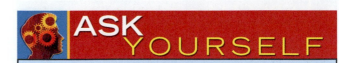

ASK YOURSELF

You and your partner arrive at the scene of a multivehicle accident. Power lines are down and arcing, and you see what appears to be gasoline on the roadway. What do you do now? Do you run to the vehicle and assist the trapped driver?

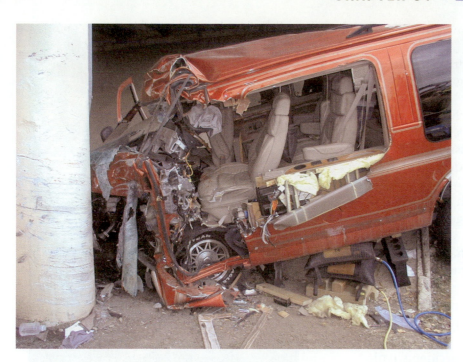

Fig. 34-6 The mechanism of injury can point to potential patient injuries.

involving the organs, brain, spine, and blood vessels. The mechanism of injury can give EMTs a clue to the potential for internal trauma.

When evaluating scene conditions, EMTs should consider the following major aspects:

- **Traffic control:** The rescue scene must be protected from traffic. The best way to do this is to place heavy equipment in the path of traffic flow. This blocks the accident scene and prevents further injury to the victims and injury to the rescuers. The police can best address the rerouting of traffic.
- **Stabilization:** This is a high priority with any accident involving a vehicle or machinery. It maximizes contact with the ground, restricts movement, and prevents further injury to the victim and injury of rescuers.
- **Hazardous materials:** Such materials must be identified and dealt with or removed before rescue operations can proceed.
- **Electrical hazards:** Rescuers should be sure to turn off involved machinery, disconnect vehicle batteries, and contact utility companies to remove or de-energize power lines. All industrial machinery should be locked out and tagged out, meaning all power has been turned off and the machinery has been locked and tagged, to prevent further injury.
- **Fire:** Fire is a major concern at vehicular accidents because of the presence of gasoline, diesel fuel, or compressed natural gas. A charged fire hose line and portable dry chemical fire extinguishers must be available at all vehicular extrications.
- **Crowd control:** Generally, the police control the crowd, because onlookers can hamper or restrict rescue activities, delaying victim extrication. Public access must be restricted.
- **Work zones:** Use of an action/extrication zone, a support/tool zone, and a limited access/command zone can help maintain order at extrications. Only those needed to perform required functions should be allowed in these areas. This improves efficiency and limits exposure of rescuers to potential hazards.
- **Octal survey:** This type of scene survey is an eight-sided evaluation: inside, outside, top, bottom, front, back, left side, and right side. Personnel in the command zone should continually re-examine these areas for developments that could alter action plans or require safety alerts.

Emergency responders should also be aware of the unique hazards associated with vehicle and machinery rescues:

- Volatile fuels, oils, battery acid, hydraulic fluids, and chemicals
- Stored energy systems, such as batteries and hood and rear hatch pistons, as well as pneu-

matic and hydraulic systems operating at extreme pressures

- Air bag systems, such as the driver's side air bag, the passenger's side air bag, and side impact air bags
- Energy absorption systems, such as bumpers, hydraulic shocks, springs, chains, and belts under extreme tension or compression
- Heavily constructed vehicles, equipment, and machinery
- Equipment and machinery with heavy rollers, sharp edges, flails, or other dangerous processing components
- Poor road or field conditions that may not allow rescue equipment access or may cause settling or shifting of equipment
- Powerful rescue tools and equipment that may injure rescuers if used improperly

Victims of vehicle and machinery accidents typically have crushing injuries, such as bone fractures, and lacerations and contusions. Head, thoracic, and pelvic injuries also should be expected, as well as internal injuries, such as hollow organ rupture, solid organ laceration, or respiratory and circulatory collapse. EMTs should always consider spinal cord injuries as a possibility. They therefore should move the victim as little as possible, using proper immobilization technique.

■ WATER RESCUE

Most jurisdictions have some type of body of water within or adjacent to them. It is essential that rescue personnel recognize the hazards associated with and common to all water rescue operations (Fig. 34-7). Before any rescue operation begins, rescue personnel who may come in contact with the water's edge must put on an appropriate **personal flotation device (PFD),** one that has been approved by the U.S. Coast Guard. Drowning obviously is a prime concern, but environmental hazards also may pose risks. Such hazards include temperature extremes, which can expose victims and rescuers to heat exhaustion, dehydration, frostbite, frost nip, and hypothermia. Body heat can be lost in still water at a rate 25 times that seen in still air. The initial effects of exposure are loss of the abilities to think clearly and to perform simple motor skills. The aquatic environment itself can present hazards, such as plants, seaweed, currents, heavy sediment, silt, reduced visibility, animals, insects, and bacteriologic or viral biohazards.

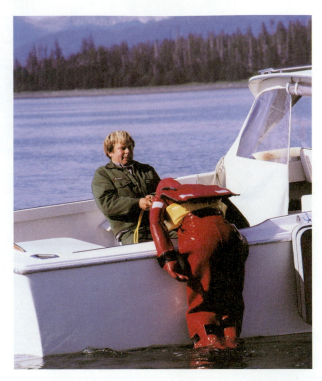

Fig. 34-7 One-person water rescue technique.

In addition, unique hazards are associated with the four specialty divisions of water rescue:

- Dive rescue
- Ice rescue
- Surf rescue
- Swift water rescue

Dive Rescue

A water rescue may require the assistance of rescue-trained and certified divers who can use a self-contained underwater breathing apparatus **(SCUBA).** SCUBA diving can be a hazardous activity. Panic or anxiety can result in decompression sickness, nitrogen narcosis, oxygen toxicity, embolism, or drowning. These may occur as a result of a diver becoming lost, trapped, or losing the air supply. Also, during underwater rescue operations, rescue divers can become trapped in a submerged vehicle, boat, rail car, or aircraft. Fatigue, exhaustion, and dehydration are other hazards associated with SCUBA diving. The protective suit that prevents hypothermia in water and the heavy diving equipment can cause heat-related stress when the diver is out of the water. Divers should have assistance putting on, taking off, and transporting their equipment. Dive rescue team guidelines and procedures should require strong leadership within the ICS structure.

Ice Rescue

Ice rescue operations often involve several victims, because would-be rescuers or untrained emergency responders often attempt emotion-driven rescues. They frequently underestimate the fast-acting hypothermic effects of ice cold water, or they may become trapped under the ice by an unseen swift water current. Rescue SCUBA divers working in this environment should also be aware of the additional difficulties that ice diving presents and should follow rescue dive team procedures for ice diving.

Surface ice rescues should only be performed by trained personnel who are also properly equipped. The EMT should be watching the clock at cold water drowning (submersion) incidents. Often victims thought to have drowned may be resuscitated if recovered promptly. When the human body is immersed in very cold water, a physiologic safety system known as the *mammalian dive reflex* is activated by the lower brain. This reflex causes the circulatory system to move oxygenated blood to critical core body areas and to slow the metabolism, reducing the need for oxygen. Cold water drowning victims have been successfully resuscitated after submersion for a prolonged period. Factors that affect the chances of survival of a near-drowning victim include age, physical condition, water temperature, submersion time, and the efficiency of the cardiopulmonary resuscitation (CPR) technique.

Surf Rescue

Surf rescue situations arise where land meets a larger body of water, such as an ocean, a sea, or a lake. As waves approach the beach and the bottom contour rises, the waves break over. Large breaking waves can produce thousands of pounds of force, crushing and destroying anything in their path. These waves can capsize watercraft and make tracking victims in the water very difficult. Storms and high winds can intensify the waves and swells, turning once-placid beaches into deathtraps. Invisible undertows, tidal surges, riptides, and currents can snatch and drown a victim without warning, even in relatively shallow water. Only personnel familiar with the coastline who are equipped and trained should perform this type of water rescue.

EMTs can expect victims of surf-related incidents to have blunt trauma injuries. The entire body may have been tumbled against rocks, coral, and the seabed or lakebed. Other common injuries are head injuries, spinal injuries, contusions, fractures, and lacerations.

Swift Water Rescue

The primary hazard associated with swift water rescue is the constant, awesome, and relentless power of moving water. Swift water in rivers, streams, flooded ravines, and washes after a rainstorm can sweep victims away with a force the victim cannot overcome. Rescuers must exercise caution around swift water, because one misstep can turn the rescuer into a victim. Swift water propels victims into stationary objects, resulting in blunt trauma. Victims of swift water incidents should try to float on their backs, keeping their feet pointed downstream so that they strike objects with the feet. Attempts to stand up may entangle the feet in objects, and as a result the victim may be pulled toward the bottom and drown. It usually is best not to try to fight the current by swimming. Instead, victims should try to guide themselves toward shore, on an angle, with the current. Only rescue personnel trained and equipped for swift water rescue should attempt it.

Low head dams can present another water rescue situation. Victims and rescuers often overlook the hazards associated with these dams. Low head dams are low dams built in rivers and streams to slow the downstream flow or create a reservoir before the dam. Another name for low head dams is "drowning machines." As water flows over a dam and falls vertically, it drives to the bottom and rises to the surface slightly downstream. At this point, some water continues downstream and some back flows toward the dam. This point, known as the *boil line,* is the entry point to the "drowning machine." The killing force in the "drowning machine" is a vertical whirlpool created by a strong water current. People who attempt a rescue or recovery from a vertical whirlpool without proper training and equipment only increase the body count. As a result of aeration of the water at the boil line, objects become less buoyant. Therefore a boat driven into the face of a low head dam will fill with water, dumping its occupants into the "drowning machine." Even rescuers wearing personal flotation devices (PFD) may be at risk of being swallowed and drowned by this force.

■ WILDERNESS SEARCH AND RESCUE

The **National Search and Rescue Plan** was published in 1956 by the National Search and Rescue Committee. This plan establishes the U.S. Air Force as the lead agency for inland search and rescue operations in the continental United States. Local Civil Air Patrol units are used for many aspects of these types of rescues. Wilderness search and rescue operations have four basic elements:

1. Locate the victim.
2. Reach the victim.
3. Stabilize the victim.
4. Evacuate the victim.

Locating the victim usually is the most time-consuming and personnel-intensive aspect of wilderness rescue. Once a search area has been established, one or more of the following search tactics can be applied:

- *Type I:* Hasty teams (teams able to respond with very little set-up time) are used, with a minimum number of experienced rescuers sent out to locate the victim.
- *Type II:* An open grid is used, involving relatively fast, high-probability search grid patterns with aircraft, search dogs, and open grid sweeps on foot. Three to seven searchers are spaced 300 to 600 feet apart.
- *Type III:* A closed grid is used, involving as many as 30 searchers spaced 15 to 20 feet apart walking in line. This type of pattern typically is used for evidence recovery.

As with any rescue operation, certain hazards may be encountered. EMTs should be aware of these hazards, because they may find themselves involved in a wilderness search group:

- **Personal hazards,** such as blisters, scrapes, scratches, falls, bruises, and dehydration

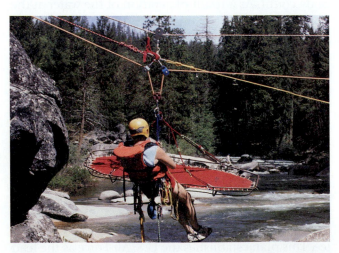

Fig. 34-8 A rescuer carries a stretcher to a patient waiting for assistance.

- **Environmental hazards,** such as insect bites and stings, poisonous plants, exposure injuries, snow blindness, altitude sickness, lightning, sunburn, windburn, and dangerous wildlife
- **Terrain hazards,** such as cliffs, avalanches, standing water, ice, moving water, caves, and high winds (Fig. 34-8)
- **Manmade hazards,** such as booby traps, mines, wells, alcohol stills, drug labs, hazardous material dumps, attack dogs, and armed criminals

Wilderness search and rescue teams should be led only by competent, experienced search personnel deployed by ICS leaders and operating within the ICS structure. Wilderness rescue can involve any of the rescue disciplines previously discussed.

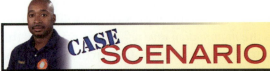

CASE SCENARIO
conclusion

After draping a blanket over the patient and Jane to protect them from shattering window glass, Elizabeth directs the fire department's rescue crew to begin opening the driver's side door. Before beginning the process, the crew confirms that no additional air bags were deployed during the crash. Although it appears that a simple pry bar tool should suffice to pop the locking mechanism, it turns out that a hydraulic spreader tool is needed to force the door away from the frame. In short order the door is pried open by the rescue crew. Elizabeth and the EMS crew quickly move the immobilized patient from the vehicle onto the waiting backboard on the gurney. ■

TEAMWORK

Rescue operations usually involve technical rescue specialists. It is important to be familiar with your local incident management protocols and guidelines so that you can work safely with law enforcement officers, firefighters, and other responders. Advance preparations for potential technical rescue incidents (i.e., identifying and planning for possible incidents in your response area) can improve a victim's chances of survival.

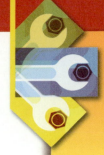
Critical Points

- You may be the first to arrive on the scene. Your personal safety is paramount. Do not attempt rescue operations for which you are not trained; leave this work to appropriately trained rescue specialists.
- Work within the structure of the incident management system and be prepared to provide emergency care for the victim.
- The mechanism of injury and the environment from which the patient is retrieved can be indicators of possible injuries.

Key Terms

A (inverted vee) collapse A type of structural collapse in which a horizontal component detaches at one or both ends of its span, creating one triangular void supported close to the center by a vertical component.

Awareness level Awareness level training is the minimum level of training a first responder should have for hazardous materials or technical rescue. Awareness level training does not allow the provider to perform HazMat or rescue operations.

Cantilever collapse A type of structural collapse characterized by limited detachment of a horizontal structure from the vertical support system, resulting in collapse usually to one side of the structure; this forms a triangular void toward the standing vertical component.

Collapse mechanism A determination of the reason for the structural failure and establishment of zones within the collapse that may prove to be more likely to promote victim survival.

Confined space entry OSHA defines two types of confined space entry. Non-permit-required confined space is a space that is large enough for a worker to perform his or her duties. However, workers in this space may have limited or restricted means of entry or exit, and the space is not designed for continuous employee occupancy. Permit-required confined space might have hazardous atmospheres, material that might engulf the entrant, or a configuration that could entrap the entrant.

Environmental hazards Insect bites and stings, poisonous plants, exposure injuries, snow blindness, altitude sickness, lightning, sunburn, windburn, and dangerous wildlife.

Extrication The process of removing a patient from entanglement in a motor vehicle or other situation in a safe and appropriate way.

Initial collapse The initial collapse is the collapse itself. By calling the collapse the *initial collapse,* it makes the point about the dangers of secondary collapse and the risk posed to rescuers.

Lean-to collapse A vertical structural component rests against another vertical structural component, creating a triangular void between the vertical components.

Manmade hazards Hazards posed or created by human beings, such as booby traps, alcohol stills, drug labs, hazardous material dumps, attack dogs, and armed criminals.

National Search and Rescue Plan The National Search and Rescue plan that was published in 1956. It establishes the U.S. Air Force as the lead coordinating agency for inland search and rescue.

Occupancy Activity performed in a structure and the number of potential occupants.

Octal survey An eight-sided scene evaluation that includes the inside, outside, top, bottom, front, back, left side, and right side.

Operations level This level of training refers to HazMat training that allows the provider to set up perimeters and safety zones while limiting the possible exposure. In regard to technical rescue, operations-level training, it allows the provider to actually perform rescue operations.

Pancake collapse A type of structural collapse in which horizontal structural components detach from vertical support systems, resulting in uniform downward collapse.

Personal flotation device (PFD) Flotation vests, suits, or other flotation devices (approved for specific applications like pools, open water, swift water, scuba) that must be worn by rescuers in order to perform water rescue.

Prior intelligence Information from occupants, the public, and local authorities that can predict the location of trapped victims.

Secondary collapse A trench rescue hazard that arises after the initial collapse. In secondary collapse, the remaining sections of the

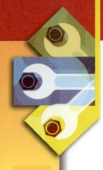

NUTS AND BOLTS

trench, which have less stability, fall, causing successive collapses. Secondary collapse is the most lethal hazard in a trench rescue.

Self-contained underwater breathing apparatus (SCUBA) Equipment specifically designed to allow for breathing underwater.

Shielding A method of creating a protected trench by placing extremely strong metal boxes inside the trench.

Shoring A method of creating a support system in a trench by exerting pressure against the trench walls to prevent soil from moving.

Sloping A method of creating a protected trench by cutting back the side walls of the trench to the angle of repose (i.e., the angle at which soil no longer slides).

Stabilization Securing an atmosphere, structure, or space, making operations within that space safe.

Structural type The type of structural materials involved and the type of collapse.

Technician level Specialized technical training allowing providers to administer technical assistance in securing hazardous environments and unsafe scenes.

Terrain hazards Hazards presented by the terrain itself. Examples would be steep hills, ravines, and water.

Trench An excavation that is less than 15 feet wide and is deeper than it is wide.

Urban search and rescue teams (USARs) Specialized, certified rescue teams that are able to respond with equipment and personnel to rescue victims of natural and man-made disasters.

Vee collapse A type of structural collapse in which a horizontal structural component close to the center of the span collapses, creating two triangular voids on either side of the collapse.

Learning Checklist

❑ Technical rescue generally consists of seven areas of specialty: structural collapse rescue, rope rescue, confined space rescue, trench and excavation rescue, vehicle and machinery rescue, water rescue, and wilderness search and rescue.

❑ All emergency medical personnel responding to a technical rescue incident should be trained at minimum to the Awareness level.

❑ Technical rescue incidents have many unique hazards that can directly affect the victim and the emergency responder.

❑ It is imperative that those responding to incident scenes be familiar with incident management and local emergency evacuation procedures and guidelines.

❑ EMTs should perform a hazard and risk assessment, as well as continuous scene size-up, because the environment can change rapidly in a technical rescue.

❑ The resources available should be considered before an event and EMTs should know how to obtain additional resources when needed.

❑ EMTs should become familiar with and practice the NIMS/ICS policies and procedures established in their area of operation. A standardized ICS greatly improves emergency personnel safety, streamlines technical rescue operations, and increases the victim's chances of survival.

❑ Structural collapses are caused by earthquakes, wind storms, floods, heavy snow or rain, substandard construction, explosions, fire, transportation accidents, and age-related decay.

❑ The four phases of a rescue response to a structural collapse are the initial spontaneous response, the planned community response, use of void space rescue forces, and use of technical experts and urban search and rescue teams.

❑ Victims of a structural collapse can suffer a wide variety of traumatic injuries, as well as exacerbations of pre-existing medical conditions.

❑ The two types of rope rescue are high angle (vertical) evacuation and low angle (slope) evacuation.

❑ EMTs should never enter a confined space unless they have obtained the proper training, resources, and authority to do so.

❑ Victims removed from a confined space are likely to have suffered various traumatic injuries, along with respiratory injuries from hazardous inhalation exposure.

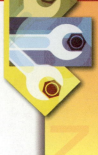

- At a trench collapse scene, rescuers should keep all vehicular traffic at a distance, limit access by unnecessary personnel, avoid foot traffic adjacent to trench walls, and eliminate vibration by shutting down all mechanical equipment.
- The establishment of a strong ICS, along with control zones, ensures rescuer safety and expedites trench rescue operations.
- EMTs should prepare for the following injuries to victims removed from trench and excavation collapses: open and closed fractures, crush syndrome, traumatic asphyxia, hypothermia, head injuries, lung injuries, spinal injuries, and hypoxia.
- The EMT's scene size-up at a vehicle or machinery rescue should evaluate environmental conditions, victim injuries, and scene conditions, such as traffic control, stabilization of the vehicle or machine, hazardous materials, electrical considerations, fire, crowd control, and work zones.
- Environmental extremes can adversely affect rescue personnel and the patient. At prolonged or complicated rescues, tarps, blankets, fans, portable heaters, and hot/cold packs may be used to reduce the effects of environmental extremes. To prevent environmental injury to rescuers, heated or cooled rest areas and fluids must be provided.
- In a motor vehicle crash rescue, injuries most often are caused by blunt force trauma from impact with the windshield, air bag, steering wheel, dashboard, side posts, rearview mirror, door, or roof. In a machinery rescue, the mechanism of injury often involves an auger, a punch press, or a conveyer belt. It is important to recognize the mechanism of injury, because it indicates the magnitude of force applied in the injury. The victim's injuries may be external, as indicated by bruises, lacerations, fractures, and amputations. They also may be internal, involving the organs, brain, spine, and blood vessels. The mechanism of injury provides a clue to possible internal trauma.
- EMTs must stay alert to the unique hazards associated with vehicle and machinery rescues.

- Typically, victims of vehicle and machinery accidents suffer crushing injuries, such as bone fractures, lacerations, and contusions. Head, thoracic, and pelvic injuries also should be expected, with internal injuries such as hollow organ rupture, solid organ laceration, or respiratory and circulatory collapse. Spinal cord injuries should always be considered. The victim should be moved as little as possible, and proper immobilization technique is a must.
- Many hazards are associated with and common to the four types of water rescue operations: dive rescue, ice rescue, surf rescue, and swift water rescue
- The four basic elements of wilderness search and rescue operations are (1) locate the victim, (2) reach the victim, (3) stabilize the victim, and (4) evacuate the victim

---

National Standard Curriculum Objectives

Cognitive Objectives

After completing this lesson, the EMT student will be able to do the following:

- Describe the purpose of extrication.
- Discuss the role of the EMT in extrication.
- Identify the equipment the EMT requires for personal safety.
- Define the fundamental components of extrication.
- State the steps that should be taken to protect the patient during extrication.
- Evaluate various methods of gaining access to the patient.
- Distinguish between simple and complex access.

Affective Objectives

No objectives identified.

Psychomotor Objectives

No objectives identified.

CHAPTER

35

CHAPTER OUTLINE

Definitions

Disaster Planning

Role of Physicians

Incident Command System

OUTLINE

LESSON GOAL

The response to a disaster involves many unique challenges for the emergency medical technician (EMT) and requires significant planning and preparation. This chapter describes the responsibilities of responders to a disaster scene and reviews the aspects of a disaster scene that responders must be familiar with and plan for accordingly. ■

GOAL

Disasters

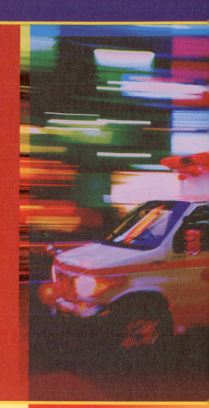

35

CHAPTER OBJECTIVES

After completing this chapter, the EMT student will be able to do the following:

1 Define a disaster and explain why a disaster in one locale may not be a disaster in another area.

2 Review the response to a disaster and the role of those first on the scene in the overall management of a disaster.

3 Discuss the performance of triage at a disaster site.

4 Review the categories of patients triaged at a disaster site and discuss how triage in a disaster situation might differ from triage in other situations.

5 Discuss the focus of medical treatment at a disaster.

6 Discuss the priorities of transport from a disaster scene and the special concerns of transporting from a disaster area.

7 Discuss the role of physicians on the scene of a disaster.

8 Review the incident command system and discuss the specific responsibilities of each section of the system.

9 Discuss communications at the scene of a disaster and where problems in communications can occur.

10 Describe resources that will be required at a disaster scene and discuss why planning must be done before a disaster occurs.

11 Discuss the importance of staging at a disaster scene and the role EMTs play in ensuring proper staging.

Continued

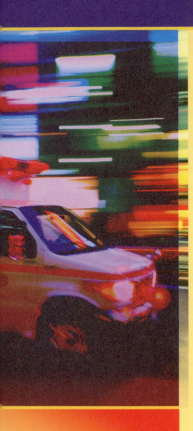

Chapter Objectives—cont'd

12 Describe the importance of proper and visible identification of the leaders at a disaster scene.

13 Discuss the importance of a call down to the hospitals once the disaster is over.

14 Discuss the role of the media at a disaster and the importance of planning ahead on how to address the needs of the media at a disaster scene.

15 Discuss the importance of a debriefing after a disaster and the role proper debriefing and incident review can play in responders' recovery from a disaster.

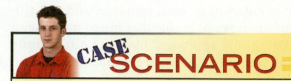

CASE SCENARIO

Ray and his partner can hear the wailing of the old town air horn in the distance, just as county communications announces the sighting of a large funnel cloud right outside the city limits. Storms had been passing through all afternoon, and the National Weather Service had been aggressive about announcing possible tornadoes. The hospital had called in additional ambulance personnel, and the crews had stocked their rigs with additional supplies in case a worst case scenario developed. Unfortunately, that's what happens. Twenty minutes after the announcement, tones begin to send fire, rescue, and emergency medical services (EMS) crews toward the industrial park in the area where the tornado was spotted.

Pulling up to the scene, Ray can see that several emergency vehicles are already there. They are in front of a commercial building that was torn apart by the tornado's heavy winds. The area is devastated.

Questions: What are Ray's priorities at this point? What forms of protective personal equipment should he be using? Who should Ray report to?

In the past 25 years, disasters, both natural and acts of terrorism, have claimed more than 3 million lives worldwide. They have adversely affected more than 800 million people and have caused billions of dollars in property damage.[1,2] Disasters have always been a part of the human experience (e.g., the San Francisco earthquake of 1906). However, the incidence of disasters or potential disasters has increased dramatically over the past decade, and all signs point to that trend continuing into the foreseeable future. In the past 10 years, the world has witnessed acts of terrorism against the World Trade Center in New York City (2001), the London subway and bus systems (2005), the U.S. embassies in Kenya and Tanzania (1998), the Alfred P. Murrah Federal Building in Oklahoma City (1995), and the Tokyo subway (1995), just to name a few. A number of natural disasters also have occurred, including Hurricane Katrina's devastation of the Gulf Coast (2005), hurricanes in Florida (2004), the tsunami in eastern Asia (2004), earthquakes in Turkey (1999), and flooding in California (1998)—a very short list of examples. Increasing population density, particularly in areas prone to flooding and hurricanes; the production and transportation of potentially toxic and hazardous materials; and a seemingly heightened risk of terrorism are all factors that suggest an increasing probability of a disaster or mass casualty situation.

The reality is that each and every person whose career involves responding to medical emergencies can expect to be involved in at least one major disaster at some point in his or her career. These professionals need to be prepared for such an event (Fig. 35-1). It could reasonably be argued that it's not possible to be completely prepared for events such as those mentioned previously. However, it may well be possible to be better prepared. Although EMTs may not be involved in every aspect of disaster management, they are a part of the team and important to the success of the response. To participate effectively, you must have an understanding of all aspects of disaster management.

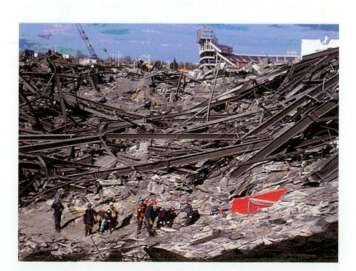

Fig. 35-1 Factors such as the increasing population density, particularly in areas prone to flooding and hurricanes; the manufacture and transportation of potentially toxic and hazardous materials; and the seemingly heightened risk of terrorism all suggest an increasing likelihood of disasters and mass casualty situations.

Emergency responders, including EMTs, usually have significant responsibilities in the management of a disaster. They therefore must be familiar with common aspects of disaster management and with local policies and protocols. This chapter reviews general aspects of disaster management and some principles that have emerged from experience in dealing with catastrophic situations. The goal is to prepare EMT students to take part in an event should they be called to do so.

It is important to note that one factor is perhaps even more crucial to effective disaster management than on-scene care: that factor is early recognition that the situation may overwhelm existing resources and communication of that fact to appropriate channels, so that the process of preparing and activating additional resources can begin. This requires a thorough knowledge of the available resources and how to activate them, as well as the protocols and capabilities of other responding agencies and local hospitals.

■ DEFINITIONS

A **disaster** can be defined as any event that overwhelms the ability of local resources to respond to that event. Thus the same event may qualify as a disaster in one area but not in another. The actual number of victims is less important than the type and degree of injuries they have suffered. For example, a two-car accident with four critical patients may be a regular occurrence and easily managed with existing resources in some areas but could quickly overwhelm local resources in another area. The term **multiple casualty incident (MCI)** often is used to describe disaster situations. However, strictly speaking, an MCI is simply an event that results in more than one victim; it does not address the local system's ability to handle it.

Keeping this definition of a disaster in mind, you can see that any disaster planning must begin

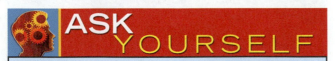

Put yourself in my shoes for a moment. As a responder to the World Trade Center disaster on September 11, 2001, many thoughts crossed my mind. When I first stepped onto ground zero, I thought, "Where on earth do we start? Will I be able to perform as expected? How do I keep myself safe?"

with an assessment of local resources and identification of the types of events that might overwhelm them. Using this approach, planners can identify how and where to access additional resources in a timely manner. It also allows earlier recognition of an event that might require those additional resources.

■ DISASTER PLANNING

Response to a Disaster

It will not always be apparent to EMTs before or even after arriving at a scene that a disaster exists. Because early recognition is critical, you must be diligent in considering the possibility of a disaster on every call. As the EMS provider, your safety is of primary importance at any scene, and a disaster or potential disaster is no exception. Always size up a scene before entering. This may be particularly challenging, given the temptations that may exist for you at the scene of a disaster. It may be very tempting to enter a scene immediately upon arrival, particularly if a victim is in sight and in need of help. Always keep in mind that you can't do your patients any good if you become a victim yourself. In fact, you may even make a bad situation worse if you do not ensure your own safety before entering the scene.

Park your vehicle in a safe spot, preferably uphill and upwind of the scene in case any hazardous materials are involved. Always wear appropriate protective equipment; at minimum, this means gloves and eye protection. As you approach a scene, always consider the possibility that a disaster exists. Once a disaster or the potential for a disaster has been recognized, the responsibilities of responders may change significantly.

First responders on the scene of a disaster have two priorities: (1) to perform an overall assessment of the situation and (2) to communicate those findings to a regional trauma center or a centralized EMS resource/communications center. The first part of this assessment should determine the following factors:

- The nature of the incident
- The extent of the damage
- The overall number of victims and the types of injuries involved
- Any hazards rescuers face in responding to the scene
- The best access to the scene, along with any known barriers to access

The second part of the overall assessment involves the organization of a command post (incident command is discussed later in the chapter).

Communication of the findings of the overall assessment to the appropriate agency can be easily overlooked; however, this is crucial to a successful response to a disaster. Just as the first response to a person suffering cardiac arrest should be to dial 911, even before cardiopulmonary resuscitation (CPR) is started, the first responders on the scene of a disaster must report their assessment of the event before they begin treating the victims. This allows the other resources needed for a proper response to be accessed and activated as soon as possible. The bigger the disaster, the more important this step becomes.

As mentioned previously, the findings of the overall assessment should be reported to the regional trauma center or a centralized EMS resource/communications center, which then relays information to other area hospitals. The regional trauma center also can obtain information from the other hospitals about emergency department capacity, critical care and operating room capabilities, and the availability

of resources. In this way, the entire system can prepare and implement the best response to a situation. Early, organized preparation by local hospitals is one of the keys to successful management of a disaster.

Once the overall assessment has been reported, the triage process can begin.

Triage

Triage is the process of sorting and classifying patients into categories based upon the severity of their illness or injuries and the likelihood of survival and then prioritizing the patients for treatment and transport. The aim is to do the most good for the greatest number of patients. Medical providers frequently are called upon to perform triage. It usually involves identifying the patient most in need of attention and then applying all available resources to that patient until the immediate needs have been addressed. In a disaster situation, however, the possibility that available resources will be overwhelmed must be considered and even assumed. If the goal is to do the most good for the largest number of people, then in a disaster you cannot simply identify one need and address that need exclusively. As tempting as it may be to begin treatment at once, it is vital to the successful management of a true disaster that triage be completed before treatment is started (Fig. 35-2).

The goal of the initial triage effort is to locate and evaluate all patients involved in the incident and to establish the priority by which patients will be treated and transported. Priority is given to patients with the most urgent conditions who are thought to have a likely chance of survival if those conditions are treated. Generally, four categories are used in triage: critical or severe, moderate or urgent, minor or delayed, and mortally wounded or dead. Many systems use triage tags (Fig. 35-3), which identify the patient and his or her triage category. The tags typically are numbered sequentially to aid the logging of victims at the scene.

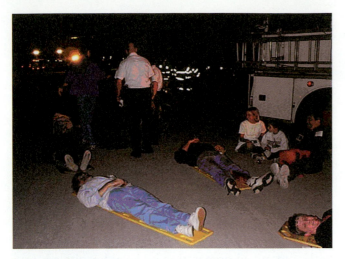

Fig. 35-2 Triage is performed before treatment is begun.

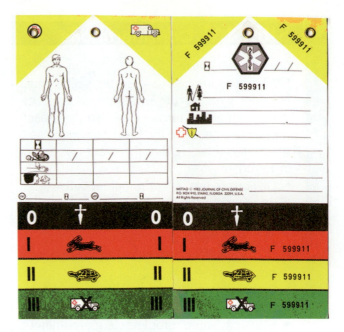

Fig. 35-3 Triage tag.

Triage tags have very little space on which to write. Therefore each category (and its tag) often has an identifying color. Clearly showing the victim's triage category is the most important function of the triage tag. The following colors usually are assigned to the four triage categories:

- *Red—critical or severe:* These patients, given available care, have a reasonable chance of survival, but without care that chance is markedly diminished. Injuries that may fall into this category include respiratory distress caused by suspected pneumothorax or an open chest wound, penetrating injuries to the abdomen, or certain head injuries. Patients in this category receive the highest priority for treatment and transport.
- *Yellow—moderate or urgent:* These patients have injuries that are not expected to lead to significant morbidity or mortality if not treated immediately but that clearly need further medical management at a hospital. Certain extremity fractures, burns, and blunt abdominal trauma may fall into this category. Patients in this category typically are treated and transported *after* the patients in the red category (critical or severe) have been managed.
- *Green—minor or delayed:* Also sometimes referred to as the "walking wounded," these patients have injuries that are not expected to lead to significant morbidity while they wait for patients in the red and yellow categories to be treated and transported. Patients with lacerations or sprains might be triaged into this category. Patients in the green category might reasonably be transported by bus or van in some situations. Therefore disaster

plans should attempt to provide alternative means of transport for these individuals, because ambulances may not be available for long intervals. Some patients in this category may not even require transport at all, but it is still important to keep track of the number and types of injuries considered minor or delayed (green category). Patients with injuries categorized as minor or delayed may leave the scene or somehow get themselves to the hospital, and they most often go to the nearest hospital. This influx may overwhelm that facility despite careful coordination of transport. Information about the number of patients in the green category can be very valuable to planning as disaster management progresses.
- *Black—mortally wounded or dead:* Patients who are either dead or deemed to be beyond saving, given available medical resources, are triaged to this category. In a disaster situation, this category includes any victims in cardiac arrest or any who are not breathing on their own. The resources needed to intubate, ventilate, defibrillate, perform CPR, and otherwise manage these patients may not be available or may be better allocated elsewhere.[3] One exception to this is an electrical injury, such as a lightning strike, in which a single procedure (defibrillation) may significantly improve the patient's condition. It is important to remember that once all patients have been triaged, treated, and transported or otherwise managed, victims

initially triaged to the black category must be re-evaluated to determine for certain whether they are dead or dying.

A newer method of determining triage categories is the *simple triage and rapid transport (START)* system.[4] With this method, all victims who can walk are directed to a site away from the primary triage area; these individuals are in the green category. All other victims are assessed for pulse, respiratory rate, and ability to follow commands; they then are categorized as immediate treatment (red), delayed treatment (yellow), or unsalvageable (black) (Fig. 35-4).

Treatment

As a general rule, limited treatment is provided at a disaster scene. Initial treatment at the triage site should be limited to performing simple airway maneuvers (e.g., a head-tilt, chin-lift or jaw thrust to open an obstructed airway) and applying pressure to areas of obvious external hemorrhage. Once all patients have been triaged and transport plans have been initiated, more extensive treatment on the scene may be appropriate as conditions dictate (Fig. 35-5). If the number of casualties is potentially overwhelming or if few hospitals are available to receive victims, it may be beneficial to keep patients at the

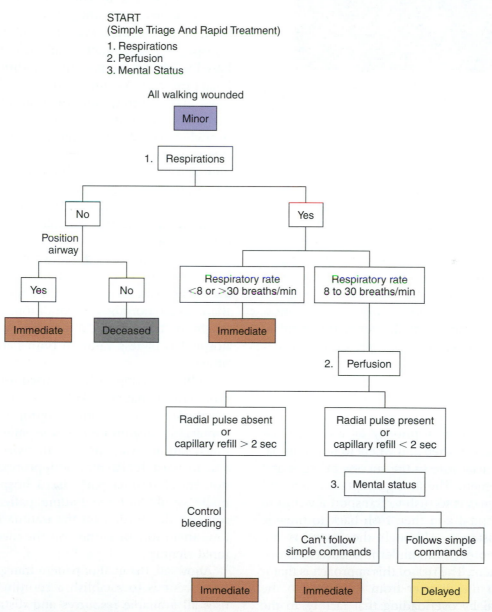

Fig. 35-4 The simple triage and rapid treatment (START) system.

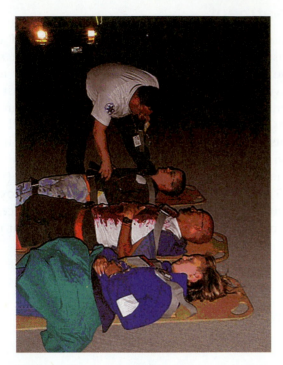

Fig. 35-5 Once all patients have been triaged and transport plans have been initiated, more extensive treatment on the scene may be appropriate as conditions dictate.

scene for a longer time. In such cases more extensive treatment at the scene may be warranted, depending on the particular situation. Disaster plans should address this possibility and provide a means of establishing field hospitals (tents) and even operating suite capabilities when the number of casualties vastly overwhelms transport capabilities. In most multiple casualty situations, however, treatment at the scene is minimal, and appropriate transport is the priority.

Transport

Although transport is a priority at most disaster scenes, decisions on when and where to transport patients play a crucial role in the success of scene and overall management. The strong temptation at multiple casualty scenes is to rush to transport a victim to the nearest hospital and then rush back to provide additional assistance. Although the intent is admirable, this approach can undermine successful disaster management. The risk of this approach is that it may transplant the disaster from the scene to the nearest hospital by overloading that facility, to the detriment of patients, Adding to this is a phenomenon known as *convergence*, in which patients who leave the scene on their own usually go to the closest hospital to seek care. The end result of these two factors is that the hospital nearest a disaster scene quickly becomes overwhelmed.

Decisions on timing of transport and destination should be as centralized and coordinated as possible to prevent this situation. Ideally, one central triage area should be set up where all victims are initially evaluated. In addition, one person at this location should be designated to coordinate the transport destinations in conjunction with the regional trauma center (or local hospital if a regional trauma center does not exist). It is not always reasonable to have a single, centralized triage process; however, it is still important to coordinate destination decisions as much as possible. This obviously is very different from normal, everyday situations in which transporting personnel decide on the destination based solely on the patient's condition, desire, and local protocols. A centralized destination process allows even, appropriate distribution of patients, thereby preventing any one hospital from being overwhelmed. When many hospitals are available, this process tracks the destination of each patient and distributes the next patients to other hospitals when possible. This also allows for greater involvement of hospitals that might not otherwise see as many patients but that can take some of the burden off the closest hospital.

Always keep in mind that when there is only one hospital in the immediate area, it may be appropriate to keep certain victims at the scene much longer than under nondisaster conditions to avoid overwhelming the only local hospital. An overwhelmed hospital is of less value to both patients and EMS providers.

Helicopters typically are used to transport the most critical patients. However, in certain disaster situations, it may be most appropriate to use helicopters to transport more stable patients to locations much farther away, which otherwise might not be able to assist. It also may be appropriate to transport noncritical trauma patients to hospitals that normally would not see trauma patients. This takes some of the burden off the trauma centers and allows them to concentrate on the more critically injured victims.

Above all, the goal of patient transport from a disaster scene is to establish a coordinated effort that uses all available resources and distributes patients equally, to the greater good of the many.

■ ROLE OF PHYSICIANS

Physicians can play a very important role at a disaster scene, in addition to their medical expertise. Local physicians may have a more extensive knowledge of local hospital capabilities, surgery capacities, and internal ability to adjust to extenuating circumstances. However, to be helpful, physicians must be familiar with prehospital care and local EMS systems and protocols. They also must be willing to work within the disaster management structure and the incident command system to ensure a coordinated effort in the management of the scene. The best time to address a role for physicians at the scene of a disaster is in the planning stages, where roles can be defined to maximize the talents and assets of physicians.

■ INCIDENT COMMAND SYSTEM

The **incident command system (ICS)** is a standard emergency management system that is used for disaster response or in any situation that calls for multiple agencies and resources to respond. ICS defines a chain of command and an organization of efforts. It is adaptable to all types of incidents that may involve a multiagency or multijurisdictional response. The five elements, or sections, of the ICS structure are incident command, operations, planning, logistics, and finance (Fig. 35-6).

- *Incident command:* The incident commander has overall responsibility for the incident. This person is responsible for defining objectives and action plans so as to best use available resources to stabilize and resolve the incident.

- *Operations section:* The director or chief of this section is responsible for the management of all incident tactical activities. The operations section sometimes is divided into law, fire, and medical branches. This section also is responsible for managing the resources assigned to staging areas (Fig. 35-7).

- *Planning section:* This section is responsible for collecting, evaluating, and disseminating information about incident operations. This includes assessing the current status of the incident and the status of resources and predicting the future needs of the incident and those involved in the response.

- *Logistics section:* This section is responsible for providing facilities, services, and materiel to support management of the incident. This includes providing for transportation needs, supplies, equipment, food, and personnel.

- *Finance section:* This section is responsible for the financial accountability of the operation, including maintaining records on personnel and equipment time, providing payments to vendors for supplies and use of equipment, and determining costs of the command objectives as well as alternatives.

Communications

Successful management of a disaster scene depends on effective communication. Yet many reviews of disaster situations have identified communications as an area where improvement is needed.[5] Experience has shown that effective communication at a disaster scene can be difficult to achieve. Radio links are commonly used, although more disaster plans are including cell phones as a means of communication

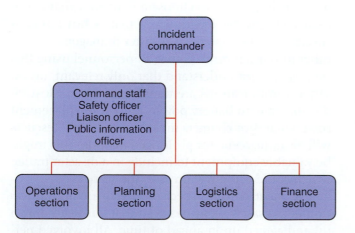

Fig. 35-6 The five elements or sections of the incident command system (ICS) are incident command, operations, planning, logistics, and finance.

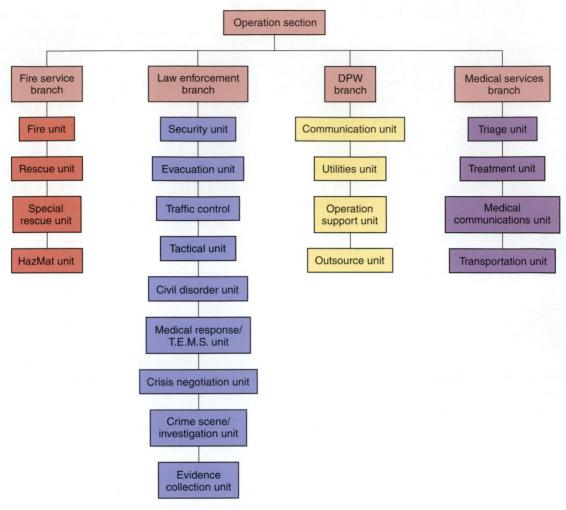

Fig. 35-7 An example of an organizational flowchart for an Incident Command System.

during disaster management. Although cell phones may be reasonable in some cases, it is important to remember that in some areas they may not get optimal reception (so-called dead spots). Even when reception is good, another problem may arise. Large crowds often gather at disaster scenes in hopes of learning more about the situation. Besides creating potential scene control problems, these individuals frequently use their cell phones to talk to other people about the event. This could limit the ability of rescuers at the scene to communicate by cell phone. This does not mean that incident leaders should never use cell phones in the management of a disaster scene. However, a backup plan should be in place. If cell phones are to be the primary mode of communication, the backup plan should ensure the availability of alternative means, such as radios, intercoms, or even runners (specially designated individuals, bystanders, or even less injured victims).

If radios are to play a role in scene communications, several issues must be addressed. What frequency will be used to communicate in the event of a disaster? Do all necessary personnel have access to this frequency, including law enforcement, EMS, and fire? It is important to choose a frequency that is not used regularly for day-to-day activities but rather is specifically designated for disaster management. Another important point is that all personnel using this frequency must understand that only relevant, necessary communications are transmitted on it. Most radios operate on battery power; therefore replacement batteries and/or chargers must be available if rescuers will be at the scene for prolonged periods. This might be valuable equipment to include in a disaster trailer, which could bring resources to the scene.

The most crucial aspect of effective communication at a disaster scene is a plan that has been drawn up and agreed upon ahead of time. All involved per-

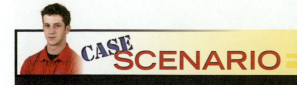

CASE SCENARIO

continued

The incident commander has already turned on the flashing green light on her vehicle, making it easy to locate her. She orders Ray to take the triage function, pointing to an open area not far from the devastated building where injured people are being directed. Ray clips on the triage tagging belt and heads over to the site.

There are at least 15 victims at the site, and more are either walking or being assisted over by helpers. Also, other rescuers are bringing their equipment and gurneys to the site. Over the next minute, Ray tags the following patients:

Patient #1: Jill is 45 years old. She has cuts on her face and arms that are bleeding. Towels seem to control the bleeding. She is quiet, alert, and breathing without difficulty.

Patient #2: James is 23 years old. He appears to have a broken arm and a broken leg, and he has a large contusion on the left side of his head. His face and arms have numerous cuts and bruises. He is anxious and breathing quickly, about 32 breaths per minute.

Patient #3: Aaron is 57 years old and a manager at the facility. He is holding his chest and complaining of crushing chest pain. He tells Ray that he has a history of heart disease. His breathing and pulse rate are normal. He looks pale.

Patient #4: Karen is 35 years old. She has a bleeding head wound and was found unconscious near the building. Two firefighters carried her over to the triage area. Her mental state is still altered, and she is breathing at a rate of 8 breaths per minute. Her pulse is slow.

More victims appear in the triage area. Ray continues to work steadily and quickly, trying to tag as many patients as possible.

Questions: *Which of the patients mentioned was in the most serious condition? Who was least injured, according to triage principles? What level of care should these patients receive on the scene?*

---

sonnel must be knowledgeable about the provisions of the plan and must have had the opportunity to contribute to it. This includes all agencies that might be called upon in a disaster situation. It is never too early to start planning all aspects of the management of a disaster scene, and communication at and from the scene is a critical element of this plan.

Resources

During a disaster, a number of critical resources and supplies must be available for immediate distribution both to the scene and to involved hospitals. As with nearly all aspects of disaster management, this must be organized and arranged in advance, before an actual disaster occurs. Disaster trailers that can be transported to the scene are one way of providing necessary resources (Fig. 35-8). When agencies prepare a trailer or other storage area for disaster resources, it is important that they consider the types of disasters for which it most likely will be used and

plan accordingly. For example, a hazardous materials spill probably will require different resources than will a motor vehicle accident with many casualties in a high-speed area. Important considerations include ensuring that the proper equipment for managing pediatric patients is stocked and determining where involved personnel will go for additional resources when current supplies are used up.

Another important element is the resources that will be required for the responders. Special clothing (e.g., for extreme cold) might be required. Food, water, and bathroom facilities often are in short supply in the area of a disaster. However, responders require these supplies so that they can continue to provide care. If a prolonged deployment is necessary, it is important to identify who will relieve the initial responders. In certain situations, the first act of some personnel playing a crucial role in a disaster plan will be to go home and get some sleep; that way, they will be refreshed and ready to replace the initial responders when those rescuers begin wearing out.

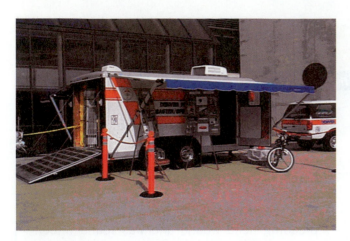

Fig. 35-8 Disaster trailers that can be transported to a scene are one means of providing necessary resources.

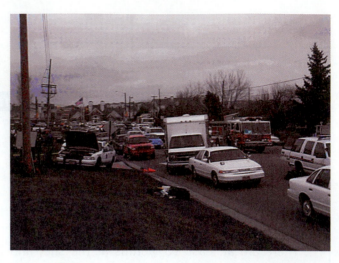

Fig. 35-9 Vehicles or other equipment can quickly clog the available ways into or out of a disaster scene.

The allocation of available resources is another factor that must be considered. It is very tempting to apply all available resources immediately to the scene of an identified disaster. However, other areas probably will need some of those resources as well. Nearly all areas will continue to require the services to which they are accustomed (e.g., adequate amount of personnel and resources), even during a disaster. Designating appropriate resources to provide these services may prevent the development of another disaster situation.

Staging

The staging section deals with equipment, vehicles, and personnel. These and similar resources are gathered in this locale so that they can be deployed to areas that need them, as indicated by the logistics section. Efficient staging of vehicles and equipment can play a crucial role in the effective management of a disaster scene. Predicting or planning for the variety of vehicles that may arrive at a disaster scene is very difficult. It may not be immediately clear what use, if any, some vehicles might have. Also, the available ways into the scene (ingress) and out of it (egress) usually are limited, particularly if a centralized command and triage area is established. These routes can quickly become clogged by vehicles or other equipment (Fig. 35-9). Unfortunately, all manner of vehicles probably will come to the scene, invited or not. It is important to plan the arrangement of these vehicles early on, to allow efficient use of the resources available and effective movement to and from the

scene. It is not uncommon for responding personnel to drive whatever vehicle they're in as close to the scene as possible, get out and lock the vehicle, and continue in on foot. This can cause clutter and confusion at a scene that can ill afford either. The most effective way to prevent this is to limit access close to the scene as much as possible and to designate a specific location to which responding personnel are directed immediately upon arrival. Effective staging also gives the command structure at the scene a better idea of some of the resources available in the form of vehicles already at the scene.

Identification

A means of identifying involved personnel at a disaster scene is a critical priority. Disaster scenes usually involve a large number of people, and identifying crucial personnel can be very difficult. A common way of addressing this is to have vests or jackets available at the scene in easily identifiable colors that clearly signal the wearer's role (Fig. 35-10). A disaster trailer or other storage area for disaster resources (e.g., triage tags, extra equipment) may be a good place to keep the identifying clothing to be used at the scene. As with any other type of equipment, personnel likely to respond to the event must be made aware of the identification equipment available to them and must know how to get it. Most equipment storage areas are kept locked when not in use, therefore information on how to get to this equipment "24/7" must be immediately available.

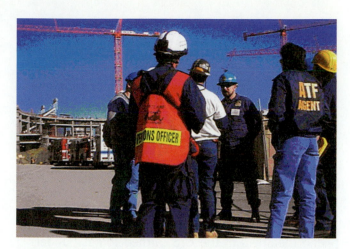

Fig. 35-10 Vests or jackets available at the scene help identify personnel and their roles.

Call Down

In order for EMS and other agencies to meet the personnel needs required to handle a disaster, protocols and processes must be in place to perform a calldown of personnel to see who is available and able to respond to help at the disaster scene.

Similarly, the response at local hospitals during a disaster generally is quite detailed and involved, just as it is at the scene. Hospitals must ready the emergency department, operating rooms, intensive care unit (ICU), and ward bed space. They also must make sure that adequate equipment and staff are available to provide the best possible care for the victims of the disaster. Frequently this means canceling elective surgeries, outpatient clinic appointments, and elective admissions. Extra staff members are called in or otherwise asked to prepare to help care for the victims arriving at the hospital. This response limits the local hospitals' ability to meet their commitments to the community, as well as their ability to provide care for those not involved in the disaster or involved to a lesser degree. It is crucial to get word to local hospitals when the immediate need is over and no more patients should be expected from the scene. This allows the hospitals to most efficiently return to "business as usual." It also may prevent the development of another crisis, one that could arise if normal health care delivery is less accessible for a long period.

Media Relations

The media play a prominent role at any disaster or potential disaster scene. In most cases they are at the scene and at the hospitals, and they may stay well beyond the event itself. Although it is easy to overlook the media in the development of a disaster plan, this is a mistake. Unquestionably they will be there, quite possibly in large numbers, looking for information. Therefore it is prudent to have personnel assigned to deal with news organizations. In most ICS models, an identified public information officer (PIO) is located close to the incident commander. This person has specific training in working with the media. News organizations can play an important role if they are addressed effectively. They can disseminate vital information to the public and get messages to the families of victims or potential victims. However, they also can prove a hindrance if they are not given information about the event. Obviously, the information released depends on the situation; this is the responsibility of those in charge. Savvy scene leaders know that attempting to just brush aside or ignore the media does not work. Reporters, too, have a job to do. If they are not given some means of obtaining information or communicating with those at the scene, they may try to obtain this information in other ways.

The best approach to dealing with the media is to assign specific individuals (perhaps public relations personnel, if available) to work with them and provide regular briefings. A specific area should be set aside for the media; it should not be too close, but cannot be too far, from the scene. The designated media liaisons must meet regularly with the gathered news organizations to provide updates and to release pertinent information that does not put victims or providers at risk and that appropriately respects their privacy. The media can play a helpful, cooperative, and even essential role at the scene of a disaster. However, they also can be a source of frustration if not handled in an efficient, organized manner.

Aftermath and Debriefing

The victims of a disaster often include the rescuers and others who responded to the event.[6] Planning for a disaster response must include addressing the needs of rescuers in the form of a debriefing. The debriefing should be available as soon as reasonably possible after the event (preferably immediately afterward) and should continue for weeks or even months. It must be open to all involved personnel, and in some cases it should be open to individuals who were not directly involved in the response but who either work with or otherwise support the responders (e.g., spouses and friends). Many systems use a format known as a *critical incident stress debriefing system (CISDS)* to accomplish this goal.

Review sessions should be held so that lessons can be learned from the event and the response. The point of these sessions is to learn, not to criticize. Those who were not involved in the response may find it easy and often tempting to find fault with those who were involved. However, the review sessions are neither the time nor the place for anything other than constructive ideas, proposed with the goal of creating learning opportunities for everyone. Disaster responses are crucial learning opportunities, but healing must occur as well. Individual sessions should be held that accomplish each of these goals

Disaster scenes can expose responders to catastrophic injuries and death, and all witnesses probably are affected to some degree. Some people may react immediately, whereas others may react months or even years later; all need support and understanding as they deal with what they have witnessed. Failure to appreciate the effect of a disaster on those involved can have devastating consequences. Sometimes a responder's regular coworkers may be in the best position to offer the necessary support. However it is to be done, and hopefully long before any catastrophic event occurs, the disaster plan must put in place a system that addresses the psychologic needs of responders and provides a support network for a group that invariably will need it.

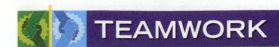

TEAMWORK

It is vital that EMTs have a basic understanding of methods of ensuring the safety of other responders and the public in a disaster situation. You may find yourself working side by side not only with local police officers, firefighters, nurses, and physicians, but also with urban search and rescue teams, Federal Bureau of Investigation (FBI) agents, U.S. Drug Enforcement Administration (DEA) officers, federal marshals, and members of the U.S. armed forces. Understanding your role in a disaster response ensures the safety of your team and everyone around you.

References

1. Mileti DS: *Disasters by design: a reassessment of natural hazards in the United States,* Washington, DC, 1999, Joseph Henry Press.
2. Noji EK: Progress in disaster management, *Lancet* 343:1239, 1994.
3. Waeckerle JF: Disaster planning and response, *N Engl J Med* 324:815, 1991.
4. Super G, Groth S, Hook R et al: *START: simple triage and rapid treatment plan,* Newport Beach, CA, 1994, Hoag Memorial Hospital Presbyterian.
5. Hayes BE, Dahlen RD, Pratt FD et al: A prehospital approach to multiple-victim incidents, *Ann Emerg Med* 15:458-462, 1986.
6. Durham TW, McCannon SL, Allison EJ: The psychological impact of disaster on rescue personnel, *Ann Emerg Med* 14:664-668, 1985.

Resources

Auf der Heide A: *Disaster response: principles of preparation and coordination,* St Louis, 1989, Mosby.
DeLorenzo RA: Mass gathering medicine: a review, *Prehospital Disaster Med* 12:68, 1997.
Michael JA, Barbera JA: Mass gathering medical care: a 25-year review, *Prehospital Disaster Med* 12:305, 1997.
Schultz CH, Koenig KL, Noji EK: Disaster preparedness. In Marx JA, editor: *Rosen's emergency medicine: concepts and clinical practice,* ed 5, St Louis, 2002, Mosby.

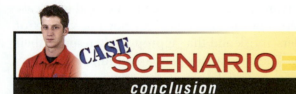

CASE SCENARIO
conclusion

Over the next hour, Ray and the other rescuers identify, treat, and transport 40 victims of the tornado. Luckily, most of the patients were not seriously injured. The few that required immediate care were transported to the regional trauma center by air and by ground ambulances. The other patients were loaded onto a county transit bus and taken to local hospitals for treatment. Unfortunately, four dead victims were recovered from the ruins of the building, a fact that saddened the rescue crews. ■

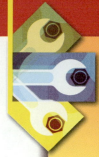

NUTS and BOLTS

Critical Points

- All health care providers should be prepared to participate in the response to a disaster.
- A disaster is any situation that overwhelms the resources available to respond.
- Scene safety is a critical factor.
- Communication of the details of the event should be done prior to your direct involvement in the current situation.
- Triage should be done before any treatment or transport occurs; triage involves separating patients into red, yellow, green, and black categories.
- Treatment at the scene of a disaster generally is limited and focuses on simple airway maneuvers and applying direct pressure to bleeding areas.
- Transport from the scene of a disaster should be centrally coordinated; the goal is to avoid transporting the disaster from the scene to the hospital.
- Planning ahead in the areas of communication at the scene, access to resources for both victims and providers, and staging of vehicles arriving at the scene is crucial for successful management of a disaster scene.
- A way to properly and clearly identify key personnel at the scene should be set up in advance.
- A strategy for dealing with the media should be carefully considered in the preplanning for a disaster response.
- A debriefing should be available for all those involved in the response to a disaster immediately after they return from the scene, or as soon as possible thereafter. Continuing counseling also should be available.
- EMTs should have a working knowledge of the NIMS/ICS structure as it is used to manage disasters across the country.
- The media can be a help at a disaster scene. However, it is important to remember that nothing is "off the record." If you are not authorized to speak for your agency, refer reporters to your public information officer.
- Responders should be urged to attend CISDS sessions after a disaster or other traumatic event. Their health and careers will benefit greatly.

Learning Checklist

- ❑ Increasing population density, particularly in areas prone to flooding and hurricanes; production and transportation of potentially toxic and hazardous materials; and a seemingly increasing risk of terrorism all suggest an increasing probability of a disaster or mass casualty situation.
- ❑ Effective management of a disaster requires both early recognition that a situation may overwhelm existing resources and communication of this potential to the appropriate agencies so that the process of preparing and activating additional resources can be started.
- ❑ A disaster is any event that overwhelms the ability of local resources to respond to that event.
- ❑ As at any scene, scene safety is of primary importance at a disaster to prevent responders from becoming victims themselves. This may be particularly challenging in a disaster, given the temptation for responders to go to work immediately.
- ❑ EMTs' priorities at the scene of a disaster are an overall assessment of the situation and communication of the findings of that assessment.
- ❑ Triage is the process of sorting and classifying patients into categories according to priority of treatment, with the aim of doing the most good for the greatest number of patients.
- ❑ Four triage categories (and identifying colors) are used at the scene of a disaster: critical or severe (red); moderate or urgent (yellow); minor or delayed (green); and mortally wounded or dead (black).
- ❑ It is vital to the successful management of a disaster that the triage process be completed before treatment is begun.

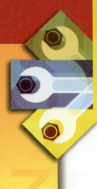

❑ As a general rule, limited treatment is provided at the scene of a disaster. Initial treatment at the triage site should be limited to simple airway maneuvers (e.g., chin lift or jaw thrust to open an obstructed airway) and applying pressure to areas of obvious external hemorrhage.

❑ At multiple casualty scenes, transport personnel often rush a victim to the nearest hospital and then rush back to help. The risk of this approach is that most of the victims may wind up at that hospital, possibly overburdening the facility. This, coupled with convergence, creates a big problem.

❑ The end result of rapid transport to the nearest hospital and convergence often is a local hospital that quickly becomes overwhelmed—and thus another disaster scene.

❑ The incident command system is a standard emergency management system that is used in disaster response or in any situation that requires multiple agencies and resources to respond.

❑ The ICS structure has five elements, or sections: incident command, operations, planning, logistics, and finance.

❑ Successful management of a disaster scene depends on effective communication.

❑ For an effective communication setup, all responding agencies must be able to use the designated method (e.g., access to a particular frequency if radios are chosen).

❑ Resource management at the scene of a disaster involves not only preparing the resources needed for victims, but also those required for responders.

❑ Efficient staging of vehicles and equipment is a crucial part of the effective management of a disaster scene.

❑ Disaster scenes usually involve a large number of people, and identifying crucial personnel can be very difficult. A common way to address this problem is to provide vests or jackets in easily identifiable colors that clearly signal the role of the wearer.

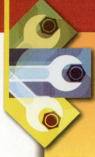
❑ The best approach to dealing with the media at a disaster scene is to assign specific personnel (perhaps public relations professionals, if available) to work with them.

❑ Before a disaster occurs, a system must be in place to address the psychologic needs of responders and to provide a support network for these individuals, who invariably will need it.

Key Terms

Disaster Any situation that overwhelms the resources available for a response to that event.

Incident Command System (ICS) A system for coordinating procedures and resources to assist in the command, control, direction, and coordination of a response to a disaster.

Multiple casualty incident (MCI) Any incident that results in multiple victims who require treatment and transport.

Triage The process of categorizing patients into treatment and transport priorities.

National Standard Curriculum Objectives

Cognitive Objectives
After completing this lesson, the EMT student will be able to do the following:

■ Describe the actions a first responder should take if there is reason to believe a hazard is present at the scene.

■ Discuss the role of the first responder in a disaster or MCI.

■ Summarize the components of basic triage.

Affective Objective
After completing this lesson, the EMT student will be able to do the following:

■ Explain the rationale for having the unit always prepared to respond to a disaster situation.

Psychomotor Objective
After completing this lesson, the EMT student will be able to do the following:

■ Given the scenario of a disaster, perform triage.

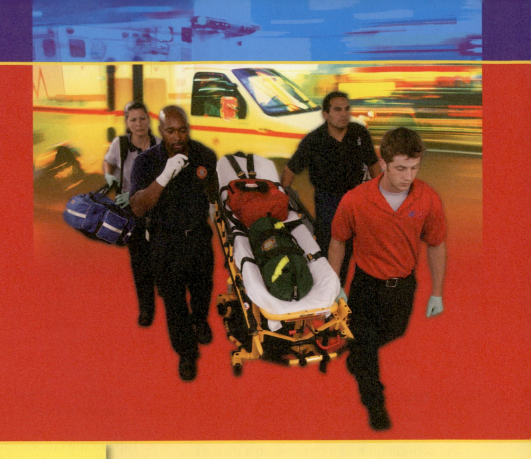

CHAPTER

36

LESSON GOAL

The goal of this chapter is to familiarize the emergency medical technician (EMT) with the methods used to identify the presence and dangers of hazardous materials (hazmat). Operations conducted by properly trained and equipped hazmat response personnel provide safe access to victims so that EMTs can provide prehospital emergency care. This chapter identifies the basic hazardous materials principles and practices used in North America. However, EMTs are well advised to seek additional hazmat training. ■

Hazardous Materials

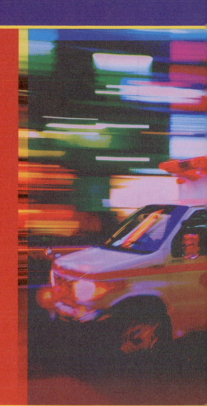

CHAPTER OBJECTIVES

After completing this chapter, the EMT student will be able to do the following:

1 List the training levels for hazardous materials responders.

2 Discuss the importance of hazardous materials identification.

3 Describe how a hazmat scene can be made safe for EMTs and bystanders.

4 Discuss the actions EMTs should take while waiting for properly trained personnel to arrive.

5 Discuss the environmental hazards that affect emergency medical services (EMS) operations.

6 Discuss the criteria that define a multiple casualty situation.

7 Discuss the importance of determining the number of victims, their location, and their injuries.

8 Explain the concept of incident command.

9 Discuss the importance of personal protective equipment and the proper disposal of contaminated material.

10 Explain the importance of the debriefing after the event.

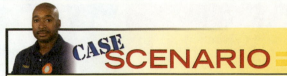

CASE SCENARIO

Jack is just getting out of his car as the garage doors to the ambulance bay open. "Strange," Jack thinks to himself as he walks quickly to Elizabeth's unit. "Why are both crews going out?"

Elizabeth, too, is moving quickly toward the ambulance. Sam, another crew chief, is heading toward the second ambulance, which is parked on the far side of the building. The other members of both crews are loading themselves into the ambulances. The building's loudspeaker crackles; Jack can hear a lot of radio traffic as he gets into the ambulance.

"What's happening?" Jack calls to Sam. Elizabeth is already on the radio, alerting county communications that they are en route.

Sam calls back over the sound of the air horn. "There's something going on down at the Aceland Market. Got some calls about shortness of breath. County just toned out the second unit because there may be more than one victim. Fire's going out on it, too."

Aceland Market is the newest and largest grocery store to open in the center of the shopping district. As her unit rolls into the parking lot, Elizabeth sees two police cruisers. Several people are standing across from the fire lane in front of the market, and more people are coming out the front doors. Many have their hands over their faces; some are holding towels or paper napkins to their noses and mouths. Picking up the microphone, Elizabeth reports to county communications, "MedComm, Community 7 arriving on scene. Single level commercial building. Large number of apparent victims. More to follow."

Questions: *What is the biggest concern for Elizabeth and her crew at this point? What other information should the crew report to the dispatch center as soon as possible? What additional resources should Elizabeth consider as she sizes up the scene?*

■ HAZARDOUS MATERIALS RESPONSE AND TRAINING

Hazardous materials response capabilities are divided into four comprehensive levels of training. These levels are described in a standard established by the National Fire Protection Association (NFPA), specifically NFPA 472: Standard for Professional Competence of Responders to Hazardous Materials Incidents:

- *Hazmat awareness:* This level of training prepares initial responders to identify a hazardous materials situation, to notify appropriate hazmat specialists, and to take precautions to isolate bystanders and rescuers from exposure to the suspected hazardous material.
- *Hazmat operations:* This level of training prepares initial responders to set up perimeters and safety zones while limiting exposure to the suspected hazardous materials.
- *Hazmat technician:* This level of training prepares responders to stop the release of and/or contain hazardous materials.

- *Hazmat specialist:* This advanced level of training allows the responder to provide command and support skills to a hazardous materials event.

Operational features of NFPA 472 have been adopted by the U.S. Environmental Protection Agency (EPA) and the U.S. Occupational Safety and Health Administration (OSHA). The elements of this standard likely are enforced in your local area by OSHA or your state Department of Labor. The basic component of NFPA 472 requires *all* emergency medical personnel responding to a hazardous materials incident to be trained at minimum to the hazmat awareness level. This specialized training usually can be obtained through local fire and rescue service organizations. The information in this chapter is provided as a reference to this awareness level training. EMTs who want to develop their skills in the hazardous materials field should seek follow-up instruction for the operations and technician training levels. EMTs may also want to explore Haz-Medic training and education, as describe in NFPA 473: Standard for Competencies for EMS Personnel Responding to Hazardous Material Incidents.

ELEMENTS OF A HAZARDOUS MATERIALS RESPONSE

Scene Safety

Hazardous materials incidents present many unique dangers that can directly affect victims and emergency responders. Emergency responders tend to be action oriented and want to help victims immediately. Normally, this is an asset. However, in a hazmat incident, it can be dangerous. When emotions take over, attempts at victim rescue often are made without the proper training, equipment, or resources needed for a successful outcome. In these haphazard attempts, the emergency responder frequently becomes another victim. It is important that all emergency responders develop a strong, competent, level-headed attitude so that they can gain control of the incident scene and prevent injury to themselves and others.

As an EMT, you will be working with other responding agencies. You should be familiar with and follow the personnel accountability system used by the agency charged with scene management. It is imperative that personnel responding to incident scenes be familiar with local emergency evacuation procedures and guidelines. The personal protective equipment that hazmat technicians should wear depends on the type of hazardous materials involved.

Risk Assessment

Emergency responders to a hazardous materials event must perform hazard and risk assessments. Scene size-up must be done continually because conditions can change rapidly. The initial hazard analysis sets the groundwork for the entire incident, but expect the follow-up analysis to be dynamic. A hazmat incident can affect a large area; in most cases, it is limited by terrain and environmental conditions.

Locating and determining the number of victims in the incident is a primary component of size-up. To make this job easier for themselves, EMTs should consider the time of day relative to the location of the incident (e.g., a packed office complex at 3 PM). Emergency responders also must ask themselves questions that analyze risk-versus-benefit factors. Will the end result justify the means? What is the acceptable level of risk to achieve the desired outcome? How will prolonged rescue efforts, coupled with extreme environmental conditions, influence victims' survival chances and rescuers' health and safety? These moral and ethical questions raise much concern among emergency responders, and there comes

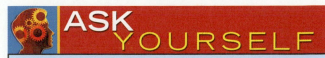

a time when, no matter what efforts you put forth, they will not change the end result.

Emergency responders can improve victims' chances of survival by identifying and planning ahead for possible **hazardous material** events in their response area. Figure out more than one way into a possible site, so that you are prepared if the event or environmental conditions close roads. Familiarize yourself beforehand with building layouts and hazardous materials locations in your community, because this can improve the emergency response to an incident. Make sure you know which resources would be immediately available and how to obtain additional resources when they are needed.

Preplanning also can help rescuers find and get to victims more quickly. Keep in mind, however, that personal safety is paramount when you are searching for and dealing with victims of a hazardous materials incident. EMTs should never enter a contaminated area or touch a contaminated victim unless they are trained in the use of specialized personal protective equipment and procedures.

INCIDENT COMMAND STRUCTURE

The Federal Emergency Management Agency's (FEMA) National Incident Management System (NIMS) has become widely accepted in North America as the basis of a standardized **incident command structure or system (ICS)**. As an EMT at a hazmat incident, you most likely will be concerned with the following elements for your response:

- Command
- Safety
- Hazmat

- Medical
- Rehabilitation/medical surveillance
- Control zones

EMTs must become familiar with and practice the NIMS/ICS policy and procedures established in their area of operation. The NFPA web site provides useful links to educational resources that can help you improve your understanding of the NIMS concept. Many local fire, rescue, and police agencies also provide NIMS/ICS training for emergency and government personnel in their region. Use of a standardized ICS structure greatly improves the safety of emergency personnel, streamlines hazardous materials operations, and increases victims' chances of survival.

■ RECOGNITION AND IDENTIFICATION OF HAZARDOUS MATERIALS

Recognition of a hazardous materials incident is of prime importance to the emergency responder. Many variables must be considered when EMTs are called to an emergency scene that may indicate the presence of a hazardous material. Precautions must be taken well before you arrive. Many times the information provided by dispatch can provide clues to the presence of a hazmat incident. Consider the following factors:

- *Nature of the call:* Have multiple victims been reported? Does the call involve fumes or an odor? Does it involve a material on the skin or in the eyes of the patient?
- *Occupancy:* Does the tenant at the incident suggest the presence and use of hazardous materials?
- *Location:* Did the incident occur in an agricultural area, an industrial district, or a transportation center, which may indicate the presence of a potential hazardous material?

Some points should pop into the EMT's mind as soon as the alarm sounds. Make sure you respond to such an event (or possible event) with extreme caution; do not become a casualty yourself. Always note the wind direction. Always approach a suspected contaminated area with the wind to your back. Approach from higher ground and avoid dips and valleys in the terrain. When you are given routing instructions by

SPECIAL Considerations

Always Consider Safety
As EMTs approach the scene of a possible hazardous materials incident, they should check for indications that the area may be unsafe to enter. The following may be clues to an unsafe scene:
- Multiple victims with medical emergencies
- Casualties that have no apparent cause
- Containers from laboratory or biologic supply houses
- Unusual numbers of sick or dying people or animals
- Numerous dead animals, including birds and fish, in one area (not just an occasional road kill)
- Absence of insect life (if normal insect activity is missing, check for dead insects)
- Dead fish or aquatic birds (check for these if the scene is near water)
- Unexplained odors (any odor that is completely out of character for the surroundings is an important clue)
- Patterns of casualties (outdoors, victims likely will be distributed downwind; indoors, victims usually will be clustered near air ventilation system outlets)
- Illness in confined areas (depending on the site of the incident, a different casualty rate may be seen for those working indoors compared with those working outdoors)
- Low-lying clouds (if this condition is not consistent with the surroundings)

other agencies already on the scene, follow those directions to the staging area without variance, to ensure a safe entry.

Scene Size-Up

In approaching a scene that potentially involves a hazardous material, EMTs should consider the presence of railcars, tank trucks, tractor trailers, shipping containers, fixed-site tank farms, and agricultural equipment to be a likely component of a hazmat incident. Survey the scene from a safe distance. Use binoculars to search for any telltale signs of a problem involving a hazardous material. These signs may include the following:

- Hazmat placards or labels
- Vapors, smoke, or fumes
- Flowing or pooled liquids
- Fire
- Dead livestock

Placard and Label Warnings

The U.S. Department of Transportation (DOT), in cooperation with the United Nations (U.N.), has developed a placard and label warning system that must be used for all modes of transportation of hazardous materials. The placard and label system is based on nine special hazard classification groups. Each class has a unique color code or design, based on the general chemical properties of the group (Figs. 36-1 and 36-2). The nine classes are as follows:

- *Class 1—Explosive:* Indicated by an orange diamond with a silhouette of an exploding ball with U.N. identification numbering.
- *Class 2—Gas:* Indicated by a green diamond (nonflammable) with a silhouette of a gas cylinder *or* by a red diamond (flammable) with a silhouette of a flame *or* by a white diamond (poison gas) with a silhouette of a skull and crossbones.
- *Class 3—Flammable liquid:* Indicated by a red diamond with a silhouette of a flame with U.N. identification numbering.
- *Class 4—Flammable solid:* Indicated by a white diamond with vertical red stripes with a silhouette of a flame *or* by a white diamond with the lower half in red (spontaneously combustible) *or* by a blue diamond (dangerous when wet). U.N. identification numbering may be present.
- *Class 5—Oxidizer:* Indicated by a yellow diamond with a silhouette of a burning ball with U.N. identification numbering.
- *Class 6—Poison:* Indicated by a white diamond with a silhouette of a skull and crossbones. U.N. identification numbering may be present.
- *Class 7—Radioactive:* Indicated by a yellow-over-white diamond with a silhouette of a propeller. U.N. identification numbering may be present.
- *Class 8—Corrosive:* Indicated by a white-over-black diamond with a silhouette of a test-tube, bar, and hand. U.N. identification numbering may be present.
- *Class 9—Miscellaneous:* Indicated by black vertical bars over a white diamond.

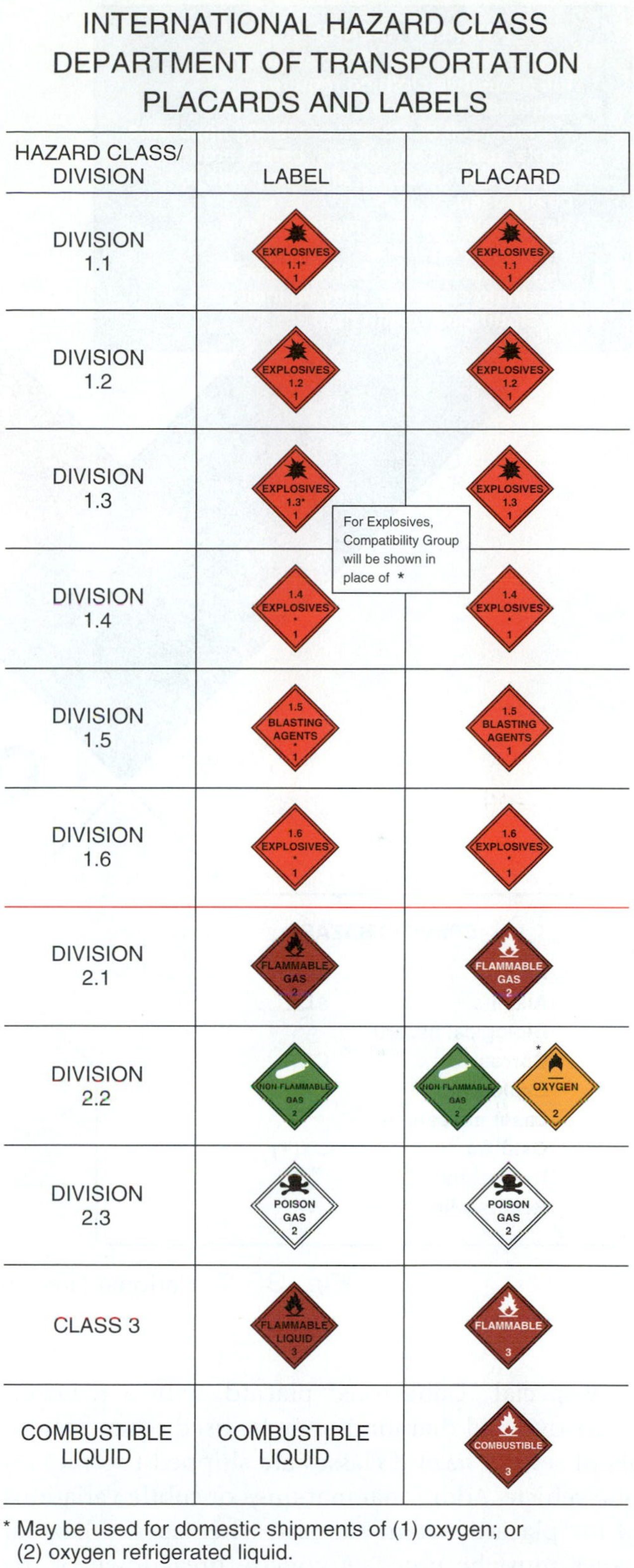

INTERNATIONAL HAZARD CLASS DEPARTMENT OF TRANSPORTATION PLACARDS AND LABELS

HAZARD CLASS/ DIVISION	LABEL	PLACARD
DIVISION 1.1		
DIVISION 1.2		
DIVISION 1.3		For Explosives, Compatibility Group will be shown in place of *
DIVISION 1.4		
DIVISION 1.5		
DIVISION 1.6		
DIVISION 2.1		
DIVISION 2.2		
DIVISION 2.3		
CLASS 3		
COMBUSTIBLE LIQUID	COMBUSTIBLE LIQUID	

* May be used for domestic shipments of (1) oxygen; or (2) oxygen refrigerated liquid.

Fig. 36-1 International class placard. Carriers of hazardous materials must display specific placards or labels designated by the U.S. Department of Transportation in cooperation with the United Nations.

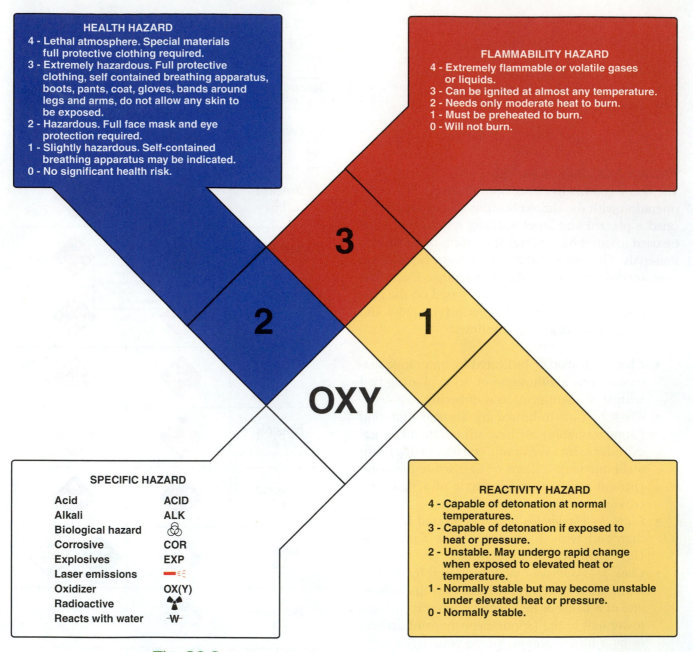

Fig. 36-2 National Fire Protection Association (NFPA) placard.

A special "Dangerous" placard, with a red-over-white-over-red diamond, may be used when materials of several hazard classes are shipped together on one vehicle. Additional markings or subtle variations of the placard system are used when special hazmat issues must be noted. A concise breakdown of the placard and label system can be found in the front section of the current *Emergency Response Guidebook* (also called the *ERG* or the *Orange Book*), which is published by the DOT (Fig. 36-3).

The U.S. military use a set of specialized placards. If an ordnance depot or military base is located in your response area, you would be wise to become familiar with these placards. For the most part, the different branches of the armed forces do not use a common symbolism. Also, information will be limited to prevent leakage of information to opposition forces. Generally, the placards signal the level of deflagration or detonation; this is indicated by five basic symbols used by the U.S. military:

- Numeral 1 inside an octagon: Mass detonation hazard
- Numeral 2 inside an X: Explosive with fragmentation hazard
- Numeral 3 inside a triangle: Mass fire or incendiary hazard

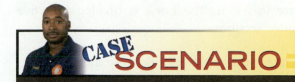

CASE SCENARIO

continued

Elizabeth quickly delegates several responsibilities to her crew.

"Jim, grab a triage kit; Jack, you work with him." She looks around the parking lot. "Let's run some yellow tape from there" she points to a light pole "to over here. Then let's do another tape line from that car's antenna back over to there." Jack can see that Elizabeth is creating a triage funnel to move possible victims in an organized fashion.

As Jack and Jim head out on their assignment, Elizabeth walks toward the police officer who seems to be directing people out of the building. She can hear Sam's unit coming down the street. As she gets closer to the front entrance of the market, she can faintly smell something unusual; an acidlike odor is coming from the store. Elizabeth stops right where she is. The police officer is covering his mouth and nose and coughing. "Hey!" she yells to him. "Move away from there!"

The police officer moves away from the door. "I think everyone's out of the store," he gasps, wiping his eyes and nose.

"Do you know what happened?" Elizabeth asks.

"The store manager says he saw a few kids drop a can in the middle of the store, and it began giv-ing off a lot of white smoke right away. The kids ran out," the police officer replies.

From earlier training exercises, Elizabeth knows that the building has several emergency exits on all four sides.

"Is there any fire that you know of?" she asks the officer.

"No report of fire, just smoke," he answers.

"Where are the other officers?" Elizabeth asks him.

"I think everyone headed to different sides of the building," he says. Elizabeth heads back to her ambulance. She can see that a few people are lining up along the tape lines. Others are lying on the ground near the back of the ambulance. Jim and Jack are already triaging people at the end of the triage funnel.

The second ambulance pulls up next to Elizabeth's unit. "What do you want us to do?" Sam calls to her.

Questions: *What roles should Sam and his crew assume at this time? Should Sam's crew transport the patients lying on the ground?*

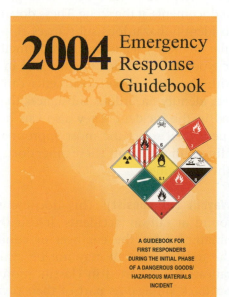

Fig. 36-3 *Emergency Response Guidebook,* published by the U.S. Department of Transportation.

- Numeral 4 inside a diamond: Moderate fire or incendiary hazard
- Circle: Chemical hazard (the circle may contain a depiction of a gas mask, BA (bottled air), or chemical suit)

The generally accepted practice is to retreat from an incident involving hazardous military cargo. It is best to let nuclear, biologic, and chemical experts or ordnance disposal specialists deal with all aspects of response and remediation when such cargo is involved in an incident (Fig. 36-4).

Emergency Response Guidebook

The *Emergency Response Guidebook* is an essential information resource that should be carried on all emergency response vehicles. It is invaluable when emergency responders are confronted with a possible hazmat situation. The ERG provides both generic and specific information that may help emergency responders in making the initial decisions at a hazmat transportation incident. All emergency responders must familiarize themselves with the ERG before

they have to use it. The book is divided into five color-coded sections:

- *White* (front and back): Because these two segments are the same color, they are considered a single section. They contain general information on emergency phone numbers, directions for use of the ERG, definitions, placards, labels, and transportation vehicle silhouettes.
- *Yellow* (second section): An index, in numeric order, of the U.N. identification numbers. It cross-references the guide number with the name of the material. (Guide numbers correspond to specific response guides for dealing with particular hazmat situations; these are presented in the orange section.)
- *Blue* (third section): An index of dangerous goods. It cross-references the guide number with the U.N. identification number.
- *Orange* (fourth section): The most important section of the ERG. It includes the response guides cross-referenced by the yellow and blue sections. Each guide provides safety information and recommendations for protecting the emergency responder and the public.
- *Green* (fifth section): A numeric index of special identification numbers for materials highly toxic to humans. It cross-references the numbers with initial safe isolation distances and safe protective action distances.

Other Hazardous Materials Information

Emergency responders may be able to gather other hazmat documents at the scene. These documents are used to identify hazardous substances shipped by a particular method. Each transportation method has a specific type of hazmat document. Used in conjunction with the ERG, these documents can help responders identify hazardous substances that may be involved in the incident. They also can help emergency personnel select the most appropriate action for dealing with the event. These other documents include the following:

- **Waybill** (or **consist**): This document can be found at railway accidents. It usually can be obtained from the engineer or conductor of the train. A waybill may not be available for railcars being sorted in classification yards or on track sidings. As part of their preplanning efforts, emergency response personnel should develop a good working relationship with rail carriers in their area.

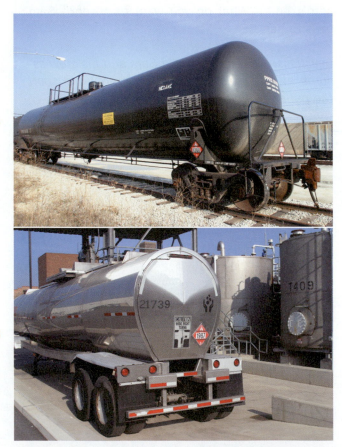

Fig. 36-4 A, U.S. Department of Transportation (DOT) placard on a railcar. **B,** DOT placards on the back of a truck.

- **Bill of lading:** This document can be found at trucking accidents. It usually can be obtained from the driver or from inside the truck cab. A bill of lading may not be available for trailers being sorted, loaded, or unloaded at trucking terminals. As part of their preplanning efforts, emergency response personnel should establish a good working relationship with area trucking terminals.
- **Air bill:** This document can be found at aircraft accidents. It can be obtained from the pilot. As part of their preplanning efforts, emergency personnel should establish procedures at local airports for obtaining this information when needed.
- **Dangerous cargo manifest:** This document is used by the marine shipping industry. It most likely can be obtained from the captain of the vessel. Inland barges may be equipped with a box where such documents are stored while the barge is moored. As part of their preplanning efforts, emergency personnel should work with port authorities and barge lines to establish procedures for obtaining this information when needed.
- **Material Safety Data Sheet (MSDS):** The MSDS is probably the most important source of information for EMTs who must determine the treatment of victims of a hazmat exposure. The MSDS is a multipage document that contains highly detailed information about a specific material. It can be found at all types of transportation incidents. It also is required at fixed-site locations where hazardous materials are stored or used. A copy of this document should be brought with a decontaminated victim to the medical facility.

Fixed-site storage facilities may not show any indication of the type of materials being stored in bulk quantity. The most reliable and accepted hazard indicators are (1) a combination of the NFPA 704 placard system and the DOT/U.N. identification numbering system or (2) a full product name stenciled on the bulk containers. The NFPA 704 placard consists of a diamond divided into quadrants: blue (health), red (flammability), yellow (reactivity), and white (Fig 36-5). A numeral (0 to 4) inside each of the colored quadrants represents the level of hazard, 4 being the highest hazard rating. The white quadrant is used to indicate special hazards, such as radioactivity or water reactivity. Special hazards are identified in the white quadrant with symbols. Manufacturers use similar

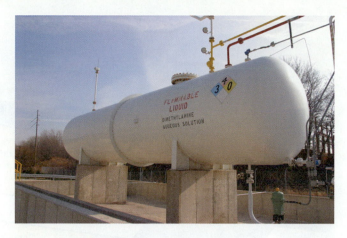

Fig. 36-5 National Fire Protection Association (NFPA) placard identifying fixed storage of a flammable liquid.

warning systems, and the layout can vary from industry to industry. As part of their preplanning efforts, emergency responders should work with the industries in their area to familiarize themselves with the identification system in use. Keep in mind that no system may be required, or none may be in use.

Interagency Cooperation for Risk Reduction

Development of a regional plan detailing the EMS response in a hazmat incident is crucial. When EMTs respond to a potential hazmat site, they must be able to work smoothly with other response agencies within the established command structure. EMS providers also must be knowledgeable about area medical facilities and their capabilities in such an event.

Victim decontamination procedures are a vital component of the regional preparedness plan. These procedures must be performed by trained hazmat personnel, usually in the warm zone (contamination reduction zone), before the victims can be turned over to EMTs for medical care. It is essential to prevent or minimize the spread of chemical, biologic, and radioactive contaminants to unprotected emergency responders. This is done by using multilevel control zone techniques, including a contamination reduction corridor (Fig. 36-6). The contamination reduction corridor ensures methodic decontamination of all exposed emergency personnel and victims, which prevents cross-contamination of personnel, vehicles, and medical facilities. Cross-contamination can make resources useless. For this reason, the regional preparedness plan should include procedures for early notification of hospitals and medical facili-

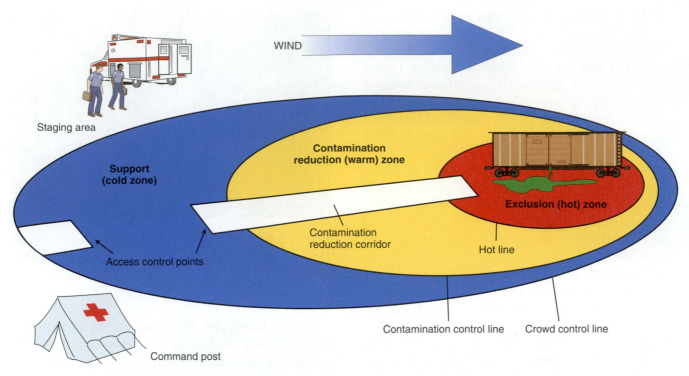

WIND

Staging area

Support
(cold zone)

Contamination
reduction (warm) zone

Exclusion (hot) zone

Contamination
reduction corridor

Hot line

Access control points

Command post

Contamination control line   Crowd control line

Fig. 36-6 Control zones established during a hazardous materials incident.

⚠ CAUTION!

Never put a patient who needs to be decontaminated in your ambulance. Once contaminated, your vehicle cannot be used to transport other patients.

ties in the event of a hazardous materials incident in their service areas. Medical facilities can be exposed to cross-contamination by *walking wounded*, victims who leave a hazmat incident by uncontrolled means. Therefore these facilities may want to activate their site-specific hazmat control plans before any potentially contaminated walking wounded arrive, or as an additional level of precaution in accepting victims EMTs may transport to them.

■ TYPES OF VICTIM EXPOSURE

The victim of a hazmat incident can be exposed by four specific routes that result in chemical injury:

- Inhalation
- Ingestion
- Absorption
- Injection

Exposure to a hazardous material can result in thermal burns, frostbite, mechanical injuries, poisoning, tissue damage from corrosives, asphyxiation, diseases caused by etiologic (infectious) materials or carcinogens, and immediate or long-term illness from radiation exposure. EMTs can also expect to encounter benign psychosomatic illness related to the hazmat event, particularly if the incident receives intense news coverage.

■ RESPONSE AND RECOVERY

Responding to and recovery from a hazardous materials incident may not end at shift change; they may be long, tedious operations. Contaminated materials must be properly disposed of or decontaminated. A medical surveillance program must be established for response personnel in case they came in contact with a hazardous material. Far too often fire, police, and EMS personnel develop illnesses or conditions from such exposure, disorders that could have been prevented if they had been acted upon early. A post-incident critique should be held after the hazmat event to examine all aspects of the operation. The lessons learned from this analysis will better prepare responders for future hazmat incidents.

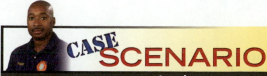

CASE SCENARIO
conclusion

Over the next 20 minutes, five more ambulances arrive on scene. One of Jack's crew members has set up a staging area where the units can park without congesting the working scene. The fire department also has several units there. The EMTs are assisting with the treatment of patients and with moving them from the treatment area to the waiting transport units. Elizabeth, the fire chief, and the police captain are standing off to the side of one of the ambulances. Working together, incident command has hammered out the details of the emergency operation, keeping in close contact with each other's services. Sometime later it is determined that the canister was a home-made weapon that triggered a large release of pepper spray. Nearly 25 patients were evaluated for minor reactions to the exposure; five patients were transported for shortness of breath and further evaluation.

TEAMWORK

Hazardous materials incidents may involve local, state, and federal responders, depending on the magnitude of the situation. EMTs, unless properly trained, must recognize their limitations. To ensure the safety of everyone involved, you need to know how to use the *Emergency Response Guidebook* correctly. Ask your local firefighters when the next hazardous materials awareness courses will be given, and attend these and other courses offered by local agencies.

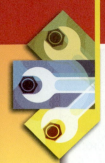

Critical Points

- EMTs must know and understand the different HAZMAT levels they may encounter in their work.
- EMTs must have a working knowledge of the DOT's *Emergency Response Guidebook.*
- When called to the scene of a transport accident involving hazardous materials, EMTs must know where to find the documents that provide information about the materials being transported.

Learning Checklist

❑ The four levels of hazmat training are hazmat awareness, hazmat operations, hazmat technician, and hazmat specialist.

❑ Hazmat incidents must be sized up continually because conditions at the scene can change rapidly.

❑ Emergency responders can improve victims' chances of surviving a hazmat incident by identifying and planning ahead for possible hazardous material events in their response area.

❑ According to NIMS, EMTs should be concerned with the following elements: command, safety, hazmat, medical, rehabilitation/medical surveillance, and control zones.

❑ In a recognized or potential hazmat incident, dispatch should inform EMTs of (1) the nature of call, (2) the occupancy, and (3) the location.

❑ EMTs must respond to a hazmat incident with extreme caution to avoid becoming casualties themselves.

❑ When approaching a questionable scene, EMTs should survey it from a safe distance. They should look for signs indicating involvement of a hazardous material, such as hazmat placards or labels, vapors, smoke or fumes, flowing or pooled liquids, fire, or dead livestock.

❑ The nine hazard classification groups are (1) explosive, (2) gas, (3) flammable liquid, (4) flammable solid, (5) oxidizer, (6) poison, (7) radioactive, (8) corrosive, and (9) miscel-

laneous. Also, the military uses a set of specialized placards.

❑ The DOT's *Emergency Response Guidebook* (ERG) provides both general and specific information that may help emergency responders who must make the initial decisions at a hazmat transportation incident. The book is divided into five sections, which are color coded (white, yellow, blue, orange, and green) according to the type of information the section contains.

❑ The most reliable hazard indicators combine the placard system established by the NFPA 704 standard with the DOT/UN identification numbering system.

❑ The EMS response to a hazmat incident must be based on a previously developed, comprehensive regional plan and on cooperation with other response agencies and with medical facilities.

❑ Hazmat exposure that causes chemical injury can occur by four specific routes: inhalation, ingestion, absorption, and injection.

Key Terms

Air bill A document used to identify hazardous substances transported by air. It can be obtained from the pilot or may be found at the scene of aircraft accidents.

Bill of lading A document used to identify hazardous substances transported by truck. It usually can be obtained from the driver or is kept in the truck cab, or it may be found at the scene of a trucking accident. Bills of lading may not be available for trailers being sorted, loaded, or unloaded at trucking terminals.

Dangerous cargo manifest A document used to identify hazardous substances shipped by water. It most likely can be obtained from the captain of the vessel. Inland barges may be equipped with a box where such documents are stored while the barge is moored.

Hazardous material Any material or substance that can pose an unreasonable risk either to a person's safety or health or to property.

Incident command structure or system (ICS) A protocol or system for coordinating proce-

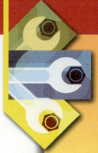

dures to assist in the command, control, direction, and coordination of emergency response resources.

Material Safety Data Sheet (MSDS) A multipage document that provides detailed, material-specific information about a hazardous substance. The MSDS probably is the most important source of information for EMTs determining the treatment of a victim of a hazardous materials exposure. MSDS are kept at the fixed storage facility or by the transporter while en route.

Placard A sign that has various symbols and numerals that help identify a hazardous material or class of materials, usually located on the back of a transporting vehicle or storage site.

Waybill (consist) A document used to identify hazardous substances transported by rail. It usually can be obtained from the engineer or conductor, or it may be found at the site of a railway accident. Waybills may not be available for railcars being sorted in classification yards or on track sidings. Emergency response personnel should establish a cooperative relationship with the rail carriers in their area before an incident occurs.

National Standard Curriculum Objectives

Cognitive Objectives
After completing this lesson, the EMT student will be able to do the following:

- Explain the role of EMTs on a call involving hazardous materials.
- Describe what EMTs should do if there is reason to believe a hazard exists at the scene.

- Describe the actions EMTs should take to ensure bystander safety.
- State what EMTs should do until appropriately trained personnel arrive at the scene of a hazardous materials situation.
- Break down the steps to the method of approaching a hazardous situation.
- Discuss the various environmental hazards that affect EMS providers.
- List the criteria that define a multiple casualty situation.
- Evaluate the role of EMTs in a multiple casualty situation.
- Define the role of EMTs in a disaster operation.
- Describe the basic concepts of incident management.
- Explain the methods of preventing contamination of oneself, equipment, and facilities.
- Review the local mass casualty incident plan.

Affective Objectives
No objectives identified.

Psychomotor Objective
After completing this lesson, the EMT student will be able to do the following:

- Perform triage, given the scenario of a mass casualty incident.

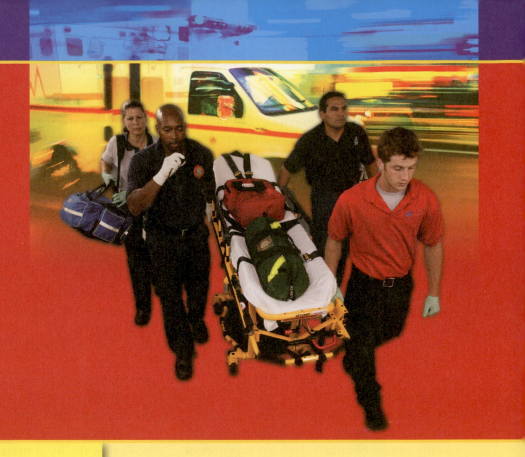

CHAPTER

37

CHAPTER OUTLINE

Fallacies of Weapons of Mass Destruction

Basic Principles

Chemical Agents

Biologic Agents

Radiologic/Nuclear Agents

Explosive Devices

OUTLINE

LESSON GOAL

The goal of this chapter is to familiarize the emergency medical technician student with the concept of weapons of mass destruction, how these weapons might be used against the U.S. population, and the type of treatment that would be appropriate for each agent. Threats to the care provider caused by these agents also are covered. The intent of this chapter also is to demystify these agents, demonstrating that, while taxing, prehospital care providers who have preparation and knowledge can handle appropriately an incident with weapons of mass destruction. ■

GOAL

Weapons of Mass Destruction

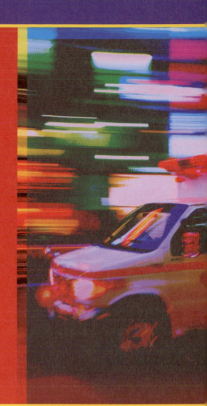

CHAPTER OBJECTIVES

After completing this chapter, the EMT student will be able to do the following:

1 Identify the potential threat of weapons of mass destruction and their threat to society.

2 Identify various weapons of mass destruction threat agents and the signs and symptoms of exposure to them.

3 Select the proper modality of treatment for various agents.

4 Identify special threats to health care providers, such as secondary contamination and potentially unsafe scenes.

5 Describe types of chemical warfare agents.

6 Recognize signs and symptoms of exposure to chemical agents or weapons of mass destruction.

7 Describe the management of victims of chemical agent attack.

8 Describe the various types of biologic warfare agents, and recognize the signs and symptoms of exposure.

9 Describe how to manage and treat infectious victims properly.

10 Determine what agents are a risk for secondary transmission and how to protect against this spread using personal protective equipment and isolation measures.

11 Describe the various types of radiologic hazards.

12 List the acute health effects from radiation contamination and exposure.

Continued

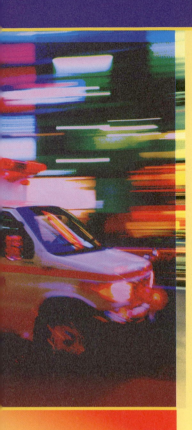

Chapter Objectives—cont'd

13 Describe the principles of diagnosis, treatment, and management of radiation casualties.

14 Describe the difference between exposure and contamination and how this affects the medical care of victims of radiation accident.

15 Describe basic radiation protection principles.

16 Outline common injuries and management strategies associated with blast injuries.

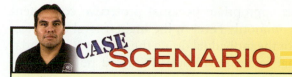

CASE SCENARIO

"Special call, Battalion Seven, Engine One-O-Seven, Engine Thirty-two, Truck Twenty, Hazmat Two, Rescue Seventeen, Rescue Ten. Explosion report, near the vicinity of Twelfth Street and Lincoln Avenue. More to follow."

Rafael and the rest of the fire crew headed out to the engine parked in the bay. Rafael felt a bit of apprehension mixed in with his excitement. There had been reports coming from the police department that violent threats had been received that had targeted several department stores and other "soft" targets over recent days. The address provided by the communications center was near one of the busier stores in their second due response district. As the engine moved quickly toward the incident, Rafael could see the captain looking at the mobile display terminal (MDT) as additional information came in. Hitting the intercom button, José advised, "Police on the scene are saying that there are a lot of victims. Battalion Seven is advising us to take additional precautions."

Questions: *What are some of the safety concerns about which the engine crew should be concerned? If this was indeed a violent act, what additional precautions should the crew take?*

What are weapons of mass destruction (WMD)? This term has multiple definitions, but WMD commonly are agents that can cause widespread illness, injury, death, or generalized panic. Agents used in this manner also tend to be relatively nonconventional; that is, they are rarely used in normal warfare. These agents usually are categorized into groups: biologic agents, chemical agents, radiologic/nuclear agents, and explosive devices. These agents sometimes are referred to as CBRNE (chemical, biologic, radiologic, nuclear, and explosive) agents. A common goal in the use of these agents is to inflict illness/injury on a large number of victims and incite fear and panic in the population at large. For example, the release of the nerve agent **sarin** by the Aum Shinrikyo cult in Tokyo, Japan, in 1995 caused 5500 victims to seek treatment, severely taxing the health care system. However, the anthrax-laden letters mailed in the United States in 2001 caused only 22 cases of anthrax, yet caused widespread fear and panic, with some individuals refusing to open their mail. Historically, WMD agents have not been part of medical or prehospital care training. However, world circumstances now unfortunately mandate that health care providers be knowledgeable in the field of WMD.

FALLACIES OF WEAPONS OF MASS DESTRUCTION

Several fallacies have arisen concerning WMD. Most notably is the belief that "it can't happen here." The unfortunate destruction of the Murrah building in Oklahoma City, Oklahoma, however, demonstrated that any locale can be a target and that terrorists are not all from foreign countries. A second fallacy is that all WMD agents are so toxic that all victims will die. The Tokyo sarin attack, although affecting many victims, resulted in only 12 chemical-related casualties, even with limited treatment. A third fallacy is that there is nothing that you as a health care provider can do to change the result of an attack. Hopefully, the student will realize after reviewing this chapter that there is much that he or she can do to improve patient outcomes in any WMD attack.

BASIC PRINCIPLES

A number of basic tenets apply to all situations involving WMD: (1) rescuer safety, (2) removal from the source of exposure, (3) ABCs (airway, breathing, circulation—no mouth to mouth resuscitation), (4) decontamination, and (5) appropriate treatment. Whether a provider is dealing with a **chemical agent**, powder that might represent a **biologic agent**, or a **radiation source**, the provider should remember and apply these five principles.

CHEMICAL AGENTS

Many chemical compounds have the potential of being used as a **chemical weapon**. They usually are divided into classes: nerve agents, vesicants (blister agents), and industrial chemicals (especially those having severe pulmonary effects).

Nerve Agents

Nerve agents are chemicals that interfere with normal nerve transmissions in the body, causing the tissues and organs controlled by the nerves to malfunction. These chemicals are in the category of organophosphate compounds,[1] some of which commonly are used in gardens for insect control. The two most commonly discussed nerve agents are sarin (also referred to as "GB" by the military) and **VX.** Tabun and soman are two additional nerve agents that were manufactured in the past.

Presentation of Nerve Agent Exposure

As mentioned previously, nerve agents affect many parts of the body. The nature and the extent of effect depend largely on the dose and method of the exposure. An easy way to remember many of the presenting symptoms and findings is by using the SLUDGE syndrome mnemonic (Box 37-1). In affected patients, symptoms include salivation (drooling), lacrimation (tearing), urination (wetting themselves), defecation (soiling themselves), gastrointestinal distress (nausea), and emesis (vomiting). Some or all of these symptoms may be present. Another common finding is constricted pupils **(miosis)**. Because of this constriction, the eye does not get enough light, and the victim may complain of dim vision, difficulty focusing, and eye pain. A major effect on the respiratory system is constriction of the airways **(bronchoconstriction)** resulting in shortness of breath, which may be severe. The effects on the muscles of the skeletal system include twitching, weakness, and inability to move (paralysis). The effects on the heart include slow heartbeat, rapid heartbeat, or irregular heartbeat. In severe exposures, the central nervous system may be affected, resulting in unconsciousness and seizures.

Diagnosis of Nerve Agent Exposure

The capability to determine a nerve agent release by testing the environment requires specialized equipment. This equipment is rarely readily available and requires appropriate personal protective equipment (PPE; commonly Level A, the highest level of protection) for the individual doing the testing. It is mandatory that rescuers without PPE avoid putting themselves in danger by entering any environment where a nerve agent may be present (e.g., do not go into a room where a large number of victims are seizing and vomiting.). The rescuer must make the potential diagnosis of potential nerve agent exposure by situational assessment (e.g., multiple casualties with similar symptoms and common time or location factors) and evaluation of the patients' presenting symptoms.

Sarin Exposure

Sarin can exist as a liquid at room temperature, but it becomes a vapor quickly (in minutes). Patients with mild exposure to the vapor have constricted pupils, runny nose, and mild shortness of breath, all of which do not progress to any significant degree over time. A moderate exposure results in severe shortness of breath (dyspnea), nausea, vomiting, diarrhea, and weakness. Severe exposure results in rapid loss of consciousness, seizures, paralysis, and cessation of breathing. These effects usually are seen within seconds of exposure, reaching their peak within minutes.

VX Exposure

VX is a nerve agent that mainly exists in a liquid form. It may persist in the environment for many hours. Exposure normally would be through skin contact. Moreover, it may take several hours for the patient to develop symptoms. VX is an extremely potent agent, with a tiny droplet being enough to cause a fatality. Mild exposure may cause localized sweating in the area in which the skin contacted the VX, with localized muscle twitching. Eye problems usually are not seen. These symptoms may be delayed for up to 18 hours after exposure. Moderate exposure also produces gastrointestinal effects. Severe exposure causes loss of consciousness within 30 minutes, followed by seizures, loss of breathing, paralysis, and death.

Treatment of Nerve Agent Exposure

Nerve agent exposure can be treated successfully by rapid administration of two drugs, atropine and pralidoxime, to the symptomatic patient. The initial dose of atropine is 2 mg. This dose is repeated as necessary (up to 20 mg) until the patient's breathing (or bag ventilation) is easy and his or her secretions have dried up. Atropine may be given intravenously, intramuscularly, or down an endotracheal tube. After the atropine has been administered, pralidoxime (1 g in

---

BOX 37-1

The SLUDGE Syndrome

Salivation (drooling)
Lacrimation (tearing)
Urination
Defecation
Gastrointestinal distress
Emesis (vomiting)

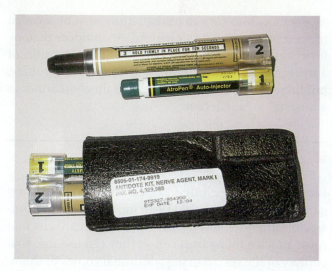

Fig. 37-1 Mark I Autoinjector. This device contains atropine and pralidoxime for treatment of nerve agent exposure.

SPECIAL Considerations

Treatment with antidotes in the field must be age and weight appropriate. For the treatment of the symptomatic patient from nerve agent exposure, this would mean the following:

Atropine

Infant (birth to 2)	0.5 mg IM
IV for infants and children	0.02 mg/kg
Child (2 to 10)	1.0 mg IM
Adolescent (>10)	2.0 mg
Elderly	1.0 mg IM

Pralidoxime

<20 kg	15 mg/kg IV
>20 kg	600-mg IM autoinjector or 1 g IV
Elderly	One half adult dose (7.5 mg/kg IV)

an adult) may be administered intravenously or intramuscularly. These antidotes are packaged together for intramuscular injection in a unit referred to as a **Mark I Autoinjector** kit (a nerve agent antidote kit, or NAAK for short), shown in Fig. 37-1. These kits were developed for the military but have been approved for civilian use. Many emergency medical services agencies have purchased these kits for their providers to use for self-treatment or partner treatment in the event of nerve agent exposure. The autoinjectors contain 2 mg of atropine and 600 mg of pralidoxime, respectively.

Patients with potential exposure to a nerve agent who are showing no symptoms do not require treatment but do require observation: 1 hour for possible vapor exposure (sarin); 18 hours for possible liquid exposure (VX). Patients with mild vapor exposure with only pupillary constriction and rhinorrhea (runny nose) require only observation. If, however, these patients develop shortness of breath, they should be treated. All patients with mild symptoms from liquid nerve agent exposure should be treated. All patients with moderate or severe symptoms, whether from vapor or liquid exposure, require treatment. Patients with severe symptoms also may be treated with a benzodiazepine (such as diazepam) to decrease the likelihood of developing seizures.

An issue of concern in dealing with any victims of potential nerve agent exposure is rescuer contamination. Patients with vapor exposure emit the vapor from their clothing (off-gassing) and from their pulmonary system. Only rescuers in PPE before decontamination should treat these patients, for decontamination entails removal of all clothing, at a minimum. Mouth-to-mouth resuscitation must not be performed on these individuals. Patients with liquid exposure represent an elevated risk of rescuer contamination because of the persistence of the liquid agent. These patients, if symptomatic, also should be treated only by rescuers in PPE before decontamination. Patient decontamination in this case should include clothing removal and a thorough washdown. All exposed patients should be decontaminated before ambulance transport.

Vesicants (Blister Agents)

Vesicants affect the skin, eyes, and other organs. They are referred to as blister agents because they can cause blisters that appear similar to those caused by a second-degree burn. They also may cause severe inflammation to the eyes, blindness, cough, shortness of breath, nausea, and vomiting. Severe exposure may result in death.

Two vesicant agents that could be used as WMD include sulfur mustard and lewisite. Both can have effects as a liquid or as a vapor. Symptoms from sulfur mustard may take hours to develop, whereas exposure to lewisite results in immediate symptoms. Initial treatment involves immediate decontamination of the victim, with attention to the concern for cross-contamination to the rescuer. Long-term care for vesicant exposure is largely supportive.

Pulmonary Toxicants

Pulmonary toxicants represent a large group of commonly used chemicals that affect mainly the respiratory system. These chemicals can cause death with significant exposure. Chemicals in this group include phosgene, chlorine, and ammonia. These exist mainly as gas and present a threat to any rescuer who is dealing with a victim in the environment of exposure. Phosgene (and isocyanate) was involved in the 1984 Bhopal, India, tragedy, resulting in 10,000 severely injured victims and 3,300 fatalities. Exposure to any of these agents produces irritation to the eyes, shortness of breath, and cough, although the symptoms from phosgene exposure may be delayed for several hours. In any of these exposures, the same basic tenets apply: (1) rescuer safety, (2) removal from the source of exposure, (3) ABCs (airway, breathing, circulation—no mouth-to-mouth resuscitation), (4) decontamination, and (5) supportive care. After phosgene exposure, any victim exertion is to be avoided because this may worsen any lung problems.

Cyanide

Several cyanide compounds could serve as WMD agents, most notably hydrogen cyanide and cyanogen chloride. Both of these agents exist as a gas, with hydrogen cyanide smelling of bitter almonds to the 50% of the population who can detect it. Both of these compounds are toxic, causing rapid onset of symptoms following any significant exposure. Low concentrations may produce symptoms of headache, weakness, dizziness, and difficulty walking. Higher concentrations may cause seizures, loss of respiration, and cardiac arrest. Treatment involves safe removal of the patient from the area of exposure, decontamination by disrobing and washdown, ABCs, supplemental oxygen at 100%, and transport to definitive care.

Again, mouth-to-mouth resuscitation must be avoided to prevent rescuer contamination. An antidote therapy for cyanide poisoning involves the administration of amyl nitrite, sodium nitrite, and sodium thiosulfate, but these must be administered in a timely manner in a hospital to be effective.

■ BIOLOGIC AGENTS

Biologic agents include (1) **bacteria**—single-cell organisms that are capable of living and dividing outside of other living cells; (2) **viruses**—organisms that must attack a living host cell so they can use that machinery of the cell to make additional copies of themselves; and (3) **toxins**—chemicals made by living organisms that are toxic to other forms of life, such as human beings. Potential biologic WMD agents have been classified by the Centers for Disease Control and Prevention into categories as to the likelihood of an agent being delivered to a large population, the health impact on a population in terms of illness, and civil disruption and preparedness needs.[2] The highest-risk agents are classified as Category A agents and are listed in Table 37-1.

The inhalation route is the most likely route for a biologic weapon attack. This method of attack has the highest likelihood of producing large numbers of seriously ill casualties. Person-to-person transmission is always a major concern when dealing with patients who may be suffering the effects of a biologic agent. This is especially problematic before the biologic agent has been identified positively. Table 37-2 lists appropriate precautions based upon the potential biologic agents.

A large-scale bioweapon attack initially may be difficult to detect, for most biologic agents in their early stages of effect cause patients to have relatively

TABLE 37-1		
Category A potential biologic weapons of mass destruction agents[2]		
Disease	**Agent Category**	**Agent**
Smallpox	Virus	Variola major
Anthrax	Bacteria	*Bacillus anthracis*
Plague	Bacteria	*Yersinia pestis*
Botulism	Bacterial toxin	*Clostridium botulinum*
Tularemia	Bacteria	*Francisella tularensis*
Viral hemorrhagic fevers	Virus	Ebola, Lassa, Marburg, and others

TABLE 37-2

Risk of spread and required precautions for Category A biologic agents*

Disease	Risk of Person-to-Person Spread	Precautions Required
Smallpox	High	Standard, airborne, contact; use N-95 mask
Anthrax	Low	Standard
Plague	High	Standard, droplet
Botulism	Very low	Standard
Tularemia	Very low	Standard
Viral hemorrhagic fevers	High	Standard, strict contact

*Standard precautions for a health care provider include hand washing, gloves, mask and eye protection, and gown when performing procedures.

SPECIAL Populations

Individuals who are immunocompromised, such as those undergoing chemotherapy or those with human immunodeficiency virus/acquired immunodeficiency syndrome, may be the first to become ill from a biologic weapons attack. These individuals also may be more prone to infection complications following a significant exposure to radiation.

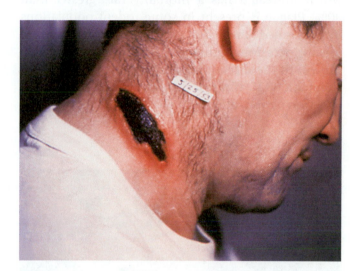

Fig. 37-2 Anthrax lesion.

mild symptoms, usually involving the respiratory tract. Clues that a bioattack is under way could include many persons being affected, often in different geographic locations, and patients who have similar symptoms that rapidly progress to severe illness. If a bioattack is suspected, several aspects of the patient's history should be emphasized: activities over the preceding days or weeks (including travel), employment history, and contact with other ill individuals. Biologic agents are covered individually as follows:

Bacterial Agents

Anthrax

Anthrax is caused by the **bacterium** *Bacillus anthracis,* an organism that historically is found in animals such as cattle and sheep. In human beings, an anthrax infection can manifest itself through skin lesions (via skin contact with the bacteria) or severe, often fatal respiratory tract infection (if the bacteria are inhaled). Gastrointestinal anthrax may be contracted if the bacteria are ingested. The skin form of the disease, cutaneous anthrax, causes black lesions to form on the skin (Fig. 37-2). Cutaneous anthrax may be spread to others if these lesions are touched without appropriate protection.

The respiratory form of the disease, inhalational anthrax, takes a few days (1 to 6) to develop after a person has inhaled the anthrax bacteria. These patients initially have some or all of the following symptoms: fever, sweats, fatigue, cough, nausea or vomiting, shortness of breath, pain on breathing, and body aches. No cases of person-to-person transmission of inhalational anthrax have ever been reported. If treated early with antibiotics, patients can survive an anthrax infection. Individuals who have been exposed to an anthrax attack should receive prophylaxis with oral antibiotics to avoid developing the disease.

Plague

Plague is caused by the bacterium *Yersinia pestis*. This is the same organism that caused massive infection and death in Europe during the fourteenth century, with up to one third of the European population dying. These pandemic infections were known as the black death and the bubonic plague. During this time, the infection was spread to human beings by fleas that would bite infected rats and then bite a human host. After the infected bite, the victim would develop greatly swollen lymph nodes called buboes (Fig. 37-3). Plague also can be spread via the respiratory route, with a victim inhaling the airborne droplets exhaled by an infected patient, resulting in a respiratory presentation called pneumonic plague, which untreated has a mortality rate greater than 90%. Plague is present in some rodent populations in the United States, including rats and prairie dogs, causing occasional human infection. The pneumonic version of the disease would be the most likely version for a WMD biologic attack. After a 2- to 3-day incubation period, affected patients have some or all of the following symptoms: high fever, chills, body aches, cough with bloody sputum, shortness of breath, and cyanosis. All patients with potential plague infection should wear a mask to minimize infection of others, with all care providers following standard precautions.

Tularemia

Tularemia is caused by the bacterium *Francisella tularensis* and most commonly is seen in ticks, rabbits, and rodents in the United States[3] (Fig. 37-4). This bacterium is one of the most infectious known and most likely would be spread via the respiratory route if it were used as a WMD agent. After a several-day incubation period, patients with tularemia have a flu-like illness consisting of symptoms of fever, headache, body aches, and cough. If the disease is not treated with antibiotics in a timely fashion, these patients have a 35% to 60% chance of dying. Oral antibiotic prophylaxis is indicated for anyone who may have been exposed to this organism. Person-to-person spread has never been reported with tularemia.

Viral Agents

Smallpox

Smallpox is caused by the **virus** variola major and until the latter part of the twentieth century was endemic in undeveloped countries. Because the smallpox virus can live only in human beings, it was possible through diligent case tracking to wipe out smallpox in the world in 1977.[4] Two samples of the smallpox virus were retained for research: one at the Centers for Disease Control and Prevention in Atlanta, the other in the Soviet Union. Unfortunately, the Soviets are al-

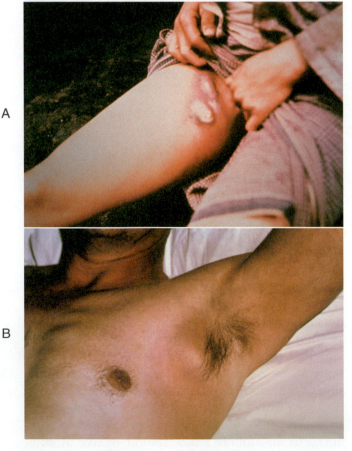

A

B

Fig. 37-3 Bubonic plague.

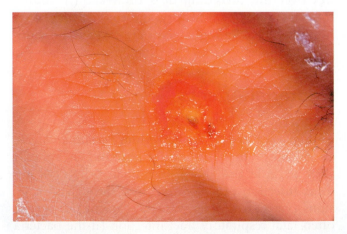

Fig. 37-4 Tularemia lesion.

leged to have manufactured large amounts of the smallpox virus for potential use as a biologic weapon.[5] Protection through smallpox vaccination had been available since Edward Jenner developed the process in the late eighteenth century. Smallpox vaccination does have a finite risk of complications, so its routine administration was discontinued in the United States shortly after smallpox was declared eradicated in the world, leaving a large proportion of the population in the United States at risk for smallpox infection. Smallpox most commonly is spread via airborne route from coughing patients, although the scabs on the smallpox rash lesions and other body fluids also may be infectious. The airborne route most likely would be used in a biologic warfare event, either through aerosolized virus particles or through exposure to an infected terrorist. Person-to-person transmission then would cause spread of the disease.

A marked rash with pustules is the most significant finding in patients with smallpox, as shown in Fig. 37-5. This rash appears 7 to 17 days after exposure. Infected patients are themselves infectious beginning 1 day before the rash erupts. Before rash development, patients may have a nonspecific, flulike illness with fever, weakness, or cough. After the rash develops, patients are infectious until the rash develops scabs and they dry up and fall off, which may take 2 to 4 weeks. Health care providers should take great care in dealing with a patient with potential smallpox. This includes standard, droplet, and contact precautions and respiratory isolation for the patient. All providers who have contact with a potential smallpox case should use N-95 (high-filtration) masks.

After exposure to a case of smallpox, significant protection can be provided to the exposed individual by smallpox vaccination, if received within 3 to 4 days of exposure. Treatment of patients who develop smallpox is otherwise just supportive. All exposed but asymptomatic individuals must be quarantined for at least 17 days after exposure. If they have not manifested aspects of the disease by that time, they will not get the disease from that exposure.

Viral Hemorrhagic Fevers

The viral hemorrhagic fevers are a diverse group of RNA viruses that share common aspects of presentation, and all attack the vascular bed of the patient. This group includes Ebola, Marburg, Rift Valley fever, dengue fever, Crimean-Congo hemorrhagic fever, and *Hantavirus*. The most probable method for spread as a WMD agent would be through aerosolization of virus particles to be inhaled by the victim. These viruses are virulent, with the fatality rate in some strains of Ebola running as high as 80%. Person-to-person spread occurs through contact with infected body fluids.

Patients with hemorrhagic fever have fever, weakness, body aches, low blood pressure, and generalized bleeding from mucous membranes and body orifices. These patients require negative pressure isolation with strict barrier precautions for care providers with gloves, masks, eye protection, gowns, and hand washing with antimicrobial soap. Unfortunately, there are no vaccines for most viral hemorrhagic fevers, and the treatment is limited to supportive care.

Toxins

Botulinum Toxin

Botulinum toxin is a toxin that attacks the nervous system in human beings. The toxin is produced by the bacterium *Clostridium botulinum*. This disease commonly is called botulism. This toxin is the most

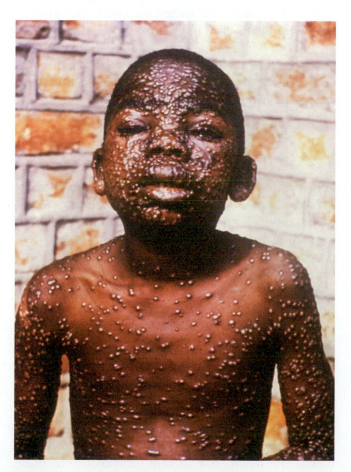

Fig. 37-5 Smallpox rash.

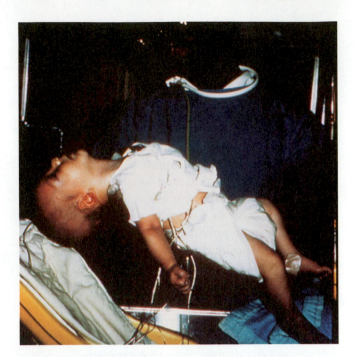

Fig. 37-6 Paralysis caused by botulism.

lethal compound per unit weight known to man, with 70 billionths of a gram being enough to kill a normal-sized adult.[6] For use as a weapon of mass destruction, botulinum toxin could be aerosolized (respiratory route) or placed in food or drink (oral route). Absorption through intact skin is minimal.

Patients exposed to botulinum toxin have neurologic complaints, usually relating to the upper part of the body, such as blurred or double vision, dilated pupils, eye pain when looking at light, difficulty swallowing, or difficulty talking. These symptoms progress until the patient is paralyzed completely and is unable to breathe (Fig. 37-6). A limited amount of antitoxin is available from the Centers for Disease Control and Prevention, but it must be administered early in the course of the disease to be effective. Treatment is otherwise supportive, with long-term mechanical ventilation necessary in severe cases until the effect of the toxin wears off, which may be many months.

Biologic Agents: Principles of Decontamination

If a patient has symptoms from a potential biologic agent attack, decontamination is not necessary because the exposure took place in the past. In these cases, however, one should use appropriate PPE to avoid person-to-person transmission. In cases in which an individual has had an acute exposure to a potential powder WMD agent, field decontamination is indicated. In these situations, prehospital personnel should not enter the area of the powder exposure. The aerosolized powder still may be present in the air. Rescuers should remove the patient to a protected area and then have his or her clothing and body wet down with water to minimize further aerosolization. Rescuers should remove the patient's clothing, cutting off upper body garments, and then bag it. Rescuers then should complete the decontamination of the patient.

■ RADIOLOGIC/NUCLEAR AGENTS

Radiologic agents are those that produce ionizing radiation, often as a result of an unstable element breaking down to a more stable element, with the subsequent release of energy in the form of ionizing radiation. This ionizing radiation can be in the form of a high-energy particle or a gamma ray (Table 37-3). This ionizing radiation is able to strip electrons off atoms in the human body, causing pathologic chemical changes to molecules, with subsequent health problems. The basic unit of measurement for an amount of radiation is the rad (radiation absorbed dose). Persons receive small amounts of radiation on an ongoing basis, on the order of about a third of a rad per year. The lethal dose of radiation over a short time for an adult is 250 to 450 rad.

Types of Radiation Exposure

Radiation exposure can take the form of external irradiation, contamination (external or internal), incorporation, or combined radiation injury. External irradiation implies that the individual has been exposed to an external source of radioactivity for a time. After the individual has been removed from the source, all chemical damage has been done to the body. The individual cannot act as a source of radiation and is not radioactive, presenting no risk to health care providers.

Contamination implies that radioactive material continues to be present on the outside of the individual (clothing or skin) or the inside, if the individual has ingested or inhaled radioactive material. This individual does emit radiation (usually at a low level) and will continue to do so until decontaminated. The health risk to care providers from these patients is usually minimal over a short period, as long as the contamination is not spread to others.

TABLE 37-3

Types of ionizing radiation

Radiation Type	Composition	Degree of Penetration	Example
Alpha particle	Two neutrons, two protons	Limited	Plutonium-238
Beta particle	Single electron	Moderate	Uranium-238
Neutron	Single neutron	Very penetrating	Neutron bomb
Gamma ray	Photon	Very penetrating	Americium-241

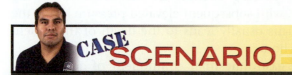

CASE SCENARIO

continued

Engine 7 and Truck 20 were parked about a block from the scene as Engine 32 pulled up. Smoke was drifting out of the damaged entrance to the department store, although Rafael could see no obvious signs of fire. As the crew hurried to don their self-contained breathing apparatuses, the captain received word from the Engine 7 officer to bring their aid equipment up to a triage and treatment area they had set up on the other side of the block from the damaged storefront.

As they moved forward into the scene, there were still victims coming out of the building, many of them holding their hands and various articles of clothing over their nose and mouth. Several were assisting other persons who appeared to have difficulty walking. A few had blood on their bodies.

More fire companies continued to arrive on scene. The hazardous materials response team also arrived with their large vehicle and were suiting up to begin their evaluation of the scene. Rafael made his way over to the treatment area with the medical bags and met up with the treatment officer.

Questions: *What type of injuries should Rafael expect to treat? What level of care should be provided during this type of event? Which patients would be transported to area hospitals first, the first treated or most injured?*

Incorporation involves organs in the body actually taking up specific radioactive elements, such as the thyroid gland taking up radioactive iodine or bone taking up radioactive strontium. This can cause ongoing radiation injury to the patient but presents little risk to care providers.

Combined radiation injury consists of any of the aforementioned types of radiation exposure with concomitant trauma to the individual.

Radiation Protection

Four basic principles determine the effect of radiation on an individual. The first is the duration of the exposure, shorter obviously being better. The second is distance from the source of radiation: the amount of exposure is related to the inverse of the square of the distance from the radiation source. That is, if you double the distance from the source, the amount of radiation decreases to a fourth (2^2) of the initial value, or if you triple the distance, the exposure decreases by a factor of 9 (3^2). The third principle is shielding: the more and the denser the material between the radioactive source and the individual, the less the exposure. The fourth is the overall quantity of the radioactive material.

Sources of Radiation Exposure

A terrorist could use five approaches to attempt to cause radiation injuries. These include a radiation point source, a **radiologic dispersion device,** a nuclear reactor breach, an improvised nuclear device, and a nuclear weapon.

Radiation Point Source

A radiation point source is simply radioactive material left in a location so that anyone in the vicinity will be exposed to radiation. This does not pose a threat to those who are not in the area or those treating individuals who were exposed.

Radiologic Dispersion Device

A radiologic dispersion device (the so-called dirty bomb) consists of radioactive material wrapped around a conventional explosive charge that then is detonated. The actual radiation injury to an individual in the vicinity usually is limited, especially over the short term. All such individuals should be assumed to be contaminated. The major impact of such a device would be the ensuing psychological effect and panic on the general population and the necessity of decontamination of the site of the blast and the surrounding area.

Nuclear Reactor Breach

Nuclear reactors could be a possible terrorist target, with the intent of violating the integrity of the shielding surrounding the reactor, with subsequent release of radiation into the atmosphere. Fortunately, reactor containment vessels are sturdily constructed, and reactor sites (in the United States) have strong security in place.

Improvised Nuclear Device

As opposed to the radiation dispersal device, an improvised nuclear device would be intended to initiate a nuclear chain reaction, resulting in a nuclear blast. Because nuclear devices are exceedingly difficult to design and construct, such a device probably would provide only a partial yield and a limited nuclear event. The degree of danger would be related to the size and efficiency of the nuclear blast.

Nuclear Weapon

A detonated nuclear weapon without doubt would cause extensive injury and illness, the degree based on the size of the weapon. The blast wave, the thermal pulse, and subsequent fires would cause injury. Survivors would run a significant risk of developing an **acute radiation syndrome** (see the following). Although thought by some to be an unlikely event, many are concerned about the fate of many suitcase-sized tactical nuclear weapons that reportedly cannot be accounted for after the breakup of the Soviet Union. These nuclear weapons are reportedly "small" but are still of the order of the nuclear bomb that was dropped on Hiroshima, Japan, bringing an end to World War II.

Acute Radiation Syndrome

Acute radiation syndrome (radiation sickness) is a group of symptoms that develop after a significant amount of whole body radiation, on the order of 100 rad or more. Three major body systems may be involved in this syndrome: the central nervous system, the gastrointestinal system, and the hematologic (blood) system. The central nervous system component of acute radiation syndrome is seen only after extremely high doses of radiation (>1000 rad) over a short period. Shortly after the exposure, these individuals develop swelling of the brain caused by edema, with subsequent elevated pressure inside the skull. This usually leads to the death of the patient within hours.

The gastrointestinal component of acute radiation syndrome is slower to develop, often after several hours. These patients have nausea and vomiting and may develop diarrhea. This is due to disruption and breakdown of the wall of the gastrointestinal tract, which may allow bacteria to leave the gut and enter the vascular system, causing infection throughout the body (sepsis). After several days, these patients may develop bloody diarrhea that usually results in death.

The hematopoietic component of radiation sickness usually takes days to develop and causes suppression of the ability of the bone marrow to produce white blood cells and platelets. This may result in subsequent infections and bleeding.

Treatment of the Radiation-Contaminated Patient

Patients contaminated with radiation ideally should be decontaminated before they are treated. However, trauma trumps radiation: life-threatening conventional injuries should be given top priority, with decontamination being performed after the patient has been stabilized. Decontamination should consist of the removal of clothing and a thorough washing with soap and water. After initial decontamination, the patient should be gone over thoroughly with a Geiger counter, searching for areas of missed radiation, necessitating further decontamination. Early presentation of patients with signs and symptoms of radiation illness indicates a large exposure to those individuals.

Health care providers working with contaminated patients should follow universal precautions for their own protection, including gown, gloves, cap, mask, and eye protection. Contaminated patients, properly handled, present little risk to health care personnel.

■ EXPLOSIVE DEVICES

Bomb detonation continues to be a favored modality of terrorist behavior, as witnessed by activity in the Middle East, Oklahoma City, the Olympics in Atlanta, and the train bombings in Madrid. A large range of devices exist that may be used, from the small improvised explosive device to the large ammonium nitrate/fuel oil bomb.

Mechanism of Blast Injury

Explosive devices produce a blast pressure wave as a result of device detonation. The magnitude of the blast pressure wave depends on the size of the bomb, the type of explosive used in the device, the environment in which it is exploded (e.g., open air versus enclosed space), the proximity of the bomb to reflecting surfaces, and the distance of the patient from the explosion. This pressure wave has two components, the initial increased pressure (positive pressure phase) followed by a smaller negative pressure wave. The blast may cause three basic types of blast injury. The first type is a primary blast injury, which is the effect of the blast wave on the tissues of the body. The second type is secondary blast injury, which is caused by objects that go airborne because of the blast and then strike the victim (similar to penetrating trauma). The third type is tertiary blast injury, which is caused by the victim being hurled into a stationary object (similar to blunt trauma). Miscellaneous injuries also may be the result of the blast, such as flash burns, chemical burns, and smoke inhalation.

Primary blast injury mainly affects organ systems with a high air-to-fluid ratio: auditory (ears), pulmonary (lungs), and gastrointestinal (bowel). Unfortunately, however, these injuries often have no external manifestations to let you know of their presence. The auditory system is the most sensitive to injury, with hearing loss and rupture of the tympanic membrane inside the ear. Following a blast, bilaterally intact tympanic membranes is a strong indicator that the individual will have no other primary blast injuries.

Blast lung injury involves damage to the walls of the air sacs (alveoli) and the outer lining of the lung. Patients with these injuries may appear normal or may have rapid breathing and evidence of lack of oxygen (hypoxia). These injuries may result in a pneumothorax (collapsed lung) or air emboli (air bubbles entering the veins leaving the lungs). The air emboli may proceed to the brain, resulting in neuro-

ASK YOURSELF

You are called to the bus station because of a possible explosion. As you exit your ambulance, you note many victims running toward you with tears streaming from their eyes and saliva drooling from their mouths, with several having vomited. In the distance, you see several persons on the ground seizing.

1. Did you park your rig too close to the scene?
2. Are you at any risk from the victims running toward you?
3. What is the first thing you should do to care for the seizing victims?

logic signs similar to a stroke, or to the heart, resulting in a myocardial infarction. If there are concerns about the possibility of an air embolus, place the patient recumbent on the left side with the head down (with appropriate spinal precautions if tertiary blast injury is present). Blast lung often may be seen as a delayed presentation up to 48 hours after the initial blast.

Blast injury to the gastrointestinal tract may involve contusions to the bowel wall, bowel rupture, or solid organ injury. A routine evaluation for abdominal trauma is appropriate for all patients suffering significant blast exposure.

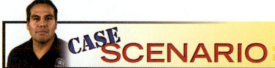

CASE SCENARIO
conclusion

Over the next hour, a small army of firefighters and paramedics rescued dozens of victims of the bombing. Although many patients had minor lacerations, ringing ears, and minimal smoke inhalation, several had critical injuries that required immediate transport. Fortunately, the police found no secondary devices that could have caused harm to the first responders. Throughout the city, emergency personnel quickly reviewed disaster response plans in case tragedy was to strike again. ■

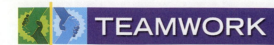
TEAMWORK

As an emergency medical technician, you will find yourself interacting with a large number of other systems at the local, state, and federal level. Understanding the incident command system and your role in a weapons of mass destruction incident will ensure safety for you, other responders, and the public.

References

1. Sidell FR: Nerve agents. In Sidell FR, Takafuji ET, Franz DR, editors: *Medical aspects of chemical and biological warfare,* Washington, DC, 1997, Office of the Surgeon General.
2. Centers for Disease Control and Prevention: Public health assessment of potential biological terrorism agents, *Emerg Infect Dis* 8:225-230, 2002.
3. Evans ME, Friedlander AM: Tularemia. In Sidell FR, Takafuji ET, Franz DR, editors: *Medical aspects of chemical and biological warfare,* Washington, DC, 1997, Office of the Surgeon General.
4. McClain DJ: Smallpox. In Sidell FR, Takafuji ET, Franz DR, editors: *Medical aspects of chemical and biological warfare,* Washington, DC, 1997, Office of the Surgeon General.
5. Alibek K: *Biohazard,* New York, 1999, Random House.
6. Middlebrook JL, Franz DR: Botulinum toxins. In Sidell FR, Takafuji ET, Franz DR, editors: *Medical aspects of chemical and biological warfare,* Washington, DC, 1997, Office of the Surgeon General.

Resources

Alibek K: *Biohazard,* New York, 1999, Random House.
Chemical Casualty Care Division, US Army Medical Research Institute of Chemical Defense: *Medical management of chemical casualties handbook,* ed 3, Aberdeen Proving Ground, MD, 2000, The Institute.
Garrett L: *The coming plague: newly emerging diseases in a world out of balance,* New York, 1995, Penguin Books.
Jarrett DG: *Medical management of radiological casualties,* Bethesda, MD, 1999, Armed Forces Radiobiology Research Institute.
Kortepeter M, Christopher G, Cieslak T, et al, editors: *USAMRIDD's medical management of biological casualties handbook,* ed 4, Fort Detrick, MD, 2001, US Army Medical Research Institute of Infectious Diseases.
Sidell FR, Takafuji ET, Franz DR, editors: *Medical aspects of chemical and biological warfare,* Washington, DC, 1997, Office of the Surgeon General.

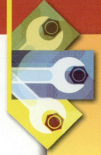

Critical Points

When dealing with a possible weapons of mass destruction attack, the importance of scene safety cannot be overemphasized. That you do not become a secondary victim is critical. You must have a high index of suspicion based on your scene size-up that a weapon of mass destruction attack may be a possibility, and you must take appropriate action. The ability to recognize the different classes of weapons of mass destruction agents based on the patient situation and presentation is necessary, because the actual agent may not be known for a significant time after the attack. Health care provider protection is important in dealing with patients who may be the victims of a biologic agent exposure. In dealing with radiation-contaminated victims, treat life-threatening injuries before attempting decontamination. Suspect clandestine lung and bowel injuries in patients who have sustained significant blast exposure.

Learning Checklist

❏ A common goal in the terrorist use of weapons of mass destruction agents is to inflict illness/injury on a large number of victims and incite fear and panic in the population at large.

❏ Health care providers can do much to improve patient outcomes in any weapons of mass destruction attack.

❏ Chemical weapons of mass destruction agents are divided into three classes: nerve agents, vesicants (blister agents), and industrial chemicals (especially those having severe pulmonary effects).

❏ Patients with a moderate exposure to nerve agents may have the SLUDGE syndrome and difficulty breathing.

❏ Patients with vapor nerve agent exposure demonstrate symptoms within seconds to minutes; symptoms from exposure to a liquid agent may be delayed for hours.

❏ Cross-contamination from a victim of nerve agent exposure is always a concern.

❏ Patients with significant symptoms from nerve agent exposure should be treated with atropine and pralidoxime in a timely fashion.

❏ Patients with exposure to blister agents should be decontaminated rapidly.

❏ Patients who are symptomatic from cyanide exposure need rapid hospital treatment with cyanide antidotes.

❏ Patients with inhalational anthrax are not contagious; those with cutaneous anthrax can spread cutaneous anthrax to others who touch their lesions.

❏ Patients with plague are infectious.

❏ Smallpox may be transmitted from patients from shortly before they break out in a rash until after the developing scabs fall off.

❏ Do not enter a room where a powdered biologic agent is present.

❏ Patients who have been exposed to radiation but have not been contaminated with radiologic material are not radioactive.

❏ Blast injury to the lungs and bowel may not be immediately obvious.

Key Terms

Acute radiation syndrome A group of symptoms that develop after a significant amount of whole body radiation, on the order of 100 rad or more. Also called *radiation sickness*.

Bacterium A single-cell organism that is capable of living and dividing outside of other living cells.

Biologic agent A general term referring to any biologic material (bacteria, virus, or toxin) that is used as a weapon, usually against a large number of persons.

Botulinum toxin A compound made by the bacterium *Clostridium botulinum* that causes neurologic dysfunction and culminates in total body paralysis.

Bronchoconstriction Constriction of the bronchi and bronchioles in the lung, causing difficulty breathing.

Chemical weapon A general term for any common chemical compound (such as chlorine gas) or any specially manufactured compound (such as sarin) that is used as a weapon, usually against a large number of persons.

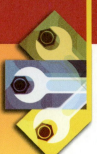

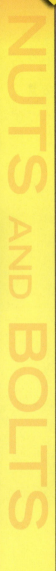

Mark I Autoinjector A self-contained unit that contains the medications atropine and pralidoxime in an injection device for administration to a victim of nerve agent exposure.

Miosis Constriction of the pupil, which limits the amount of light reaching the eye.

Radiologic dispersion device A device usually made by packing radioactive material around an explosive device. Detonation of such a device usually results in relatively low-level radiologic contamination but would cause extensive public panic and potentially extensive need for decontamination of the affected area.

Sarin A chemical compound specifically developed to serve as a weapon of mass destruction nerve agent. Sarin also goes by the military term *GB* and in the lay press may be

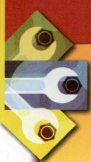

referred to as "nerve gas." Sarin is rapid acting. It may be a liquid but usually is dispersed as a gas at room temperature.

Toxins Chemicals made by living organisms that are toxic to other forms of life.

Virus An organism that must attack a living host cell so that it can use the machinery of the cell to replicate.

VX A nerve agent that normally exists as a liquid at room temperature. The onset of symptoms following exposure to this agent may be delayed up to 18 hours.

National Standard Curriculum Objectives

No objectives were identified.

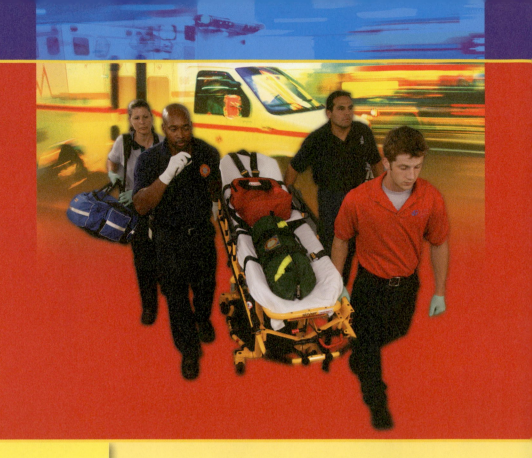

38

CHAPTER OUTLINE

Airway Anatomy

Assessment

Management Techniques

OUTLINE

LESSON GOAL

GOAL

The purpose of this chapter is to introduce the emergency medical technician (EMT) to the principles and techniques of advanced airway management. Many of the anatomic, physiologic, and clinical concepts pertinent to advanced airway management are discussed in Chapter 7; the student should review these before proceeding through this chapter. This chapter focuses predominantly on the proper performance of orotracheal intubation for infants, children, and adult patients. The chapter also covers adjunctive procedures of laryngeal mask airway insertion, tracheal-esophageal Combitube (Kendall-Sheridan Catheter Corp., Argyle, New York) placement, and nasogastric tube insertion.

Continuous practice and reeducation regarding advanced airway skills are fundamental responsibilities of anyone who may be called upon to perform them in the field. ∎

Advanced Airway Management

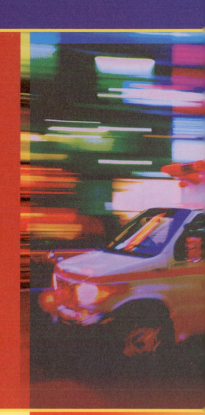

CHAPTER OBJECTIVES

After completing this chapter, the EMT student will be able to do the following:

1 Define those portions of upper airway anatomy pertinent to the performance of advanced airway management.

2 Describe how changes in the anatomy and the physiology of the upper respiratory tract through the stages of infant/child to adult development influence the approach to advanced airway management.

3 Explain in detail the step-by-step procedure for orotracheal intubation in the infant, child, and adult patient.

4 List the potential complications of orotracheal intubation.

5 Describe the rationale and the means by which proper endotracheal tube placement must be confirmed.

6 Explain the importance of properly securing a correctly placed endotracheal tube.

7 Explain the indications, method, and contraindications for inserting a nasogastric tube.

8 Describe the correct methods of inserting alternative airway devices like the Combitube and the laryngeal mask airway.

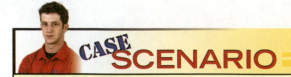

Ray could hear the police officer's automated external defibrillator going through its verbal commands as he climbed the stairs to the victim's bedroom. The call had come in for a "man down, unconscious" at a trailer park complex not far from the hospital. The communicator dispatched two police officers to the scene as well. They reported that they had what appeared to be an older female in cardiac arrest, and they were beginning cardiopulmonary resuscitation. As Ray entered the room, one of the officers discharged the automated external defibrillator, causing the patient's limbs to jerk once. A second shock was not indicated, and the officers continued cardiopulmonary resuscitation.

Ray had just completed the oral intubation training just a week earlier. The medical director felt that a secured airway would be beneficial to managing the unconscious patient's airway, and all of the emergency medical technicians in the service went through extensive training to develop skill proficiency. Ray finished his operating room time last week at the university hospital, and the medical director signed him off on the skill.

Ray began to unroll the intubation kit that was stored in the side pouch of the jump kit.

Questions: *What are the different pieces of equipment that Ray will need to assemble before attempting the intubation? What will Ray be concerned about as he begins the procedure? In addition to the intubation equipment, what other device should Ray have immediately with him?*

■ AIRWAY ANATOMY

A thorough understanding of the anatomy of the **upper respiratory tract** is fundamental to successful airway management. Chapter 7 discusses the anatomy of the entire respiratory system. This chapter reviews the specific structures of the upper airway, with an emphasis on the manner in which those structures relate to one another in terms of position and function. The importance of identifying the anatomic landmarks of the upper airway during the performance of the advanced management techniques covered in this chapter cannot be overemphasized. Failure to do so correctly carries with it a high likelihood that the attempted procedure will fail, with potentially disastrous consequences for the patient.

Normal Upper Airway Anatomy in the Adult

The upper airway consists of the nose, the mouth, the **pharynx,** the **larynx,** and the upper portion of the **trachea**. Air inhaled via the nose or the mouth passes into the pharynx, the cavity commonly referred to as the throat. The pharynx may be subdivided into the **nasopharynx,** that portion directly behind the nose; the **oropharynx,** or the space immediately posterior to the mouth; and the **hypopharynx.** The hypopharynx is the inferior portion of the pharynx. Because it lies behind and below the base of the tongue, the hypopharynx is typically not visible when one is simply looking through the open mouth to the back of the throat. Instead, directly visualizing the hypopharynx often requires the use of a **laryngoscope,** a handled device with an attached blade and distal light source that, when used properly, exposes and illuminates this portion of the airway.

The openings to the larynx and the **esophagus** are situated at the lowermost portion of the hypopharynx. The esophagus is a muscular tube located immediately behind (posterior) the larynx and trachea. It serves as the conduit through which swallowed food and liquid passes into the stomach. The opening of the larynx lies anterior to that of the esophagus, making it more difficult than the esophagus to visualize directly even with the assistance of a laryngoscope (Fig. 38-1). Understanding this anatomic relationship is crucial when one is attempting to pass an **endotracheal tube** through the larynx and into the trachea. Mistaking the esophageal opening for that of the larynx will lead to the erroneous intubation of the esophagus, and if unrecognized, death of the patient.

Visualizing and identifying the structures of the upper larynx enable an easy differentiation between the laryngeal opening and the esophagus and thus are a fundamental component of direct endotracheal intubation. Attempting to pass an endotracheal tube

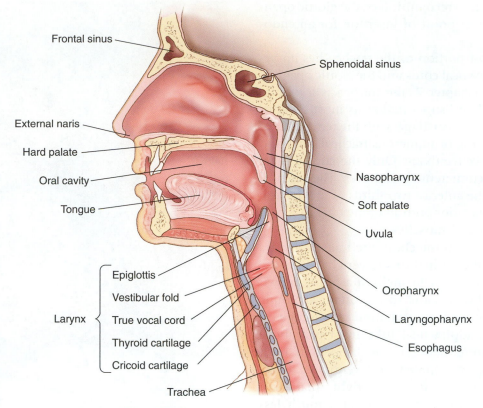

Fig. 38-1 Anatomy of the upper airway.

without seeing and recognizing these structures, however, is extremely dangerous because of the risk for esophageal intubation. When viewed with the assistance of a laryngoscope from a position behind the patient's head and through the open mouth, the most anterior—or from the perspective of the intubator, the most superior—visible structure is the base of the tongue (Fig. 38-2). Immediately behind the base of the tongue lies the **epiglottis,** a flap of soft tissue that folds over to cover the opening to the larynx during the mechanical act of swallowing and thus prevents food or liquid from passing into the trachea.

The epiglottis is separated from the base of the tongue by the **vallecula,** a recessed area that is an important landmark for intubation by direct visualization. Within the vallecula the **glossoepiglottic ligament** tethers the epiglottis to the anterior wall of the hypopharynx. When placed properly into the vallecula, the tip of the laryngoscope is used to exert traction on the glossoepiglottic ligament and lift the epiglottis off the opening of the larynx to facilitate intubation. When the epiglottis is retracted in this fashion, the **glottic opening,** or **glottis,** becomes visible. The glottis is the actual point of entry into the trachea. Its border is formed by the **true vocal**

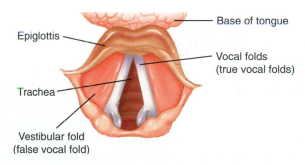

Fig. 38-2 Anatomy of the upper larynx as viewed from above.

cords, pearly white cartilaginous structures with thin muscular attachments. Movement of the true vocal cords controls airflow into the trachea and the pitch of vibration when they are used for speech. The **arytenoids** are pyramid-shaped structures that attach each of the true vocal cords to the posterior aspect of the cricoid ring of the trachea. A number of other soft tissue structures surround the true vocal cords, including the **vestibular folds,** or **false vocal cords,** and the **cuneiform** and **corniculate cartilages.** Successfull identification of these structures allows for easy recognition of the glottic opening and the correct point of insertion for an endotracheal tube.

The uppermost portion of the trachea lies immediately below the vocal cords and the glottic opening. As discussed in Chapter 7, the trachea is a tubular structure formed and supported at its most superior aspect by the **cricoid cartilage,** with the remainder of its length consisting of numerous tracheal rings and interposed connective tissue. Only the cricoid cartilage is fully circumferential, however. The tracheal rings surround the anterior two thirds of the trachea; support of the posterior portion of the trachea is provided by the **tracheal muscle.**

As it descends into the chest, the trachea divides at the level of the fifth thoracic vertebra into the right and left mainstem **bronchi** at a point known as the **carina.** The carina is an important anatomic structure in endotracheal intubation because the tip of an inserted endotracheal tube must rest above this dividing point between the bronchi if both lungs are to be oxygenated and ventilated effectively. Moreover, because the right mainstem bronchus departs from the carina at a much less acute angle than does the left mainstem bronchus, an endotracheal tube inserted beyond the level of the carina enters the right bronchus far more often than it does the left.

Anatomy of the Upper Airway in Infants and Children

A number of important anatomic differences exist between the adult airway and that of infants and children. These differences reflect changes that occur, as normal growth and development progress, in the size, proportions, and position of many of the structures discussed in this chapter. Understanding these differences is vital to successful management of the pediatric airway.

Among infants and children the head is proportionately much larger in relation to the body than it is in the adult. As a result, when a pediatric patient is supine, pressure on the occiput tilts the head and the plane of the face forward. As discussed in Chapter 7, this can compress and thereby obstruct portions of the upper airway. This also can render direct visualization of the structures of the hypopharynx with a laryngoscope more difficult. For this reason, it is often helpful to place a folded towel or similar structure behind the patient's shoulders to return the head to a neutral position,

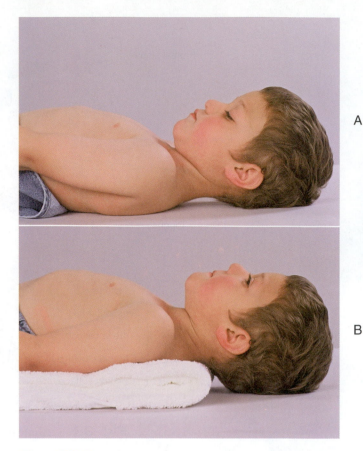

Fig. 38-3 A, Flexion of the pediatric neck in the supine position. **B,** Return of the head and neck to neutral position with padding beneath the shoulders.

with the face parallel to the flat surface on which the patient lies (Fig. 38-3).

The passageways of the nose, mouth, and pharynx are smaller in children and infants and are therefore more susceptible to obstruction from swelling or the presence of a foreign body. The tongue, moreover, occupies a proportionately greater space in the oropharynx and hypopharynx. The potential for the tongue to obstruct the upper airway of the supine pediatric patient is therefore even greater than it is in the adult, and the greater relative tongue size also can interfere with insertion of a laryngoscope and adequate visualization of the structures of the hypopharynx.

The larynx occupies a more superior and anterior position in the hypopharynx in the pediatric patient (Fig. 38-4). This is important to remember when attempting to locate and visualize the glottic opening of an infant or child and may dictate which type of laryngoscope blade is best for accomplishing this purpose. The epiglottis is proportionately larger among infants and small children, and its support by the glossoepiglottic ligament is not as taut as in

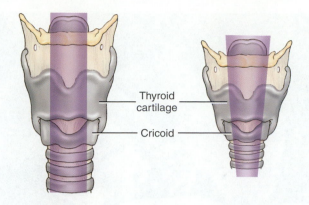

Fig. 38-4 Anterior and superior position of the pediatric larynx relative to that of the adult.

adults. As a result, even a laryngoscope that has been well placed into the vallecula may be ineffective in lifting the epiglottis to expose the glottic opening.

In contrast to adults, in whom the glottic opening forms the narrowest portion of the upper airway, among infants and children the cricoid cartilage is the most constrictive segment of this portion of the respiratory tract. Consequently, an endotracheal tube that passes through the vocal cords of a pediatric patient may meet resistance at the level of the cricoid cartilage and proceed no farther. Therefore, having tubes of various sizes readily available when attempting to intubate an infant or small child is important.

Lastly, the fact that the trachea and bronchi are shorter in smaller pediatric patients renders the correct placement of an endotracheal tube with its tip just above the carina more difficult. The potential for inadvertently advancing the tube into the right mainstem bronchus is greater. At the same time, a properly placed tube is much more susceptible to dislodgment with the slightest flexion, extension, or rotation of the patient's neck. This may result in the unexpected removal of the endotracheal tube from the upper airway entirely or, worse, an unrecognized withdrawal of the endotracheal tube tip from the larynx and reinsertion into the esophagus. For that reason, the placement of an endotracheal tube in a pediatric patient mandates that it be properly secured and frequently reassessed for correct positioning.

■ ASSESSMENT

Chapter 7 discusses the signs and symptoms of respiratory compromise and distress that signal the need for basic airway management and assisted ventilation. The patient who is responsive to some degree or

who has an intact gag reflex will not tolerate many of the advanced airway interventions covered in this chapter without first being administered sedating and paralyzing medications that are generally not available in the prehospital setting. Such patients are therefore best supported with basic airway management and assisted ventilation until arrival at a medical facility. Advanced airway intervention by the emergency medical technician generally is limited to those patients who are found to be completely unresponsive or apneic or who become so after all other supportive modalities have failed.

■ MANAGEMENT TECHNIQUES

Proper airway management begins with careful attention to the opening, suctioning, and assisted ventilation techniques discussed in Chapter 7. When these have failed, however, it may become necessary to perform more invasive procedures designed to ensure uncompromised airflow through the upper respiratory tract and adequate oxygenation and ventilation of the patient. Procedures of this type likely to be performed by the emergency medical technician include endotracheal intubation, placement of a **laryngeal mask airway** (LMA), or insertion of a dual-lumen esophageal/tracheal tube **(Combitube)**. The successful performance of these interventions requires proper equipment, skilled technique, careful confirmation of correct placement for the device used, proper securing of the device after placement, and vigilance for signs of the serious complications that may occur during or after these procedures. Once upper airway control is established, further supportive techniques, such as decompression of the gastrointestinal tract with a **nasogastric tube,** are important to maintain adequate and continued ventilation of the patient.

Orotracheal Intubation of the Adult

Endotracheal intubation is the most secure means of controlling the airway. The correct placement of an endotracheal tube into the trachea guarantees a patent conduit for airflow through the upper respiratory tract, and an appropriate seal around the tube prevents the aspiration of blood and gastric contents into the lower respiratory passages. The most effective method of endotracheal intubation is **orotra-**

BOX 38-1

Proper Orotracheal Intubation Equipment

1. Gloves
2. Mask
3. Eye protection
4. Laryngoscope blades and handles
5. An assortment of endotracheal tubes
6. A stylet
7. Water-soluble lubricant
8. A 10-mL syringe
9. A suction unit with catheter attachments
10. Tape or a commercially available endotracheal tube-securing device
11. Bag respirator

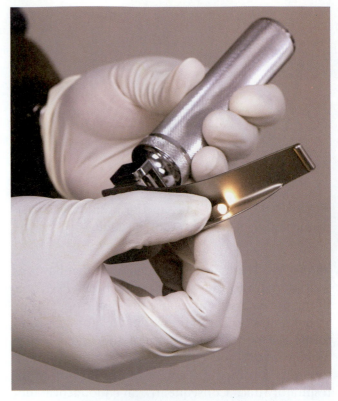

Fig. 38-5 Laryngoscope with functioning light source.

cheal intubation, or the passage of an endotracheal tube between the vocal cords and into the trachea under direct visualization through the patient's mouth with the aid of a laryngoscope.

One must assemble the proper equipment before any attempt at orotracheal intubation (Box 38-1). The laryngoscope is a two-piece instrument that consists of a handle and a detachable blade with a light source at its tip. When the blade is attached to the handle and locked in the 90-degree position, the light source is illuminated (Fig. 38-5). Batteries for the light source are housed in the laryngoscope handle, and it is essential to assemble the laryngoscope and check for proper functioning of the batteries and light source regularly.

Two varieties of laryngoscope blades exist: the curved and the straight (Fig. 38-6). Both are designed to provide a direct line of sight through the patient's open mouth to the vocal cords by compressing the tongue and pushing it to one side while at the same time lifting the epiglottis to expose the glottic opening. Both are available in a variety of lengths to accommodate patients of different sizes. The curved blade has a side flange running along most of its length that is designed to help sweep the tongue to one side to allow for a better view of the hypopharynx. The curve of the blade allows its tip to be placed in the vallecula, where upward and forward traction in the supine patient exerts tension on the glossoepiglottic ligament and thus indirectly lifts the epiglottis to expose the glottic opening (Fig. 38-7). The straight blade provides a direct line of sight to the laryngeal structures by compressing the tongue. Its tip is placed between the epiglottis and the glottis, where upward and forward traction di-

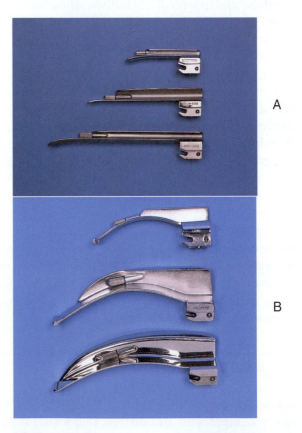

Fig. 38-6 Straight **(A)** and curved **(B)** laryngoscope blades.

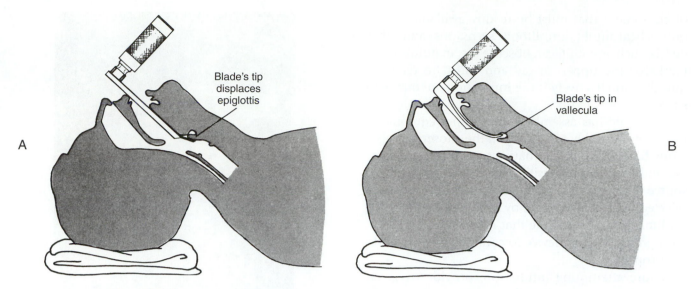

Fig. 38-7 Correct positioning of the straight (A) versus the curved (B) laryngoscope blade in relation to the vallecula and the epiglottis.

rectly elevates the epiglottis to reveal the glottic opening (see Fig. 38-2).

Endotracheal tubes are hollow, translucent, and pliable. Endotracheal tubes are designated by size and whether an inflatable cuff is present at the distal end. Tube size is defined by the internal diameter in millimeters and can range from 2.5 for small infants to 9 for large adults. Typically, a 7.5-mm tube is adequate for most adults. Regardless of the tube size selected, alternative tubes one size larger and one size smaller must be readily available in case they are needed during the intubation attempt.

When a cuff is present, a one-way inflation valve and pilot balloon are attached to the proximal end of the tube. Inflation with 5 to 10 mL of air at the proximal valve expands the distal cuff to create an airtight seal between the tube and inner lining of the trachea. Cuffed tubes are used for adults and older children; infants and small children (less than 8 years of age) do not require a cuffed tube because the narrowing at the cricoid cartilage usually establishes an airtight seal.

All endotracheal tubes must have a 15-mm adaptor at the proximal end as a standard attachment to connect to other airway equipment such as a bagmask. Centimeter markings on the side of the tube indicate length from the tip of the tube and are thus useful for quantifying the depth to which the tube has been inserted.

The **stylet** is a thin, semirigid rod inserted into the endotracheal tube to provide stiffness and allow the tube to be bent to a desired angle (Fig. 38-8). This

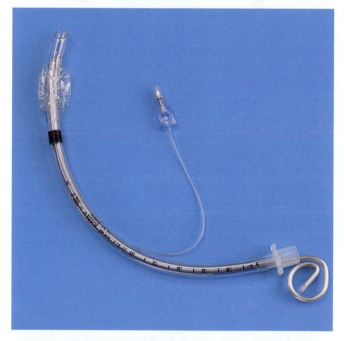

Fig. 38-8 Endotracheal tube with stylet.

can be helpful in guiding the tube during attempted insertion. If the stylet is used, one must take great care to ensure that the tip of the stylet does not extend beyond the distal opening of the tube because an exposed tip may puncture or lacerate the airway as the tube is inserted.

A functioning suction device with a rigid catheter attachment as described in Chapter 7 is another piece of equipment that must be readily available during orotracheal intubation. Blood, secretions, and other debris, such as vomit, can obscure the anatomic landmarks of the upper airway and must be removed quickly and effectively if the intubation attempt is to succeed.

Once one has assembled the proper equipment, one should quickly test it. Attach the chosen laryngoscope blade plus an alternative selection to the handle and lock it into position to verify that the light source is functioning adequately. If cuffed, test each selected endotracheal tube by inflating the cuff with a 10-mL syringe to ensure that no air leak is present. Turn on the suction device to confirm that it is working properly.

Before attempting intubation, provide oxygenation and ventilation for the patient using a bag-mask with an oropharyngeal airway in place to prevent the tongue from occluding the upper airway according to basic airway management techniques. Remove impediments to orotracheal intubation such as dentures, debris, or foreign bodies. The application of a small amount of water-soluble lubricant to the distal end of the endotracheal tube before the intubation attempt may facilitate passage of the tube through the glottis. Ideally, the patient should be supine, and if trauma is suspected, in-line cervical spine immobilization should be provided at all times during the procedure by an assistant whose hands are placed on either side of the patient's head. Another assistant should stand by to hand the endotracheal tube to the rescuer performing the intubation when needed.

A designated assistant also may help by performing the **Sellick maneuver.** The Sellick maneuver, also known as *cricoid pressure,* is performed by locating the cricoid cartilage immediately below the thyroid cartilage, or Adam's apple, on the anterior neck. Because the cricoid cartilage is a fully circumferential and rigid ring within the upper trachea, applying pressure to the cartilage with a thumb and forefinger pushes the entire larynx posteriorly. This may help to bring the structures of the larynx into view for the rescuer attempting intubation. In addition, because the esophagus lies immediately behind the cricoid cartilage, posterior displacement of the cartilaginous ring compresses the esophagus and thereby prevents the regurgitation of gastric contents that can obscure visualization of the glottic opening and cause complications if aspirated into the lower respiratory tract (Fig. 38-9).

When the proper equipment has been assembled and tested, the patient has received ventilation and

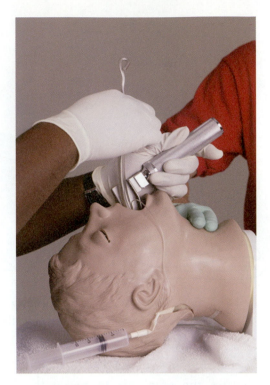

Fig. 38-9 The Sellick maneuver.

oxygenation to the degree that circumstances allow, and any available assistants have been assigned supportive roles as described previously, the rescuer attempting the intubation should take a position behind the patient's head. The rescuer should wear proper personal protective equipment, including gloves, a mask, and eye shielding at all times.

Once these preparatory measures have been taken, the rescuer may attempt orotracheal intubation (Skill 38-1). As an assistant initiates the Sellick maneuver, the rescuer should hold the laryngoscope in the left hand while using the right hand to open the patient's mouth. This is best done with the scissoring or cross-fingered technique. From a position above and behind the patient's head, the rescuer inserts the middle finger of the right hand into the mouth along the patient's upper right molars. The rescuer then places the thumb of the right hand against the right front teeth of the patient's jaw. Scissoring the thumb and middle finger opens the jaw, allowing for optimal insertion of the laryngoscope and visualization of the hypopharynx.

With the patient's mouth opened, the rescuer inserts the laryngoscope into the right corner of the mouth with the left hand. One must take great care to avoid damaging the patient's teeth or lacerating the lips during insertion. Use the laryngoscope blade to sweep the tongue to the left while advancing the tip

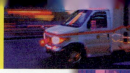

SKILL 38-1

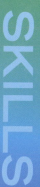

Orotracheal Intubation

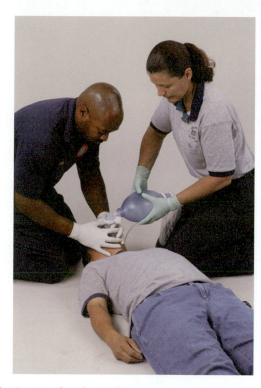

Adult Orotracheal Intubation

1. Maintain assisted ventilation with high-flow supplemental oxygen for the patient.

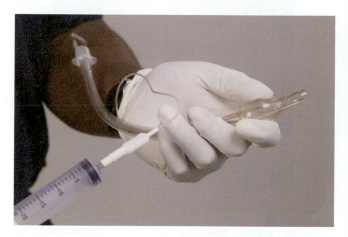

2. Assemble the proper equipment listed in Box 38-1.
3. Test the equipment by assessing chosen laryngoscope blades for a working light source, endotracheal tubes for cuff inflation, and available suction for proper function.

Continued

SKILL 38-1
Orotracheal Intubation—cont'd

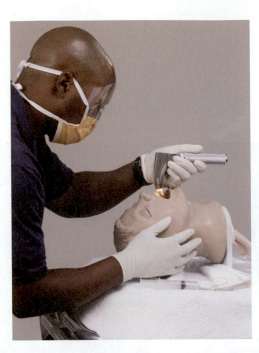
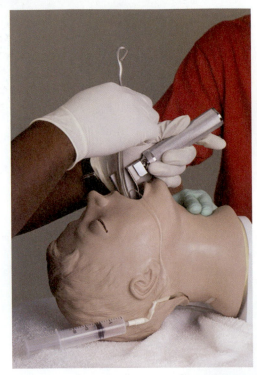

4. Insert a stylet into the chosen endotracheal tube, taking care that the distal end of the stylet does not protrude from the distal opening of the tube. The proximal end of the stylet should be bent to an angle greater than 90 degrees against the 15-mm adapter to prevent the stylet from inadvertently slipping further into the endotracheal tube.

5. Designate available assistants to provide in-line cervical spine immobilization, perform the Sellick maneuver, and hold the endotracheal tube until it is called for.

6. Remove any obstructing items such as dentures, dislodged teeth, or foreign bodies from the patient's mouth.

7. Hold the selected laryngoscope in the left hand with the blade in the locked and "on" position.

8. If the patient's jaw is relaxed, insert the fingers of the right hand into the right side of the patient's mouth. Open the jaw widely using a scissoring maneuver with the thumb and middle finger.

9. Gently insert the laryngoscope blade through the right side of the mouth and deep into the hypopharynx while sweeping the tongue to the left.

10. Identify the epiglottis. If using a curved blade, position its tip immediately above the epiglottis and within the vallecula. If using a straight blade, position its tip on the underside of the epiglottis.

11. Pull the handle of the laryngoscope upward and away to lift the epiglottis and expose the vocal cords and the glottic opening. *Do not allow the back of the laryngoscope to touch the patient's teeth, because any force that is levered against the teeth will damage or dislodge them.*

12. While maintaining sight of the glottic opening at all times, with the right hand take the endotracheal tube from the assistant and insert its tip through the glottic opening to the desired depth.

SKILL 38-1
◉ *Orotracheal Intubation—cont'd*

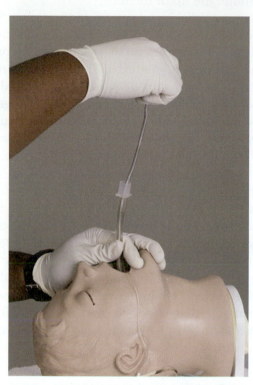

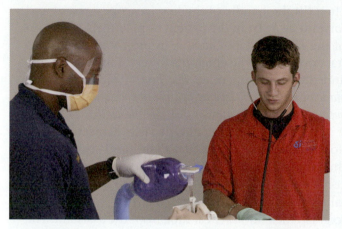

13. Gently remove the laryngoscope while continuing to hold the endotracheal tube with the right hand.

14. Keep a firm grip on the inserted endotracheal tube while removing the stylet.

15. While maintaining a firm grip on the endotracheal tube, inflate the cuff with 5 to 10 mL of air.

16. Attach the 15-mm adapter to a bag-mask device and deliver breaths.

17. Confirm tube placement by auscultating over the right and left lung fields and the epigastrium *and* using an end-tidal carbon dioxide detector or an esophageal intubation detection device.

18. Once proper tube placement has been confirmed, secure the endotracheal tube at the opening of the mouth with tape or a commercially available securing device.

Pediatric Orotracheal Intubation

Visualized orotracheal intubation can be performed successfully on patients of all ages; however, the emergency medical technician should be aware of some modifications that occur when the patient is an infant. First, use only a straight laryngoscope blade. The infant's vocal cords are located more anteriorly than an adult's, and a curved blade is harder to use and more likely to traumatize the infant's oropharynx. Second, use only uncuffed endotracheal tubes. The infant's trachea narrows at its proximal end, providing a close enough margin effectively to hold air below the vocal cords without the need for a pressurized cuff on the tube. A cuff also could be an additional agent for traumatizing the infant's trachea when it is inflated. Finally, whereas an adult's head and neck are hyperextended (except in trauma patients) in preparation for visualized orotracheal intubation, the infant's cervical alignment must remain in no more than mild extension because of the potential for crimping and collapsing the immature tracheal cartilaginous rings.

Also note that because of the incomplete formation of the cranium in infants and small children (particularly of the cribriform plate), do not attempt the "blind nasal" intubation procedure in such patients. Similarly, because of the child's small mouth size and anterior positioning of the vocal cords, do not use the digital-tactile technique in infants and small children.

deep into the hypopharynx. This should allow for the visualization and identification of the anatomic structures of the upper larynx described earlier. If a curved blade has been selected, insert its tip into the vallecula. If a straight blade is used, position its distal end immediately beneath (posterior to) the epiglottis. Then lift the handle of the laryngoscope upward and forward away from the patient's upper teeth. If the tip of the laryngoscope blade is in proper position, this traction will lift the epiglottis to reveal the vocal cords and the glottic opening. *The heel of the laryngoscope blade must never be levered against the patient's front teeth because this will fracture or dislodge the teeth.*

Once the glottic opening is visible, insert the endotracheal tube. The rescuer's left hand should hold the laryngoscope in the position, exposing the vocal cords, with direct sight of the glottis being maintained at all times. The right hand then should be free to grasp the endotracheal tube from the assistant. The rescuer should direct the tip of the tube through the glottic opening and advance it. In a normal-size adult, advance the endotracheal tube until the tip lies 3 to 5 cm above the carina. This position is best estimated by inserting the tube until the markings along its length align with the patient's front teeth at about the 22-cm line. Then gently remove the laryngoscope from the patient's mouth. If used, remove the stylet at this point and inflate the cuff with 5 to 10 mL of air. Then connect a bag-mask to the adapter of the tube and deliver breaths.

Because inadvertent insertion of the endotracheal tube in the esophagus is a serious, life-threatening complication of intubation, immediate confirmation of proper tube positioning in the trachea after placement is mandatory. Ideally, two or three methods of verifying correct tube placement should be used to minimize the chances of failing to identify an esophageal intubation. Direct visualization of the endotracheal tube passing between the vocal cords is the most important indicator of correct tracheal intubation. Further affirmation can be obtained by observing the chest for symmetric rise and fall and auscultation of breath sounds over both lung fields with each delivered breath. Also auscultate the epigastrium because gurgling sounds in this location signify esophageal intubation. If this occurs, immediately remove the endotracheal tube and provide the patient with ventilation by basic airway management techniques.

An **esophageal intubation detection device** is a syringe that fits the adapter of the endotracheal tube. When it is attached to the tube and suction is applied, the device can indicate whether placement is in the trachea or the esophagus. Easy aspiration of air signifies tracheal placement. Difficulty drawing air into the device, however, means that the end of the tube is in the esophagus, because the applied suction is causing a collapse of the more pliable esophageal wall around the tip of the tube.

The most reliable means of confirmation, however, is to document the presence of end-tidal carbon dioxide ($ETCO_2$) at the end of each exhalation during assisted ventilation. Air exhaled from the lungs is laden with carbon dioxide, whereas air forced into the esophagus and stomach and then expunged by way of an improperly placed endotracheal tube is not. Detection of carbon dioxide in air exiting by way of the endotracheal tube therefore indicates that the lungs, not the gastrointestinal tract, are being ventilated by a tube in proper position. Detection may be done with an $ETCO_2$ detection device that can be interposed between the adaptor at the proximal end of the endotracheal tube and the bag-mask (Fig. 38-10). When $ETCO_2$ is present, an indicator changes color on the device, confirming that the endotracheal tube is in the trachea. Quantitative $ETCO_2$ monitors are also available that trace the level of $ETCO_2$ in real time, generating a distinctive waveform that reflects the ventilatory cycle.

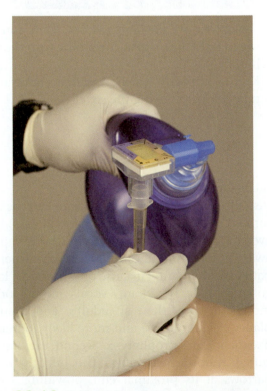

Fig. 38-10 End-tidal carbon dioxide detector. A change in color as the patient exhales indicates the presence of carbon dioxide, confirming proper endotracheal tube placement.

Throughout these maneuvers the rescuer must maintain a firm grip on the endotracheal tube at all times. Inattention to this detail can result in the tube becoming dislodged at any moment. If this occurs, the end of the endotracheal tube may be removed from the trachea and oropharynx entirely or, more disastrous, may slip unnoticed into the esophagus. The tube can be released only after it has been fastened securely at the opening of the patient's mouth with tape or a commercially available attachment device.

Recognition of the potential complications of attempted endotracheal intubation is important. The most serious of these is unrecognized esophageal intubation, because this results in the patient receiving no

assisted ventilation whatsoever. If not promptly appreciated and corrected, this is often fatal for the patient.

Multiple, prolonged, and unsuccessful attempts at intubation may deprive the patient of oxygen for a dangerously extended time. For that reason, no single attempt should exceed 30 to 45 seconds, and the patient should be given oxygen and ventilation with basic airway techniques before any repeat effort is made. If intubation is not successfully achieved after two or three tries, one should make no further attempts. Instead, the patient should be transported with assisted ventilation en route.

Insertion of a laryngoscope into the hypopharynx can cause complications as well. Manipulation of the structures of the hypopharynx with a laryngoscope blade can stimulate the autonomic nervous system, which in turn can cause abnormal acceleration or deceleration of the heart rate. Careful monitoring of vital signs before and after intubation is therefore important. Vomiting following such stimulation is also common, and in the supine, unresponsive patient, this may result in aspiration of gastric contents into the lungs. The Sellick maneuver therefore is recommended as an adjunct to orotracheal intubation, and adequate suction should be immediately available at all times during the procedure. Lastly, trauma to the teeth, gingivae, and lips can occur if the laryngoscope is inserted, used, or removed carelessly.

If the endotracheal tube is inserted too far into the trachea, it usually enters the right mainstem bronchus (Fig. 38-11). When this occurs, the left lung cannot be

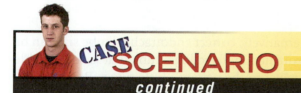

CASE SCENARIO *continued*

The light of the laryngoscope was "bright, white, and tight." Ray carefully set the tool down on the clean pad and instructed the officer working the bag-mask to increase the respiratory rate to one breath every 3 seconds in order to hyperoxygenate the patient. Ray quickly assembled the endotracheal tube, stylet, and 10-mL syringe while maintaining sterile precautions. The pilot balloon inflated with a push of the syringe and held its air, indicating that the obturator cuff would do its job. Looking at the anatomic appearance of the patient, Ray estimated that the procedure should be fairly straightforward: the neck was not unusually large in proportion to the rest of the jaw line and head, and the lower mandible was not recessed. Ray asked the officer to stop giving the patient ventilation and remove the oropharyneal airway. He moved to a prone position and adjusted the patient's head into an optimal position. Ray began to slip in the tip of the laryngoscope blade into the patient's mouth.

Questions: *What is the optimal position of the patient's head for an intubation procedure? How should Ray manipulate the laryngoscope in order to displace the tongue and visualize the glottic opening? What should he do if he cannot see the vocal cords? If Ray can visualize the glottic opening, how far should he insert the endotracheal tube?*

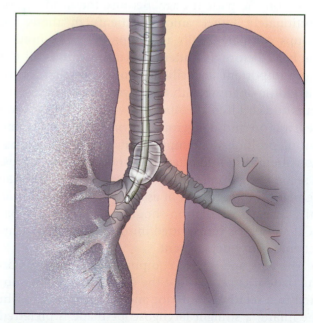

Fig. 38-11 Right mainstem bronchus intubation.

ventilated and oxygenated effectively. For this reason, it is essential to auscultate over both lung fields immediately after the tube has been placed. If breath sounds are present on the right but not across the left lung field, deflate the cuff and slowly withdraw the tube until air movement can be heard bilaterally. Take care not to remove the endotracheal tube from the trachea entirely, however. Once the cuff has been reinflated and symmetric bilateral breath sounds are present, then secure the tube.

Dislodgment of the endotracheal tube from the trachea can occur whenever there is movement of the patient or the tube. When this occurs, control of the airway has been lost and effective oxygenation and ventilation of the patient ceases. This is best prevented by adequately securing the tube in place once proper positioning has been confirmed. Whenever a patient is moved from one position or from one surface to another, auscultate breath sounds to reconfirm that the tube remains properly situated. Lastly, patients who are capable of movement after intubation may try to remove the tube because of discomfort; in such a situation, careful restraint of the patient's hands can prevent self-extubation.

Orotracheal Intubation of the Infant or Child

Because of the special anatomic features of the upper airway present among infants and children, one must keep several important considerations in mind when performing endotracheal intubation on patients in these age groups. Carefully select and size equipment based on the patient's age. Because the head is proportionately larger among patients of these age groups compared with adults, properly positioning the head before any attempted intubation is all the more important to facilitate proper visualization of the glottic opening with the laryngoscope. Lastly, infants and children are especially vulnerable to oxygen deprivation and dangerous slowing of the heart rate during prolonged attempts at intubating. No intubation attempt should extend beyond 15 to 30 seconds. A second attempt lasting no longer than the first may be made after a period of assisted ventilation. If this fails, assisted ventilation should resume and the patient should be transported immediately to the nearest emergency department.

The type and size of equipment used depends on the patient's age. Because the glottic opening is situated in a relatively anterior and superior position in the infant, a straight laryngoscope blade is preferred when one is intubating patients of this age group because it compresses the base of the tongue and provides a direct line of sight to the vocal cords. The curved blade is superior for older children because its greater width and its flange facilitate sweeping the proportionately larger tongue to the side to provide an unobstructed view of the hypopharynx.

Patient age likewise determines the size and type of endotracheal tube best suited for attempted intubation. Small or premature newborns usually require a 3- to 3.5-mm endotracheal tube. For older infants and children, the best means of estimating the correct endotracheal tube size is to use the following formula:

$$\text{Endotracheal tube size} = \frac{\text{Age in years} + 16}{4}$$

Alternatively, correct endotracheal tube size can be approximated by selecting a tube that is comparable in diameter to the patient's little finger. Regardless of the method used, tubes one size larger and one size smaller than the one initially chosen should be readily available before the intubation attempt. Use uncuffed tubes for patients less than 8 years of age.

If trauma has occurred and the potential for cervical spine injury exists, the patient's head and cervical spine must remain properly aligned and supported during intubation. Usually, little force is necessary when attempting to visualize the vocal cords of a pediatric patient with a laryngoscope. If no trauma is suspected, place the patient's head in the "sniffing position" by placing a small folded towel behind the occiput while keeping the face in a plane that is parallel to the underlying surface. This will assist in providing a direct line of sight from the opening of the mouth to the glottic opening.

When passing the endotracheal tube through the vocal cords, remember the short length of the trachea. A common mistake is to insert the tube too deeply, resulting in intubation of the right mainstem bronchus. The depth to which the tube should be inserted as measured from the distal tip of the endotracheal tube to the front teeth varies by age (Table 38-1). A quick means of estimating the correct distance from the teeth to the midtrachea is to use the following formula:

$$\text{Depth (in centimeters)} = 3 \times \text{Endotracheal tube size (in millimeters)}$$

Once the tube is in place, give the patient ventilation and confirm proper tube placement by the

TABLE 38-1

Estimated endotracheal tube insertion depth based on age

Patient Age	Insertion Depth (cm)
6 months to 1 year	12
2-4 years	14
4-6 years	16
6-10 years	18
10-12 years	20

TABLE 38-2

Age-appropriate nasogastric tube sizes

Patient Age	Tube Size
Newborn or infant	8F
Toddler or preschool child	10F
School-age child	12F
Adolescent or adult	14F to 16F

presence of equal and clear breath sounds bilaterally. If the tube is properly positioned but only minimal chest wall rise occurs with bagging or if an air leak is heard emanating from the oropharynx, the seal between the uncuffed tube and glottic opening is inadequate. Remove the tube and insert the next largest size. Further confirmation of correct tube placement with an $ETCO_2$ detection device is indicated.

The importance of adequately securing the endotracheal tube cannot be overemphasized. Because the endotracheal tube and the trachea in which it sits are much shorter in infants and small children, even the slightest movement can dislodge the tube, causing catastrophic loss of airway control.

Nasogastric Tube Placement

Distention of the stomach is common following assisted mask ventilation because air forced into the hypopharynx passes into the esophagus and the trachea. As the stomach enlarges, it restricts the movement of the diaphragm, making ventilation more difficult even if the patient has been intubated with an orotracheal tube. Gastric distention also increases the likelihood of vomiting. Placing a nasogastric tube after the airway has been managed appropriately and connecting the tube to a suction device decompresses the stomach, lessening the risk for these complications.

Necessary equipment includes a properly sized nasogastric tube, water-soluble lubricant, a 60-mL syringe with a tip that will insert into the proximal opening of the nasogastric tube, a compatible suction device, tape, and an emesis basin. Sizes of nasogastric tubes range from 8F to 16F, with the appropriate size varying according to patient age (Table 38-2).

Once one has assembled the proper equipment, one can estimate the length of the nasogastric tube that will need to be inserted to position the distal tip in the stomach by measuring the distance from the end of the nose, around the back of the ear, to the xiphoid process. Then lubricate the tip of the nasogastric tube and insert it into the larger of either nostril and advance it (Skill 38-2). If there is no indication for cervical spine immobilization, flexing the patient's neck slightly may help direct the tube into the esophagus. Once the premeasured length of the nasogastric tube has been inserted, confirm proper placement by a return of gastric contents through the tube or by using the syringe to inject air into the stomach while listening for the resultant gurgling over the epigastrium with a stethoscope. Once correct placement has been verified, secure the tube firmly to the nose with tape while attaching the proximal end to a suction device.

Nasogastric tube insertion can cause complications. Passing the nasogastric tube into the nasopharynx when major facial trauma and the potential for basilar skull fracture exist is contraindicated because of the danger that the tube may penetrate a fractured cribriform plate and enter the cranial vault. For that reason, when major facial trauma is present, insert the tube through the mouth as an **orogastric tube.** Other potential complications include induced epistaxis during the insertion, vomiting, and inadvertent passage of the tube into the trachea.

Laryngeal Mask Airway

The LMA is an effective alternative for airway management when endotracheal intubation is not possible and basic airway techniques are impractical or ineffective. The airway consists of a semirigid tube attached to an inflatable mask designed to fit over the

SKILL 38-2
Nasogastric Tube Placement

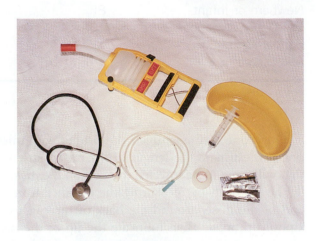

1. Assemble the equipment described in the text.

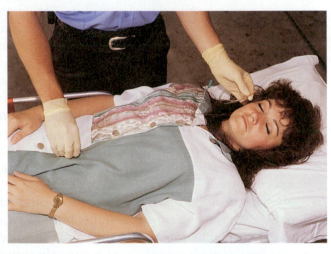

2. Check for evidence of facial trauma and potential fractures that may preclude placement of a nasogastric tube.
3. Estimate the insertion length of the chosen nasogastric tube by measuring from the nose and around the ear to below the xiphoid process.

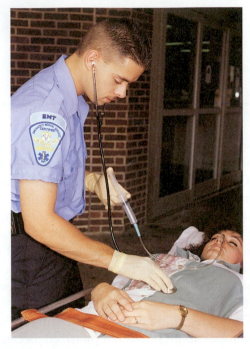

4. Apply water-soluble lubricant to the distal tip of the nasogastric tube.
5. Insert the tip of the nasogastric tube into the larger of the patient's nostrils.
6. Advance the tube to the premeasured length.
7. Confirm placement in the stomach by insufflating with approximately 10 to 20 mL of air through the proximal port of the nasogastric tube while listening for gurgling over the patient's epigastrium.

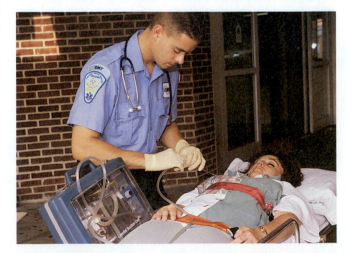

8. Once proper placement has been confirmed, securely tape the nasogastric tube to the patient's nose and face.

SKILLS

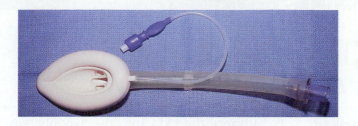

Fig. 38-12 The laryngeal mask airway.

glottic opening in the hypopharynx (Fig. 38-12). When properly placed and inflated, the mask creates a seal over the superior larynx, enabling assisted ventilation with a bag-mask attached to the proximal end of the device. Available LMA sizes range from 1 (for infants) to 5 (for large adults).

Insertion requires a properly sized LMA, water-soluble lubricant, and a 20-mL syringe (Skill 38-3). Inflate the mask to ensure that no air leak is present and then deflate it before insertion. Applying lubricant to the back of the mask greatly eases passage into the hypopharynx. Then hold the LMA in one hand like a pencil while an assistant pulls the patient's jaw and tongue forward and downward. A black line running along the posterior length of the attached tube should be aligned with the center of the patient's nose, and the opening of the mask should face the floor of the patient's mouth. Then insert the LMA blindly in this alignment until resistance is met in the hypopharynx. Do not turn or rotate the tube. Inflate the mask and confirm proper positioning by auscultating for symmetric breath sounds over the chest and absent sounds over the epigastrium with bagging. Then firmly secure the proximal end of the tube.

One important note is that placement of the LMA does not protect against the aspiration of gastric contents, because there is no partitioning between the glottic and esophageal openings beneath the mask. For that reason, it does not provide the same definitive airway control as that accomplished with endotracheal intubation. This is important to remember because insertion of the LMA may trigger vomiting. Also, misalignment of the inserted device within the hypopharynx may cause airway obstruction. Lastly, ineffective ventilation may result if the mask is not inflated properly or has not formed a complete seal over the glottic opening.

Esophageal/Tracheal Combitube

The esophageal/tracheal Combitube is a double-lumen tube that, similar to the LMA, can be inserted blindly to provide assisted ventilation when orotracheal intubation is not feasible (Fig. 38-13). A pharyngeal and a

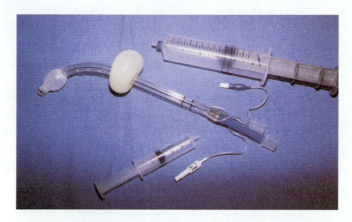

Fig. 38-13 The esophageal/tracheal Combitube.

tracheal lumen, each with its own attachment port at the proximal end, are separated by a partition along the length of the device. The tracheal lumen opens at the distal end of the device, similar to a standard endotracheal tube. Air enters and exits the distal pharyngeal lumen through multiple fenestrations along a section of the tube that separates two inflatable balloons and rests near the glottic opening. The larger, proximal balloon inflates to secure the device in the back of the oropharynx, while the smaller, distal balloon inflates to form a seal between the device and the surrounding walls of the esophagus or the trachea, depending on where the device has been placed.

The Combitube is designed for use in adult patients only. The Combitube is contraindicated for the airway management of children less than 16 years of age or less than 5 feet in height. Sizes of the Combitube range from 37F for small adults to 41F for larger patients. The Combitube should not be used in patients with an intact gag reflex, those who have known esophageal disease, or patients who have ingested corrosive substances. The Combitube also is contraindicated when the presence of a foreign body obstructing the upper airway is suspected.

To insert the Combitube, first inflate the balloons of the device to confirm that no air leaks are present, and then deflate them (Skill 38-4). Apply water-soluble lubricant to the distal end. While pulling the patient's tongue and jaw forward and downward, in-

Text continued on p. 780

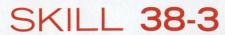

SKILL 38-3
Insertion of a Laryngeal Mask Airway

1. Select an appropriately sized laryngeal mask airway (LMA).
2. Inflate the mask to detect any air leak. If no leakage is present, deflate the mask.
3. Apply a water-soluble lubricant to the back of the mask.
4. While holding the LMA like a pencil in the dominant hand, use the other hand to grasp the patient's tongue and jaw and pull them forward and downward.
5. Insert the LMA with the black line along the posterior length of the device aligned with the middle of the patient's nose.

6. Advance the LMA into the hypopharynx until resistance is met.
7. Inflate the mask.
8. Attach the proximal end of the LMA to a bag-mask and deliver breaths.
9. Confirm adequate placement by listening for breath sounds over the lung fields and observing for symmetric chest wall rise with each delivered breath.
10. Secure the proximal end of the LMA.

SKILLS

SKILL 38-4
◉ *Insertion of the Combitube (Multi-lumen Airway Insertion)*

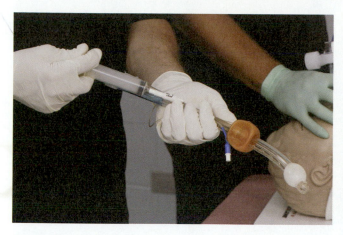

1. Inflate both balloons to detect any air leak. If no leakage is present, deflate the balloons.

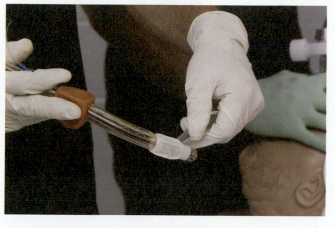

2. Apply a water-soluble lubricant to the distal end of the device.

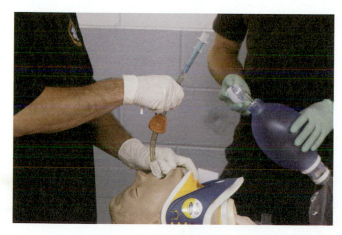

3. While holding the Combitube in the dominant hand, use the other hand to grasp the patient's tongue and jaw and pull them forward and downward.

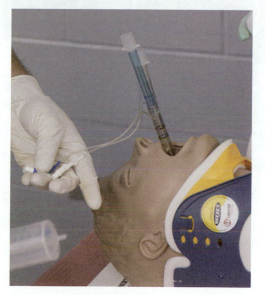

4. Insert the Combitube up to the two black ring markings on the tube. Align with the patient's front teeth.

Continued

SKILL 38-4
◎ *Insertion of the Combitube—cont'd*

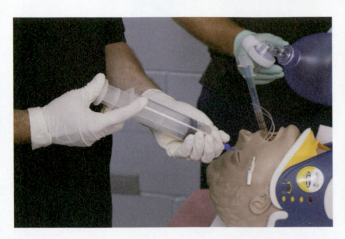

5. Inflate the oropharyngeal balloon first.

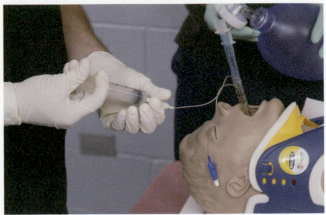

6. Inflate the distal balloon.

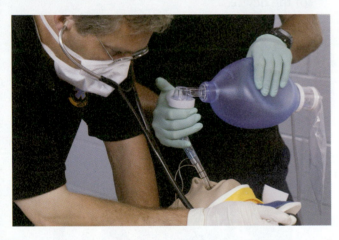

7. Attach a bag-mask to the pharyngeal lumen and deliver breaths.

SKILL 38-4
Insertion of the Combitube—cont'd

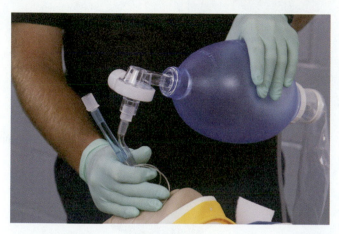

8. Listen for breath sounds and observe for symmetric chest expansion. If present, confirm proper placement further by using an end-tidal carbon dioxide detector and secure the proximal end of the tube. If no breath sounds are present, proceed to step 9.
9. Attach the bag-valve-mask to the tracheal lumen and deliver breaths.
10. Listen for breath sounds and observe for symmetric chest expansion. If present, confirm placement further with an end-tidal carbon dioxide detector or an esophageal intubation detection device.
11. Secure the proximal end of the Combitube.

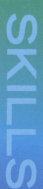

SKILLS

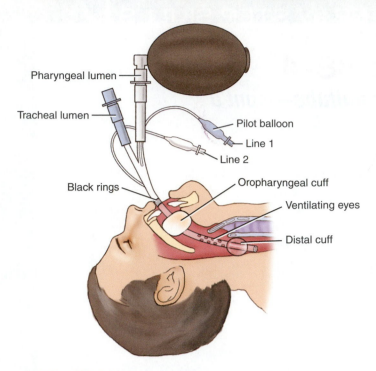

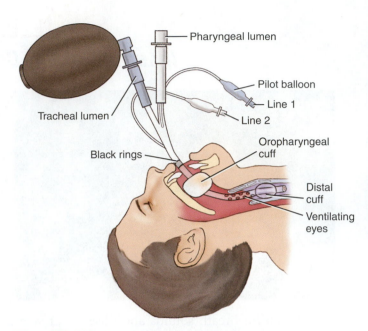

Fig. 38-14 The Combitube in the esophageal position.

Fig. 38-15 The Combitube in the tracheal position.

sert the Combitube through the mouth and into the hypopharynx until the patient's front teeth are aligned between two black rings imprinted on the proximal portion of the device. With blind insertion, it is highly likely that the distal end of the Combitube will enter the esophagus. Inflate the proximal, oropharyngeal balloon first with 100 mL of air. When the device has been secured by this means, inflate the distal, esophageal cuff with 15 mL of air.

Attach a bag-mask device first to the pharyngeal lumen. If symmetric breath sounds are heard over the chest and no sounds are present over the epigastrium, the tip of the Combitube rests in the esophagus; the patient may be given ventilation successfully through the pharyngeal lumen because air is passing into and out of the trachea through the fenestrations above the sealed-off esophagus (Fig. 38-14). If no breath sounds are heard, the chest wall does not rise with delivered ventilations, or gurgling sounds are present over the epigastrium, the tip of the Combitube has entered the trachea and air delivered via the fenestrations of the pharyngeal lumen is being forced into the esophagus. Remove the bag-mask device and attach it instead to the tracheal lumen. The patient then may be given ventilation as if a standard endotracheal tube were present (Fig. 38-15). Confirm proper placement by auscultating breath sounds, observing chest wall expansion, and using an ETCO$_2$ detection device, if available.

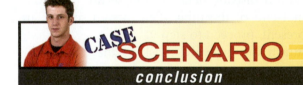

CASE SCENARIO
conclusion

Ray quickly inserted the distal end of the endotracheal tube past the vocal cords. The hours of training he had received in the operating room really helped him determine the depth of placement. When he had placed the tube to the correct depth, Ray removed the stylet, inflated the cuff with enough air to occlude the trachea around the tube, attached an end-tidal carbon dioxide detector, and slid the bag-mask back onto the tube opening. As he squeezed the bag, Ray could see the chest rise noticeably. He asked the officer to take over the bag-mask and placed the tips of the stethoscope into his ears. Listening carefully over the chest walls, Ray determined that he could hear breath sounds equally across the chest and that sounds in the epigastric area were absent, indicating successful placement. The colorimetric carbon dioxide detector provided secondary confirmation of tube placement by changing color as the expired air passed through the device. Smiling inwardly, he began to secure the tube with a commercial holder.

TEAMWORK

When the emergency medical technician is performing advanced airway management, it is usually because he or she is the first responder on the scene. Adequate accomplishment of the techniques described in this chapter demand not only skill on the part of the person performing the procedure but also the ability to communicate effectively with other emergency medical personnel and to instruct them as to how and why they may assist with managing the airway.

The emergency medical technician also must be able to explain the rationale for any advanced airway intervention during base contact and on arrival to a receiving facility. A detailed account of the procedure performed, along with any difficulties or complications encountered, is vitally important to provide the health care providers assuming care of the patient with information that is accurate and useful for continued care.

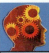

ASK YOURSELF

You are the first responder on the scene for a patient who has suffered a cardiopulmonary arrest. Your patient is a large 58-year-old man who is apneic with no pulse palpated. As your partner begins chest compressions, you attempt assisted ventilation with a bag-mask but do not observe any chest wall rise with delivered breaths despite multiple attempts to open and reposition the airway. You prepare to intubate the patient via the orotracheal route, but as you test the largest curved laryngoscope blade in your kit to its handle, the light source fails to illuminate. The largest straight blade, however, is functioning.

1. What problems might be encountered in using a straight laryngoscope blade in a large adult patient?
2. Describe in detail the alternative airway management techniques that might be used if endotracheal intubation using the straight laryngoscope blade is unsuccessful.

Resources

Butler KH, Clyne B: Management of the difficult airway: alternative airway techniques and adjuncts, *Emerg Med Clin North Am* 21(2):259-289, 2003.

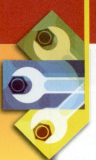

NUTS AND BOLTS

Critical Points

The emergency medical technician must be thoroughly familiar with and well practiced in the techniques of advanced airway management if these procedures are to be performed in the field. If performed decisively and correctly, these techniques can be lifesaving. If not, the patient's life may be jeopardized. Appropriate advanced airway management requires detailed knowledge of upper airway anatomy and an appreciation of how age-related variations in that anatomy determine the optimal approach to securing the airway. Likewise, familiarity with the potential complications of advanced airway management is mandatory if serious errors are to be avoided.

Learning Checklist

❏ Describe in detail the anatomy of the upper respiratory tract as it pertains to advanced airway management.

❏ Explain the anatomic and physiologic factors that differentiate advanced airway management for infants and children from advanced airway management for adults.

❏ Describe in detail endotracheal intubation in infant, child, and adult patients.

❏ Explain the method and rationale for confirming proper endotracheal tube placement.

❏ Explain the rationale for properly securing the endotracheal tube once it is in place.

❏ List the most serious complications of endotracheal intubation.

❏ Describe in detail the proper placement of a nasogastric tube.

❏ Explain the indications for placing an orogastric tube.

❏ Describe in detail the proper use of alternative advanced airway devices, such as the laryngeal mask airway and the Combitube.

Key Terms

Arytenoids Pyramid-shaped structures attaching the posterior aspect of the true vocal cords to the cricoid ring.

Bronchi Large air passages that divide off of the trachea in the lower respiratory tract.

Carina The point at which the trachea divides into the left and right mainstem bronchi.

Combitube An alternative airway device that consists of a dual-lumen tube with two inflatable balloons and is inserted blindly through the oropharynx.

Cricoid cartilage Ring-shaped cartilaginous structure at the junction of the larynx with the trachea.

Cuneiform and corniculate cartilages Cartilaginous structures that anchor the vestibular folds and the true vocal cords of the larynx.

Endotracheal tube A translucent and pliable tube passed through the glottic opening and into the trachea to provide a secure conduit for air passage through the upper respiratory tract.

Epiglottis A curved flap of tissue that covers the opening of the trachea when swallowing occurs to prevent food or liquid from entering the lower respiratory tract.

Esophageal intubation detection device A syringe attached to the proximal end of an inserted endotracheal tube. Easy aspiration of a large volume of air with the syringe confirms proper placement of the endotracheal tube in the trachea rather than in the esophagus.

Esophagus A muscular tube that is situated immediately behind the larynx and trachea and connects the hypopharynx with the stomach.

False vocal cords Cartilaginous folds surrounding the true vocal cords of the larynx when viewed from above.

Glossoepiglottic ligament The ligament by which the epiglottis is suspended from the superior aspect of the larynx. Traction on the glossoepiglottic ligament with the tip of a curved laryngoscope blade properly inserted into the vallecula lifts the epiglottis to reveal the glottic opening.

Glottic opening See *glottis*.

Glottis The opening between the true vocal cords that marks the transition from the hypopharynx to the upper trachea.

Hypopharynx The inferior portion of the larynx; it contains the superior openings of the larynx and the esophagus.

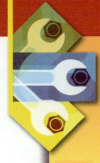

Laryngeal mask airway An alternative airway device consisting of a tube connected to an inflatable mask designed to form a seal over the larynx and the glottic opening.

Laryngoscope A lighted device designed to assist in visualizing the structures of the hypopharynx, particularly the vocal cords and the glottic opening.

Larynx Cartilaginous structure in the anterior neck connecting the posterior pharynx with the trachea in the upper airway. Also known as the *voice box.*

Nasogastric tube A long, pliable tube inserted through the nostril and the esophagus into the stomach. Applying suction to a properly placed nasogastric tube decompresses the stomach, lessening the risk for aspiration and facilitating assisted ventilation.

Nasopharynx The cavity or air passage that lies immediately posterior to the nose and forms the upper portion of the pharynx.

Orogastric tube A long, pliable tube inserted through the mouth and esophagus into the stomach for decompression of the latter. The passage of an orogastric tube is preferred when significant facial trauma precludes the safe passage of a nasogastric tube.

Oropharynx The air cavity/passageway situated at the back of the mouth.

Orotracheal intubation The passage of an endotracheal tube through the glottic opening and into the trachea under direct visualization with the aid of a laryngoscope.

Pharynx The cavity or open space above the larynx and posterior to the nose and mouth. It may be subdivided further into the nasopharynx and the oropharynx.

Sellick maneuver The application of posterior-directed pressure to the cricoid cartilage with the thumb and forefinger, thereby occluding the esophagus to prevent regurgitation of gastric contents during attempted intubation.

Stylet A thin, semirigid rod inserted into an endotracheal tube to prevent bending or kinking during insertion and to allow its user to bend the tube to a desired angle.

Trachea The air conduit that extends from the lower portion of the larynx into the chest, where it then divides into the right and left mainstem bronchi.

Tracheal muscle A long strip of muscle that forms the posterior wall of the trachea.

True vocal cords Thin strips of connective tissue attached to the muscles of phonation within the upper portion of the larynx. These important landmarks for endotracheal intubation form the border of the glottic opening.

Upper respiratory tract A system of air passages formed by the nose and mouth, the pharynx, and the larynx.

Vallecula The recessed area in the hypopharynx that separates the base of the tongue from the epiglottis. Insertion of the tip of a curved laryngoscope blade into this recess allows for retraction of the epiglottis and visualization of the glottic opening.

Vestibular folds Cartilaginous folds surrounding the true vocal cords of the larynx when viewed from above.

National Standard Curriculum Objectives

Cognitive Objectives

After completing this lesson, the EMT student will be able to do the following:

- Identify and describe the airway anatomy in the infant, child, and the adult.
- Differentiate between the airway anatomy in the infant, child, and the adult.
- Explain the pathophysiology of airway compromise.
- Describe the proper use of airway adjuncts.
- Review the use of oxygen therapy in airway management.
- Describe the indications, contraindications, and technique for insertion of nasal gastric tubes.
- Describe how to perform the Sellick maneuver (cricoid pressure).
- Describe the indications for advanced airway management.
- List the equipment required for orotracheal intubation.

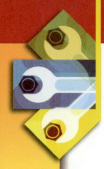

NUTS AND BOLTS

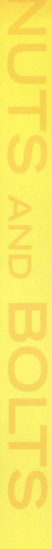

- Describe the proper use of the curved blade for orotracheal intubation.
- Describe the proper use of the straight blade for orotracheal intubation.
- State the reasons for and proper use of the stylet in orotracheal intubation.
- Describe the methods of choosing the appropriate size of endotracheal tube in an adult patient.
- State the formula for sizing a endotracheal tube for an infant or child.
- List complications associated with advanced airway management.
- Define the various alternative methods for sizing the endotracheal tube for an infant or child.

- Describe the skill of orotracheal intubation in the adult patient.
- Describe the skill of orotracheal intubation in the infant and child patient.
- Describe the skill of confirming endotracheal tube placement in the adult, infant, and child patient.
- State the consequence of and the need to recognize unintentional esophageal intubation.
- Describe the skill of securing the endotracheal tube in the adult, infant, and child patient.

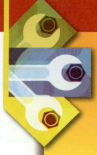

Affective Objectives

After completing this lesson, the EMT student will be able to do the following:

- Recognize and respect the feelings of the patient and family during advanced airway management.
- Explain the value of performing advanced airway procedures.
- Describe the need for the emergency medical technician to perform advanced airway procedures.
- Explain the rationale for the use of a stylet.
- Explain the rationale for having a suction unit immediately available during intubation attempts.
- Explain the rationale for confirming breath sounds.
- Explain the rationale for securing the endotracheal tube.

Psychomotor Objectives

After completing this lesson, the EMT student will be able to do the following:

- Demonstrate how to perform the Sellick maneuver (cricoid pressure).
- Demonstrate the skill of orotracheal intubation in the adult patient.
- Demonstrate the skill of orotracheal intubation in the infant and child patient.
- Demonstrate the skill of confirming endotracheal tube placement in the adult patient.
- Demonstrate the skill of confirming endotracheal tube placement in the infant and child placement.
- Demonstrate the skill of securing the endotracheal tube in the adult patient.
- Demonstrate the skill of securing the endotracheal tube in the infant and child patient.

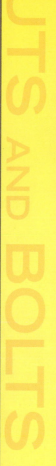

Appendix A
Assisting Advanced Life Support Providers

■ ASSEMBLING AN INTRAVENOUS SETUP

1. Determine the fluid and quantity, and needles or needleless catheters. Open the IV kit.
2. Check the name, quantity, and clarity of the IV solution, as well as the expiration date.
3. Remove the protective seal from the port, and insert the tube from the drip chamber into the IV bag.

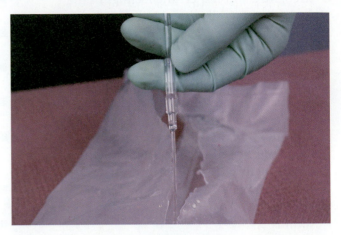

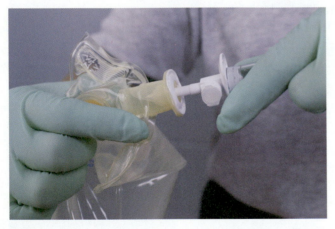

4. Prime the pump and run fluid through tubing to distal end.

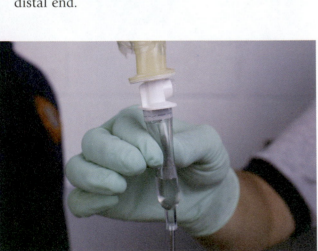

5. Continue to flush tubing until no air bubbles are present.

6. Hang the IV bag, and run the solution into the drip chamber and IV tubing. Shut off the line and protect the end of the tubing from contamination.

■ SETTING UP A CARDIAC MONITOR

1. Identify the need for cardiac monitoring, and identify electrode placement based on the monitor cable system.
2. Expose the patient's skin in the area of electrode placement to ensure it is dry and free of excess hair. Shave the patient's chest if necessary.
3. Remove the protective cover from the electrode and apply it to the patient's skin.

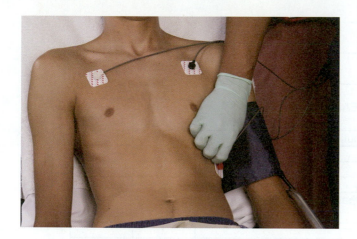

4. Connect the electric cables. Turn the monitor on and make sure the appropriate monitoring view is selected.

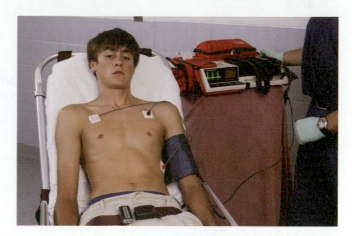

Appendix B
NREMT Skills Sheets

AIRWAY, OXYGEN AND VENTILATION SKILLS
UPPER AIRWAY ADJUNCTS AND SUCTION

Start Time: _____

Stop Time: _____ Date: _____

Candidate's Name: _____

Evaluator's Name: _____

OROPHARYNGEAL AIRWAY	Points Possible	Points Awarded
Takes, or verbalizes, body substance isolation precautions	1	
Selects appropriately sized airway	1	
Measures airway	1	
Inserts airway without pushing the tongue posteriorly	1	
Note: The examiner must advise the candidate that the patient is gagging and becoming conscious		
Removes the oropharyngeal airway	1	

SUCTION

Note: The examiner must advise the candidate to suction the patient's airway		
Turns on/prepares suction device	1	
Assures presence of mechanical suction	1	
Inserts the suction tip without suction	1	
Applies suction to the oropharynx/nasopharynx	1	

NASOPHARYNGEAL AIRWAY

Note: The examiner must advise the candidate to insert a nasopharyngeal airway		
Selects appropriately sized airway	1	
Measures airway	1	
Verbalizes lubrication of the nasal airway	1	
Fully inserts the airway with the bevel facing toward the septum	1	
Total:	13	

Critical Criteria

_____ Did not take, or verbalize, body substance isolation precautions

_____ Did not obtain a patent airway with the oropharyngeal airway

_____ Did not obtain a patent airway with the nasopharyngeal airway

_____ Did not demonstrate an acceptable suction technique

_____ Inserted any adjunct in a manner dangerous to the patient

BAG-VALVE-MASK
APNEIC PATIENT

Start Time: _____

Stop Time: _____ Date: _____

Candidate's Name: _____

Evaluator's Name: _____	Points Possible	Points Awarded
Takes, or verbalizes, body substance isolation precautions	1	
Voices opening the airway	1	
Voices inserting an airway adjunct	1	
Selects appropriately sized mask	1	
Creates a proper mask-to-face seal	1	
Ventilates patient at no less than 800 ml volume **(The examiner must witness for at least 30 seconds)**	1	
Connects reservoir and oxygen	1	
Adjusts liter flow to 15 liters/minute or greater	1	
The examiner indicates arrival of a second EMT. The second EMT is instructed to ventilate the patient while the candidate controls the mask and the airway		
Voices re-opening the airway	1	
Creates a proper mask-to-face seal	1	
Instructs assistant to resume ventilation at proper volume per breath **(The examiner must witness for at least 30 seconds)**	1	
Total:	11	

Critical Criteria

_____ Did not take, or verbalize, body substance isolation precautions

_____ Did not immediately ventilate the patient

_____ Interrupted ventilations for more than 20 seconds

_____ Did not provide high concentration of oxygen

_____ Did not provide, or direct assistant to provide proper volume/breath
(more than two (2) ventilations per minute are below 800 ml)

_____ Did not allow adequate exhalation

BLEEDING CONTROL/SHOCK MANAGEMENT

Start Time: _____

Stop Time: _____ Date: _____

Candidate's Name: _____

Evaluator's Name: _____	Points Possible	Points Awarded
Takes, or verbalizes, body substance isolation precautions	1	
Applies direct pressure to the wound	1	
Elevates the extremity	1	
Note: The examiner must now inform the candidate that the wound continues to bleed.		
Applies an additional dressing to the wound	1	
Note: The examiner must now inform the candidate that the wound still continues to bleed. The second dressing does not control the bleeding.		
Locates and applies pressure to appropriate arterial pressure point	1	
Note: The examiner must now inform the candidate that the bleeding is controlled		
Bandages the wound	1	
Note: The examiner must now inform the candidate the patient is now showing signs and symptoms indicative of hypoperfusion		
Properly position the patient	1	
Applies high concentration oxygen	1	
Initiates steps to prevent heat loss from the patient	1	
Indicates the need for immediate transportation	1	
Total:	10	

Critical Criteria

_____ Did not take, or verbalize, body substance isolation precautions

_____ Did not apply high concentration oxygen

_____ Applied a tourniquet before attempting other methods of bleeding control

_____ Did not control hemorrhage in a timely manner

_____ Did not indicate a need for immediate transportation

CARDIAC ARREST MANAGEMENT/AED

Start Time: _____

Stop Time: _____ Date: _____

Candidate's Name: _____

Evaluator's Name: _____	Points Possible	Points Awarded
ASSESSMENT		
Takes, or verbalizes, body substance isolation precautions	1	
Briefly questions the rescuer about arrest events	1	
Directs rescuer to stop CPR	1	
Verifies absence of spontaneous pulse **(skill station examiner states "no pulse")**	1	
Directs resumption of CPR	1	
Turns on defibrillator power	1	
Attaches automated defibrillator to the patient	1	
Directs rescuer to stop CPR and ensures all individuals are clear of the patient	1	
Initiates analysis of the rhythm	1	
Delivers shock (up to three successive shocks)	1	
Verifies absence of spontaneous pulse **(skill station examiner states "no pulse")**	1	
TRANSITION		
Directs resumption of CPR	1	
Gathers additional information about the arrest event	1	
Confirms effectiveness of CPR (ventilation and compressions)	1	
INTEGRATION		
Verbalizes or directs insertion of a simple airway adjunct (oral/nasal airway)	1	
Ventilates, or directs ventilation of the patient	1	
Assures high concentration of oxygen is delivered to the patient	1	
Assures CPR continues without unnecessary/prolonged interruption	1	
Re-evaluates patient/CPR in approximately one minute	1	
Repeats defibrillator sequence	1	
TRANSPORTATION		
Verbalizes transportation of the patient	1	
Total:	21	

Critical Criteria

_____ Did not take, or verbalize, body substance isolation precautions

_____ Did not evaluate the need for immediate use of the AED

_____ Did not direct initiation/resumption of ventilation/compressions at appropriate times

_____ Did not assure all individuals were clear of patient before delivering each shock

_____ Did not operate the AED properly (inability to deliver shock)

_____ Prevented the defibrillator from delivering indicated stacked shocks

IMMOBILIZATION SKILLS
JOINT INJURY

Start Time: _____

Stop Time: _____ Date: _____

Candidate's Name: _____

Evaluator's Name: _____	Points Possible	Points Awarded
Takes, or verbalizes, body substance isolation precautions	1	
Directs application of manual stabilization of the shoulder injury	1	
Assesses motor, sensory and circulatory function in the injured extremity	1	
Note: The examiner acknowledges "motor, sensory and circulatory function are present and normal."		
Selects the proper splinting material	1	
Immobilizes the site of the injury	1	
Immobilizes the bone above the injured joint	1	
Immobilizes the bone below the injured joint	1	
Reassesses motor, sensory and circulatory function in the injured extremity	1	
Note: The examiner acknowledges "motor, sensory and circulatory function are present and normal."		
Total:	8	

Critical Criteria

_____ Did not support the joint so that the joint did not bear distal weight

_____ Did not immobilize the bone above and below the injured site

_____ Did not reassess motor, sensory and circulatory function in the injured extremity before and after splinting

IMMOBILIZATION SKILLS
LONG BONE INJURY

Start Time: _____

Stop Time: _____ Date: _____

Candidate's Name: _____

Evaluator's Name: _____

	Points Possible	Points Awarded
Takes, or verbalizes, body substance isolation precautions	1	
Directs application of manual stabilization of the injury	1	
Assesses motor, sensory and circulatory function in the injured extremity	1	
Note: The examiner acknowledges "motor, sensory and circulatory function are present and normal"		
Measures the splint	1	
Applies the splint	1	
Immobilizes the joint above the injury site	1	
Immobilizes the joint below the injury site	1	
Secures the entire injured extremity	1	
Immobilizes the hand/foot in the position of function	1	
Reassesses motor, sensory and circulatory function in the injured extremity	1	
Note: The examiner acknowledges "motor, sensory and circulatory function are present and normal"		
Total	10	

Critical Criteria

_____ Grossly moves the injured extremity

_____ Did not immobilize the joint above and the joint below the injury site

_____ Did not reassess motor, sensory and circulatory function in the injured extremity before and after splinting

IMMOBILIZATION SKILLS
TRACTION SPLINTING

Start Time: _____

Stop Time: _____ Date: _____

Candidate's Name: _____

Evaluator's Name: _____	Points Possible	Points Awarded
Takes, or verbalizes, body substance isolation precautions	1	
Directs application of manual stabilization of the injured leg	1	
Directs the application of manual traction	1	
Assesses motor, sensory and circulatory function in the injured extremity	1	
Note: The examiner acknowledges "motor, sensory and circulatory function are present and normal"		
Prepares/adjusts splint to the proper length	1	
Positions the splint next to the injured leg	1	
Applies the proximal securing device (e.g..ischial strap)	1	
Applies the distal securing device (e.g..ankle hitch)	1	
Applies mechanical traction	1	
Positions/secures the support straps	1	
Re-evaluates the proximal/distal securing devices	1	
Reassesses motor, sensory and circulatory function in the injured extremity	1	
Note: The examiner acknowledges "motor, sensory and circulatory function are present and normal"		
Note: The examiner must ask the candidate how he/she would prepare the patient for transportation		
Verbalizes securing the torso to the long board to immobilize the hip	1	
Verbalizes securing the splint to the long board to prevent movement of the splint	1	
Total:	14	

Critical Criteria

_____ Loss of traction at any point after it was applied

_____ Did not reassess motor, sensory and circulatory function in the injured extremity before and after splinting

_____ The foot was excessively rotated or extended after splint was applied

_____ Did not secure the ischial strap before taking traction

_____ Final immobilization failed to support the femur or prevent rotation of the injured leg

_____ Secured the leg to the splint before applying mechanical traction

Note: If the Sagar splint or the Kendricks Traction Device is used without elevating the patient's leg, applicatic of manual traction is not necessary. The candidate should be awarded one (1) point as if manual traction were applied.

Note: If the leg is elevated at all, manual traction must be applied before elevating the leg. The ankle hitch m be applied before elevating the leg and used to provide manual traction.

MOUTH TO MASK WITH SUPPLEMENTAL OXYGEN

Start Time: _____

Stop Time: _____ Date: _____

Candidate's Name: _____

Evaluator's Name: _____	Points Possible	Points Awarded
Takes, or verbalizes, body substance isolation precautions	1	
Connects one-way valve to mask	1	
Opens patient's airway or confirms patient's airway is open (manually or with adjunct)	1	
Establishes and maintains a proper mask to face seal	1	
Ventilates the patient at the proper volume and rate (800-1200 ml per breath/10-20 breaths per minute)	1	
Connects the mask to high concentration or oxygen	1	
Adjusts flow rate to at least 15 liters per minute	1	
Continues ventilation of the patient aT the proper volume and rate (800-1200 ml per breath/10-20 breaths per minute)	1	
Note: The examiner must witness ventilations for at least 30 seconds		
Total:	8	

Critical Criteria

_____ Did not take, or verbalize, body substance isolation precautions

_____ Did not adjust liter flow to at least 15 liters per minute

_____ Did not provide proper volume per breath
(more than 2 ventiliations per minute were below 800 ml)

_____ Did not ventilate the patient at a rate of 10-20 breaths per minute

_____ Did not allow for complete exhalation

OXYGEN ADMINISTRATION

Start Time: _____

Stop Time: _____ Date: _____

Candidate's Name: _____

Evaluator's Name: _____	Points Possible	Points Awarded
Takes, or verbalizes, body substance isolation precautions	1	
Assembles the regulator to the tank	1	
Opens the tank	1	
Checks for leaks	1	
Checks tank pressure	1	
Attaches non-rebreather mask to oxygen	1	
Prefills reservoir	1	
Adjusts liter flow to 12 liters per minute or greater	1	
Applies and adjusts the mask to the patient's face	1	
Note: The examiner must advise the candidate that the patient is not tolerating the non-rebreather mask. The medical director has ordered you to apply a nasal cannula to the patient.		
Attaches nasal cannula to oxygen	1	
Adjusts liter flow to six (6) liters per minute or less	1	
Applies nasal cannula to the patient	1	
Note: The examiner must advise the candidate to discontinue oxygen therapy		
Removes the nasal cannula from the patient	1	
Shuts off the regulator	1	
Relieves the pressure within the regulator	1	
Total:	15	

Critical Criteria

_____ Did not take, or verbalize, body substance isolation precautions

_____ Did not assemble the tank and regulator without leaks

_____ Did not prefill the reservoir bag

_____ Did not adjust the device to the correct liter flow for the non-rebreather mask
(12 liters per minute or greater)

_____ Did not adjust the device to the correct liter flow for the nasal cannula
(6 liters per minute or less)

Patient Assessment/Management - Medical

Start Time: _____

Stop Time: _____ Date: _____

Candidate's Name: _____

Evaluator's Name:							Points Possible	Points Awarded
Takes, or verbalizes, body substance isolation precautions							1	
SCENE SIZE-UP								
Determines the scene is safe							1	
Determines the mechanism of injury/nature of illness							1	
Determines the number of patients							1	
Requests additional help if necessary							1	
Considers stabilization of spine							1	
INITIAL ASSESSMENT								
Verbalizes general impression of the patient							1	
Determines responsiveness/level of consciousness							1	
Determines chief complaint/apparent life threats							1	
Assesses airway and breathing	Assessment						1	
	Indicates appropriate oxygen therapy						1	
	Assures adequate ventilation						1	
Assesses circulation	Assesses/controls major bleeding						1	
	Assesses pulse						1	
	Assesses skin (color, temperature and condition)						1	
Identifies priority patients/makes transport decisions							1	
FOCUSED HISTORY AND PHYSICAL EXAMINATION/RAPID ASSESSMENT								
Signs and symptoms (Assess history of present illness)							1	

Respiratory	Cardiac	Altered Mental Status	Allergic Reaction	Poisoning/ Overdose	Environmental Emergency	Obstetrics	Behavioral
*Onset? *Provokes? *Quality? *Radiates? *Severity? *Time? *Interventions?	*Onset? *Provokes? *Quality? *Radiates? *Severity? *Time? *Interventions?	*Description of the episode. *Onset? *Duration? *Associated Symptoms? *Evidence of Trauma? *Interventions? *Seizures? *Fever?	*History of allergies? *What were you exposed to? *How were you exposed? *Effects? *Progression? *Interventions?	*Substance? When did you ingest/become exposed? *How much did you ingest? *Over what time period? *Interventions? *Estimated weight?	*Source? *Environment? *Duration? *Loss of consciousness? *Effects-general or local?	*Are you pregnant? *How long have you been pregnant? *Pain or contractions? *Bleeding or discharge? *Do you feel the need to push? *Last menstrual period?	*How do you feel? *Determine suicidal tendencies. *Is the patient a threat to self or others? Is there a medical problem? Interventions?

		Points Possible	
Allergies		1	
Medications		1	
Past pertinent history		1	
Last oral intake		1	
Event leading to present illness (rule out trauma)		1	
Performs focused physical examination (assesses affected body part/system or, if indicated, completes rapid assessment)		1	
Vitals (obtains baseline vital signs)		1	
Interventions (obtains medical direction or verbalizes standing order for medication interventions and verbalizes proper additional intervention/treatment)			
Transport (re-evaluates the transport decision)		1	
Verbalizes the consideration for completing a detailed physical examination		1	
ONGOING ASSESSMENT (verbalized)			
Repeats initial assessment		1	
Repeats vital signs		1	
Repeats focused assessment regarding patient complaint or injuries		1	
Critical Criteria Total:		30	

Critical Criteria

_____ Did not take, or verbalize, body substance isolation precautions when necessary

_____ Did not determine scene safety

_____ Did not obtain medical direction or verbalize standing orders for medical interventions

_____ Did not provide high concentration of oxygen

_____ Did not find or manage problems associated with airway, breathing, hemorrhage or shock (hypoperfusion)

_____ Did not differentiate patient's need for transportation versus continued assessment at the scene

_____ Did detailed or focused history/physical examination before assessing the airway, breathing and circulation

_____ Did not ask questions about the present illness

_____ Administered a dangerous or inappropriate intervention

Patient Assessment/Management - Trauma

Start Time: _____

Stop Time: _____ Date: _____

Candidate's Name: _____

Evaluator's Name: _____

		Points Possible	Points Awarded
Takes, or verbalizes, body substance isolation precautions		1	
SCENE SIZE-UP			
Determines the scene is safe		1	
Determines the mechanism of injury		1	
Determines the number of patients		1	
Requests additional help if necessary		1	
Considers stabilization of spine		1	
INITIAL ASSESSMENT			
Verbalizes general impression of the patient		1	
Determines responsiveness/level of consciousness		1	
Determines chief complaint/apparent life threats		1	
Assesses airway and breathing	Assessment	1	
	Initiates appropriate oxygen therapy	1	
	Assures adequate ventilation	1	
	Injury management	1	
Assesses circulation	Assesses/controls major bleeding	1	
	Assesses pulse	1	
	Assesses skin (color, temperature and conditions)	1	
Identifies priority patients/makes transport decision		1	
FOCUSED HISTORY AND PHYSICAL EXAMINATION/RAPID TRAUMA ASSESSMENT			
Selects appropriate assessment (**focused or rapid assessment**)		1	
Obtains, or directs assistance to obtain, baseline vital signs		1	
Obtains S.A.M.P.L.E. history		1	
DETAILED PHYSICAL EXAMINATION			
Assesses the head	Inspects and palpates the scalp and ears	1	
	Assesses the eyes	1	
	Assesses the facial areas including oral and nasal areas	1	
Assesses the neck	Inspects and palpates the neck	1	
	Assesses for JVD	1	
	Assesses for tracheal deviation	1	
Assesses the chest	Inspects	1	
	Palpates	1	
	Auscultates	1	
Assesses the abdomen/pelvis	Assesses the abdomen	1	
	Assesses the pelvis	1	
	Verbalizes assessment of genitalia/perineum as needed	1	
Assesses the extremities	1 point for each extremity includes inspection, palpation, and assessment of motor, sensory and circulatory function	4	
Assesses the posterior	Assesses thorax	1	
	Assesses lumbar	1	
Manages secondary injuries and wounds appropriately **1 point for appropriate management of the secondary injury/wound**		1	
Verbalizes re-assessment of the vital signs		1	
	Total:	40	

Critical Criteria

_____ Did not take, or verbalize, body substance isolation precautions
_____ Did not determine scene safety
_____ Did not assess for spinal protection
_____ Did not provide for spinal protection when indicated
_____ Did not provide high concentration of oxygen
_____ Did not find, or manage, problems associated with airway, breathing, hemorrhage or shock (hypoperfusion)
_____ Did not differentiate patient's need for transportation versus continued assessment at the scene
_____ Did other detailed physical examination before assessing the airway, breathing and circulation
_____ Did not transport patient within (10) minute time limit

SPINAL IMMOBILIZATION
SEATED PATIENT

Start Time: _____

Stop Time: _____   Date: _____

Candidate's Name: _____

Evaluator's Name: _____

	Points Possible	Points Awarded
Takes, or verbalizes, body substance isolation precautions	1	
Directs assistant to place/maintain head in the neutral in-line position	1	
Directs assistant to maintain manual immobilization of the head	1	
Reassesses motor, sensory and circulatory function in each extremity	1	
Applies appropriately sized extrication collar	1	
Positions the immobilization device behind the patient	1	
Secures the device to the patient's torso	1	
Evaluates torso fixation and adjusts as necessary	1	
Evaluates and pads behind the patient's head as necessary	1	
Secure the patient's head to the device	1	
Verbalizes moving the patient to a long board	1	
Reassesses motor, sensory and circulatory function in each extremity	1	
Total:	12	

Critical Criteria

_____ Did not immediately direct, or take, manual immobilization of the head

_____ Released, or ordered release of, manual immobilization before it was maintained mechanically

_____ Patient manipulated, or moved excessively, causing potential spinal compromise

_____ Device moved excessively up, down, left or right on the patient's torso

_____ Head immobilization allows for excessive movement

_____ Torso fixation inhibits chest rise, resulting in respiratory compromise

_____ Upon completion of immobilization, head is not in the neutral position

_____ Did not assess motor, sensory and circulatory function in each extremity after voicing immobilization to the long board

_____ Immobilized head to the board before securing the torso

SPINAL IMMOBILIZATION
SUPINE PATIENT

Start Time: _____

Stop Time: _____ Date: _____

Candidate's Name: _____

Evaluator's Name:	Points Possible	Points Awarded
Takes, or verbalizes, body substance isolation precautions	1	
Directs assistant to place/maintain head in the neutral in-line position	1	
Directs assistant to maintain manual immobilization of the head	1	
Reassesses motor, sensory and circulatory function in each extremity	1	
Applies appropriately sized extrication collar	1	
Positions the immobilization device appropriately	1	
Directs movement of the patient onto the device without compromising the integrity of the spine	1	
Applies padding to voids between the torso and the board as necessary	1	
Immobilizes the patient's torso to the device	1	
Evaluates and pads behind the patient's head as necessary	1	
Immobilizes the patient's head to the device	1	
Secures the patient's legs to the device	1	
Secures the patient's arms to the device	1	
Reassesses motor, sensory and circulatory function in each extremity	1	
Total:	14	

Critical Criteria

_____ Did not immediately direct, or take, manual immobilization of the head

_____ Released, or ordered release of, manual immobilization before it was maintained mechanically

_____ Patient manipulated, or moved excessively, causing potential spinal compromise

_____ Patient moves excessively up, down, left or right on the device

_____ Head immobilization allows for excessive movement

_____ Upon completion of immobilization, head is not in the neutral position

_____ Did not assess motor, sensory and circulatory function in each extremity after immobilization to the device

_____ Immobilized head to the board before securing the torso

VENTILATORY MANAGEMENT
DUAL LUMEN DEVICE INSERTION FOLLOWING
AN UNSUCCESSFUL ENDOTRACHEAL INTUBATION ATTEMPT

Start Time: _____

Stop Time: _____ Date: _____

Candidate's Name: _____

Evaluator's Name: _____

	Points Possible	Points Awarded
Continues body substance isolation precautions	1	
Confirms the patient is being properly ventilated with high percentage oxygen	1	
Directs the assistant to hyper-oxygenate the patient	1	
Checks/prepares the airway device	1	
Lubricates the distal tip of the device (may be verbalized)	1	
Note: the examiner should remove the OPA and move out of the way when the candidate is prepared to insert the device		
Positions the patient's head properly	1	
Performs a tongue-jaw lift	1	
USES COMBITUBE / **USES THE PTL**		
Inserts device in the mid-line and to the depth so that the printed ring is at the level of the teeth / Inserts the device in the mid-line until the bite block flange is at the level of the teeth	1	
Inflates the pharyngeal cuff with the proper volume and removes the syringe / Secures the strap	1	
Inflates the distal cuff with the proper volume and removes the syringe / Blows into tube #1 to adequately inflate both cuffs	1	
Attaches/directs attachment of BVM to the first (esophageal placement) lumen and ventilates	1	
Confirms placement and ventilation through the correct lumen by observing chest rise, auscultation over the epigastrium and bilaterally over each lung	1	
Note: The examiner states, "You do not see rise and fall of the chest and hear sounds only over epigastrium"		
Attaches/directs attachment of BVM to the second (endotracheal placement) lumen and ventilates	1	
Confirms placement and ventilation through the correct lumen by observing chest rise, auscultation over the epigastrium and bilaterally over each lung	1	
Note: The examiner states, "You see rise and fall off the chest, there are no sounds over the epigastrium and breath sounds are equal over each lung"		
Secures device or confirms that the device remains properly secured	1	
Total:	15	

Critical Criteria

_____ Did not take or verbalize body substance isolation precautions

_____ Did not initiate ventilations within 30 seconds

_____ Interrupted ventilations for more than 30 seconds at any time

_____ Did not hyper-oxygenate the patient prior to placement of the dual lumen airway device

_____ Did not provide adequate volume per breath (maximum 2 errors/minute permissable)

_____ Did not ventilate the patient at a rate of at least 10 breaths per minute

_____ Did not insert the dual lumen airway device at a proper depth or at the proper place within 3 attempts

_____ Did not inflate both cuffs properly

_____ **Combitube** - Did not remove the syringe immediately following inflation of each cuff

_____ **PTL** - Did not secure the strap prior to cuff inflation

_____ Did not confirm, by observing chest rise and auscultation over the epigastrium and bilaterally over each lung that the proper lumen of the device was being used to ventilate the patient

_____ Inserted any adjunct in a manner that was dangerous to the patient

VENTILATORY MANAGEMENT
ENDOTRACHEAL INTUBATION

Start Time: _____

Stop Time: _____ Date: _____

Candidate's Name: _____

Evaluator's Name: _____

	Points Possible	Points Awarded
Note: If a candidate elects to initially ventilate the patient with a BVM attached to a reservoir and oxygen, full credit must be awarded for steps denoted by "**" provided first ventilation is delivered within the initial 30 seconds		
Takes, or verbalizes, body substance isolation precautions	1	
Opens the airway manually	1	
Elevates the patient's tongue and inserts a simple airway adjunct (Oropharyngeal/nasopharyngeal airway)	1	
Note: **The examiner must now inform the candidate "no gag reflex is present and the patient accepts the airway adjunct"**		
**Ventilates the patient immediately using a BVM device unattached to oxygen	1	
**Hyperventilates the patient with room air	1	
Note: **The examiner must now inform the candidate that ventilation is being properly performed without difficulty**		
Attaches the oxygen reservoir to the BVM	1	
Attaches the BVM to high flow oxygen (15 liter per minute)	1	
Ventilates the patient at the proper volume and rate (800-1200 ml/breath and 10-20 breaths/minute)	1	
Note: **After 30 seconds, the examiner must auscultate the patient's chest and inform the candidate that breath sounds are present and equal bilaterally and medical direction has ordered endotracheal intubation. The examiner must now take over ventilation of the patient.**		
Directs assistant to hyper-oxygenate the patient	1	
Identifies/selects the proper equipment for endotracheal intubation	1	
Checks equipment — Checks for cuff leaks	1	
Checks laryngoscope operation and bulb tightness	1	
Note: **The examiner must remove the OPA and move out of the way when the candidate is prepared to intubate the patient.**		
Positions the patient's head properly	1	
Inserts the laryngoscope blade into the patient's mouth while displacing the patient's tongue laterally	1	
Elevates the patient's mandible with the laryngoscope	1	
Introduces the endotracheal tube and advances the tube to the proper depth	1	
Inflates the cuff to the proper pressure	1	
Disconnects the syringe from the cuff inlet port	1	
Directs assistant to ventilate the patient	1	
Confirms proper placement of the endotracheal tube by auscultation bilaterally and over the epigastrium	1	
Note: **The examiner must ask, "If you had proper placement, what would you expect to hear?"**		
Secures the endotracheal tube (may be verbalized)	1	
Total:	21	

Critical Criteria

_____ Did not take or verbalize body substance isolation precautions when necessary

_____ Did not initiate ventilation within 30 seconds after applying gloves or interrupts ventilations for greater than 30 seconds at a time

_____ Did not voice or provide high oxygen concentrations (15 liter/minute or greater)

_____ Did not ventilate the patient at a rate of at least 10 breaths per minute

_____ Did not provide adequate volume per breath (maximum of 2 errors per minute permissible)

_____ Did not hyper-oxygenate the patient prior to intubation

_____ Did not successfully intubate the patient within 3 attempts

_____ Used the patient's teeth as a fulcrum

_____ Did not assure proper tube placement by auscultation bilaterally over each lung **and** over the epigastrium

_____ The stylette (if used) extended beyond the end of the endotracheal tube

_____ Inserted any adjunct in a manner that was dangerous to the patient

_____ Did not immediately disconnect the syringe from the inlet port after inflating the cuff

VENTILATORY MANAGEMENT
ESOPHAGEAL OBTURATOR AIRWAY INSERTION FOLLOWING AN UNSUCCESSFUL ENDOTRACHEAL INTUBATION ATTEMPT

Start Time: _____

Stop Time: _____ Date: _____

Candidate's Name: _____

	Points Possible	Points Awarded
Evaluator's Name: _____		
Continues body substance isolation precautions	1	
Confirms the patient is being ventilated with high percentage oxygen	1	
Directs the assistant to hyper-oxygenate the patient	1	
Identifies/selects the proper equipment for insertion of EOA	1	
Assembles the EOA	1	
Tests the cuff for leaks	1	
Inflates the mask	1	
Lubricates the tube (may be verbalized)	1	
Note: The examiner should remove the OPA and move out of the way when the candidate is prepared to insert the device		
Positions the head properly with the neck in the neutral or slightly flexed position	1	
Grasps and elevates the patient's tongue and mandible	1	
Inserts the tube in the same direction as the curvature of the pharynx	1	
Advances the tube until the mask is sealed against the patient's face	1	
Ventilates the patient while maintaining a tight mask-to-face seal	1	
Directs confirmation of placement of EOA by observing for chest rise and auscultation over the epigastrium and bilaterally over each lung	1	
Note: The examiner must acknowledge adequate chest rise, bilateral breath sounds and absent sounds over the epigastrium		
Inflates the cuff to the proper pressure	1	
Disconnects the syringe from the inlet port	1	
Continues ventilation of the patient	1	
Total:	17	

Critical Criteria

_____ Did not take or verbalize body substance isolation precautions
_____ Did not initiate ventilations within 30 seconds
_____ Interrupted ventilations for more than 30 seconds at any time
_____ Did not direct hper-oxygenation of the patient prior to placement of the EOA
_____ Did not successfully place the EOA within 3 attempts
_____ Did not ventilate at a rate of at least 10 breaths per minute
_____ Did not provide adequate volume per breath (maximum 2 errors/minute permissible)
_____ Did not assure proper tube placement by auscultation bilaterally and over the epigastrium
_____ Did not remove the syringe after inflating the cuff
_____ Did not successfully ventilate the patient
_____ Did not provide high flow oxygen (15 liters per minute or greater)
_____ Inserted any adjunct in a manner that was dangerous to the patient

Glossary

A (inverted vee) collapse A type of structural collapse in which a horizontal component detaches at one or both ends of its span, creating one triangular void supported close to the center by a vertical component.

Abandonment Loosely defined as a total lack of supervision leading to a safety hazard for the child or infant.

Abdomen The part of the body between the hips and chest.

Abdominal aortic aneurysm Dilation of the wall of the abdominal aorta producing a pulsating sac on the artery that may be full of fluid or clotted blood.

Abdominal quadrants The four sections into which the abdomen is divided to aid in assessment.

Abnormal behavior Behavior exhibited by a person that is outside of the norm for the situation and is socially unacceptable; this behavior may result in harm to the person or to others.

Abortion Loss of a pregnancy before 20 weeks of gestation.

Abrasion Open soft tissue injury characterized by scraping.

Absorbed toxin A toxin that enters the body through the skin.

Accessory muscles Muscles of the anterior neck and intercostal spaces that pull the anterior portion of the rib cage upward and outward, expanding intrathoracic volume. Use of these muscles often signifies respiratory distress.

Accessory organs An organ or other distinct collection of tissues that contributes to the function of another similar organ.

Acetabulum Large, cup-shaped articular cavity that contains the head of the femur.

Acetaminophen A nonprescription drug with analgesic and antipyretic effects similar to aspirin. The trade name for acetaminophen is Tylenol.

Acetylsalicylic acid Chemical name for aspirin.

Activated charcoal Substance used to adsorb toxins from the gastrointestinal tract.

Acute mountain sickness The mildest form of altitude illness.

Acute radiation syndrome A group of symptoms that develop after a significant amount of whole body radiation, on the order of 100 rad or more. Also called *radiation sickness*.

Administration The route or how a drug is delivered.

Administrative information Information that relates to the call but not specifically to the patient, such as date and time of dispatch.

Adolescent A child 12 to 18 years of age.

Adrenaline See *epinephrine*.

Advance directive A legal document that allows individuals to provide directions regarding their health care in the event they cannot communicate. The usual examples are a living will or a durable power of attorney for health care.

Aerobic metabolism Metabolism that occurs in the presence of oxygen.

Aerosol Medicinal particles suspended in a gas or in air.

Agonal respirations Short, irregular, and gasping breaths interspersed with long periods of apnea, usually signifying imminent death.

Air bag A woven bladder that fills with an inert gas to cushion the occupant from hitting hard objects.

Air bill A document used to identify hazardous substances transported by air. It can be obtained from the pilot or may be found at the scene of aircraft accidents.

Air embolism An air bubble introduced into the circulatory system through, for example, an open wound that can result in an obstruction of blood flow.

Air splint A splint that has a cavity that is filled with air, thus providing support for an injured extremity.

Airway The respiratory system structures through which air passes.

Alkali A chemical that has a high pH; the opposite of an acid.

Allergen An antigenic substance.

Allergic reaction An exaggerated immune response in an individual to any substance.

Alpha particle A positively charged particle consisting of two protons and two neutrons.

Altered mental status Any mental state that differs from a conscious person's normal state of awareness or competence.

Alveolar air spaces The gas-filled spaces of the alveoli.

Alveoli Small air sacs within the lungs formed by elastic, highly vascularized membrane. Oxygen delivered to the alveoli during inspiration diffuses across the membrane and into the bloodstream. In the bloodstream, oxygen is taken up by red blood cells, bound to hemoglobin, and transported to tissues throughout the body. At the same time, carbon dioxide dissolved in the blood diffuses in the opposite direction, crossing the membrane and accumulating within the alveoli to be exhaled.

Amniotic sac (bag of waters) The fluid-filled protective sac that surrounds the fetus inside the uterus.

Amputation Complete avulsion where a body part has been removed from the body.

Anaerobic metabolism Metabolism that occurs in the absence of oxygen.

Analgesic A medication given to relieve pain.

Anaphylaxis A severe, life-threatening hypersensitivity reaction to a previously encountered antigen that results in vasodilation and subsequent hypotension.

Anatomic dead space The amount of inhaled air in the trachea and mainstem bronchi, which therefore is not available for exchange (approximately 150 mL in adults).

Anatomic splint A splint in which the body is used as a self-splint.

Anatomy The structure of the body.

Anemic A decrease in hemoglobin in the blood to levels below the normal range of 12 to 16 g/dL for women and 13.5 to 18 g/dL for men.

Angina Chest discomfort felt upon exertion and usually relieved when resting.

Angioedema Localized edematous reaction of the deep dermis or submucosal tissues.

Angulation An injury that is deformed (bent) at the wound.

Antegrade amnesia The loss of memory for events that occurred immediately after the event that precipitated the amnesia.

Anterior Toward the front of the body.

Antibodies Proteins that react with antigens.

Anticholinergic medications Drugs that block the action of acetylcholine (neurotransmitter) at receptor sites. Symptoms produced by these drugs can include dry mouth, hot skin, delirium, flushed skin, and big pupils.

Antidote A remedy that counteracts a poison.

Antigen Any substance that induces a state of hypersensitivity when it comes into contact with appropriate cells.

Antihistamine A drug that blocks the action of histamine, thus preventing or alleviating the major symptoms of an allergic response.

Antipyretic A medication given to treat a fever.

Antivenin A product that neutralizes or lessens the effect of the injected toxic venom.

Anxiety A fearful emotional state characterized by increased nervousness, tension, pacing, hand wringing, and trembling.

Aorta The largest artery in the body. It originates from the heart and lies in front of the spine in the thoracic and abdominal cavity.

Apgar score A system of quickly evaluating an infant's heart rate, respiratory effort, muscle tone, reflex irritability, and color at birth. The score is determined at 1 minute after birth, and the evaluation is repeated 5 minutes after the birth.

Apices of the lungs The tops of the lungs, lying just under the clavicles bilaterally.

Apnea The absence of spontaneous respiration.

Apneic A term referring to patients who are not breathing.

Apneustic respirations Respiratory pattern represented by long, deep breaths with periods of apnea between each breath.

Arc injuries Burns caused by exposed skin being too close to two contact points of electricity.

Arch of driver safety The components that ensure safe operation of an emergency vehicle, including the physical and mental abilities of the driver, knowledge of traffic laws, and driver attitude.

Arrhythmia Any cardiac rhythm other than normal sinus, including bradycardias and tachycardias, of either atrial or ventricular origin.

Arterial bleeding Bleeding characterized by pumping or spurting of bright red blood.

Arteries Blood vessels that carry oxygenated blood out to the body.

Arterioles Smallest arteries of the body.

Arteriosclerosis Progressive disease of the arteries that results in narrowing of the lumen caused by deposits of fat and hardening of the arterial wall.

Artery A muscular blood vessel that carries blood away from the heart.

Arytenoids Pyramid-shaped structures attaching the posterior aspect of the true vocal cords to the cricoid ring.

Assault To create the fear of injury.

Assisted ventilation Provision of breaths to a patient with inadequate or absent ventilatory effort.

Asthma A respiratory disorder characterized by recurring episodes of dyspnea and wheezing caused by constriction of the bronchi, coughing, and viscous mucous secretions.

Asystole Event in which the heart has no rhythm and has ceased all activity.

Ataxic respirations Respiratory pattern represented by irregularly shallow and deep a respirations with no pattern. Also known as *Biot's respirations.*

Atelectasis Collapse of underventilated areas of lung because of inadequate chest motion and lung expansion.

Atherosclerosis The narrowing of the blood vessels that occurs secondary to the buildup of fatty deposits.

Atrial fibrillation A chaotic heart rhythm that results in an unusually irregular pulse; the condition is seen in many elderly patients.

Atrium Upper chamber of the heart. The heart has a right atrium that receives oxygen-depleted blood from the body and a left atrium that receives oxygen-enriched blood from the lungs.

Atrophy The wasting away, deterioration, or shrinking of a body organ, tissue, or part.

Auscultate To examine by listening to the body with a stethoscope.

Auscultation An assessment technique that involves listening to sounds inside the body with a stethoscope.

Automated implanted cardioverter-defibrillator An automated device implanted in a person's chest that delivers a number of low-energy shocks directly to the myocardium.

Automatic external defibrillator Machine that is designed to deliver a shock for defibrillation of a cardiac rhythm known as ventricular fibrillation.

Autonomy Self-rule; patients have the right to determine for themselves what medical treatment they do or do not want.

AVPU A mnemonic assessment tool used to determine a person's mental status. The acronym stands for *a*lert (the person is alert, awake, and oriented); *v*erbal (the person responds to voice); *p*ainful stimuli (the person responds only to a painful stimulus); *u*nresponsive (the person is not awake and is completely unresponsive to any type of stimulation).

Avulsion Open soft tissue injury characterized by skin being torn and leaving a flap or being removed completely.

Axial loading Vertical compression of the spine.

Bacterium A single-cell organism that is capable of living and dividing outside of other living cells.

Bag-valve-mask Device used to provide assisted ventilation, consisting of a face mask connected by a one-way valve to a self-inflating bag and an oxygen reservoir.

Ball-and-socket joints Joints in which the head of one bone (the ball) fits into a socket in the articulating bone (the socket), allowing a wide range of motion in almost any direction. The hip and shoulder joints are examples of this type of joint.

Bandages Devices used to hold a dressing in place or provide pressure to an injury.

Barotrauma Illness or injury caused by a sudden change in pressure.

Base station Radio at a fixed location, such as a dispatch center, hospital, or emergency medical services station, that cannot be moved from place to place. This type of radio is the most powerful radio in the emergency medical services communication system.

Baseline mental status The mental status that is normal for the particular patient.

Bases of the lungs The bottoms of the lungs, lying approximately at the level of the sixth rib.

Basilar skull fracture A fracture of the base of the skull.

Basket stretcher A type of stretcher that is useful for removing patients on rough terrain or during high-angle rescues where a patient must be lowered from a height or lifted, as from a ditch or well.

Battery Touching a person without permission.

Battle's sign Bruising or bluish discoloration to the bone behind the ear, indicating a basilar skull fracture.

Behavior The manner in which a person acts or performs including any or all of one's physical and mental activities.

Behavioral emergency Any situation in which the patient exhibits abnormal behavior that is unacceptable or intolerable to oneself, one's family, or one's community.

Benzodiazepines A group of medications used to treat seizures and calm patients. Examples include diazepam, midazolam, and lorazepam.

Beta particles Negatively or positively charged particles that have the mass of an electron.

Beta-blockers Drugs that cause blood flow to increase and blood pressure to decrease. Beta-blockers also can slow heart rate.

Bilateral Occurring or appearing on two sides.

Bilaterally Pertaining to both sides of the body.

Bill of lading A document used to identify hazardous substances transported by truck. It usually can be obtained from the driver or is kept in the truck cab, or it may be found at the scene of a trucking accident. Bills of lading may not be available for trailers being sorted, loaded, or unloaded at trucking terminals.

Biologic agent A general term referring to any biologic material (bacteria, virus, or toxin) that is used as a weapon, usually against a large number of persons.

Biotelemetry Transmission of biologic data via a radio or other form of communication to a distant location such as a hospital.

Birth canal That part of the female reproductive tract through which the fetus is delivered; it includes the lower part of the uterus, the cervix, and the vagina.

Bladder The membranous sac that serves as a receptacle for secretions; the urinary bladder collects urine.

Blanket drag A rescue evacuation technique in which a blanket is used to drag the patient from the hazardous situation.

Blast injuries Created by explosions of all types, these injuries can create penetration by any involved materials. The patient even may become a projectile and be injured by impact with fixed objects. Additionally, any nearby materials may be accelerated by the blast and strike nearby victims.

Blood The fluid in the body that is made up of red blood cells, white blood cells, platelets, and plasma.

Blood pressure The pressure the blood exerts against the walls of the blood vessels.

Bloody show Blood and mucus discharged from the vagina, often an early sign of labor.

Blow-by oxygen Method of oxygen delivery for infants and children without placing the mask on the face.

Body mechanics The most effective way to use your body to lift or move a patient.

Body of the sternum The central part of the sternum between the manubrium and xiphoid process.

Body substance isolation Protective equipment worn to prevent exposure to blood-borne pathogens or body fluids.

Body surface area Amount of body skin damaged by burns, abrasions, or other injury. Body surface area is expressed in terms of percentage.

Botulinum toxin A compound made by the bacterium *Clostridium botulinum* that causes neurologic dysfunction and culminates in total body paralysis.

Brachial artery The major artery of the upper arm.

Brachial pulse The pulse felt over the brachial artery in the upper arm.

Bradyasystole A rhythm that is either slowed (brady) or completely absent (asystole).

Bradycardia A slow heart rate.

Brainstem The lower part of the brain responsible for a variety of vital functions and regulatory activities, including respiration and circulation.

Breach of duty A negligent act or omission that violates the standards of care expected from an emergency medical technician under the circumstances.

Breath sounds The sounds of air moving in and out of the lungs.

Breath-holding spells Episodes in which children hold their breath for approximately 30 to 60 seconds, resulting in cyanosis and sometimes syncope. This is rare before 6 months of age.

Breech presentation Presentation of the buttocks or feet of the fetus as the first part of the infant's body to enter the birth canal.

Bronchi Large air passages that divide off of the trachea in the lower respiratory tract.

Bronchioles Smaller air passages within the lungs that divide off of the main bronchi and ultimately terminate in clusters of alveoli.

Bronchitis Acute or chronic inflammation of the mucous membranes of the tracheobronchial tree.

Bronchoconstriction Constriction of the bronchi and bronchioles in the lung causing difficulty breathing.

Cesarean section A surgical delivery in which the muscles of the abdomen are cut and the baby is delivered through the abdomen.

Calcaneus One of seven tarsals in the foot; the heel bone.

Calcium-channel blockers Drugs that cause blood flow to increase through vasodilation and decrease the myocardial ability of the cell to respond to electric stimulation. Patients with angina at rest and/or occasional rapid heart rates may be prescribed this medication.

Cantilever collapse A type of structural collapse characterized by limited detachment of a horizontal structure from the vertical support system, resulting in collapse usually to one side of the structure; this forms a triangular void toward the standing vertical component.

Capillaries Tiny vessels that allow the exchange of oxygen and carbon dioxide and nutrients and waste to occur.

Capillary bleeding Bleeding characterized by the oozing of blood.

Capillary refill The time it takes for the capillary bed to refill after it is compressed and the pressure is released.

Carbon monoxide poisoning Poisoning caused by the inhalation of carbon monoxide.

Cardiac arrest The halting of all functioning heart activity.

Cardiac compromise A term used for harmful cardiac conditions.

Cardiac contusion Injury to the heart muscle from a direct blow; bruising.

Cardiac ischemia A condition of inadequate oxygenation of the heart muscle, which results in heart dysfunction. It may be caused by decreased oxygen delivery or excessive cardiac demands.

Cardiac monitor A machine that reads the electrical activity of the heart.

Cardiac muscle One of three muscle types; the specialized striated muscle of which the heart is composed.

Cardiac output The amount of blood expelled by the ventricles of the heart with each beat (the stroke volume) multiplied by the heart rate.

Cardiac syncope A syncopal episode caused by reduced cardiac output and resulting hypotension, which occur secondary to tachycardia or bradycardia; the most dangerous cause of syncope in the elderly patient.

Cardiac tamponade Mechanical compression of the heart by large amounts of fluid or blood within the pericardial space.

Cardiogenic shock Shock caused by dysfunction of the heart.

Cardiopulmonary arrest Cessation of blood flow and respiratory function, either from a primary heart or lung event.

Carina The point at which the trachea divides into the left and right mainstem bronchi.

Carotid arteries Arteries that supply the head and neck with blood.

Carotid pulse The pulse felt on either side of the neck.

Carpals Eight bones that make up the structure of the wrist.

Carry Supporting all or part of the patient's weight while moving him or her.

Cartilage A spongy material on the ends of bones that provides cushioning and prevents bone ends from rubbing together.

Cartilaginous joints One of three major classes of joints; cartilaginous joints have limited motion.

Cataract Common eye condition caused by clouding of the lens, which decreases vision.

Catatonia A disturbance characterized by physical and emotional symptoms. These symptoms may include rigidity, negativity, stupor, and noncommunicative states.

Causal connection A clear connection between the patient's injuries and actions taken or omitted by a health care provider.

Cavitation The shock wave–created space in tissues struck by a bullet. This space can be many times the diameter of the bullet that causes it.

Cellular metabolism The process by which cells use the nutrients and oxygen to produce energy. Also called *cellular respiration.*

Centers for Disease Control and Prevention An agency of the U.S. government that provides resources and equipment for the investigation, identification, prevention, and control of infectious disease.

Central access dispatch A form of dispatch that coordinates numerous emergency medical services units in a given region.

Central cyanosis Cyanosis that manifests as a bluish discoloration of the central areas of the body, indicating a more profound degree of hypoxia, or low-oxygen state.

Central lines Intravascular lines surgically placed near the heart for long-term use.

Central neurogenic hyperventilation Respiratory pattern represented by continuous deep breaths; the rate may be slow or fast.

Central pulse A pulse point in or near the trunk.

Cephalic The presentation of the baby's head first in delivery.

Cerebellum An outpocketing of the brain located behind or posterior to the brainstem. It is concerned primarily with coordination of movement and balance.

Cerebrovascular accident An abnormal condition of the brain caused by occlusion of a blood vessel by an embolus, thrombus, or hemorrhage or vasospasm; also known as a *stroke.*

Cerebrum The largest and most superior portion of the brain responsible for intellectual activity, motor control, sensory perception, visual stimuli, smell, hearing, and other body functions.

Cervical collar Rigid collar that provides partial immobilization and prevents some movement of the cervical spine.

Cervical spinal immobilization device A device used to maintain immobilization of the head and neck; commonly called a *cervical collar*.

Cervical vertebrae The first seven vertebrae of the spinal column.

Cervix The lowest part of the uterus; it connects to the vagina as part of the birth canal. The cervix must shorten and dilate during labor for the fetus to pass into the vagina.

Chain of evidence An accountability of evidence at a crime scene. Any evidence should be accounted for from the time it came into your possession until it is turned over to the authorities.

Chain of survival A term used by the American Heart Association to define a series of actions that include early access to emergency medical services, early cardiopulmonary resuscitation, early defibrillation, and early advanced cardiac life support.

Chemical weapon A general term for any common chemical compound (such as chlorine gas) or any specially manufactured compound (such as sarin) that is used as a weapon, usually against a large number of persons.

CHEMTREC The Chemical Transportation Emergency Center, continuously accessible via phone (1-800-424-9300). CHEMTREC provides immediate online advice to emergency and rescue personnel on site at hazardous materials incidents.

Cheyne-Stokes respirations Respiratory pattern represented by respirations that start slow and shallow and increase in rate and depth and then decrease in rate and depth with periods of apnea between.

Chief complaint The patient's initial or primary statement of what the problem is.

Chilblain Redness or swelling of the skin caused by excessive exposure to cold.

Child abuse An improper or excessive action by parents, guardians, or caretakers that injures or causes harm to children.

Cholinergic substances Substances that have physiologic effects similar to those of acetylcholine. These substances cause symptoms such as diarrhea, lacrimation, bronchorrhea, drooling, vomiting, seizures, weakness, and a slow heart rate.

Chronic bronchitis A disease characterized by a productive cough for at least 3 months out of the year for at least 2 consecutive years. The condition is caused by inflammation of the bronchi with repeated attacks of coughing and sputum production.

Chronic obstructive pulmonary disease A progressive and irreversible condition characterized by diminished capacity of the lungs caused by dilation and mucous obstruction. Chronic bronchitis, emphysema, and asthma are forms of the disease.

Cincinnati Stroke Scale A type of screening device used to identify stroke patients rapidly.

Circulatory system The network of channels through which blood circulates.

Circumferential pressure Application of pressure completely around an extremity to control bleeding.

Classic heatstroke A form of heatstroke that has a slower onset, possible occurring over several days during a heat wave

Clavicles The bones that extend from the sternum and join with scapulae to form the pectoral girdle; the collar bones.

Cleaning Washing something thoroughly with soap and water.

Clear the patient A phrase used to describe the action an emergency medical technician must take to ensure that no bystander is touching the patient while the emergency medical technician is analyzing or shocking with an automatic external defibrillator.

Closed or direct questions Closed questions are those that can be answered with a "yes" or "no" response. If used, options should be provided for the patient, and the question should not be phrased in a manner that leads him or her to a specific answer.

Closed skeletal injury Type of injury that does not breach the outer surface of the skin.

Clothes drag A rescue evacuation technique that uses the patient's clothing to drag the patient along the long axis of the body from a hazardous situation.

Cocaine A crystalline alkaloid used medically as a local anesthetic and illegally for its euphoric effects.

Coccygeal One of four bones that fuse together to form the single bone, the coccyx; the most distal part of the spinal column.

Coccyx The most distal part of the spinal column; it is composed of four or five coccygeal vertebrae that fuse.

Coercion Forcing or pressuring a person to make a decision that may not be of the individual's own choice.

Cold urticaria Wheals caused by exposure to cold.

Cold zone The clean zone where emergency medical services personnel can assess the patient further, ensure that adequate decontamination is performed before transport, and perform patient care functions as required.

Collapse mechanism (au: please provide definition)

Colostomy bag A bag placed over the opening of a colostomy (an opening made into the abdomen where the bowel is brought to the surface, allowing bowel contents to empty into the bag).

Combitube An alternative airway device that consists of a dual-lumen tube with two inflatable balloons and is inserted blindly through the oropharynx.

Communicable A classification of disease in which the causative agent may pass or be carried from one person to another directly or indirectly.

Communicable period The time period during which a person can transmit an infectious disease to others.

Communication The transmission of information, ideas, and skills through language, body movements, gestures, and expressions.

Communication barrier A condition that interferes with standard communication, such as a language barrier or a patient who cannot hear you. When faced with these situations, the emergency medical technician must do whatever is necessary to overcome the barrier.

Communication system A system composed of radios, computers, and other equipment that allows the emergency medical technician to communicate with others from remote sites.

Communications center The part of the communication system that coordinates receiving calls, triage, dispatch, and other activities of an emergency medical services system.

Compensated shock Shock characterized by a normal systolic blood pressure with signs and symptoms of inadequate tissue perfusion.

Compensation The body's ability to use negative feedback mechanisms to try to correct an underlying disorder (e.g., compensated shock).

Competency A judicial determination as to an individual's ability to care and make decisions for himself or herself. A guardian is appointed if the person is ruled incompetent.

Complex access Gaining access to the patient with the use of tools or specialized equipment.

Complex febrile seizure A febrile seizure that is focal and/or lasts longer than 15 minutes.

Compliance A measure of the elasticity of the lungs.

Compression forces The driving of one spinal vertebra into another by a force transmitted from above (the head) or from below the spinal column.

Computerized mobile data terminals Terminals located in the ambulance that allow the emergency medical technicians to communicate with the dispatcher via computer screen. Tracking of units also can be done.

Concussion Damage to the brain caused by a violent jarring or shaking, such as a blow or an explosion.

Conduction The transfer of heat energy from a warmer object to a cooler one as a result of direct contact.

Cone of damage Amount of internal damage caused by the movement of an impaled object, such as a knife.

Cone of injury Any internal tissues within reach of a knife inserted at the point of entry. This can be far more distant and extensive than evident at first.

Confined space entry (au: please provide definition)

Confrontation A communication technique used to point out something about the patient's actions or behavior that is not consistent with what he or she is telling you.

Conjunctiva Membrane that lines the interior surface of the eyelids and covers the anterior surface of the sclera of the eye.

Constrict To decrease in size or get smaller.

Contamination Radiation injury caused by radioactive particles that are physically present. The contaminated patient can pass radioactive materials to others.

Continuity of care Care that is continued by other health care providers after the patient has been released from your care.

Continuous quality improvement Continual evaluation of system response and patient care with the purpose of maintaining or obtaining the highest standard of care possible.

Contraction interval The time from the beginning of one contraction to the beginning of the next contraction.

Contraction time The time from the beginning to the end of a single uterine contraction.

Contractions Episodes of tightening of the muscular uterine wall that occur rhythmically during normal labor. This leads to expulsion of the fetus and placenta from the uterus.

Contraindications Reasons or factors that prohibit administration of a drug.

Control zones Geographic areas at a hazardous materials incident that are designated based on safety and the degree of hazard.

Contusion A closed soft tissue injury characterized by discoloration beneath the surface of the skin; a bruise.

Convection The transfer of heat through a gas or liquid by the circulation of heated particles.

Convergence The rapid gathering of onlookers, rescuers, and members of the press at a scene of a disaster.

Convulsion Hyperexcitation of neurons in the brain, leading to sudden, violent, involuntary contractions of muscles; also known as a *seizure*.

Costal cartilage Cartilaginous tissue that connects the eighth, ninth, and tenth ribs to the sternum.

Coumadin The trade name for the most often prescribed blood thinner medication (warfarin). The drug is a common cause of bleeding problems.

Coxae The hip bones; the hip bone is composed of the ilium, ischium, and pubis.

Crackles Crackling sounds heard in the lungs that are caused by the alveoli popping open, usually the result of fluid accumulating in the lungs.

Crepitation The sound made when bone ends rub together or there is air inside the tissue.

Crepitus A crunching or grating sound heard when broken bone ends rub together.

Cribbing Materials or devices, including wood or airbags, used to support a large amount of weight during rescue operations.

Cricoid cartilage Ring-shaped cartilaginous structure at the junction of the larynx with the trachea.

Cricoid pressure (Sellick maneuver) Pressure around the cricoid cartilage that presses the esophagus against the spine, preventing regurgitation and aspiration.

Cricoid ring A cartilaginous ring at the junction of the larynx and the trachea.

Cricothyroid membrane Thin sheet of connective tissue spanning the space between the anterior portions of the thyroid cartilage and the cricoid cartilage.

Crisis An overwhelming event.

Critical incident A particularly overwhelming incident that results in emotional stress.

Critical incident stress A stress reaction that normally occurs after a person has experienced a particularly difficult situation.

Critical incident stress debriefing A function of the critical incident stress management system. The debriefing uses specific techniques to help individuals express their feelings and recover more quickly from a stressful incident.

Critical incident stress management A comprehensive system devised to help professionals recover from critical incidents.

Critique Evaluation of an emergency medical services call through documentation.

Croup An acute viral infection of the upper and lower airway that may cause partial obstruction and a barking cough. Croup usually is seen in children 3 months to 3 years old.

Crowing High, shrill sound heard during breathing.

Crowning The appearance of the head of the infant at the vaginal opening during delivery.

Crush injury Closed soft tissue injury where a body part is compressed between two sources with densities that are greater than that of the skin.

Cuboid bone The most lateral of the seven tarsals of the foot.

Cuneiform and corniculate cartilages Cartilaginous structures that anchor the vestibular folds and the true vocal cords of the larynx.

Cuneiform bones Three tarsals (medial, lateral, and intermediate) that make up part of the foot.

Cyanosis Blue discoloration of the skin signifying poor oxygen delivery to the tissues. The oxygen-carrying molecule in red blood cells, hemoglobin, takes on a bluish color when not bound to oxygen. Thus when a high proportion of hemoglobin in the blood delivered to the tissues is not bound to oxygen, the tissues appear blue.

Cyanotic Characterized by bluish skin discoloration caused by low oxygen saturation of the blood.

Dangerous cargo manifest A document used to identify hazardous substances shipped by water. It most likely can be obtained from the captain of the vessel. Inland barges may be equipped with a box where such documents are stored while the barge is moored.

DCAPBTLS A mnemonic used to identify injury to the body. The acronym stands for *d*eformity, *c*ontusions, *a*brasions, *p*uncture, *b*urns, *t*enderness, *l*aceration, and *s*welling.

Dead space Volume of gas that remains stagnant in the respiratory tract with each ventilation, usually about 150 mL in a normal-sized adult.

Debriefing A review of a stressful event that allows discussion between the people involved. It usually is held 24 to 72 hours after the event.

Decision-making capacity A medical determination as to a patient's ability to understand and to accept or refuse treatment.

Decoding The process by which the intended receiver interprets the meaning of the message sent by another individual.

Decompensated shock The end stage of shock when hypotension is present.

Decompensation A state in which the body is no longer able to use feedback mechanisms to correct an underlying disorder (e.g., decompensated shock).

Decompression sickness A painful, sometimes fatal condition caused by the formation of nitrogen bubbles in the tissue of divers, caisson workers, and aviators who move too rapidly from environments of higher to those of lower atmospheric pressure.

Decontaminate The physical or chemical process of reducing, removing, and preventing the spread of contaminants from persons at a hazardous material incident.

Defibrillation Administering a shock to a patient in ventricular defibrillation in order to cause the heart to regain function.

Defibrillator Name for a machine that defibrillates specific cardiac arrhythmias.

Deformity A structural distortion or bend that alters the normal appearance of the body or a body part.

Defusing Another form of review of stressful events that allows discussion between the people involved, but shorter and less formal than a debriefing. It usually is held within a few hours of the event.

Dehydration The decrease of fluid in the body caused by problems such as vomiting, diarrhea, or excessive sweating.

Delirium An acute, temporary state of confusion that may result in illusions, hallucinations, and misinterpretations. Delirium has many causes and is often reversible.

Delusions False beliefs.

Dementia A progressive alteration of mental status associated with deterioration of at least one other cognitive function. It may be associated with emotional disturbances and emotional changes. Dementia has many causes and is often not reversible.

Dependent lividity The discoloration of body tissues in the lower or dependent areas of the body, caused by the collection of coagulated blood.

Depression A mental state characterized by feelings of loneliness, sadness, low self-esteem, and self-reproach.

Dermal (skin) absorption Uptake of a substance into or across the skin.

Dermis Middle layer of the skin serving as the "control center" of the skin.

Detailed physical exam The process of systematically evaluating the body, starting at the head and progressing to the toes.

Detergent A chemical that binds a molecule and allows it to be dissolved in water. Detergents are categorized as cationic or anionic depending on the type of molecules they bind.

Deviate To move to one side.

Diabetes A disease that results from failure of the pancreas to produce sufficient amounts of insulin.

Diabetes mellitus A disease that prevents insulin from being produced. Without insulin, the body cannot breakdown sugar into usable forms of energy.

Diabetic ketoacidosis Diabetic coma; an acute, life-threatening complication of uncontrolled diabetes.

Diaphragm Thin, dome-shaped muscle that forms the inferior border of the thoracic cavity and separates the contents of the chest from those of the abdomen. Flattening of the diaphragm with contraction expands the intrathoracic volume and draws air into the lungs. Relaxation of the diaphragm lessens intrathoracic volume and allows for exhalation.

Diastolic pressure The pressure applied to the blood vessels during the relaxation phase of cardiac contractions. Represented as the bottom number of a blood pressure reading.

Diffusion The process by which particles in a fluid move from an area of higher concentration to an area of lower concentration in an effort to equalize distribution.

Digestive tract The musculomembranous tube extending from the mouth to the anus; the tube is lined with mucous membrane and is part of the digestive system. The mouth, pharynx, esophagus, stomach, small intestine, and large intestine compose the digestive tract.

Digoxin A cardiac medication that helps to control cardiac rate and helps strengthen cardiac contraction.

Dilate To increase in size or get larger.

Dilation Spontaneous opening of the cervix that occurs as part of labor.

Direct contact burns Injuries sustained from coming in contact with electricity.

Direct force Force applied directly to a body as a result of contact.

Direct injury An injury that results from a force that comes into direct contact with an area of the body.

Direct laryngoscopy The process of placing an endotracheal tube into the trachea while visualizing the glottic opening with a laryngoscope.

Direct medical control Real-time communication between prehospital care personnel and medical control. This can take place in person, on the phone, or over the radio; also called *online medical control*.

Direct medical direction Medical direction in which a physician speaks directly with emergency medical technicians in the field; also referred to as *online medical direction*.

Direct pressure Bleeding control technique that involves applying pressure; the best way to control active bleeding.

Disaster Any situation that overwhelms the resources available to respond to that event.

Disentanglement Removal of structures or obstructions from around the patient to provide access to the patient and a path from the vehicle or other structures.

Disinfectant The process of killing microorganisms on a surface or item. High-level disinfection destroys all microorganisms except large numbers of bacterial spores; it is used for equipment that has contacted mucous membranes. Intermediate-level disinfection destroys the tuberculosis bacteria, most viruses, and fungi, but it does not destroy bacterial spores; it is used for disinfecting surfaces that contact skin and have been visibly contaminated with body fluids. Low-level disinfection destroys most bacteria and some fungi and viruses but not tuberculosis or bacterial spores; it is used for routine cleaning or removing of soiling when no body fluids are visible.

Disinfecting In addition to cleaning, using alcohol or bleach to kill contaminants.

Dislocation A medical diagnosis indicating the disruption in the integrity of a joint in which one or more bones separate from each other.

Disorganization Interruptions in normal thought process or randomization of thought process.

Disorientation Loss of familiarity with one's surroundings.

Dispatch center A centralized location where personnel obtain information about an incident and assign resources and emergency medical services workers to manage it.

Dispatcher The individual who receives the call for help and dispatches the appropriate resources through the emergency medical services system.

Disruptive behavior Any behavior that is deemed inappropriate for the environment or that others find disturbing.

Distal Away from the trunk of the body.

Distal pulses Pulses taken at a point farther from the midline of the body, such as the pedal or radial pulse.

Distance When one is speaking with a patient, a distance of 2 to 5 feet should be maintained for patient comfort.

Distention A state of swelling or enlargement; the term usually is used to describe the abdomen.

Distributive shock Shock caused by a pathologic dilation of the blood vessels.

Diverticular disease Outpouchings of the colon, which can bleed, become infected, or cause intestinal obstruction.

Do not resuscitate A physician's order indicating that cardiopulmonary resuscitation is not to be performed in the event of cardiopulmonary arrest. It may not apply to medical treatment up until this event.

Domestic dispute A form of violence that results from a family argument and may result in abuse of spouse or children.

Domestic violence Intentionally inflicted injury caused by family members or those of close relation.

Dorsal Toward the back (or ventral) surface.

Dorsalis pedis artery Artery that supplies the foot with blood.

Dosage Amount of a medication that should be administered.

Dosimeter Radiation-measuring device used to monitor the total accumulation of radiation.

Dressing Sterile material placed over an open wound.

Drowning Asphyxiation caused by submersion in a liquid.

Drug Any medicinal substance, or to administer a medicinal substance.

Drug actions The means by which a drug exerts a desired effect.

Due regard The principle that a reasonable and careful person in similar circumstances would act in a way that is safe and considerate for others, such as an ambulance providing enough notice of approach to prevent a collision.

Durable power of attorney for health care A legal, signed document in which a person designates who will be empowered to make medical decisions on the individual's behalf if he or she cannot.

Duty to act The legal requirement to evaluate and treat a patient.

Dyspnea The sensation of difficulty breathing.

Ecchymosis Bluish discoloration of an area of skin or mucous membrane caused by the leakage of blood into the subcutaneous tissues as a result of trauma.

Ecstasy A drug similar to amphetamine that causes mild hallucinations as well as stimulant effects. The chemical name is methylenedioxymethamphetamine (MDMA).

Ectopic pregnancy A pregnancy that implants outside the uterus, usually in the fallopian tube.

Edema An abnormal accumulation of fluid in tissues; swelling.

Electrodes The remote pads that are attached to the defibrillator with lead wires attached to the patient to monitor the electric activity within the heart.

Ellipsoid joint Modified ball-and-socket joint in which the bones are elliptical rather than round. An ellipsoid joint is similar to a hinge joint; its range of motion is limited, but movement takes place on two planes. The joint where the occipital bone of the skull converges with the first vertebra is an example of this type of joint.

Emancipated minor A child who is released from the control of parents or guardians.

Embolus A mass (liquid, solid, or gas) that occludes a blood vessel.

Embryo The developing egg from about 2 weeks after fertilization until about 8 weeks of pregnancy.

Emergency An unexpected, life-threatening situation.

Emergency drags Using the patient's clothing or extremities to pull him or her along the floor or ground in a critical situation.

Emergency medical dispatch A nationally recognized method for training dispatchers in the systematic questioning of persons who call 911 and, when necessary, provision of instructions over the phone.

Emergency medical dispatcher An emergency medical services dispatcher who has received special education for giving medical care instructions to patients and others over the phone before emergency medical technicians arrive.

Emergency medical services system The network of services that handles prehospital medical and trauma emergencies. Emergency medical services systems can be organized at a local, regional, state, or national level.

Emergency medical technician A medical provider who performs prehospital care. The term typically refers to the emergency medical technician level of qualification but may be used to denote any level of prehospital care. Emergency medical technicians are part of the organized emergency medical services system.

Emergency moves Any lift, drag, or carry to remove a patient from a potentially dangerous environment.

Empathetic responses A communication technique that acknowledges the patient's feelings and lets him or her know those feelings are acceptable.

Emphysema A respiratory condition characterized by overinflation and destructive changes to alveolar walls, resulting in a loss of lung elasticity and decreased gas exchange.

EMT-Basic A basic prehospital life support provider trained to the National Highway Traffic Safety Administration guidelines for emergency medical technician, basic level.

EMT-Intermediate An emergency medical technician with the additional education in one or more advanced techniques such as vascular access and intubation.

EMT-Paramedic An emergency medical technician with the additional education to the level of full advanced life support.

Encoders and decoders A process that blocks out radio transmissions not intended for that unit.

Encoding The process by which the sender of a message places the message into a format that the receiver can understand.

Endotracheal tube A translucent and pliable tube passed through the glottic opening and into the trachea to provide a secure conduit for air passage through the upper respiratory tract.

Enhanced 911 A computerized dispatch system that automatically identifies a caller's location when the 911 system is accessed and allows for computer documentation of special information about patients based on their telephone number.

Epidermis Outermost layer of the skin, made up mostly of dead skin cells.

Epidural hematoma An accumulation of blood in the epidural space caused by damage to and leakage of blood from the middle meningeal artery; this causes compression of the dura mater and therefore of the brain.

Epigastric A term that refers to the upper midabdomen, just below the sternum.

Epigastrium The area over the stomach.

Epiglottis A curved flap of tissue that covers the opening of the trachea when swallowing occurs to prevent food or liquid from entering the lower respiratory tract.

Epiglottitis Inflammation of the epiglottis, usually bacterial, causing marked airway obstruction and requiring rapid definitive intervention.

Epilepsy A group of neurologic disorders characterized by recurrent episodes of convulsive seizures, sensory disturbances, abnormal behavior, loss of consciousness, or all of these.

Epinephrine A catecholamine hormone secreted by the adrenal medulla. It is also a neurotransmitter. Epinephrine is also the generic name of a synthetic pharmacologic agent used to treat severe allergic reactions. This agent counteracts the actions that cause respiratory distress and hypoperfusion.

Epinephrine autoinjector A prefilled syringe of epinephrine for use in anaphylaxis.

Epistaxis Bleeding from the nose.

Equality A term used for comparing the body side to side to determine sameness.

Erythrocytes Red blood cells. These cells contain molecules of hemoglobin that bind oxygen diffusing into the bloodstream across the alveolar membranes in the lung for delivery to the tissues throughout the body.

Escorts The use of police vehicles to direct the movements of an ambulance from the scene of an emergency to the hospital.

Esophageal intubation detection device A syringe attached to the proximal end of an inserted endotracheal tube. Easy aspiration of a large volume of air with the syringe confirms proper placement of the endotracheal tube in the trachea rather than in the esophagus.

Esophagus A muscular tube that is situated immediately behind the larynx and trachea and connects the hypopharynx with the stomach.

Ethanol Drinking alcohol; the most common drug of abuse.

Evaporation Change of a substance from a liquid to a gas.

Evisceration Protrusion of abdominal contents through a wound in the abdominal wall.

Exertional heatstroke A form of heatstroke that occurs during muscular activity, often in otherwise fit or well-conditioned individuals.

Expose To remove the clothing to assess a patient.

Exposure The process of coming in contact with, but not necessarily being infected by, a disease-causing agent.

Expressed consent (informed consent) Consent given by a patient for treatment to be performed. This consent may be given verbally or through an affirming gesture such as a nod of the head.

Extension Straightening of a joint.

Extremity carry A rescue evacuation technique in which one rescuer supports the patient's legs and the other rescuer supports the torso to remove the patient from the hazardous situation.

Extrication The process of removing a patient from entanglement in a motor vehicle or other situation in a safe and appropriate way.

Extrication sector The sector in the incident management system responsible for dealing with extrication of patients who are trapped at the scene. This responsibility includes rescue, the initial assessment, and sorting patients for transport to the treatment sector.

Extubation The removal of a tube.

Facilitation A communication technique that encourages the patient to provide more information or continue with his or her response.

Fallopian tube One of the paired structures that extend from each side of the uterus to each ovary. The tubes provide a way for the egg to reach the uterus.

False vocal cords Cartilaginous folds surrounding the true vocal cords of the larynx when viewed from above.

Fascia Fibrous tissue covering a muscle.

Febrile seizure A seizure caused by a rapid rise in body temperature.

Federal Communications Commission An agency of the federal government that is responsible for governing all radio transmissions in the United States.

Feedback An integral part of the communications process that determines whether the message intended was actually the message received.

Femoral artery Artery that supplies the upper and lower leg with blood.

Femur The longest bone in the body; the thigh bone.

Fetus The term used for an infant from about 8 weeks of pregnancy until birth.

Fibrous joint One of three major classes of joints; fibrous joints have little or no motion.

Fibula A non–weight-bearing bone of the lower leg located next to the tibia.

First responder The first person at the scene of a medical or trauma emergency who is trained in medical care. First responders are part of the organized emergency medical services system.

First-degree burns Minor burns characterized by reddened skin.

Flail chest A condition in which several ribs are broken in two places, causing a floating segment; it may also occur if the sternum breaks free from the rib cage.

Flash burns Burns from an open electrical source to exposed tissue.

Flat bones A bone classification; flat bones characteristically are more flat than round (e.g., the ribs).

Flexible stretcher A type of stretcher that can be used to carry a patient through narrow corridors or over difficult terrain.

Flexion Bending of a joint.

Flexion forces Bending of fixed and mobile vertebrae to the point of fracture.

Floating ribs The eleventh and twelfth ribs, which connect to the spinal column but do not attach anywhere else.

Flow-restricted, oxygen-powered ventilation device Ventilator that, when triggered, delivers airflow through a face mask at a maximum flow rate of 40 L/min and a maximum inspiratory pressure of 60 cm H_2O.

Focused history Information obtained from a patient regarding the person's medical history.

Foley A tube placed in the bladder to drain urine.

Fontanels Openings or spaces between the bones of the skull in infants and small children. The openings close as the child grows.

Foot drag A rescue evacuation technique that uses the patient's feet to drag the patient along the long axis of the body from a hazardous situation.

Forensics The science of studying the evidence, living or dead, to determine mechanism and cause of death or the circumstances of the crime.

Formable splint A soft splint that can be shaped to fit the contours of the area being splinted.

Fossa A large depression formed by the juncture of two bones.

Fowler's position Placing a patient on a wheeled stretcher with the head of the stretcher raised to 45 to 60 degrees.

Fracture A medical diagnosis indicating the interruption of the continuity or integrity of a bone.

Frenulum A small, midline flap of mucosal tissue on inside of the lip or bottom of the tongue.

Frontal bone One of the main bones of the skull; it forms the forehead.

Frostbite The traumatic effect of extreme cold on skin and subcutaneous tissues. The first sign is a distinct pallor of exposed skin surfaces, particularly the nose, ears, fingers, and toes.

Frostnip Superficial frostbite.

Full-thickness burns Burns that penetrate all three layers of the skin and into the tissue below.

Function The assessment factor that pertains to normal movement and function.

Gag reflex The occurrence of gagging or vomiting as a result of stimulation of the posterior oropharynx.

Gain access The part of the extrication process in which the rescuers gain entry to trapped patients.

Gamma hydroxybutyrate (GHB) An illicit "rave drug" originally used as an anesthetic and muscle-building aid. It now is abused for its euphoric effects. It also is used as one of the "date rape" drugs, used for its ability to rapidly incapacitate after small doses.

Gamma rays High-energy electromagnetic radiation rays similar to x-rays but more energetic.

Gas The form of a drug or element that is neither liquid nor solid; a gas has no definite shape, and its volume is determined by its container and by temperature and pressure.

Gasping Short breaths with a rapid inspiratory phase associated with respiratory distress and fatigue.

Gastric distention The accumulation of air in the stomach, which places pressure on the diaphragm, making artificial ventilation difficult and increasing the possibility of vomiting.

Gastric tube A tube placed directly into the stomach for feeding.

Gel A substance that is firm in consistency although containing much liquid; a gelatinous substance.

General impression The first impression formed by the emergency medical technician on arrival at the scene.

Generalized seizure A tonic-clonic or grand mal seizure.

Generic name The name assigned to a drug during development of the pharmacologic agent.

Glasgow Coma Scale A quick, practical, standardized system for assessing the degree of impairment of consciousness in critically ill patients. It also is used to predict the duration and ultimate outcome of coma. The scale is used primarily in patients with head injuries.

Glaucoma A chronic eye disease usually affecting elderly patients and causing decreased vision and ultimately blindness unless treated because of increase in the pressure within the eye.

Glossoepiglottic ligament The ligament by which the epiglottis is suspended from the superior aspect of the larynx. Traction on the glossoepiglottic ligament with the tip of a curved laryngoscope blade properly inserted into the vallecula lifts the epiglottis to reveal the glottic opening.

Glottic opening See *glottis.*

Glottis The opening between the true vocal cords that marks the transition from the hypopharynx to the upper trachea.

Glucagon A substance secreted by the pancreas that can cause stored forms of glucose to be released and glucose to be made from other molecules.

Glucometer A device for measuring the amount of glucose in blood.

Glucose A simple sugar found in certain foods, especially fruits. It is a major source of energy that can be measured in the blood.

Glucose gel Concentrated glucose in a paste form.

Glucose monitor A battery-powered instrument used to calculate blood glucose levels from as little as one drop of blood.

Good Samaritan A person who offers help when not specifically on call or obligated to do so.

Grand mal seizure A condition characterized by generalized involuntary muscle contractions and cessation of respiration, followed by tonic and clonic muscle spasms. Breathing returns with noisy respirations. The condition also is known as a *tonic-clonic seizure.*

Great vessels Aorta and inferior and superior venae cavae and their largest branches.

Grunting A gruntlike sound heard at the end of respirations. Common in infants with respiratory distress.

Guarding Tensing of the muscles or other body parts to protect an area.

Gunshot wounds Wounds resulting in penetrating trauma and organ injury from a gunshot.

Gurgling When a patient attempts to breathe, a sound made from the accumulation of fluids in the airway.

Hallucinations Perception of an event, often auditory or visual, that actually is not occurring in reality.

Hallucinogens Drugs that cause hallucinations (e.g., MDMA, lysergic acid diethylamide [LSD], and psilocybin mushrooms).

Halo test A test in which a small amount of fluid is placed on a piece of gauze to determine whether cerebrospinal fluid is present.

Hazardous material Any material or substance that can pose an unreasonable risk to either a person's safety or health or to property.

HAZMAT An abbreviation used to describe a hazardous materials incident.

Head and foot method Hoisting or lowering a transportation device where one emergency medical technician is at the patient's head while the other is at the patient's feet.

Head tilt–chin lift Simple airway-opening maneuver accomplished with one hand placed on the patient's forehead and two or three fingers of the other hand positioned beneath the chin. The chin then is lifted gently upward as the head is tilted backward. Flexing the neck and pulling the mandible forward in this manner will pull the tongue out of the posterior pharynx. This technique is contraindicated if the potential for a cervical spine injury exists.

Health care proxy The legal empowerment of a third party to make decisions regarding the health care of an individual.

Heart failure Reduction in the power of cardiac contractions because of destruction of heart muscle.

Heart rate The number of times the heart beats in a minute.

Heat cramps Any cramp or painful spasm of the voluntary muscles in the arms, legs, or abdomen that occurs after several hours of sustained activity in hot environments with excessive sweating.

Heat exhaustion A heat-related emergency that involves the excessive loss of water or salts.

Heat index The combination of heat and humidity.

Heatstroke The severest but rarest form of heat illness. It results from failure of the temperature-regulating capacity of the body, which can be caused by prolonged exposure to sun or to high temperatures.

Hematoma Closed soft tissue injury characterized by blood pooling at the injury site, producing swelling.

Hemithorax Half of the chest cavity.

Hemoglobin The chemical that carries oxygen in the blood and releases it when it reaches the tissues.

Hemorrhage The loss of a large amount of blood volume in a short period, either externally or internally.

Hemorrhagic shock Hypoperfusion that results from bleeding.

Hemothorax Injury to blood vessels of the lungs or rib cage and subsequent bleeding into the chest cavity.

High altitude cerebral edema The severest form of acute high altitude illness. It is characterized by a progression of global cerebral signs in the presence of acute mountain sickness.

High altitude pulmonary edema A form of pulmonary edema that occurs in people who move rapidly to higher altitudes. Fluid accumulates in the lungs as atmospheric pressure decreases.

High-efficiency particulate air mask A special mask designed to decrease the spread of infection of airborne disease, such as tuberculosis.

Hinge joints Joints in which a concave bone and a convex bone merge; this type of joint flexes and extends on one plane. The knee and elbow are examples of this type of joint.

HIPAA Abbreviation of Health Insurance Portability and Accountability Act.

Histamine A chemical released by the immune system during an allergic reaction that causes many of the signs and symptoms of the reaction.

History Information gathered about a patient's medical condition.

History of the present illness The portion of the history that clarifies the chief complaint or presenting problem through a series of questions (e.g., OPQRST [onset, provocation, quality, radiation, severity, time]).

Hollow organs Intestinal organs through which materials pass, such as the stomach, small intestines, large intestines, ureters, and bladder.

Homeopathic remedies Small doses of medicines or herbs or both that are believed to stimulate the immune system.

Homicidal patient A person who has the intention of harming another person.

Hormones Body chemicals secreted by glands in the endocrine system that regulate body activities and functions in many body systems.

Host An animal or plant that harbors and provides sustenance for another organism (the parasite); recipient of an organ or other tissue derived from another organism (the donor).

Hot zone The area in which contamination occurs.

Huffing (glue sniffing) Deliberate inhalation of hydrocarbons to produce intoxication.

Humerus The bone of the upper arm.

Hyoid bone A free-floating bone in the neck (i.e., it is not attached to any other bone).

Hyperglycemia A greater than normal amount of glucose in the blood.

Hypersensitivity An inappropriate immune response to a generally harmless antigen.

Hypertension Increased blood pressure.

Hyperthermic The condition in which the body temperature is above normal (98.6° F or 37° C).

Hypertrophy An increase in the size of the cells of a tissue in response to an increased workload.

Hyperventilation Rapid and deep breathing resulting in a decrease in carbon dioxide retention.

Hypoglycemia A state of low blood sugar.

Hypoperfusion Decreased or inadequate perfusion that results in insufficient delivery of oxygen and nutrients necessary for normal tissue and cellular function; also known as *shock*.

Hypopharynx The inferior portion of the larynx; it contains the superior openings of the larynx and the esophagus.

Hypothermia Abnormal and dangerous condition in which the body temperature falls below 95° F (35° C) and the body's normal functions are impaired. This occurs because heat loss to the environment exceeds heat production by metabolism.

Hypoventilation Inadequate volume of gas exchange in the lungs.

Hypovolemia An abnormally low circulating blood volume.

Hypovolemic shock Shock caused by a lack of adequate circulating volume. This can occur secondary to gastrointestinal losses, such as with vomiting and diarrhea, blood loss, or inadequate fluid intake.

Hypoxemia A deficiency in the concentration of oxygen in arterial blood.

Hypoxia Inadequate cellular oxygenation.

Hypoxic drive The low arterial oxygen pressure stimulus to respiration.

Hysteria A disorder in which a loss of physical functioning occurs. It is often the sign of a psychological conflict or need.

Iliac arteries Arteries that supply the lower extremities with oxygen and nutrient-enriched blood.

Iliac wings The anterior/superior aspect of the pelvis.

Ilium One of three bones that make up half of the pelvis. The superior end of the ilium is known as the *iliac crest*.

Immune system The system responsible for protecting the body from disease.

Immunity The ability of the body to resist infection after exposure to an infectious agent. The state of being protected from (immune to) disease.

Impaled object Pointed object that has penetrated the skin.

Implied consent A type of consent in which verbal or written consent is not possible but circumstances warrant that a reasonable person would want and expect emergency treatment to be rendered.

Incident command system A system for coordinating procedures and resources to assist in the command, control, direction, and coordination of a response to a disaster.

Incident management system A disaster response system in which one central management team coordinates resources to ensure a systematic and efficient approach.

Incontinence Involuntary loss of urine or stool.

Incorporation The take up of radioactive materials by the body cells, tissues, and organs.

Incubation period The time between contact with an infectious agent and occurrence of signs and symptoms of infection.

Index of suspicion An anticipation that certain types of situations result in specific types of injuries.

Indications Conditions in which administering a specific drug may benefit the patient.

Indirect force Force that travels through the body and causes damage in an area or areas away from the contact site.

Indirect injury An injury in one body area that results from a force that comes into contact with a different part of the body.

Indirect medical control The use of standing orders, or written protocols, to provide care. This type of medical control does not involve actual communication with a medical director at the time of the incident; also called *off-line medical control*.

Indirect medical direction Any direction provided by physicians that is not direct, including system design, protocol development, education, and quality improvement; also referred to as *off-line medical direction*.

Infant A child less than 1 year of age.

Infection control The practice of actions to block the spread of infectious agents.

Inferior Toward the feet or bottom of the body.

Inferior vena cava Large vein that carries oxygen-poor blood from the lower extremities and torso.

Informed consent Consent made when the patient has been made fully aware of the risks, benefits, and consequences of the care being provided and any alternatives to that care.

Informed refusal The process of informing a patient of risks versus benefits in refusing medical treatment. The patient should clearly understand the risks and benefits, and the process should be well documented.

Ingested toxin A toxin that is consumed orally.

Ingestion Taking food, medicines, or drink into the body by mouth.

Inhalation Drawing air or other substances into the body by way of the nose and trachea.

Inhaled medications Medications that are introduced into the body by breathing in by the mouth or nose.

Inhaled toxin A toxin that is breathed into the lungs, where it is absorbed into the bloodstream.

Inhaler An apparatus for administering aerosol medication through inhalation.

Initial assessment The early part of assessment devoted to identifying and treating life-threatening conditions related to airway, breathing, circulation, and mental status.

Initial collapse (au: please provide definition)

Injectable medication A medication that is administered by injection beneath the skin or into a vein.

Injected toxin A toxin that enters the body through a puncture in the skin.

Injection Forcing a liquid into a body part, such as into the subcutaneous tissues, the vascular tree, or an organ.

Inspect To look for injuries or problems.

Inspection An assessment technique that involves looking for injuries or problems.

Insufflation Taking a drug by inhaling it. The drug then is absorbed from the tissue lining the nose into the bloodstream.

Insulin A naturally occurring hormone, secreted by the pancreas, that regulates the metabolism of glucose.

Insulin-dependent A diabetic patient who requires injections of insulin for the body to use sugar. Not all diabetic patients require insulin injections.

Intercostal muscles The muscles that lie between the ribs and assist respiration by raising and lowering the adjacent ribs with each breath.

Intercostal retractions The use of accessory muscles to increase the work of breathing, which appears as the sucking in of the muscles between the ribs.

Interference A component of the communication model that is responsible for most instances of miscommunication.

Interstitium or interstitial fluid The space between cells.

Intracellular space The fluid space within a cell.

Intracerebral hematoma A localized collection of extravasated blood within the cerebrum, associated with a cerebral laceration caused by a contusion.

Intramuscular Within the muscular substance.

Intramuscular injection An injection of medication or toxin that enters the muscle.

Intramuscular medication A medication that is administered by injection into a muscle.

Intravascular fluid space The fluid space within a blood vessel.

Intravenous medication A medication that is delivered by injection directly into a vein.

Involuntary muscles Muscles that move without conscious effort.

Ipecac syrup A substance used to induce vomiting with overdose and certain poisonings.

Irradiation Caused by radioactive energy in wave or ray form that passes through but is not physically present on the body. The irradiated patient cannot spread radioactive materials to others.

Irregular bones A bone classification; irregular bones are characterized by their nonspecific shape (e.g., the facial bones).

Ischemia When an area of the heart muscle is not receiving enough oxygen.

Ischemic chest pain Characteristic pain resulting from inadequate blood supply to the myocardium.

Ischium One of three bones that make up half of the pelvis.

Jaundice A yellowish color to the skin caused by liver disease.

Jaw thrust Airway-opening technique best suited for the supine patient with a possible cervical spine injury. One hand is placed on either side of the patient's head to provide neutral, in-line cervical spine stabilization, while fingers of each hand are positioned behind the angle of the mandible. Forward pressure thrusts the jaw outward, lifting the tongue off of the wall of the posterior pharynx.

Joint The convergence of two or more bones.

Joint capsule Layered tissue that surrounds and protects a joint. The joint capsule is composed of a tough, outer fibrous capsule and an inner membrane that produces synovial fluid.

Jugular vein distention Enlargement of the jugular veins on the sides of the neck.

Kendrick extrication device A semirigid, short device that is used to immobilize and extricate victims of vehicle crashes who are found in the sitting position.

Kidneys The pair of bean-shaped organs that filter the blood and eliminate wastes in urine.

Kussmaul's respirations Respiratory pattern represented by continuous deep breaths; the rate may be slow or fast. Associated with diabetic ketoacidosis.

Kyphosis An abnormal outward curvature of the spine that creates a dorsal hump.

Labor The process by which the fetus and placenta are expelled from the uterus. It usually is divided into three stages, starting from the first contraction and ending with delivery of the placenta.

Labored respirations Difficulty breathing represented by the use of accessory muscles and an increase in the work of breathing.

Laceration Open soft tissue injury characterized by a jagged cutting of the skin.

Ladder splint A durable, lightweight splint made of metal that can be bent to conform to the shape of long bones.

Laryngeal mask airway An alternative airway device consisting of a tube connected to an inflatable mask designed to form a seal over the larynx and the glottic opening.

Laryngectomy Surgical removal of part of the larynx.

Laryngoscope A lighted device designed to assist in visualizing the structures of the hypopharynx, particularly the vocal cords and the glottic opening.

Larynx Cartilaginous structure in the anterior neck connecting the posterior pharynx with the trachea in the upper airway. Also known as the *voice box.*

Lateral Away from the midline of the body.

Laterally recumbent position Placing the patient on his or her side. A patient lying on his or her left side is said to be "left laterally recumbent."

Leading questions Questions that are phrased in such a way that they lead the patient to an answer that may not necessarily be the most correct answer.

Level of consciousness A degree of cognitive function involving arousal mechanisms in the brain. Levels of consciousness range from unconsciousness to full attention.

Life threat Injuries or medical problems that threaten the patient's life.

Ligaments Tough, elastic, cordlike tissues that connect bone to bone.

Limb presentation When one of the baby's extremities is the presenting part at birth.

Linear laceration A laceration in a straight line.

Living will A legal document prepared by a patient that gives direction to the person's physicians regarding end-of-life care. Usually not relevant to the prehospital setting.

Locked-in position A technique by which the back is maintained in straight alignment during the lift so as not to cause strain or injury.

Logroll A rotation technique used to slide an immobilization device under a patient with minimal flexion, extension, or rotation of the spinal column.

Long backboard (full body spinal immobilization device) A device used to maintain immobilization of the head, neck, torso, pelvis, and extremities.

Long bones A bone classification; long bones characteristically are longer than they are wide (e.g., the femur).

Long spine board A flat wooden, plastic, or metal device used to maintain spinal immobilization or to transport a patient.

Los Angeles Prehospital Stroke Screen A type of screening device used to identify stroke patients rapidly.

Lower gastrointestinal tract Area of the gastrointestinal tract distal to the duodenum.

Lower respiratory tract Air passages formed by the trachea, bronchi, and bronchioles, and terminating in the alveoli.

LSD The street name for lysergic acid or "acid"; a potent hallucinogen.

Lumbar vertebrae Five vertebrae of the spinal column (L20 to L24).

Mainstem bronchi The two main branches to the lungs from the trachea.

Malpractice Any wrong or injurious treatment that results in harm to a patient.

Mandible The lower jawbone.

Mania An emotional disorder characterized by euphoria, irritability, and grandiose thoughts.

Man-made hazards Hazards posed or created by human beings, such as booby traps, alcohol stills, drug labs, hazardous material dumps, attack dogs, and armed criminals.

Manual in-line stabilization Holding of a patient's head in a neutral position that is in line with the rest of the body.

Manubrium Uppermost section of the sternum.

Marijuana A crude preparation of the leaves and flowering tops of *Cannabis* plants. It usually is made into cigarettes and inhaled as smoke for its euphoric effects.

Mark I Autoinjector A self-contained unit that contains the medications atropine and pralidoxime in an injection device for administration to a victim of nerve agent exposure.

Marrow A spongy material in the center of bones. Yellow marrow is mostly fat cells. Red marrow produces red blood cells.

Material safety data sheet A multipage document that provides detailed, material-specific information about a hazardous substance. The material safety data sheet probably is the most important source of information for emergency medical technicians determining the treatment of a victim of a hazardous materials exposure.

Maxilla The upper jawbone.

Mechanism of action How a medication affects the body.

Mechanism of injury The cause of the injuries or damage to the patient.

Meconium A dark green substance that represents the infant's first bowel movement.

Medial Toward the midline of the body.

Medical direction The active participation of physicians in all phases of the emergency medical services system, including protocol development, needs assessment of the system, education, quality improvement, and outcome studies and on-line medical direction. Also called *medical control*.

Medical director A physician who develops guidelines and protocols for the prehospital treatment of patients. The medical director is responsible for the prehospital medical care delivered by emergency medical services providers.

Medication A drug or remedy for a certain condition.

Meningitis Inflammation of the membranes surrounding the brain.

Mental status An assessment of how the patient responds mentally to the situation around him or her.

Mesentery A fold of tissue that attaches organs to the body wall. Mesentery usually refers to small bowel mesentery, which anchors the small intestine to the back of the abdominal wall. Blood vessels, nerves, and lymphatic vessels branch through the mesentery to supply the intestine.

Metacarpals Five bones that form the structure of the hand.

Metatarsals Five bones that form the structure of the foot.

Metered dose inhaler An instrument used to deliver a medication through inhalation that allows a controlled and precise dose to be given.

Methamphetamine A derivative of amphetamine used both medically and illicitly as a central nervous system stimulant.

Microorganisms Organisms not visible to the naked eye.

Midaxillary An imaginary line on the body that extends from the armpit down through the lower chest wall.

Midclavicular An imaginary line on the body that extends from the middle section of the clavicle down through the lower chest wall.

Midline An imaginary vertical line drawn through the middle of the body.

Minimum data set Data that include patient information and administrative information documented on the patient care report. This information is used for statistical purposes.

Minute ventilation The tidal volume of an average breath multiplied by the number of times the individual breathes over 1 minute.

Minute volume The amount of air available for alveolar exchange each minute. The minute volume (MVa) is determined by subtracting the physiologic dead space (VD) from the tidal volume (TV) and multiplying the result by the respiratory rate (RR): $MVa = (TV - VD) \times RR$.

Miosis Constriction of the pupil, which limits the amount of light reaching the eye.

Miscarriage (spontaneous abortion) Loss of the products of conception before the fetus can survive on its own.

Mobile radio A radio that is mounted in a vehicle.

Monitoring-defibrillation electrode pads Pads that connect an automatic external defibrillator or other device to the patient to monitor the patient's electrocardiogram and deliver shock.

Motor function The ability to move.

Mottled Blotchy appearance of the skin caused by a decrease in circulation.

Mouth-to-mask ventilation Form of assisted ventilation in which the rescuer places a mask over the face of the victim, maintains an airtight seal against the face, and delivers breaths directly to the patient by blowing directly through a port in the mask.

Mucous membranes Layer of membranes of the respiratory and digestive tracts.

Multiple casualty incident Any incident that results in multiple victims who will require treatment and transport.

Multisystem trauma Significant trauma involving more than one system of the body.

Multitiered response systems Combination of basic life support and advanced life support providers responding to calls.

Murphy's eye A small hole in the side of an endotracheal tube that provides a passage of air if the tip of the tube becomes clogged.

Mutual aid A prearranged response system that is established with neighboring communities to ensure a large-scale response of emergency personnel and vehicles, including police, firefighters, and ambulances during a catastrophic incident.

Myocardial Referring to cardiac muscle.

Myocardial infarct Heart attack; caused when an artery of the heart is blocked partially or completely, causing damage to the heart.

Nasal cannula Oxygen tubing with two small prongs that are inserted into either nostril. A relatively inefficient means of delivering supplemental oxygen.

Nasal flaring A characteristic flaring of the nostrils in infants and small children; it suggests the presence of respiratory distress.

Nasogastric tube A long, pliable tube inserted through the nostril and the esophagus into the stomach. Applying suction to a properly placed nasogastric tube decompresses the stomach, lessening the risk for aspiration and facilitating assisted ventilation.

Nasopharyngeal (nasal) airway Flexible tube inserted through one nostril into the posterior pharynx as a means of preserving the passage of air through the posterior pharynx.

Nasopharynx The cavity or air passage that lies immediately posterior to the nose and forms the upper portion of the pharynx.

Nasotracheal intubation Intubation of the trachea through the nose.

National EMS Education and Practice Blueprint A consensus document that establishes a core content for the scope of practice for the four levels of prehospital care providers.

National Incident Management System (au: please provide definition)

National Search and Rescue Plan (au: please provide definition)

Nature of illness A determination of the patient's illness from findings.

Navicular bone The most medial of the seven tarsal bones.

Near drowning An episode in which a patient survives at least 24 hours after submersion, whether or not the patient ultimately survives.

Nebulizer A device for producing a fine spray or mist that includes medication to be inhaled.

Needle decompression Insertion of a large intravenous-style needle between the ribs to relieve a tension pneumothorax.

Neglect Insufficient attention to or respect for someone who has a claim to that attention.

Negligence A deviation from the accepted standard of care resulting in injury to the patient. For negligence to occur, there must be a duty to act, a breach of duty, injury to the patient, and a causal connection.

Nerves Fibers and connective tissue located outside the brain that send and receive signals from the brain.

Neurogenic shock A form of shock that results from peripheral vascular dilation.

Newborn An infant from birth to 1 month of age.

Newton's law of motion A body in motion will stay in motion and a body at rest will stay at rest until acted on by an outside force.

Nitroglycerin The generic name for a drug that acts to dilate the blood vessels, decreasing the workload of the heart.

Noisy respirations Any noise coming from the patient's airway; it indicates a respiratory problem.

Nonemergency moves Any lift, drag, or carry used when the scene is safe or the patient is not in critical condition.

Non-rebreather mask Combination of a face mask, a bag reservoir, and a one-way flow valve that allows oxygen to flow from the reservoir into the mask without letting exhaled air into the reservoir. This ensures that a high concentration of oxygen is contained within the reservoir at all times, in turn delivering a high concentration of oxygen with each inhalation.

Nonstriated muscles Muscles characterized by the absence of lines in the muscle tissue.

Nonurgent move A patient move used when there is no present or anticipated threat to the patient's life and care can be administered adequately and safely.

Nonverbal communication An important element of communication in which messages are relayed through movements, posture, gestures, and the eyes.

Normal anatomic position The position of a human body standing upright, facing forward, with arms at the side and the palms turned forward.

Normal respirations Respirations occurring without airway noise or effort from the patient, usually occurring at a rate of 12 to 20 breaths per minute in an adult.

Nuclear radiation Energy emitted from the nucleus of an unstable atom.

Nuclear, biological, chemical Three major terrorist threats with which emergency medical services providers must be prepared to deal in the event of an attack.

Nystagmus Continuous movement or shaking back and forth of the eye.

Objective assessment Information obtained regarding the patient's condition by what you find during physical assessment.

Objective information Factual information that is based on observations of the emergency medical technician.

Obstetrics kit A prepackaged kit of equipment and items needed to prepare for and assist with the delivery of a baby.

Occipital bone A major (and the most posterior) bone of the skull.

Occiput The back of the skull.

Occupancy Activity performed in a structure and the number of potential occupants.

Occlusive Referring to protection from the air. An occlusive dressing will not let air into the wound.

Occupational Health and Safety Administration A federal agency that has developed guidelines to protect health care workers.

Octal survey An eight-sided scene evaluation that includes the inside, outside, top, bottom, front, back, left side, and right side.

Off-line medical direction The accountability by a physician of emergency medical services providers through the use of protocols, quality improvement activities, educational endeavors, and other measures to ensure effective field care.

One-handed carrying technique A carrying technique used when multiple personnel are available for the carry and rescuers are placed strategically around the device.

Ongoing assessment The process of monitoring a patient over time. It includes repeating the initial assessment, reassessing and recording vital signs, repeating the focused assessment, and checking interventions.

Online medical direction The accountability of field care by a physician though the use of radio or telephone communications.

Onset An event that causes a symptom to occur.

Open skeletal injury Trauma that breaches the integrity of the outer surface of the skin.

Open pneumothorax A pneumothorax associated with a punctured chest wall.

Open-ended questions Questions that cannot be answered with a "yes" or "no" response. These questions provide the most information because they allow the patient free reign in response as the patient tells you what he or she is experiencing. They also allow the emergency medical technician the most insight into the patient's condition.

Operations level (au: please provide definition)

Opiates Drugs or substances that contain opium or an opium derivative (e.g., heroin, morphine, codeine, and fentanyl).

OPQRST An acronym used in collecting a patient history about a specific sign or symptom. The letters stand for *o*nset, *p*rovocation, *q*uality, *r*adiation, *s*everity, and *t*ime.

Oral glucose A form of glucose gel that is administered orally to patients with suspected diabetic emergencies.

Oral medication A medication that is delivered by mouth.

Oral mucosa The lining of the mouth.

Orientation A person's awareness of person, place, and time.

Orogastric tube A long, pliable tube inserted through the mouth and esophagus into the stomach for decompression of the latter. The passage of an orogastric tube is preferred when significant facial trauma precludes the safe passage of a nasogastric tube.

Oropharyngeal (oral) airway Rigid, curved instrument that, when properly placed, maintains an open conduit for air passage between the tongue and the posterior wall of the oropharynx in the supine patient.

Oropharynx The air cavity/passageway situated at the back of the mouth.

Orotracheal intubation The passage of an endotracheal tube through the glottic opening and into the trachea under direct visualization with the aid of a laryngoscope.

Orthopnea Respiratory difficulty when supine. Breathing is much easier sitting upright or standing.

Orthostatic hypotension A fall in blood pressure of 20 mm Hg or more or an increase in heart rate of 20 beats per minute or more that results from a change in position; it often occurs secondary to hypovolemia.

Osteoporosis A decrease in the amount of bone tissue occurring in older persons as a result of more bone breakdown than bone formation, which leads to weaker bones.

Ovaries The paired female reproductive organs found on each side of the lower abdomen.

Overdose Taking of a drug in excess or in combination with other agents to the point where poisoning occurs.

Pacemakers A group of cells in the heart that initiates the electric impulses of the heart; a mechanical device implanted to control certain dysrhythmias or provide a backup if the natural pacemaker of the heart fails.

Painful, swollen extremity A descriptive emergency medical services field observation.

Palliative That which makes the patient's condition better.

Palpate To feel for injuries during patient assessment.

Palpation An assessment technique that involves feeling for injuries during the patient assessment.

Pancake collapse A type of structural collapse in which horizontal structural components detach from vertical support systems, resulting in uniform downward collapse.

Paradoxical breathing "See-saw" movement of the chest and abdominal wall muscles with breathing in an effort to augment expansion of the thoracic cavity with inspiration. Often a sign of respiratory distress, particularly among infants and children.

Paradoxical movement Movement associated with a flail chest in which the chest wall moves in on inspiration and out on expiration.

Paramedic The most advanced level of prehospital emergency medical care. Paramedics are part of the organized emergency medical services system.

Paranoia A disorder in which a person is plagued with bizarre thoughts of persecution.

Parietal bone A major bone of the skull; it constitutes the top of the skull.

Partial seizure A seizure in which only part of the body is affected.

Partial-thickness burn Burn that penetrates the epidermis and part of the dermis.

Passive immunity Immunity that is introduced into a body (not produced by it), such as injection of an antibody against tetanus.

Patella The kneecap.

Pathogens Microorganisms capable of causing disease.

Patient assessment The process of systematically evaluating a patient for injuries or illness.

Patient confidentiality The legal right of patients to have their medical information protected and not shared.

Patient data Data about the call that are specific to the patient.

Patient information Information that relates specifically to the patient, such as age and gender.

Patient narrative The section of the prehospital care report that allows emergency medical technicians to document patient information using a standard medical reporting format.

Patient refusal form Specific form to document a patient's refusal of treatment and transport.

Patient trends Evaluation of a sequence of patient vital signs and assessments that indicate improvement or deterioration of the patient's condition.

Pectoral girdle The union of the clavicle and scapula where the upper extremity attaches to the body.

Pedal edema Swelling of the ankles and feet.

Pelvic girdle The union of the ilium, the ischium, and the pubis where the lower extremity attaches to the body.

Pelvis The lower part of the trunk of the body.

Penetrating trauma Stabbing, gunshot wounds, or other injuries created by the entry of a sharp object into the body.

Penetration or puncture An open soft tissue injury caused by an object being pushed into or through the skin.

Perfusion The circulation of blood to the tissues of the body.

Perineum The tissue between the mother's vaginal and rectal openings. This tissue may be torn during delivery.

Peripheral Away from the center of the body.

Peripheral pulses Pulse points in an extremity.

Peritoneum Membrane lining a body cavity.

Personal flotation device (au: please provide definition)

Personal hazards (au: please provide definition)

Personal protective equipment Equipment used to isolate a health care worker from a patient's body substances. Also refers to specialty equipment used by emergency providers during the course of a rescue or a fire.

Pertinent negatives Findings that are not present that may be expected given the scenario.

Petit mal seizure A seizure during which the patient usually has a blank stare with no obvious muscle contractions; it usually lasts for seconds to minutes. This type of seizure also is known as an *absence seizure.*

Phalanges The fourteen bones in each hand and foot that make up the structures of the fingers and toes, respectively. Each thumb and great toe consists of two phalanges; each other finger or toe has three.

Pharmacology The science of drugs and study of their origin, ingredients, uses, and actions on the body.

Pharynx The cavity or open space above the larynx and posterior to the nose and mouth. It may be subdivided further into the nasopharynx and the oropharynx.

Phencyclidine (PCP) A stimulant drug that also induces a state in which the pain sensation is diminished.

Phobia An irrational fear.

Physiologic dead space A combination of the anatomic dead space and the amount of air in the alveoli that is not available for exchange. This amount of air varies from person to person based on the number of nonfunctional alveoli.

Physiology The function of the body.

Pin index safety system A safety system of gas cylinders that allows tanks of different types of gas to accept special regulators designed specifically for that gas.

Pivot joints Round bones that rotate within a ring of bone and ligament. The forearm near the elbow, where the radius and ulna meet, is an example of a pivot joint.

Placard A sign that has various symbols and numerals that help identify a hazardous material or class of materials.

Placenta (afterbirth) The organ inside the uterus that serves the function of exchanging nutrition and waste between the mother and the fetus.

Placenta previa Placement of the placenta such that it partially or completely covers the cervix.

Placental abruption (abruptio placentae) Separation of part of the placenta away from the wall of the uterus.

Plain English The preferred method of emergency medical services radio communication in which information is stated directly and not coded in any manner.

Plane (gliding) joints Joints formed by two flat-surfaced bones.

Plasma Fluid in the blood that helps move the blood cells and platelets.

Platelets Cells that cause the blood to clot in order to stop bleeding.

Pleuritic chest pain Pain made worse by breathing.

Pneumatic (air) splint Plastic splints filled with air to provide circumferential support to an injured extremity.

Pneumatic antishock garment A garment designed to produce pressure on the lower part of the body, thereby preventing the pooling of blood in the legs and abdomen.

Pneumothorax Development of air in the normally empty space between the lung and the chest wall.

Point tenderness Pain in a specific location to which a patient usually can point.

Poison A substance that on ingestion, inhalation, absorption, or injection may cause structural damage or functional disturbance.

Poison control center A service that provides data on all aspects of poisonings, keeps records of poisonings, and refers patients to treatment centers.

Portable radio A portable radio can be taken wherever the emergency medical technician goes. These are generally low-power handheld radios with limited transmission distance.

Portable stretcher A type of stretcher that can be carried easily to and from the scene of an emergency.

Position of comfort Placing the patient in his or her most comfortable position when there is no need for emergency procedures such as immobilization.

Position of function The natural position of the hand (i.e., with the fingers slightly curled).

Positive pressure ventilation The act of forcing air into the lungs.

Posterior Toward the back of the body.

Posterior tibial artery The artery passing just behind the ankle bone, where it is palpable between the medial malleolus and the Achilles tendon.

Postictal period Period immediately after a generalized seizure; it manifests as confusion, agitation, or somnolence.

Post-traumatic stress disorder An anxiety disorder that is caused by exposure to an extremely traumatic event. Affected individuals may relive the event in nightmares or flashbacks; symptoms may include avoidance of stimuli associated with trauma, hyperalertness, and difficulty sleeping, remembering, or concentrating.

Postural vital signs Vital signs obtained when the patient is supine and then is moved to a sitting position or when the patient is sitting and then is moved to an erect or standing position.

Power grip The correct hand placement for hoisting or lowering a transportation device. For hoisting, the hands should be spaced approximately 10 inches apart, with the fingers facing up. For lowering, the hands should be spaced the same distance apart, with the fingers facing down.

Power lift The most effective way to lift a heavy object.

Preeclampsia A complication of pregnancy that includes hypertension, swelling of the extremities, and in its most severe form, seizures.

Prehospital care report The standard form used for documenting patient care in emergency medical services systems, also referred to as a *patient care report* or *PCR*.

Preschool child A child from 3 to 6 years of age.

Presenting part The first part of the infant to appear at the vaginal opening; this is usually the head.

Pressure dressing Dressing applied to help reduce swelling or control excessive bleeding.

Pressure point Common pulse location where pressure can be applied to collapse an artery and thereby reduce or stop blood flow to a wound.

Preterm (premature) delivery Delivery before the thirty-seventh week of pregnancy.

Priapism Persistent erection of the penis associated with spinal cord injury or other medical conditions.

Prior intelligence Information from occupants, the public, and local authorities that can predict the location of trapped victims.

Privacy In a private setting, patients are more comfortable and more likely to provide complete answers to questions asked. If your initial interview was conducted in a public setting, ask questions again when privacy may allow more open responses.

Prolapsed cord Slipping of the umbilical cord down past the presenting part.

Prone The body lying face down.

Protocol A written procedure for a clinical treatment.

Provocation An action that causes a symptom to change or intensify.

Proximal Toward the trunk of the body.

Proximal pulse point pressure Bleeding control technique that involves applying manual pressure to the most proximal pulse of an injury site.

Psilocybin The chemical found in some mushrooms that causes hallucinations.

Psychosis A mental disorder in which there is often disorganization of thought to the point that the person may be unable to care for himself or herself.

Psychotic Behavior by a person who has lost touch with reality.

Pubis One of three major bones that make up half the pelvis.

Public access defibrillation Laypersons trained to use an automated external defibrillator in public areas.

Public safety dispatch point Commonly referred to as a dispatch center, these points receive calls for service from the public and assign resources to each incident. Public safety dispatch points also track the movement of emergency equipment and may provide prearrival instructions to callers.

Pulmonary arrest Cessation of respiratory function.

Pulmonary artery Artery that carries deoxygenated blood from the right ventricle of the heart to the lungs.

Pulmonary contusion Lung injury that results in fluid or blood seeping into the alveolar air spaces, preventing that area from exchanging oxygen and carbon dioxide with the blood.

Pulmonary edema The accumulation of extravascular fluid in the lung tissues and alveoli, caused mostly by congestive heart failure.

Pulmonary embolism The blockage of a pulmonary artery by foreign matter.

Pulmonary vein Vein that carries oxygenated blood from the lungs to the left atrium of the heart.

Pulsation A rhythmic beating or pulsing.

Pulse Area where an artery can be felt over a bony prominence in the body when the heart contracts.

Pulse oximeter A device for measuring the oxygen saturation of hemoglobin.

Pulse oximetry Measurement of the saturation of hemoglobin with oxygen via a pulse oximeter, read as a percentage of saturation.

Pulse rate The number of times the heart beats in 1 minute.

Pulseless electrical activity A condition in which the heart has an organized electric rhythm but with no palpable pulse.

Puncture Penetrating injury caused by a sharp, pointed object.

Puncture wound Open soft tissue injury resulting from a pointed object penetrating the skin.

Pupil The black center or opening into the eye.

Quadrants The four quarters of an anatomic area.

Quality The assessment factor that pertains to the description of a symptom.

Quality assurance Method of ensuring quality patient care and system response.

Quality improvement Methods of ensuring a high level of patient care.

Quality of life An individual belief in what constitutes a meaningful existence.

Quarantine The isolation of patients exposed to or having a contagious disease for a period until they are incapable of developing or transmitting the disease.

Raccoon's eyes Bilateral bruising around the eyes; often associated with a basilar skull fracture.

Radial artery Artery located on the thumb side of the wrist.

Radial pulse The pulse felt on the thumb side of the wrist.

Radiation Movement to another area; the term often is used to describe pain that moves from one location to another.

Radiological dispersion device A device usually made by packing radioactive material around an explosive device. Detonation of such a device usually results in relatively low-level radiologic contamination but would cause extensive public panic and potentially extensive need for decontamination of the affected area.

Radius Larger of the two bones of the forearm.

Rales Fine crackling sounds generated when fluid-filled or collapsed alveoli suddenly reexpand with inspiration.

Range of motion An extremity's normal ability to move based on the type of joint involved. Injuries limit range of motion.

Rapid assessment A quick evaluation of the medical patient from head to toe, usually accomplished in 60 to 90 seconds.

Rapid extrication The rapid removal of a patient in critical condition from a vehicle.

Rapid trauma assessment A rapid, orderly, head to toe assessment of a patient.

Ration To specifically or arbitrarily determine which patients will receive the treatment or resources available.

Reactive to light The constriction of the pupil when light is shined into the eye.

Reasonable force The force necessary to keep a person from injuring himself or herself or others.

Receiving operator The individual who receives the call for assistance.

Recovery position Placing an unresponsive, breathing, nontrauma victim on his or her side to allow access to the airway to keep it open.

Red blood cells Cells that carry oxygen and are transported in the blood.

Referred pain Pain that is felt at a site different from that of an injured or diseased organ or body part.

Regression A relapse or return of symptoms.

Repeater A piece of radio equipment that receives low-power radio transmissions and rebroadcasts them at a higher power. Repeaters may be vehicle mounted, freestanding, or associated with a base station.

Reperfusion acidosis A form of acidosis that results when circulation is restored and the acidic substances are washed into the central circulation.

Rescue breathing Artificially breathing for a patient who cannot breathe on his or her own.

Respiration The physiologic process by which oxygen that is drawn into the lungs is delivered to tissues and cells throughout the body and is exchanged for the waste products of cell metabolism.

Respiratory arrest Cessation of breathing.

Respiratory distress An increase in the work of breathing. It may involve tachypnea (increased rate of breathing), hyperpnea (increased depth of breathing), nasal flaring, accessory muscle use, and retractions.

Respiratory failure A deterioration from respiratory distress when the provider must intervene and take over the work of breathing for the patient.

Respiratory rate The number of times a patient breathes in 1 minute.

Retractions The drawing in of soft tissues between the ribs, above the clavicle, and below the sternum. Retractions reflect increased work of breathing.

Retrograde amnesia The loss of memory of events that occurred before a particular time in a person's life, usually before the event that precipitated the amnesia.

Rhonchi Abnormal, coarse sounds heard over the upper airways as air moves through thick mucous secretions. Rhonchi often clear with coughing.

Ribs Flat bones of the thoracic cavity that protect the lungs, heart, great vessels, and diaphragm.

Rigid splint A splint that cannot be bent or conformed to the body. Rigid splints are used to stabilize long bones; also called a *board splint*.

Rigor mortis A state of body stiffness caused by the depletion of proteins in muscles after death.

Route of drug administration The method by which a drug is administered to a patient, such as intramuscular, oral, and intravenous.

Rule of nines Method of determining the amount of damage done to body surface area as a result of burns, abrasions, or other injury.

Run data Data about the call that do not include the patient element.

Sacrum A distal part of the spinal column; it consists of five sacral vertebrae that fuse as the body ages.

Saddle joints Joints in which two saddle-shaped bones converge at a 90-degree angle, allowing movement on two planes. The thumb joint is an example of this type of joint.

SAMPLE The mnemonic used to assist in collecting a patient history (S, signs and symptoms; A, allergies; M, medications; P, past medical history; L, last oral intake; E, events preceding).

Sarin A chemical compound specifically developed to serve as a weapon of mass destruction nerve agent. Sarin also goes by the military term *GB* and in the lay press may be referred to as "nerve gas." Sarin is rapid acting. It may be a liquid but usually is dispersed as a gas at room temperature.

Scapulae Large, flat bones that form the structure of the back and pectoral girdle.

Scene safety The first step in the scene size-up phase of patient assessment; a procedure that ensures safety to the emergency medical technician, the patient, and bystanders by effectively securing the scene.

Scene size-up The first phase of patient assessment that includes scene safety, the appropriate use of personal protective equipment, and the determination of the mechanism of injury or the nature of illness.

Schizophrenia A psychotic disorder characterized by distortions of reality. Disturbances in language and communication may occur. The patient also may have bizarre thoughts, including those of persecution, paranoia, and hallucinations.

Scoop stretcher A specialized device consisting of an aluminum frame and a rectangular tube with shovel-type lateral flaps for sliding under the patient.

Scope of practice The parameters and limitations of a given medical provider.

Secondary collapse A trench rescue hazard that arises after the initial collapse. In secondary collapse, the remaining sections of the trench, which have less stability, fall, causing successive collapses. Secondary collapse is the most lethal hazard in a trench rescue.

Secondary drowning The rapid deterioration of respiratory status from several to 96 hours after resuscitation.

Second-degree burns Partial- to full-thickness burns characterized by pain and the formation of blisters.

Seesaw breathing A physical finding in small children and infants characterized by alternate use of the abdominal and chest wall muscles and indicating respiratory distress.

Seizure Hyperexcitation of neurons in the brain, leading to sudden, violent, involuntary contractions of muscles; also known as a *convulsion*.

Self-contained breathing apparatus Specialized mask and regulator used by rescue personnel in environments that may be dangerous, such as those containing smoke, carbon monoxide, or other hazardous materials.

Self-contained underwater breathing apparatus (au: please provide definition)

Self-extubation The patient's intentional or unintentional removal of a tube.

Sellick maneuver The application of posterior-directed pressure to the cricoid cartilage with the thumb and forefinger, thereby occluding the esophagus to prevent regurgitation of gastric contents during attempted intubation.

Semiautomatic external defibrillator Type of automatic external defibrillator that requires operator direction to analyze and shock.

Semi-Fowler position An inclined position with the upper half of the body raised by elevating the head of the stretcher about 30 degrees.

Sensation The ability to feel.

Sepsis A systemic response to a blood infection that results in hemodynamic instability, usually manifested by tachycardia and hypotension.

Septum The wall that divides the right side of the heart and the left side of the heart.

Severity The assessment factor that pertains to qualification of a symptom's intensity.

Shallow respirations Respirations that have low volumes of air in inspiration and expiration.

Sharps container A special container designed for the disposal of needles and other sharp instruments used in the care of a patient.

Shielding A method of creating a protected trench by placing extremely strong metal boxes inside the trench.

Shock A condition characterized by inadequate delivery of oxygen and nutrients to cells, resulting in organ system malfunction. Eventually shock is detectible with abnormal vital signs. It can lead to death. Five types of shock are cardiogenic shock, compensated shock, decompensated shock, distributive shock, and hypovolemic shock.

Shock position Placement of a patient supine with the legs elevated 8 to 12 inches to facilitate venous return.

Shoring A method of creating a support system in a trench by exerting pressure against the trench walls to prevent soil from moving.

Short bones A bone classification; short bones characteristically have an approximately equal length and width (e.g., the bones of the wrists and ankles).

Short spine board A device used to immobilize and extricate patients who are found in a sitting position.

Shoulder dystocia Impaction of the baby's anterior shoulder underneath the mother's pubic bone such that delivery is slowed or prevented.

Shunt A tube running from the brain to the abdomen to drain excess cerebrospinal fluid.

Side effects Any reaction to or consequence of a medication of therapy.

Side-to-side method Hoisting or lowering a transportation device where the emergency medical technicians are on either side of the device.

SIDS (sudden infant death syndrome) The sudden, unexpected death of a previously healthy infant.

Sign A patient finding you can see, feel, hear, smell, or measure.

Simple access Gaining access to the patient without the use of any tools or specialized equipment.

Simple febrile seizure A single tonic-clonic febrile seizure lasting less than 15 minutes.

Six *P*s of musculoskeletal assessment Assessment factors for evaluating musculoskeletal trauma; they are pain, pallor, pulse, paresthesia, paralysis, and puffiness or pressure.

Skeletal muscle One of three muscle classifications; skeletal muscle is *striated*, which means the muscle tissue appears to have lines running through it.

Skin tear A traumatic injury to an elderly person's skin that can be caused by minor circumstances. It occurs because of the loss of elasticity and the thinning of the skin that take place with aging.

Sling and swathe An immobilization technique for an upper extremity injury in which the forearm is placed in a sling and a bandage, and the swathe secures the humerus to the body.

Sloping A method of creating a protected trench by cutting back the side walls of the trench to the angle of repose (i.e., the angle at which soil no longer slides).

Smooth (visceral) muscle A major class of muscle that includes involuntary muscles, such as the muscles that move food through the digestive tract.

Snoring The noise made during breathing as the tongue partially obstructs the airway.

Solid organs Organs including the heart, lungs, kidneys, pancreas, and liver.

Somatic pain Pain that is sharp and easily localized

Source A person, insect, object, or another substance that carries or is contaminated by an infectious agent.

Special situation report A special report used to document unusual occurrences, such as an injury to the patient during transport.

Sphygmomanometer The cuff and gauge used to measure the blood pressure.

Spinal column A series of 26 bones that support most of the body's weight and protect the spinal cord. It is the main nerve pathway to and from the brain; also called the *vertebral column*.

Sprain An injury to a tendon or ligament.

Stabilization (au: please provide definition)

Staging sector The sector in the incident management system that coordinates with the transportation sector for the movement of vehicles to and from the transportation sector.

Stair chair A folding chair used to carry patients who can assume the sitting position.

Standard of care The body of knowledge, laws, policies, common practices, standards, and guidelines that provide the basis for care.

Standard precautions Precautions used in all situations to avoid transmission of infection from recognized and unrecognized sources. Standard precautions apply to the blood, body fluids, secretions, excretions (except sweat), nonintact skin, and mucous membranes. Standard precautions incorporate the older universal precautions and body substance isolation procedures.

Standing backboard techniques Placing a standing patient with a suspected neck or spinal injury onto a long backboard, while the patient remains standing. These are two- or three-person techniques.

Standing orders A document that describes the patient care to be performed when medical control is not contacted or is unavailable.

Status epilepticus A condition marked by seizures that persist or intermittently continue, without a return to a normal level of consciousness, for longer than 30 minutes.

Stellate laceration Laceration that is jagged.

Sterilizing Using chemicals and superheated steam to kill all microorganisms.

Sternal notch The anatomic notch created by the clavicles and the sternum.

Sternum The breast bone.

Stimulant A drug or medication that causes an increase in the activity of the sympathetic nervous system (fight or flight). Common stimulants include cocaine, amphetamine, and PCP.

Stoma Opening on the anterior surface of the neck that connects the trachea directly to the outside air.

Strain An injury to a muscle.

Stress Bodily or mental tension caused by a physical, chemical, emotional, or other factors.

Striated muscles Muscles in which the tissue appears to have lines.

Stridor A high-pitched, harsh respiratory sound that is a sign of upper airway obstruction.

Stroke An abnormal condition of the brain caused by occlusion of a blood vessel by an embolus, thrombus, or hemorrhage or vasospasm; also known as a *cerebrovascular accident*.

Stroke volume The amount of blood ejected by the heart with each contraction.

Structural cardiac abnormalities A condition marked by a grossly abnormal heart structure, including valve, muscle, and vessel positioning irregularities.

Structural type The type of structural materials involved and the type of collapse.

Stylet A thin, semirigid rod inserted into an endotracheal tube to prevent bending or kinking during insertion and to allow its user to bend the tube to a desired angle.

Subcutaneous emphysema A condition characterized by leakage of air into the chest wall, which produces a crackling feeling under the skin on palpation; it often is caused by an injury to the lung.

Subcutaneous tissue Innermost layer of the skin.

Subdural hematoma An accumulation of blood in the subdural space, usually caused by an injury.

Subjective assessment Information obtained about the patient's condition by questioning the patient, family members, or bystanders.

Subjective information Information that is perceived by the patient or bystanders and not by the emergency medical technician.

Sublingual Under the tongue.

Sublingual route Placement of a medication under the patient's tongue.

Submandibular Indicates the area under the mandible, or lower jaw.

Submental Indicates the area under the chin.

Submersion episode Any submersion into water that requires field care and transport to a hospital for treatment or observation.

Suction devices Devices used to suction secretions and fluids from the mouth and oropharynx of unresponsive patients.

Sudden infant death syndrome The sudden, unexpected death of a previously healthy infant.

Suicide An attempt by a person to end his or her life.

Superficial On the surface of the body.

Superficial burns First-degree burns that affect only the outermost layers of skin.

Superior Toward the head or top of the body.

Superior vena cava Large vein that carries oxygen-poor blood from the head and arms.

Supine The body lying on its back.

Supine hypotensive syndrome A physiologic phenomenon in which the enlarged uterus compresses the inferior vena cava in the abdomen and impedes the return of blood to the heart. This can happen during the second half of pregnancy when a woman lies supine.

Support or supply sector The sector in the incident management system responsible for obtaining additional resources including disposable supplies, personnel, and equipment for others sectors.

Supraclavicular retractions The use of accessory muscles to increase the work of breathing, which appears as the sucking in of the muscles above the clavicles.

Surrogate An individual placed in the position to make decisions for another person; an advocate or alternate.

Suspension A preparation of a finely divided, undissolved substance dispersed in a liquid medium.

Sutures Joints between the skull bones.

Swathe A folded triangular bandage or roller bandage used to bind the upper arm to the chest wall.

Swelling Abnormal enlargement of a body part or organ caused by an increased volume of fluid in blood vessels or between cells.

Symptom A patient finding that the patient describes such as pain. It cannot be observed or measured by another person.

Synchronized time recording The act of matching your time device (wristwatch) with that of other time devices (wall clock).

Syncope Fainting; a brief lapse in consciousness. Syncope may be preceded by a sensation of light-headedness.

Synovial fluid Fluid produced in the joint capsule to lubricate the bone ends of a joint.

Synovial joints One of the major classes of joints; synovial joints allow a wide range of motion.

Systolic pressure The pressure applied to the blood vessels during the contraction phase of the cardiac cycle. Represented as the top number of a blood pressure reading.

Tachypnea Rapid breathing.

Talus One of seven tarsals; the ankle bone.

Tarsals Seven bones that make up the ankle and proximal aspect of the foot.

Technician level (au: please provide definition)

Temporal bone A major bone of the skull; it forms the side of the skull.

Tenderness Pain elicited on palpation.

Tendons Durable, elastic tissues that join muscle to muscle and muscle to bone.

Tension pneumothorax Pressure increase inside the chest from a natural one-way valve that allows air into the chest cavity but with no escape. Eventually this pressure increase can result in compression of the heart and the unaffected lung to the point of circulatory failure and death.

Terrain hazards (au: please provide definition)

Therapeutic dose The dose of a medication required to have the desired effect on a patient.

Thermoregulation The body's ability to regulate temperature despite changes in the environment. The hypothalamus is responsible for this process.

Thermoregulatory emergency Any emergency involving a change in the temperature of the body.

Third-degree burns Full-thickness burns characterized by charred, white, or gray skin, with no pain involved.

Third-spacing Loss of fluid from the blood vessels (first space) and even the cells (second space) to be trapped uselessly in the tissues between cells and organs. In this location, the fluid is of no physiologic value to the patient.

Thoracic vertebrae The 12 central vertebrae of the spinal column (T8 to T19).

Thorax The chest.

Thyroid cartilage Cartilaginous structure of the larynx commonly known as the Adam's apple.

Tibia The long bone of the lower leg; the shin bone.

Tibial artery Artery located in the lower extremities.

Tidal volume Volume of air inspired and exhaled with each breath, usually about 500 mL in an average-sized adult.

Tier Action of continued care when a prehospital emergency medical services system continues care with an advanced prehospital emergency medical services system.

Time The duration of the chief complaint and significant associated complaints.

Toddler A child 1 to 3 years of age.

Tonic-clonic seizure A seizure characterized by generalized involuntary muscle contracts and cessation of respiration followed by tonic and clonic muscle spasms. Breathing returns with noisy respirations. The condition is also known as a *grand mal seizure.*

Tourniquet Constricting band placed above an injured extremity to stop the flow of blood. Tourniquets should be used only as a last resort.

Toxic Poisonous.

Toxicology The study of poisons.

Toxidrome A constellation of signs and symptoms characteristic of intoxication with a specific poison.

Toxins Chemicals made by living organisms that are toxic to other forms of life.

Trachea The air conduit that extends from the lower portion of the larynx into the chest, where it then divides into the right and left mainstem bronchi.

Tracheal deviation Position of the trachea to either side of the midline of the neck.

Tracheal muscle A long strip of muscle that forms the posterior wall of the trachea.

Tracheal stoma A permanent artificial opening in the trachea.

Tracheostomy Surgical procedure by which a channel is created in the anterior neck connecting the upper portion of the trachea to the outside air.

Traction splint A special splint for midshaft fractures of the femur that applies gentle but constant pressure to keep the lower extremity aligned.

Trade name The name given to a drug by the manufacturer.

Traffic delineation devices Devices used to alter traffic flow around an emergency scene.

Tragus The tonguelike cartilage found at the ventral opening of the external acoustic meatus.

Transdermal medication A medication that is delivery by being applied to the skin; the drug is absorbed through the skin.

Transient ischemic attack An episode of cerebrovascular insufficiency, usually associated with partial obstruction of a cerebral artery by plaque or an embolus.

Transmission The method by which an infectious agent travels from the source to its host.

Transmission-based precautions Special precautions over and above standard precautions that are used for patients documented or suspected to be infected with highly transmissible disease.

Transportation device Any equipment, such as stretchers, stair chair, long backboards, or vacuum backboards, used to move a patient from one location to another.

Transportation sector A sector in the incident management system that coordinates resources including receiving hospitals, air medical resources, and ambulances.

Trauma center A specialized hospital equipped with personnel and resources to provide immediate, advanced care for a critically injured trauma patient.

Trauma system A system that helps identify the appropriate hospital or specialized center to which a trauma patient should be transported.

Treatment sector The sector in the incident management system that provides care to patients received from the triage and extrication sectors.

Trench An excavation that is less than 15 feet wide and is deeper than it is wide.

Trench foot Moist gangrene of the foot that is caused by the freezing of wet skin; also known as *immersion foot.*

Trend The collection of several vital signs readings and comparing of the values for patterns.

Trendelenburg's position A position in which the body is supine with the feet elevated and head down.

Trending The process of monitoring findings over time to identify patterns.

Triage The process of sorting or prioritizing patients into treatment and transport categories.

Tripod position A position characterized by sitting upright and leaning forward with the head and neck thrust forward; it generally is associated with respiratory distress.

True vocal cords Thin strips of connective tissue attached to the muscles of phonation within the upper portion of the larynx. These important landmarks for endotracheal intubation form the border of the glottic opening.

Tunnel vision Focusing on horrific-looking injuries instead of identifying possible life-threatening injuries.

Turnout gear Heavy clothing that is puncture resistant and gives some protection from hazardous materials and materials at extremes of temperature.

Twisting force Force applied where a body part acts as a pivot point and twists beyond the normal range of motion.

Twisting injury An injury that results from a turning motion of the body in opposite directions.

Type I ambulance An ambulance designed with a modular box patient compartment mounted on a truck-style chassis.

Type I diabetes A type of diabetes in which the body is unable to metabolize carbohydrates because of insulin deficiency. The condition usually develops during childhood and requires the patient to take insulin shots.

Type II ambulance Van-style ambulance.

Type II diabetes A type of diabetes in which patients are not insulin dependent or prone to ketosis, although insulin may be used to correct symptoms and persistent hyperglycemia. The onset usually occurs during adulthood. The condition often is associated with obesity.

Type III ambulance An ambulance designed with a modular box patient compartment mounted on a van chassis.

Ulna The smaller of the two bones in the forearm.

Umbilical cord The cord containing blood vessels that connects the fetus to the placenta.

Umbilical cord prolapse Appearance of the umbilical cord in front of the presenting part, usually with compression of the cord and interruption of blood supply to the baby.

United States Pharmacopeia The official publication including all drugs officially recognized by the federal Food, Drug, and Cosmetic Act.

Universal precautions Measures taken to prevent contamination by body substances and fluids that may carry blood-borne pathogens such as human immunodeficiency virus, hepatitis B virus, or hepatitis C virus.

Upper gastrointestinal tract Most common area of gastrointestinal bleeding; it involves areas proximal to the duodenum.

Upper respiratory tract A system of air passages formed by the nose and mouth, the pharynx, and the larynx.

Urban search and rescue teams (au: please provide definition)

Ureter One of a pair of tubes that carries urine from the kidney into the bladder.

Urgent move A patient move used when the patient's condition may become life-threatening.

Urinary system All organs and ducts involved in the secretion and elimination of urine from the body.

Urticaria Red, raised, circular lesions on the skin; also called *hives*.

Uterus The hollow, pear-shaped internal female reproductive organ in which the fertilized ovum is planted and develops.

Vaccination Inoculation with a vaccine to establish immunity to a particular disease.

Vacuum splint An extremity or full body splint; air is drawn out of the splint so that the splint contracts and conforms to the body to maintain immobilization.

Vagina The lower part of the birth canal, extending from the uterus to the outside of the body.

Vallecula The recessed area in the hypopharynx that separates the base of the tongue from the epiglottis. Insertion of the tip of a curved laryngoscope blade into this recess allows for retraction of the epiglottis and visualization of the glottic opening.

Vasculature Blood vessels.

Vasovagal syncope A sudden loss of consciousness generated by a transient vascular and neurogenic reaction; may be triggered by pain, fright, or trauma.

Vector Insects, animals, or inanimate objects that carry and transmit disease. For example, malaria is transmitted by mosquitoes (the vector).

Vee collapse A type of structural collapse in which a horizontal structural component close to the center of the span collapses, creating two triangular voids on either side of the collapse.

Veins Vessels that carry deoxygenated blood back to the heart.

Venae cavae Major veins that carry blood back to the right atrium of the heart from the body.

Venous bleeding Active bleeding characterized by large amounts of dark red blood steadily flowing from a wound site.

Venous system System of veins in the body.

Ventilation Mechanical process of inspiration and exhalation by which air rich in oxygen is breathed into the lungs and an equal volume of gas is expired, eliminating carbon dioxide from the body.

Ventral Toward the abdomen or anterior.

Ventricle Lower chamber of the heart. The heart has a right ventricle that pumps deoxygenated blood to the lungs and a left ventricle that pumps oxygenated blood to the body.

Ventricular fibrillation A rapid, chaotic cardiac rhythm in which the heart "quivers" with electrical impulses but fails to contract.

Ventricular tachycardia Rapid heartbeat that does not allow the heart time to fill and pump blood properly.

Venules Smallest size of vein.

Verbal report An essential component of the patient transfer to the hospital. The verbal report should contain the patient's name. It also should inform the receiving medical professional of the chief complaint, pertinent history, patient condition, details of the physical assessment, your treatment, and the response to treatment.

Vertebrae The irregular bones that form the spinal column.

Vestibular folds Cartilaginous folds surrounding the true vocal cords of the larynx when viewed from above.

Vial of life A container that holds medical information about a patient.

Virus An organism that must attack a living host cell so that it can use that machinery of the cell to replicate.

Visceral pain Abdominal pain that is caused by any abnormal condition of the viscera; it is usually severe, diffuse, and difficult to localize.

Vital signs The specific measurements or assessments of a patient's skin, breathing, pulse, blood pressure, and pupil size and response.

Vocal cords Thin strips of connective tissue attached to the muscles of phonation within the upper portion of the larynx. Variations in the vibration of the vocal cords caused by air passing through the upper airway generate the sounds necessary for speech.

Voluntary muscles Muscles that move as a result of conscious effort or direction.

VX A nerve agent that normally exists as a liquid at room temperature. The onset of symptoms following exposure to this agent may be delayed up to 18 hours.

Warm zone Area immediately surrounding the hot zone and the place where decontamination occurs.

Waybill (consist) A document used to identify hazardous substances transported by rail. It usually can be obtained from the engineer or conductor, or it may be found at the site of a railway accident. Waybills may not be available for railcars being sorted in classification yards or on track sidings. Emergency response personnel should establish a cooperative relationship with the rail carriers in their area before an incident occurs.

Weapons of mass destruction Nuclear, biological, and chemical agents intended to do harm.

Wheeled stretcher The primary transport stretcher used by prehospital providers. The stretcher has a wheeled base and comes in a variety of types.

Wheezes A whistling sound heard in the lungs that is caused by air moving through narrowed bronchioles.

Wheezing High-pitched expiratory breath sounds caused by narrowing of the small air passages (bronchioles) in the lungs that most commonly is a result of an acute asthmatic episode.

White blood cells Cells in the blood that help the body fight infection.

Xiphoid process Cartilaginous tissue at the distal end of the sternum.

Zygomatic arch A bony structure that forms the lateral aspect of the eye socket.

Illustration Credits

Chapter 1

Figs. 1-1 to 1-5, 1-7 to 1-11: Chapleau W: *Emergency first responder: making the difference*, St. Louis, 2004, Mosby.

Fig. 1-3: the National Center for Health Statistics (NCHS) Vital Statistics System.

Fig. 1-6: Henry MC, Stapleton ER: *EMT prehospital care*, ed 2, Philadelphia, 1997, WB Saunders.

Chapter 2

Figs. 2-1 to 2-4, 2-6 to 2-10: Chapleau W: *Emergency first responder: making the difference*, St. Louis, 2004, Mosby.

Chapter 4

Fig. 4-1, 4-4: Drake R, Vogl R, Mitchell A: *Gray's anatomy for students*, London, 2004, Churchill Livingstone.

Fig. 4-2, 4-3: Modified from Drake R, Vogl R, Mitchell A: *Gray's anatomy for students*, London, 2004, Churchill Livingstone.

Figs. 4-5 to 4-14, 4-16, 4-18: Herlihy B, Maebius NK: *The human body in health and illness*, ed 2, St. Louis, 2003, Saunders.

Fig. 4-15, 4-17, 4-23: McSwain NE, Paturas JL: *The basic EMT: comprehensive prehospital patient care*, ed. 2, St. Louis, 2003, Mosby

Fig. 4-19: Thibodeau GA, Patton KT: *Anthony's textbook of anatomy and physiology*, ed 16, St. Louis, 1999, Mosby.

Fig. 4-20: Chapleau W: *Emergency first responder: making the difference*, St. Louis, 2004, Mosby.

Fig. 4-21: Thibodeau GA, Patton KT: *Anatomy and physiology*, ed 3, St. Louis, 1996, Mosby.

Fig. 4-22: Seeley R: *Anatomy and physiology*, ed 3, St. Louis, 1995 Mosby.

Figure 4-23: McSwain NE, Paturas JL: *The basic EMT: comprehensive prehospital patient care*, ed. 2, St. Louis, 2003, Mosby

Chapter 5

Fig. 5-4: Jarvis C: *Physical examination and health assessment*, ed 3, Philadelphia, 2000, WB Saunders.

Figs. 5-6 to 5-11, Skill 5-1 and 5-2: Chapleau W: *Emergency first responder: making the difference*, St. Louis, 2004, Mosby.

Chapter 6

Fig. 6-4: McSwain NE, Paturas JL: *The Basic EMT*, ed 2, St. Louis, 2003, Mosby.

Figs. 6-13, 6-14, 6-17, 6-18, Skill 6-6, Skill 6-12: Chapleau W: *Emergency first responder: making the difference*, St. Louis, 2004, Mosby.

Fig. 6-15: Stoy/Center for Emergency Medicine: *Mosby's EMT-Basic textbook*, St Louis, 1996, Mosby Lifeline.

Chapter 7

Figs. 7-1, 7-2, 7-4, 7-7, 7-13: Herlihy B, Maebius NK: *The human body in health and illness*, ed 2, St. Louis, 2003, Saunders.

Fig. 7-3, 7-5, 7-15: McSwain NE, Paturas JL: *The basic EMT: comprehensive prehospital patient care*, ed. 2, St. Louis, 2003, Mosby

Fig. 7-6: Applegate EJ: *The anatomy and physiology learning system.* Philadelphia, 1995, Saunders.

Fig. 7-8: NAEMT: *PHTLS: Basic and advanced prehospital trauma life support*, ed 4, St. Louis, 1999, Mosby.

Chapter 8

Fig. 8-8: US Department of Transportation. National Standard Curriculum for EMT-Basics, 1994.

Chapter 9

Fig. 9-1: US Department of Transportation. National Standard Curriculum for EMT-Basics, 1994.

Chapter 10

Fig 10-3, Skill 10-1: Chapleau W: *Emergency first responder: making the difference*, St. Louis, 2004, Mosby.

Chapter 12

Fig. 12-1, 12-4, 12-5: Sanders M: *Mosby's paramedic textbook*, ed 3, St. Louis, 2006, Mosby.

Figs. 12-2, 12-3: London PS: *A colour atlas for diagnosis after recent injury*, Epswich, England, 1990, Wolf Medical Publications, Ltd.

Skill 12-1: Chapleau W: *Emergency first responder: making the difference*, St. Louis, 2004, Mosby.

Chapter 14

Fig. 14-4, *B*: Henry MC, Stapleton ER: *EMT prehospital care*, ed 2, Philadelphia, 1997, WB Saunders.

Chapter 15

Fig. 15-1: Courtesy Greater Community Hospital Ambulance, Creston, Iowa.

Fig. 15-2: From SirenPro®, courtesy Digital Objectives, Inc.

Fig. 15-3: Courtesy Greater Community Hospital Ambulance, Creston, Iowa.

Chapter 17

Fig. 17-1: Herlihy B, Maebius N: *The human body in health and illness*, Philadelphia, 2000, Saunders.

Fig. 17-2: Thibodeau and Patton: *Structure and function of the body*, ed. 11, St. Louis, 2000, Mosby.

Fig. 17-3: Henry MC, Stapleton ER: *EMT prehospital care*, ed 2, Philadelphia, 1997, WB Saunders.

Figs. 17-5, 17-6: Chapleau W: *Emergency first responder: making the difference*, St. Louis, 2004, Mosby.

Chapter 18

Figs. 18-1, 18-2: Herlihy B, Maebius NK: *The human body in health and illness*, ed 2, Philadelphia, 2003, Saunders.

Fig. 18-4: Aehlert B: *ECGs made easy*, ed. 2, St. Louis, 2002, Mosby.

Fig. 18-5, 18-8: Chapleau W: *Emergency first responder: making the difference*, St. Louis, 2004, Mosby.

Figs. 18-6, 18-7: Aehlert B: *ECGs made easy*, ed. 2, St. Louis, 2002, Mosby.

Fig. 18-9: Medtronic Inc.

Chapter 19

Figs. 19-1, 19-2, 19-3: Drake R, Vogl R, Mitchell A: *Gray's anatomy for students*, London, 2004, Churchill Livingstone.

Figs. 19-4, 19-5, 19-7: Chapleau W: *Emergency first responder: making the difference*, St. Louis, 2004, Mosby.

Fig 19-6: Herlihy B, Maebius NK: *The human body in health and illness*, ed, St. Louis, 2003, Mosby.

Fig 19-8: Lewis SM, Heitkemper MM, and Dirksen SR: *Medical-surgical nursing: assessment and management of clinical problems*, ed 5, St. Louis, 2000, Mosby.

Chapter 21

Fig. 21-1: Epstein O, Cookson J, Perkin GS, et al: *Clinical examination*, ed 3, St. Louis, 2003, Mosby.

Fig. 21-2. Zietelli BJ, Davis HW: *Atlas of pediatric physical diagnosis*, ed 4, St. Louis, 2002, Mosby.

Chapter 22

Fig. 22-1, 22-3, 22-5 to 22-7: Sanders MJ: *Mosby's paramedic textbook*, ed. 3, St. Louis, 2006, Mosby.

Fig. 22-2, 22-4, 22-8, 22-9: Auerbach PS: *Wilderness medicine*, ed. 4, St. Louis, 2001, Mosby.

Chapter 23

Fig 23-1: McSwain N, Paturas J. *The Basic EMT*, ed 2, St. Louis, 2003, Mosby.

Fig 23-2: Redrawn from the National Weather Service Forecast Office. http://www.wrh.noaa.gov/lkn/windchill.php Accessed July 7, 2005.

Fig 22-3: Redrawn from the National Weather Service Forecast Office. http://www.crh.noaa.gov/pub/heat.php Accessed July 7, 2005.

Fig 23-5: Auerbach P: *Wilderness medicine*, ed 4, St. Louis, 2001, Mosby. A-D: (a) Courtesy Murray P. Hamlet, DVM, (b) Courtesy Cameron Bangs, MD, (c) Courtesy Murray P. Hamlet, DVM, (d) Courtesy Cameron Bangs, MD.

Chapter 25

Fig. 25-1, 25-6, 25-7, *B*, 25-8: Stoy W, Platt T, Lejeune D: *Mosby's EMT-Basic textbook*, ed 2, St. Louis, 2005, Mosby.

Fig. 25-2 *A*, *B*, 25-5, 25-5 McSwain N, Paturas J: *The basic EMT: comprehensive prehospital patient care*, ed 2, St. Louis, 2003, Mosby.

Fig. 25-3: Henry M, Stapleton E: *EMT prehospital care*, ed 3, St. Louis, 2004, Mosby.

Fig. 25-7, *A*: From London PS: *A colour atlas of diagnosis after recent injury*, London, 1990, Wolfe.

Chapter 26

Figs. 26-3, 26-4, 26-11: *NAEMT: PHTLS prehospital trauma life support*, ed 5, St. Louis, 2003, Mosby.

Figs. 26-6, 26-9: Williams J: *Color atlas for injury in sport*, ed 2, Chicago, 1990, Mosby-Yearbook.

Fig. 26-7, 26-21, 26-22: Henry MC, Stapleton ER: *EMT prehospital care*, ed 3, St Louis, 2004, Mosby.

Fig. 26-13: Chapleau W: *Emergency first responder, making the difference.* St. Louis, 2004, Mosby.

Fig. 26-20: McSwain NE, Paturas JL: *The basic EMT*, ed 2, St. Louis, 2003, Mosby.

Chapter 27

Fig. 27-1: A, Seidel HM, Ball JW, Dains JE, Benedict GW: *Mosby's guide to physical examination*, ed 5, St. Louis, 2003, Mosby. B, Drake R, Vogl R, Mitchell A: *Gray's anatomy for students*, London, 2004, Churchill Livingstone.

Fig. 27-2: Redrawn from NAEMT: *PHTLS: basic and advanced prehospital trauma life support*, ed 5, St. Louis, 2003, Mosby.

Figs. 27-3 to 27-10, 27-12: NAEMT: *PHTLS: basic and advanced prehospital trauma life support*, ed 5, St. Louis, 2003, Mosby.

Fig. 27-11: Courtesy Dr. Greg Schmunk.

Fig. 27-13: Courtesy Dr. Greg Schmunk.

Fig. 27-14: London PS: *A colour atlas of diagnosis after recent injury*, London, 1990, Wolfe.

Fig. 27-15: McSwain NE, Paturas JL: *The basic EMT*, ed 2, St. Louis, 2003, Mosby.

Chapter 28

Figure 28-1, 28-4, 28-5: Pre-Hospital Trauma Life Support Committee of the National Association of Emergency Medical Technicians in Cooperation with the Committee on Trauma of the American College of Surgeons: Pre-hospital Trauma Life Support, ed 5, St. Louis, 2003, Mosby.

Fig. 28-2, 28-11, 28-13, 28-15, 28-22: McSwain N, Paturas J: *The basic EMT*, ed 2, St. Louis, 2003, Mosby.

Fig. 28-3, 28-16, 28-17: London PS: *A colour atlas of diagnosis after recent injury*, London, 1990, Wolfe.

Fig. 28-6 Sanders M: *Mosby's paramedic textbook*, ed 3, St. Louis, 2005, Mosby.

Fig. 28-7, 28-14: Henry M, Stapleton E: *EMT prehospital care*, ed 3, St. Louis, 2004, Mosby.

Figs. 28-8, 28-9, 28-10: Sanders M: *Mosby's paramedic textbook*, ed 3, St. Louis, 2005, Mosby.

Fig. 28-12: Herlihy B, Maebius N: *The human body in health and illness*, ed 2, 2003, St. Louis, Saunders.

Figs. 28-18 to 28-21, 28-23, 28-24: Chapleau W: *Emergency first responder: making the difference*, St. Louis, 2004, Mosby.

Chapter 29

Fig. 29-1: Herlihy B, Maebius N: *The human body in health and illness*, ed 2, 2003, St. Louis, Saunders.

Fig. 29-2, 29-6, 29-11: NAEMT: *PHTLS: Basic and advanced prehospital trauma life support*, ed. 5, St. Louis, 2003, Mosby.

Fig. 29-3, 29-14, 29-15: London PS: *A colour atlas of diagnosis after recent injury*, Ipswich, England, 1990, Wolfe.

Fig. 29-4, 29-16: Sanders MJ: *Mosby's paramedic textbook*, rev ed 2, St. Louis, 2001, Mosby.

Fig. 29-7: Thibodeau GA, Patton KT: *Anatomy and physiology*, ed 2, St. Louis, 1993, Mosby.

Fig. 29-8: NAEMT: *PHTLS: Basic and advanced prehospital trauma life support*, ed 4, St. Louis, 1999, Mosby.

Fig 29-10, 29-13: Henry MC, Stapleton ER: *EMT prehospital care*, ed 3, St. Louis, 2004, Mosby.

Fig: 29-12, Skill 29-2: Chapleau W: *Emergency first responder: making the difference*, St. Louis, 2004, Mosby.

Fig. 29-17: NAEMT: *PHTLS: Basic and advanced prehospital trauma life support*, ed 5, St. Louis, 2003, Mosby.

Fig. 29-19: Courtesy Life Support Products Inc., Irvine, Calif.

Chapter 30

Fig. 30-1: LeFleur Brooks: *Exploring medical language*, ed 4, St. Louis, 1998, Mosby.

Fig. 30-2, 30-5, 30-6, 30-10, Skill 30-1: McSwain N, Paturas J: *The basic EMT*, ed 2, St. Louis, 2003, Mosby.

Figs. 30-3, 30-5, 30-9, 30-10: Chapleau W: *Emergency first responder: making the difference*, St. Louis, 2004, Mosby.

Fig. 30-8: Aehlert B: Pediatric Advanced Life Support Study Guide, ed 2, St. Louis, 2005, Mosby.

Chapter 31

Fig. 31-3: Cote CJ, Todres ID, Goudsouzian NG, et al: A *practice of anesthesia for infants and children*, ed 3, Philadelphia, 2001, Saunders.

Chapter 32

Fig. 32-4: Epstein O, Cookson J, Perkin GS, et al: *Clinical examination*, ed 3, St. Louis, 2003, Mosby.

Chapter 33

Fig 33-2, 33-3, 33-5 to 33-8: Chapleau W: *Emergency first responder: making the difference*, St. Louis, 2004, Mosby.

Chapter 34

Fig. 34-1: Vines T, Hudson S: *High angle rescue technique*, ed 3, St. Louis, 2004, Mosby.

Fig. 34-2, 34-4, 34-5, 34-7, 34-8: Smith B: *Rescuers in action*, St. Louis, 1996, Mosby.

Fig. 34-3: Courtesy Peter Escobedo.

Fig. 34-6: Moore R: *Vehicle rescue and extrication*, ed 2, St. Louis, 2003, Mosby.

Chapter 35

Figs. 35-1 to 35-3, Figs. 35-5 to 35-7, 35-9: Courtesy Craig Gravitz.

Fig. 35-4 Adapted from the Simple Triage and Rapid Treatment (S.T.A.R.T.) Algorithm developed by Hoag Hospital and Newport Beach Fire Department

Fig. 35-8: Courtesy Craig Gravitz and Chris Colwell.

Chapter 36

Fig. 36-1: Currance, PL: *Medical response to weapons of mass destruction*, St Louis, 2005, Mosby.

Fig. 36-2, 36-4 to 36-6: Chapleau W: *Emergency first responder: making the difference*, St. Louis, 2004, Mosby.

Fig. 36-3: US Department of Transportation. National Standard Curriculum for EMT-Basics, 1994.

Chapter 37

Fig. 37-1: Currance PL: *Medical response to weapons of mass destruction*, St. Louis, 2005, Mosby.

Fig. 37-2, 37-5, 37-6: Department of Health and Human Services Centers for Disease Control and Prevention.

Fig. 37-3: A, Department of Health and Human Services Centers for Disease Control and Prevention. B, Department of Health and Human Services Centers for Disease Control and Prevention/Margaret Parsons, Dr. Karl F. Meyer

Fig. 37-4: Department of Health and Human Services Centers for Disease Control and Prevention/ Dr. Brachman.

Chapter 38

Figure 38-1, 38-2: From McSwain N, Paturas J: *The basic EMT*, ed 2, St. Louis, 2003, Mosby.

Figure 38-3: Prehospital Trauma Life Support Committee of the National Association of Emergency Medication Technicians in Cooperation with the Committee on Trauma of The American College of Surgeons: Prehospital Trauma Life Support: Basic and Advanced Prehospital Trauma Life Support, ed 5, St. Louis, 2003, Mosby.

Figure 38-6, 36-8: From Sanders M: *Mosby's paramedic textbook*, ed 3, St. Louis, 2005, Mosby.

Figure 38-7: From Henry M, Stapleton E: *EMT prehospital care*, ed. 3, St. Louis, 2004, Mosby.

Figure 38-11: Courtesy Kristen Burke.

Figure 38-12: Prehospital Trauma Life Support Committee of the National Association of Emergency Medicaion Technicians in Cooperation with the Committee on Trauma of The American College of Surgeons: Prehospital Trauma Life Support: Basic and Advanced Prehospital Trauma Life Support, ed 5, St. Louis, 2003, Mosby.

Figure 38-13: Courtesy Robert D. White, MD.

Index